MANAGEMENT OF SLEEP DISORDERS IN PSYCHIATRY

MANAGEMENT OF SLEEP DISORDERS IN PSYCHIATRY

EDITED BY

AMIT CHOPRA, MD, FAPA

PIYUSH DAS, MD, DABSM

KARL DOGHRAMJI, MD

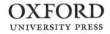

OXFORD
UNIVERSITY PRESS

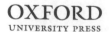

Oxford University Press is a department of the University of Oxford. It furthers
the University's objective of excellence in research, scholarship, and education
by publishing worldwide. Oxford is a registered trade mark of Oxford University
Press in the UK and certain other countries.

Published in the United States of America by Oxford University Press
198 Madison Avenue, New York, NY 10016, United States of America.

Library of Congress Cataloging-in-Publication Data
Names: Chopra, Amit, editor. | Das, Piyush, editor. |
Doghramji, Karl, editor.
Title: Management of sleep disorders in psychiatry / [edited by] Amit Chopra,
Piyush Das, Karl Doghramji.
Description: New York, NY : Oxford University Press, [2020] |
Includes bibliographical references and index. |
Identifiers: LCCN 2019040663 (print) | LCCN 2019040664 (ebook) |
ISBN 9780190929671 (pb) | ISBN 9780190929695 (epub) | ISBN 9780190929688 (updf)
Subjects: MESH: Sleep Wake Disorders—therapy | Psychiatry—methods
Classification: LCC RC547 (print) | LCC RC547 (ebook) | NLM WL 108 |
DDC 616.8/4980068—dc23
LC record available at https://lccn.loc.gov/2019040663
LC ebook record available at https://lccn.loc.gov/2019040664

9 8 7 6 5 4 3 2
Printed by Marquis, Canada

I dedicate this book to my parents, Sunita and Ramesh Chopra, for their hard work, love, and support that has been the greatest source of inspiration for me.

—Amit Chopra

To my wife Harsh Das and 4-year-old twin daughters, Prajna Das and Pragya Das. Thank you for allowing me time out of "your time with me" to contribute to this book. You people are my whole world!

—Piyush Das

I dedicate this book to my wife Laurel, son Mark, and daughter Leah; to my parents Peter and Mary for their loving encouragement and support; and to all my patients from whom I have learned some of the most valuable lessons in clinical medicine.

—Karl Doghramji

CONTENTS

CONTRIBUTORS

Salih Aleissi, MD
University Sleep Disorders Center,
College of Medicine, King Saud University,
Riyadh, Saudi Arabia and the Strategic
Technologies Program of the National Plan for
Sciences and Technology and Innovation,
Saudi Arabia

Sulaiman Alhifzi, MD
University Sleep Disorders Center, College of
Medicine, King Saud University, Riyadh, Saudi
Arabia; the Strategic Technologies Program of
the National Plan for Sciences and Technology
and Innovation, Saudi Arabia

Aljohara S. Almeneesier, MD
University Sleep Disorders Center, College of
Medicine, King Saud University, Riyadh, Saudi
Arabia; the Strategic Technologies Program of
the National Plan for Sciences and Technology
and Innovation, Riyadh, Saudi Arabia; Family
and Community Medicine, King Saud University,
Riyadh, Saudi Arabia

Chi-Hung Au, MBChB, FHKCPsych
Department of Psychiatry, Queen Mary Hospital,
Hong Kong SAR, China

Ramya Bachu, MD
Psychiatry and Behavioral Health Institute,
Allegheny Health Network, Pittsburgh, PA

Ahmed S. BaHammam, MD
Professor of Medicine, Director, Sleep Disorders
Center, College of Medicine, King Saud
University, Riyadh, Saudi Arabia; the Strategic
Technologies Program of the National Plan
for Sciences and Technology and Innovation,
Riyadh, Saudi Arabia

Raman Baweja, MD, MS
Associate Professor, Department of Psychiatry
& Behavioral Health, Penn State College of
Medicine, Hershey, PA

Fee Benz, MSc
Department of Clinical Psychology and
Psychophysiology, Medical Center–University
of Freiburg, Faculty of Medicine, University of
Freiburg Freiburg, Germany

Gregory M. Brown, MD, PhD, FRCPC, FRSC
Professor Emeritus, Department of Psychiatry,
University of Toronto, Affiliate Scientist,
Molecular Brain Science, Centre for Addiction
and Mental Health, Toronto, ON, Canada

Janeese A. Brownlow, PhD
Department of Psychiatry, Perelman School
of Medicine at the University of Pennsylvania,
Philadelphia, PA

Deepa Burman, MD
Co-Director, Pediatric Sleep Evaluation Center,
UPMC Children's Hospital of Pittsburgh Visiting
Associate Professor, Pediatrics, University of
Pittsburgh, Pittsburgh, PA

Vincent F. Capaldi II
Walter Reed Institute for Army Research,
Silver Spring, MD

Daniel P. Cardinali, MD, PhD
BIOMED-UCA-CONICET and Department
of Teaching and Research, Faculty of Medical
Sciences, Pontificia Universidad Católica
Argentina, Buenos Aires, Argentina

Man-Sum Chan, MBChB, FHKCPsych
Maternal Mental Health, Waitemata District
Health Board, Takapuna, Auckland, NZ

Amit Chopra, MD, FAPA
Medical Director, Center for Treatment-Resistant
Depression, Medical Director, Center for
Psychiatric Neuromodulation, Sleep Specialist,
Center for Sleep Medicine, Allegheny Health
Network, Pittsburgh, PA

Ka-Fai Chung, MBBS, MRCPsych
Clinical Associate Professor, Department of
Psychiatry, University of Hong Kong, Hong Kong
SAR, China; and Corporal Michael J. Crescenz
Veterans Affairs Medical Center,
Philadelphia, PA

Piyush Das, MD, DABSM
Department of Sleep Medicine, Saint Cloud
Hospital and Centracare Health Plaza, Saint
Cloud, MN

Brett J. Davis, BA
University of California, Los Angeles,
Los Angeles, CA

Jacob G. Dinerman, BA
Department of Psychiatry, Massachusetts General
Hospital, Boston, MA

Karl Doghramji, MD
Professor of Psychiatry, Neurology, and
Medicine, Medical Director, Jefferson Sleep
Disorders Center, Program Director, Fellowship
in Sleep Medicine, Thomas Jefferson University,
Philadelphia, PA

Jessica Duis, MD
University of North Carolina, Chapel Hill, NC

Beverly Fang, MD
Department of Psychiatry, University of
Maryland School of Medicine, Baltimore, MD;
Sleep Disorders Center, Division of Pulmonary
and Critical Care Medicine, University of
Maryland School of Medicine, Baltimore, MD

Benjamen Gangewere, MD
Associate Medical Director for Behavioral
Health, Penn Highlands Health Care,
Dubois, PA

Sheila N. Garland, PhD
Department of Psychology, Faculty of
Science, Memorial University, St. John's, NL,
Canada; Division of Oncology, Faculty of
Medicine, Memorial University, St. John's,
NL, Canada

Philip R. Gehrman, PhD
Associate Professor, Department of Psychiatry,
Perelman School of Medicine, University of
Pennsylvania, Philadelphia, PA

Thomas Gossard, MD, MS
Co-Director, Mayo Center for Sleep Medicine,
Division of Pulmonary and Critical Care
Medicine, Departments of Neurology and
Medicine, Mayo Clinic College of Medicine and
Science, Rochester, MN

Michael A. Grandner, PhD, MTR
Department of Psychiatry, University of Arizona,
Tucson, AZ

Ravi Gupta, MD, PhD
Additional Professor, Department of
Psychiatry, All India Institute of Medical
Sciences, Rishikesh, India

Kotaro Hatta, MD, PhD
Department of Psychiatry, Juntendo University
Nerima Hospital, Tokyo, Japan

Elisabeth Hertenstein, PhD
University Hospital for Psychiatry and
Psychotherapy, Bern, Switzerland

Anna Ivanenko, MD, PhD
Professor of Clinical Psychiatry and
Behavioral Sciences, Northwestern University,
Feinberg School of Medicine, and Division of
Child and Adolescent Psychiatry, Ann
and Robert H. Lurie Children's Hospital,
Chicago, IL

William C. Jangro, DO
Assistant Professor, Department of Psychiatry
and Human Behavior, Sidney Kimmel
Medical College, Thomas Jefferson University,
Philadelphia, PA

Jessica A. Janos, BA
Department of Psychiatry, Massachusetts
General Hospital, Boston, MA

Anna Johann, MSc
Department of Psychiatry and Psychotherapy,
Medical Center–University of Freiburg, Faculty
of Medicine, University of Freiburg, Germany

Kyle P. Johnson, MD
Professor, Division of Child and Adolescent
Psychiatry, Oregon Health and Science
University, Portland, OR

Daniel S. Joyce, PhD
The Stanford Center for Sleep Sciences and Medicine, Stanford University, Stanford, CA; Department of Psychiatry and Behavioral Sciences, School of Medicine, Stanford University, Stanford, CA

Jessica Jung, MD
Noran Neurological Clinic, Minneapolis, MN

Alicia Kaplan, MD
Associate Professor of Psychiatry, Temple University SOM, Department of Psychiatry, Allegheny General Hospital, Pittsburgh, PA

Bhanu Prakash Kolla, MD, MRCPsych
Department of Psychiatry and Psychology, Mayo Clinic College of Medicine and Science, Rochester, MN; Center for Sleep Medicine, Mayo Clinic College of Medicine and Science, Rochester, MN

Muruga Loganathan, MD
Department of Behavioral Medicine and Psychiatry, West Virginia University, Morgantown, WV

Erik K. St. Louis, MD, MS
Co-Director, Mayo Center for Sleep Medicine, Division of Pulmonary and Critical Care Medicine, Departments of Neurology and Medicine, Mayo Clinic College of Medicine and Science, Rochester, MN

Beth Malow, MD, MS
Vanderbilt University Medical Center, Nashville, TN

Erika Manis, MD
Promedica Physicians Group within Promedica Health Systems in Toledo, Psychiatry and Sleep Medicine, Wright State University, Toledo, OH

Meghna P. Mansukhani, MD
Center for Sleep Medicine, Mayo Clinic College of Medicine and Science, Rochester, MN

Rebecca Marshall, MD, MPH
Assistant Professor, Division of Child and Adolescent Psychiatry, Oregon Health and Science University, Portland, OR

Katherine E. Miller, PhD
Mental Illness Research, Education and Clinical Center, Corporal Michael J. Crescenz VA Medical Center, Philadelphia, PA

Hiren Muzumdar, MD
Director, Pediatric Sleep Evaluation Center, UPMC Children's Hospital of Pittsburgh Associate Professor, Pediatrics, University of Pittsburgh, Pittsburgh, PA

Anoop Narahari, MD
Psychiatry and Behavioral Health Institute, Allegheny Health Network, Pittsburgh, PA

Daniel A. Neff, MD
Psychiatry Fellow, Department of Psychiatry and Human Behavior, Perelman School of Medicine, University of Pennsylvania, Philadelphia, PA

Seithikurippu R. Pandi-Perumal, Msc
President and CEO of Somnigen Inc., Toronto, ON, Canada

Rikinkumar S. Patel, MD, MPH
Department of Psychiatry, Griffin Memorial Hospital, Norman, OK

Philippe Peigneux, PhD
Neuropsychology and Functional Neuroimaging Research Unit at Centre de Recherches Cognition et Neurosciences and UNI–ULB Neurosciences Institute, Université Libre de Bruxelles, Bruxelles, Belgium

Michael L. Perlis, PhD
Department of Psychiatry, University of Pennsylvania, Philadelphia, PA, and Center for Sleep and Circadian Neurobiology, University of Pennsylvania, Philadelphia, PA

Michael J. Peterson, MD, PhD, DFAPA, FACLP
Department of Psychiatry, University of Wisconsin School of Medicine and Public Health, Madison, WI

Mark R. Pressman, PhD
Sidney Kimmel Medical College of Thomas Jefferson University, Philadelphia, PA; Lankenau Institute of Medical Research, Wynnewood, PA; and Villanova University Law School, Villanova, PA

Dieter Riemann, PhD
Department of Psychiatry and Psychotherapy, Medical Center–University of Freiburg, Faculty of Medicine, University of Freiburg, Freiburg, Germany

Timothy Roehrs, PhD
Sleep Disorders and Research Center,
Henry Ford Health System,
Detroit, MI

Bruce Rohrs, PhD
Assistant Professor of Psychiatry, Temple
University School of Medicine; and Psychologist,
Psychiatric and Behavioral Health Institute,
Allegheny Health Network, Pittsburgh, PA

Lilia Roshchupkina
UR2NF-Neuropsychology and
Functional Neuroimaging Research Unit at
CRCN-Centre de Recherches Cognition
et Neurosciences and UNI-ULB Neurosciences
Institute, Université Libre de Bruxelles
(ULB), Belgium

Richard J. Ross, MD, PhD
Department of Psychiatry, Perelman School
of Medicine at the University of Pennsylvania,
Philadelphia, PA

Thomas Roth, PhD
Department of Psychiatry and Behavioral
Neuroscience, Wayne State University,
School of Medicine, Detroit, MI

David P. Shaha, MD
Sleep Disorders Center, Womack Army Medical
Center, Fort Bragg, NC

Anita Valanju Shelgikar, MD, MHPE
Department of Sleep Medicine, University of
Michigan, Ann Arbor, MI

Althea Robinson Shelton, MD, MPH
Vanderbilt University Medical Center,
Nashville, TN

Shirshendu Sinha, MBBS
Department of Psychiatry and Psychology, Mayo
Clinic College of Medicine and Science,
Rochester, MN

Louisa G. Sylvia, PhD
Dauten Family Center for Bipolar Treatment
Innovation, Massachusetts General Hospital,
Boston, MA; Department of Psychiatry, Harvard
Medical School, Boston, MA; and Department
of Psychiatry, Massachusetts General Hospital,
Boston, MA

Ivan Vargas, PhD
Department of Psychiatry, University of
Pennsylvania, Philadelphia, PA; and
Center for Sleep and Circadian
Neurobiology, University of Pennsylvania,
Philadelphia, PA

Samantha L. Walsh, BS
Department of Psychiatry, Massachusetts General
Hospital, Boston, MA

Clarence Watson, JD, MD
Perelman School of Medicine, University of
Pennsylvania, Philadelphia, PA

Kenneth J. Weiss, MD
Perelman School of Medicine, University of
Pennsylvania, Philadelphia, PA

Emerson M. Wickwire, PhD
Department of Psychiatry, University of
Maryland School of Medicine, Baltimore,
MD; and Sleep Disorders Center, Division
of Pulmonary and Critical Care Medicine,
University of Maryland School of Medicine,
Baltimore, MD

Scott G. Williams, MD
Department of Medicine, Fort Belvoir
Community Hospital, Fort Belvoir, VA

Nevin Zaki, MD
Sleep Research Unit Department of Psychiatry,
Faculty of Medicine, Mansoura University,
Mansoura, Egypt

Jamie M. Zeitzer, PhD
The Stanford Center for Sleep Sciences and
Medicine, Stanford University, Stanford, CA;
Department of Psychiatry and Behavioral
Sciences, School of Medicine, Stanford
University, Stanford, CA; and VA Mental Illness
Research, Education and Clinical Center,
Veterans Affairs Palo Alto Health, Care System,
Palo Alto, CA

PART 1

Introduction to Sleep Medicine

1

Sleep Medicine and Psychiatry

The Inseparable Two

PIYUSH DAS, ANOOP NARAHARI, AND AMIT CHOPRA

INTRODUCTION

Virtually every biological function in humans depends on normal sleep homeostasis to maintain normalcy. As will be evidenced throughout this volume, sleep and its disturbance are intimately linked to normal brain function and psychiatric disorders, respectively. The monoamine neurotransmitters like serotonin, epinephrine, and dopamine that are involved in regulation of sleep and wakefulness [1] are also the ones that are known to be dysregulated in psychiatric disorders. This likely explains the significant comorbidity of sleep symptoms in most, if not all, psychiatric disorders. In the field of clinical psychiatry, a simplistic way of visualizing this relationship is the knowledge that sleep disturbances are defining and diagnostic features of a number of psychiatric disorders. However, the emerging view is that this relationship is more complex and bidirectional, which defies the long-standing view that treating the psychiatric disorder corrects the sleep disturbance. Perhaps, this complex bidirectional relationship stems from common neurochemistry between sleep and emotional function [2].

Sleep disturbances precede, accompany, or follow psychiatric symptoms across a wide spectrum of psychiatric disorders [3–7]. Additionally, medications used to treat psychiatric conditions can lead to sleep disturbances [8]. Ohayon et al. observed the incidence of insomnia in the course of mood and anxiety disorders and noted that insomnia appeared prior to (~40%) or simultaneously with (~22%) mood disorder symptoms, whereas insomnia appeared at the same time (~38%) or after (~34%) the onset of the anxiety disorder [9]. Sleep is also impaired in individuals with alcohol and substance abuse problems. Acute alcohol intake increases slow wave sleep (SWS) and decreases rapid eye movement (REM) sleep during the first half of sleep while the opposite effects are observed in the second half of sleep resulting in sleep fragmentation due to reduced SWS and vivid dreaming due to increase in REM sleep [10]. Patients develop tolerance to sedative effects of alcohol quickly, leaving them at risk of chronic sleep disturbances. The sleep disturbances stemming from chronic alcohol use can last for months to years after discontinuation of alcohol [11].

A recent systematic review showed insomnia to be a major risk factor for new onset of many different psychiatric conditions, with the strongest association seen with depression [12]. Sleep disturbance is a biomarker of genetic vulnerability in nonaffected first-degree relatives of patient with psychiatric illness. For example, short REM sleep latency seen in a significant percentage of patients with major depressive disorder (MDD) is also increasingly seen in first-degree relatives of patients with MDD in whom this finding seems to predict an increased risk for not just developing depression but also increased risk for relapse following response to antidepressant medication [13–15].

A study indicated that administration of eszopiclone, a hypnotic medication along with antidepressant fluoxetine resulted in greater reduction in depressive symptomatology and faster onset of antidepressant action, and not just improvement in sleep measures compared to fluoxetine plus placebo [16]. The same group conducted a follow-up study and showed that discontinuation of eszopiclone after 8 weeks of co-administration with fluoxetine did not result in significant central nervous system or benzodiazepine withdrawal symptoms, rebound insomnia, or rebound depression, and improvements in sleep and depressive symptoms were maintained [17]. These findings exemplify the importance of treating both the sleep and psychiatric symptoms to improve overall treatment outcomes.

Suicidality represents a major concern in patients with depression. A systematic review provided evidence for sleep disturbances as a risk factor for suicidal behaviors in depressed individuals [18]. A study by Bernert et al. suggested association of polysomnography-defined reduction in SWS and higher nocturnal wakefulness with suicidal ideation independent of severity of depression [19]. A subsequent study linked objective and subjective sleep disturbances with acute suicidal ideations independent of depressed mood and suggested sleep as a potential biomarker of suicide risk and a therapeutic target [20].

The ample evidence described here confirms that sleep and psychiatry are indeed inseparable; however, not many psychiatric providers receive adequate education and training in sleep medicine, and as a result, sleep disturbances remain underdiagnosed and undertreated in clinical psychiatric practice. This book aims to prepare the readers for comprehensive evaluation and evidence-based management of sleep disorders in psychiatric patients, which is an area of urgent clinical need and an opportunity for growth in research and academics within psychiatric specialty to improve patient care outcomes.

This chapter, as a prelude to the book, highlights the landmark developments in the fields of sleep medicine and its integration with psychiatry in the last century and opens the window toward broader understanding of the neurobiological and clinical implications of the relationship between sleep and psychiatric disorders.

HISTORICAL PERSPECTIVE

The sleep disturbances are known to exist in patients with psychiatric disorders since antiquity. Hippocratic writers mentioned that sleeplessness was one of the features of melancholia. Although the history of sleep medicine dates back many centuries, the last century has seen major advances in the field leading to what we know as modern sleep medicine. The discovery of electroencephalography (EEG) by Hans Berger in Germany in 1929 was harbinger of the advances in sleep medicine. Less than 10 years later, Alfred Loomis in United States discovered electrophysiological correlates of non-REM (NREM) sleep including vertex waves, sleep spindles, K-complexes, and delta waves. He also characterized varying depths of NREM sleep using these correlates with increasing percentage of delta waves signaling increasing depth of NREM

sleep. Eugene Aserinsky, William Dement, and Nathaniel Kleitman serendipitously discovered REM (REM sleep) in a laboratory at University of Chicago in 1952 [21] and conceptualized its association with dreaming. In 1957, Dement and Kleitman characterized human sleep cycling between NREM and REM multiple times throughout the night and proposed classification of sleep into NREM sleep with its four stages of varying depth and REM sleep [22]. All these electrophysiological discoveries laid foundation for further landmark discoveries in the field of clinical sleep medicine.

In 1970, Stanford University developed the first comprehensive sleep center with an ability to perform nocturnal polysomnography (sleep study). Up till 1975, there were five sleep centers in the United States and sleep medicine was still viewed as an "experimental specialty" with insurance companies routinely denying reimbursement claims [23]. However, that year, Blue Shield of California began reimbursing for clinical sleep services thus recognizing the field of sleep medicine [23]. Around the same time the Association of Sleep Disorders Centers (ASDC) was founded, with a focus on developing sleep centers and providing recommendations for clinical work and research in sleep medicine. In 1976, ASDC formed a nosology committee to develop a diagnostic system for a range of sleep and arousal disorders that are seen clinically. The sleep center at Montefiore Hospital in New York was the first to be accredited by ASDC in 1977. A year later, the first issue of the journal Sleep was published [23].

In 1984, the ASDC announced the formation of a new organization, the Clinical Sleep Society (CSS), for individuals interested in the clinical aspects of sleep and sleep disorders [23]. The CSS Steering Committee then launched a recruitment drive directed primarily at pulmonologists, neurologists, and psychiatrists. In 1987, the ASDC-CSS reorganized to form the American Sleep Disorders Association (ASDA) with two branches of membership including the sleep centers and individuals. In 1988, the Sleep Medicine Fellowship Training Committee was formed with a focus on developing formal guidelines for the comprehensive and standardized training of physicians and fellowship accreditation was provided to its first two programs, Stanford University in California and the Center for Sleep and Wake in New York, in 1989 [23]. In 1999, the ASDA changed its name to the American Academy of Sleep Medicine (AASM) [23].

The classic experiments done by Rechtschaffen and colleagues catapulted the importance of sleep for good health and life and recognition as an important clinical specialty [23].These experiments illustrated that total sleep deprivation resulted in the death of all rats within 2 to 3 weeks. Additionally, selective deprivation of NREM and REM sleep resulted in the death of the animals over a slightly longer period of time. The rats became hypermetabolic and lost weight with progressive sleep deprivation, despite increasing food intake. Due to sleep deprivation, the rats developed skin lesions and erosions of the gastrointestinal tract, with development of hypothermia just prior to death [24]. The authors concluded that the rats died of sepsis, which indicated that sleep deprivation may impair the ability of the body's immune system to deal with infection [25]. Based on findings from a large prospective epidemiological study, it has been shown that mortality rates after 6 years of follow-up were significantly increased for subjects reporting less than 4 hours or more than 10 hours of sleep per night at baseline [26]. In humans, there now exists substantial evidence documenting the adverse consequences of short-term total or partial sleep deprivation on cognition, mood, behavior, performance, and organ-system function [27–30]. Major sleep disorders including obstructive sleep apnea, narcolepsy, restless leg syndrome (RLS), REM sleep behavior disorder (RBD), circadian rhythm sleep–wake disorder, and insomnia have undergone meticulous elucidation of underlying mechanisms and developments of treatment modalities in parallel to advances made in electrophysiological advancements in the field of sleep medicine during the last century.

Probably, one of the most important advance in the history of sleep medicine was the discovery of obstructive sleep apnea in 1966 when Gastaut and colleagues conducted polysomnography studies of obese patients with excessive daytime sleepiness (previously characterized as having Pickwickian syndrome) [31]. Repetitive episodes of upper airway obstruction terminated by short arousals that fragmented sleep (which we now know as obstructive sleep apnea) were attributed to be the underlying cause of excessive daytime sleepiness in these individuals. In late 1970s, Remmers et al. implicated elevated genioglossus muscle activity in pathophysiology of obstructive sleep apnea resulting in recognition of tracheostomy as an effective treatment [32]. A few years later (1980), Collin Sullivan invented nasal continuous

positive airway pressure (CPAP) as an effective method of preventing upper airway collapse, consolidating sleep and alleviating excessive daytime sleepiness [33]. The invention of CPAP in 1980 was a revolutionary advancement in the field of sleep medicine and still recognized as gold standard treatment for obstructive sleep apnea. Since that time, our understanding of the features and consequences of obstructive sleep apnea has progressed significantly, and it is now recognized as a major health issue having an association with not just medical disorders like systemic arterial hypertension, ischemic heart disease, arrhythmia, heart failure, and stroke, but also psychiatric conditions like depression and anxiety [34, 35].

The scientific progress made in the field of chronobiology or study of circadian rhythms in body functions deserves a special mention in terms of advancements in the field of sleep medicine in the past half century. In 1972, suprachiasmatic nucleus (SCN) of anterior hypothalamus was discovered to be the master circadian clock after destruction of SCN was shown to wipe out circadian rhythms in adrenal corticosterone, and drinking and locomotor activity in rats [36]. In the same year, the retino-hypothalamic tract that connects SCN with environmental light was identified [37]. These discoveries were followed by elucidation of molecular and genetic mechanisms regulating the circadian rhythms beginning in 1990s, with resultant isolation of clock genes including *clock, per, Bmal*1, and *cry*, among others [38]. Other research studies linked circadian disruption at the molecular and systemic levels to sleep disorders, obesity and diabetes, heart disease, cancer, and psychiatric disorders [39].

In 1880, Gelineau, a French neurologist, recognized narcolepsy and cataplexy as a condition associated with sudden sleep attacks [40]. A major breakthrough occurred in 1998 when narcolepsy was attributed to disrupted hypocretin neurotransmission an year after independent discovery of hypocretin/orexin by two separate groups of scientists around the same time in two different parts of the world. Luis de Lecea, Thomas Kilduff, and colleagues coined the term *hypocretin* based on its hypothalamic origin and structural similarity with secretin [41], whereas Takeshi Sakurai, Akira Amemiya, and colleagues named the same neuropeptide *orexin* due to its appetite-boosting effect [42]. Orexins or hypocretins, the neuropeptides that are thought to have central importance in regulation of sleep–wake cycle and stabilization of wakeful state were first implicated in pathophysiology of psychiatric disorders in 2002 when orexin levels in schizophrenic patients were found to positively and significantly correlate with sleep latency, one of the most consistent sleep abnormalities seen in schizophrenia in a study by Nishino and colleagues [43]. Later research studies suggested that orexins may play a role in the pathophysiology of multitude of psychiatric conditions, including MDD, anxiety, schizophrenia, and even substance use disorders [44–47].

Earliest description of restless legs was written by Thomas Willis in 1600s; however, it was not named RLS until Karl-Axe Ekbom published a report on eight patients with restless legs in 1944 and his doctoral thesis in 1945: "Restless Legs—a clinical study of hitherto overlooked disease in the legs characterized by peculiar paresthesia ('Anxietas Tibiarum'), pain and weakness occurring in two forms, asthenia crurum paresthetica and asthenia crurum dolorosa" [48]. Later, a dopamine–iron connection was found to be central tenet in many patients with RLS [49]. A possible explanation for this hypothesis is that iron is a necessary cofactor for the function of tyrosine hydroxylase, a rate-limiting step in dopamine synthesis [23]. Dopamine-receptor agonists are effective therapies for RLS thus indicating that RLS is associated with a decrease in dopaminergic function in the brain [23]. Studies have revealed that RLS severity correlates with serum ferritin concentrations below 45 to 50 mg/L [50, 51]. Low cerebrospinal fluid (CSF) ferritin concentration has been demonstrated in RLS patients with normal serum ferritin concentrations, as compared to controls, which suggests that low iron stores in the brain may be associated with RLS [52]. In a magnetic resonance imaging study, reduced brain iron in the substantia nigra (proportionate to disease severity) has been described in RLS patients as compared to controls [53]. Approximately 50% of RLS patients have a positive family history of this condition [54], and a linkage to chromosome 12q has been reported in familial RLS [55]. RLS symptoms have been associated with depression and prevalence of RLS symptoms increasing with the severity of depressive symptoms based on findings from a large cross-sectional study [56].

REM sleep behavior disorder, characterized by dream enactment behaviors and REM sleep without atonia (RSWA), was first described in 1985 by Mark Mahowald and Carlos Schenck at the University of Minnesota [57]. RBD has been associated with neurodegenerative disorders characterized by alpha-synuclein positive inclusion bodies such as Parkinson's disease, multiple system atrophy, or Lewy body dementia [58]. RBD has been found to be a harbinger of neurodegenerative diseases such as Parkinson's disease as supported by radionuclide studies that show neurologically normal RBD patients have reduced striatal dopamine activity, a finding suggestive of these patients having presymptomatic stages of Parkinson's disease [59, 60]. This insight has a potential to develop preventative therapies for neurodegenerative diseases in the future [23, 61].

Finally, significant advancements have been made in understanding of the epidemiology, phenomenology, and treatment of insomnia, the most prevalent of all sleep disorders. Based on epidemiologic data, the prevalence of insomnia symptoms in the prior year has been reported to be 30% to 45% [62–64], whereas the prevalence of insomnia disorders has been estimated to be 10% to 15% [65]. The risk factors associated with insomnia include a prior history of insomnia, increasing age, female gender, psychiatric symptoms and disorders, medical symptoms and disorders, impaired activities of daily living, anxiolytic and hypnotic medication use, and low socioeconomic status [23]. Additionally, between 50% and 80% of individuals with insomnia at baseline report persistent complaint of insomnia after follow-up intervals of 1 to 3.5 years thus suggesting chronicity of this disorder [62, 66, 67]. The concept of psychophysiological arousal as a cause of insomnia emerged and supported by findings of elevated heart rate, elevated temperature and muscle tone at sleep onset, elevated whole body metabolic rate during both day and night, higher rates of self-reported ruminations and intrusive thoughts, and EEG studies showing hyperarousal in individuals with insomnia compared to healthy controls [68]. Pharmacological treatments [69, 70] and cognitive-behavioral treatments [71] have developed significantly over the past few decades to address this highly prevalent sleep disorder.

INTEGRATION OF SLEEP MEDICINE AND PSYCHIATRY

This section briefly describes the history of integration of the fields of sleep medicine and psychiatry. Freud may be considered one of the pioneers in integrating sleep and psychiatry in the last century as he explained dreaming as a key concept in the psychoanalytic theory of mind [72]. Freud viewed dreaming as an unconscious mental process through which the dreamer edits the unacceptable unconscious material that would otherwise invade conscious state and cause distress in its original form. He conceptualized that people with mental illness could be cured by bringing their unconscious thoughts and motivations into their conscious state as that would result in gaining "insight." However, research by prominent research-ers like Eugene Aserinsky, William Demente, and Nathaniel Kleitman led to discovery of REM sleep in 1953, and work done by Michel Jouvet led to localization of REM generation in pons thereby redefining dreaming as a physi-ological process of brain [73]. Furthermore, the activation-synthesis model developed by J. Allan Hobson and Robert McCarley reinforced that brain rather than mind was the dream state generator [74] and proposed that dreams are created by changes in neuronal activity that acti-vates the brainstem during REM sleep.

The *Diagnostic and Statistical Manual* (DSM) of sleep disorders was first introduced in 1968 under the category of "Disorders of Sleep" in DSM-II. In 1980, sleep disorders including sleep walking and sleep terror disorder were included in DSM-III classification. The categories of dys-somnia (including insomnia, hypersomnia, sleep wake schedule disorder) and parasomnia (sleep walking, sleep terror, nightmare disorder) were subsequently included in the DSM-III R version in 1987. Significant changes were noted in DSM-IV TR in 2005 as it included additional categories of sleep disorders such as breathing-related sleep

---

TABLE 1.1 SLEEP-WAKE DISORDERS
IN DSM-V

- Insomnia disorder
- Hypersomnolence disorder
- Narcolepsy
- Obstructive sleep apnea hypopnea
- Central sleep apnea
- Sleep-related hypoventilation
- Circadian rhythm sleep-wake disorders
- Nonrapid eye movement (NREM) sleep arousal disorders
- Nightmare disorder
- Rapid eye movement (REM) sleep behavior disorder
- Restless legs syndrome
- Substance-/medication-induced sleep disorder

---

disorders, circadian rhythm sleep disorders, sleep disorders related to another mental disorder, and other sleep disorders.

DSM-V offers the most comprehensive classification of sleep wake disorders (see Table 1.1) that is synchronous with other classification systems such as *International Classification of Sleep Disorders* (ICSD-3). DSM-V classification underscores the need for independent clinical attention of a sleep disorder regardless of the co-existing mental or other medical problems. DSM-V no longer has the distinction between primary and secondary insomnia as noted in DSM-IV. The diagnostic criteria for insomnia disorder in DSM-V are more specific in terms of frequency of symptoms (at least 3 times per week) and the duration has been changed to 3 months. The DSM-V has eliminated the distinction of primary hypersomnia and replaced it with hypersomnolence disorder, which now has (a) duration criteria, defined as acute (less than a month), subacute (1–3 months), and chronic (longer than 3 months) and (b) a dimensional approach of specifying the severity (mild, moderate, severe). DSM-V incorporates hypocretin deficiency, polysomnography, and multiple sleep testing criteria as a diagnostic criteria for narcolepsy with more specificity in symptoms frequency (3 times per week) and duration (3 months). DSM-V recognizes that coexisting medical conditions, mental disorders, and sleep disorders are interactive and bidirectional in nature. Additionally, two previous diagnoses, including sleep disorder related to another mental disorder and sleep disorder related to another medical condition, have been eliminated in this version.

Sleep disturbances are inherent in a range of psychiatric disorders including mood, anxi-ety, and psychotic disorders. Since the mid-20th century, researchers have tried to systematically examine this association to advance the under-standing of neurobiology and treatment of psychiatric disorders. The advent of the psycho-physiological study of sleep, which started in the 1950s (sleep studies in schizophrenic patients at the Manteno State Hospital), allowed the scien-tific approach of sleep disturbance in psychiatric disorders as well as role of psychopathology in the course of various sleep disorders [75]. Since 1970s, extensive research on EEG markers in patients with MDD has revealed that individuals with MDD and those in remission exhibit increased REM density and shortened SWS. Interestingly, high-risk probands with no history of MDD share similar EEG findings with those having

MDD and those in remission from MDD. These EEG features in combination may represent a genetic biomarker of MDD [76]. Circadian rhythm dysfunction may be considered trait marker of bipolar disorder, and it may act as predictor for the first onset and the relapse of mood episodes in bipolar disorder [77]. It has been postulated that treatments focusing on sleep disturbances and circadian rhythm dysfunction in combination with pharmacological and psychosocial interventions are likely to help relapse prevention in bipolar disorder [77]. Slow wave sleep (SWS) deficit has been described in patients with schizophrenia (duration >3 years), while sleep onset latency was increased in medication-naïve, medication-withdrawn, and medicated patients [78]. These findings highlight the importance of understanding, recognizing, and treating the comorbid sleep disturbances in patients with psychiatric disorders for optimal clinical outcomes. This book aims to synthesize the currently available scientific evidence that examines the comorbidity, neurobiology, and treatment of sleep disturbances comorbid with psychiatric disorders based on DSM-V classification. This book identifies the lack of and thus the need for further research and systematic evidence and provides future directions to advance the fields of sleep medicine and psychiatry.

CONCLUSIONS

As clearly evident in this chapter, sleep medicine and psychiatry are intertwined medical specialties. The majority of psychiatric patients have sleep complaints, and therefore understanding of patient's sleep is an important part of comprehensive psychiatric assessment. The intriguing relationship between sleep disturbances and psychiatric disorders raises several questions. First, does the sleep disturbance herald or result from psychiatric disorder, or is this relationship bidirectional? Second, do sleep disruption and psychiatric disorders share common brain structures or neurochemical processes? Third, is there a cause-and-effect relationship between the two, or are the two simply comorbid? Finally, do the treatments of comorbid sleep disturbances positively affect psychiatric outcomes in a broad spectrum of psychiatric disorders? This book synthesizes the current literature to understand the crucial relationship answer the intriguing queries in regards to these two inseparable clinical specialties.

KEY CLINICAL PEARLS

- Sleep disturbances are almost universal in patients suffering from psychiatric disorders.
- Psychiatric symptoms seem to precede, accompany, or follow sleep disturbances with this sequence existing across wide range of psychiatric disorders.
- A bidirectional relationship seems to exist between sleep and psychiatric disorders.
- It is crucial to separately address the sleep disturbance comorbid to psychiatric condition, rather than relying on sole treatment of the psychiatric condition, to optimize treatment outcome.
- There is a significant need for psychiatric providers to train in evaluation and management of comorbid sleep disorders in patients with psychiatric condition(s).

SELF-ASSESSMENT QUESTIONS

1. Which of the following statements is false?
   a. The treatment of MDD with SSRI often leads to resolution of insomnia complaint in patients with MDD.
   b. Insomnia is a common ancillary symptom of MDD.
   c. Insomnia can lead to new-onset depression.
   d. Insomnia is a predictor of relapse of depression.

Answer: a

2. What marked the beginning of modern sleep science?
   a. The discovery of REM sleep
   b. The discovery of electrophysiological correlates of NREM sleep including vertex waves, sleep spindles, K-complexes, and delta waves
   c. Electroencephalogram (EEG)
   d. The discovery of orexins

Answer: c

3. Which landmark discovery in the last quarter century revolutionized our understanding of pathophysiology of narcolepsy?
   a. The discovery of REM sleep
   b. The discovery of orexin/hypocretin
   c. The discovery of clock genes
   d. The discovery of dopamine–iron connection

Answer: b

4. Which one of these statements is true about effects of acute alcohol consumption on sleep?
   a. Alcohol increases REM sleep during the first half of sleep.
   b. Alcohol reduces REM sleep during the second half of sleep.
   c. Alcohol leads to vivid dreaming during the second half of sleep.
   d. Alcohol increases slow wave sleep during the second half of sleep.

Answer: c

5. Which of the following primary sleep disorders are included in DSM-5 classification of sleep-wake disorders?
   a. Obstructive sleep apnea hypopnea
   b. Central sleep apnea
   c. Sleep-related hypoventilation
   d. All of above

Answer: d

REFERENCES

1. McCarley, R.W., *Neurobiology of REM and NREM sleep.* Sleep Med, 2007. **8**(4): p. 302–330.
2. Murphy, M.J. and M.J. Peterson, *Sleep Disturbances in Depression.* Sleep Med Clin, 2015. **10**(1): p. 17–23.
3. Ford, D.E. and D.B. Kamerow, *Epidemiologic study of sleep disturbances and psychiatric disorders. An opportunity for prevention?* JAMA, 1989. **262**(11): p. 1479–1484.
4. Soehner, A.M., K.A. Kaplan, and A.G. Harvey, *Prevalence and clinical correlates of co-occurring insomnia and hypersomnia symptoms in depression.* J Affect Disord, 2014. **167**: p. 93–97.
5. Breslau, N., et al., *Sleep disturbance and psychiatric disorders: a longitudinal epidemiological study of young adults.* Biol Psychiatry, 1996. **39**(6): p. 411–418.
6. Geoffroy, P.A., et al., *Insomnia and hypersomnia in major depressive episode: Prevalence, sociodemographic characteristics and psychiatric comorbidity in a population-based study.* J Affect Disord, 2018. **226**: p. 132–141.
7. Dealberto, M.J., *[Sleep disorders in psychiatric diseases. Epidemiological aspects].* Encephale, 1992. **18**(4): p. 331–340.
8. DeMartinis, N.A. and A. Winokur, *Effects of psychiatric medications on sleep and sleep disorders.* CNS Neurol Disord Drug Targets, 2007. **6**(1): p. 17–29.
9. Ohayon, M.M. and T. Roth, *Place of chronic insomnia in the course of depressive and anxiety disorders.* J Psychiatr Res, 2003. **37**(1): p. 9–15.
10. Abad, V.C. and C. Guilleminault, *Sleep and psychiatry.* Dialogues Clin Neurosci, 2005. **7**(4): p. 291–303.
11. Stein, M.D. and P.D. Friedmann, *Disturbed sleep and its relationship to alcohol use.* Subst Abus, 2005. **26**(1): p. 1–13.
12. Pigeon, W.R., T.M. Bishop, and K.M. Krueger, *Insomnia as a Precipitating Factor in New Onset Mental Illness: a Systematic Review of Recent Findings.* Curr Psychiatry Rep, 2017. **19**(8): p. 44.
13. Giles, D.E., et al., *Risk factors in families of unipolar depression. I. Psychiatric illness and reduced REM latency.* J Affect Disord, 1988. **14**(1): p. 51–59.
14. Giles, D.E., et al., *Polysomnographic parameters in first-degree relatives of unipolar probands.* Psychiatry Res, 1989. **27**(2): p. 127–136.
15. Emslie, G.J., et al., *Sleep polysomnography as a predictor of recurrence in children and adolescents with major depressive disorder.* Int J Neuropsychopharmacol, 2001. **4**(2): p. 159–168.
16. Fava, M., et al., *Eszopiclone co-administered with fluoxetine in patients with insomnia coexisting with major depressive disorder.* Biol Psychiatry, 2006. **59**(11): p. 1052–1060.
17. Krystal, A., et al., *Evaluation of eszopiclone discontinuation after cotherapy with fluoxetine for insomnia with coexisting depression.* J Clin Sleep Med, 2007. **3**(1): p. 48–55.
18. Bernert, R.A., et al., *Sleep disturbances as an evidence-based suicide risk factor.* Curr Psychiatry Rep, 2015. **17**(3): p. 554.
19. Bernert, R.A., et al., *Sleep architecture parameters as a putative biomarker of suicidal ideation in treatment-resistant depression.* J Affect Disord, 2017. **208**: p. 309–315.
20. Bernert, R.A., et al., *Objectively assessed sleep variability as an acute warning sign of suicidal ideation in a longitudinal evaluation of young adults at high suicide risk.* J Clin Psychiatry, 2017. **78**(6): p. e678–e687.
21. Aserinsky, E. and N. Kleitman, *Regularly occurring periods of eye motility, and concomitant phenomena, during sleep.* Science, 1953. **118**(3062): p. 273–274.
22. Dement, W. and N. Kleitman, *Cyclic variations in EEG during sleep and their relation to eye movements, body motility, and dreaming.* Electroencephalogr Clin Neurophysiol, 1957. **9**(4): p. 673–690.
23. Shepard, J.W., Jr., et al., *History of the development of sleep medicine in the United States.* J Clin Sleep Med, 2005. **1**(1): p. 61–82.
24. Rechtschaffen, A., et al., *Sleep deprivation in the rat: X. Integration and discussion of the findings.* Sleep, 1989. **12**(1): p. 68–87.

25. Everson, C.A., *Sustained sleep deprivation impairs host defense.* Am J Physiol, 1993. **265**(5 Pt 2): p. R1148–R1154.

26. Kripke, D.F., et al., *Short and long sleep and sleeping pills. Is increased mortality associated?* Arch Gen Psychiatry, 1979. **36**(1): p. 103–116.

27. Satterfield, B.C., et al., *Unraveling the genetic underpinnings of sleep deprivation-induced impairments in human cognition.* Prog Brain Res, 2019. **246**: p. 127–158.

28. Riemann, D., et al., *Sleep, insomnia, and depression.* Neuropsychopharmacology, 2019.

29. Dorrian, J., et al., *Self-regulation and social behavior during sleep deprivation.* Prog Brain Res, 2019. **246**: p. 73–110.

30. Kaufmann, T., et al., *The brain functional connectome is robustly altered by lack of sleep.* Neuroimage, 2016. **127**: p. 324–332.

31. Gastaut, H., C.A. Tassinari, and B. Duron, *Polygraphic study of the episodic diurnal and nocturnal (hypnic and respiratory) manifestations of the Pickwick syndrome.* Brain Res, 1966. **1**(2): p. 167–186.

32. Remmers, J.E., et al., *Pathogenesis of upper airway occlusion during sleep.* J Appl Physiol Respir Environ Exerc Physiol, 1978. **44**(6): p. 931–938.

33. Sullivan, C.E., et al., *Reversal of obstructive sleep apnoea by continuous positive airway pressure applied through the nares.* Lancet, 1981. **1**(8225): p. 862–865.

34. Bahammam, A., *Obstructive sleep apnea: from simple upper airway obstruction to systemic inflammation.* Ann Saudi Med, 2011. **31**(1): p. 1–2.

35. Garbarino, S., et al., *Association of Anxiety and Depression in Obstructive Sleep Apnea Patients: A Systematic Review and Meta-Analysis.* Behav Sleep Med, 2018: p. 1–23.

36. Weaver, D.R., *The suprachiasmatic nucleus: a 25-year retrospective.* J Biol Rhythms, 1998. **13**(2): p. 100–112.

37. Moore, R.Y. and N.J. Lenn, *A retinohypothalamic projection in the rat.* J Comp Neurol, 1972. **146**(1): p. 1–14.

38. Rosenwasser, A.M. and F.W. Turek, *Neurobiology of Circadian Rhythm Regulation.* Sleep Med Clin, 2015. **10**(4): p. 403–412.

39. Touitou, Y., A. Reinberg, and D. Touitou, *Association between light at night, melatonin secretion, sleep deprivation, and the internal clock: Health impacts and mechanisms of circadian disruption.* Life Sci, 2017. **173**: p. 94–106.

40. Schenck, C.H., et al., *English translations of the first clinical reports on narcolepsy and cataplexy by Westphal and Gelineau in the late 19th century, with commentary.* J Clin Sleep Med, 2007. **3**(3): p. 301–311.

41. de Lecea, L., et al., *The hypocretins: hypothalamus-specific peptides with neuroexcitatory activity.* Proc Natl Acad Sci U S A, 1998. **95**(1): p. 322–327.

42. Sakurai, T., et al., *Orexins and orexin receptors: a family of hypothalamic neuropeptides and G protein-coupled receptors that regulate feeding behavior.* Cell, 1998. **92**(4): p. 573–585.

43. Nishino, S., et al., *CSF hypocretin-1 levels in schizophrenics and controls: relationship to sleep architecture.* Psychiatry Res, 2002. **110**(1): p. 1–7.

44. Shariq, A.S., et al., *Evaluating the role of orexins in the pathophysiology and treatment of depression: A comprehensive review.* Prog Neuropsychopharmacol Biol Psychiatry, 2019. **92**: p. 1–7.

45. Borgland, S.L. and G. Labouebe, *Orexin/hypocretin in psychiatric disorders: present state of knowledge and future potential.* Neuropsychopharmacology, 2010. **35**(1): p. 353–354.

46. Chen, Q., et al., *The hypocretin/orexin system: an increasingly important role in neuropsychiatry.* Med Res Rev, 2015. **35**(1): p. 152–197.

47. Deutch, A.Y. and M. Bubser, *The orexins/hypocretins and schizophrenia.* Schizophr Bull, 2007. **33**(6): p. 1277–1283.

48. Kirsch, D.B., *There and back again: a current history of sleep medicine.* Chest, 2011. **139**(4): p. 939–946.

49. Earley, C.J., et al., *Insight into the pathophysiology of restless legs syndrome.* J Neurosci Res, 2000. **62**(5): p. 623–628.

50. O'Keeffe, S.T., K. Gavin, and J.N. Lavan, *Iron status and restless legs syndrome in the elderly.* Age Ageing, 1994. **23**(3): p. 200–203.

51. Sun, E.R., et al., *Iron and the restless legs syndrome.* Sleep, 1998. **21**(4): p. 371–377.

52. Earley, C.J., et al., *Abnormalities in CSF concentrations of ferritin and transferrin in restless legs syndrome.* Neurology, 2000. **54**(8): p. 1698–1700.

53. Allen, R.P., et al., *MRI measurement of brain iron in patients with restless legs syndrome.* Neurology, 2001. **56**(2): p. 263–265.

54. Winkelmann, J., et al., *Clinical characteristics and frequency of the hereditary restless legs syndrome in a population of 300 patients.* Sleep, 2000. **23**(5): p. 597–602.

55. Desautels, A., et al., *Identification of a major susceptibility locus for restless legs syndrome on chromosome 12q.* Am J Hum Genet, 2001. **69**(6): p. 1266–1270.

56. Auvinen, P., et al., *Prevalence of restless legs symptoms according to depressive symptoms and depression type: a cross-sectional study.* Nord J Psychiatry, 2018. **72**(1): p. 51–56.

57. Schenck, C.H., et al., *Chronic behavioral disorders of human REM sleep: a new category of parasomnia.* Sleep, 1986. **9**(2): p. 293–308.

58. Olson, E.J., B.F. Boeve, and M.H. Silber, *Rapid eye movement sleep behaviour disorder: demographic, clinical and laboratory findings in 93 cases*. Brain, 2000. **123** (Pt 2): p. 331–339.

59. Eisensehr, I., et al., *Reduced striatal dopamine transporters in idiopathic rapid eye movement sleep behaviour disorder. Comparison with Parkinson's disease and controls*. Brain, 2000. **123**(Pt 6): p. 1155–1160.

60. Albin, R.L., et al., *Decreased striatal dopaminergic innervation in REM sleep behavior disorder*. Neurology, 2000. **55**(9): p. 1410–1412.

61. Boeve, B.F., et al., *Association of REM sleep behavior disorder and neurodegenerative disease may reflect an underlying synucleinopathy*. Mov Disord, 2001. **16**(4): p. 622–630.

62. Ganguli, M., C.F. Reynolds, and J.E. Gilby, *Prevalence and persistence of sleep complaints in a rural older community sample: the MoVIES project*. J Am Geriatr Soc, 1996. **44**(7): p. 778–784.

63. Mellinger, G.D., M.B. Balter, and E.H. Uhlenhuth, *Insomnia and its treatment. Prevalence and correlates*. Arch Gen Psychiatry, 1985. **42**(3): p. 225–232.

64. Foley, D.J., et al., *Sleep complaints among elderly persons: an epidemiologic study of three communities*. Sleep, 1995. **18**(6): p. 425–432.

65. Ohayon, M.M., *Prevalence of DSM-IV diagnostic criteria of insomnia: distinguishing insomnia related to mental disorders from sleep disorders*. J Psychiatr Res, 1997. **31**(3): p. 333–346.

66. Foley, D.J., et al., *Incidence and remission of insomnia among elderly adults: an epidemiologic study of 6,800 persons over three years*. Sleep, 1999. **22**(Suppl 2): p. S366–S372.

67. Katz, D.A. and C.A. McHorney, *Clinical correlates of insomnia in patients with chronic illness*. Arch Intern Med, 1998. **158**(10): p. 1099–1107.

68. Bonnet, M.H., G.G. Burton, and D.L. Arand, *Physiological and medical findings in insomnia: implications for diagnosis and care*. Sleep Med Rev, 2014. **18**(2): p. 111–122.

69. Nowell, P.D., et al., *Benzodiazepines and zolpidem for chronic insomnia: a meta-analysis of treatment efficacy*. Jama, 1997. **278**(24): p. 2170–2177.

70. Holbrook, A.M., et al., *Meta-analysis of benzodiazepine use in the treatment of insomnia*. Cmaj, 2000. **162**(2): p. 225–233.

71. Morin, C.M., et al., *Nonpharmacologic treatment of chronic insomnia. An American Academy of Sleep Medicine review*. Sleep, 1999. **22**(8): p. 1134–1156.

72. Zhang, W. and B. Guo, *Freud's Dream Interpretation: A Different Perspective Based on the Self-Organization Theory of Dreaming*. Front Psychol, 2018. **9**: p. 1553.

73. Luppi, P.H., *Jouvet's animal model of RBD, clinical RBD, and their relationships to REM sleep mechanisms*. Sleep Med, 2018. **49**: p. 28–30.

74. Hobson, J.A. and R.W. McCarley, *The brain as a dream state generator: an activation-synthesis hypothesis of the dream process*. Am J Psychiatry, 1977. **134**(12): p. 1335–1348.

75. Dement, W.C., *History of sleep medicine*. Neurol Clin, 2005. **23**(4): p. 945–965, v.

76. Pillai, V., D.A. Kalmbach, and J.A. Ciesla, *A meta-analysis of electroencephalographic sleep in depression: evidence for genetic biomarkers*. Biol Psychiatry, 2011. **70**(10): p. 912–919.

77. Takaesu, Y., *Circadian rhythm in bipolar disorder: A review of the literature*. Psychiatry Clin Neurosci, 2018. **72**(9): p. 673–682.

78. Chan, M.S., et al., *Sleep in schizophrenia: A systematic review and meta-analysis of polysomnographic findings in case-control studies*. Sleep Med Rev, 2017. **32**: p. 69–84.

2

Sleep Architecture and Physiology

DEEPA BURMAN AND HIREN MUZUMDAR

INTRODUCTION

Sleep is a dynamic physiologic process with a critical impact on health and daytime well-being. It is an integral component of neurological functioning that is often disrupted by psychiatric disorders, and, conversely, sleep disruptions can exacerbate psychiatric conditions. In addition, many widely prescribed psychotropic medications exert their effects through modulation of different monoamines and interactions with receptors such as histamine and muscarinic cholinergic receptors, impacting sleep in both beneficial and harmful ways. Understanding sleep physiology and architecture is critical to the understanding and management of sleep perturbations commonly associated with psychiatric disorders. Sleep structure itself is complex and evolves with age, and the effects of sleep on various physiologic systems can vary with age and the stages of sleep. In this chapter, we discuss sleep architecture in a normal adult and its changes across the lifespan. We also discuss physiological changes during sleep in various organ systems in healthy and disease states.

SLEEP ARCHITECTURE

Sleep is a nonhomogenous process. Normal human sleep is comprised of two distinct alternating states—rapid eye movement (REM) and non-REM (NREM) sleep. Polysomnography is the gold standard tool for assessing sleep and categorizing sleep in to various stages. This staging of sleep on a polysomnogram occurs in 30-second periods known as epochs using electroencephalography (EEG), muscle tone by electromyography (EMG) and eye movements by electrooculography (EOG). NREM sleep is marked by a variably synchronous cortical EEG including sleep spindles, K complexes and slow waves, and is associated with low muscle tone and minimal psychological activity. It is further divided into three stages: stage N1, stage N2, and stage N3 (older rules differentiated deep sleep into stages 3 and 4) based on amplitude and frequencies of brain waves. Stage N1 is a transition stage from wakefulness to sleep characterized by low amplitude mixed frequencies with slow, rolling eye movements. It is the lightest stage of sleep, and patients awakened from it do not perceive that they were actually asleep. Stage 2 comprises of the largest percentage of total sleep in an average adult. Two distinct features of this stage are sleep spindles (short burst of neural oscillatory activity with a frequency of 11–16 Hz lasting at least 0.5 seconds) and K complexes (negative sharp waves immediately followed by a positive component that last greater than 0.5 seconds). Stage N3 is also referred to as "slow wave or deep sleep" and is characterized by low frequency (0.5–2 Hz), high amplitude EEG (>75 microvolts) in at least 20% of the epoch. In REM sleep, EEG is desynchronized with low voltage mixed frequency, muscles are atonic with intermittent phasic eye movements and dreaming is noted. Sawtooth waves are seen and REMs are the defining feature of this stage. Inhibition of alpha motor neurons also results in atonia of all voluntary muscles (except extraocular and diaphragm).

Average human adults manifest several consistent architectural features during their sleep period. Sleep begins in NREM stage N1 and progresses through the deeper NREM stages N2 and N3. REM sleep (stage R) occurs approximately 80 to 100 minutes after sleep onset. Subsequently, NREM and REM sleep cycle with a period of approximately 90 to 110 minutes. N3 sleep (deep sleep or slow-wave sleep [SWS]) is concentrated in the first half of the night. REM sleep episodes lengthen across the night and are longer toward the second half of the night. In addition to staging information, several sleep architectural parameters, which are commonly included in a polysomnography report, are noted in Table 2.1.

TABLE 2.1. COMMON SLEEP ARCHITECTURE PARAMETERS REPORTED IN A SLEEP STUDY

Sleep Architecture Parameters	Definition
Total Recording time (min)	Total time from lights out to lights on
Total sleep time (TST) (min)	Time spent in different stages of sleep
Sleep latency (min)	Time from start of recording, "lights out", to the start of first epoch of sleep.
REM latency (min)	Time from first epoch of sleep to first epoch of stage REM
Wake after sleep onset (WASO)	Stage wake recorded after sleep onset until end of recording, "lights on."
Arousal Index	Total number of arousals × 60/TST (min)
Sleep efficiency (%)	TST × 100/Total recording time

TABLE 2.2. TIME IN EACH STAGE AS A PERCENTAGE OF TOTAL SLEEP TIME IN ADULTS

Stage	Percentage
Wakefulness in sleep	5% of the night
Stage N1	2%–5% of sleep
Stage N2	45%–55% of sleep
Stage N3	5%–15% of sleep
Stage R (4–6 episodes)	20%–25% of sleep

Normal Sleep across Life Span

Sleep duration and architecture vary across life span like many other biological phenomena. Infants who are 3 months or younger normally enter sleep through REM which is abnormal in normal adults. The amount of **sleep required to feel refreshed** changes across lifespan reducing from about 16 to 18 hours at birth to 10 hours in children, 9 hours in adolescence, about 8 hours in early adulthood, and 6 to 7 hours in older people. Some data even suggest that the breakdown of sleep with age might reflect physiologic age and reflect alterations in function present at the genomic level. Table 2.2 summarizes sleep at different stages of life.

Infants (Younger Than 3 Months) and Children

Newborns sleep for 16 to 18 hours a day without a clear circadian phase. There are data that the circadian melatonin rhythm appears at the end of the neonatal period and circadian rhythm of wakefulness and sleep is clearly set up as early as 4 months of age and consolidates between 6 and 7 months. It is *abnormal* for an adult to start sleep in REM, but infants start sleep in REM until around 3 months of age when they begin to develop a night/

day cycle. Until 36 weeks, postconceptional age "trace discontinue" pattern is seen on EEG of a developing brain, which comprises bursts of high-amplitude mixed-frequency waves interspersed with periods of flat, attenuated activity. This pattern is replaced by "trace alternant," in which brief bursts of high-amplitude delta waves are interspersed among periods of low-amplitude waves (25–50 μV) up to 46 weeks postconceptional age.[1]

NREM is staged as quiet sleep and REM as active sleep in infants. Indeterminate or transitional sleep is an EEG waveform that is not clearly quiet or active sleep in infants and disappears with maturation. When brain structure and function achieve a level that can support high-voltage, slow-wave EEG activity, N3 or SWS become prominent. Sleep spindles begin to appear around 6 to 8 weeks of age,[1,2] but NREM cannot be clearly demarcated into specific stages until around 3 to 6 months of age. In children older than 3 months, sleep starts as NREM sleep, and REM sleep does not occur until 80 minutes or longer after sleep onset. The cycles of NREM–REM sleep last approximately 50 to 60 minutes in the newborn compared with approximately 90 to 110 minutes in the adult.

SWS is maximal in young children and decreases with age. SWS in young children is both qualitatively and quantitatively different from that of older adults. For example, it is very difficult to wake youngsters in the SWS of the night's first sleep cycle. SWS has its largest decline during the second decade of life while at the same time stage N2 increases to its adult level of around 45% to 55% of sleep.[3] The proportion of REM sleep reduces from 50% during early infancy to 30% at 6 months of age and to adult levels of 20% at approximately 2 years of age.

Adults

Stage N1 is the transition stage from wakefulness to sleep and usually persists for a few (1–7) minutes at the onset of sleep. N1 is the lightest stage with a low arousal threshold and is easily interrupted by low intensity stimuli such as softly calling a person's name, touching a person lightly, and quietly closing a door. Stage N1 sleep occurs as a transitional stage throughout the night, and a common sign of disrupted sleep is an increase in the amount and percentage of stage N1 sleep. Stage N2 comprises the largest percentage of sleep time in a normal adult. It is marked by sleep spindles or K complexes in the EEG. A more intense stimulus is required to produce arousal in this stage of sleep. High-voltage (greater than 75 µV) slow-wave activity gradually appears in the EEG (for more than 20% the epoch), as stage N2 progresses to stage N3.

Stage R (REM sleep) comprises of low voltage, mixed frequency EEG. Sawtooth waves are commonly seen in the EEG. REM (phasic REM) and atonia of voluntary muscles (tonic REM) are notable with variable arousal threshold. REM in the first cycle of the night is usually short-lived (1–5 minutes). The percentage of REM sleep usually increases across the night in each cycle while the SWS is dominant in the early part of the sleep cycle (the first one-third) and diminishes as the sleep period progresses. Table 2.3 summarizes time spent in each stage as a percentage of the total sleep time in adults.

Elderly

Although there is a clear age-dependent decline in sleep efficiency up to and beyond age 90 years, the vast majority of age-dependent changes in sleep architecture occur before age 60 years.[4] Some variables (total sleep time, REM) are characterized by a linear decline, whereas others (SWS, wake after sleep onset) follow a more exponential course. REM sleep, as a percentage of total sleep, is maintained until a later age, after which a small linear decline occurs. This decline ceases with advancing age and between ages of 75 and 85, there may be small increases in REM percentage. The absolute amount of REM sleep at night has been correlated with intellectual functioning.[5] It declines markedly with organic brain dysfunctions of the elderly.[5] Arousals during sleep increase markedly with age, but healthy adults have no difficulty falling back to sleep.[6] K complex and spindle density decrease with age[7] but the most prominent change in sleep with age is the decline in SWS. Feinberg[1,8] hypothesized that this age-related decline might parallel loss of cortical synaptic density. SWS might no longer be present after age 60 years in men, but women appear to maintain SWS later than men.

TABLE 2.3. SLEEP AT DIFFERENT STAGES OF LIFE

Stage of Life	Key Features
Newborns	16–18 hours including 5–10 hours of napping Polyphasic (sleeping multiple times in 24 hours) Comprised of 50% REM
2–3 months	Spindles start to appear
3–6 months	Major sleep period is at night Stage 1, 2, and 3 can be ascertained K complexes start to appear
1–3 years	12–14 hours of sleep including 1.5–2 hours of napping 25% REM sleep
3–5 years	11–13 hours of sleep including naps, 0-2.5 hours is napping
5–12 years	9–12 hours of sleep and no naps
13–20 years	8–10 hours of sleep, no naps Delay in sleep phase may occur
20–65 years	Large decline in slow wave sleep amplitude Progressive decline in SWS percentage
65 years and older	Napping returns Advance sleep phase may occur Increased sleep fragmentation

However, the most notable finding regarding sleep in the elderly is the profound increase in interindividual variability.

SLEEP PHYSIOLOGY

Sleep is a state of relative external unresponsiveness that has predictable cycling and reversal of unresponsiveness that distinguishes it from other states of unconsciousness. It is a complex process that is controlled by many areas of the brain and results from inhibition of wake promoting systems by homeostatic sleep factors such as adenosine and GABAergic neurons. Further discussion of sleep wake neuro-regulation is beyond the scope of this chapter and is covered elsewhere in the textbook. Table 2.4 demonstrates key physiological changes during sleep in various organ systems.

Sleep and wake are determined by the circadian process (Process C) and the homeostatic sleep process (Process S) and various physiologic parameters are differentially affected by the two

TABLE 2.4. OVERVIEW OF VARIOUS ORGAN SYSTEM PHYSIOLOGY
IN SLEEP

Organ System	Key Changes
Endocrine function	Sleep deprivation: increases ghrelin, decreases leptin, also results in insulin resistance
Thermoregulation	Homeostasis is present in NREM with decreased hypothalamic temperature set point
	Homeostasis inhibited in REM sleep
Cardiovascular system	Autonomic stability is present in NREM sleep and relative instability in REM sleep.
	Lower blood pressure and slow regular heart rate in NREM sleep.
	Irregular heart rate and transient increases in blood pressure in REM sleep.
	Increased heart rate is present in phasic REM and coronary blood flow decreases in patients with coronary artery disease
	Cerebral blood flow decreases in NREM and increases in REM
Gastrointestinal system	Maximal acid secretion between 10 PM to 2 AM
	Esophageal sphincter tone is lower in NREM compared to REM
Autonomic Nervous System	Increased parasympathetic tone in NREM
	Brief surges in sympathetic activity during phasic REM and parasympathetic activity during tonic REM sleep
Respiratory System	Decreased respiratory rate with mild decrease in ventilatory drive in response to hypoxia and hypercapnia in NREM sleep
	Increased respiratory rate with significantly decreased ventilatory drive in response to hypercapnia and hypoxia during REM sleep
Reproductive system	Presence of penile erections and increased vaginal blood flow in REM sleep

Abbreviation: NREM, nonrapid eye movement; REM, rapid eye movement.

processes. The circadian process or rhythm is an approximately 24-hour cycle in the biochemical, physiological, or behavioral processes of living entities including each cell of the body. These rhythms are synchronized by a master clock located in the suprachiasmatic nuclei (SCN) in the anterior hypothalamus in humans. Cells throughout the human body contain endogenous circadian oscillators operating via transcription-translation feedback loops. These peripheral clocks are susceptible to adjustment from the SCN clock via circulating hormones such as melatonin, other metabolic cues, and systemic changes such as body temperature. The master internal clock has mechanisms that allow it to synchronize itself with external time (such as sunrise and sunset). This process of synchronization is called entrainment. Light is the strongest entrainment signal that keeps the specific time of the body's clock (also called phase) aligned with external time. The lowest body temperature, time of melatonin secretion, and spontaneous wake-up time are

some markers of body's internal clock time. When internal wake-up time is shifted earlier (e.g., from 8 AM local time to 6 AM local time), it is termed "phase advance." Conversely, when internal time is shifted later, it is termed "phase delay." Light exposure induces variable changes in the internal clock depending on the time of the internal clock at which light exposure occurs. Light exposure late in the evening leads to later wake-up time (phase delay) while light exposure in the morning leads to earlier wake-up time (phase advance). Sensitivity to shift in timing from light exposure is least at internal mid-day.

Homeostatic sleep drive, in contrast to the circadian drive, is a physiologic drive similar to hunger or thirst, and all stages of normal sleep are under homeostatic control; that is, sleep deprivation leads to subsequent rebound of sleep stage. Like the circadian period, an individual's sleep requirement is hard-wired and cannot be "trained" by practicing sleep restriction. Normal sleep requirements are higher during early life and steadily decline with age (Table 2.3). When sleep requirements are not met, a "sleep debt" ensues and results in sleepiness. Sleep restriction impairs vigilance, cognition, learning, and emotional health. During wakefulness, cortical energy consumption is significant; rejuvenation of cortical energy stores and clearance of metabolites are majors feature of sleep. Sleep is also implicated in learning such that learning followed by sleep has been shown to promote longer memory formation, and learning during states of sleep deprivation is impaired.

The balance of the circadian drive and the homeostatic sleep drive determines wakefulness. The circadian drive is lowest about 2 hours before the natural wake time and increases in preparation of waking up. Circadian drive builds through the day with a natural dip in the afternoon that promotes napping. Sleep drive builds up through the day with wakefulness and is balanced by the increase in circadian drive. Approximately 2 hours before bedtime, the pineal gland releases the sleep-promoting hormone melatonin into the bloodstream, and melatonin receptors in the SCN then suppress the firing of SCN neurons and sleep eventually ensues. Of note, the hours before sleep onset can be highly resistant to sleep because of high circadian alertness signal. Circadian drive drops through the night to balance the reduction of sleep drive as sleep is "consumed" through the night. Thus, in the morning after optimal duration of sleep, circadian drive is low, but alertness is high because sleep requirement for that night is met.

Like sleep requirements that change with age, circadian phase can also vary with age. There is a tendency for sleep phase delay starting in early teens and progressively increasing until late teens and early 20s. As a result, adolescents prefer to wake up later in the morning, and evidence suggests that they function better with later onset of school. The exact mechanism is not understood, but a longer circadian period, slower development of sleep pressure during the day, and greater resistance to sleep pressure in inducing sleep have been considered as potential mechanisms. In contrast, there is evidence for more advanced sleep phase in the elderly with better performance of tasks in the morning as compared to later in the day.

Respiratory Physiology in Sleep

A basic knowledge of functional anatomy of breathing is vital to understand control of breathing during sleep. The respiratory center/oscillator/signal generator or respiratory pacemaker is located in the medulla. It receives and responds to three general types of information:

1. chemical information (from chemoreceptors responding to partial pressure of oxygen [PaO_2], partial pressure of carbon dioxide [$PaCO_2$], and pH),
2. mechanical information (from receptors in the respiratory tract and chest wall), and
3. behavioral information (from higher cortical centers) to allow breathing to be altered during speech, swallowing, and other activities.

Two principal groups of neurons in the medulla are responsible for central control of ventilation: the dorsal respiratory group located in the region of the nucleus tractus solitarus is principally but not exclusively responsible for inspiration, and the ventral respiratory group located in the region of nucleus ambiguus and retroambigualis is responsible for both inspiration and expiration.[2,9] The ventral group also includes the Botzinger complex and pre-Botzinger region that have intrinsic pacemaker activity and control respiratory rhythmicity.

During sleep (especially NREM), breathing is only under metabolic control. Breathing during wakefulness is controlled by voluntary and behavioral elements, chemical factors, including partial pressure of oxygen (PO_2), partial pressure of carbon dioxide (PCO_2) and acidemia, and mechanical signals from the lung, chest wall, and airway.[3,10]

There are three interrelated controllers of breathing:

1. central controllers located in the medulla aided by supramedullary structures, including forebrain influence, central and peripheral chemoreceptors, and pulmonary and upper airway receptors;
2. the thoracic bellows, which consists of respiratory and other thoracic muscles, their innervation, and bones; and
3. the lungs and airways.[4,11]

During sleep, there is loss of voluntary control and a decrease in the usual ventilatory responses to both low oxygen (hypoxemia) and high carbon dioxide (hypercapnia) levels. Both hypoxemic and hypercapnic responses are most depressed in REM sleep. The higher brain centers efferent pathways can bypass the respiratory center in the medulla; thus, nonrespiratory activities can override the metabolic homeostatic function of the respiratory control system.

The function of ventilation is optimal gas exchange to maintain normal arterial PCO_2 and PO_2. PCO_2 is the primary determinant of chemical control of ventilation and depends predominantly on the central chemoreceptors with some influence from the peripheral chemoreceptors (carotid and aortic bodies). In normal individuals, ventilatory responses to arterial PCO_2 are linear, with ventilation increasing with hypercapnia. However, when PCO_2 falls below a certain level (called the apnea threshold), ventilation is inhibited. Normal individuals exhibit an increase in the carbon dioxide (CO_2) set point during sleep (the level at which CO_2 is maintained) leading to an increase in arterial PCO_2 by 2 to 8 mmHg. While CO_2 production drops during sleep with reduction in metabolic rate, there is a relatively greater reduction in alveolar ventilation causing the rise in PCO_2. The ventilatory response to CO_2 retention also decreases 20% to 50% during NREM sleep and decreases further during REM sleep due to decrease in tone of the respiratory muscles.

The ventilatory response to arterial PO_2 depends almost entirely on the peripheral chemoreceptors. Ventilatory responses to oxygen are hyperbolic with a sudden increase in ventilation when arterial PO_2 falls below 60 mmHg. When PaO_2 drops acutely below 30 to 40 mmHg, the medulla may be depressed by the hypoxemia; thus, ventilation may decrease.

Normal individuals exhibit mild hypoxemia during sleep due to reduction in alveolar ventilation (arterial PO_2 decreases by 3–10 mmHg, and oxygen saturation decreases about 2%). The ventilatory response to hypoxia falls during sleep in healthy adults. The hypoxic ventilatory response is lower during NREM sleep than during wakefulness in men.[5,12] The responses are similar in wakefulness and NREM sleep in the studies in which women predominated.[5,12] When the upper airway is occluded in normal people during experimental studies, arousal occurs more rapidly in REM than NREM sleep. This contrasts with the situation with obstructive sleep apnea, in which arousal response to occlusion is faster in NREM sleep.[6,13]

Changes in the load of the respiratory system lead to increased respiratory effort. Receptors in the lung respond to irritation, inflation (stretch), deflation, and congestion of blood vessels. The information from these sensors is transmitted centrally via the vagus nerve resulting in shortened inspiration and reduced tidal volume to cause a rapid, shallow breathing pattern. Mechanisms that are likely to contribute to decreased ventilatory responses during sleep include the following:

1. The drop in basal metabolic rate during sleep, with no major difference in the different sleep stages,[7,14] is probably a factor in the decreased chemosensitivity during sleep. However, it cannot explain the further reduction in ventilatory response from NREM to REM sleep. Brain metabolism in REM sleep is similar to that in wakefulness.
2. The mild hypercapnia that results from hypoventilation[15] results in a 4% to 25% increase in brain blood flow in SWS compared with wakefulness. It is probable that the hypoventilation and decreased responses to chemical and mechanical stimuli in NREM sleep partially reflect the loss of the "wakefulness" drive to ventilation.[11]
3. In addition to loss of the wakefulness drive to ventilation, increase in airflow resistance probably contributes to decrease in ventilatory responses during NREM sleep. The further reduction of ventilator responses during REM sleep is likely to result from altered central nervous system function during REM sleep resulting in withdrawal of excitatory noradrenergic and serotonergic inputs to upper airway motor neurons.
4. Muscle tone is maximal during wakefulness, slightly decreased in NREM sleep, and markedly decreased or absent in REM sleep. The intercostal muscles are hypotonic during NREM sleep and atonic during REM sleep. This reduction in tone may contribute to decreased ventilatory response during sleep.

CARDIOVASCULAR PHYSIOLOGY AND AUTONOMIC NERVOUS SYSTEM DURING SLEEP

Autonomic control of circulation is pivotal in ensuring an adequate cardiac output to the vital organs through continuous and rapid adjustments of heart rate (HR), arterial blood pressure (BP), and redistribution of blood flow. A broad range of autonomic changes that occur during a typical night of sleep provide both respite and stress to the cardiovascular system.

HR briefly increases during inspiration in synchrony with increased venous return resulting in increased cardiac output. During expiration, a progressive slowing in HR occurs. This normal sinus variability (sinus arrhythmia) in HR is indicative of cardiac health and is particularly noted during NREM sleep. Lack of this intrinsic variability has been associated with cardiac pathology and advancing age.

NREM sleep is associated with autonomic stability. HR, cardiac output, and BP decrease during NREM sleep with further reductions during tonic REM, but during phasic REM sleep, these parameters transiently increase due to increase in sympathetic tone. In a severely compromised heart, there is potential for impaired blood flow through stenotic coronary vessels when BP decreases. Increased surges in autonomic activity during phasic REM sleep provoke accelerations and pauses in heart rhythm that are well tolerated in normal individuals, but those with heart disease may be at risk. Similar pauses in heart rhythm and frank asystole with bursts of vagal nerve activity are also seen during transitions from NREM to REM sleep.

There is a progressive fall in cardiac output during sleep, with the maximum decrement occurring during the early morning in the last REM cycle.[16]

Dipping Phenomenon

Systolic pressure at night is around 10% less than systolic BP[17] during the day. Individuals that exhibit this are called "dippers." However, if the nocturnal systolic BP does not fall by 10% during sleep, these individuals are known as "nondippers." There are also individuals in whom BP does not drop but increases during sleep periods, and they are called "reverse dippers." Individuals who are considered "extreme dippers" (excessive BP decrease, >20%), as well as nondippers and reverse dippers, are at higher risk for stroke than dippers.[18]

The autonomic and cardiovascular changes occurring during NREM and REM sleep are briefly outlined in Table 2.4.

ENDOCRINE PHYSIOLOGY

Sleep impacts peripheral endocrine function via the pathways affecting the activity of the hypothalamic releasing and inhibiting factors that govern pituitary hormone release and the autonomic nervous system control of endocrine glands. Reduced sleep quality and quantity adversely affects these processes. Table 2.5 outlines common hormones and their relation to sleep or circadian rhythm.

Growth hormone (GH) secretion is closely associated with sleep. There is a combined and possibly synergistic role of GH-releasing hormone (GHRH) stimulation, elevated nocturnal ghrelin levels, and decreased somatostatinergic tone in the control of GH secretion during sleep.[19]

TABLE 2.5. HORMONAL CONTROL IN SLEEP

Hormone	Sleep Parameter
Adrenocorticotropic hormone (ACTH)	Circadian rhythm linked
Growth hormone	Increased secretion in slow-wave sleep
Prolactin	Secreted during sleep
Thyroid-stimulating hormone	Inhibited by sleep

In healthy adults, the most reproducible GH pulse occurs shortly after sleep onset.[20] The 24-hour plasma GH secretion profile consists of stable low levels abruptly interrupted by bursts of secretion. GH pulses before sleep may reflect the presence of a sleep debt, occurring consistently after recurrent experimental sleep restriction.[21] Maximal GH release occurs within minutes of the onset of slow-wave sleep.

Circadian rhythmicity controls the 24-hour periodicity of corticotropic activity. ACTH secretion peaks in the early morning, drops through the day to a nadir late at night. Sleep onset is reliably associated with a short-term inhibition of cortisol secretion[22] except when sleep is initiated in the morning.[23] This suggests that sleep suppresses cortisol release only within a limited range of entrainment. Sleep deprivation delays the normal return of corticotropic axis. The nadir of cortisol levels is higher when morning sleep occurs because of the absence of the inhibitory effects of the first hours of sleep, and the morning maximum is lower because of the absence of the stimulating effects of morning awakening.

Thyroid-stimulating hormone (TSH) levels increase through the course of the day and peak shortly before sleep onset. Sleep has an inhibitory effect on TSH secretion at habitual bedtime but that same effect on TSH is not seen during daytime sleep indicating a role of circadian timing in TSH regulation. Sleep deprivation is associated with an elevation of TSH secretion.[24] But when SWS rebounds following a period of sleep deprivation this increase is not as remarkable.

Prolactin levels undergo a major nocturnal elevation starting shortly after sleep onset and culminating around mid-sleep. Awakenings interrupting sleep inhibit nocturnal prolactin release.[25]

Luteinizing hormone and follicle-stimulating hormone are secreted in a pulsatile pattern before onset of puberty and an increase of pulsatile activity is associated with sleep onset in a majority of girls and boys. An increase in the amplitude of gonadotropin release during sleep is one of the hallmarks of puberty.[26] In pubertal girls, a diurnal variation of circulating estradiol levels is seen with higher concentrations during the daytime instead of the nighttime. In pubertal boys, the rise of testosterone at night coincides with the elevation of gonadotropins. The nocturnal rise of testosterone seems to be temporally linked to the latency of the first REM episode.[27] A robust increase in testosterone may also be observed during daytime sleep, suggesting that sleep, irrespective of time of day, stimulates gonadal hormone release.[28] In young adults, the concentration of androgens decreases significantly during periods of total sleep deprivation and recover promptly once the sleep is restored.[29]

Orexin-containing neurons are active during wakefulness and quiescent during sleep. They are located in the lateral hypothalamus and project directly to the locus coeruleus and other brainstem and hypothalamic arousal areas. There, they interact with the leptin-responsive neuronal network involved in balancing food intake and energy expenditure. Orexin is inhibited by leptin, a satiety hormone, and stimulated by ghrelin, an appetite promoting hormone.[30] The 24-hour leptin profile shows a marked increase at night, partly dependent on meal intake.[31] Prolonged total sleep deprivation causes a decrease in the amplitude of the diurnal variation[32] of leptin. Plasma ghrelin levels are primarily regulated by food intake: levels rise sharply before each designated meal time and fall to trough levels within 1 to 2 hours after eating. SWS is associated with increased ghrelin levels.

Melatonin production is controlled by a polysynaptic pathway originating from the retinal ganglion cells and transmitted via retinohypothalamic tract to the suprachiasmatic nucleus. These efferents then come to the superior cervical ganglia, thereafter transmitting impulses to the pineal gland. This pathway is activated during the night and suppressed by exposure to bright light. Melatonin reaches its maximal value between 3 AM and 5 AM and is decreased during the day. Maximal nocturnal secretion of melatonin has been noted in young children aged 1 to 3 years after which the secretion begins to fall around puberty and decreases significantly in the elderly.[33]

Sleep disruption can perturb hormonal secretion. Nocturnal release of GH and PRL is decreased in patients with untreated obstructive sleep apnea, presumably due to sleep disruption but is increased following continuous positive airway pressure (CPAP) treatment. The shift work–related increased incidence of infertility in women is thought to be related to a sleep-associated inhibitory effect on gonadotropin release during the follicular phase of the menstrual cycle.

GASTROINTESTINAL PHYSIOLOGY

The activity of gastrointestinal system during sleep is controlled by autonomic and enteric nervous system. Basal gastric acid secretion shows a clear circadian rhythm.[34] A peak in acid secretion generally occurs between 10:00 PM and 2:00 AM. In the absence of meal stimulation, the basal acid secretion in the waking state is minimal.

Peristaltic amplitude and a swallowing rate decrease with sleep along with prolongation of esophageal acid clearance. Transient lower esophageal sphincter and upper esophageal sphincter pressures are also decreased during sleep. As a result, sleep is a very vulnerable time for patients with reflux; conversely, sleep disturbances are common in patients with peptic ulcer disease due to higher levels of gastric acid secretion after sleep onset.[35]

MISCELLANEOUS: RENAL, MUSCULOSKELETAL, IMMUNE SYSTEM

Renal blood flow is decreased during sleep. Urine volume also decreases because of a reduction in the renal glomerular filtration rate and increased renal tubular reabsorption of water in normal individuals. Sleep deprivation and nocturnal patterns can affect chronic kidney disease and cause a faster decline in renal function. OSA has been linked to proteinuria and a decline in glomerular filtration rate. Conversely, patients with chronic renal failure can have a rostral fluid shift resulting in excess fluid in the neck and increasing upper airway collapsibility. In patients with obstructive sleep apnea syndrome, sodium and urinary output normalizes following CPAP treatment, which may be related to restoration of normal plasma renin activity and aldosterone oscillations, as well as decreased release of atrial natriuretic peptide.

Adenosine is a neural sleep factor in the basal forebrain that results in the somnogenic effects of prolonged wakefulness by acting through the A_1 and A_{2A} receptors. Caffeine causes its effects via antagonism of all types of adenosine receptors[36] primarily A_1 and A_{2A}. This enables its strategic use in daytime sleepiness and shift work.

Cytokines are important in the pathogenesis of excessive daytime sleepiness in a variety of sleep disorders and in sleep deprivation.[37] Interleukin (IL), interferon-α, and tumor necrosis factor-α (TNF-α) promote sleep. Viral or bacterial infections can cause increased NREM sleep and excessive sleepiness due to the increased production of proinflammatory cytokines.

Sleep acts as a host defense against infection (with bacterial, viral, and fungal infections enhancing NREM while suppressing REM sleep) and facilitates the healing process. It is responsible for immunological homeostasis and for improving immune responses. Sleep deprivation can alter immune functions.

Thus, several physiological changes occur during sleep in the autonomic and somatic nervous systems and other organ systems that may affect many disease processes and have clinical implications.

CONCLUSIONS

This chapter outlines the progression of normal sleep architecture across the lifespan, processes that control the sleep–wake cycle and physiological changes occurring during sleep. Psychiatric disorders underlie many sleep problems and sleep problems, in turn, are experienced by many patients with psychiatric disorders. Knowledge of sleep physiology and physiologic changes associated with sleep is relevant to understanding and managing sleep-related issues in patients with psychiatric disorders. Sleep physiology informs ongoing research that explores molecular and genetic targets for the treatment of sleep and psychiatric problems while providing an understanding of efficacy of currently available pharmacological and behavioral interventions. We expect that these developments will provide new treatment options and better definition of current treatments in alleviating sleep disorders, both primary and secondary to mental health disorders.

KEY CLINICAL PEARLS

- Sleep in adults consists of cycles of NREM and REM sleep with deep sleep predominating early in sleep and duration of Stage R lengthening in the second part of the night.
- Sleep needs vary across the life span with newborns needing 16 to 18 hours of sleep including naps, which decreases gradually to average adult needing 7 to 9 hours of sleep without naps and return of napping in individuals older than 65 years of age.
- Sleep requirements cannot reduced by "training"

- Sleep and wake are determined by the circadian process (Process C) and the homeostatic sleep process (Process S)
- Alterations in gas exchange can occur during sleep due to normal physiological effects on ventilation. Fall in ventilation can occur due to increased upper airway resistance and decreased chemosensitivity along with loss of the wakefulness stimulus to breathe.
- Systolic pressure at night is around 10% less than systolic pressure during the day called the "dipping phenomenon."
- GH secretion occurs around the first cycle of stage N3 sleep and prolactin secretion also increases during sleep.
- Satiety-promoting hormone leptin decreases during sleep loss and can lead to an increased risk for obesity.
- Normal defense mechanisms against gastroesophageal reflux disease are decreased during sleep.
- Caffeine increases alertness by antagonizing adenosine receptors and can be used strategically in shift workers.
- Sleep acts as a host defense against infection (with bacterial, viral, and fungal infection enhancing NREM sleep and suppressing REM sleep) and facilitates the healing process.

SELF-ASSESSMENT QUESTIONS

1. Which of the following sleep architectural parameters decreases with age?
   a. Stage N1
   b. Arousal Index
   c. Sleep Efficiency
   d. REM latency

Answer: c

2. Sleep deprivation can cause which of the following?
   a. Increase in response to immunizations
   b. Increase in Growth Hormone
   c. Increase in Ghrelin
   d. Increase in pain tolerance

Answer: c

3. Which is true for relative hypercapnic ventilatory response?
   a. REM < NREM < Wake
   b. REM < Wake < NREM
   c. NREM < REM < Wake
   d. NREM < Wake < REM

Answer: a

4. Cortisol secretion is
a. closely tied to sleep timing.
b. increased at night by sleep deprivation.
c. lowest in the morning.
d. highest during REM sleep.

Answer: b

5. Which chemical is involved in both regulation of hunger and arousal?
a. Leptin
b. Ghrelin
c. Adenosine
d. Orexin

Answer: d

REFERENCES

1. Scraggs TL. EEG maturation: viability through adolescence. *Neurodiagn J*. 2012;52(2):176–203.
2. Hughes JR. Development of sleep spindles in the first year of life. *Clin Electroencephalogr*. 1996;27(3):107–115.
3. McLaughlin Crabtree V, Williams NA. Normal sleep in children and adolescents. *Child Adolesc Psychiatr Clin N Am*. 2009;18(4):799–811. doi:10.1016/j.chc.2009.04.013.
4. Ohayon MM, Carskadon MA, Guilleminault C, Vitiello MV. Meta-analysis of quantitative sleep parameters from childhood to old age in healthy individuals: developing normative sleep values across the human lifespan. *Sleep*. 2004;27(7):1255–1273.
5. Prinz PN, Peskind ER, Vitaliano PP, et al. Changes in the sleep and waking EEGs of nondemented and demented elderly subjects. *J Am Geriatr Soc*. 1982;30(2):86–93.
6. Klerman EB, Davis JB, Duffy JF, Dijk D-J, Kronauer RE. Older people awaken more frequently but fall back asleep at the same rate as younger people. *Sleep*. 2004;27(4):793–798.
7. Crowley K, Trinder J, Kim Y, Carrington M, Colrain IM. The effects of normal aging on sleep spindle and K-complex production. *Clin Neurophysiol*. 2002;113(10):1615–1622.
8. Feinberg I. Schizophrenia: caused by a fault in programmed synaptic elimination during adolescence? *J Psychiatr Res*. 1982;17(4):319–334.
9. Mitchell RA, Berger AJ. Neural regulation of respiration. *Am Rev Respir Dis*. 1975;111(2):206–224. doi:10.1164/arrd.1975.111.2.206.
10. Berger AJ, Mitchell RA, Severinghaus JW. Regulation of respiration: (second of three parts). *N Engl J Med*. 1977;297(3):138–143. doi:10.1056/NEJM197707212970305.
11. Phillipson EA. Control of breathing during sleep. *Am Rev Respir Dis*. 1978;118(5):909–939. doi:10.1164/arrd.1978.118.5.909.
12. Douglas NJ, White DP, Weil JV, et al. Hypoxic ventilatory response decreases during sleep in normal men. *Am Rev Respir Dis*. 1982;125(3):286–289. doi:10.1164/arrd.1982.125.3.286.
13. Issa FG, Sullivan CE. Arousal and breathing responses to airway occlusion in healthy sleeping adults. *J Appl Physiol Respir Environ Exerc Physiol*. 1983;55(4):1113–1119. doi:10.1152/jappl.1983.55.4.1113.
14. White DP, Weil JV, Zwillich CW. Metabolic rate and breathing during sleep. *J Appl Physiol*. 1985;59(2):384–391. doi:10.1152/jappl.1985.59.2.384.
15. Santiago TV, Guerra E, Neubauer JA, Edelman NH. Correlation between ventilation and brain blood flow during sleep. *J Clin Invest*. 1984;73(2):497–506. doi:10.1172/JCI111236.
16. Khatri IM, Freis ED. Hemodynamic changes during sleep. *J Appl Physiol*. 1967;22(5):867–873. doi:10.1152/jappl.1967.22.5.867.
17. Pandian JD, Wong AA, Lincoln DJ, et al. Circadian blood pressure variation after acute stroke. *J Clin Neurosci*. 2006;13(5):558–562. doi:10.1016/j.jocn.2005.09.003.
18. Brotman DJ, Davidson MB, Boumitri M, Vidt DG. Impaired diurnal blood pressure variation and all-cause mortality. *Am J Hypertens*. 2008;21(1):92–97. doi:10.1038/ajh.2007.7.
19. van der Lely AJ, Tschöp M, Heiman ML, Ghigo E. Biological, physiological, pathophysiological, and pharmacological aspects of ghrelin. *Endocr Rev*. 2004;25(3):426–457. doi:10.1210/er.2002-0029.
20. Van Cauter E, Plat L, Copinschi G. Interrelations between sleep and the somatotropic axis. *Sleep*. 1998;21(6):553–566.
21. Spiegel K, Leproult R, Colecchia EF, et al. Adaptation of the 24-h growth hormone profile to a state of sleep debt. *Am J Physiol Regul Integr Comp Physiol*. 2000;279(3):R874–R883. doi:10.1152/ajpregu.2000.279.3.R874.
22. Born J, Muth S, Fehm HL. The significance of sleep onset and slow wave sleep for nocturnal release of growth hormone (GH) and cortisol. *Psychoneuroendocrinology*. 1988;13(3):233–243.
23. Weibel L, Follenius M, Spiegel K, Ehrhart J, Brandenberger G. Comparative effect of night and daytime sleep on the 24-hour cortisol secretory profile. *Sleep*. 1995;18(7):549–556.
24. Brabant G, Prank K, Ranft U, et al. Physiological regulation of circadian and pulsatile thyrotropin secretion in normal man and woman. *J Clin Endocrinol Metab*. 1990;70(2):403–409. doi:10.1210/jcem-70-2-403.
25. Spiegel K, Luthringer R, Follenius M, et al. Temporal relationship between prolactin secretion and slow-wave electroencephalic activity during sleep. *Sleep*. 1995;18(7):543–548.

26. Wu FC, Butler GE, Kelnar CJ, Huhtaniemi I, Veldhuis JD. Ontogeny of pulsatile gonadotropin releasing hormone secretion from midchildhood, through puberty, to adulthood in the human male: a study using deconvolution analysis and an ultrasensitive immunofluorometric assay. *J Clin Endocrinol Metab.* 1996;81(5):1798–1805. doi:10.1210/jcem.81.5.8626838.

27. Luboshitzky R, Herer P, Levi M, Shen-Orr Z, Lavie P. Relationship between rapid eye movement sleep and testosterone secretion in normal men. *J Androl.* 1999;20(6):731–737.

28. Axelsson J, Ingre M, Akerstedt T, Holmbäck U. Effects of acutely displaced sleep on testosterone. *J Clin Endocrinol Metab.* 2005;90(8):4530–4535. doi:10.1210/jc.2005-0520.

29. Akerstedt T, Palmblad J, la Torre de B, Marana R, Gillberg M. Adrenocortical and gonadal steroids during sleep deprivation. *Sleep.* 1980;3(1):23–30.

30. Adamantidis A, de Lecea L. The hypocretins as sensors for metabolism and arousal. *J Physiol (Lond).* 2009;587(1):33–40. doi:10.1113/jphysiol.2008.164400.

31. Schoeller DA, Cella LK, Sinha MK, Caro JF. Entrainment of the diurnal rhythm of plasma leptin to meal timing. *J Clin Invest.* 1997;100(7):1882–1887. doi:10.1172/JCI119717.

32. Mullington JM, Chan JL, Van Dongen HPA, et al. Sleep loss reduces diurnal rhythm amplitude of leptin in healthy men. *J Neuroendocrinol.* 2003;15(9):851–854.

33. Brzezinski A. Melatonin in humans. *N Engl J Med.* 1997;336(3):186–195. doi:10.1056/NEJM199701163360306.

34. Moore JG, Englert E. Circadian rhythm of gastric acid secretion in man. *Nature.* 1970;226(5252):1261–1262.

35. Feldman M, Richardson CT. Total 24-hour gastric acid secretion in patients with duodenal ulcer. Comparison with normal subjects and effects of cimetidine and parietal cell vagotomy. *Gastroenterology.* 1986;90(3):540–544.

36. O'Callaghan F, Muurlink O, Reid N. Effects of caffeine on sleep quality and daytime functioning. *Risk Manag Healthc Policy.* 2018;11:263–271. doi:10.2147/RMHP.S156404.

37. Kapsimalis F, Basta M, Varouchakis G, Gourgoulianis K, Vgontzas A, Kryger M. Cytokines and pathological sleep. *Sleep Med.* 2008;9(6):603–614. doi:10.1016/j.sleep.2007.08.019.

3

Neurobiology of Sleep and Wakefulness

AMIT CHOPRA, RIKINKUMAR S. PATEL, AND PIYUSH DAS

INTRODUCTION

Historically, it has been thought that the wakefulness is due to sensory inputs to the brain and sleep is caused by cessation of sensory inputs [1, 2]. However, approximately 100 years ago during the epidemic of encephalitis lethargica in Europe, Viennese neurologist Constantin von Economo discovered that lesions in posterior hypothalamus (PH) result in hypersomnolence, whereas, anterior hypothalamus and preoptic (PO) area lesions result in insomnia [3]. These findings suggested that both sleep and wakefulness are controlled by intrinsic neural systems. Later, Moruzzi and Magoun [1] demonstrated that electrical stimulation of the reticular formation in anesthetized cats shifted the EEG from the slow activity, typical of anesthesia, to fast activity similar to that seen during wakefulness. These findings gave rise to the concept of ascending reticular activating system (ARAS) and further studies in 1970s and 1980s confirmed that ascending reticular system originated from a series of well-defined cell groups with identified neurotransmitters [2].

During 1980s and 1990s, researchers identified a cell group of sleep-active neurons, the ventrolateral PO nucleus (VLPO), that inhibits major arousal pathways during sleep and contained the inhibitory neurotransmitters including GABA and galanin [3–6]. In 1998, two groups of investigators simultaneously discovered a pair of closely related neuropeptides, produced exclusively by a cluster of neurons in the posterior half of the lateral hypothalamus (LH) [2]. These neuropeptides were named orexin by one group and hypocretin by the other group [7, 8]. Shortly after, these two groups of investigators again simultaneously discovered that a lack of orexin or their type 2 receptor caused symptoms of narcolepsy in experimental animals [9, 10]. Within a year, the mysterious nature of human narcolepsy was identified as patients with narcolepsy and cataplexy were noted to have fewer orexin neurons in the LH area in addition to low orexin levels in the cerebrospinal fluid (CSF).

In addition to c-Fos technique, that measures neuronal activity, more recent advances in the field of neurosciences, including optogenetics and chemogenetics, have led to substantial improvements in our understanding of the neural mechanisms that selectively regulate the occurrence and timing of wakefulness, nonrapid eye movement (NREM), and rapid eye movement (REM) sleep. Optogenetics uses the light-sensitive proteins, including channelrhodopsin (ChR2) and halorhodopsin (NpHR), to either active or inhibit the activity of target neurons [11]. Chemogenetics, a complimentary technique to optogenetics, uses a drug-based approach to control neuronal activity instead of light [12]. Despite the previously mentioned advancements in neuroscience, the precise mechanisms of sleep–wakefulness control still remain to be elusive. In this chapter, we review the current understanding of neurobiological basis of sleep and wakefulness in mammals with an emphasis on the role of specific neural networks and neurotransmitters; circadian, homeostatic, allostatic and other factors; and sleep–wake switching mechanisms in the causation and maintenance of sleep and wakefulness.

OVERVIEW OF SLEEP AND WAKEFULNESS

Wakefulness, NREM, and REM sleep are three distinct states representing the continuum of normal range of consciousness. Each state is characterized by specific behavioral and physiological patterns, and neurophysiological mechanisms associated with its generation and control [13]. Neurobiologists define wakefulness as a spectrum of behavioral states characterized by voluntary motor activation and responsiveness to internal and external stimuli. During wakefulness, there is increased sympathetic tone and decreased parasympathetic tone that maintains most organ systems in a state of action or readiness [13]. During NREM sleep, there is a state of reduced activity due to decreased sympathetic tone and increased parasympathetic activity. REM sleep is characterized

TABLE 3.1. PHYSIOLOGICAL CRITERIA FOR
WAKEFULNESS AND SLEEP

Criterion	Wakefulness	NREM sleep	REM sleep
EEG	Desynchronized; alpha waves	Synchronized	Desynchronized; theta or saw-tooth waves
EMG	Normal	Mildly reduced	Moderate to severely reduced or absent
EOG	Waking eye movements	Slow-rolling eye movements	Rapid eye movements

Abbreviations: EEG, electroencephalography; EMG, electromyography; EOG, electrooculography

by increased parasympathetic activity and variable sympathetic activity associated with increased activation of certain brain functions.

The states of wakefulness and sleep are characterized as stages that are defined by stereotypical neurophysiological patterns of electroencephalography (EEG), electromyography (EMG), and electrooculography [13]. During wakefulness, the EEG shows low amplitude and fast frequencies, and the EMG shows variable amounts of muscle activity. During quiet waking, low-amplitude gamma (30–120 Hz) and beta (15–30 Hz) frequency rhythms are a prominent feature of the EEG [14]. Transition from wakefulness to NREM sleep is generally mediated by wakeful drowsiness that is characterized by dominant posterior alpha rhythm (8–13 Hz).

Once NREM sleep occurs, it is further subdivided in to three stages: N1, N2, and N3. The levels of arousal varies within NREM sleep as an individual can be aroused easily from N1 sleep (light sleep), but much stronger stimuli are required to wake from N3 sleep (deep sleep) [13]. With the onset of N1 sleep, the alpha rhythm attenuates, and an EEG pattern of relatively low voltage and mixed frequency is noted with slow-rolling eye movements. N2 sleep is characterized by the appearance of sleep spindles (7–15 Hz) and K complexes. Further progression to N3 sleep is defined by the occurrence of high-amplitude, low-frequency delta (0–4 Hz) EEG activity [13].

NREM sleep alternates with REM sleep every 90 to 110 minutes during sleep cycle. In REM sleep, theta activity (4–7 Hz) is present, particularly in the hippocampus, but the dominant cortical frequencies are faster with lower voltage, and there is almost complete loss of tone in skeletal muscles, except those used for breathing and eye movements. An individual may switch back and forth from NREM to REM sleep, with occasional transitions to periods of wakefulness [15].

Table 3.1 summarizes the physiological characteristics of wakefulness, NREM, and REM sleep.

REGULATION OF WAKEFULNESS

The brain actively generates and maintains arousal via different neural structures and utilizing different neurotransmitters. These brain arousal systems comprise of the ascending networks projecting to the cerebral cortex, which stimulate cortical activation as reflected by fast EEG activity, and the descending networks projecting to the spinal cord, which stimulate sensory-motor activation as reflected by high EMG activity [16]. Neuronal discharge in these arousal systems declines rapidly at sleep onset [17]. These arousal systems are comprised of neuronal aggregates within the brainstem reticular formation, thalamus, PH, and basal forebrain (BF) [16].

Brainstem Arousal Systems

Early animal studies highlight the importance of the reticular brainstem region for maintenance of sustained wakefulness [1, 18]. The ARAS originates in the brainstem and integrates majority of the sleep-regulating stimuli [2, 16]. High activity of the ARAS during active wakefulness forms a wake-promoting "bottom–up" system [19]. The main afferents to ARAS include the wake-promoting orexinergic neurons from the LH and the sleep-promoting GABAergic neurons from the VLPO [6, 20, 21]. These two afferent projections integrate the circadian and homeostatic sleep–wake signals and channel this information to the ARAS [2]. The reticular neurons also receive converging inputs from other sources including peripheral sensory systems that relay somatic or visceral sensory, auditory, vestibular, or visual inputs, and the cerebral cortex that relays sensory and motor-related outputs [16].

The ARAS pathway has two major efferent branches including a dorsal ascending pathway to the thalamus and a ventral ascending pathway that extends to the hypothalamus and forebrain [2, 16]. The acetylcholine (Ach)-producing cell groups including pedunculopontine (PPT) and laterodorsal tegmental (LDT) nuclei are the major source of upper brainstem input to the thalamic-relay nuclei, as well as to the reticular nucleus of the thalamus [22]. The neurons in the PPT/LDT fire most rapidly during wakefulness and REM sleep [23]; however, these cells are much less active during NREM sleep, a sleep stage characterized by slow cortical activity [2].

Reticular neurons, concentrated within the caudal pontine and medullary reticular formation, also send descending projections into the spinal cord [16]. Depending upon state of arousal or sleep, reticular neurons may exert facilitatory or inhibitory influences upon sensory and motor transmission in the spinal cord [24]. The majority of the neurons in the reticular formation likely utilize excitatory neurotransmitter glutamate [16] as reticular neurons have the capacity to package and thus release glutamate as a neurotransmitter [25]. The reticular projection neurons are also under inhibitory control by local GABAergic neurons; however, this control could be exerted differentially during different states such as arousal or sleep [16]. Additionally, many anesthetic agents act by blocking glutamatergic transmission [26, 27] thus blocking the action of the ARAS and descending reticulo-spinal facilitatory system. On the other hand, anesthetic agents such as barbiturates act by enhancing GABAergic transmission through $GABA_A$ receptors [28] and thus could act by inhibiting the projection neurons of ARAS [16].

The ventral nonthalamic pathway comprises of activating monoaminergic projections from noradrenergic (NA) locus coeruleus (LC), serotoninergic dorsal (DR), and median raphe nuclei, dopaminergic ventral periaqueductal grey matter (PAG) and histaminergic (HA) tuberomammillary neurons [2]. Neurons in each of these monoaminergic projections are most active during wakefulness, slow down during NREM sleep, and stop altogether during REM sleep [29, 30]. During REM sleep, the monoaminergic neurons remain silent, whereas the cholinergic pathway is selectively activated [19].

Thalamo-Cortical Activating System

The thalamo-cortical projection system comprises of midline, medial, and intralaminar thalamic nuclei that commonly project to multiple cortical regions [16]. These thalamic nuclei receive ascending input from the reticular, cholinergic (Ach), NA, and serotonergic neurons (5-hydroxytryptamine [5-HT]) [9]. Glutamate, Ach, and NA have an excitatory effect on thalamic neurons, while 5-HT may have an inhibitory effect [31, 32]. The early physiological studies indicate that the stimulation of the nonspecific thalamo-cortical projection system evokes widespread and prolonged cortical activation by release of glutamate [33–35]. The thalamo-cortical projection nuclei discharge spontaneously in association with cortical activation during wakefulness and REM sleep [36].

The thalamic reticular nucleus (TRN) is an inhibitory shell positioned between the thalamus and the cortex that influences the cortical activity by modulating cortico-thalamo-cortical transmission [37]. TRN neurons receive input from brainstem arousal systems and project upon the thalamo-cortical projection neurons. At sleep onset, the firing patterns of brainstem arousal systems decrease and TRN neurons become hyperpolarized and consequently release GABA, thereby inhibiting the thalamo-cortical projection neurons to facilitate sleep onset and continuation [32, 38]. TRN neurons also participate in the propagation of sleep spindles (12–14 Hz) and delta (1–3 Hz) or slower (<1 Hz) waves during slow-wave sleep (SWS) within thalamo-cortical circuits [39].

Hypothalamic Arousal Systems

Hypothalamic neurons control autonomic and neuroendocrine function, and the neurons in the PH region are important for activation of the sympathetic nervous system and the hypothalamo–pituitary–adrenal (HPA) axis during arousal [16]. The PH comprises of multiple nuclei and regions, including the LH, and it may be responsive to multiple collateral inputs from brainstem and forebrain arousal systems [16]. LH neurons project directly to the cerebral cortex [40], and other PH neurons project into the brainstem and spinal cord thus innervating reticular, monoamine and sympathetic neurons [41, 42]. PH neurons probably utilize glutamate as the primary neurotransmitter [43] and tend to fire maximally during wakefulness and decrease their discharge during SWS [44]. HA neurons, located in the posterior hypothalamic tuberomammillary nucleus (TMN), receive multiple inputs from the brainstem and forebrain systems and project diffusely through the brain, including the cerebral cortex [45]. HA neurons are presumed to be wake-active neurons and cease discharge during NREM and REM sleep. Additionally, anti-HA drugs are known to produce somnolence [46, 47].

Orexin-producing neurons in the PH region (including the LH area) are crucial for maintenance of wakefulness as lack of orexin function results in narcolepsy, a sleep disorder characterized by excessive daytime sleepiness and cataplexy [48]. These orexin-producing neurons have excitatory projections to other arousal systems including the LC, the nonspecific thalamo-cortical projection system, the HA neurons, and the cholinergic BF neurons [21, 49–53]. There are mutual projections between the VLPO neurons and the orexin neurons [54–56]; however, the VLPO neurons lack orexin receptors [57]. Therefore, orexin neurons reinforce the arousal systems and likely do not directly inhibit the VLPO. Orexin receptors have been researched as a target for treatment of insomnia. Suvorexant, a dual orexin receptor antagonist, is US Food and Drug (FDA)-approved for the treatment of both sleep onset and sleep maintenance at 10 to 20 mg dose range [58].

Basal Forebrain Wake-Promoting Systems

The cholinergic BF neurons receive input from all the brainstem and hypothalamic arousal systems [16]. These neurons are excited by glutamate [59], NA [60], histamine [61], orexin [53], and inhibited by serotonin [62]. These neurons project widely to the cerebral cortex, and stimulation of the BF suppresses delta activity and SWS, elicits cortical stimulation [63], and increases REM sleep [64]. Release of Ach is high during both wakefulness and REM sleep, relative to NREM sleep, in the cerebral cortex, and it is actually highest during REM sleep [65–67].

The noncholinergic BF neurons are co-distributed with the cholinergic cells and include glutamatergic as well as GABAergic neurons [16]. Evidence suggests that the cortically projecting magnocellular basal neurons include glutamatergic, GABAergic, and cholinergic cells [68–70] that receive input from brainstem reticular formation and other arousal systems and comprise of the important BF relay to the cerebral cortex [16]. In particular, GABAergic BF neurons may promote SWS as evident from early experiments showing induction of SWS with stimulation of the BF [71–72] and loss of SWS with lesions of the BF [73].

REGULATION OF NREM SLEEP

Sleep spindles and K complexes are the defining features of N2 sleep in humans. K complexes represent a combination of one cycle of the neocortical slow oscillation followed by a sleep spindle in thalamo-cortical neurons [74–76]. Current evidence suggests that spindles are generated in the thalamic GABAergic reticular and perigeniculate nuclei [77]. In vivo, extracellular and intracellular recording studies reveal that thalamic reticular neurons fire in a tonic pattern during wakefulness and switch to burst firing patterns during NREM sleep, which is similar to thalamo-cortical relay neurons [78, 79]. Tonic firing and inhibition of spindle bursts during wakefulness is likely due to excitation of the thalamic reticular neurons by norepinephrine and serotonin [80]. Spindles can also be inhibited by input from other ARAS systems such as brain stem cholinergic [81] and BF cholinergic and GABAergic inputs [82, 83]. The mechanism underlying inhibition of spindle activity during REM sleep is less clear; however, it has been proposed that inhibitory input from REM on cholinergic neurons may play a role [84, 85].

Preoptic Region and BF

Based on early studies involving lesions or stimulation, the PO region and BF have been known to exert a sleep-promoting influence. While lesions in these areas have been associated with insomnia [73], the stimulation can cause a predominance of parasympathetic responses, including decreased heart rate, blood pressure, respiration, and temperature along with decreased activity and sleep [71]. PO/BF regions contain a large number of neurons that utilize the neurotransmitter GABA and exert sleep-on, wake-off firing patterns [14]. Neurons in the PO/BF discharge maximally during NREM sleep as revealed by single-unit recording studies [6, 86, 87]. Current evidence strongly suggests that the neurons concentrated in the VLPO and median PO nucleus (MnPO) exert NREM sleep promoting effect [3, 88], and lesions of these nuclei lead to significant and long-lasting reductions in sleep [89, 90]. It has been demonstrated that the majority of sleep-active neurons in the PO and BF areas contain the synthetic enzyme, glutamic acid decarboxylase, for synthesis of GABA [91, 92]. However, evidence from both c-Fos and juxtacellular recording studies suggests that many GABAergic neurons in these regions are active during waking and cortical activation [92, 93]. These findings suggest that the sleep-active GABAergic neurons must be different in other ways from the wake-active GABAergic neurons.

In vitro pharmacological studies, performed in the BF and VLPO, suggest that cholinergic neurons are depolarized and excited by NA through α1-adrenergic receptors, whereas, a small contingent of GABAergic cells in the VLPO are hyperpolarized and inhibited by NA through α2-adrenergic receptors [60, 94, 95]. Moreover, data from studies based on juxtacellular recording and labeling of neurons, which discharge maximally during slow-wave activity (SWA), is suggestive that a large proportion of these neurons are GABAergic in nature and bear α2-adrenergic receptors [96]. Therefore, it may be conceptualized that sleep-active GABAergic neurons in the BF and PO area, which are inhibited by NA, would thus be active with a decline in NA release from LC neurons during the state of decreasing arousal [97]. Additionally, these sleep-active GABAergic neurons can inhibit cortical or subcortical systems promoting cortical activation or behavioral arousal, including NA, HA, and orexinergic neurons [3, 98, 99]. Conversely, these sleep-active neurons are innervated by arousal-promoting brain regions [54] as Ach, NE, and 5-HT all directly inhibit VLPO neurons; histamine suppresses VLPO activity via local GABAergic interneurons [100], and orexins may have similar effects. Adenosine (AD) in the BF maintains sleep homeostasis, as extracellular AD concentration increase during wakefulness leading to increased sleep pressure and consequently rebound sleep. Sleep-active neurons in VLPO and MnPO may help mediate the homeostatic response to sleep deprivation as neurons in both these regions fire faster during the sleep deprivation period and during the subsequent sleep period [88]. This surge in VLPO activity can be blocked by an AD antagonist, and in vitro electrophysiological studies reveal that AD excites VLPO neurons by direct and indirect mechanisms [101, 102].

Parafacial Zone

Evidence from early transection studies suggests that the caudal brainstem also contains neurons that promote NREM sleep [103]. Parafacial zone (PZ), a region just dorsal and lateral to the facial nerve in the rostral medulla, has been identified as a cluster of NREM sleep-active neurons [104]. These neurons utilize GABA and glycine as neurotransmitters and express Fos during NREM sleep. Cell specific lesions or disruption of GABA/glycinergic transmission in PZ has been associated with increase in wakefulness [105]. Additionally, chemogenetic activation, a process by which macromolecules interact with unrecognized small molecules, of these neurons rapidly induces sustained periods of NREM sleep associated with high EEG delta power, which is similar to the

observations after sleep deprivation. On the other hand, chemogenetic inhibition of PZ GABAergic neurons strongly decreases NREM sleep, even during times of high sleep drive. It is possible that PZ may also promote sleep via inhibition of additional wake-promoting systems [104].

Cortical Sleep-Active nNOS Neurons

A small subset of the broader population of GABAergic cortical interneurons that produce neuronal nitric oxide (NO) synthase (nNOS) is especially active during NREM sleep [104]. c-Fos expression in cortical nNOS neurons has been correlated with the amounts of NREM sleep and SWA during NREM sleep [106, 107]. These nNOS neurons, which release GABA and NO, respond to homeostatic sleep drive and synchronize slow cortical rhythms via long-range intracortical projections. These hypotheses are supported by the evidence that mice, constitutively lacking nNOS, have shorter bouts of NREM sleep, decreased total NREM sleep, and a blunted homeostatic response to sleep deprivation [107].

REGULATION OF REM SLEEP

Except muscle atonia during REM sleep, it has many similarities to wakefulness including desynchronized cortical activity, eye movements, high cortical metabolism, and complex mental activity. It has been proven that neural circuits in the pons are required for REM sleep [104]. Early animal studies have demonstrated that the transections at the caudal edge of the pons are associated with the usual low amplitude, fast EEG activity but without the muscle atonia during REM sleep whereas transections at the rostral edge of the pons eliminate the fast EEG activity but preserve the atonia of REM sleep [108, 109]. Based on these findings, REM sleep was thought to be controlled by reciprocal connections between REM sleep-promoting cholinergic neurons in the PPT/LDT nuclei, and REM sleep-suppressing monoaminergic neurons in the LC and dorsal raphe (DR) nucleus [13, 110]. However, more recent evidence suggests a central role of glutamatergic neurons in the sublaterodorsal nucleus (SLD) of the pons in generation of REM sleep [104].

Pedunculopontine and Laterodorsal Tegmental Nuclei

Similar to wakefulness, Ach levels are high during REM sleep [104]. Additionally, microinjection of cholinergic agonist, carbachol, into laterodorsal pons has been associated with long-lasting REM sleep like state in animal studies [111]. Contrary to the prior notion, the cholinergic neurons in the PPT/LDT area are now considered as modulators rather than central elements of the pontine REM sleep generator [104]. The photo-stimulation of PPT/LDT cholinergic neurons has been shown to promote transitions from NREM to REM sleep [112]. More recent evidence supports the role of non-cholinergic neurons of the PPT/LDT in generation of REM sleep [113, 114]. It is apparent that most glutamatergic neurons in PPT/LDT region fire just before and during REM sleep, and many of these neurons also fire during wakefulness. The GABAergic neurons in the PPT/LDT region seem to be predominantly wake-active, but some of these neurons may be more active during REM as compared to NREM sleep. The exact mechanisms of REM sleep regulation involving these three neurotransmitter systems in PPT/LDT region remains to be an important area for future research [104].

Sublaterodorsal Nucleus
Seminal research work has established that glutamatergic neurons of the SLD, a region that lies just ventral to the caudal LDT and LC, are essential for generating the muscle atonia during REM sleep [104]. SLD neurons fire in a tonic pattern and are active during REM sleep as evident by c-Fos immunoreactivity and by single unit recordings [115, 116]. Additionally, pharmacological activation of the SLD region rapidly produces a long-lasting REM sleep-like state characterized by a low voltage EEG, prominent EEG theta activity, and continuous muscle atonia [117]. SLD is probably activated by cholinergic neurons of the PPT/LDT. SLD is the most sensitive region for the promotion of REM sleep by carbachol, a cholinergic agonist [111]. On the other hand, animals with focal lesions of the SLD or deletion of glutamate signaling in the SLD demonstrate a REM sleep-like state but without atonia, which is characterized by complex motor behaviors during sleep. SLD lesions that extend into adjacent regions can also shorten the bouts and the total amount of REM sleep [118, 115].

REM Sleep-Suppressing Neurons in the Pons
During wakefulness, several neuronal groups in the pons, including the monoaminergic neurons of the LC and DRN, are thought to suppress REM sleep [104]. These neurons are nearly silent during REM sleep but are very active during wakefulness

and suppress REM sleep by inhibiting REM sleep-active neurons in SLD region [119]. Additionally, NE and 5-HT inhibit cholinergic neurons of the PPT/LDT region [120, 121]. Hence, antidepressants that increase monoamine levels often have REM suppressant effect [104].

Ventro-lateral PAG (vlPAG) and the lateral pontine tegmentum (LPT) are another set of REM sleep-suppressing neurons that are active during wake and NREM sleep and probably silent during REM sleep [122]. The vlPAG/LPT neurons send GABAergic projections to the SLD, and lesions or pharmacological inactivation of the vlPAG/LPT region increase REM sleep [115, 122]. On the other hand, chemogenetic activation of GABAergic vlPAG/LPT neurons reduces REM sleep [123]. These findings, taken together, suggest that the vlPAG/LPT inhibits REM sleep via GABAergic projections to the SLD [104]. Conversely, REM sleep-active GABAergic neurons in SLD innervate the vlPAG/LPT [115, 124], thus suggesting that the vlPAG/LPT and SLD may form a mutually inhibitory circuit that regulates REM sleep [104].

Medullary Reticular Formation
The ventromedial medulla (VMM) contains neurons that fire fastest in REM sleep, slower in NREM sleep, and very little during wake, and these firing patterns correlate with the amount of muscle atonia [125]. Glutamate levels in the VMM tend to increase as animals enter REM sleep, and blockade of glutamatergic signaling onto these neurons leads to REM sleep without muscle atonia [104]. These findings suggest that glutamatergic input, probably from the SLD, activates the VMM neurons to produce muscle atonia [126]. Additionally, lesions of VMM can partially disrupt the atonia of REM sleep [127, 128].

Other medullary neurons, residing in the dorsal paragigantocellular reticular (DPGi) and lateral paragigantocellular (LPGi) nuclei, may also promote REM sleep by inhibiting REM sleep-suppressing neurons of the pons such as the LC, DRN, and vlPAG/LPT. Photostimulation of GABAergic neurons in the LPGi and adjacent regions or their projections to the vlPAG tend to prolong REM sleep or trigger transitions into REM sleep, whereas chemogenetic inhibition of these neurons has been associated with decrease in REM sleep [129]. These findings suggest a greater role of medullary neurons than simply to generate atonia of REM sleep, and further research is needed to determine whether REM sleep is mainly driven by the pons, medulla, or the two regions together [104].

Hypothalamic Control of REM Sleep

Two specific groups of neurons in hypothalamic area generate and regulate REM sleep. One cluster of REM sleep-active neurons is located in a region referred to as the extended VLPO that is just dorsal and medial to the VLPO. These neurons, which release GABA and galanin, are active during REM sleep, whereas the lesions of the extended VLPO have been associated with reduction in REM sleep [130]. The extended VLPO neurons may promote REM sleep by inhibiting brainstem neurons that suppress REM sleep including DR, LC, and ventral periaqueductal gray [104].

Another group of REM sleep-promoting neurons in hypothalamus is scattered across the LH and PH. These neurons produce the neuropeptide melanin-concentrating hormone (MCH) and fire maximally during REM sleep [131]. Several authors have reported that photo-activation or chemo-activation of the MCH neurons increases REM sleep [132, 133, 134]. In addition to SLD, MCH neurons densely innervate the REM sleep-suppressing neurons of the LC, DRN, and vlPAG/LPT. It is plausible that release of excitatory glutamate from MCH neurons directly activates pontine REM sleep-promoting neurons, whereas the release of MCH and GABA inhibits REM sleep-suppressing neurons [104].

The orexin neurons of LH are intermixed with the MCH neurons, but these neurons have completely opposite effects on REM sleep. Intracerebroventricular (ICV) injection of orexin-A reduces REM sleep for many hours [135], and photo-activation of the orexin neurons awakens mice from REM sleep [136]. Similarly, chemogenetic activation of the orexin neurons robustly suppresses REM sleep [137], whereas orexin antagonists increase REM sleep and decrease REM sleep latency. Chronic loss of the orexin neurons in rodents and people with narcolepsy results in very poor regulation of REM sleep characterized by intrusion of REM sleep into wakefulness at any time of day leading to muscle atonia and dream-like hallucinations [104]. The precise mechanisms through which orexin inhibit REM sleep are still being explored, but the orexin neurons heavily innervate REM sleep-suppressing regions such as the LC, DR, vlPAG/LPT, and the absence of orexin signaling in 5-HT DR neurons accounts for reduced episodes of atonia during wakefulness [138]. Since the orexin neurons are mainly active while awake, it is probable that orexin suppresses REM sleep in a tonic pattern during wakefulness [104].

Activation-Synthesis Hypothesis of Dream Generation

Another key and most fascinating aspect of REM sleep is its close association with dreaming. Interpretation of dreams has gained significant attention in many cultures and predates modern science [14]. Based on the work of Freud and his counterparts, the notion that dreams provided insights in to "psychic disturbance" gained widespread acceptance in Western cultures [14]. However, modern neuroscience offers a different view that dreams arise from internally generated patterns of brain activation and dream content does not imply specific meaning or message for the individual [14, 139–142].

Hobson and McCarley laid out activation-synthesis hypothesis of dream generation that entails activation of sensory (particularly visual systems), vestibular, emotional, and memory formation areas of the brain [14]. Hippocampus and amygdala are "reactivated" during REM sleep, which explains memory consolidation processes [143, 144] and emotional content of the dream [14]. Dream experience is influenced by sensations and feedback from neural command signals for muscular activity; however, the motor activity is inhibited by brainstem muscle atonia generating systems during REM sleep [14].

Neuroimaging studies, including positron emission tomography (PET) and functional magnetic resonance imaging (fMRI), have reported increased blood flow/oxygen utilization in a network of interconnected regions including the pontine tegmentum, thalamus, amygdala, basal ganglia, anterior cingulate, and occipital cortex during REM sleep [145–147]. Decreased activity of dorsolateral prefrontal cortex, parietal cortex, posterior cingulate cortex, and precuneus has been reported, which likely accounts for the lack of insight, distortion of time perception, and difficulty in remembering dreams upon waking [145, 148]. In contrast, amygdala activation is likely responsible for the high percentage of dreams featuring negative emotions such as anxiety and fear [14].

OTHER MECHANISMS

Homeostatic Regulation of Sleep

As proposed by Borbely [149], the timing, depth, and duration of sleep are controlled by interaction of time of the day (circadian control, Process C) and the duration of prior wakefulness (homeostatic control, Process S). Homeostatic regulation of sleep implies that a period of sleep deprivation is followed by compensatory increase in the amount of sleep in an individual. Prolonged periods of wakefulness are associated with exhaustion of brain glycogen reserves and degradation of adenosine 5′-triphosphate (ATP) levels [150, 151]. Since ATP is degraded to AD, the levels of extracellular AD rise in some parts of the brain, including the BF, during periods of wakefulness [152]. Halassa and colleagues [153] demonstrated that a genetic deletion, blocking the rise in AD in mice, prevented rebound recovery sleep after sleep deprivation.

AD has been proposed to be the accumulator of the homeostatic need to sleep [23, 154, 155]. There are two major classes of AD receptors in the brain: AD A1 receptors, which are predominantly inhibitory, and A2a receptors, which are excitatory in nature [15]. Caffeine, the most commonly consumed stimulant in the world, blocks AD receptors and attenuates the consequences of sleep deprivation on arousal, vigilance, and attention [156]. Caffeine presumably acts through blockade of A2a receptors as it loses its wake-promoting effect in A2a receptor knockout mice [157]. In cats, injection of AD or an AD A1 receptor agonist into the BF causes sleep [23]. Similarly, in rats, injection of an AD A2a receptor agonist near the VLPO causes sleep and also results in expression of Fos (a marker of neuronal activity) in VLPO neurons [158]. Additionally, AD probably disinhibits the VLPO via presynaptic A1 receptors by reducing inhibitory GABAergic inputs [101]. Therefore, accumulation of a sleep-promoting substance that enhances the activity of sleep-promoting cells and reduces the activity of wake-promoting neurons may be one of the underlying mechanisms of homeostatic sleep drive [2]. After a period of sleep deprivation, NREM sleep is typically repleted first, and this probably implies that NREM and REM sleep have separate homeostatic mechanisms [2].

Circadian Regulation of Sleep

The circadian system synchronizes sleep–wake cycles with the light/dark cycle of the earth spanning over a 24-hour period [104]. In mammals, circadian timing is regulated by the suprachiasmatic nucleus (SCN), which serves as a biological clock to orchestrate the timing of sleep–wake behavior, metabolism, and physiology in synchrony with the changes in the light/dark cycle [159, 160]. SCN is a pair of compact nuclei in the most ventral and medial part of the hypothalamus that receives a major retinal input via the retinohypothalamic tract [161]. SCN has few outputs to sleep-regulatory systems, and it mainly projects to other hypothalamic nuclei, especially to

the subparaventricular zone (SPZ), a region just above the SCN, and the dorsomedial nucleus of the hypothalamus (DMH) [2].

Neurons in the ventral SPZ relay necessary information for organizing daily sleep-wake cycles, whereas dorsal SPZ neurons are crucial for rhythms of body temperature [2]. Outputs from the ventral SPZ are integrated in the DMH, which seems to be the origin of projections to the VLPO for circadian cycles of sleep [2]. Ventral SPZ appears to be an important circadian relay as cell-specific lesions of this region has been associated with severe reduction in circadian rhythms of wake and NREM and REM sleep in rats [162]. Additionally, cell-specific lesions of the DMH also eliminate circadian rhythms of sleep–wake behavior [163]. It has been shown that glutamatergic DMH neurons strongly innervate wake-promoting brain regions (orexin neurons, TMN, LC, VTA, DR and LDT), whereas, GABAergic DMH neurons innervate sleep-promoting regions (VLPO and MnPO) [15, 164]. Thus, the DMH likely plays an important role integrating circadian signals to actively promote wakefulness at certain times and sleep at others [104].

Allostatic Regulation of Sleep

McEwen and colleagues [165] described certain situations as allostatic loads whereby animals require urgent alterations of specific physiological responses, including sleep–wake states, in response to the conditions in their environment. These include stressful situations such as confronting a predator, encountering a potential mate, seasonal changes, or the need for migration that may require an adjustment of sleep–wake behavior [166, 167]. Lack of food is a common stressor in the wild, and the effects of food deprivation on sleep in small animals that can carry minimal energy reserves are dramatic [15]. Marked increases in wakefulness and locomotor activity have been reported in food-deprived mice; however, mice lacking in orexin-producing neurons show very little arousal or increase in locomotion during periods of food deprivation, which suggests that orexin neurons are required for the arousing effects of hunger [168]. Whereas, mice lacking MCH, a peptide with exact opposite activity profile and neurotransmitter action as compared to orexin, show exaggerated increases in locomotion, more wakefulness, and much less REM sleep than normal mice during food deprivation [169]. Therefore, orexin and MCH neurons have opposite effects on sleep–wake pathways in response to the stress of insufficient food [15].

Behavioral stress is another common allostatic factor that affects sleep and frequently causes insomnia [15]. In a study of mice, exposed to foot shock, the authors proposed that increased levels of corticotrophin-releasing factors (CRH) may cause arousal in mice by exciting orexin neurons via CRH-1 receptors [170]. In another study, Cano and colleagues [171] observed that stressed rats took twice as long to fall asleep as compared to controls. Rats with insomnia expressed Fos in a surprising pattern such that both sleep-promoting neurons (VLPO) and wake promoting neurons (LC and TMN) were active. This pattern of dual activation of sleep and wake activity is likely suggestive that both homeostatic and circadian drives activated the VLPO, whereas allostatic stress activated the LC and TMN [171]. Thus, stress-induced insomnia may represent an unusual state characterized by inability of wake- and sleep-promoting neurons to overcome each other, due to both receiving strong excitatory stimuli [15].

Furthermore, these stressed rats expressed Fos in the brain regions including infralimbic cortex, the central nucleus of amygdala, and the bed nucleus of stria terminalis [171]. These cortico-limbic sites project to the wake-promoting neurons in LC and TMN, and areas in the upper pons that regulate REM sleep switching [172–174]. These inputs may play an important role in maintaining a waking state during periods of high behavioral arousal; however, in stress-induced insomnia, their activation by residual stress or anxiety may contribute to inability to sleep. Additionally, Nofzinger and colleagues [175] reported increased activation of these corticolimbic sites in human subjects with insomnia. The activation of medial prefrontal and amygdaloid circuitry can increase arousal, despite sleep-promoting action of VLPO, thus leading to a state of hyperarousal. This co-activation can result in high frequency EEG during NREM sleep, which explains the condition of "sleep-state misperception" in people with insomnia who describe being awake despite the EEG being suggestive of NREM sleep [15].

Other Neurochemicals and Peptides
Peptides
Two core components of the HPA axis, corticotrophin-releasing factor (CRF) [176, 177] and adrenocorticotrophic hormone (ACTH) [178], are known to promote wakefulness, possibly mediated by CRF activation of CRF receptor-1 on orexin neurons [179]. Thyrotropin-releasing hormone (TRH) and TRH analogs have been shown to have wake-promoting effect in canines with narcolepsy [180, 181]; however, in a clinical study, TRH only exerted a "weak" effect on sleep efficiency [182]. Neuropeptide Y (NPY), a potent inducer of

feeding behavior, exerts varied sleep effects ranging from sleep suppression to alterations in EEG spectral power in rodents [183, 184]. However, in humans, intravenous administration of NPY has been shown to reduce sleep latency in young men [185] and older men and women [186]. Growth hormone (GH)-releasing hormone (GHRH) is another sleep-promoting peptide that has been extensively studied [176, 187, 188], partly due to the fact that pharmacological stimulation of SWS results in increased GH release [189]. However, varying results on sleep have been reported in studies of peptides related to the GH system [190, 191]. MCH is a hypothalamic neuropeptide that has profound effects on both SWS and REM sleep [192]. Based on results from optogenetic studies, MCH neurons have been implicated in the control of REM sleep [132, 134] as well as sleep onset [193]. Other peptides including prolactin [194], vasoactive intestinal polypeptide [195] and pituitary adenylate cyclase-activating polypeptide [196] seem to have REM-promoting activity.

Cytokines
Among cytokines, interleukin-1 (IL-1) and tumor necrosis factor alpha (TNFα) have been most studied in terms of their effects on sleep and may exert their effects through direct receptor-mediated modulation of the hypothalamus and serotonergic raphe nuclei [192]. Injection of IL-1 or TNFα enhances NREM sleep, whereas, inhibition of either IL-1 or TNFα inhibits spontaneous sleep and rebound sleep following a period of sleep deprivation [197].

Prostaglandins
Concentration of prostaglandin D2 (PGD2) tends to exhibit circadian alteration in rats [198]. CSF levels of PGD2 increase in response to increasing propensity toward sleep under normal conditions and sleep deprivation [199]. Additionally, inhibition of PGD synthase (PGDS), an enzyme responsible for PGD2 synthesis, leads to marked suppression of sleep in rats [200, 201], and blockade of PGD2 receptors inhibits physiological sleep in mice [202]. A PGD2 sensitive sleep-promoting zone (PGD2-SZ) has been identified in the ventral surface of the rostral BF in rats [203]. Furthermore, administration of a selective AD A2a-R agonist (CGS21680) to the PGD2-SZ has been shown to induce sleep in rats [204]. On the contrary, the SWS-promoting effect of PGD2 is blunted in AD A2a-R–deficient mice [205], and it is inhibited by pretreatment with KF17837, a highly selective A2a-R antagonist [204]. Based on these findings, it is plausible that PGD2 is coupled

to A2a-R adenosinergic signaling and that the PGD2-SZ plays an important role as an interface between these two systems [192].

Gonadal Hormones

Sex and sex hormones modulate sleep as women exhibit increased subjective sleep disturbance, particularly insomnia [206], and increased spindle activity and SWA compared to men [207–209]. Factors such as sleep deprivation, aging, and major depression account for the sex differences in SWA [207, 210]. Variation in sleep spindle activity and REM sleep, but not SWA, has been noted across the menstrual cycle [211, 212]. Circulating ovarian steroids, particularly estradiol and progesterone, play a role in sleep differences across the menstrual cycle [213–215]. It has been shown that sex differences in sleep appear to be developmentally determined by a combination of genetic sex and gonadal hormone exposure [216]. Estradiol downregulates the synthetic enzyme for PGD2 [217], increases orexin and orexin receptor expression levels [218], and modulates Fos expression in the VLPO and TMN [219].

SLEEP–WAKE TRANSITION

Flip-Flop Switch

One of the remarkable features of sleep-state control systems is that both wake- and sleep-promoting neurons appear to be mutually inhibitory [15]. Flip-flop switches are incorporated into electrical circuits to ensure rapid and complete state transitions. Similarly in the brain, due to mutually inhibitory action of neurons on the neurons on other side of circuit, if the either side gains a small advantage over other, then it turns off the neurons on the other side, thus causing a rapid collapse in neuronal activity and a change in state [15]. As compared to electric flip-flop switch, which contains single element and acts almost instantly, the state-switching phenomenon in the brain takes seconds to minutes (depending upon the type of species) due to mutual antagonism of large populations of neurons [15]. Sleep-promoting VLPO neurons inhibit many wake-promoting brain regions, and these regions, in turn, inhibit the VLPO. Saper and colleagues [2] proposed that this mutual inhibition generates patterns of activity akin to an electrical flip-flop switch. During sleep, the inhibition of wake-promoting neurons lessens any inhibition of the VLPO by the wake-promoting systems, thus enabling high levels of activity in the VLPO. Just the opposite of this phenomenon likely occurs during wake, and

this dynamic interaction enables rapid transitions between sleep and wakefulness states with little time spent in intermediate drowsy states [104]. Other sleep-promoting neurons, including BF and cortical sleep-active neurons, may have similar relations with wake-promoting neurons [104].

CONCLUSIONS

Modern neuroscience has significantly helped our understanding of the phenomenon of sleep and wakefulness, which are regulated by intricate neural networks and neurotransmitter systems in conjunction with circadian, homeostatic, allostatic, and other factors as outlined in this chapter. Knowledge of these mechanisms has led to significant clinical discoveries such as the origins of rare sleep disorders, like narcolepsy, and also paved the way for therapeutic interventions for common sleep disturbances such as insomnia and hypersomnia. The significant comorbidity of sleep disturbances and psychiatric disorders provides an opportunity to both understand the sleep-related neurobiological mechanisms and develop effective treatments of a range of psychiatric disorders.

FUTURE DIRECTIONS

Deep brain imaging is one of the newest technologies in neuroscience that measures changes in calcium channels in neurons in the intact brain during behavior, by using fluorescent probes [220, 221]. This technology has already proven useful to identify the potential REM sleep generator neurons in the pons as it has been found that found that glutamate cells in pons region are most active during REM sleep, whereas GABA cells are most active during wakefulness [114]. The CRISPR-Cas system is a new genetic tool that allows researchers to silence, delete, enhance, or insert specific genes at a precise location within a genome [222, 223]. CRISPR is an acronym for "clustered regularly interspaced short palindromic repeats," and it contains segments of DNA containing short repetitions of base sequences with each repetition followed by spacer DNA [12]. Cas protein is used to manipulate the genome by removing or adding genes with the help of Cas 9 nuclease and guide RNA [12]. Recently, CRISPR-Cas system has been used to identify the role of N-methyl-D-aspartate receptors in sleep-regulation in mice [224]. Finally, new histological techniques are emerging [12] that focus on making the neural tissue transparent, scanning the tissue with a laser from light-sheet microscope, and then compiling 3D image of scanned images using software [225–227]. This technology allows visualization of the cytoarchitecture of neurons in significant detail such that it can helpful in reconstructing visual maps of sleep–wake circuitry and understanding the interaction between different neural circuits [12]. The development and implementation of these new technologies is likely to consolidate our understanding of why and how we sleep.

KEY CLINICAL PEARLS

- Wakefulness is maintained by monoaminergic systems of the brainstem, cholinergic neurons in the brainstem and BF, and hypocretin/orexin cells of the hypothalamus.
- Loss of hypocretin/orexinergic neurons is associated with hypersomnolence disorders such as narcolepsy.
- Caffeine presumably acts through blockade of adenosine (A2a) receptors to promote wakefulness.
- Circadian pacemaker, located in the SCN of hypothalamus, and sleep homeostatic mechanisms interact to determine the timing of sleep and wakefulness across a 24 hour cycle.
- GABAergic neurons concentrated in the VLP) and MnPO exert NREM sleep promoting effect.
- Similar to wakefulness, Ach levels are high during REM sleep.
- Antidepressants that increase monoamine levels often have REM suppressant effect as norepinephrine (NE) and serotonin (5-HT) suppress REM sleep-promoting cholinergic neurons in pons.
- Emerging evidence suggests that periaqueductal gray and descending projections from hypothalamus control pontine REM generators.
- Women exhibit increased subjective sleep disturbance, particularly insomnia, and increased spindle activity and SWA compared to men.
- Factors such as sleep deprivation, aging and major depression account for the sex differences in SWA.

SELF-ASSESSMENT QUESTIONS

1. Caffeine acts at which of the following receptors to promote wakefulness?
   a. Adenosine
   b. Serotonin
   c. Norepinephrine
   d. Dopamine

Answer: a

2. All of the following neurotransmitters have wake promoting effect *except*
   a. orexin.
   b. dopamine.
   c. GABA.
   d. histamine.

Answer: c

3. All of the following brain regions have NREM promoting effect *except*
   a. sublaterodorsal nucleus.
   b. ventrolateral preoptic area (VLPO).
   c. median preoptic nucleus (MnPO).
   d. parafacial Zone (PZ).

Answer: a

4. All of the following neurotransmitters have REM promoting effect *except*
   a. acetylcholine.
   b. melanin-concentrating hormone.
   c. glutamate.
   d. serotonin.

Answer: d

5. Suvorexant, an FDA approved medication for insomnia, targets which of the following receptors?
   a. Histamine
   b. Orexin
   c. Glutamate
   d. Norepinephrine

Answer: b

REFERENCES

1. Moruzzi, G. and H.W. Magoun, *Brain stem reticular formation and activation of the EEG. 1949.* J Neuropsychiatry Clin Neurosci, 1995. **7**(2): p. 251–267.
2. Saper, C.B., T.E. Scammell, and J. Lu, *Hypothalamic regulation of sleep and circadian rhythms.* Nature, 2005. **437**(7063): p. 1257–1263.
3. Sherin, J.E., et al., *Activation of ventrolateral preoptic neurons during sleep.* Science, 1996. **271**(5246): p. 216–219.
4. Gaus, S.E., et al., *Ventrolateral preoptic nucleus contains sleep-active, galaninergic neurons in multiple mammalian species.* Neuroscience, 2002. **115**(1): p. 285–294.
5. Sherin, J.E., et al., *Innervation of histaminergic tuberomammillary neurons by GABAergic and galaninergic neurons in the ventrolateral preoptic nucleus of the rat.* J Neurosci, 1998. **18**(12): p. 4705–4721.
6. Szymusiak, R., et al., *Sleep-waking discharge patterns of ventrolateral preoptic/anterior hypothalamic neurons in rats.* Brain Res, 1998. **803**(1-2): p. 178–188.

7. Sakurai, T., et al., *Orexins and orexin receptors: a family of hypothalamic neuropeptides and G protein-coupled receptors that regulate feeding behavior.* Cell, 1998. **92**(5):573–585.

8. de Lecea, L., et al., *The hypocretins: hypothalamus-specific peptides with neuroexcitatory activity.* Proc Natl Acad Sci U S A, 1998. **95**(1): p. 322–327.

9. Lin, L., et al., *The sleep disorder canine narcolepsy is caused by a mutation in the hypocretin (orexin) receptor 2 gene.* Cell, 1999. **98**(3): p. 365–376.

10. Chemelli, R.M., et al., *Narcolepsy in orexin knockout mice: molecular genetics of sleep regulation.* Cell, 1999. **98**(4): p. 437–451.

11. Yizhar, O., et al., *Optogenetics in neural systems.* Neuron, 2011. **71**(1): p. 9–34.

12. Shiromani, P.J. and J.H. Peever, *New Neuroscience Tools That Are Identifying the Sleep-Wake Circuit.* Sleep, 2017. **40**(4).

13. Harris, C.D., *Neurophysiology of sleep and wakefulness.* Respir Care Clin N Am, 2005. **11**(4): p. 567–586.

14. Brown, R.E., et al., *Control of sleep and wakefulness.* Physiol Rev, 2012. **92**(3): p. 1087–1187.

15. Saper, C.B., et al., *Sleep state switching.* Neuron, 2010. **68**(6): p. 1023–1042.

16. Jones, B.E., *Arousal systems.* Front Biosci, 2003. **8**: p. s438–s451.

17. Szymusiak, R. and D. McGinty, *Hypothalamic regulation of sleep and arousal.* Ann N Y Acad Sci, 2008. **1129**: p. 275–286.

18. Magoun, H.W., *An ascending reticular activating system in the brain stem.* AMA Arch Neurol Psychiatry, 1952. **67**(2): p. 145–154; discussion 167–171.

19. Krone, L., et al., *Top-down control of arousal and sleep: Fundamentals and clinical implications.* Sleep Med Rev, 2017. **31**: p. 17–24.

20. Mileykovskiy, B.Y., L.I. Kiyashchenko, and J.M. Siegel, *Behavioral correlates of activity in identified hypocretin/orexin neurons.* Neuron, 2005. **46**(5): p. 787–798.

21. Peyron, C., et al., *Neurons containing hypocretin (orexin) project to multiple neuronal systems.* J Neurosci, 1998. **18**(23): p. 9996–10015.

22. Hallanger, A.E., et al., *The origins of cholinergic and other subcortical afferents to the thalamus in the rat.* J Comp Neurol, 1987. **262**(1): p. 105–124.

23. Strecker, R.E., et al., *Adenosinergic modulation of basal forebrain and preoptic/anterior hypothalamic neuronal activity in the control of behavioral state.* Behav Brain Res, 2000. **115**(2): p. 183–204.

24. Magoun, H.W. and R. Rhines, *An inhibitory mechanism in the bulbar reticular formation.* J Neurophysiol, 1946. **9**: p. 165–171.

25. Stornetta, R.L., C.P. Sevigny, and P.G. Guyenet, *Vesicular glutamate transporter DNPI/VGLUT2 mRNA is present in C1 and several other groups of brainstem catecholaminergic neurons.* J Comp Neurol, 2002. **444**(3): p. 191–206.

26. Yamamura, T., et al., *Is the site of action of ketamine anesthesia the N-methyl-D-aspartate receptor?* Anesthesiology, 1990. **72**(4): p. 704–710.

27. MacIver, M.B., et al., *Volatile anesthetics depress glutamate transmission via presynaptic actions.* Anesthesiology, 1996. **85**(4): p. 823–834.

28. Schulz, D.W. and R.L. Macdonald, *Barbiturate enhancement of GABA-mediated inhibition and activation of chloride ion conductance: correlation with anticonvulsant and anesthetic actions.* Brain Res, 1981. **209**(1): p. 177–188.

29. Aston-Jones, G. and F.E. Bloom, *Activity of norepinephrine-containing locus coeruleus neurons in behaving rats anticipates fluctuations in the sleep-waking cycle.* J Neurosci, 1981. **1**(8): p. 876–886.

30. Fornal, C., S. Auerbach, and B.L. Jacobs, *Activity of serotonin-containing neurons in nucleus raphe magnus in freely moving cats.* Exp Neurol, 1985. **88**(3): p. 590–608.

31. Monckton, J.E. and D.A. McCormick, *Neuromodulatory role of serotonin in the ferret thalamus.* J Neurophysiol, 2002. **87**(4): p. 2124–2136.

32. McCormick, D.A., *Neurotransmitter actions in the thalamus and cerebral cortex and their role in neuromodulation of thalamocortical activity.* Prog Neurobiol, 1992. **39**(4): p. 337–388.

33. Starzl, T.E. and H.W. Magoun, *Organization of the diffuse thalamic projection system.* J Neurophysiol, 1951. **14**(2): p. 133–146.

34. Kaneko, T. and N. Mizuno, *Immunohistochemical study of glutaminase-containing neurons in the cerebral cortex and thalamus of the rat.* J Comp Neurol, 1988. **267**(4): p. 590–602.

35. Fremeau, R.T., Jr., et al., *The expression of vesicular glutamate transporters defines two classes of excitatory synapse.* Neuron, 2001. **31**(2): p. 247–260.

36. Glenn, L.L. and M. Steriade, *Discharge rate and excitability of cortically projecting intralaminar thalamic neurons during waking and sleep states.* J Neurosci, 1982. **2**(10): p. 1387–1404.

37. Young, A. and R.D. Wimmer, *Implications for the thalamic reticular nucleus in impaired attention and sleep in schizophrenia.* Schizophr Res, 2017. **180**: p. 44–47.

38. Steriade, M. and R.R. Llinas, *The functional states of the thalamus and the associated neuronal interplay.* Physiol Rev, 1988. **68**(3): p. 649–742.

39. Steriade, M., D. Contreras, and F. Amzica, *Synchronized sleep oscillations and their paroxysmal developments.* Trends Neurosci, 1994. **17**(5): p. 199–208.

40. Saper, C.B., *Organization of cerebral cortical afferent systems in the rat. II. Hypothalamocortical projections.* J Comp Neurol, 1985. **237**(1): p. 21–46.

41. Saper, C.B., L.W. Swanson, and W.M. Cowan, *An autoradiographic study of the efferent connections of the lateral hypothalamic area in the rat.* J Comp Neurol, 1979. **183**(4): p. 689–706.

42. Holstege, G., *Some anatomical observations on the projections from the hypothalamus to brainstem and spinal cord: an HRP and autoradiographic tracing study in the cat.* J Comp Neurol, 1987. **260**(1): p. 98–126.

43. Ziegler, D.R., W.E. Cullinan, and J.P. Herman, *Distribution of vesicular glutamate transporter mRNA in rat hypothalamus.* J Comp Neurol, 2002. **448**(3): p. 217–229.

44. Steininger, T.L., et al., *Sleep-waking discharge of neurons in the posterior lateral hypothalamus of the albino rat.* Brain Res, 1999. **840**(1-2): p. 138–147.

45. Panula, P., et al., *Histamine-immunoreactive nerve fibers in the rat brain.* Neuroscience, 1989. **28**(3): p. 585–610.

46. Lin, J.S., K. Sakai, and M. Jouvet, *Evidence for histaminergic arousal mechanisms in the hypothalamus of cat.* Neuropharmacology, 1988. **27**(2): p. 111–122.

47. Monti, J.M., T. Pellejero, and H. Jantos, *Effects of H1- and H2-histamine receptor agonists and antagonists on sleep and wakefulness in the rat.* J Neural Transm, 1986. **66**(1): p. 1–11.

48. Ono, D. and A. Yamanaka, *Hypothalamic regulation of the sleep/wake cycle.* Neurosci Res, 2017. **118**: p. 74–81.

49. Horvath, T.L., et al., *Hypocretin (orexin) activation and synaptic innervation of the locus coeruleus noradrenergic system.* J Comp Neurol, 1999. **415**(2): p. 145–159.

50. Bayer, L., et al., *Selective action of orexin (hypocretin) on nonspecific thalamocortical projection neurons.* J Neurosci, 2002. **22**(18): p. 7835–7839.

51. Bayer, L., et al., *Orexins (hypocretins) directly excite tuberomammillary neurons.* Eur J Neurosci, 2001. **14**(9): p. 1571–1575.

52. Eriksson, K.S., et al., *Orexin/hypocretin excites the histaminergic neurons of the tuberomammillary nucleus.* J Neurosci, 2001. **21**(23): p. 9273–9279.

53. Eggermann, E., et al., *Orexins/hypocretins excite basal forebrain cholinergic neurones.* Neuroscience, 2001. **108**(2): p. 177–181.

54. Chou, T.C., et al., *Afferents to the ventrolateral preoptic nucleus.* J Neurosci, 2002. **22**(3): p. 977–990.

55. Sakurai, T., et al., *Input of orexin/hypocretin neurons revealed by a genetically encoded tracer in mice.* Neuron, 2005. **46**(2): p. 297–308.

56. Yoshida, K., et al., *Afferents to the orexin neurons of the rat brain.* J Comp Neurol, 2006. **494**(5): p. 845–861.

57. Marcus, J.N., et al., *Differential expression of orexin receptors 1 and 2 in the rat brain.* J Comp Neurol, 2001. **435**(1): p. 6–25.

58. Patel, K.V., A.V. Aspesi, and K.E. Evoy, *Suvorexant: a dual orexin receptor antagonist for the treatment of sleep onset and sleep maintenance insomnia.* Ann Pharmacother, 2015. **49**(4): p. 477–483.

59. Khateb, A., et al., *Rhythmical bursts induced by NMDA in guinea-pig cholinergic nucleus basalis neurones in vitro.* J Physiol, 1995. **487 (Pt 3)**: p. 623–638.

60. Fort, P., et al., *Noradrenergic modulation of cholinergic nucleus basalis neurons demonstrated by in vitro pharmacological and immunohistochemical evidence in the guinea-pig brain.* Eur J Neurosci, 1995. **7**(7): p. 1502–1511.

61. Khateb, A., et al., *Cholinergic nucleus basalis neurons are excited by histamine in vitro.* Neuroscience, 1995. **69**(2): p. 495–506.

62. Khateb, A., et al., *Pharmacological and immunohistochemical evidence for serotonergic modulation of cholinergic nucleus basalis neurons.* Eur J Neurosci, 1993. **5**(5): p. 541–547.

63. Cape, E.G. and B.E. Jones, *Effects of glutamate agonist versus procaine microinjections into the basal forebrain cholinergic cell area upon gamma and theta EEG activity and sleep-wake state.* Eur J Neurosci, 2000. **12**(6): p. 2166–2184.

64. Cape, E.G., et al., *Neurotensin-induced bursting of cholinergic basal forebrain neurons promotes gamma and theta cortical activity together with waking and paradoxical sleep.* J Neurosci, 2000. **20**(22): p. 8452–8461.

65. Marrosu, F., et al., *Microdialysis measurement of cortical and hippocampal acetylcholine release during sleep-wake cycle in freely moving cats.* Brain Res, 1995. **671**(2): p. 329–332.

66. Jasper, H.H. and J. Tessier, *Acetylcholine liberation from cerebral cortex during paradoxical (REM) sleep.* Science, 1971. **172**(3983): p. 601–602.

67. Celesia, G.G. and H.H. Jasper, *Acetylcholine released from cerebral cortex in relation to state of activation.* Neurology, 1966. **16**(11): p. 1053–1063.

68. Gritti, I., et al., *GABAergic and other noncholinergic basal forebrain neurons, together with cholinergic neurons, project to the mesocortex and isocortex in the rat.* J Comp Neurol, 1997. **383**(2): p. 163–177.

69. Manns, I.D., L. Mainville, and B.E. Jones, *Evidence for glutamate, in addition to acetylcholine and GABA, neurotransmitter synthesis in basal forebrain neurons projecting to the entorhinal cortex.* Neuroscience, 2001. **107**(2): p. 249–263.

70. Henny, P. and B.E. Jones, *Vesicular glutamate (VGlut), GABA (VGAT), and acetylcholine (VACht) transporters in basal forebrain axon terminals innervating the lateral hypothalamus.* J Comp Neurol, 2006. **496**(4): p. 453–467.

71. Sterman, M.B. and C.D. Clemente, *Forebrain inhibitory mechanisms: sleep patterns induced by basal forebrain stimulation in the behaving cat.* Exp Neurol, 1962. **6**: p. 103–117.

72. Sterman, M.B. and C.D. Clemente, *Forebrain inhibitory mechanisms: cortical synchronization induced by basal forebrain stimulation.* Exp Neurol, 1962. **6**: p. 91–102.

73. McGinty, D.J. and M.B. Sterman, *Sleep suppression after basal forebrain lesions in the cat.* Science, 1968. **160**(3833): p. 1253–1255.

74. Amzica, F. and M. Steriade, *The K-complex: its slow (<1-Hz) rhythmicity and relation to delta waves.* Neurology, 1997. **49**(4): p. 952–959.

75. Amzica, F. and M. Steriade, *Cellular substrates and laminar profile of sleep K-complex.* Neuroscience, 1998. **82**(3): p. 671–686.

76. Cash, S.S., et al., *The human K-complex represents an isolated cortical down-state.* Science, 2009. **324**(5930): p. 1084–1087.

77. Fuentealba, P. and M. Steriade, *The reticular nucleus revisited: intrinsic and network properties of a thalamic pacemaker.* Prog Neurobiol, 2005. **75**(2): p. 125–141.

78. Marks, G.A. and H.P. Roffwarg, *Spontaneous activity in the thalamic reticular nucleus during the sleep/wake cycle of the freely-moving rat.* Brain Res, 1993. **623**(2): p. 241–248.

79. Steriade, M. and M. Deschenes, *The thalamus as a neuronal oscillator.* Brain Res, 1984. **320**(1): p. 1–63.

80. McCormick, D.A. and Z. Wang, *Serotonin and noradrenaline excite GABAergic neurones of the guinea-pig and cat nucleus reticularis thalami.* J Physiol, 1991. **442**: p. 235–255.

81. Pare, D., et al., *Projections of brainstem core cholinergic and non-cholinergic neurons of cat to intralaminar and reticular thalamic nuclei.* Neuroscience, 1988. **25**(1): p. 69–86.

82. Asanuma, C. and L.L. Porter, *Light and electron microscopic evidence for a GABAergic projection from the caudal basal forebrain to the thalamic reticular nucleus in rats.* J Comp Neurol, 1990. **302**(1): p. 159–172.

83. Parent, A., et al., *Basal forebrain cholinergic and noncholinergic projections to the thalamus and brainstem in cats and monkeys.* J Comp Neurol, 1988. **277**(2): p. 281–301.

84. Carden, W.B. and M.E. Bickford, *Location of muscarinic type 2 receptors within the synaptic circuitry of the cat visual thalamus.* J Comp Neurol, 1999. **410**(3): p. 431–443.

85. McCormick, D.A. and D.A. Prince, *Acetylcholine induces burst firing in thalamic reticular neurones by activating a potassium conductance.* Nature, 1986. **319**(6052): p. 402–405.

86. Szymusiak, R. and D. McGinty, *Sleep-related neuronal discharge in the basal forebrain of cats.* Brain Res, 1986. **370**(1): p. 82–92.

87. Alam, M.N., D. McGinty, and R. Szymusiak, *Preoptic/anterior hypothalamic neurons: thermosensitivity in wakefulness and non rapid eye movement sleep.* Brain Res, 1996. **718**(1-2): p. 76–82.

88. Alam, M.A., et al., *Neuronal activity in the preoptic hypothalamus during sleep deprivation and recovery sleep.* J Neurophysiol, 2014. **111**(2): p. 287–299.

89. John, J. and V.M. Kumar, *Effect of NMDA lesion of the medial preoptic neurons on sleep and other functions.* Sleep, 1998. **21**(6): p. 587–598.

90. Lu, J., et al., *Effect of lesions of the ventrolateral preoptic nucleus on NREM and REM sleep.* J Neurosci, 2000. **20**(10): p. 3830–3842.

91. Gong, H., et al., *Activation of c-fos in GABAergic neurones in the preoptic area during sleep and in response to sleep deprivation.* J Physiol, 2004. **556**(Pt 3): p. 935–946.

92. Modirrousta, M., L. Mainville, and B.E. Jones, *Gabaergic neurons with alpha2-adrenergic receptors in basal forebrain and preoptic area express c-Fos during sleep.* Neuroscience, 2004. **129**(3): p. 803–810.

93. Manns, I.D., A. Alonso, and B.E. Jones, *Discharge profiles of juxtacellularly labeled and immunohistochemically identified GABAergic basal forebrain neurons recorded in association with the electroencephalogram in anesthetized rats.* J Neurosci, 2000. **20**(24): p. 9252–9263.

94. Fort, P., et al., *Pharmacological characterization and differentiation of non-cholinergic nucleus basalis neurons in vitro.* Neuroreport, 1998. **9**(1): p. 61–65.

95. Gallopin, T., et al., *Identification of sleep-promoting neurons in vitro.* Nature, 2000. **404** (6781): p. 992–995.

96. Manns, I.D., et al., *Alpha 2 adrenergic receptors on GABAergic, putative sleep-promoting basal forebrain neurons.* Eur J Neurosci, 2003. **18**(3): p. 723–727.

97. Jones, B.E., *From waking to sleeping: neuronal and chemical substrates.* Trends Pharmacol Sci, 2005. **26**(11): p. 578–586.

98. Steininger, T.L., et al., *Subregional organization of preoptic area/anterior hypothalamic projections to arousal-related monoaminergic cell groups.* J Comp Neurol, 2001. **429**(4): p. 638–653.

99. Henny, P. and B.E. Jones, *Projections from basal forebrain to prefrontal cortex comprise cholinergic, GABAergic and glutamatergic inputs to pyramidal cells or interneurons.* Eur J Neurosci, 2008. **27**(3): p. 654–670.

100. Williams, R.H., et al., *Optogenetic-mediated release of histamine reveals distal and autoregulatory mechanisms for controlling arousal.* J Neurosci, 2014. **34**(17): p. 6023–6029.

101. Chamberlin, N.L., et al., *Effects of adenosine on gabaergic synaptic inputs to identified ventrolateral preoptic neurons.* Neuroscience, 2003. **119** (4): p. 913–918.

102. Gallopin, T., et al., *The endogenous somnogen adenosine excites a subset of sleep-promoting neurons via A2A receptors in the ventrolateral preoptic nucleus.* Neuroscience, 2005. **134**(4): p. 1377–1390.

103. Batini, C., et al., *Persistent patterns of wakefulness in the pretrigeminal midpontine preparation.* Science, 1958. **128**(3314): p. 30–32.

104. Scammell, T.E., E. Arrigoni, and J.O. Lipton, *Neural Circuitry of Wakefulness and Sleep.* Neuron, 2017. **93**(4): p. 747–765.

105. Anaclet, C., et al., *The GABAergic parafacial zone is a medullary slow wave sleep-promoting center.* Nat Neurosci, 2014. **17**(9): p. 1217–1224.

106. Gerashchenko, D., et al., *Identification of a population of sleep-active cerebral cortex neurons.* Proc Natl Acad Sci U S A, 2008. **105**(29): p. 10227–10232.

107. Morairty, S.R., et al., *A role for cortical nNOS/NK1 neurons in coupling homeostatic sleep drive to EEG slow wave activity.* Proc Natl Acad Sci U S A, 2013. **110**(50): p. 20272–20277.

108. Jouvet, M., *[Research on the neural structures and responsible mechanisms in different phases of physiological sleep].* Arch Ital Biol, 1962. **100**: p. 125–206.

109. Siegel, J.M., R. Nienhuis, and K.S. Tomaszewski, *REM sleep signs rostral to chronic transections at the pontomedullary junction.* Neurosci Lett, 1984. **45**(3): p. 241–246.

110. Hobson, J.A., R.W. McCarley, and P.W. Wyzinski, *Sleep cycle oscillation: reciprocal discharge by two brainstem neuronal groups.* Science, 1975. **189**(4196): p. 55–58.

111. Kubin, L., *Carbachol models of REM sleep: recent developments and new directions.* Arch Ital Biol, 2001. **139**(1-2): p. 147–168.

112. Van Dort, C.J., et al., *Optogenetic activation of cholinergic neurons in the PPT or LDT induces REM sleep.* Proc Natl Acad Sci U S A, 2015. **112**(2): p. 584–589.

113. Boucetta, S., et al., *Discharge profiles across the sleep-waking cycle of identified cholinergic, GABAergic, and glutamatergic neurons in the pontomesencephalic tegmentum of the rat.* J Neurosci, 2014. **34**(13): p. 4708–4727.

114. Cox, J., L. Pinto, and Y. Dan, *Calcium imaging of sleep-wake related neuronal activity in the dorsal pons.* Nat Commun, 2016. **7**: p. 10763.

115. Lu, J., et al., *A putative flip-flop switch for control of REM sleep.* Nature, 2006. **441**(7093): p. 589–594.

116. Sakai, K., S. Crochet, and H. Onoe, *Pontine structures and mechanisms involved in the generation of paradoxical (REM) sleep.* Arch Ital Biol, 2001. **139**(1-2): p. 93–107.

117. Boissard, R., et al., *The rat ponto-medullary network responsible for paradoxical sleep onset and maintenance: a combined microinjection and functional neuroanatomical study.* Eur J Neurosci, 2002. **16**(10): p. 1959–1973.

118. Krenzer, M., et al., *Brainstem and spinal cord circuitry regulating REM sleep and muscle atonia.* PLoS One, 2011. **6**(10): p. e24998.

119. Crochet, S. and K. Sakai, *Effects of microdialysis application of monoamines on the EEG and behavioural states in the cat mesopontine tegmentum.* Eur J Neurosci, 1999. **11**(10): p. 3738–3752.

120. Luebke, J.I., et al., *Serotonin hyperpolarizes cholinergic low-threshold burst neurons in the rat laterodorsal tegmental nucleus in vitro.* Proc Natl Acad Sci U S A, 1992. **89**(2): p. 743–747.

121. Williams, J.A. and P.B. Reiner, *Noradrenaline hyperpolarizes identified rat mesopontine cholinergic neurons in vitro.* J Neurosci, 1993. **13**(9): p. 3878–3883.

122. Sapin, E., et al., *Localization of the brainstem GABAergic neurons controlling paradoxical (REM) sleep.* PLoS One, 2009. **4**(1): p. e4272.

123. Hayashi, Y., et al., *Cells of a common developmental origin regulate REM/non-REM sleep and wakefulness in mice.* Science, 2015. **350**(6263): p. 957–961.

124. Maloney, K.J., L. Mainville, and B.E. Jones, *c-Fos expression in GABAergic, serotonergic, and other neurons of the pontomedullary reticular formation and raphe after paradoxical sleep deprivation and recovery.* J Neurosci, 2000. **20**(12): p. 4669–4679.

125. Chase, M.H., et al., *Role of medullary reticular neurons in the inhibition of trigeminal motoneurons during active sleep.* Exp Neurol, 1984. **84**(2): p. 364–373.

126. Lai, Y.Y. and J.M. Siegel, *Medullary regions mediating atonia.* J Neurosci, 1988. **8**(12): p. 4790–4796.

127. Holmes, C.J. and B.E. Jones, *Importance of cholinergic, GABAergic, serotonergic and other neurons in the medial medullary reticular formation for sleep-wake states studied by cytotoxic lesions in the cat.* Neuroscience, 1994. **62**(4): p. 1179–1200.

128. Schenkel, E. and J.M. Siegel, *REM sleep without atonia after lesions of the medial medulla.* Neurosci Lett, 1989. **98**(2): p. 159–165.

129. Weber, F., et al., *Control of REM sleep by ventral medulla GABAergic neurons.* Nature, 2015. **526**(7573): p. 435–438.

130. Lu, J., et al., *Selective activation of the extended ventrolateral preoptic nucleus during rapid eye movement sleep.* J Neurosci, 2002. **22**(11): p. 4568–4576.

131. Hassani, O.K., M.G. Lee, and B.E. Jones, *Melanin-concentrating hormone neurons discharge in a reciprocal manner to orexin neurons across the sleep-wake cycle.* Proc Natl Acad Sci U S A, 2009. **106**(7): p. 2418–2422.

132. Jego, S., et al., *Optogenetic identification of a rapid eye movement sleep modulatory circuit in*

the hypothalamus. Nat Neurosci, 2013. **16**(11): p. 1637–1643.

133. Vetrivelan, R., et al., *Melanin-concentrating hormone neurons specifically promote rapid eye movement sleep in mice.* Neuroscience, 2016. **336**: p. 102–113.

134. Tsunematsu, T., et al., *Optogenetic manipulation of activity and temporally controlled cell-specific ablation reveal a role for MCH neurons in sleep/wake regulation.* J Neurosci, 2014. 34(20): p. 6896–6909.

135. Mieda, M., et al., *Differential roles of orexin receptor-1 and -2 in the regulation of non-REM and REM sleep.* J Neurosci, 2011. **31**(17): p. 6518–6526.

136. Adamantidis, A.R., et al., *Neural substrates of awakening probed with optogenetic control of hypocretin neurons.* Nature, 2007. **450**(7168): p. 420–424.

137. Sasaki, K., et al., *Pharmacogenetic modulation of orexin neurons alters sleep/wakefulness states in mice.* PLoS One, 2011. **6**(5): p. e20360.

138. Hasegawa, E., et al., *Orexin neurons suppress narcolepsy via 2 distinct efferent pathways.* J Clin Invest, 2014. **124**(2): p. 604–616.

139. Hobson, J.A., *REM sleep and dreaming: towards a theory of protoconsciousness.* Nat Rev Neurosci, 2009. **10**(11): p. 803–813.

140. Hobson, J.A. and R.W. McCarley, *The brain as a dream state generator: an activation-synthesis hypothesis of the dream process.* Am J Psychiatry, 1977. **134**(12): p. 1335–1348.

141. McCarley, R.W., *Dreams: disguise of forbidden wishes or transparent reflections of a distinct brain state?* Ann N Y Acad Sci, 1998. **843**: p. 116–133.

142. McCarley, R.W. and J.A. Hobson, *The neurobiological origins of psychoanalytic dream theory.* Am J Psychiatry, 1977. **134**(11): p. 1211–1221.

143. Ji, D. and M.A. Wilson, *Coordinated memory replay in the visual cortex and hippocampus during sleep.* Nat Neurosci, 2007. **10**(1): p. 100–107.

144. Walker, M.P. and R. Stickgold, *Sleep, memory, and plasticity.* Annu Rev Psychol, 2006. **57**: p. 139–166.

145. Hobson, J.A. and E.F. Pace-Schott, *The cognitive neuroscience of sleep: neuronal systems, consciousness and learning.* Nat Rev Neurosci, 2002. **3**(9): p. 679–693.

146. Lovblad, K.O., et al., *Silent functional magnetic resonance imaging demonstrates focal activation in rapid eye movement sleep.* Neurology, 1999. **53**(9): p. 2193–2195.

147. Maquet, P., et al., *Functional neuroanatomy of human rapid-eye-movement sleep and dreaming.* Nature, 1996. **383**(6596): p. 163–166.

148. Schwartz, S. and P. Maquet, *Sleep imaging and the neuro-psychological assessment of dreams.* Trends Cogn Sci, 2002. **6**(1): p. 23–30.

149. Borbely, A.A., *A two process model of sleep regulation.* Hum Neurobiol, 1982. **1**(3): p. 195–204.

150. Kong, J., et al., *Brain glycogen decreases with increased periods of wakefulness: implications for homeostatic drive to sleep.* J Neurosci, 2002. **22**(13): p. 5581–5587.

151. Shepel, P.N., et al., *Purine level regulation during energy depletion associated with graded excitatory stimulation in brain.* Neurol Res, 2005. **27**(2): p. 139–148.

152. Porkka-Heiskanen, T., R.E. Strecker, and R.W. McCarley, *Brain site-specificity of extracellular adenosine concentration changes during sleep deprivation and spontaneous sleep: an in vivo microdialysis study.* Neuroscience, 2000. **99**(3): p. 507–517.

153. Halassa, M.M., et al., *Astrocytic modulation of sleep homeostasis and cognitive consequences of sleep loss.* Neuron, 2009. **61**(2): p. 213–219.

154. Radulovacki, M., et al., *Adenosine analogs and sleep in rats.* J Pharmacol Exp Ther, 1984. **228**(2): p. 268–274.

155. Benington, J.H. and H.C. Heller, *Restoration of brain energy metabolism as the function of sleep.* Prog Neurobiol, 1995. **45**(4): p. 347–360.

156. Urry, E. and H.P. Landolt, *Adenosine, caffeine, and performance: from cognitive neuroscience of sleep to sleep pharmacogenetics.* Curr Top Behav Neurosci, 2015. **25**: p. 331–366.

157. Huang, Z.L., et al., *Adenosine A2A, but not A1, receptors mediate the arousal effect of caffeine.* Nat Neurosci, 2005. **8**(7): p. 858–859.

158. Scammell, T.E., et al., *An adenosine A2a agonist increases sleep and induces Fos in ventrolateral preoptic neurons.* Neuroscience, 2001. **107**(4): p. 653–663.

159. Marcheva, B., et al., *Circadian clocks and metabolism.* Handb Exp Pharmacol, 2013(217): p. 127–155.

160. Welsh, D.K., J.S. Takahashi, and S.A. Kay, *Suprachiasmatic nucleus: cell autonomy and network properties.* Annu Rev Physiol, 2010. **72**: p. 551–577.

161. Morin, L.P., *Neuroanatomy of the extended circadian rhythm system.* Exp Neurol, 2013. **243**: p. 4–20.

162. Lu, J., et al., *Contrasting effects of ibotenate lesions of the paraventricular nucleus and subparaventricular zone on sleep-wake cycle and temperature regulation.* J Neurosci, 2001. **21**(13): p. 4864–4874.

163. Chou, T.C., et al., *Critical role of dorsomedial hypothalamic nucleus in a wide range of behavioral circadian rhythms.* J Neurosci, 2003. **23**(33): p. 10691–10702.

164. Vujovic, N., et al., *Projections from the subparaventricular zone define four channels of output from the circadian timing system.* J Comp Neurol, 2015. **523**(18): p. 2714–2737.

165. McEwen, B.S., *Allostasis and allostatic load: implications for neuropsychopharmacology.* Neuropsychopharmacology, 2000. **22**(2): p. 108–124.

166. Palchykova, S., T. Deboer, and I. Tobler, *Seasonal aspects of sleep in the Djungarian hamster.* BMC Neurosci, 2003. **4**: p. 9.

167. Rattenborg, N.C., et al., *Migratory sleeplessness in the white-crowned sparrow (Zonotrichia leucophrys gambelii).* PLoS Biol, 2004. **2**(7): p. E212.

168. Yamanaka, A., et al., *Hypothalamic orexin neurons regulate arousal according to energy balance in mice.* Neuron, 2003. **38**(5): p. 701–713.

169. Willie, J.T., et al., *Abnormal response of melanin-concentrating hormone deficient mice to fasting: hyperactivity and rapid eye movement sleep suppression.* Neuroscience, 2008. **156**(4): p. 819–829.

170. Winsky-Sommerer, R., B. Boutrel, and L. de Lecea, *Stress and arousal: the corticotrophin-releasing factor/hypocretin circuitry.* Mol Neurobiol, 2005. **32**(3): p. 285–294.

171. Cano, G., T. Mochizuki, and C.B. Saper, *Neural circuitry of stress-induced insomnia in rats.* J Neurosci, 2008. **28**(40): p. 10167–10184.

172. Dong, H.W., et al., *Basic organization of projections from the oval and fusiform nuclei of the bed nuclei of the stria terminalis in adult rat brain.* J Comp Neurol, 2001. **436**(4): p. 430–455.

173. Hurley, K.M., et al., *Efferent projections of the infralimbic cortex of the rat.* J Comp Neurol, 1991. **308**(2): p. 249–276.

174. Van Bockstaele, E.J., J. Peoples, and R.J. Valentino, *A.E. Bennett Research Award. Anatomic basis for differential regulation of the rostrolateral peri-locus coeruleus region by limbic afferents.* Biol Psychiatry, 1999. **46**(10): p. 1352–1363.

175. Nofzinger, E.A., et al., *Functional neuroimaging evidence for hyperarousal in insomnia.* Am J Psychiatry, 2004. **161**(11): p. 2126–2128.

176. Ehlers, C.L., T.K. Reed, and S.J. Henriksen, *Effects of corticotropin-releasing factor and growth hormone-releasing factor on sleep and activity in rats.* Neuroendocrinology, 1986. **42**(6): p. 467–474.

177. Opp, M., F. Obal, Jr., and J.M. Krueger, *Corticotropin-releasing factor attenuates interleukin 1-induced sleep and fever in rabbits.* Am J Physiol, 1989. **257**(3 Pt 2): p. R528–R535.

178. Chastrette, N., R. Cespuglio, and M. Jouvet, *Proopiomelanocortin (POMC)-derived peptides and sleep in the rat. Part 1--Hypnogenic properties of ACTH derivatives.* Neuropeptides, 1990. **15**(2): p. 61–74.

179. Winsky-Sommerer, R., et al., *Interaction between the corticotropin-releasing factor system and hypocretins (orexins): a novel circuit mediating stress response.* J Neurosci, 2004. **24**(50): p. 11439–11448.

180. Nishino, S., et al., *Effects of thyrotropin-releasing hormone and its analogs on daytime sleepiness and cataplexy in canine narcolepsy.* J Neurosci, 1997. **17**(16): p. 6401–6408.

181. Riehl, J., et al., *Chronic Oral Administration of CG-3703, a Thyrotropin Releasing Hormone Analog, Increases Wake and Decreases Cataplexy in Canine Narcolepsy.* Neuropsychopharmacology, 2000. **23**(1): p. 34–45.

182. Hemmeter, U., et al., *Effects of thyrotropin-releasing hormone on the sleep EEG and nocturnal hormone secretion in male volunteers.* Neuropsychobiology, 1998. **38**(1): p. 25–31.

183. Zini, I., et al., *Actions of centrally administered neuropeptide Y on EEG activity in different rat strains and in different phases of their circadian cycle.* Acta Physiol Scand, 1984. **122**(1): p. 71–77.

184. Szentirmai, E. and J.M. Krueger, *Central administration of neuropeptide Y induces wakefulness in rats.* Am J Physiol Regul Integr Comp Physiol, 2006. **291**(2): p. R473–R480.

185. Antonijevic, I.A., et al., *Neuropeptide Y promotes sleep and inhibits ACTH and cortisol release in young men.* Neuropharmacology, 2000. **39**(8): p. 1474–1481.

186. Held, K., et al., *Neuropeptide Y (NPY) shortens sleep latency but does not suppress ACTH and cortisol in depressed patients and normal controls.* Psychoneuroendocrinology, 2006. **31**(1): p. 100–107.

187. Obal, F., Jr., et al., *Growth hormone-releasing factor enhances sleep in rats and rabbits.* Am J Physiol, 1988. **255**(2 Pt 2): p. R310–R316.

188. Steiger, A., *Neurochemical regulation of sleep.* J Psychiatr Res, 2007. **41**(7): p. 537–552.

189. Van Cauter, E., et al., *Simultaneous stimulation of slow-wave sleep and growth hormone secretion by gamma-hydroxybutyrate in normal young Men.* J Clin Invest, 1997. **100**(3): p. 745–753.

190. Havlicek, V., M. Rezek, and H. Friesen, *Somatostatin and thyrotropin releasing hormone: central effect on sleep and motor system.* Pharmacol Biochem Behav, 1976. **4**(4): p. 455–459.

191. Rezek, M., et al., *Cortical administration of somatostatin (SRIF): effect on sleep and motor behavior.* Pharmacol Biochem Behav, 1976. **5**(1): p. 73–77.

192. Schwartz, M.D. and T.S. Kilduff, *The Neurobiology of Sleep and Wakefulness.* Psychiatric Clinics of North America, 2015. **38**(4): p. 615–644.

193. Konadhode, R.R., et al., *Optogenetic stimulation of MCH neurons increases sleep.* J Neurosci, 2013. **33**(25): p. 10257–10263.

194. Roky, R., J.L. Valatx, and M. Jouvet, *Effect of prolactin on the sleep-wake cycle in the rat.* Neurosci Lett, 1993. **156**(1-2): p. 117–120.

195. Obal, F., Jr., et al., *Prolactin, vasoactive intestinal peptide, and peptide histidine methionine elicit selective increases in REM sleep in rabbits.* Brain Res, 1989. **490**(2): p. 292–300.

196. Fang, J., L. Payne, and J.M. Krueger, *Pituitary adenylate cyclase activating polypeptide enhances*

rapid eye movement sleep in rats. Brain Res, 1995. **686**(1): p. 23–28.

197. Krueger, J.M., et al., *The role of cytokines in physiological sleep regulation.* Ann N Y Acad Sci, 2001. **933**: p. 211–221.

198. Pandey, H.P., et al., *Concentration of prostaglandin D2 in cerebrospinal fluid exhibits a circadian alteration in conscious rats.* Biochem Mol Biol Int, 1995. **37**(3): p. 431–437.

199. Ram, A., et al., *CSF levels of prostaglandins, especially the level of prostaglandin D2, are correlated with increasing propensity towards sleep in rats.* Brain Res, 1997. **751**(1): p. 81–89.

200. Matsumura, H., R. Takahata, and O. Hayaishi, *Inhibition of sleep in rats by inorganic selenium compounds, inhibitors of prostaglandin D synthase.* Proc Natl Acad Sci U S A, 1991. **88**(20): p. 9046–9050.

201. Takahata, R., et al., *Intravenous administration of inorganic selenium compounds, inhibitors of prostaglandin D synthase, inhibits sleep in freely moving rats.* Brain Res, 1993. **623**(1): p. 65–71.

202. Qu, W.M., et al., *Lipocalin-type prostaglandin D synthase produces prostaglandin D2 involved in regulation of physiological sleep.* Proc Natl Acad Sci U S A, 2006. **103**(47): p. 17949–17954.

203. Matsumura, H., et al., *Prostaglandin D2-sensitive, sleep-promoting zone defined in the ventral surface of the rostral basal forebrain.* Proc Natl Acad Sci U S A, 1994. **91**(25): p. 11998–12002.

204. Satoh, S., et al., *Promotion of sleep mediated by the A2a-adenosine receptor and possible involvement of this receptor in the sleep induced by prostaglandin D2 in rats.* Proc Natl Acad Sci U S A, 1996. **93**(12): p. 5980–5984.

205. Urade, Y., et al., *Sleep regulation in adenosine A2A receptor-deficient mice.* Neurology, 2003. **61**(11 Suppl 6): p. S94–S96.

206. Zhang, B. and Y.K. Wing, *Sex differences in insomnia: a meta-analysis.* Sleep, 2006. **29**(1): p. 85–93.

207. Armitage, R., et al., *Slow-wave activity in NREM sleep: sex and age effects in depressed outpatients and healthy controls.* Psychiatry Res, 2000. **95**(3): p. 201–213.

208. Manber, R. and R. Armitage, *Sex, steroids, and sleep: a review.* Sleep, 1999. **22**(5): p. 540–555.

209. Mourtazaev, M.S., et al., *Age and gender affect different characteristics of slow waves in the sleep EEG.* Sleep, 1995. **18**(7): p. 557–564.

210. Armitage, R. and R.F. Hoffmann, *Sleep EEG, depression and gender.* Sleep Med Rev, 2001. **5**(3): p. 237–246.

211. Driver, H.S., et al., *Sleep and the sleep electroencephalogram across the menstrual cycle in young healthy women.* J Clin Endocrinol Metab, 1996. **81**(2): p. 728–735.

212. Shechter, A., F. Varin, and D.B. Boivin, *Circadian variation of sleep during the follicular and luteal phases of the menstrual cycle.* Sleep, 2010. **33**(5): p. 647–656.

213. Paul, K.N., A.D. Laposky, and F.W. Turek, *Reproductive hormone replacement alters sleep in mice.* Neurosci Lett, 2009. **463**(3): p. 239–243.

214. Colvin, G.B., D.I. Whitmoyer, and C.H. Sawyer, *Circadian sleep-wakefulness patterns in rats after ovariectomy and treatment with estrogen.* Exp Neurol, 1969. **25**(4): p. 616–625.

215. Deurveilher, S., B. Rusak, and K. Semba, *Estradiol and progesterone modulate spontaneous sleep patterns and recovery from sleep deprivation in ovariectomized rats.* Sleep, 2009. **32**(7): p. 865–877.

216. Cusmano, D.M., M.M. Hadjimarkou, and J.A. Mong, *Gonadal steroid modulation of sleep and wakefulness in male and female rats is sexually differentiated and neonatally organized by steroid exposure.* Endocrinology, 2014. **155**(1): p. 204–214.

217. Mong, J.A., et al., *Estradiol differentially regulates lipocalin-type prostaglandin D synthase transcript levels in the rodent brain: Evidence from high-density oligonucleotide arrays and in situ hybridization.* Proc Natl Acad Sci U S A, 2003. **100**(1): p. 318–323.

218. Silveyra, P., et al., *Gonadal steroids modulated hypocretin/orexin type-1 receptor expression in a brain region, sex and daytime specific manner.* Regul Pept, 2009. **158**(1-3): p. 121–126.

219. Hadjimarkou, M.M., et al., *Estradiol suppresses rapid eye movement sleep and activation of sleep-active neurons in the ventrolateral preoptic area.* Eur J Neurosci, 2008. **27**(7): p. 1780–1792.

220. Hamel, E.J., et al., *Cellular level brain imaging in behaving mammals: an engineering approach.* Neuron, 2015. **86**(1): p. 140–159.

221. Gobel, W. and F. Helmchen, *In vivo calcium imaging of neural network function.* Physiology (Bethesda), 2007. **22**: p. 358–365.

222. Hsu, P.D., E.S. Lander, and F. Zhang, *Development and applications of CRISPR-Cas9 for genome engineering.* Cell, 2014. **157**(6): p. 1262–1278.

223. Ran, F.A., et al., *Double nicking by RNA-guided CRISPR Cas9 for enhanced genome editing specificity.* Cell, 2013. **154**(6): p. 1380–1389.

224. Sunagawa, G.A., et al., *Mammalian Reverse Genetics without Crossing Reveals Nr3a as a Short-Sleeper Gene.* Cell Rep, 2016. **14**(3): p. 662–677.

225. Hama, H., et al., *Scale: a chemical approach for fluorescence imaging and reconstruction of transparent mouse brain.* Nat Neurosci, 2011. **14**(11): p. 1481–1488.

226. Erturk, A., et al., *Three-dimensional imaging of solvent-cleared organs using 3DISCO.* Nat Protoc, 2012. **7**(11): p. 1983–1995.

227. Tomer, R., et al., *Advanced CLARITY for rapid and high-resolution imaging of intact tissues.* Nat Protoc, 2014. **9**(7): p. 1682–1697.

4

Circadian Rhythms

DANIEL S. JOYCE AND JAMIE M. ZEITZER

INTRODUCTION

Life on Earth has been evolving under a regular solar cycle for the last ~3.7 billion years. All organisms, including humans, are sensitive to this 24-hour light/dark cycle caused by the Earth's rotation about its axis. Our **circadian rhythm** is the repeated cycling of physiological processes that occurs in all bodily tissues with a cycle length of about 24-hours and is controlled by our **central circadian pacemaker** (also known as the body clock or master circadian pacemaker) located in the suprachiasmatic nucleus in the hypothalamic region of the brain. In combination with the **sleep homeostat** (a mechanism tracking time awake in relation to time asleep), circadian rhythms dictate our **sleep/wake cycles**. Under normal circumstances, our circadian rhythm remains **entrained** or synchronized to environmental and behavioral cues, while **circadian desynchrony** is a phenomenon in which one's central circadian pacemaker is misaligned with these cues. You have probably experienced this in the form of **jetlag** when crossing time zones. You may have had some combination of difficulty sleeping at night, excessive daytime sleepiness, fatigue, reduced cognitive performance, suppressed appetite, and mood lability. Thankfully, most jetlag is relatively short-lived, and your pacemaker will re-entrain itself to this shifted light cycle in a matter of days. For individuals who have circadian-based sleep disorders, such as irregular or non-24 sleep–wake disorder, these symptoms can be chronic, even lifelong. Clearly, a well-entrained circadian rhythm is crucial for healthy functioning in day-to-day life. This chapter will provide an overview to circadian clocks within the body, their normal functioning and relationship to sleep, how we quantify circadian rhythmicity and dysfunction, and the effects of circadian dysfunction with respect to human health.

WHY CIRCADIAN RHYTHMS?

From an evolutionary standpoint, it is useful to understand why we have circadian rhythms that have given rise to the complex behaviors that dictate our daily lives. Every organism that has ever been studied, be it single-celled or multicellular, possesses circadian rhythms. This includes those that live in seemingly constant environments, such as extremophiles that live in volcanic vents deep in the ocean,[1] and even bacteria that do not live for a full 24 hours.[2–4] Thus, it seems likely that circadian rhythms are the optimal adaptation to the periodic cycling of environmental variables and confer a selective advantage upon organisms that have a synchronous and robust temporal organization. The selective advantage of circadian rhythms may be related to the anticipatory, rather than reactive, form of homeostasis that knowing the geophysical time of day confers. Because the majority of life evolved under adverse and temporally cyclical environmental conditions,[5] a mechanism that can anticipate environmental changes, and take advantage of temporal resource niches, can be primed by upregulating and downregulating genes and processes in advance, rather than responding to changing environmental events as they occur. In conjunction with this, circadian rhythms may also be advantageous because they lead to the temporal organization of biochemical processes. For example, as upregulation and downregulation of genes and their resulting protein synthesis are tuned temporally to the anticipated environment, energy is conserved as not all proteins are required to be produced all of the time.

WHAT ARE CIRCADIAN RHYTHMS?

Chronobiology is the study of biological temporal patterns, including daily, tidal, seasonal and annual rhythms. From the Latin *circa dies*, "about one day," circadian rhythms are an organism's endogenous rhythmicity in physiological processes that follow an approximately 24-hour cycle. It is important to note that many oscillations can be diurnal (i.e., they demonstrate 24-hour rhythms), but that these rhythms are not necessarily *circadian* rhythms as they are not endogenously generated. As an example, a plank of wood may expand and contract in response to changes in temperature that appear to be circadian in nature, but the changes are caused by an external source and are not endogenously maintained in its absence. A rhythm must therefore persist in an organism even without any external cues for it to be considered circadian.

Circadian rhythms are difficult to measure in humans. While useful as a marker of the circadian rhythms of many rodents, rest/activity cycles in humans are inadequate markers of circadian rhythms as our activity patterns may be greatly influenced by social (e.g., deciding to stay awake late) or external (e.g., taking sleep medication, drinking coffee in the evening) factors that will mask the underlying circadian drive on sleep/wake patterns.[6] To examine human circadian rhythms, paradigms such as "constant routine" and "forced desynchrony" have been developed that can hold constant or even mathematically decouple environmental influences and physiologic processes (e.g., sleep) for endogenous rhythmicity to be measured or inferred.[7,8] In general, there are three mathematical components of a circadian rhythm that are computed: cycle length (period or tau, τ), timing (phase or phi, ϕ), and amplitude.

In humans, the average period length of the nonentrained ("free running," possible only in rare disorders or under tightly controlled laboratory conditions) circadian rhythm is 24.2 hours in adults[9] and about 6 minutes longer in men than women.[10] It has been hypothesized that the length of the period may be longer in individuals with delayed sleep phase disorder[11] and in totally blind individuals.[12] We are, however, typically entrained to external signals that synchronizes our internal clock with the external world. These external signals are collectively known as *zeitgebers* (from the German "time giver").[13,14] Zeitgebers include both natural and artificial light, feeding, activity, and temperature. In humans, light is the strongest zeitgeber.[15]

CIRCADIAN CLOCKS WITHIN THE BODY

Circadian clocks are self-sustained **oscillators**; that is, a cell that rhythmically generates an autonomous, repeated signal—in this case, one with a near 24-hour rhythm. In humans, the central circadian clock is the suprachiasmatic nuclei (SCN), part of the basal hypothalamus in the brain. The ~20,000 cells of the SCN are arranged into two nuclei located at the base of the third ventricle above the optic chiasm, and express GABA

(γ-aminobutyric acid) as a primary neurotransmitter.[16] The SCN can act as a circadian clock when isolated from the rest of the brain[17] or even if its cells are isolated ex vivo in culture, independent of physical or chemical contact from other cells.[18]

Individual SCN neurons produce a 24-hour rhythm through a molecular clock that is comprised of a transcriptional-translational feedback loop (TTFL).[19,20] In the canonical circadian clock mechanism, CLOCK and BMAL1 are transcriptional regulators in humans that dimerize to initiate transcription of the *Period 1-2* (*Per1-2*) and *Cryptochrome 1-2* (*Cry1-2*) genes via an E-box enhancer. PER and CRY proteins then dimerize in the cytoplasm and translocate to the nucleus where their presence inhibits the transcriptional drive of CLOCK and BMAL1. Reduction of CLOCK/BMAL1 activity in turn inhibits the transcription of *Per* and *Cry* genes, leading to a decrease in PER and CRY protein expression that then disinhibits CLOCK and BMAL1. Many additional clock genes are involved in this process, as well as posttranslational modifications. This general TTFL mechanism is conserved across eukaryotes (organisms that contain a nucleus in their cells), although the precise genes involved differ considerably, suggesting that circadian rhythms may have evolved differently within the phylogenetic tree.[5]

Our body also contains peripheral oscillators. Unlike the central clock, the oscillators within peripheral cells are only self-sustaining under ideal ex vivo laboratory conditions and will drift out of alignment with one another in the absence of a central clock signal.[21] Peripheral oscillators are thus under the control of the central circadian clock, which in turn synchronizes us with the external world. The precise nature of the relationship between central and peripheral oscillators has not been confirmed. The classical model posits that output from the SCN is able to reset peripheral oscillators through a "Master-Slave" model.[22] In this model, the central clock is the master pacemaker to which peripheral oscillators are attuned, and they in turn provide a local rhythmic coordinating signal for peripheral tissues. This model is highly hierarchical as zeitgebers are unable to act directly on peripheral oscillators. A newer alternative model is that of the "Orchestra," whereby the primary circadian pacemaker provides a master signal (the "conductor"), while peripheral oscillators are the "musicians" with varying levels of independence that may themselves be influenced by local or external stimuli.[23] The precise mechanism(s) linking peripheral oscillators to the central clock is unknown but is thought to include neural, humoral, and temperature cues.[23,24]

RELATIONSHIP BETWEEN CIRCADIAN RHYTHMS AND SLEEP

The impact of circadian rhythms (in combination with an appetitive sleep process) is apparent in the cycling of alertness across the day. As seen in Figure 4.1, a two-process model[25–27] describes the interplay between circadian rhythms (Process C) and the sleep homeostat (Process S). In healthy individuals entrained to the solar day, the circadian drive for wake increases throughout the day and peaks in the hours just before normal bedtime and does so independently of sleep behavior. The sleep drive of Process S, however, builds monotonically throughout the waking day until it is dissipated by the act of sleeping. A behavioral consequence of this interplay is the familiar "postlunch dip" in the early afternoon, in which sleep may occur due to the relatively low circadian drive for wake in conjunction with a relatively moderate sleep drive. This afternoon siesta, common in some cultures, is likely an adaptation to take advantage of this interplay between Processes C and S, as well as concurrent environmental factors.[28,29] While the homeostatic need for sleep is dissipated during sleep, the circadian drive to sleep is highest at the end of the normal sleep period. The impact of the paradoxical timing of the circadian drive for sleep may be experienced most acutely as a "second wind," the increased alertness you feel during sleep deprivation once you have passed the peak circadian drive for sleep. Thus, people are less

tired after 36 hours of sleep deprivation (the time of peak circadian wake drive) than they are after 22 hours of sleep deprivation (the time of peak circadian sleep drive). This interplay between circadian drive for sleep and wake and the sleep homeostat enables the consolidation of sleep and wake into a single daily episode, a feature present in humans, but in few other mammals.[30]

Circadian rhythms also manifest in the quality and staging of sleep itself. The amount of wake during sleep, rapid eye movement (REM) sleep, non-REM sleep (stage N1 and N2) and sleep spindles all show substantial circadian variation.[7] In contrast, slow wave non-REM sleep remains relatively unimpacted by circadian time and is mostly driven by time awake.[7] While we do not understand the exact functional roles of the different stages of sleep, the circadian variation in these stages could lead to less restorative sleep if sleep occurs at a nonoptimal circadian phase (i.e., during the day).

MEASURING CIRCADIAN RHYTHMS

Given that the SCN is a very small (1 mm³) structure deep inside the brain, in humans it is not possible to examine its molecular or cellular rhythms in vivo using current technology. In many nonhuman mammals, the timing of the daily onset of wake-related locomotion under controlled conditions acts as a sensitive marker of the timing of the circadian clock.[31] In humans, however, sleep and wake activity are not valid markers of this timing as they can be altered through external and internal factors that will mask the underlying rhythm. As demonstrated

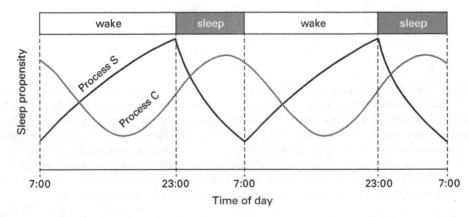

FIGURE 4.1. The two-process model of sleep/wake regulation. Consolidated sleep/wake behavior is facilitated by the interplay of the circadian Process C and homeostatic sleep drive Process S. Process C is cyclical and typically entrained to the solar day, while Process S can only be dissipated by the act of sleeping.

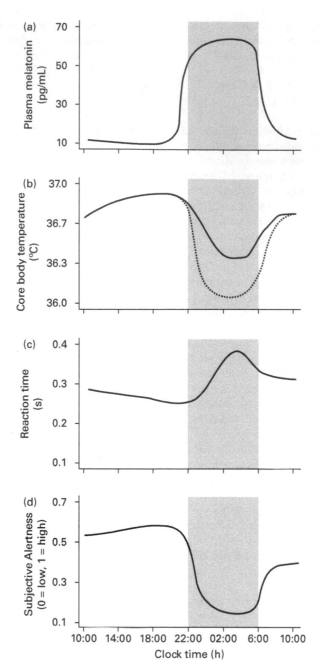

FIGURE 4.2. Circadian rhythms occur in a variety of physiologic measures. When properly unmasked through techniques such as constant routine, endogenous circadian rhythms in a variety of measures can be observed. Melatonin (a) is expressed during typical hours of sleep (darkness is permissive for melatonin expression), with a rapid rise just before normal bed time and fall coinciding with normal wake time. Core body temperature (b) has a pseudosinusoidal waveform with a peak in the afternoon and a nadir late in the sleep period (under constant routine, solid line) or in the middle of the typical sleep time (under entrained conditions, dashed line). Objective (c) and subjective (d) measures of alertness coincide with minimum core body temperature, but are often too noisy to be used as accurate markers of circadian timing. Gray shading indicates normal timing of sleep.

in Figure 4.2a,b, various markers have been validated as being representative of internal circadian timing in humans.

Melatonin

Projections originating in the SCN innervate the pineal gland, which produces the hormone melatonin, under control of the sympathetic nervous system.[32] Darkness is permissive for melatonin production while nocturnal light exposure can acutely inhibit its production. Thus, melatonin plasma levels are low during the biological day and high during the biological night, in a near square-wave form (Figure 4.2a).[33] Light is a strong suppressor of melatonin production with even relatively modest light intensities (180 lux, equivalent to indoor lighting) sufficient to inhibit melatonin production.[34] Some drugs, such as beta-blockers, are also known to reduce melatonin production[35,36] as they interfere with the sympathetic stimulation of pinealocyte adrenergic receptors. As melatonin production is under tight circadian control, if light exposure is managed properly, variation in melatonin concentrations is a robust expression of the timing of the central circadian clock and is considered the gold standard marker of the timing of the central circadian clock.[37] As it is a small, highly lipophilic molecule, melatonin readily passes from blood to saliva and is easily measured in either tissue. Typically, melatonin has a rapid rise in the evening, sustained levels throughout the normal sleep period, and a rapid decline in the morning. As such, melatonin onset (the so-called dim light melatonin onset [DLMO]) or peak are robust markers of circadian timing.[37] There is a significant range of peak melatonin values among individuals,[38,39] but the functional significance of this variance is unknown. The absolute amount of melatonin, however, is not commensurate with the amplitude of the circadian clock.[40]

Core Body Temperature

Core body temperature, as typically monitored through ingestible capsules or rectal thermistors, has a pseudo-sine wave form, with a minimum typically occurring during the latter half of the normal sleep period and a maximum during the afternoon (Figure 4.2b).[41] Under proper conditions,[42] the circadian variation of core body temperature is an accurate reflection of both the timing and amplitude of the central circadian clock.[43] Core body temperature is the only well-validated marker of the amplitude of the central circadian clock of humans (a measure of the robustness of the rhythm). To examine the circadian rhythm of core body temperature, factors such as activity, sleep, diet, ambient temperature, stress, and light must all be tightly controlled as they can mask the underlying circadian component of the daily oscillation of core body temperature. As controlling each of these masking agents is laborious and expensive and requires a specialized in-patient laboratory, the use of core body temperature as a marker of circadian timing is limited in practice.

Cortisol

As with melatonin, cortisol is a robust marker of the timing of the central circadian clock.[37] It can be readily measured in saliva or blood and has a characteristic sinusoidal oscillation over the course of the day, with peak concentrations around normal wake time and its nadir in the evening. The circadian contribution to cortisol is likely mediated through a direct control of corticotropin-releasing hormone, which in turn regulates adrenocorticotrophic hormone, which stimulates cortisol production from the adrenal cortex. To measure cortisol accurately, light and stress must be controlled, as well as large postural shifts. Cortisol, however, is highly pulsatile and statistically noisier than melatonin to assess.[37]

Other Circadian Rhythms

Both objective and subjective measures of neurobehavior can have circadian variation (Figure 4.2c,d). However, unlike physiological measures, these measures are more readily influenced by cognitive factors including arousal/sleepiness and emotional states, thereby making them unreliable markers of circadian timing. There are many different kinds of objective quantitation of neurobehavior. These include measures of changes in waking EEG spectral composition, counting slow eye movements, and performance in sustained attention tasks. Cognitive factors also demonstrate circadian changes,[44,45] wherein inhibitory information processing in particular is impaired while excitatory information processing remains relatively invariant.[46] Aspects of attention, memory, and executive functioning can be evaluated, and, in general, performance is found to be high when core body temperature is high and to degrade at melatonin onset, when core body temperature begins to lower.[47,48] These variations in cognitive performance are most notable when they lead to workplace or motor vehicle accidents, which often occur during the early morning hours when the circadian clock has a strong sleep-promoting signal.[49]

ENTRAINMENT

While the solar day is 24 hours, the average endogenous period of the central circadian clock in humans is 24.2 hours.[9] Thus, without a mechanism to synchronize our internal circadian clock with the outside day, our internal clock would slowly drift out of alignment. In essence, every five days our internal circadian clock would move a time zone (0.2 hours per day × 5 days = 1 hour) while we try to maintain a regular schedule. Light is the main stimulus by which the endogenous body clock remains synchronized with the outside world.[15] Photoentrainment is the term used to describe the synchronization of the internal clock with an external light signal. All photoentrainment in mammals occurs through the eyes; their removal results in a complete loss of photoentrainment.[50] As such, people who have had their eyes removed will be unable to photoentrain and will likely experience non-24 hour sleep–wake disorder.

In the eye, environmental light energy is transduced by rod, cone, and intrinsically photosensitive retinal ganglion cell (ipRGCs) photoreceptors. The classical rod and cone photoreceptors have high temporal resolution and primarily detect light for image-forming vision, while the slower, more sustained signaling of ipRGCs suggests a primary role of integrating long durations of light over many hours such as occurs with the rhythmic light/dark cycle. The ipRGCs are a unique class of retinal ganglion cells that capture light via the intrinsic chromophore melanopsin.

Melanopsin is sensitive to blue wavelength light (predominant in oceans and the atmosphere), but ipRGCs themselves also receive extrinsic rod and cone inputs.[51] The precise manner in which intrinsic (melanopsin) and extrinsic (rods and cones) ipRGC components interact is currently an area of intense research. It is notable that ipRGCs are intimately entwined with healthy brain function: in animal models, they project to over a dozen efferent brain targets for nonimage-forming vision as well as modulating circadian rhythms; they may also be important for diverse functions including regulating pupil size, mood, and alertness.[52–55]

Many different aspects of light moderate its impact on circadian rhythms. Notably, the timing, intensity, history (i.e., previous exposure), color, duration, and pattern of light exposure all can change how light interacts with circadian timing. The relationship between the *timing* of light and its impact on circadian rhythms can be visualized as a phase response curve (PRC).[56] Each PRC is defined for a specific stimulus (zeitgeber) but, in general, can be used to show that, in humans, light in the early part of the biological night delays circadian rhythms (i.e., events will occur later the next day) while light in the late part of the biological night advances circadian rhythms (i.e., events will occur earlier the next day). One can also imagine this as light in the evening as an artificially late sunset while light in the morning acts as an artificially early sunrise. Light during the daytime has relatively little direct impact on circadian phase.[57]

The relationship between the *intensity* of light and its impact on circadian rhythms can be visualized as a dose response curve.[34] The relationship between light intensity and circadian response is sigmoidal, such that very low intensities have relatively little impact, high intensities saturate the system, and intensities in between have logarithmically greater impact on the timing of the human circadian clock. The exact intensities at which these transitions occur is likely moderated by the *history* of light exposure such that greater light exposure during the daytime leads to less sensitivity at night.[58,59] This is a nontrivial point as most of the laboratory studies that examine the impact of light on human circadian function are done on an artificially low background light that is highly sensitizing. From these studies, it has been interpreted that the light emitted from personal electronic devices (e.g., e-readers or mobile phones) can have a significant impact on sleep and circadian function.[60] However, the normal (nonlaboratory) light intensities to which people are exposed to during the day would be more than sufficient to minimize the direct impact of light on circadian rhythms.[58,59] Rather, the indirect impact of light, in providing a permissive environment for cognitively engaging activities, is of significant concern for sleep.[61] The *color* (wavelength) of light can also have an impact on the effectiveness of the light stimulation. While conscious visual perception is maximally sensitive to green light (555 nm), the circadian system is more sensitive to shorter wavelengths (blue).[62–64] The precise nature of this sensitivity, however, is an ongoing topic of research as there is likely an interaction between the *duration* of light and the color of light,[65] such that as light exposure continues for hours or minutes, the sensitivity of the circadian system to different colors will also vary. Likewise, the impact of the temporal *pattern* of light exposure is also an evolving area of research, but also important in considering the effects of light on circadian timing.[66]

Other Phase-Shifting Agents

It is important to note that in contemporary society we are exposed to many agents that exert pressure upon our circadian rhythms. While light is the strongest zeitgeber, other zeitgebers include caffeine[67] and exogenous melatonin.[68] Melatonin is commonly used as a chronobiotic (i.e., a drug impacting the circadian system) in relief of the symptoms of jetlag. The impact of melatonin is dependent upon both the dose and the timing of ingestion. The PRC for melatonin is antiphase to that of light—melatonin taken in the evening causes phase advances and melatonin taken in the morning causes phase delays.[68] Low doses are generally recommended as higher doses (>300 µg) will remain in circulation for many hours,[69] potentially inducing both phase delays and phase advances for a net neutral impact on circadian timing. Exogenous melatonin is also used as a mild hypnotic, especially when ingested during the daytime. These two (chronobiotic, hypnotic) impacts of exogenous melatonin are likely mediated through different mechanisms.[70] While the chronobiotic impact of melatonin is likely mediated by activation of melatonin MT_2 receptors on the SCN, there are several, nonexclusive mechanisms that have been posited to explain the hypnotic properties of melatonin.[70] These include inhibition of SCN firing, modulation of thermoregulation via influence on peripheral vasculature, or potentially through direct activation of melatonin receptors in the hypothalamus.

CHRONOTYPE

Although we share the same physiological pathways for photoentrainment, there are substantial differences in individuals' circadian phase preferences when it comes to sleep and waking activities. Chronotype is an individual's circadian expression as determined by activity preferences and timing of sleep and is readily measured by morningness–eveningness questionnaires.[71,72] The chronotype spectrum runs from extreme larks ("morning people") through intermediate chronotypes to extreme owls ("evening people"). Extreme larks have a strong preference for morning activity: they rise with or before the sun and prefer to get the bulk of their daily activities completed while the day is young, typically going to bed in the early evening. Extreme owls tend to rise in the late morning and prefer to engage in strenuous mental or physical activity later into the day or evening. Intermediate

chronotypes fall in between these two bounds and adhere to more normative sleep/wake timing and behavioral patterns.

Physiologic and performance measures support the existence of chronotypes, with temperature, melatonin expression, and sleepiness aligning with self-reported chronotype preference.[73] Chronotype has a strong genetic component (approximately 54%),[74] although its expression changes with age. Because of this high chronotype preference stability, owls in particular can suffer due to the mismatch between their circadian preference (going to sleep "late") and typical work hours (being forced to wake "early"), resulting in curtailed sleep. Sleep behavior shows differences between work and nonwork days for lark, intermediate, and owl chronotypes; larks tend to maintain their sleep patterns across work and nonwork days while intermediate and especially owl chronotypes demonstrate sleep debt accumulated from the working week being dispelled during free days.[72] This results in substantial sleep rebound of several hours on free days for owl chronotypes. While the acute effects of chronotype-activity misalignment include fatigue, reduced cognitive performance, and mood lability, the chronic effects are not well understood regarding health, longevity, and quality of life. A mismatch between chronotype and sleep timing, however, has been shown to be associated with a more rapid progression of breast cancer.[75]

CIRCADIAN RHYTHMS, AGING, AND SEX

Aging

The timing and amplitude of circadian rhythms change throughout the lifespan and are intimately linked to aging. SCN neurons have been shown in fetuses at weeks 18 to 20 of gestation, and circadian rhythms can be detected at the start of the third trimester, at 30 weeks of gestation.[76] As the prenatal SCN is not innervated by the retina,[77] fetal SCN rhythms are attuned to those of the mother's melatonin and cortisol expression, rest–activity patterns, and body temperature.[78] In newborn infants, the maturation of circadian rhythms and entrainment to zeitgebers is not immediate, but rather can take months to stabilize. During this time, there is a poorly understood transition from responding to maternal signals (e.g., melatonin in breast milk) to responding to light.[79]

There is another age-related shift in circadian rhythms that typically occurs during the transition from childhood to adolescence. Adolescents demonstrate a preference for delayed sleep onset in conjunction with a later wake time as compared to preadolescents. This shift in the timing of sleep preference is accompanied by a commensurate phase delay in their melatonin, a delay that increases as pubertal stage increases.[80] Adolescents have a period length (tau) that is, on average, 9 minutes longer than that of adults and also exhibit increased dim light sensitivity.[81] This endogenous delay in circadian timing is reinforced with later, technology-based socializing, resulting in stable, late bed times, protracted sleep deprivation[82,83] and the occurrence of sleep at suboptimal circadian phases.[30]

As adulthood progresses, circadian rhythms continue to change. Older individuals may have a lower circadian amplitude and a lengthening of their period,[84] with an accompanying circadian phase advance.[85] Shifts in chronotype occur as suggested by the fact that only 7% of young adults are morning types compared to 75% of older adults.[46] Some of these changes in circadian physiology may be secondary to the reduction of the number of SCN neurons that is observed in older individuals.[86] Neurodegenerative disorders linked to aging such as Alzheimer's disease are associated with even greater cell loss through unknown pathomechanisms,[86,87] and behaviorally, individuals with such disorders exhibit severe fragmentation of sleep across the day and night.[88] More generally, because the regular pattern of sleep/wake states is, in part, a key manifestation of Process C,[30,89] age-related sleep disorders may reflect a dampened impact of circadian rhythms on the pattern of sleep, leading to the observed shift in the temporal organization of sleep.[84,90]

Sex

Relatively little has been studied concerning sex differences in human circadian rhythms. Period length is approximately 6 minutes shorter in women compared to men,[10] possibly due to the expression of estrogen in women. The net effect of these sex differences appear to be minor, with only a small effect on circadian rhythms that are unlikely to be clinically relevant.

Circadian Rhythms and Health

Because circadian rhythms are intimately tied to our physiology and behaviors, dysfunction of the circadian system can have severe consequences in the short- and long-term. Circadian dysfunction can be broken down into two categories: dysfunction due to external influences and dysfunction due to endogenous factors.

External factors (e.g., zeitgebers) can influence the timing of the circadian system in an otherwise healthy individual, such that an individual's phase is no longer optimally attuned to the solar day. While jetlag is the most abrupt and obvious form of exogenously imposed circadian desynchrony, there are other more insidious forms, including what has been coined "social jetlag" (shifting sleep/wake rhythms several hours between weekend and weekday),[91] increased exposure to artificial light during the solar night,[92] and decreased natural light exposure during the solar day.[93] In all of these situations, the clock itself and its entrainment mechanisms function correctly, but the consequent behavior has a negative impact on health or well-being. Endogenous circadian dysfunction occurs when the circadian mechanism is itself dysfunctional. Such a situation is much less common, but can result in a chronic and debilitating disease such as delayed sleep–wake phase disorder, in which people go to sleep and awaken very late relative to societal norms (prevalence of ~0.15% of adults)[94–97] or in non-24-hour sleep–wake rhythm disorder, in which the timing of the circadian clock is no longer controlled by light and will run at or near its endogenous period, such as occurs in certain types of blindness.[98]

Regardless of the source of the dysfunction, misalignment of daily activity with the central circadian pacemaker can have serious behavioral consequences including impaired reasoning, emotion, and psychomotor skills. Extremely serious industrial accidents have been at least partly attributed to circadian misalignment,[49] including the Chernobyl nuclear incident of 1986 and the grounding of the Exxon Valdez oil tanker in 1989.[99,100] Despite the inherent dangers of misalignment of the body clock with work schedules, shift work is common, with 20% of workers engaged in shifting work schedules in the United States.[101] In particular, the military, security and policing, acute health care, and ground and air transportation sectors perform shift work[102–106] where impaired cognitive and psychomotor abilities could have serious consequences. As an example, nurses who do night shift work are two to three times more likely to both misdiagnose and incorrectly treat patients as compared to nurses on the day shift.[107]

The long-term health risks of misalignment of the body clock, light exposure, and activity are only now beginning to be understood. Aside from the implications for psychiatric disorders, such factors are linked to increased metabolic risks, obesity, diabetes,[108] breast cancer,[109] and multiple sclerosis.[110] Relatedly, the relationship between the relative timing between therapeutics administration and sleep timing and the efficacy of the therapeutics has been noted in cancer.[111] While the precise relationship between circadian rhythms and both physiology and psychology is incompletely understood, future research should help to illuminate these connections and lead to improvements in human health.

CONCLUSIONS

Circadian rhythms are ubiquitous in nature and touch upon all aspects of human brain function. The most observable role of the circadian clock is its involvement in the timing and consolidation of sleep. Although individuals demonstrate differences in their preferred timing of sleep/wake activities (chronotype), optimal human sleep/wake health requires stable entrainment to the solar day such that an individual is typically awake during the day and asleep at night. In today's society however, a variety of environmental and social pressures mean that we are less well synchronized to this solar day than ever before, which results in chronically unstable or shifting circadian rhythms and suppressed circadian amplitude. The long-term negative effects of such phenomenon remain largely unknown but likely contribute to the causes and symptoms of psychiatric disorders.

FUTURE DIRECTIONS

While circadian disruption can be a feature of psychiatric disorders, there is relatively little *direct* evidence for the role of the circadian clock in the etiology of psychiatric conditions. Future research will need to be centered on elucidating the exact role the circadian clock has in psychiatric disorders and the manner in which circadian rhythms could be manipulated to mitigate psychiatric symptoms or, potentially, the core pathophysiology. One important consideration for future work will be to develop new paradigms to accurately measure ambulatory, real-time circadian rhythms. The gold-standard measure, the timing of salivary or blood melatonin concentrations, is too complex to measure over weeks or months in the real world; however, such information will be necessary to understand the role of circadian rhythms in psychiatric disorders.

KEY PEARLS

- Circadian rhythms influence all aspects of mental and physical health.
- Light is the most potent influence on the timing of circadian rhythms.
- Irregular lighting exposure, especially at night, can lead to negative impacts on the circadian clock and the downstream rhythms that it influences.
- Minimization of nighttime light and regular, bright morning light are generally appropriate for a robust circadian rhythm.
- Research is ongoing into the contribution of circadian rhythms to the etiology of psychiatric disorders.

MULTIPLE CHOICE QUESTIONS

1. Circadian oscillations are best described as
   a. endogenous and unentrainable.
   b. exogenous and unentrainable.
   c. endogenous and entrainable.
   d. exogenous and entrainable.

Answer: c

2. After unexpectedly having to work through the night, you still find it hard to sleep in the morning. This is because your sleep propensity due to which of the following?
   a. Process S is high and circadian sleep drive is high.
   b. Process S is high and circadian sleep drive is low.
   c. Process S is low and circadian sleep drive is high.
   d. Process S is low and circadian sleep drive is low.

Answer: b

3. In humans, the strongest zeitgeber is
   a. social interactions.
   b. light.
   c. locomotor activity.
   d. sleep.

Answer: b

4. For people who work an 8 AM to 5 PM, Monday to Friday work week; the duration of sleep rebound on weekends will typically be greatest for
   a. extreme larks.
   b. larks.

c. owls.

d. extreme owls.

Answer: d

5. A dampened circadian rhythm amplitude may be due to

a. aging.

b. disease.

c. travel across time zones.

d. any of the above

Answer: d

REFERENCES

1. Cuvelier D, Legendre P, Laes A, Sarradin P-M, Sarrazin J. Rhythms and community dynamics of a hydrothermal Tubeworm assemblage at Main Endeavour Field—A multidisciplinary deep-sea observatory approach. *PLoS One*. 2014;9(5):e96924.
2. Kondo T, Mori T, Lebedeva NV, Aoki S, Ishiura M, Golden SS. Circadian rhythms in rapidly dividing Cyanobacteria. *Science*. 1997;275(5297):224–227.
3. Mori T, Binder B, Johnson CH. Circadian gating of cell division in Cyanobacteria growing with average doubling times of less than 24 hours. *Proc Natl Acad Sci U S A*. 1996;93(19):10183–10188.
4. Beale AD, Whitmore D, Moran D. Life in a dark biosphere: A review of circadian physiology in "arrhythmic" environments. *J Comp Physiol [B]*. 2016;186(8):947–968.
5. Wulund L, Reddy AB. A brief history of circadian time: The emergence of redox oscillations as a novel component of biological rhythms. *Perspec Sci*. 2015;6:27–37.
6. Mrosovsky N. Masking: History, definitions, and measurement. *Chronobiol Int*. 1999;16(4):415–429.
7. Dijk D, Czeisler C. Contribution of the circadian pacemaker and the sleep homeostat to sleep propensity, sleep structure, electroencephalographic slow waves, and sleep spindle activity in humans. *J Neurosc*. 1995;15(5):3526–3538.
8. Wyatt JK, Cecco AR-D, Czeisler CA, Dijk D-J. Circadian temperature and melatonin rhythms, sleep, and neurobehavioral function in humans living on a 20-h day. *Am J Physiol Regul Integr Comp Physiol*. 1999;277(4):R1152–R1163.
9. Czeisler CA, Duffy JF, Shanahan TL, et al. Stability, precision, and near-24-hour period of the human circadian pacemaker. *Science*. 1999;284(5423):2177–2181.
10. Duffy JF, Cain SW, Chang A-M, et al. Sex difference in the near-24-hour intrinsic period of the human circadian timing system. *Proc Natl Acad Sci U S A*. 2011;108(Suppl 3):15602–15608.
11. Micic G, de Bruyn A, Lovato N, et al. The endogenous circadian temperature period length (tau) in delayed sleep phase disorder compared to good sleepers. *J Sleep Res*. 2013;22(6):617–624.
12. Sack RL, Lewy AJ, Blood ML, Keith LD, Nakagawa H. Circadian rhythm abnormalities in totally blind people: Incidence and clinical significance. *J Clin Endocrinol Metab*. 1992;75(1):127–134.
13. Rajaratnam SMW, Arendt J. Health in a 24-h society. *The Lancet*. 2001;358(9286):999–1005.
14. Roenneberg T, Foster RG. Twilight times: Light and the circadian system. *Photochem Photobiol*. 1997;66(5):549–561.
15. Czeisler CA, Wright KP. Infuence of circadian rhythmicity in humans. In: Turek FW, Zee PC, eds. *Neurobiology of Sleep and Circadian Rhythms*. New York: Marcel Dekker; 1999:149–180.
16. Moore RY, Speh JC. GABA is the principal neurotransmitter of the circadian system. *Neurosci Lett*. 1993;150(1):112–116.
17. Inouye ST, Kawamura H. Persistence of circadian rhythmicity in a mammalian hypothalamic "island" containing the suprachiasmatic nucleus. *Proc Natl Acad Sci U S A*. 1979;76(11):5962–5966.
18. Welsh DK, Takahashi JS, Kay SA. Suprachiasmatic nucleus: Cell autonomy and network properties. *Annu Rev Physiol*. 2010;72(1):551–577.
19. Reppert SM, Weaver DR. Coordination of circadian timing in mammals. *Nature*. 2002;418:935.
20. Ko CH, Takahashi JS. Molecular components of the mammalian circadian clock. *Hum Mol Genet*. 2006;15(Suppl 2):R271–R277.
21. Yoo S-H, Yamazaki S, Lowrey PL, et al. PERIOD2::LUCIFERASE real-time reporting of circadian dynamics reveals persistent circadian oscillations in mouse peripheral tissues. *Proc Natl Acad Sci U S A*. 2004;101(15):5339–5346.
22. Pittendrigh CS. Circadian rhythms and the circadian organization of living systems. *Cold Spring Harb Symp Quant Biol*. 1960;25:159–184.
23. Dibner C, Schibler U, Albrecht U. The mammalian circadian timing system: Organization and coordination of central and peripheral clocks. *Annu Rev Physiol*. 2010;72(1):517–549.
24. Buhr ED, Yoo S-H, Takahashi JS. Temperature as a universal resetting cue for mammalian circadian oiscillators. *Science*. 2010;330(6002):379–385.
25. Borbély AA. A two process model of sleep regulation. *Hum Neurobiol*. 1982;1(3):195–204.
26. Borbély AA, Daan S, Wirz-Justice A, Deboer T. The two-process model of sleep regulation: A reappraisal. *J Sleep Res*. 2016;25(2):131–143.
27. Daan S, Beersma DG, Borbely AA. Timing of human sleep: recovery process gated by a circadian pacemaker. *Am J Physiol Regul Integr Comp Physiol*. 1984;246(2):R161–R183.

28. Dinges DF. Napping patterns and effects in human adults. In: Dinges DF, Broughton RJ, eds. *Sleep and alertness: chronobiological, behavioral, and medical aspects of napping*. New York: Raven Press; 1989:171–204.

29. Campbell S, Zulley J. Ultradian components of human sleep/wake patterns during disentrainment. *Exp Brain Res*. 1985(Suppl 12).

30. Dijk DJ, Czeisler CA. Paradoxical timing of the circadian rhythm of sleep propensity serves to consolidate sleep and wakefulness in humans. *Neurosci Lett*. 1994;166(1):63–68.

31. Daan S, Aschoff J. Circadian rhythms of locomotor activity in captive birds and mammals: Their variations with season and latitude. *Oecologia*. 1975;18(4):269–316.

32. Zeitzer JM, Ayas NT, Shea SA, Brown R, Czeisler CA. Absence of detectable melatonin and preservation of cortisol and thyrotropin rhythms in tetraplegia1. *J Clin Endocrinol Metab*. 2000;85(6):2189–2196.

33. Rajaratnam SMW, Dijk D-J, Middleton B, Stone BM, Arendt J. Melatonin phase-shifts human circadian rhythms with no evidence of changes in the duration of endogenous melatonin secretion or the 24-hour production of reproductive hormones. *J Clin Endocrinol Metab*. 2003;88(9):4303–4309.

34. Zeitzer JM, Dijk D-J, Kronauer RE, Brown EN, Czeisler CA. Sensitivity of the human circadian pacemaker to nocturnal light: Melatonin phase resetting and suppression. *J Physiol*. 2000;526(3):695–702.

35. Cowen PJ, Bevan JS, Gosden B, Elliott SA. Treatment with beta-adrenoceptor blockers reduces plasma melatonin concentration. *Br J Clin Pharmacol*. 1985;19(2):258–260.

36. Arendt J, Bojkowski C, Franey C, Wright J, Marks V. Immunoassay of 6-Hydroxymelatonin Sulfate in Human Plasma and Urine: Abolition of the Urinary 24-Hour Rhythm with Atenolol. *J Clin Endocrinol Metab*. 1985;60(6):1166–1173.

37. Klerman EB, Gershengorn HB, Duffy JF, Kronauer RE. Comparisons of the variability of three markers of the human circadian pacemaker. *J Biol Rhythms*. 2002;17(2):181–193.

38. Zeitzer JM, Daniels JE, Duffy JF, et al. Do plasma melatonin concentrations decline with age? *Am J Med*. 1999;107(5):432–436.

39. Arendt J. Melatonin. *Clin Endocrinol (Oxf)*. 1988;29(2):205–229.

40. Shanahan TL, Kronauer RE, Duffy JF, Williams GH, Czeisler CA. Melatonin rhythm observed throughout a three-cycle bright-light stimulus designed to reset the human circadian pacemaker. *J Biol Rhythms*. 1999;14(3):237–253.

41. Brown EN, Czeisler CA. The statistical analysis of circadian phase and amplitude in constant-routine core-temperature data. *J Biol Rhythms*. 1992;7(3):177–202.

42. Duffy JF, Dijk D-J. Getting through to circadian oscillators: Why use constant routines? *J Biol Rhythms*. 2002;17(1):4–13.

43. Jewett ME, Kronauer RE, Czeisler CA. Phase-amplitude resetting of the human circadian pacemaker via bright light: A further analysis. *J Biol Rhythms*. 1994;9(3-4):295–314.

44. Aschoff J, Wever R. Human circadian rhythms: a multioscillatory system. *Fed Proc*. 1976;35(12):232–236.

45. Wever RA. *The circadian system of man: Results of experiments under temporal isolation*. Berlin: Springer; 1979.

46. Yoon C, May CP, Hasher L. Aging, circadian arousal patterns, and cognition. In: Park D, Schwartz N, eds. *Cognitive aging: A primer*. Philadelphia, PA: Psychology Press; 2000:151–170.

47. Schmidt C, Collette F, Cajochen C, Peigneux P. A time to think: Circadian rhythms in human cognition. *Cogn Neuropsychol*. 2007;24(7):755–789.

48. Cajochen C, Khalsa SBS, Wyatt JK, Czeisler CA, Dijk D-J. EEG and ocular correlates of circadian melatonin phase and human performance decrements during sleep loss. *Am J Physiol Regul Integr Comp Physiol*. 1999;277(3):R640–R649.

49. Mitler MM, Carskadon MA, Czeisler CA, Dement WC, Dinges DF, Graeber RC. Catastrophes, sleep and public policy: Consensus report. *Sleep*. 1988;11(1):100–109.

50. Underwood H, Groos G. Vertebrate circadian rhythms: Retinal and extraretinal photoreception. *Experientia*. 1982;38(9):1013–1021.

51. Dacey DM, Liao H-W, Peterson BB, et al. Melanopsin-expressing ganglion cells in primate retina signal colour and irradiance and project to the LGN. *Nature*. 2005;433:749–754.

52. Schmidt TM, Chen SK, Hattar S. Intrinsically photosensitive retinal ganglion cells: Many subtypes, diverse functions. *Trends Neurosci*. 2011;34(11):572–580.

53. Do MTH, Yau KW. Intrinsically photosensitive retinal ganglion cells. *Physiol Rev*. 2010;90(4):1547–1581.

54. Hattar S, Kumar M, Park A, et al. Central projections of melanopsin-expressing retinal ganglion cells in the mouse. *J Comp Neurol*. 2006;497(3):326–349.

55. Hattar S, Liao H-W, Takao M, Berson DM, Yau K-W. Melanopsin-containing retinal ganglion cells: Architecture, projections, and intrinsic photosensitivity. *Science*. 2002;295(5557):1065–1070.

56. Czeisler C, Kronauer R, Allan J, et al. Bright light induction of strong (type 0) resetting of the human circadian pacemaker. *Science.* 1989;244(4910):1328–1333.

57. Jewett ME, Rimmer DW, Duffy JF, Klerman EB, Kronauer RE, Czeisler CA. Human circadian pacemaker is sensitive to light throughout subjective day without evidence of transients. *Am J Physiol Regul Integr Comp Physiol.* 1997;273(5):R1800–R1809.

58. Chang A-M, Scheer FAJL, Czeisler CA. The human circadian system adapts to prior photic history. *J Physiol.* 2011;589(5):1095–1102.

59. Hébert M, Martin SK, Lee C, Eastman CI. The effects of prior light history on the suppression of melatonin by light in humans. *J Pineal Res.* 2002;33(4):198–203.

60. Chang A-M, Aeschbach D, Duffy JF, Czeisler CA. Evening use of light-emitting eReaders negatively affects sleep, circadian timing, and next-morning alertness. *Proc Natl Acad Sci U S A.* 2015;112(4):1232–1237.

61. Zeitzer JM. Real life trumps laboratory in matters of public health. *Proc Natl Acad Sci U S A.* 2015;112(13):E1513–E1513.

62. Lockley SW, Brainard GC, Czeisler CA. High sensitivity of the human circadian melatonin rhythm to resetting by short wavelength light. *J Clin Endocrinol Metab.* 2003;88(9):4502–4505.

63. Cajochen C, Münch M, Kobialka S, et al. High sensitivity of human melatonin, alertness, thermoregulation, and heart rate to short wavelength light. *J Clin Endocrinol Metab.* 2005;90(3):1311–1316.

64. Zaidi FH, Hull JT, Peirson SN, et al. Short-wavelength light sensitivity of circadian, pupillary, and visual awareness in humans lacking an outer retina. *Curr Biol.* 2007;17(24):2122–2128.

65. Gooley JJ, Rajaratnam SMW, Brainard GC, Kronauer RE, Czeisler CA, Lockley SW. Spectral responses of the human circadian system depend on the irradiance and duration of exposure to light. *Sci Transl Med.* 2010;2(31):31ra33–31ra33.

66. Najjar RP, Zeitzer JM. Temporal integration of light flashes by the human circadian system. *J Clin Invest.* 2016;126(3):938–947.

67. Burke TM, Markwald RR, McHill AW, et al. Effects of caffeine on the human circadian clock in vivo and in vitro. *Sci Transl Med.* 2015;7(305):305ra146.

68. Lewy AJ, Ahmed S, Jackson JML, Sack RL. Melatonin shifts human circadian rhythms according to a phase-response curve. *Chronobiol Int.* 1992;9(5):380–392.

69. Dollins AB, Zhdanova IV, Wurtman RJ, Lynch HJ, Deng MH. Effect of inducing nocturnal serum melatonin concentrations in daytime on sleep, mood, body temperature, and performance. *Proc Natl Acad Sci U S A.* 1994;91(5):1824–1828.

70. Dubocovich ML, Markowska M. Functional MT1 and MT2 melatonin receptors in mammals. *Endocrine.* 2005;27(2):101–110.

71. Horne JA, Östberg O. A self-assessment questionnaire to determine morningness-eveningness in human circadian rhythms. *Int J Chronobiol.* 1976;4:97–110.

72. Roenneberg T, Wirz-Justice A, Merrow M. Life between clocks: Daily temporal patterns of human chronotypes. *J Biol Rhythms.* 2003;18(1):80–90.

73. Lack L, Bailey M, Lovato N, Wright H. Chronotype differences in circadian rhythms of temperature, melatonin, and sleepiness as measured in a modified constant routine protocol. *Nat Sci Sleep.* 2009;1:1–8.

74. Hur Y-M, Jr TJB, Lykken DT. Genetic and environmental influence on morningness-eveningness. *Pers Individ Dif.* 1998;25(5):917–925.

75. Hahm B-J, Jo B, Dhabhar FS, et al. Bedtime misalignment and progression of breast cancer. *Chronobiol Int.* 2014;31(2):214–221.

76. Mirmiran M, Kok JH, Boer K, Wolf H. Perinatal development of human circadian rhythms: Role of the foetal biological clock. *Neurosci Biobehav Rev.* 1992;16(3):371–378.

77. Stanfield B, Cowan WM. Evidence for a change in the retino-hypothalamic projection in the rat following early removal of one eye. *Brain Res.* 1976;104(1):129–136.

78. Mirmiran M, Lunshof S. Perinatal development of human circadian rhythms. In: Buijs RM, Kalsbeek A, Romijn HJ, Pennartz CMA, Mirmiran M, eds. *Progress in Brain Research.* Vol 111. New York: Elsevier; 1996:217–226.

79. Lewy A. Melatonin and human chronobiology. *Cold Spring Harb Symp Quant Biol.* 2007;72:623–636.

80. Carskadon MA, Acebo C, Richardson GS, Tate BA, Seifer R. An approach to studying circadian rhythms of adolescent humans. *J Biol Rhythms.* 1997;12(3):278–289.

81. Carskadon MA, Acebo C, Jenni OG. Regulation of adolescent sleep: Implications for behavior. *Ann N Y Acad Sci.* 2004;1021(1):276–291.

82. Calamaro CJ, Mason TBA, Ratcliffe SJ. Adolescents living the 24/7 lifestyle: Effects of caffeine and technology on sleep duration and daytime functioning. *Pediatrics.* 2009; 123(6):e1005–e1010.

83. Van den Bulck J. Television viewing, computer game playing, and internet use and self-reported time to bed and time out of bed in secondary-school children. *Sleep.* 2004;27(1):101–104.

84. Weitzman ED, Moline ML, Czeisler CA, Zimmerman JC. Chronobiology of aging: temperature, sleep-wake rhythms and entrainment. *Neurobiol Aging*. 1982;3(4): 299–309.

85. Leutz MJ. Circadian temperature rhythms in healthy young and old men. *Sleep Res*. 1984;13:222.

86. Swaab DF, Fliers E, Partiman TS. The suprachiasmatic nucleus of the human brain in relation to sex, age and senile dementia. *Brain Res*. 1985;342(1):37–44.

87. Stopa EG, Volicer L, Kuo-Leblanc V, et al. Pathologic evaluation of the human Suprachiasmatic Nucleus in severe dementia. *J Neuropathol Exp Neurol*. 1999;58(1):29–39.

88. Prinz PN, Peskind ER, Vitaliano PP, et al. Changes in the Sleep and Waking EEGs of Nondemented and Demented Elderly Subjects. *J Am Geriatr Soc*. 1982;30(2):86–92.

89. Dijk D-J, Duffy JF, Riel E, Shanahan TL, Czeisler CA. Ageing and the circadian and homeostatic regulation of human sleep during forced desynchrony of rest, melatonin and temperature rhythms. *J Physiol*. 1999;516(2):611–627.

90. Miles LE, Dement WC. Sleep and aging. *Sleep*. 1980;3(2):1.

91. Wittmann M, Dinich J, Merrow M, Roenneberg T. Social jetlag: Misalignment of biological and social time. *Chronobiol Int*. 2006;23(1-2):497–509.

92. Gooley JJ, Chamberlain K, Smith KA, et al. Exposure to room light before bedtime suppresses melatonin onset and shortens melatonin duration in humans. *J Clin Endocrinol Metab*. 2011;96(3):E463–E472.

93. Wright Kenneth P, McHill Andrew W, Birks Brian R, Griffin Brandon R, Rusterholz T, Chinoy Evan D. Entrainment of the human circadian clock to the natural light-dark cycle. *Curr Biol*. 2013;23(16):1554–1558.

94. Yazaki M, Shirakawa S, Okawa M, Takahashi K. Demography of sleep disturbances associated with circadian rhythm disorders in Japan. *Psychiatry Clin Neurosci*. 1999;53(2):267–268.

95. Schrader H, Bovim G, Sand T. The prevalence of delayed and advanced sleep phase syndromes. *J Sleep Res*. 1993;2(1):51–55.

96. Pelayo R. Prevalence of delayed sleep phase syndrome among adolescence. *Sleep Res*. 1988;17:391.

97. Barion A, Zee PC. A clinical approach to circadian rhythm sleep disorders. *Sleep Med*.8(6):566–577.

98. Lockley S, Skene D, James K, Thapan K, Wright J, Arendt J. Melatonin administration can entrain the free-running circadian system of blind subjects. *J Endocrinol*. 2000;164(1):R1–R6.

99. Folkard S. Circadian performance rhythms: some practical and theoretical implications. *Philos Trans R Soc Lond B Biol Sci*. 1990; 327(1241):543–553.

100. National Transportation Safety Board. Grounding of U.S. tankship Exxon Valdez on Bligh Reef, Prince William Sound near Valdez, AK, March 24, 1989. 1990.

101. McMenamin TM. A time to work: recent trends in shift work and flexible schedules. *Mon Labor Rev*. 2007;130:3.

102. Caldwell JA. Fatigue in the aviation environment: An overview of the causes and effects as well as recommended countermeasures. *Aviat Space Environ Med*. 1997;68(10):932–938.

103. Cruz C, Della Rocco P, Hackworth C. Effects of quick rotating shift schedules on the health and adjustment of air traffic controllers. *Aviat Space Environ Med*. 2000;71(4):400–407.

104. Goh VH-H, Tong TY-Y, Lim C-L, Low EC-T, Lee LK-H. Circadian disturbances after night-shift work onboard a naval ship. *Obstet Gynecol Surv*. 2000;55(10):610–611.

105. Häkkänen H, Summala H. Sleepiness at work among commercial truck drivers. *Sleep*. 2000;23(1):49–57.

106. Luna TD, French J, Mitcha JL. A study of USAF air traffic controller shiftwork: Sleep, fatigue, activity, and mood analyses. *Aviat Space Environ Med*. 1997;68(1):18–23.

107. Gold DR, Rogacz S, Bock N, et al. Rotating shift work, sleep, and accidents related to sleepiness in hospital nurses. *Am J Public Health*. 1992;82(7):1011–1014.

108. Delezie J, Challet E. Interactions between metabolism and circadian clocks: reciprocal disturbances. *Ann N Y Acad Sci*. 2011;1243(1):30–46.

109. Hansen J. Increased breast cancer risk among women who work predominantly at night. *Epidemiology*. 2001;12(1):74–77.

110. Hedström AK, Akerstedt T, Hillert J, Olsson T, Alfredsson L. Shift work at young age is associated with increased risk for multiple sclerosis. *Ann Neurol*. 2011;70(5):733–741.

111. Lévi F, Focan C, Karaboué A, et al. Implications of circadian clocks for the rhythmic delivery of cancer therapeutics. *Adv Drug Deliv Rev*. 2007;59(9):1015–1035.

5

Sleep and Cognition

LILIA ROSHCHUPKINA AND PHILIPPE PEIGNEUX

INTRODUCTION

To understand the cost of sleep, just spend one night without it.

One often wonders why we spend a third of our lives sleeping, and what the fundamental functions subtended by what is subjectively perceived as a cessation of waking activity are. To elucidate these functions is increasingly crucial in the context of production-oriented modern societies, in which the number of hours devoted to sleep constantly and dramatically decreases. Among other factors, reduced dependency on daylight, extended shift work and 24/7 activities, social media availability, and other social conditions may lead to an artificial shortening in sleep time duration at all ages, often falling outside the recommendations for healthy individuals [1]. Evidence from various fields including molecular genetics, behavioral, and cognitive neurosciences provide converging evidence that sleep exerts a beneficial role to regulate brain activity and cognitive processes, besides other non-exclusive functions such as for instance cerebral and body restitution [2]. This chapter aims at explaining the contribution of sleep to the processes that form and enable thinking abilities and help individuals to operate efficiently in daily life. We will first focus on the impact of sleep on key cognitive functions in the waking state, including executive functions (EF) and inhibitory control, attention, and working memory (WM). We will then explore the sleep-dependent information processing and transformations that support higher order cognitive processes, such as long-term memory (LTM) consolidation, gist extraction, insight, and the ability to create inferential judgments.

SLEEP AND EXECUTIVE FUNCTIONS

In its popular acceptance, cognition refers to thinking and knowing. More precisely, cognition can be seen as the global ability to process and integrate the information received as a result of perception, learning, or experience and converting it into knowledge. These cognitive actions are to a large extent supported by an EF system that encompasses cognitive control abilities and relates to a family of top–down mental processes. Inhibitory control, attentional flexibility, and WM in particular are three core EF subsystems that govern goal-directed actions and adaptive responses to novel, complex, or ambiguous situations [3]. High order cognitive executive processes (such as language, reasoning, prospective planning, problem-solving, decision-making) build up on core EFs [4, 5] and play a fundamental role to support goal achievement. EFs are nonexclusively associated with frontal lobes activity [6]. Neurophysiological (e.g., electroencephalography [EEG]) and neuroimaging (e.g., positron emission tomography (PET] and functional resonance imaging [fMRI]) studies showed that frontal lobes efficiency is highly sensitive to the effect of sleep. For instance, increased sleep pressure during total sleep deprivation (TSD), operationalized by increased theta power density in the waking EEG and increased slow-wave activity (SWA) in the sleeping EEG in the first sleep cycle [7], is most prominent in frontal areas [8, 9]. After TSD, metabolism also more markedly decreases in these areas [10]. Considering the impact of sleep restriction on frontal activity and the tight (but nonexclusive) association between frontal activity and EFs, it is logical to hypothesize that sleep restriction will impair performance mostly on cognitive tasks that involve EFs, although there are large interindividual differences in the vulnerability to the effects of sleep deprivation (SD) [11].

REGULATION OF INHIBITORY CONTROL

Inhibition is an important component of cognitive control. It can be defined as a set of mechanisms allowing the suppression of inappropriate actions and the resistance to interference from irrelevant stimuli [12]. According to Barkley [13], inhibition comprises three interrelated processes: (i) inhibition of a prepotent or dominant response (*response inhibition*), (ii) *stopping of an ongoing response*, and (iii) distractibility (*interference control*). The first two functions are commonly tested with tasks that require frequent automatic responses to stimuli and the need to withhold the response (response inhibition) or to interrupt the ongoing response (stopping) when presented with a specific stimulus. Two paradigmatic examples are the Go/NoGo [14] and the stop-signal [15,16] tasks. In the Go/NoGo task, participants are presented with a continuous stream of stimuli and have to respond as fast as possible to Go stimuli or to refrain responding to the NoGo stimuli. In the stop-signal task, fast responses are required for all stimuli, but a "stop" stimulus sometimes appears very shortly after the imperative one, in which case the ongoing action must be inhibited. After 36 hours of TSD, participants fail more often to inhibit a to-be-refrained response and produce more incorrect responses in the Go/NoGo task [17]. Two nights of TSD are associated with difficulties in withholding an inappropriate motor response, *slower* reaction times to Go stimuli, and increased false positives [18]. These deficits are restored following a single night of recovery sleep, indicating that the negative consequences of acute SD are temporary and easily reversed by sleep itself.

A paradigmatic *interference control* task is the Stroop test, in which color names are presented in various ink colors. Participants must name the color of the ink, which can be congruent (same ink color than the name; e.g., "green" in green ink) or incongruent (e.g., "green" in red ink) with the word. In the latter case, processing time is slowed down and/or ink color naming errors are made due to the interference between the automatic name reading reflex and the actual ink color to report. Studies initially found preserved interference effects after SD, despite overall increased reaction times [19, 20]. However, further investigations showed that SD selectively impairs the top–down adaptation mechanisms supporting cognitive control, whereas seemingly preserved interference effects at the behavioral level are only supported by bottom–up, automatic mechanisms [21]. From a neurophysiological level standpoint, successful response inhibition (NoGo/stop trials) was associated with right dorsolateral prefrontal cortex (DLPFC) activity [22, 23], whereas commission errors (NoGo/stop errors) were associated with anterior cingulate cortex (ACC) and medial frontal gyrus activity [24, 25]. These brain regions are considered crucial for high-order cognitive control, especially the ACC for conflict monitoring [26] and the prefrontal cortex (PFC) for the suppression of irrelevant responses [27]. Similarly, in the Stroop task, the PFC is involved in the attentional maintenance of task-relevant information (color identification; [28, 29]), and the ACC supports conflict resolution between competing responses (i.e. responding to the color or to the word; [28]).

ATTENTIONAL PROCESSES

Attention is a transversal component, impacting most other cognitive functions. Different types of attention can be distinguished, among others:

1. *vigilant (sustained) attention*—the ability to keep ready to react in a monotonous environment over extended periods of time.
2. *selective attention*—the ability to focus on a specific stimulus in the face of distractors.
3. *divided attention*—the ability to simultaneously process different types stimuli.
4. *orienting (switching) attention*—the mental flexibility ability that allows individuals to shift the focus of their attention between tasks or stimuli sets.

SD exerts a dramatic impact on vigilance [30], which is mostly investigated using the psychomotor vigilance task (PVT). In the PVT, visual or auditory stimuli are presented at irregular long (2–10 seconds) interstimulus intervals during 10 minutes [31]. Reaction times and response omissions (lapses) are modulated both by time spent awake [32] and circadian factors [33]. SD also enhances time-on-task effects, with performance worsening across the course of the task. Although best evidenced in tasks lasting 30 minutes or more, time-on-task effects have been also evidenced within the first minutes of performance in SD individuals [30]. SD also increases the propensity of individuals to experience "lapses" or "microsleep" states, eventually leading to abnormally slow responses (>500 ms) and commission errors (i.e., a response in the absence of the stimulus) [30, 34]. Behavioral performance in other attentional domains tends to be accompanied by changes in vigilance, probably because all forms of attention generally recruit similar cognitive control areas [35].

Accordingly, early studies showed that SD is accompanied by reduced metabolic activity within a network of brain regions essential for attention and information processing (including the PFC, ACC, thalamus, basal ganglia, and cerebellum), correlated with alertness and cognitive performance [36]. SD also drives reduced activation in fronto-parietal attentional networks especially in the right hemisphere [37]. In healthy individuals undergoing 36 hours of TSD, faster responses in the PVT were associated with increased activity within a cortical sustained attention network (including prefrontal, motor, and parietal cortical areas) and subcortical structures such as the basal ganglia. Abnormally slow responses were associated with a greater activation of medial prefrontal regions implicated in the default mode network (DMN), which tends to be most active in nondirected tasks conditions when the brain is in a resting state [38]. It suggests that sleep loss may result in inappropriate activation of the DMN (i.e., in on-task conditions) and/or lead to a failure to effectively allocate resources to task-relevant brain regions. Additionally, acute SD modulates superior parietal lobule (SPL) and inferior parietal sulcus (IPS) activity in most attentional tasks, including sustained [38–39], selective [40, 41], divided [42], and orienting [43] attention. Likewise, SD reduces thalamic activity and increases attentional lapses in vigilant attention (for review, see Krause et al. [44]), suggesting that the thalamus is a pivotal gating hub through which alterations in brainstem ascending arousal signals affect cortical attentional networks under SD conditions. Thus, neuroimaging results suggest that sleep loss significantly alters the normal functioning of attentional networks and promotes increased disengagement from external sensory inputs.

WORKING MEMORY AND SLEEP

Working memory can be defined as the hypothetical limited capacity system that permits the temporary storage and manipulation of information necessary for performing a wide range of cognitive activities, hence a mental workspace that temporarily stores important information subtending ongoing mental activities. WM comprises two short-term memory (STM) components, the

phonological loop (acoustic-auditory information) and the *visuospatial sketchpad* (visual-spatial information), coupled with an *episodic buffer* that bridges WM with available LTM information; all these elements are supervised and organized by a *central executive* attentional control system [45]. Attention and WM (especially its central executive component) are often interrelated due to their common reliance on a limited amount of simultaneously available cognitive resources [46]. Consistently, SD adversely impacts both accuracy and response time in WM tasks, especially in tasks featuring a high cognitive load [47]. The phonological loop and visuospatial sketchpad are also altered under chronic sleep restriction condition (e.g. 4 hours of sleep per day during 5 days, [48]) with a reduced percentage of correct responses and increased reaction time. In this latter study, performance decrease was especially marked for the visuospatial component, tentatively associated with additional efforts to process, store, and use spatial stimuli. As for the phonological component, it decreased only on the fifth day of partial sleep reduction, but remained at low level even after the recovery night, at variance with the immediate restoration of the visuospatial function. These results are in line with previous findings that daily sleep restriction to 4 hours during several days reduces the ability to respond to verbal stimuli [49]. It suggests that partial SD has a stronger effect on visuospatial WM storage in terms of speed and accuracy, but that the phonological component requires more time to recover after chronic sleep restriction condition. Looking at capacity and filtering efficiency, two main components of WM, Drummond and colleagues [50] showed that visual WM capacity was not significantly affected neither by total or partial SD (4 hours sleep per day), whereas total SD (but not partial SD) impaired performance in the filtering task. Thus, there are differences in the vulnerability of visual WM elements to different forms of SD. To the best of our knowledge, no studies reported SD effects on the WM episodic buffer.

The functional neuroanatomy of WM greatly overlaps with the attention system; hence, SD affects both. Increased brain activation in SD conditions was found associated with relatively preserved performance, whereas decreased activation was associated with performance decline [51]. Accordingly, SD-related deficits in both WM and attention tasks were found to correlate with reduced activity in the DLPFC and posterior parietal cortex [50]. Interestingly, greater task complexity can paradoxically result in a more preserved performance in the SD condition [52]. More difficult tasks that require higher cognitive load may result in a greater prefrontal and thalamic activation, acting as a compensatory mechanism. Using a verbal n-back (memory updating) paradigm in an fMRI study, Chee and Choo [53] tested participants at three cognitive load levels, under rested and 24-hour SD conditions. Results evidenced a load-dependent modulation of activity in the left PFC and in the thalamus in the SD state. Reduced activity in occipital areas extending to the inferior parietal cortex was consistently found at all WM loads, echoing previous experiments [52, 54], suggesting that reduced parieto-occipital activation may be an effect of SD, however task- and load-independent. Additionally, altered DMN activation [50, 53] and thalamic activity fluctuations [53] have been reported during WM performance in the SD condition, suggesting compensatory adaptation mechanisms [52]. Accordingly, the amplitude of the WM decline was correlated with the degree of deviant on-task DMN activity in SD individuals [50, 53]. Thus, inadequate activation of the DMN during on-task cortical activity might be a common mechanism underlying SD-related deficits in both attention and WM. Furthermore, increased connectivity between the hippocampus, the thalamus, and the DMN was correlated with WM performance decline under SD conditions [55]. In turn, increased connectivity between the thalamus and the precuneus under SD predicted partial recovery of WM performance. These findings suggest that different brain regions exhibit varying degrees of vulnerability to the deleterious effects of SD and that compensatory neural activity mechanisms support partial recovery or preservation of performance in specific cognitive conditions.

SLEEP-DEPENDENT LEARNING AND MEMORY PROCESSES

Memory is the cognitive system that retains information about previously experienced events (sensations, impressions, ideas, etc.). Memory is not unitary, and memory systems differ in terms of storage time, capacity, and type of the information to be remembered. From a temporal perspective, *sensory memory* represents the shortest memory element. It retains impressions of sensory information up to a few seconds only. Sensory information can then pass into the STM system, where information can be kept for a few tens of seconds

and manipulated in WM. STM capacity is limited (around 7 ± 2 items simultaneously), and new information must be transferred and linked with prior knowledge in LTM systems, whose storage capacity and duration are theoretically unlimited. LTM can be also defined according to the type of stored information. *Declarative memory* ("knowing what") is the memory for facts and events and is typically explicitly accessible by active verbal recall. *Procedural* memory ("knowing how") stores automated skills and habits that are mostly gradually acquired through repeated experience and are most often reported by action than verbal description. Long-term declarative memory further includes *episodic memories* for experiences and events acquired in a specific spatiotemporal context and *semantic memories* for fact-based information. These memory systems are partially subtended by distinctive brain systems, although not independent (i.e., the acquisition of such skills as language learning and finger sequence tapping may involve both declarative and procedural memory components [56, 57]). Memories undergo three main processing phases: (i) *encoding*—the formation of a new memory trace, susceptible to forgetting; (ii) *consolidation*—the post-acquisition processes eventually leading to the stabilization and the gradual integration of new memory traces into pre-existing knowledge networks; and (iii) *retrieval*—the reactivation (recall) of stored memories. Prior sleep quality may impact performance at the memory encoding (e.g., [58]) and retrieval (e.g., [59]) phases, also given the potential implication of attentional and executive systems and their susceptibility to SD, as previously discussed. We will here focus on the postlearning consolidation phase.

SLEEP AND DECLARATIVE MEMORY CONSOLIDATION

A dominant account for the consolidation of hippocampus-dependent declarative memories is the *standard memory consolidation model* proposing that new memories are initially encoded within hippocampal regions then gradually transferred over days or even weeks to months toward more permanent neocortical stores. Regarding the role of sleep, the active system consolidation hypothesis [60] proposes that events experienced during wakefulness are encoded in neocortical and hippocampal networks in parallel. During subsequent sleep episodes, newly acquired hippocampal memory traces are repeatedly reactivated during slow-wave sleep (SWS). Decreased cholinergic activity in SWS [61] favors a gradual transfer of hippocampal information toward neocortical stores, eventually strengthening the new traces into more persistent memory representations. Reactivation and redistribution of memories during SWS is subtended by a hippocampal-neocortical dialogue linking hippocampal ripples and thalamo-cortical spindles, synchronized by neocortical slow oscillations (SO; ~0.75 Hz) [62] (for a review see Rasch and Bonn [63]). Supporting this proposal, studies have shown that postlearning SWS is required to protect memory from future interference and improve memory performance [64, 65]. A key role for SWS in declarative memory consolidation was also highlighted in studies directly manipulating SOs during sleep (i.e., increasing or reducing SWA) to eventually enhance or suppress hippocampus-related memory representations. For instance, transcranial direct current stimulation was found to increase the number of SOs and improve memory performance [66, 67], whereas SO suppression by auditory tones impaired execution of the task [68]. Importantly, auditory stimulation must be delivered in phase with SOs to increase their rhythm and phase-coupled sleep spindle activity, which in turn positively correlate with declarative memory consolidation [69]. Given the assumption of a repeated reactivation of memory traces during SWS, researchers logically tried boosting this reactivation process using *targeted (cue-induced) memory reactivation* (TMR), in which learning-related stimulations are delivered during SWS. Typically in TMR experiments, paired associates are presented during wakefulness, for example two words [70], a word and a sound [71], or visuospatial information associated with odors [72–74]. Participants are then re-exposed to the cue related to learning (i.e., word, sound, odor, etc.) during subsequent SWS, and memory performance is assessed next morning. Results consistently showed better memory retrieval for cued associations, as compared to noncued ones. TMR during rapid eye movement (REM) sleep was not found successful [72]. Importantly, the benefit of TMR is abolished when additional auditory stimulation is provided less than ±1.3 seconds after the initial one. This deleterious effect is linked to the suppression of cue-induced spindle-related sigma activity [75, 76] suggesting that sleep spindles subtend the successful integration of cues into previously learned information.

Neuroimaging studies in humans also supported the assumption that newly acquired memories are reactivated during postlearning sleep, like in the animal. PET studies evidenced the reactivation of learning-related regional brain activity during posttraining SWS after hippocampus-dependent spatial navigation learning [77]. Hippocampal reactivation during SWS also correlated with the overnight gain in navigation performance. In an fMRI study, re-exposure to learning-related odors during SWS was found to increase activity in hippocampal areas activated in response to odor stimulation during wakefulness [72]. Spontaneous reactivation of the neural correlates of learning also takes place during postlearning wakefulness [78], however, with potentially different functional effects. In an fMRI study, participants were exposed to a learning-related odor either during wakefulness or SWS [73]. The odor induction episode was followed by an interference task to test memory stability. Reactivation during wakefulness led to memory destabilization associated with increased prefrontal cortical activity, whereas exposure during SWS stabilized the memory trace, and was associated with hippocampal and posterior cortical activity. Although these results may suggest that only postlearning SWS would provide the optimal reactivation conditions to successfully stabilize and integrate associated memories into LTM stores, it remains to be clarified whether reactivation during posttraining wakefulness is a necessary component in the creation of the novel memory trace.

SLEEP AND CONSOLIDATION OF PROCEDURAL MEMORIES

The role of sleep in the consolidation of procedural memories has been often investigated using motor sequence learning as a model for the learning of complex motor actions that applies to many instances in daily life (e.g., articulatory speech, typing, playing instruments) [79]. The dynamics of motor skills follow two main phases. First, a fast-learning phase in which performance quickly improves online, during the initial practice. Second, a slow, covert consolidation process during which performance slowly continues improving offline [80]. There is consistent evidence for offline performance gains when motor sequence learning is followed by a night of sleep, as compared to a wakefulness period, suggesting that the first posttraining sleep period is critical for initiating the long-lasting storage of new motor skills [81–83]. Consolidation of motor skills also benefits from postlearning sleep in the form of daytime naps [84–86]. However, the beneficial role of napping might be transitory, since performance after a subsequent night of sleep was found similar between participants who had a nap opportunity and those who stayed awake during the same period of time [87]. Overnight sleep was also found to result in a more robust offline improvement than daytime napping [88].

From a neurophysiological standpoint, the learning and subsequent consolidation phases of motor skills are accompanied by functional and structural reorganizations within dedicated neuronal networks, mostly in motor [89–91] and premotor areas, basal ganglia, cerebellum, and parietal cortex [92–94]. From one perspective, new motor memories would be stored in the motor cortex where representations of learned actions are progressively strengthened in specific neuronal networks, eventually resulting in practice-related plastic changes in motor maps [95]. Cortico-cerebellar and cortico-striatal loops would play a complementary role in the development and consolidation of sequential motor memories [95, 96]. Besides a motor account of sequence learning however, it must be taken into account that the so-called declarative and procedural memory systems are not fully independent and may both contribute to acquisition and consolidation processes [97, 98]. Accordingly, neuroimaging (fMRI) studies have disclosed hippocampal activity during motor sequence learning [99, 100], predictive of both subsequent performance and the successful instatement of offline consolidation [100, 101]. Conversely, activity in brain circuits usually associated with procedural learning may predict subsequent memory consolidation in declarative memory [102, 103].

It was initially thought that the division between memory systems would parallel the dissociation between sleep states. That is, REM sleep would support procedural memory consolidation processes, whereas non-REM (NREM) sleep would subtend declarative memory consolidation (for a critical review, see Peigneux et al. [104]). In line with this proposal, performance in a procedural mirror-tracing task improved after sleep in the second half of the night (richest in REM) but not after sleep in the first part of the night (richest in SWS) [105]. PET studies showed that visuomotor sequence learning-related brain activity patterns are replayed during subsequent REM sleep [106, 107] and that learning levels are correlated with cortical activity during posttraining REM sleep [107]. Additionally, overnight performance improvement was found associated with post-training REM sleep amounts [108], and pharmacological REM sleep suppression impaired consolidation [109]. However, other studies do not support the hypothesis of a dedicated and exclusive role of REM sleep in the consolidation of procedural memories. Rather, they point out an important role for NREM sleep and sleep spindles in particular. For instance, intensive training on a sequential finger-tapping task resulted in increased spindle density and NREM sleep stage N2 duration [110], and overnight performance improvement positively correlated with the amount of N2 [111], no changes being observed in other stages of sleep. In a TMR study, participants exposed to an odor during motor sequence learning then re-exposed to this odor during postlearning N2 sleep improved performance (and increased sleep spindle activity) as compared to participants re-exposed to the odor during NREM sleep or not exposed at all [112]. Likewise, representation during NREM sleep periods of melodies that participants learned to play during daytime resulted in improved performance the subsequent day [113, 114]. Although reactivation during REM sleep was not tested in these latter studies, these findings indicate an important role for NREM sleep in the consolidation of procedural memories. Noticeably, a role of NREM sleep in these studies using repeated motor sequences might be explained by the involvement of hippocampus-related declarative memory components in the learning and consolidation processes [100]. Further investigations are thus needed to more clearly delineate the respective, and likely complementary, contributions of REM and NREM sleep stages. In an fMRI study [115], participants learned two different motor sequences, each being associated with different auditory tones. The tones associated with one out of the two sequences were then represented during posttraining SWS, resulting in improved performance for the cued sequence. Results also disclosed that time spent in SWS was associated with increased activity in hippocampus and bilateral caudate nucleus for the cued sequence, whereas REM sleep was linked with enhanced cerebellar and cortical motor activity. These results suggest that modulated functional activity in key cognitive and motor circuits subtend the consolidation of procedural memories and that these processes are differentially mediated by both REM and NREM sleep stages.

SLEEP AND MEMORY TRANSFORMATIONS: INSIGHT, GIST EXTRACTION, AND INFERENTIAL JUDGMENT

Besides consolidation in itself, sleep was also shown to promote generalization (e.g., abstracting regularities from specific examples to apply in future situations), reorganization (transformation of memory traces), and subsequent integration of new memories into existing knowledge networks [116]. History tells us that great scientists woke up from sleep with the solution in mind for problems they were trying to solve (e.g., Albert Einstein's equations). Comforting folk psychology that advises us sleeping on a problem to solve it, and experimental studies indicate a facilitating role of sleep in extracting rules and generalizing knowledge. For example, in one study [117], participants were trained in a numbers problem-solving task in which a sequence of operations had to be applied to reach the solution. Alternatively, however, participants could abruptly realize (i.e., have an insight) that the number at a given position in the series of numbers directly provide the solution, thus shortcutting the need for computations. Results showed that participants exposed to the task then allowed to sleep got the insight for this hidden rule two times faster than participants who did not sleep, suggesting that sleep facilitates insight and problem-solving. Similarly, sleep benefits have been reported for rule-dependent memory tasks using probabilistic learning [107, 118] musical sequences [119] and language acquisition [120]. Furthermore, cross-modal auditory-visual transfer of statistical knowledge following a 24 hour consolidation interval including sleep was positively correlated with the amount of SWS [121]. Altogether, these results suggest a facilitating role of sleep for abstracting and generalizing information. Thus, it allows accessing general rules and shortcuts leading to solve problems rehearsed during wakefulness. In this respect, sleep-dependent generalization processes may exert a positive effect on other cognitive activities such as inferential judgments and decision-making. Accordingly, the ability to make relational inference judgments derived from a set of elements with a hidden hierarchy was found to strikingly develop over time, and even more so when sleep was present during the retention episode [122]. Interestingly, sleep benefits were not correlated with subjective confidence for these judgments, indicating that inferential judgments operate below conscious awareness levels. Other studies showed that postexposure sleep facilitate inferential judgments for transitional relations between elements—for example, a face (A) associated with an object (B), which is later associated with another face (C), thus creating an indirect relation between A and C [123, 124]. Additionally, when participants must encode lists of semantically related words (e.g., DOOR, GLASS, OPEN, etc.) but are not presented with the related list's gist word (e.g., WINDOW), participants tend more to recognize the gist word as having been learned after a postlearning sleep than wake episode [125, 126]. This result reflects the associative nature of semantic memory and paradoxically indicates that sleep favors the integration of information within pre-existing networks.

COGNITIVE CHANGES ASSOCIATED WITH PRIMARY SLEEP DISORDERS

Considering that sleep in sufficient quality and quantity is required for normal cognitive functioning, any alteration of the sleep–wake equilibrium (e.g., resulting from sleep restrictions or/and sleep disorders) leads to a number of negative outcomes. Although major primary sleep disorders such as insomnia, sleep-disordered breathing (SDB), narcolepsy, and hypersomnia have different physiological causes, they all lead to sleep disturbances and fragmentations, in turn associated with cognitive impairment and difficulties to keep sufficient vigilance levels during the day. Experimental data suggest that insomnia is associated with mild to moderate impairments on specific cognitive functions [127]. For instance, individuals with insomnia exhibit worsened performance on tasks assessing working and episodic memory, attention, and problem-solving. Interestingly, performance decline in insomniac patients can be quite selective as cognitive abilities such as alertness, perceptual, and psychomotor processes; verbal functions; and general cognitive functioning may be not be significantly different form normal sleepers. These findings are in line with recent studies indicating that insomnia mostly affects performance on complex rather than simple tasks [128, 129], probably, because complex cognitive tasks heavily rely on the integrity of the PFC [130, 131], highly sensitive to the effects of SD. Similar negative cognitive outcomes are typical for SDB disorders such as the obstructive sleep apnea/hypopnea syndrome (OSAHS) characterized by recurrent episodes of partial or complete upper airway collapse during sleep, eventually resulting in sleep fragmentation and a temporary reduction in cerebral oxygenation. Meta-analytic reviews provide solid evidence that OSAHS impacts all aspects of executive functioning, including the ability to shift between tasks or mental sets, inhibition of behavioral responses, efficiently accessing semantic LTM stores and fluid reasoning or problem-solving [132]. As OSAHS is associated with frontal lobe and subcortical damage, researchers suggest that it could increase the risk of developing dementia [133]. Other disorders such as narcolepsy (characterized by the early occurrence of REM and daytime sleep attacks, particularly in monotonous situations) and hypersomnia (inability to stay awake during the day) share excessive daytime sleepiness (ESD) as a core symptom, but not due to SD, insomnia, OSAHS, or medical issues. By itself, EDS is described as persistent sleepiness and tiredness during the day even if the overnight sleep duration was sufficient. It may be a life-threatening situation as a patient can fell asleep during driving, crossing a road, or even bathing or swimming. Additionally, EDS itself might be linked to the risk of cognitive decline and /or Alzheimer's disease in the elderly population [134]. Experimental investigations revealed an executive control deficit in narcolepsy, which might be bounded to the limitation of available cognitive processing resources due to the need for continuous resources allocation for maintenance of vigilance [135]. Still, similarly to insomniacs, narcoleptic patients exhibited more deficits in demanding attention and EF tests whereas relatively routine alertness tasks were just mildly impaired. However, patients might be able to cope with complex tasks, allocating more efforts to keep up high arousal levels but in this case would perform less accurately or slower than control subjects. In the memory domain, the encoding phase is mostly affected, apparently in relation to sleep patterns disturbances and NREM sleep reduction [136]. Other higher cognitive functions such as decision-making and reward-associated behaviors are only beginning to be investigated in narcolepsy. Cognitive scarcity in narcolepsy might be explained by the fact that compensatory and task-specific processes engage the same neuronal systems, creating competition around a limited pool of resources.

To sum up, primary sleep disorders may affect normal cognitive functioning in daily life, be potentially life-threatening in specific circumstances, and be an associated factor in future cognitive decline.

CONCLUSIONS

To sum up, we have seen in this chapter that sleep closely interplays with human cognition, seen as a complex information processing system allowing us to adapt and develop appropriate behaviors in an ever-changing environment. On the one hand, adequate sleep prior to wakefulness is an essential condition for appropriate cognitive functioning. Indeed, sleep restrictions or acute SD negatively impact on key executive and attentional functions, leading to dramatic drops in our capacity to keep on high-cognitive load tasks and maintain our attentional focus and eventually accounting for difficulties in learning and decision-making abilities. On the other hand, postlearning sleep plays a crucial role for the effective consolidation of both declarative and procedural memories. Efficient sleep-dependent memory consolidation processes are subtended by a set of neurophysiological mechanisms associated both with NREM and REM sleep stages. Additionally, sleep contributes to transformational processes that may, among others, facilitate problem-solving and drawing inferences and, consequently, optimize behaviour. Finally, sleep restrictions/fragmentations as a result of SD/sleep-related disorders may significantly affect cognitive functions and quality of life, potentially increasing the risk of development neurodegenerative disorders and dementia.

FUTURE DIRECTIONS

In this chapter, we have rapidly touched upon the vast amount of research investigating the relationships between sleep and various cognitive processes. Sleep restrictions due to a fast-paced modern life's rhythm take a toll on normal cognitive functioning and may, for instance, lead to productivity drops and potentially serious errors at the working place. Primary sleep disorders, in turn, are breaking down our normal sleep patterns, resulting in numerous cognitive and behavioral abnormalities. Future research is required to precisely understand the mechanisms and associations involved in the relations between sleep and cognition. Additionally, the relationships between the physiology of recovery (compensatory) sleep and the restoration of cognitive functions are still vastly understudied. Further studies in this direction would help to develop sleep treatment techniques and methods for recuperation from sleep-related symptoms during daytime, measurably enhancing daytime cognitive efficiency, which in turn may provide a similar wealth of benefits for subsequent sleep.

ACKNOWLEDGMENTS

LR was supported by a PhD Research Grant "Mini-ARC" from the Université Libre de Bruxelles (ULB), Belgium, and is currently a Research Fellow at the Belgian Fonds de la Recherche Scientifique (FRS-FNRS).

KEY CLINICAL PEARLS

- Inappropriate sleep quality and quantity negatively impacts cognitive control functions not only by complicating everyday tasks but also by endangering one's life s as well as the lives of people around them.
- Proper sleep hygiene practices should be reviewed with people experiencing sleep issues, including avoidance of late caffeine, establishing an appropriate sleep environment (dark, cool, and no electronic devices), setting sleep-onset and sleep-offset times to allow for decent sleep, etc.
- Timely diagnostic and treatment of sleep problems is paramount to help improving the patient's live, and reduce negative outcomes in the future.

SELF-ASSESSMENT QUESTIONS

1. Sleep deprivation impacts executive functions as follows:
   a. Increased time-on-task effect and micro sleep events due to impaired circadian drive.
   b. Improved responsiveness, time-on-task and homeostatic drive effects.
   c. Global slowing and impaired inhibition due to reduced top–down control abilities.
   d. Systematic deficits in short-duration cognitively demanding tasks.

Answer: c

2. According to the active system consolidation hypothesis, the sleep-dependent consolidation of declarative memory relies on
   a. hippocampus-cerebellar dialogue under top down control of slow oscillations.
   b. hippocampal-neocortical dialogue under top down control of slow oscillations.
   c. medial temporal lobe activation associated with increased spindles density in REM sleep.

   d. modifications in the striato-cerebellar system

Answer: b

3. Sleep-dependent consolidation for declarative memory mostly benefits from post-training sleep periods spent in
   a. only SWS.
   b. only S2.
   c. only S2 and SWS.
   d. mostly NREM (S2 and SWS), but a role for REM sleep cannot be excluded.

Answer: d

4. Which of the following statements is true?
   a. Sleep protects recent memories from interference by promoting offline consolidation processes.
   b. Motor memories are strengthened in wakefulness and sleep plays no passive role in their consolidation.
   c. Targeted memory reactivation during sleep weakens cued memories.
   d. Consolidation of complex motor tasks relies on NREM sleep only, whereas simple motor tasks are consolidated at wake.

Answer: a

5. The mechanisms underlying accelerated insight after sleep are likely due to
   a. conscious rumination during the N1 sleep phase.
   b. transformations of memory traces and creation of "false memories."
   c. abstraction and generalization of information during sleep.
   d. creation of conflicting representations during REM sleep.

Answer: c

REFERENCES

1. Hirshkowitz M, Whiton K, Albert S, et al. National Sleep Foundation's sleep time duration recommendations: methodology and results summary. *Sleep Health*. 2015;1:40–43.
2. Peigneux P, Leproult R. The functions of sleep. In: Bassetti C, Dogas, Peigneux P, ed. *Sleep Medicine*. Regensburg, Germany: European Sleep Research Society;2014:39–48.
3. Hughes C, Jaffee SR, Happé F, Taylor A, Caspi A, Moffitt TE. Origins of individual differences in theory of mind: from nature to nurture? *Child Development*. 2005;76(2):356–370.

4. Collins A, Koechlin E. Reasoning, learning, and creativity: frontal lobe function and human decision-making. *PLoS Biol.* 2012;10(3):e1001293.
5. Lunt L, Bramham J, Morris RG, et al. Prefrontal cortex dysfunction and "jumping to conclusions": bias or deficit? *Neuropsychol.* 2012 6(1):65–78.
6. Friedman NP, Miyake A. Unity and diversity of executive functions: individual differences as a window on cognitive structure. *Cortex.* 2017;86:186–204.
7. Borbely A A, Daan S, Wirz-Justice A, Deboer, T. The two-process model of sleep regulation: a reappraisal. *J Sleep Res.* 2016;25(2):131–143.
8. Cajochen C, Knoblauch V, Kräuchi K, Renz C, Wirz-Justice A. Dynamics of frontal EEG activity, sleepiness and body temperature under high and low sleep pressure. *Neuroreport.* 2001;12(10):2277–2281.
9. Finelli LA, Baumann H, Borbély AA, Achermann P. Dual electroencephalogram markers of human sleep homeostasis: correlation between theta activity in waking and slow-wave activity in sleep. *Neuroscience.* 2000;101(3):523–529.
10. Wu JC, Christian JG, Buchsbaum MS, et al. Frontal lobe metabolic decreases with sleep deprivation not totally reversed by recovery sleep. *Neuropsychopharmacology.* 2006;31:2783–2792.
11. Cui J, Tkachenko O, Gogel H., et al. Microstructure of frontoparietal connections predicts individual resistance to sleep deprivation. *Neuroimage.* 2015;106:123–133.
12. Bjorklund DF, Harnishfeger KK. The evolution of inhibition mechanisms and their role in human cognition and behavior. In: Dempster FN, Brainerd CJ, ed. *Interference and Inhibition in Cognition.* San Diego: Academic Press; 1995:142–173.
13. Barkley RA. Behavioral inhibition, sustained attention, and executive functions: Constructing a unifying theory of ADHD. *Psychological Bulletin.* 1997;121(1):65–94.
14. Trommer BL, Hoeppner JA, Lorber R, Armstrong KJ. The go-no-go paradigm in attention deficit disorder. *Ann Neurol.* 1988;24(5):610–614.
15. Logan GD, Cowan WB, Davis KA. On the ability to inhibit simple and choice reaction time responses: a model and a method. *J Exp Psychol Hum Percept Perform.* 1984;10(2):276–291.
16. Logan, GD. On the ability to inhibit thought and: A users guide to the stop signal paradigm. In Dagenbach D, Carr TH, ed. *Inhibitory processes in attention, memory, and language* San Diego, CA: Academic Press;1994:189–239.
17. Anderson C, Platten CR. Sleep deprivation lowers inhibition and enhances impulsivity to negative stimuli. *Behav Brain Res.* 2011;217:463–466.
18. Drummond SP, Paulus MP, Tapert SF J. Effects of two nights sleep deprivation and two nights recovery sleep on response inhibition. *Sleep Res.* 2006;15(3):261–265.
19. Sagaspe P, Sanchez-Ortuno M, Charles A, et al. Brain effects of sleep deprivation on Color-Word, Emotional, and Specific Stroop interference and on self-reported anxiety. *Brain Cogn.* 2006;60(1):76–87.
20. Cain SW, Silva EJ, Chang A-M, Ronda JM, Duffy JF. One night of sleep deprivation affects reaction time, but not interference or facilitation in a Stroop task. *Brain and Cognition.* 2011;76(1):37–42.
21. Gevers W, Deliens G, Hoffmann S, Notebaert W, Peigneux P. Sleep deprivation selectively disrupts top-down adaptation to cognitive conflict in the Stroop test. *J Sleep Res.* 2015;24(6):666–672.
22. Konishi S, Nakajima K, Uchida I, et al. Transient activation of inferior prefrontal cortex during cognitive set shifting. *Nat Neurosci.* 1998;1(1):80–84.
23. Garavan H, Ross TJ, Stein EA. Right hemispheric dominance of inhibitory control: an event-related functional MRI study. *Proc Natl Acad Sci U S A.* 1999;96(14):8301–8306.
24. Garavan H, Ross TJ, Kaufman J, Stein EA. A midline dissociation between error-processing and response-conflict monitoring. *Neuroimage.* 2003;20(2):1132–1139.
25. Hester R, Foxe JJ, Molholm S, Shpaner M, Garavan H. Neural mechanisms involved in error processing: A comparison of errors made with and without awareness. *NeuroImage.* 2005;27(3):602–608.
26. Fan J, McCandliss BD, Fossella J, Flombaum JI, Posner MI. The activation of attentional networks. *NeuroImage.* 2005; 26(2):471–479.
27. Aron AR, Robbins TW, Poldrack RA. Inhibition and the right inferior frontal cortex. *Trends Cogn Sci.* 2004;8(4):170–177.
28. MacDonald AW, Cohen JD, Stenger VA, Carter CS. Dissociating the role of the dorsolateral prefrontal and anterior cingulate cortex in cognitive control. *Science.* 2000;288(5472):1835–1838.
29. Banich MT, Milham MP, Atchley R, fMri studies of Stroop tasks reveal unique roles of anterior and posterior brain systems in attentional selection. *J Cogn Neurosci.* 2000;12(6):988–1000.
30. Lim J, Dingers D. Sleep deprivation and vigilant attention. *Ann. N.Y. Acad. Sci.* 2008;1129:305–322.
31. Dinges, DF, Powell, JW. Microcomputer analyses of performance on a portable, simple visual RT task during sustained operations. *Behav Res Methods Instr Computers.* 1985;17:652–655.
32. Van Dongen HP, Maislin G, Mullington JM, Dinges DF. The cumulative cost of additional wakefulness: dose-response effects on neurobehavioral functions and sleep physiology from

chronic sleep restriction and total sleep deprivation. *Sleep.* 2003;26(2):117–126.

33. Wyatt JK, Ritz-De Cecco A, Czeisler CA, Dijk DJ. Circadian temperature and melatonin rhythms, sleep, and neurobehavioral function in humans living on a 20-h day. *Am J Physiol.* 1999;277(4 Pt 2):R1152–R1163.

34. Doran SM, Van Dongen HP, Dinges DF. Sustained attention performance during sleep deprivation: evidence of state instability. *Arch Ital Biol.* 2001;139(3):253–267.

35. Lim J, Dinges DF. A meta-analysis of the impact of short-term sleep deprivation on cognitive variables. *Psychol Bull.* 2010;136(3):375–389.

36. Thomas M, Sing H, Belenky G. Neural basis of alertness and cognitive performance impairments during sleepiness. I. Effects of 24 h of sleep deprivation on waking human regional brain activity. *Journal of Sleep Research.* 2000;9:335–352.

37. Sarter M, Givens B, Bruno J. The cognitive neuroscience of sustained attention: where top-down meets bottom-up. *Brain Research Reviews.* 2001;35(2):146–160.

38. Drummond SP, Bischoff-Grethe A, Dinges DF, Ayalon L, Mednick SC, Meloy MJ. The neural basis of the psychomotor vigilance task. *Sleep.* 2005;28:1059–1068.

39. Muto V, Shaffii-le Bourdiec A, Matarazzo L, et al. Influence of acute sleep loss on the neural correlates of alerting, orientating and executive attention components. *J Sleep Res.* 2012;(6):648–658.

40. Chee MW, Tan JC, Parimal S, Zagorodnov V. Sleep deprivation and its effects on object-selective attention. *NeuroImage.* 2010;49(2):1903–1910.

41. Kong DY, Soon CS, Chee MWL. Functional imaging correlates of impaired distractor suppression following sleep deprivation. *NeuroImage.* 2012;61:50–55.

42. Jackson ML, Hughes ME, Croft RJ, et al. The effect of sleep deprivation on BOLD activity elicited by a divided attention task. *Brain Imaging Behav.* 2011;5(2):97–108.

43. Mander BA, Reid KJ, Davuluri VK, et al. Sleep deprivation alters functioning within the neural network underlying the covert orienting of attention. *Brain Res.* 2008;1217:148–156.

44. Krause AJ, Simon EB, Mander BA, et al. The sleep-deprived human brain. *Nature Rev. Neurosci.* 2017;18:404–418.

45. Baddeley A. Working memory: theories, models, and controversies. *Annu Rev Psychol.* 2012;63:1–29.

46. Kiyonaga A, Egner T. Working memory as internal attention: toward an integrative account of internal and external selection processes. *Psychon Bull Rev.* 2013;20(2): 228–242.

47. Smith ME, McEvoy LK, Gevins A. The impact of moderate sleep loss on neurophysiologic signals during working-memory task performance. *Sleep.* 2002; 25(7):784–794.

48. Angel J, Cortez J, Juárez J, et al. Effects of sleep reduction on the phonological and visuospatial components of working memory. *Sleep Sci.* 2015;8(2):68–74.

49. Lo JC, Groeger J, Santhi N, et al. Effects of partial and acute total sleep deprivation on performance across cognitive domains, individuals and circadian phase. *PLoS One.* 2012;7(9):e45987.

50. Drummond SP, Anderson DE, Straus LD, Vogel EK, Perez VB. The effects of two types of sleep deprivation on visual working memory capacity and filtering efficiency. *PLoS One.* 2012;7(4):e35653.

51. Chee MW, Chuah LY, Venkatraman V, Chan WY, Philip P, Dinges DF. Functional imaging of working memory following normal sleep and after 24 and 35 h of sleep deprivation: correlations of fronto-parietal activation with performance. *NeuroImage.* 2006;31:419–428.

52. Chee MW, Choo WC. Functional imaging of working memory after 24 hr of total sleep deprivation. *J Neurosci.* 2004;24(19):4560–4567.

53. Choo WC, Lee WW, Venkatraman V, Sheu FS, Chee MW. Dissociation of cortical regions modulated by both working memory load and sleep deprivation and by sleep deprivation alone. *NeuroImage.* 2005;25(2):579–587.

54. Bell-McGinty S, Habeck C, Hilton HJ, et al. Identification and differential vulnerability of a neural network in sleep deprivation. *Cereb. Cortex.* 2004;14:496–502.

55. Chengyang L, Daqing H, Jianlin Q, Short-term memory deficits correlate with hippocampal-thalamic functional connectivity alterations following acute sleep restriction. *Brain Imaging Behav.* 2017;(4):954–963.

56. Albouy G, Sterpenich V, Vandewalle G, et al. Interaction between hippocampal and striatal systems predicts subsequent consolidation of motor sequence memory. *PLoS ONE.* 2013;8(3):e59490.

57. Peigneux P, Fogel S, Smith C. Memory processing in relation to sleep. In Kryger M, Roth T, ed. *Principles and Practice of Sleep Medicine.* 6th ed. Philadelphia: Elsevier; 2015:229–238.

58. Van Der Werf YD, Altena E., Schoonheim MM, et al. Sleep benefits subsequent hippocampal functioning. *Nat Neurosci.* 2009;12(2):122–123.

59. Alberca-Reina E, Cantero JL, Atienza M. Impact of sleep loss before learning on cortical

dynamics during memory retrieval. *NeuroImage.* 2015;123: 51–62.

60. Diekelmann S, Born J. The memory function of sleep. *Nature Rev. Neurosci.* 2010;11:114–126.

61. Hasselmo ME. Neuromodulation: acetylcholine and memory consolidation. *Trends in Cognitive Sciences.* 1999;3(9):351–359.

62. Buzsaki G. The hippocampo-neocortical dialogue. *Cerebral Cortex.*1996;6(2): 81–92.

63. Rasch B, Born J. About sleep's role in memory. Physiol Rev. 2013;93(2):681–766.

64. Alger SE, Lau H, Fishbein W. Slow wave sleep during a daytime nap is necessary for protection from subsequent interference and long-term retention. *Neurobiol Learn Mem.* 2012;98:188–96.

65. Diekelmann S, Biggel S, Rasch B, Born J. Offline consolidation of memory varies with time in slow wave sleep and can be accelerated by cuing memory reactivations. *Neurobiol Learn Mem.* 2012;98:103–11.

66. Marshall L, Mölle M, Hallschmid M, Born J. Transcranial direct current stimulation during sleep improves declarative memory. *J Neurosci.* 2004;24(44):9985–9992.

67. Marshall L, Helgadóttir H, Mölle M, Born J. Boosting slow oscillations during sleep potentiates memory. *Nature.* 2006;444:610–613.

68. Van Der Werf YD, Altena E, Schoonheim MM, et al. Sleep benefits subsequent hippocampal functioning. *Nat Neurosci.* 2009;12:122–123.

69. Ngo HV, Martinetz T, Born J, Mölle M. Auditory closed-loop stimulation of the sleep slow oscillation enhances memory. *Neuron.* 2013;78(3):545–553.

70. Schreiner T, Rasch B. Boosting vocabulary learning by verbal cueing during sleep. *Cerebral Cortex.* 2015; 25(11):4169–4179.

71. Breton J, Robertson EM. Memory processing: the critical role of neuronal replay during sleep. *Curr. Biol.* 2013;23(18):836–838.

72. Rasch B, Büchel C, Gais S, Born J. Odor cues during slow-wave sleep prompt declarative memory consolidation. *Science.* 2007;315(5817):1426–1429.

73. Diekelmann S, Büchel C, Born J, Rasch B. Labile or stable: opposing consequences for memory when reactivated during waking and sleep. *Nat Neurosci.* 2011;14(3):381–386.

74. Rihm JS, Diekelmann S, Born J, Rasch B. Reactivating memories during sleep by odors: odor specificity and associated changes in sleep oscillations. *J Cogn Neurosci.* 2014;26(8):1806–1818.

75. Farthouat J, Gilson M, Peigneux P. New evidence for the necessity of a silent plastic period during sleep for a memory benefit of targeted memory reactivation. *Sleep Spindles & Cortical Up States.* 2017;1(1):14–26.

76. Schreiner T, Lehmann M, Rasch B. Auditory feedback blocks memory benefits of cueing during sleep. *Nat Commun.* 2015;6:8729.

77. Peigneux P, Laureys S, Fuchs S, et al. Are spatial memories strengthened in the human hippocampus during slow wave sleep? *Neuron.* 2004;44(3):535–545.

78. Peigneux P, Orban P, Balteau E, et al. Offline persistence of memory-related cerebral activity during active wakefulness. *PLoS Biol.* 2006;4(4):e100.

79. Clegga BA, DiGirolamob GJ, Keelea SW. Sequence learning. *Trends in Cognitive Sciences.* 1998;2(8):275–281.

80. Karni A, Sagi D. The time course of learning a visual skill. *Nature.* 1993;365(6443):250–252.

81. Karni A, Meyer G, Rey-Hipolito C. The acquisition of skilled motor performance: Fast and slow experience-driven changes in primary motor cortex. *PNAS.* 1998;95(3):861–868.

82. Gais S, Plihal W, Wagner, Born J. Early sleep triggers memory for early visual discrimination skills. Nat Neurosci. 2000;3:1335–1339.

83. Schonauer M, Gratsch M, Gais S. Evidence for two distinct sleep-related long-term memory consolidation processes. *Cortex.* 2015;63: 68–78.

84. Korman M, Doyon J, Doljansky J, Carrier J, Dagan Y, Karni A. Daytime sleep condenses the time course of motor memory consolidation. *Nat Neurosci.* 2007;10(9):1206–1213.

85. Nishida M, Walker MP. Daytime naps, motor memory consolidation and regionally specific sleep spindles. *PLoS ONE.* 2007;2:e341.

86. PereiracSI, Beijamini F, Vincenzi RA, Louzada FM. Re-examining sleep's effect on motor skills: How to access performance on the finger tapping task? *Sleep Sci.* 2015;8(1):4–8.

87. Albouy G, King BR, Schmidt C, et al. Cerebral activity associated with transient sleep-facilitated reduction in motor memory vulnerability to interference. *Sci Rep.* 2016;6:34948.

88. Sugawara SK, Koike T, Kawamichi H, et al. Qualitative differences in offline improvement of procedural memory by daytime napping and overnight sleep: An fMRI study. *Neurosci Res.* 2018;132:37–45.

89. Censor N, Sagi D, Cohen LG. Common mechanisms of human perceptual and motor learning. *Nat Rev Neurosci.* 2012;13(9):658–664.

90. Karni A, Meyer G, Jezzard P, et al. Functional MRI evidence for adult motor cortex plasticity during motor skill learning. *Nature.* 1995;377(6545):155–158.

91. Robertson EM, Press DZ, Pascual-Leone A. Off-line learning and the primary motor cortex. *Journal of Neuroscience.* 2005;25(27):6372–6378.

92. Doyon J, Benali H. Reorganization and plasticity in the adult human brain during learning of motor skills. *Curr Opin Neurobiol.* 2005;15:161–7.

93. Hikosaka O, Nakamura H, Sakai K, Nakahara H. Central mechanisms of motor skill learning. *Curr Opin Neurobiol.* 2002;12:217–22.

94. Shadmehr R, Krakauer J. A computational neuroanatomy for motor control. *Exp Brain Res.* 2008;185:359–81.

95. Penhune BV, Steele CJ. Parallel contributions of cerebellar, striatal and M1 mechanisms to motor sequence learning, *Behav Brain Res.* 2012;226(2):579–591.

96. Doyon J, Bellec P, Amsel R, et al. Contributions of the basal ganglia and functionally related brain structures to motor learning. *Behav Brain Res.* 2009;199:61–75.

97. Henke. K. A model for memory systems based on processing modes rather than consciousness. *Nat Rev Neurosci.* 2010;(7):523–532.

98. Cabeza R, Moscovitch M. Memory systems, processing modes, and components: functional neuroimaging evidence. *PNAS.* 2013;8(1):49–55.

99. Schendan HE, Searl MM, Melrose RJ, Stern CE. An FMRI study of the role of the medial temporal lobe in implicit and explicit sequence learning. *Neuron.* 2003;37:1013–1025.

100. Albouy GV, Sterpenich V, Balteau E, et al. Both the hippocampus and striatum are involved in consolidation of motor sequence memory. *Neuron.* 2008;58(2):261–272.

101. Albouy G, Fogel S, King BR. Maintaining vs. enhancing motor sequence memories: Respective roles of striatal and hippocampal systems. *NeuroImage.* 2015,108:423–434.

102. Ben-Yakov A, Dudai Y. Constructing realistic engrams: poststimulus activity of hippocampus and dorsal striatum predicts subsequent episodic memory. *J Neurosci.* 2011;31(24):9032–9042.

103. Reber PJ. The neural basis of implicit learning and memory: A review of neuropsychological and neuroimaging research. *Neuropsychologia.* 2013;51(10):2026–2042.

104. Peigneux P, Laureys S, Delbeuck X, Maquet P. Sleeping brain, learning brain. The role of sleep for memory systems. *Neuroreport.* 2001;12(18):A111–A124.

105. Plihal W, Born J. Effects of early and late nocturnal sleep on declarative and procedural memory. *J Cogn Neurosci.* 1997;9(4):534–547.

106. Maquet P, Laureys S, Peigneux P, et al. Experience-dependent changes in cerebral activation during human REM sleep. *Nat Neurosci.* 2003;(8):831–836.

107. Peigneux P, Laureys S, Fuchs S, et al. Learned material content and acquisition level modulate cerebral reactivation during posttraining rapid-eye-movements sleep. *NeuroImage.* 2003;20(1):125–134.

108. Fischer S, Hallschmid M, Elsner AL, Born J. Sleep forms memory for finger skills. *PNAS.* 2002;99(18):11987–11991.

109. Rasch B, Gais S, Born J. Impaired off-line consolidation of motor memories after combined blockade of cholinergic receptors during REM sleep-rich sleep. *Neuropsychopharmacology.* 2009;34:1843–53.

110. Fogel SM, Smith C. Learning-dependent changes in sleep spindles and Stage 2 sleep. *J Sleep Res.* 2006;15(3):250–255.

111. Walker MP, Brakefield T, Morgan A, Hobson JA, Stickgold R. Practice with sleep makes perfect sleep-dependent motor skill learning. *Neuron.* 2002; 35(1):205–211.

112. Laventure S, Fogel S, Lungu O, et al. NREM2 and sleep spindles are instrumental to the consolidation of motor sequence memories. *PLoS Biol.* 2016;14(3):e1002429.

113. Schönauer M, Geisler T, Gais S. Strengthening procedural memories by reactivation in sleep. *J Cogn Neurosci.* 2014;26(1):143–153.

114. Antony JW, Gobel EW, O'Hare JK, Reber PJ, Paller KA. Cued memory reactivation during sleep influences skill learning. *Nat Neurosci.* 2012;15:1114–6.

115. Cousins JN, El-Deredy W, Parkes LM, Hennies N, Lewis PA. Cued reactivation of motor learning during sleep leads to overnight changes in functional brain activity and connectivity. *PLoS Biol.* 2016;14(5):e1002451.

116. Stickgold R, Walker MP. Sleep-dependent memory triage: evolving generalization through selective processing. *Nat Neurosci.* 2013;16(2):139–145.

117. Wagner U, Gais S, Haider H, Verleger R, Born J. Sleep inspires insight. *Nature.* 2004;(427):352–355.

118. Fischer S, Drosopoulos S, Tsen J, Born J. Implicit learning—explicit knowing: a role for sleep in memory system interaction. *J Cogn Neurosci.* 2006;18(3):311–319.

119. Durrant SJ, Taylor C, Cairney S, Lewis PA. Sleep-dependent consolidation of statistical learning. *Neuropsychologia.* 2011;49(5):1322–1331.

120. Batterink LJ, Oudiette D, Reber PJ, Paller KA. Sleep facilitates learning a new linguistic rule. *Neuropsychologia.* 2014;65:169–179.

121. Durrant SJ, Cairney SA, Lewis PA. Cross-modal transfer of statistical information benefits from sleep. *Cortex.* 2016; 78:85–99.

122. Ellenbogen JM, Hu PT, Payne JD, Titone D, Walker MP. Human relational memory requires time and sleep. *PNAS.* 2007;104(18):7723–7728.

123. Lau EY, Eskes GA, Morrison DL, Rajda M, Spurr KF. Executive function in patients with obstructive sleep apnea treated with continuous positive airway pressure. *J Int Neuropsychol Soc.* 2010;16(6):1077–1088.

124. Alger SE, Payne JD. The differential effects of emotional salience on direct associative and relational memory during a nap. *Cogn Affect Behav Neurosci.* 2016;16(6):za1150–1163.

125. Payne JD, Schacter DL, Propper RE, et al. The role of sleep in false memory formation. *Neurobiol Learn Mem.* 2009;92(3):327–334.

126. McKeon S, Pace-Schott EF, Spencer RM. Interaction of sleep and emotional content on the production of false memories. *PLoS ONE.* 2012;7(11):e49353.

127. Fortier-Brochu E, Beaulieu-Bonneau S, Ivers H, et al. Insomnia and daytime cognitive performance: A meta-analysis. *Sleep Medicine Reviews.* 2012;16:83e94.

128. Altena E, Van Der Werf YD, Strijers RL, et al. Sleep loss affects vigilance: effects of chronic insomnia and sleep therapy. *J Sleep Res.* 2008;17(3):335e43.

129. Edinger JD, Means MK, Carney CE, Krystal AD. Psychomotor performance deficits and their relation to prior nights' sleep among individuals with primary insomnia. *Sleep.* 2008;31(5):599e607.

130. Braver TS, Barch DM, Kelley WM, et al. Direct comparison of prefrontal cortex regions engaged by working and long term memory tasks. *Neuroimage.* 2001;14(1 Pt 1):48e59.

131. Unterrainer JM, Rahm B, Kaller CP, et al. When planning fails: individual differences and error-related brain activity in problem solving. *Cerebral Cortex.* 2004;14:1390e7.

132. Olaithe M, Bucks RS. Executive dysfunction in OSA before and after treatment: a meta-analysis. *Sleep.* 2013; 36:1297–305.

133. Jaussent I, Bouyer J, Ancelin M, et al. Excessive Sleepiness is Predictive of Cognitive Decline in the Elderly. *Sleep.* 2012;35:9:1201–1207.

134. Bubu OM, Brannick M, Mortimer J. Sleep, cognitive impairment, and Alzheimer's disease: a systematic review and meta-analysis. *Sleep.* 2017; 40(1) zsw032.

135. Naumann A, Bellebaum C, Daum I. Cognitive deficits in narcolepsy. *Send to J Sleep Res.* 2006;15(3):329–338.

136. Aguirre, M., Broughton, R. and Stuss, D. Does memory impairment exist in narcolepsy-cataplexy. *J. Clin. Exp. Neuropsychol.*, 1985;7:14–24.

6

Office-Based Evaluation of Sleep Disordered Patients

KARL DOGHRAMJI

INTRODUCTION

As in other disciplines, the history and examination are the cornerstones of the sleep-related evaluation. Various guidelines have been proposed for history-taking in sleep disorders.[1,2] This chapter will present a systematic approach to the psychiatric patient with sleep-related complaints. To a large extent, these are consistent with recommendations of major publications in the field.

The chief complaint determines, in large part, the specific questions and areas of exploration. The complaint generally falls within the realm of insomnia, excessive daytime sleepiness, or parasomnias. However, in addition to the complaint-related historical questions, there are components of a sleep history that should be ascertained in all patients with any sleep-related complaint. It is useful, for example to construct a 24 hour pattern of the patient's sleep/wake activities beginning with the time and activities occurring before a patient prepares for bed, followed by bedtime, sleep latency, occurrences during the night, wake time, time out of bed, daytime symptoms, patterns, and activities (including naps), and then concluding back at the time at which the inquiry began. Once the typical pattern is established, deviations (e.g., sleeping in late on the weekends) can also be determined. Other important parameters include

1. Bedtime;
2. Sleep latency (time to fall asleep after lights out);
3. Nocturnal awakenings; number and duration;
4. Time of final morning awakening;
5. Rising time (i.e., time out of bed);
6. Number, time, and duration of daytime naps; and
7. Daytime symptoms including levels of sleepiness and fatigue over the course of the day

These patterns can also be assessed with sleep logs or diaries that track sleep–wake patterns over time. The following sections pertain to the clinical approach for each of the three cardinal presenting symptoms of sleep disorders.

INSOMNIA

Insomnia is a repeated difficulty with sleep initiation, duration, consolidation, or quality that occurs despite adequate opportunity for sleep and results in some form of daytime impairment.[3] From the standpoint of diagnosis and treatment, it is important to identify the portions of the time spent in bed (beginning, middle, or end) that are affected.

The time of onset and duration of symptoms also should be determined. Insomnia of long duration is thought to have greater impact on daytime functioning. Although such beliefs seem to be clinically supported, they have yet to be confirmed by systematic studies. Additionally, there is considerable variability in the definition of the time course for acute and long-term insomnia, with acute insomnia generally defined as lasting less than 30 days, yet minimum durations for chronic insomnia ranging from 30 days to 6 months.[4]

The longitudinal pattern of insomnia is also an important component of the history. Symptoms of insomnia typically change over the passage of time, as a complaint of initial insomnia, for example, can progress after years or months into one of a difficulty in sleep maintenance, with the nature of symptoms changing over the course of 4 months in majority of patients with insomnia.[5] The temporal relationship between insomnia and comorbid illnesses can also indicate what factors may have caused insomnia and provide a basis for treatment.

The frequency of nights affected per week or month during each episode can be a useful indicator of severity. Approximately a quarter of insomniacs suffer from the disturbance occasionally, and 9% report having it on a frequent basis; insomnia episodes typically lasted 4.7 days. Patients with chronic insomnia report that sleep problems affect over half of the nights in an average month (16.4 days).[6]

Precipitants of the insomnia complaint need to be determined. These can include job loss, engaging in shift work or travel across time zones, breaches in relationships or loss of relatives, onset of medical and psychiatric illness, and introduction of new medications or changes in dosages and times of administration of existing medications, among others. Medications likely to precipitate insomnia in psychiatric practice are antidepressants and stimulants, among others. Perpetuating factors of insomnia should also be identified. Following the onset of insomnia, these factors can transform insomnia into a chronic disorder. They include the development of poor sleep hygiene practices and anticipatory anxiety with the approach of bedtime. From the standpoint of future treatment, it is additionally useful to understand the type of interventions that have already been attempted for insomnia and the effectiveness and side effects of each of these.

Daytime Symptoms

Insomnia can have a profound impact on daytime functioning, with the severity of daytime symptoms generally co-varying with the degree of impairment in the quality and quantity in nocturnal sleep. Although patients with insomnia generally obtain less sleep, as compared to individuals without complaints of insomnia, they usually do not have an exaggerated tendency to fall asleep during the day, unlike their excessively sleepy counterparts. In fact, most patients with insomnia complain that they are unable to fall asleep during attempts at napping as well as during multiple sleep latency testing.[7] The inability to fall asleep during day in patients with insomnia is thought to be a correlate of hyperarousal in multiple biological and psychological systems including cognition, the hypothalamic pituitary axis, sympathetic nervous system, metabolic rate, and electroencephalographic frequency. Patients with insomnia exhibit faster electroencephalography (EEG) frequencies during sleep than healthy controls. Insomnia should also be distinguished from sleep deprivation or curtailment, where decrements in nocturnal sleep duration are directly related to the tendency to fall asleep during the day (i.e., the level of daytime sleepiness).

Despite these findings, patients with insomnia do more frequently report a variety of daytime psychological symptoms, including feeling depressed, hopeless, helpless, worried, tense, anxious, irritable, lonely, and lacking in self-confidence, than do control subjects.[8] Individuals with insomnia also report feeling tired, physically fatigued, anergic, and unmotivated. They also report cognitive difficulties such as memory impairment, difficulty with focus and attention, and mental slowing. Patients with insomnia can also report impairments in coping, accomplishing tasks, and maintaining family and social relationships and occupational function.[3]

Inventories can assist in the quantification of the severity of insomnia; although many are available, the Insomnia Severity Index (ISI)[9] is the most widely utilized screening tool that takes into account subjective symptoms and consequences of insomnia and the degree of concern or distress caused by the sleep disturbance.

Daytime Behaviors

Daytime behaviors can adversely affect nocturnal sleep and aggravate insomnia and should be systematically explored. Intense exercise too close to bedtime can disrupt sleep.[10] Long periods of bedrest, inactivity, and excessive napping can foment circadian rhythm disturbances and aggravate insomnia. Exposure to bright light close to bedtime can delay sleep onset, potentially further aggravating an insomnia characterized by a prolonged sleep latency. Circadian cycling can also be affected in the same disruptive way by lack of sufficient light exposure during the morning hours. Frequent travel and shift work can also disrupt sleep and contribute to both insomnia and daytime sleepiness.

Sleep-Related Behaviors and Cognitions

Typical behaviors during the few hours prior to bedtime, during bedtime hours, and just after morning awakening can cause or significantly intensify existing insomnia. These include caffeine and alcohol consumption prior to bedtime, large meals or excessive fluid intake within 3 hours of bedtime, exercising within 3 hours of bedtime, staying in bed while awake for extended periods of time, clock-watching prior to sleep onset or during nocturnal awakenings, exposure to bright light prior to bedtime or during awakenings, keeping the bedroom too hot or too cold, and excessive noise, among others.

Dysfunctional beliefs and attitudes can perpetuate and exacerbate insomnia. Therefore, information about the dysfunctional cognitions of patients with insomnia such as catastrophic attributions of the effects of insomnia, the time of day that they begin to worry about sleep, and their state of mind while awake during the night should all be inquired in detail.

Sleep Patterns

Ideally, individuals retire and emerge from bed at consistent times day to day, including weekends. The time spent in bed between retiring and falling asleep would preferably be less than 20 minutes, and individuals would emerge from bed soon after awakening in the morning. Additionally, awakenings in good sleepers are typically limited to one or two, and time spent in bed following awakenings kept to a minimum (i.e. less than 15 minutes). Of note, these variables may be affected by age.[11] In the elderly, it is not unusual to find more than five awakenings per night; the complaint most commonly ascribed to these awakenings is nocturia.

In delayed sleep phase disorder, the time of falling asleep and the time of awakening are consistently delayed, and in advanced sleep phase disorder, the sleep-onset times are consistently advanced, relative to the desired night/day schedule. Multiple nocturnal awakenings and prolonged sleep latencies are not specific for any one disorder, yet keeping track of these parameters can help to quantify the severity of insomnia and determining the effectiveness of treatment measures. Determining these patterns can also suggest the utility of certain behavioral and pharmacological interventions to improve sleep, such as restriction of overall time spent in bed. The assessment of variability between workdays/schooldays, weekends, and vacations can also be useful. Patients with insomnia characteristically do not maintain rigorous sleep/wake schedules, and introducing such regularity into their lives is one of the primary elements of sleep hygiene education and other cognitive-behavioral techniques.[10]

EXCESSIVE SLEEPINESS

Sleepiness, the tendency to fall asleep, is a normal phenomenon when it occurs at the desired time of the day. Excessive sleepiness (ES) is the tendency to fall asleep at inappropriate times or settings.[3]

ES should be distinguished from fatigue, which is classically defined as the inability to sustain performance over time and is typically associated with subjective reports of tiredness, weariness, exhaustion, and lack of energy.[12] Fatigue is a symptom of a wide variety of medical, psychiatric, and neurological disorders such as multiple sclerosis, autoimmune disorders, and psychiatric conditions.

The age of onset, temporal pattern, duration, and daily pattern of ES should be determined. ES onset in early life is more consistent with narcolepsy, whereas onset in middle age is more consistent with obstructive sleep apnea (OSA). ES that is episodic over time is consistent with periods of sleep restriction due to social and occupational needs. However, ES that is constant and unremitting may be more consistent with narcolepsy, OSA, or potentially affective disorders. ES that is most prominent in the morning hours, especially when accompanied by a prolonged sleep latency and complaint of initiation insomnia, can be due to delayed sleep phase syndrome, whereas ES that is most prominent in the late evening hours and associated with early morning awakening can be due to advanced sleep phase syndrome. ES that is most prominent in the morning hours and gradually resolves as the day progresses is also consistent with the carryover effects of a sedating bedtime medication. Afternoon sleepiness is commonly associated with disturbances of the quality and quantity of nocturnal sleep, and the extent of sleepiness in the afternoon is proportional to the extent of these disturbances.

The severity of ES needs to be quantified. Rating one's perceived level of sleepiness on a numerical scale, the approach utilized by the Stanford Sleepiness Scale,[13] has greater validity and reliability than direct questioning regarding how sleepy an individual feels. Behavioral indicators of ES can also be useful, such as yawning, ptosis, reduced activity, lapses in attention, and head nodding. The patient can also be questioned about his or her tendency to fall asleep in situations of everyday life; milder levels of daytime sleepiness result in falling asleep in passive situations such as while reading, watching television, and attending meetings. In severe cases, individuals fall asleep while actively engaged in complex tasks such as driving, speaking, writing, or even eating. Highly sleepy patients may also experience sleep attacks, episodes of sleep that strike without warning, whose occurrence mandates rapid clinical intervention, in part due to significantly increased risk of motor vehicle accidents. However, all patients with a complaint of ES should be cautioned about the risks of drowsy driving. The most widely utilized validated inventory for the quantification of the tendency to fall asleep is the Epworth Sleepiness Scale (ESS),[14] described in more detail elsewhere in this book. A score of 10 or above is considered to represent an abnormally high level of daytime sleepiness.

Related Symptoms

Napping should be explored in all patients. Narcolepsy patients report refreshing naps that are brief in duration or accompanied by dreams. Naps are also refreshing in individuals who are sleep deprived. In contrast, the naps tend to not be refreshing in OSA and idiopathic hypersomnia. The timing of naps should also be determined as this may alert the physician to the possibility of circadian rhythm disorders. Typically, patients with delayed sleep phase syndrome take the bulk of their naps in the morning hours, whereas those with advanced sleep phase syndrome take the bulk of their naps in the early evening hours.

ES can cause slower response times, cognitive slowing, performance errors, decline in both short-term recall and working memory, reduced learning of new tasks, increased response perseveration on ineffective solutions, increased neglect of nonessential activities (loss of situational awareness), increased compensatory effort to maintain the same performance, and diminished insight into subtle meanings. ES is associated with an increased risk for accidents at work and while driving. ES can also contribute to depressed mood.[15,16]

PARASOMNIAS

Parasomnias are undesirable physical events or experiences that occur during entry into sleep, within sleep, or during arousals from sleep.[3] The behavioral characteristics of the disturbance, the time of night that they occur, the presence or absence of memory for the event and associated dreaming, and age of onset should be evaluated. For example, disorders of arousal such as sleepwalking and night terrors usually occur during the first third of night since they arise from slow-wave sleep, are associated with amnesia for the event or a vague sense of imminent danger, are not associated with reports of dreaming, are common in childhood, and decrease in incidence with increasing age. On the other hand, rapid eye movement (REM) sleep behavior disorder (RBD)

is more likely to occur in the latter portions of the night since it arises from REM sleep, is often associated with intense dreaming and later memory for the dream and associated behaviors, and is more common in middle and older age.[3] Parasomnias are associated with an increased risk of harm to self and others; for example, RBD sufferers may strike out in response to dreams and injure themselves or a bedpartner. Therefore, an understanding of the extent of such injurious behavior in the past can be important in determining the urgency of treatment and the implementation of safety precautions.

BEDPARTNERS AND FAMILY MEMBER INTERVIEWS

Useful areas of information from family members and bedpartners include snoring; breathing pauses during sleep; unusual behaviors during sleep such as walking, talking, thrashing, head banging, body rocking, and limb movements; the tendency to fall asleep unintentionally during the day; and the extent and frequency of naps.

PAST MEDICAL, PSYCHIATRIC, AND SURGICAL HISTORY

Comorbid medical, neurological, and psychiatric disorders should be reviewed, along with their dates of onset, types of treatment, and results of treatment. Surgeries and hospitalizations should also be evaluated. Major medical and psychiatric disorders can affect sleep by virtue of their psychological impact, through pain and discomfort, as well as direct effects on sleep and wakefulness.

MEDICATIONS

A history of current and prior medications is an integral part of the sleep history. The list should include not only prescribed medications, but also over-the-counter agents, nutraceuticals, herbals substances, dietary supplements, and even foods. Their effects, side effects, dosages or quantities, and timing of administration should be recorded. If the use of a medication correlates temporally with the onset of the sleep complaint, a medication-induced sleep disorder should be suspected. Medications can also have secondary effects by virtue of their exacerbation of underlying conditions. For example, weight gain associated with medication use can lead to the development of symptoms of OSA, such as ES, snoring, and breathing pauses during sleep.

Allergies to medications should also be recorded as a component of comprehensive history taking and evaluation.[17]

SUBSTANCE USE

Stimulants such as caffeine, amphetamines, and cocaine classically disrupt sleep. Sedatives such as opiates and analgesics cause ES. Alcohol, at low dosages, can help with sleep initiation, yet chronic and excessive use can lead to disturbed sleep and the complaint of insomnia.[18]

FAMILY HISTORY

Sleep disorders tend to run in families; thus, obtaining family history is essential. For example, in restless legs syndrome (RLS), 50% of primary RLS patients have a positive family history.[19] Sleepwalking and sleep terror are 10 times greater in incidence in first-degree relatives than in the general population.[20] Additionally, OSA may have a familial basis.[21]

SOCIAL AND OCCUPATIONAL HISTORY

ES and insomnia are more common in shift workers and frequent travelers. Chronic exposure to industrial toxins and chemicals can also produce sleep/wake symptoms. Recent retirement is a strong predictor of insomnia.[10]

SYMPTOMS OF SPECIFIC DISORDERS

Defining symptoms of specific sleep disorders should be systematically explored. Examples include an irresistible urge to move the extremities in RLS; excessive daytime sleepiness, cataplexy, sleep paralysis, and hypnopompic hallucinations in narcolepsy; snoring, breathing pauses during sleep, choking and gasping during sleep, and morning dry mouth in OSA; and a prolonged sleep latency and late awakening time in delayed sleep phase syndrome.

PHYSICAL EXAMINATION

The measurement of neck circumference should be a routine part of the sleep disorders examination; a thick and/or muscular neck, as well as a neck circumference of 16 inches or greater in women and 17 inches or greater in men, are associated with an increased risk for sleep-related breathing disorders.[22] Body habitus revealing obesity with fat distribution around the neck or midriff suggests the diagnosis of OSA. Other contributors to sleep-related breathing disorders include nasal obstruction, mandibular hypoplasia, and retrognathia. Oropharyngeal abnormalities can also be involved, including enlarged tonsils and tongue, an elongated uvula and soft palate, diminished pharyngeal patency, and redundant pharyngeal mucosa. The Mallampati Airway Classification score should be determined,[23] which is useful in assessing the risk for OSA. On an average, for every 1 point increase in the Mallampati score, the odds of having OSA increases more than twofold. The chest examination should be scrutinized for expiratory wheezes and kyphoscoliosis, indicative of, among others, asthma and restrictive lung disease respectively, which, in turn, can be associated with the complaint of insomnia. Signs of right heart failure should be noted; heart failure can cause abnormalities of breathing during sleep, which, in turn, can be associated with the complaint of frequent nocturnal awakenings and unrefreshing sleep. A basic neurological examination should be performed to rule out neurological disorders that may mimic certain sleep disorders or which may coexist with them. For example, the presence of increased resting muscle tone, cogwheel rigidity and tremor can indicate the presence of Parkinson's disease, which can share some of the behavioral and sensory disturbances of RBD. The mental status examination should include an evaluation of affect, mood, anxiety, psychomotor agitation or slowing, cognition, the possibility of reduced alertness and slurred speech, and perceptual disturbances.

SCALES AND INVENTORIES

A few of the more commonly utilized inventories have already been described, including the ISI, the Fatigue Severity Scale, the ESS, sleep diaries, and the Mallampati Airway Classification. The STOP-BANG scoring model[22] is a method that was recently introduced, which strives to predict the risk of OSA without the use of polysomnography, the gold-standard procedure for the diagnosis of the disorder. It includes elements of the history and physical examination, and it has been validated for OSA screening in preoperative patients. "Yes" answers to three or more questions place the patient at high pretest probability for OSA. The questionnaire was validated in a mixed group of preoperative patients against in-lab polysomnography. Sensitivities and specificities of the questionnaire are, respectively, as follows: for mild OSA (Apnea–Hypopnea Index [AHI] between 5 and 15), 83.6% and 56.4%; for moderate OSA

(AHI between 16 and 29), 92.9% and 43.0%; for severe OSA (AHI greater than 30), 100% and 37%.

TESTS AND CONSULTATIONS: SERUM LABORATORY TESTS

RLS is more common in iron deficiency states and conditions associated with iron deficiency such as pregnancy and anemia.[24] The level of serum ferritin is inversely correlated with severity of RLS symptoms and iron supplementation has been shown to reduce RLS symptoms. Therefore, serum ferritin should be obtained in patients suspected of having RLS.[24] Sleep laboratory tests will be addressed in detail in the next chapter.

CONCLUSIONS AND RECOMMENDATIONS

Insomnia, ES, and parasomnias are commonly encountered in psychiatric practice. They are the hallmark symptoms of a variety of sleep disorders, many of which will be discussed in greater detail in the ensuing chapters. This chapter has focused on the critical first steps in bridging symptom with disorder, namely, the history and examination. These represent the cornerstones of the sleep evaluation process.

KEY PEARLS
- Develop a systematic process to address sleep related complaints.
- Organize the clinical history around a typical 24-hour sleep/wake pattern beginning with bedtime and ending back at the time at which the inquiry began and determine deviations from the normal patterns.
- Obtain the nocturnal or diurnal pattern, onset, and longitudinal course and severity of the chief complaint.
- Understand the temporal relationship between the chief complaint and potential precipitants such as psychosocial disruption, comorbid illnesses, and prior treatments.
- Systematically explore sleep-related habits and behaviors and maladaptive psychological reactions and cognitions that may foment and perpetuate sleep/wake disturbances.
- Appreciate the nature and extent of consequences of the chief complaint on daytime functioning.

- Obtain collateral information from bedpartners.
- Ask for symptoms of specific sleep disorders.
- Complete the essential elements of a general medical and psychiatric history gathering process and examination.
- Utilize inventories, tests, and consultations to complete the diagnostic picture.
- Arrive at a diagnostic formulation prior to resorting to treatment.

SELF-ASSESSMENT QUESTIONS

1. Which of the following inventories are useful in the evaluation of sleep/wake disorders?
   a. Epworth Sleepiness Scale
   b. STOP-Bang Scoring Model
   c. Fatigue Severity Scale
   d. All of the above

Answer: d

2. Excessive sleepiness is defined as
   a. the tendency to spend prolonged times in bed.
   b. the tendency to fall asleep at inappropriate times.
   c. the sensation of mental and physical slowing.
   d. excessive times spent napping.
   e. None of the above

Answer: b

3. Which of the following statements regarding insomnia is true?
   a. The pattern of insomnia symptoms during the night typically change over time.
   b. The establishment of clinically significant insomnia does not require the presence of daytime impairment.
   c. Insomnia of long term duration generally has greater impact on daytime functioning.
   d. Bouts of insomnia in chronic sufferers typically last more than a month.

Answer: a

4. Serum ferritin should be considered in diagnostic evaluation of which of the following primary sleep disorders?
   a. Obstructive sleep apnea
   b. Restless legs syndrome
   c. Delayed-sleep phase syndrome
   d. Narcolepsy

Answer: b

5. STOP-BANG questionnaire is a commonly used screening tool for which of the following primary sleep disorders?

a. Narcolepsy
b. Restless legs syndrome
c. Obstructive sleep apnea
d. Circadian rhythm sleep–wake disorders

Answer: c

REFERENCES

1. Sateia MJ, Doghramji K, Hauri PJ, Morin CM. Evaluation of chronic insomnia. an American academy of sleep medicine review. *Sleep.* 2000;23(2):243–308.
2. Schutte-Rodin S, Broch L, Buysse D, Dorsey C, Sateia M. Clinical guideline for the evaluation and management of chronic insomnia in adults. *J Clin Sleep Med.* 2008;4(5):487–504.
3. American Academy of Sleep Medicine. *International classification of sleep disorders: a diagnostic and coding manual.* 3rd ed. Darien, IL: American Academy of Sleep Medicine; 2014.
4. National Institutes of Health. National institutes of health state of the science conference statement on manifestations and management of chronic insomnia in adults. *Sleep.* 2005;28(9):1049–1057.
5. Hohagen F, Rink K, Kappler C, et al. Prevalence and treatment of insomnia in general practice. a longitudinal study. *Eur Arch Psychiatry Clin Neurosci.* 1993;242(6):329–336.
6. Ancoli-Israel S, Roth T. Characteristics of insomnia in the united states: results of the 1991 national sleep foundation survey. I. *Sleep.* 1999;22 Suppl 2:347.
7. Stepanski E, Zorick F, Roehrs T, Young D, Roth T. Daytime alertness in patients with chronic insomnia compared with asymptomatic control subjects. *Sleep.* 1988;11(1):54–60.
8. Kales JD, Kales A, Bixler EO, et al. Biopsychobehavioral correlates of insomnia, V: Clinical characteristics and behavioral correlates. *Am J Psychiatry.* 1984;141(11):1371–1376.
9. Bastien CH, Vallieres A, Morin CM. Validation of the insomnia severity index as an outcome measure for insomnia research. *Sleep Med.* 2001;2(4):297–307.
10. Hauri PJ. Sleep/wake lifestyle modifications: sleep hygiene. In: Barkoukis TJ, Matheson JK, Ferber R, Doghramji K, eds. *Therapy in sleep medicine.* Philadelphia: Elsevier Saunders; 2012:151–160.
11. Cooke JR, Ancoli-Israel S. Sleep and its disorders in older adults. *Psychiatr Clin North Am.* 2006;29(4):xi. doi:10.1016/j.psc.2006.08.003.
12. Krupp LB, LaRocca NG, Muir-Nash J, Steinberg AD. The fatigue severity scale. application to patients with multiple sclerosis and systemic lupus erythematosus. *Arch Neurol.* 1989;46(10):1121–1123.
13. Hoddes E, Zarcone V, Smythe H, Phillips R, Dement WC. Quantification of sleepiness: a new approach. *Psychophysiology.* 1973;10(4):431–436. doi:10.1111/j.1469-8986.1973.tb00801.x.
14. Johns MW. A new method for measuring daytime sleepiness: the Epworth Sleepiness Scale. *Sleep.* 1991;14(6):540–545.
15. Banks S, Dinges DF. Chronic sleep deprivation. In: Kryger M, Roth T, Dement WC, eds. *Principles and practice of sleep medicine.* 5th ed. Philadelphia: Elsevier Saunders; 2011.
16. Mitler MM, Carskadon MA, Czeisler CA, Dement WC, Dinges DF, Graeber RC. Catastrophes, sleep, and public policy: consensus report. *Sleep.* 1988;11(1):100–109.
17. Roehrs T. *Medications and sleep, an issue of sleep medicine clinics.* Amsterdam: Elsevier Health Sciences; 2010.
18. Johnson EO, Roehrs T, Roth T, Breslau N. Epidemiology of alcohol and medication as aids to sleep in early adulthood. *Sleep.* 1998;21(2):178–186.
19. Montplaisir J, Boucher S, Poirier G, Lavigne G, Lapierre O, Lesperance P. Clinical, polysomnographic, and genetic characteristics of restless legs syndrome: a study of 133 patients diagnosed with new standard criteria. *Mov Disord.* 1997;12(1):61–65. doi:10.1002/mds.870120111.
20. Kales A, Soldatos CR, Bixler EO, et al. Hereditary factors in sleepwalking and night terrors. *Br J Psychiatry.* 1980;137:111–118.
21. Casale M, Pappacena M, Rinaldi V, Bressi F, Baptista P, Salvinelli F. Obstructive sleep apnea syndrome: from phenotype to genetic basis. *Curr Genomics.* 2009;10(2):119–126. doi:10.2174/138920209787846998.
22. Chung F, Yegneswaran B, Liao P, et al. STOP questionnaire: A tool to screen patients for obstructive sleep apnea. *Anesthesiology.* 2008;108(5):812–821. doi:10.1097/ALN.0b013e31816d83e4.
23. Nuckton TJ, Glidden DV, Browner WS, Claman DM. Physical examination: Mallampati score as an independent predictor of obstructive sleep apnea. *Sleep.* 2006;29(7):903–908.
24. Aurora RN, Kristo DA, Bista SR, et al. The treatment of restless legs syndrome and periodic limb movement disorder in adults--an update for 2012: practice parameters with an evidence-based systematic review and meta-analyses: an American academy of sleep medicine clinical practice guideline. *Sleep.* 2012;35(8):1039. doi:10.5665/sleep.1988.

7

Clinical Applications of Technical Procedures in Sleep Medicine

ERIKA MANIS AND ANITA VALANJU SHELGIKAR

INTRODUCTION

The *International Classification of Sleep Disorders* (third edition; ICSD-3) is the diagnostic text referenced by sleep medicine providers.[1] The *Diagnostic and Statistical Manual of Mental Disorders* (fifth edition; DSM-5) includes a chapter dedicated to sleep–wake disorders.[2] The DSM-5 offers a classification scheme intended for use primarily by mental health practitioners. The inclusion of a chapter represents the comorbidity of sleep–wake disorders seen with psychiatric conditions. Sleep complaints associated with schizophrenia, bipolar, depression, anxiety, posttraumatic stress disorder, substance-related disorders, and neurocognitive disorders can overlap with primary sleep disorders. Appropriate diagnosis of a sleep disorder in a patient with psychiatric disease provides an opportunity to optimize treatment.

Once the clinician has established a clinical suspicion for a sleep disorder based on a detailed history, subjective screening tools, and physical exam, there arises a need for diagnostic sleep testing.[3] Review of the comprehensive sleep history and physical exam are covered in Chapter 6 of this volume on office-based evaluation of patients with sleep disorders and are outside the scope of this chapter. A detailed discussion of primary sleep disorders, including prevalence data, pathophysiology, and clinical management will be included in other chapters of this book (Section 2) and thus are not covered here. Subjective screening tools for primary sleep disorders are adjunctive to the clinical evaluation and are never used as a substitute for objective diagnostic testing.

This chapter focuses solely on the clinical indications and appropriate patient selection for diagnostic procedures used in clinical sleep medicine in psychiatric settings. Diagnostic procedures used in the evaluation and management of sleep disorders include polysomnography (PSG), the home sleep apnea test (HSAT), the multiple sleep latency test (MSLT), the maintenance of wakefulness test (MWT), and actigraphy. The evaluation of certain sleep disorders may include laboratory testing; these laboratory tests will be discussed in the diagnosis-specific chapters and will not be covered in this chapter on sleep diagnostic procedures.

TECHNICAL PROCEDURES

Polysomnography

Polysomnography, also commonly known as a sleep study, incorporates the monitoring and recording of multiple physiologic variables during sleep. A minimum of seven channels including electrooculography (EOG), electroencephalography (EEG), chin and leg electromyography (EMG), electrocardiography (ECG), airflow, respiratory effort, and oxygen saturation (determined by pulse oximetry) are recorded during the study.[4] Type I and Type II studies include at least seven monitoring channels; the difference is that a Type I study is attended by a sleep technologist, whereas a Type II study is unattended (see Table 7.1).[4]

The EEG and ECG montages routinely used in PSG have limited roles in comparison to the diagnostic applications of these procedures in the disciplines of neurology and cardiology, respectively; standard EEG recording on PSG includes only three derivations or electrode pairs (frontal, central, and occipital with mastoid references) and standard PSG ECG includes a modified Lead II recording.[5] Additional EEG derivations may be added if there is concern for sleep-related epilepsy. Arm EMG leads may be added for further evaluation of atypical or dangerous parasomnia behaviors.

Digital PSG acquisition, processing, and recording have become standard, and these digital approaches have replaced traditional

TABLE 7.1. SUMMARY OF PARAMETERS USED IN TYPES I TO IV AND PERIPHERAL ARTERIAL TONOMETRY STUDIES

	Type I	Type II	Type III	Type IV	PAT
Attended or Unattended	Attended	Unattended	Unattended	Unattended	Unattended
Location	Lab	Lab or Home	Home	Home	Home
Minimum number of channels	7	7	4	1	NA
EOG	x	x			
EEG	x	x			
EMG	x	x			
Airflow	x	x	x	x	
Respiratory effort	x	x	x	x	
ECG or HR	x	x	x	x	x
Oxygen saturation	x	x	x	x	x
CO_2 monitoring	x				
Body position	x	x	x		x
Audio/video	x				
Snore	x	x	x		x

Abbreviations: PAT, peripheral arterial tonometry; EOG, electro-oculogram; EEG, electroencephalogram; EMG, electromyogram; ECG, electrocardiogram; HR, heart rate.

analog amplifiers and paper tracings. Audio/visual recordings that are synchronized with EEG and respiratory channels are also now available. Sleep staging is done with assessment of EEG patterns, eye movements using EOG channels, and muscle tone using EMG channels. By convention, sleep is staged at 30-second intervals called epochs. Staging criteria and nomenclature for nonrapid eye movement (NREM) and rapid eye movement (REM) sleep, as well as criteria for scoring respiratory events, are based on guidelines by the American Academy of Sleep Medicine (AASM) Manual for the Scoring of Sleep and Associated Events.[5] Figure 7.1 shows a 30-second epoch of wakefulness from a Type I study, and Figure 7.2 shows a 1-minute epoch during REM sleep.

Cycles of NREM sleep (N1, N2, and N3) followed by stage R or REM sleep occur every 90 to 120 minutes throughout the night during normal adult sleep.[4] Of note, older scoring classification schemes separated slow-wave sleep into stages 3 and 4; the current classification scheme combines these two categories into stage N3 sleep. Each sleep stage has characteristic features. Compared to occipital alpha or posterior dominant rhythm EEG frequency (8–13 Hz) in closed-eye wakefulness, low-amplitude mixed-frequency (LAMF) activity (4–7 Hz) with slow eye movements (SEMs) is seen in N1, sleep spindles and K complexes in N2, slow-wave activity (SWA; 0.5–2 Hz) in N3, and rapid eye movements with low chin tone and sawtooth waves are seen in REM sleep.[5] Figures 7.3–7.7 show examples of different stages of sleep.

Respiratory events are identified by decrements in airflow using a nasal pressure transducer or an oro-nasal thermal airflow sensor during a diagnostic study and positive airway pressure (PAP) device flow during a titration study.[5] Respiratory disturbances are classified as apneas (at least 90% decrement in flow) or hypopneas (at least 30% decrement in flow associated with either a cortical arousal captured on EEG or ≥3% oxygen desaturation [American Academy of Sleep Medicine criteria] or ≥4% oxygen desaturation [Centers for Medicare & Medicaid Services]).[5] The nasal pressure transducer can monitor snoring; a microphone or piezoelectric sensor may alternatively be used.[5] Dual thoraco-abdominal

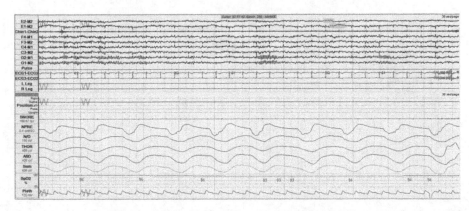

FIGURE 7.1. A 30-second epoch of wakefulness taken from a Type I study. M1/M2 = mastoid referential leads. E2-M1/E1-M2 = right/left electro-oculogram; Chin1-Chin2 = submental electromyogram (EMG); F4-M1/F3-M2 = right/left frontal EEG; C4-M1/C3-M2 = right/left central electroencephalogram (EEG); O2-M1/O1-M2 = right/left occipital EEG; ECG1-ECG2/ECG2-ECG3 = electrocardiogram; L Leg-R Leg = left/right anterior tibialis EMG;

Abbreviations: EEG, electroencephalogram; EMG, electroencephalogram; NPRE, nasal pressure transducer; N/O, oronasal thermistor; THOR, thoracic respiratory inductance plethysmography (RIP); ABD, abdominal RIP; Sum, summation of thoracic and abdominal RIP; SpO_2, oxygen saturation; Pleth, plethysmography.

belts reflect respiratory effort, aiding in the delineation of respiratory events as obstructive, central, or mixed (in the case of apneas).[5] Esophageal pressure (Pes) monitoring can be used for further quantification of the respiratory effort if needed.

Carbon dioxide (CO_2) monitoring may be added to studies as clinically indicated to assess for sleep-related hypoventilation, which can be seen in patients with obesity and underlying pulmonary conditions and is suggested by a body mass index (BMI) greater than 30 kg/m^2 (although most patients with hypoventilation have BMI over 40 kg/m^2) and serum bicarbonate at or greater than 27 mEq/L.[6] Of note, CO_2 monitoring is required for pediatric sleep studies where end-tidal CO_2 ($ETCO_2$) is used for diagnostic studies and

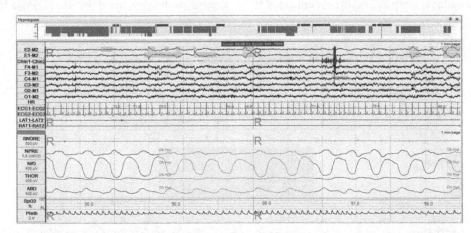

FIGURE 7.2. A 1 minute epoch during REM sleep taken from a Type I study. A hypopnea identified by at least 30% decrement in airflow using a nasal pressure transducer during a diagnostic study associated with a cortical arousal captured on EEG. M1/M2 = mastoid referential leads; E2-M1/E1-M2 = right/left electro-oculogram; Chin1-Chin2 = submental EMG; F4-M1/F3-M2 = right/left frontal EEG; C4-M1/C3-M2 = right/left central electroencephalogram (EEG); O2-M1/O1-M2 = right/left occipital EEG; ECG1-ECG2/ECG2-ECG3 = electrocardiogram; L Leg-R Leg = left/right anterior tibialis EMG.

Abbreviations: EEG, electroencephalogram; electromyogram, EMG NPRE, nasal pressure transducer; N/O, oronasal thermistor; THOR, thoracic respiratory inductance plethysmography (RIP); ABD, abdominal RIP; Sum, summation of thoracic and abdominal RIP; SpO_2, oxygen saturation; Pleth, plethysmography.

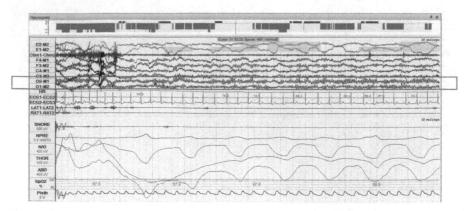

FIGURE 7.3. A 30-second epoch of occipital alpha or posterior dominant rhythm EEG frequency (8–13 Hz) in closed-eye wakefulness taken from a Type I study. M1/M2 = mastoid referential leads; E2-M1/E1-M2 = right/left electro-oculogram; Chin1-Chin2 = submental EMG; F4-M1/F3-M2 = right/left frontal EEG; C4-M1/C3-M2 = right/left central EEG; O2-M1/O1-M2 = right/left occipital EEG; ECG1-ECG2/ECG2-ECG3, electrocardiogram; L Leg-R Leg = left/right anterior tibialis EMG.

Abbreviations: EEG, electroencephalogram; EMG, electromyogram; NPRE, nasal pressure transducer; N/O, oronasal thermistor; THOR, thoracic respiratory inductance plethysmography (RIP); ABD, abdominal RIP; Sum, summation of thoracic and abdominal RIP; SpO$_2$, oxygen saturation; Pleth, plethysmography.

transcutaneous CO$_2$ is used for PAP titration studies. An ETCO$_2$ greater than 50 mmHg, (i.e., at least 10 mmHg above wakeful baseline values) or greater than 55 mmHg for greater than or equal to 10 minutes meets criteria for sleep-related hypoventilation.[5] In children, ETCO$_2$ must be greater than 50 mmHg for at least 25% of the total sleep time to meet criteria for sleep-related hypoventilation.[5]

The most common indication for a PSG is evaluation and treatment of sleep-related breathing-related sleep disorders (SRBD) such as obstructive sleep apnea (OSA) (see Table 7.2).[7] Of note, the term "sleep-related breathing disorders" is used by the American Academy of Sleep Medicine and in the ICSD-3 whereas the term "breathing-related sleep disorders" is used by the DSM-5.[1,2] For

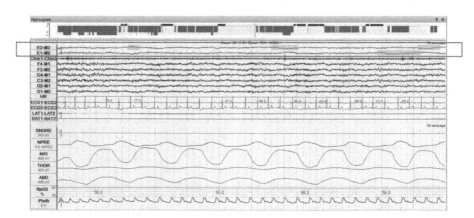

FIGURE 7.4. A 30-second epoch of low-amplitude mixed-frequency (LAMF) activity (4-7 Hz) with slow eye movements (SEMs) in stage N1 sleep taken from a Type I study. M1/M2 = mastoid referential leads; E2-M1/E1-M2 = right/left electro-oculogram; Chin1-Chin2 = submental electromyogram (EMG); F4-M1/F3-M2 = right/left frontal EEG; C4-M1/C3-M2 = right/left central electroencephalogram (EEG); O2-M1/O1-M2 = right/left occipital EEG; ECG1-ECG2/ECG2-ECG3, electrocardiogram; L Leg-R Leg = left/right anterior tibialis EMG.

Abbreviations: EEG, electroencephalogram; EMG, electromyogram; NPRE, nasal pressure transducer; N/O, oronasal thermistor; THOR, thoracic respiratory inductance plethysmography (RIP); ABD, abdominal RIP; Sum, summation of thoracic and abdominal RIP; SpO$_2$, oxygen saturation; Pleth, plethysmography.

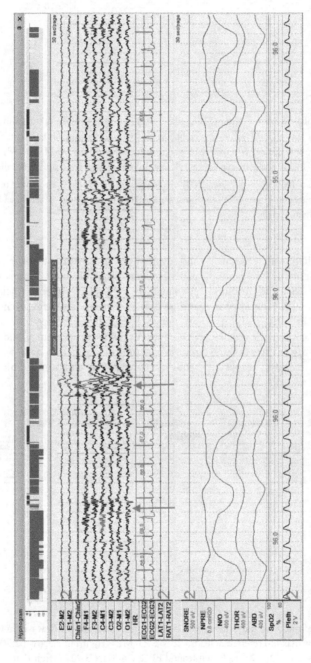

FIGURE 7.5. A 30-second epoch of sleep spindles and K complexes in stage N2 sleep taken from a Type I study. M1/M2 = mastoid referential leads; E2-M1/E1-M2 = right/left electro-oculogram; Chin1-Chin2 = submental electromyogram (EMG); F4-M1/F3-M2 = right/left frontal EEG; C4-M1/C3-M2 = right/left central electroencephalogram (EEG); O2-M1/O1-M2 = right/left occipital EEG; ECG1-ECG2/ECG2-ECG3, electrocardiogram; L Leg-R Leg = left/right anterior tibialis EMG.

Abbreviations: EEG, electroencephalogram; EMG, electromyogram; NPRE, nasal pressure transducer; N/O, oronasal thermistor; THOR, thoracic respiratory inductance plethysmography (RIP); ABD, abdominal RIP; Sum, summation of thoracic and abdominal RIP; SpO₂, oxygen saturation; Pleth, plethysmography.

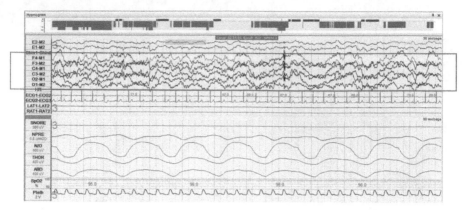

FIGURE 7.6. A 30-second epoch of slow wave activity (SWA) (0.5-2 Hz) in stage N3 sleep taken from a Type I study. M1/M2 = mastoid referential leads; E2-M1/E1-M2 = right/left electro-oculogram; Chin1-Chin2 = submental EMG; F4-M1/F3-M2 = right/left frontal EEG; C4-M1/C3-M2 = right/left central EEG; O2-M1/O1-M2 = right/left occipital EEG; ECG1-ECG2/ECG2-ECG3 = electrocardiogram; L Leg-R Leg = left/right anterior tibialis EMG.

Abbreviations: EEG, electroencephalogram; EMG, electromyogram; NPRE, nasal pressure transducer; N/O, oronasal thermistor; THOR, thoracic respiratory inductance plethysmography (RIP); ABD, abdominal RIP; Sum, summation of thoracic and abdominal RIP; SpO$_2$, oxygen saturation; Pleth, plethysmography.

purposes of this chapter, this diagnostic category will be referred to as SRBDs. Diagnostic PSG evaluates the presence and severity of OSA, and titration PSG studies assess the efficacy of PAP therapy for treatment of sleep-disordered breathing.[7] Other OSA related indications of PSG include the assessment of sleep apnea prior to surgical treatments (such as adenotonsillectomy or bariatric surgery) and evaluation of treatment response in OSA patients using non-PAP interventions such as oral appliance or surgical treatments (including nasal and/or palatal surgery, jaw surgery, and hypoglossal nerve stimulation therapy).[7-9] Additionally, OSA patients with insufficient clinical response, return of symptoms, and 10% body weight change require further PSG evaluation.[7] Clinical suspicion

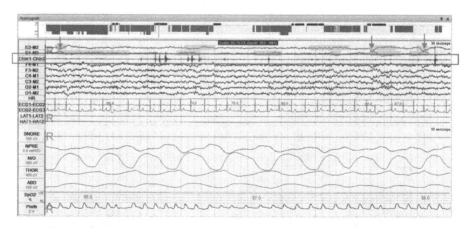

FIGURE 7.7. A 30-second epoch of rapid eye movements with low chin tone and saw-tooth waves in REM sleep taken from a Type I study. M1/M2 = mastoid referential leads; E2-M1/E1-M2 = right/left electro-oculogram; Chin1-Chin2 = submental EMG; F4-M1/F3-M2 = right/left frontal EEG; C4-M1/C3-M2 = right/left central EEG; O2-M1/O1-M2 = right/left occipital EEG; ECG1-ECG2/ECG2-ECG3 = electrocardiogram; L Leg-R Leg = left/right anterior tibialis EMG.

Abbreviations: EEG, electroencephalogram; EMG, electromyogram; NPRE, nasal pressure transducer; N/O, oronasal thermistor; THOR, thoracic respiratory inductance plethysmography (RIP); ABD, abdominal RIP; Sum, summation of thoracic and abdominal RIP; SpO$_2$, oxygen saturation; Pleth, plethysmography.

TABLE 7.2. KEY CLINICAL INDICATIONS
FOR POLYSOMNOGRAPHY

Diagnosis of sleep-related breathing disorders

Positive airway pressure titration in patients with
breathing-related sleep disorders

Assessment of treatment outcome in some cases with
obstructive sleep apnea

Prior to multiple sleep latency test in the evaluation
of suspected narcolepsy/idiopathic hypersomnia

Parasomnias with violent or potentially injurious
sleep-related behaviors

Neuromuscular disorders with sleep-related symptoms

To assist in the diagnosis of sleep disruptions thought
to be seizure related

Parasomnia or sleep related seizure disorder that
does not respond to therapy

Periodic limb movement sleep disorder

of other SRBDs like central sleep apnea syndromes,
sleep-related hypoventilation, and hypoxemia
(including significant cardiopulmonary disease,
respiratory muscle weakness due to a neuromuscular condition, or chronic opioid medication use)
is another common indication of PSG.[7]

A split-night PSG, with diagnostic monitoring followed by PAP titration during the same
recording, may underestimate the severity of OSA
as REM sleep may not be observed during the
baseline portion of the study. PAP titration may
be done as part of a split-night PSG if moderate to
severe OSA is observed during the first 2 hours of
recording and at least 3 hours remain during the
recording for titration.[3]

Other than for SRBDs, PSG is also utilized for
diagnostic evaluation of a range of primary sleep
disorders. PSG followed by MSLT is indicated for
evaluation of hypersomnolence disorders such as
narcolepsy and idiopathic hypersomnia.[7] PSG is
indicated for evaluation of REM and NREM parasomnia behaviors that are violent or potentially
injurious.[7] These may include NREM parasomnias such as confusional arousals, sleepwalking,
and sleep terrors, and REM parasomnias such
as REM behavior disorder (RBD).[1] Parasomnias
with unusual or atypical presentations raise suspicion for sleep-related epilepsy that can occur in
15% to 20% of the epilepsy patients with seizures
occurring mostly or exclusively during sleep.[7]
If the clinical evaluation and standard EEG are
inconclusive and sleep disruption is thought to be

seizure related, a PSG with full EEG is indicated to
assist in diagnosis and treatment of sleep-related
epilepsy. PSG is not indicated for common,
uncomplicated, and noninjurious parasomnias
such as nightmares, enuresis, sleepwalking, or
bruxism unless there is suspicion for OSA as a
trigger for these parasomnias.[7] PSG is not routinely indicated for insomnia assessment with or
without depression. [7]

Home Sleep Apnea Testing (HSAT)

Home sleep apnea testing is a limited channel study as it has a minimum of four channels,
which include two channels of respiratory movement or respiratory movement and airflow, heart
rate or ECG, and oxygen saturation.[4] Some HSATs
additionally have a body position sensor. Prior
nomenclature includes "out-of-center sleep test" or
"portable monitor," with HSAT being the currently
favored term. HSATs do not require the attendance
of a sleep technologist and thus can be administered in the home, outside of the sleep laboratory.

HSAT has lower sensitivity than a PSG as
it lacks EEG monitoring, which is used in the
detection of sleep and hypopneas associated with
cortical arousal. This may lead to false-negative
studies and an overall underestimation of the
severity of sleep-disordered breathing. For this
reason, it should only be considered in uncomplicated patients with a high pretest probability for
having moderate to severe OSA. A high pretest
probability for having moderate to severe OSA is
indicated by excessive daytime sleepiness in the
presence of at least two of the three following
criteria: habitual loud snoring, witnessed apneas
or gasping or choking, or diagnosed hypertension.[3] An uncomplicated patient does not have
risk factors for nonobstructive sleep disordered
breathing, nonrespiratory sleep disorders, or
environmental or personal factors that would
interfere with the accuracy of the study and preclude the acquisition and interpretation of data
from the study.[3]

Various measures can be reported on PSG or
HSAT for assessment of sleep-disordered breathing.
PSG reports typically include the Apnea–Hypopnea
Index (AHI), which takes into account the number
of apneas and hypopneas *per hour of sleep* along
with the Respiratory Distress Index (RDI), which
is the AHI plus respiratory event related arousals
(RERAs) *per hour of sleep*.[1,5] HSAT reports typically
include the Respiratory Event Index (REI), which
is the number of apneas and hypopneas associated
with oxygen desaturation *per hour of monitoring*

time.[1,5] The ICSD-3 includes use of the AHI, RDI, or REI in the diagnostic criteria for OSA.[1]

Other Types of Respiratory Monitoring during Sleep

A Type IV study measures one to two parameters.[4] These measures may include oxygen saturation, airflow, heart rate, or chest movements. An overnight pulse oximetry test is an example of a Type IV study. Type IV studies may have a role in screening for SRBDs or to assess adequate oxygenation for patients on OSA treatment. Type IV studies should not be used for diagnostic purposes.

Summary of Study Types Used in Evaluation of Sleep-Related Breathing Disorders

The traditional classification of sleep studies (Types I–IV) does not incorporate new technology such as peripheral arterial tonometry (PAT), thus alternative classification SCOPER (sleep, cardiovascular, oximetry, position, effort, and respiratory) was proposed.[3,4] The SCOPER scheme was developed to encompass other types of emerging technologies, but this more detailed classification scheme is not used in routine clinical practice. PAT devices are worn on the finger and measure blood volume in lieu of airflow as well as oxygen saturation, which is determined by pulse oximetry. A respiratory event is scored when a decrease in the PAT signal from a sympathetically mediated vasoconstriction occurs along with an increase in heart rate and simultaneous decrease in oxygen saturation.[4] For this reason, PAT should not be used for individuals who take alpha-blocking agents. Due to relative ease of use and provider familiarity, traditional classification continues to be more widely used than the SCOPER classification scheme. Generally, PAT is regarded as a Type III study with special notation.

Multiple Sleep Latency Test

MSLT is indicated for objective assessment of excessive daytime sleepiness in patients with hypersomnolence disorders such as narcolepsy and idiopathic hypersomnia, and in OSA patients with residual sleepiness despite effective therapy.[10] A clinical history revealing cataplexy, sleep attacks, sleep paralysis, and hypnopompic or hypnogogic hallucinations in addition to excessive daytime sleepiness may be suggestive of narcolepsy type 1.[1] MSLT includes a total of five nap opportunities that are spaced 2 hours apart and each nap lasts at least 20 minutes in duration.[10] MSLT is done 1.5 to 3 hours after an overnight PSG that confirms a minimum of 6 hours of sleep and excludes other primary sleep disorders that can potentially lead to hypersomnolence.[10] If the patient has a known history of sleep disordered breathing and is on PAP therapy, this is continued for the PSG and MSLT.

Standard EEG derivations and chin EMG monitoring used during PSG are recorded during the MSLT. Sleepiness is assessed by measurement of sleep onset latency (SOL) and the presence of sleep-onset rapid eye movement periods (SOREMPs). The SOL is defined as the time from lights-out to the first epoch of any stage of sleep.[10] SOL on a nap in the absence of sleep is recorded as 20 minutes, after which the nap is terminated.[10] If sleep occurs, the nap is continued for 15 minutes to assess for the occurrence of REM sleep.[10] The mean SOL is calculated as the average sleep latency across all nap opportunities.

REM latency is defined as the time from the first epoch of sleep until the first epoch of REM.[10] A SOREMP is noted when REM onset within 15 minutes of sleep onset.[10] Normal individuals may have zero to 1 SOREMPs during the MSLT. Diagnostic criteria for specific disorders of hypersomnolence, along with other conditions that may mimic central disorders of hypersomnolence, will be discussed in the specific chapters on these clinical conditions.

REM suppressant medications such as antidepressants and stimulant medications should be held (if clinically feasible) for a minimum of two weeks prior to MSLT as continuous use of these medications or withdrawal can alter the test outcomes.[10] Those medications with longer half-life may need a longer taper and discontinuation period; for example, once-daily fluoxetine should be held (if clinically feasible) for at least 5 weeks prior to MSLT. Such a scenario (sleepy patients taking psychotropic medications) can initiate a referral for psychiatric evaluation from the sleep physician to ensure psychiatric stability of the patient undergoing MSLT without psychotropic medications. If the treating psychiatrist deems discontinuation of psychiatric medications to be too dangerous (such as high suicide risk), the MSLT may still be performed, but the results need to be interpreted in the context of the patient's medication use as the mean sleep latency and presence of SOREMPs may be influenced by psychotropic medications.

Patients are advised to maintain sleep diaries and/or wear an actigraph (see the following discussion) for a period of 7 to 14 days to ensure regular sleep patterns with sufficient sleep and to rule out other sleep disorders potentially causing daytime sleepiness.[10] Complete abstinence from alcohol and potentially confounding substance use (prescription, over-the-counter, or recreational) is recommended and urine drug testing on the day of MSLT should be done for verification. MSLT interpretation can additionally be complicated by the presence of untreated mood or anxiety disorders which may prolong sleep latency and reduce REM latency. There are also age-related differences in mean sleep latency values; specifically, values for young adults are lower than for older adults. However, sensitivity and specificity of two or more SOREMPs for a diagnosis of narcolepsy has been documented as 0.73 and 0.93, respectively.[10]

Maintenance of Wakefulness Test (MWT)

In comparison to MSLT, the MWT is used to assess an individual's ability to stay awake. The MWT is to assess treatment response for daytime hypersomnolence in patients, particularly those with safety-sensitive occupations such as public transportation.[10] The room should be insulated from external light. MWT includes four successive trials to stay awake at 2-hour intervals during the daytime.[10] Each trial lasts until sleep occurs, as defined by three consecutive epochs of stage N1 sleep or one epoch of any other sleep stage, or if no sleep occurs after a period of 40 minutes.[10] Overnight PSG is not needed for MWT, unlike MSLT. Overall mean sleep latency among normal controls was 30.4 ± 11.20 minute latency to first epoch of sleep; however, there is a paucity of studies that provide well defined normative data.[10] Staying awake for the duration of all nap opportunities is the best possible outcome. However, a minimum acceptable result should be based on risk tolerance. The MWT is used as a tool to objectively measure alertness and attempts to predict daytime functionality. Mean sleep latency less than 8 minutes on MWT is clearly abnormal. Mean sleep latency between 8 and 40 minutes has uncertain significance. Staying awake for at least 40 minutes during *all* four sessions is a strong objective evidence that an individual can stay awake. However, test results do not necessarily determine the risk of mistakes or accidents/injuries in the work environment or safety in real-life circumstances.

Actigraphy

An actigraph is a portable device, usually worn on the wrist, that estimates sleep duration and sleep patterns over an extended period of time (see Figure 7.8).[11] It uses activity, as measured by limb movement, as a surrogate measure of sleep.[11] Actigraphy does not directly measure sleep as it does not include EEG monitoring. In comparison to PSG, actigraphy overestimates total sleep time and sleep efficiency by underestimating SOL and wake after sleep onset due to periods of inactive wakefulness. Actigraphy is indicated primarily in the diagnostic work-up of circadian rhythm sleep–wake disorders (delayed sleep–wake phase disorder, advanced sleep–wake phase disorder, non-24-hour sleep–wake rhythm disorder, shift work disorder, jetlag disorder); however, it can also be used in evaluation of refractory insomnia (paradoxical insomnia or sleep-state misperception, behaviorally induced insufficient sleep syndrome), and hypersomnolence disorders.[10,11]

CONCLUSIONS

Primary sleep disorders are frequently comorbid with a range of psychiatric conditions. As such, psychiatrists should be familiar with the technical procedures available for the evaluation of primary sleep disorders. A focused sleep history and physical exam are needed to establish the clinical suspicion for a sleep disorder in patients with psychiatric disease. Screening questionnaires for sleep disorders are also available, although these have variable sensitivities and specificities and are only intended to be used in addition to a clinical history and exam. Objective sleep tests such as PSG, HSAT, and MSLT can then be used, in the appropriate clinical context, for diagnostic confirmation of primary sleep disorders. PSG is most commonly ordered for diagnostic assessment of SRBDs or PAP titration for SRBDs such as OSA, but may be additionally helpful in the evaluation of disorders of central hypersomnolence, parasomnias, suspected periodic limb movement disorder, or nocturnal seizures. HSAT offers added flexibility in the evaluation of OSA, but provides a more limited assessment and therefore should only be used in carefully selected patients. Assessment of hypersomnolence and treatment response may be done with MSLT and MWT. Actigraphy can be used as part of the evaluation for disorders of hypersomnolence, insomnia, or circadian rhythm sleep–wake disorders. Psychiatric providers' familiarity with the use and application of diagnostic procedures in sleep medicine will improve their comfort in terms of explaining and interpreting these diagnostic sleep modalities to their patients. In turn, quality of care of psychiatric patients will likely improve with assessment and subsequent treatment of comorbid primary sleep disorders.

Actogram:

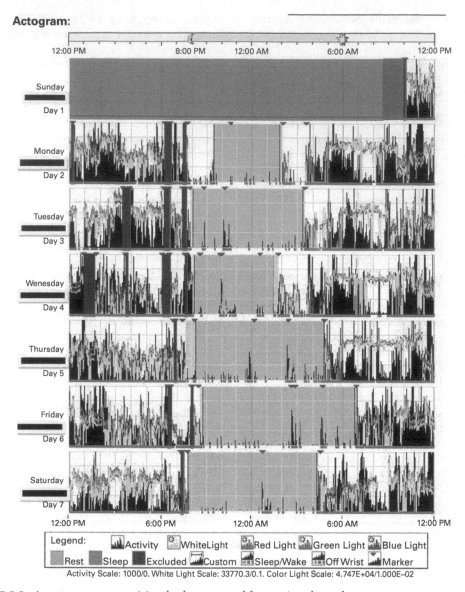

FIGURE 7.8. An actogram, summarizing the data generated from actigraphy study.

FUTURE DIRECTIONS

Future research in psychiatric patients with comorbid sleep disorders should aim to identify new treatment options and enhance currently available therapy with the intention to improve sleep and mood-related outcomes. This process begins with increased awareness that sleep complaints may be potentially more than part of a constellation of symptoms commonly seen with certain psychiatric diagnoses. Promptly eliciting a sleep-specific history and physical examination can help the psychiatrist determine if diagnostic testing through a sleep laboratory is indicated. Integrated approaches including the use of co-therapy, such as with the use of hypnotics, sedating or nonsedating antidepressants, or the optimal timing for initiation of cognitive-behavioral therapy for insomnia in the setting of depression or anxiety, are being studied, as well as investigations into the pathophysiology behind the interconnectedness between psychiatry and sleep. Future developments in sleep medicine diagnostic procedures may add to their clinical utility; however, new technologies will need to be validated as they become more widely available for clinical use.

The use of the patient-centered medical home model and incorporation of psychiatry is becoming more widespread to improve quality of delivered care and access to specialty services. New care models may expand further to similarly include the use of additional subspecialty services such as sleep medicine, in which care may or may not be delivered by a provider with a primary specialty within psychiatry. In the medical home model, there may be a role for assessment and treatment by sleep-specific physician extenders in appropriate cases and circumstances. This could also provide for an opportunity for interaction with behavioral sleep medicine (i.e., sleep psychologists) or ancillary support services such as respiratory therapists, sleep technologists, or durable medical equipment providers, if needed, similar to what is already present within or near many of the larger sleep disorder centers.

KEY CLINICAL PEARLS

- There are specific indications for PSG study and it is not routinely performed for insomnia.
- HSAT study can be helpful for ruling in OSA, but a negative study cannot rule out OSA. A negative home study should be followed by a "gold standard" PSG study for added sensitivity.
- MSLT is performed with a preceding overnight PSG along with prior 7 to 14 days of patient-recorded data for the diagnosis of central disorders of hypersomnolence such as narcolepsy and idiopathic hypersomnia.
- Holding REM suppressants (i.e., stimulants and antidepressants) for accurate MSLT testing (2 weeks generally and at least 5 weeks for fluoxetine) is ideal if able to be safely done; otherwise, the study must be interpreted in the context of the medication use (these medications may influence the presence of REM sleep and thus affect the MSLT results).
- Maintenance of wakefulness test (MWT) is used to assess an individual's ability to stay awake. MWT can be performed to assess treatment response for patients of central disorders of hypersomnolence, particularly those patients with safety-sensitive occupations such as public transportation.
- Actigraphy uses activity measured by limb movement as a surrogate measure of sleep. Actigraphy can be used in the evaluation of circadian rhythm sleep–wake disorders, refractory insomnia and central disorders of hypersomnolence.

SELF-ASSESSMENT QUESTIONS

1. A 56-year old male patient with major depressive disorder, single episode in full remission presents with persistent sleep disturbance. On further questioning, he gives a history of regular and loud snoring, witnessed apneas, nocturnal awakenings, nonrestorative sleep, and daytime tiredness. He has a history of hypertension and congestive heart failure that are well managed currently. What is the best next step to evaluate his clinical complaint?
   a. Polysomnography
   b. Home sleep apnea test
   c. Actigraphy
   d. Multiple sleep latency test (MSLT)

Answer: a

2. A 66-year-old man with severe recurrent major depressive disorder without psychotic features is admitted for suicidal ideation. He reports difficulty maintaining asleep despite use of trazodone and melatonin. He has gained 25 pounds in the past year and has a current body mass index of 39 kg/m². What other comorbid condition would raise your suspicion for obstructive sleep apnea?
   a. Hypertension
   b. Chronic obstructive pulmonary disease (COPD)
   c. Benign prostatic hyperplasia
   d. Migraine headaches
   e. Insomnia

Answer: a

3. A 19-year-old first semester college student presents with excessive daytime sleepiness including falling asleep during classes. The Epworth Sleepiness Scale score is 18/24. Physical exam reveals no abnormalities and body mass index of 21kg/m². A urine drug screen is negative for all substances tested. Sleep logs and actigraphy reveal a regular sleep–wake time and sufficient sleep of 9 hours per night. Which test will help to quantify daytime sleepiness?
   a. Home sleep apnea test
   b. Maintenance of wakefulness test
   c. Polysomnography
   d. Polysomnography followed by multiple sleep latency test

Answer: d

4. A 75-year-old patient with history of unspecified neurocognitive disorder presents with insomnia and reports a regular inability to stay asleep beyond 3 AM. She does not use an alarm and follows appropriate sleep hygiene and stimulus control recommendations. She has difficulty staying awake later than 7 PM. She reports a consistent sleep–wake schedule but notes that her sleep and wake times interfere with her ability to socialize with family and friends, and this is bothersome to her. She denies snoring or observed apneas and excessive daytime sleepiness. Which diagnostic tool could be used to confirm your provisional diagnosis?
   a. Polysomnogram
   b. Actigraphy
   c. Home sleep apnea test
   d. Maintenance of wakefulness test
   e. Multiple sleep latency test

Answer: b

6. Which of the following patients and clinical scenarios would be appropriate for use of home sleep apnea testing?
   a. 75-year-old male with heart failure and daytime sleepiness
   b. 55-year-old female with COPD and snoring
   c. 50-year-old male with hypertension and class I obesity
   d. 25-year-old female with intellectual disability and hypersomnia

Answer: c

REFERENCES

1. American Academy of Sleep Medicine. *International Classification of Sleep Disorders.* 3rd ed. Darien, IL: American Academy of Sleep Medicine; 2014.
2. American Psychiatric Association. *Diagnostic and Statistical Manual of Mental Disorders.* 5th ed. Arlington, VA: American Psychiatric Association; 2013.
3. Kapur VK, Auckley DH, Chowdhuri S, et al. Clinical practice guideline for diagnostic testing for adult obstructive sleep apnea: an American Academy of Sleep Medicine clinical practice guideline. *J Clin Sleep Med.* 2017;13(3):479–504.
4. Berry RB, Wagner MH. *Sleep Medicine Pearls.* 3rd ed. Philadelphia, PA: Elsevier Saunders; 2015.
5. Berry RB, Brooks R, Gamaldo CE, et al. *The AASM Manual for the Scoring of Sleep and Associated Events: Rules, Terminology and Technical Specifications.* Version 2.5. Darien, IL: American Academy of Sleep Medicine; 2018.
6. Mokhlesi B, Taulaimat A, Baibussowitsch I, et al. Obesity hypoventilation syndrome: prevalence and predictors in patients with obstructive sleep apnea, *Sleep Breath.* 2007;11:117–124.
7. Kushida CA, Littner MR, Morgenthaler T, et al. Practice parameters for the indications for polysomnography and related procedures: an update for 2005. *SLEEP* 2005;28(4):499–521.
8. Aurora RN, Chowdhuri S, Ramar K, et al. The treatment of central sleep apnea syndromes in adults: practice parameters with an evidence-based literature review and meta-analyses. *SLEEP* 2012;35(1):17–40.
9. Caples SM, Rowley JA, Prinsell JR, et al. Surgical modifications of the upper airway for obstructive sleep apnea in adults: a systematic review and meta-analysis. *SLEEP* 2010;33(10):1396–1407.
10. Standards of Practice Committee of the American Academy of Sleep Medicine. Practice parameters for clinical use of the multiple sleep latency test and the maintenance of wakefulness test. *SLEEP* 2005;28(1):113–121.
11. Smith MT, McCrae CS, Cheung J, et al. Use of actigraphy for the evaluation of sleep disorders and circadian rhythm sleep-wake disorders: an American Academy of Sleep Medicine clinical practice guideline. *J Clin Sleep Med.* 2018;14(7):1231–1237.
12. Krystal AD. Sleep and psychiatric disorders: Future directions. *Psychiatric Clinics of North America.* 2006;29(4):1115–1130.

PART 2

Sleep–Wake Disorders

8

Insomnia Disorder—Pathophysiology

FEE BENZ, ELISABETH HERTENSTEIN, ANNA JOHANN,
AND DIETER RIEMANN

INTRODUCTION

Insomnia disorder (ID) is defined as a subjective report of difficulty with initiating or maintaining sleep or early morning awakening occurring at least three times per week over a period of 3 months. In addition, at least one associated daytime symptom, such as fatigue, cognitive impairment or mood disturbance, has to be present (*Diagnostic and Statistical Manual of Mental Disorders* [DSM] fifth edition; DSM-5[1]). In comparison to the DSM fourth edition (DSM-IV) definition, the distinction between primary and secondary insomnia, indicating whether the insomnia is comorbid with or caused by other disorders, was replaced by the term "insomnia disorder" (ID) in DSM-5. This reflects the change in perspective where insomnia is now recognized as a distinct, and often independent, disorder.[2] ID affects a large segment of the population with prevalence rates ranging from 3.9% to 22.1% depending on the diagnostic criteria applied.[3] Whereby complaints of insomnia can be situational or recurrent, its course is often chronic.[2] Furthermore, insomnia leads to high societal costs.[4] The disorder is associated with reduced quality of life[5,6] and increased risk for developing cardio-metabolic diseases[7,8] as well as psychiatric disorders, especially depression.[9] Despite the high prevalence and its global burden, the pathophysiology of ID is still not fully clear.[2] Several models have been proposed, and this chapter aims at presenting an overview of such models. Relevant models explaining how insomnia develops, and how it becomes chronic and self-perpetuating will be described, and their evidence will be summarized. Finally, integrative approaches dealing with the pathophysiology of ID will be presented.

THE 3P MODEL

General Description

The 3P model[10] which is also known as the behavioral model, the Spielman model, or the three-factor model, is a specification of the diathesis-stress model that explains how acute insomnia develops and becomes chronic. The model describes the interaction of three factors. *Predisposing factors* such as genetics, certain personality traits (perfectionism, neuroticism), and the tendency to ruminate excessively make individuals vulnerable to develop insomnia. *Precipitating factors* include stressful life events that can trigger an acute episode of insomnia. Actually, acute insomnia is very common but usually remits after the cessation of the stressor.[11] *Perpetuating factors* explain how acute insomnia becomes chronic and refer to maladaptive strategies adopted to cope with the sleep loss such as spending excessive time in bed or napping during the day. In fact, these strategies lead to a reduced homeostatic sleep pressure[12] and therefore reinforce the sleep problem. Spielman et al.[13] updated the original version of the 3P model: original version illustrates the temporal course of the three factors while updated version introduces a fourth P factor (4 P model), namely, Pavlovian (classical) conditioning. More specifically, sleep-related stimuli (e.g., the bed) are repeatedly coupled with wakefulness. Over time, the bed becomes a conditioned stimulus eliciting arousal and wakefulness. This explains why patients with ID often report getting sleepy in the evening but feel wide awake again as soon as they are in bed. The original 3P model can also serve as a framework for other models due to its heuristic and practical value.[14] In fact, most other models of insomnia are explicitly or implicitly based on this model.[15]

Evidence

Evidence concerning predisposing factors suggests an aggregation of insomnia in families.[16] This may be due to genetic reasons as well as to process of learning where children acquire sleep-related behavior from their parents. The studies examining monozygotic and dizygotic twins estimate the heritability of insomnia between 30% and 60%[17-20] suggesting that a hereditary factor indeed exists. Although some candidate genes have been proposed,[21-23] there is no consensus about which genes are relevant for insomnia. A longitudinal study by Drake and colleagues[20] found that sleep reactivity, defined as a tendency to react to stressful events with resultant sleep disturbances, is a predisposing factor for insomnia.

Concerning precipitating factors, both retrospective and prospective studies have shown an association between life stressors and the development of new-onset insomnia.[24] For example, in a retrospective study, Bastien and colleagues[25] identified stressful life events with a negative valence related to health, family relationships, work, or school as the most frequently reported precipitating factors. A prospective study by Jansson-Fröjmark and colleagues[26] suggests that perceived work stressors are significantly, but rather weakly, associated with the development and maintenance of insomnia. Morin and colleagues[27] proposed that the appraisal of and the perceived lack of control over stressors rather than the number of stressful life events increase the vulnerability to develop insomnia. All in all, precipitating factors of insomnia have been mainly investigated retrospectively. Since this research method is prone to memory bias, further research is needed to determine which stressful events reliably precede acute insomnia.

A comprehensive review[28] on mediators of cognitive-behavioral therapy for insomnia suggests that therapeutic effects of sleep restriction, a core component of the first-line treatment of insomnia, are mediated by reduced time in bed. This finding supports the role of maladaptive strategies, such as extending time in bed to compensate for sleep loss, as perpetuating factors of insomnia. Still, longitudinal studies are necessary to investigate whether the transition from acute to chronic insomnia is mediated by extended time in bed.[29]

STIMULUS CONTROL MODEL

General Description

Stimulus control was originally described by Bootzin.[30] According to this model, the process of falling asleep can be viewed as an "instrumental act emitted to produce reinforcement."[31] External and internal sleep-onset–related cues become discriminative stimuli for the occurrence of reinforcement (sleep). Therefore, difficulties in falling asleep may be a consequence of stimulus dyscontrol. In addition, classical conditioning plays an important role.[31] In patients with insomnia, cues that are normally associated with sleep, such as the bed or the bedroom, are often paired with wakefulness, frustration, and behaviors other than sleep. Thus, sleep-related stimuli like bed or bedroom become conditioned stimuli eliciting conditioned responses of wakefulness and arousal. The classical conditioning model fits well with the observation that patients with insomnia often report being tired and sleepy in the evening, but feeling wide awake again when in the bedroom that they usually describe as having "a second wind." The goal of stimulus control therapy is to restrengthen the association between the sleeping environment, sleepiness, and sleep.

Evidence

Stimulus control therapy is a widely used behavioral treatment for insomnia and its efficacy is well documented.[32,33] However, stimulus control therapy also includes components that can influence homeostatic and circadian regulation of sleep, for example, avoiding daytime napping or getting up at the same time every morning. Hence, the success of stimulus control therapy does not provide sufficient evidence for the stimulus control model. To identify the critical components that account for the efficacy of stimulus control therapy, dismantling studies comparing discrete components of the therapy with the total multicomponent treatment are needed.[29]

COGNITIVE MODELS

Using the 3P model as a framework, cognitive models posit that cognitive arousal (rumination and worry) predispose individuals to develop insomnia, precipitate acute insomnia, and perpetuate the ID.[14] Among the most prominent cognitive models are those by Lundh and Broman,[34] Harvey,[35] and Espie and colleagues.[36]

Lundh and Broman
General Description

According to Lundh and Broman,[34] two distinct, yet interacting psychological processes contribute to the development of insomnia. *Sleep-interfering processes* (e.g., rumination) lead to arousal and sleep disturbances. *Sleep-interpreting processes* (e.g., dysfunctional sleep-related beliefs) refer to an individual's appraisal of sleeplessness and daytime impairment. Vulnerability factors that may contribute to the sleep-interfering processes include personality characteristics such as arous- ability (i.e., emotional sensitivity), a tendency to worry, slow recuperation after stress, and emo- tional conflicts in important personal relation- ships. Variables that may predispose people to engage in dysfunctional sleep-interpreting pro- cesses include perfectionism concerning sleep and daytime functioning, and sleep-related beliefs (e.g. "To function well during the day, you have to sleep 8 hours per night"). Thus, the more per- fectionistic a person is or the more dysfunctional sleep-related beliefs a person has, the more severe the condition of insomnia is perceived. In sum- mary, the authors suggest a model explaining how ruminative thinking and dysfunctional sleep- related beliefs contribute to the development of insomnia.

Evidence

Several other pathophysiological theories focus on what Lundh and Broman[34] call sleep-interfering processes, for example, stressful life events (pre- cipitating factors in the 3P model), and worries and rumination (Harvey Model), which cause emotional, cognitive, and physiological arousal (Harvey model, hyperarousal model) thereby interfering with sleep. Evidence for these pro- cesses is summarized under the corresponding theories. According to the Lundh and Broman model, patients with insomnia also engage in dys- functional sleep-interpreting processes, and there is evidence supporting this idea.[37,38] For example, Carney and colleagues[38] found that patients with insomnia held stronger dysfunctional beliefs about sleep than good sleepers. To find out if appraisal and interpretation moderate insomnia sever- ity, studies are needed that evaluate the extent to which cognitive therapeutic approaches address- ing appraisal and interpretation lead to additive effects when combined with behavioral interven- tions. The model also suggests that individual vulnerability factors may predispose insomnia patients to respond with sleep-interfering process (rumination) and to engage in sleep-interpreting processes. Lundh and Broman[34] review evidence for these factors. However, most of the reviewed data come from cross-sectional studies; so no conclusions about causality can be drawn. Taken together, there is evidence for some components proposed in the model, but not all causal links have been tested. The authors emphasize that their aim was not to capture all relevant variables but instead to provide a basic model that may be further developed as new evidence emerges.

Harvey
General Description

According to Harvey's model,[35] patients with insomnia suffer from excessive negatively toned cognitive activity. In contrast to healthy people with occasional sleep disturbances, they are afraid of the consequences of sleep loss on their daytime functioning and health. This negatively toned cognitive activity triggers autonomic arousal and emotional distress. Due to this anxious state, an increased selective attention toward sleep-related threat cues such as indicators for insufficient sleep or daytime deficits occurs. Thus, patients moni- tor their internal environment (e.g., body sensa- tions) as well as their external environment (e.g., the bedroom clock) for sleep-related threats. This monitoring increases the probability of detecting random cues that are meaningless but are inter- preted as a threat. For example, a momentary dif- ficulty of not remembering a name is interpreted as a result of sleep loss although good sleepers do sometimes not remember a name, too. Detection of such a threat reinforces rumination and wor- rying. That way, a self-perpetuating vicious circle arises. The model posits that the anxious state and the selective attention lead to an overestimation of sleep loss and its consequences for daytime func- tioning (distorted perception). Finally, erroneous beliefs about sleep and counterproductive safety behaviors (e.g., extended time in bed, napping during the day, avoiding work) contribute to the maintenance of the disorder by increasing worry- ing and rumination. Safety behaviors also prevent falsification of erroneous beliefs about sleep.

Evidence

Empirical data support some of the components proposed by this model. For instance, research has shown that people with insomnia experience excessive cognitive activity during the presleep period,[39] that this cognitive activity is more nega- tive in comparison to good sleepers,[40] and that the content of this presleep cognitive activity is related to sleeplessness.[41] Several studies using different methodologies support the assumption that patients with insomnia, compared to healthy sleepers, show an increased attention to inter- nal and external sleep-related cues and suggest that this bias is not conducive to sleep (see next section The Attention Intention Effort Model). Furthermore, a large body of research supports an underestimation of sleep by patients with insom- nia compared to controls, that is, a discrepancy between subjective estimates of total sleep time and objectively measured sleep.[42–45] Patients with insomnia do engage in a wide range of safety behaviors to prevent feared outcomes.[46] Woodley and Smith[47] found that depression and dysfunctional beliefs about sleep predicted sleep-related safety behaviors. Jansson and Linton[48] examined the association of arousal, anxiety, depression, and beliefs regarding the long-term negative consequences of insomnia with the maintenance of insomnia. Comparing a group with insomnia with a good sleeper control group, the four variables explained 50% of the variance while the belief in the long-term consequences of insomnia explained the largest amount of variance. While there is evidence for some of the components of the model, few of the suggested causal links have been tested; so further research is needed.[35]

The Attention Intention Effort Model
General Description
The central assumption of this model is that sleep is an automatic and involuntary process and that direct attempts to control this process lead to the inhibition of sleep.[36] Besides the homeostatic and the circadian processes involved in the regulation of sleep,[49] Espie and colleagues[36] suggest a third implicit process, namely "automaticity," that is associated with the regulation of sleep–wake patterns in healthy sleepers. While healthy sleepers are passive and do not really do anything to sleep, the patients with insomnia are very concerned about their sleep. Therefore, patients with insomnia show an attentional bias toward sleep-related stimuli, they explicitly intend to fall asleep, and this intention triggers effort being put into the sleep process. According to the model, this attention–intention–effort (A-I-E) pathway inhibits the sleep-wake automaticity.[36]

Evidence
As previously mentioned, a large body of research supports an attentional bias toward sleep.[50–57] Different methodologies involving questionnaire data, real-world experiments and experiments using computerized tasks have been used.[36] Compared to questionnaire data, computerized experimental studies (e.g., the emotional Stroop task) measure objective reaction times and do not rely on self-report. In real-world experiments, attention is manipulated and its role in changing insomnia symptoms is measured. For example, Tang and colleagues[52] instructed poor and good sleepers to monitor or not monitor a clock when they were trying to fall asleep. Those who monitored the clock, both poor *and* good sleepers, showed prolonged sleep onset latencies (SOL) as well as higher worry ratings compared to the control group. Such findings support the hypothesis that an attentional bias toward sleep-related stimuli may contribute to insomnia.

While there is substantial support for the attentional bias hypothesis, there is less evidence for the second (intention) and the third (effort) components of the model. Studies using the multiple sleep latency test (MSLT), consisting of five nap opportunities (20 minutes) with electroencephalography (EEG) sleep monitoring indicating daytime sleepiness, provide indirect evidence for the intention and effort components inhibiting sleep. Against expectation, patients with insomnia show prolonged rather than reduced SOL during MSLT.[58,59] This could possibly be explained by the demand characteristics of the MSLT (i.e., patients are explicitly instructed to try to fall asleep). Furthermore, the effectiveness of paradoxical intention as a single therapy[32,60] may also indirectly support the inhibitory characteristic of an explicit intention to fall asleep. In paradoxical intention therapy, patients are encouraged to try to stay awake and to take an accepting role.[61] In an experimental trial investigating the effect of paradoxical intention on sleep effort and SOL, Broomfield and colleagues[62] suggested that paradoxical intention may operate by eliminating sleep effort. This finding also supports the third component of the model. In a study by Ansfield and colleagues[63] investigating good sleepers, two factors were experimentally manipulated: sleep intention (instruction to fall asleep as fast as possible vs. whenever desired) and "cognitive load" (stirring, marching band music vs. sleep-conducive, restful outdoor sounds). Under high cognitive load, SOL was higher for participants instructed to fall asleep as fast as possible, and under low cognitive load the other group fell asleep more quickly. The cognitive load in terms of marching band music used in this study may resemble the cognitive activity experienced in the presleep period by many insomnia patients. Results suggest that the interaction of sleep intention and cognitive load is important in insomnia.[36] Studies using the Glasgow Sleep Effort Scale (GSES)[64,65] have shown that this scale can discriminate insomnia patients from good sleepers, suggesting that sleep effort is an important component in insomnia. In the light of preliminary evidence, more research is necessary especially concerning the intention and effort components of A-I-E model.

HYPERAROUSAL MODEL

General Description

With respect to the pathophysiology of insomnia, the hyperarousal model[66] has gained great attention. The hyperarousal model is an integrative approach presuming interplay between psychological and physiological factors in the development and perpetuation of ID. As the name suggests, the hyperarousal model posits a heightened arousal in the cognitive, emotional, and physiological domains during night time and daytime in patients with insomnia. The model is based on the 3P model, whereby increased arousal represents both a predisposing *and* perpetuating factor.[66–68] Thus, as a result of classical conditioning, the sleep environment becomes a conditioned stimulus for arousal instead of relaxation and sleep, and this resultant arousal (conditioned response) can perpetuate the disorder. The cortical arousal is hypothesized to promote (a) enhanced sensory information processing during sleep onset and sleep and (b) enhanced memory formation during sleep onset and for arousals during sleep, which, in both cases, can help to explain the sleep state misperception (i.e., underestimation of actual sleep time). The concept of hyperarousal fits well with neurobiological models of sleep–wake regulation like the flip-flop switch model of Saper and colleagues.[69] This model summarizes the current knowledge about the neurobiology and neurochemistry of the reciprocal interactions between sleep-inducing and wake-promoting brain areas (flip-flop switch). Hence, hyperarousal may be seen as a consequence of a dominance of arousal and wake-inducing brain pathways in comparison to sleep-inducing areas suggesting a malfunction of the "key switch" between activation and deactivation.

Evidence

Perlis and colleagues[67,70] conducted a review of the hyperarousal literature suggesting a "neurocognitive model" of insomnia. Later, Riemann and colleagues[66] published a second review of the hyperarousal perspective integrating these findings with neuroscientific knowledge on sleep–wake regulation. The finding that patients with insomnia show increased rather than reduced sleep latencies in the MSLT[58,59] supports the idea of a 24-hour hyperarousal in insomnia patients. In a meta-analysis of polysomnographic studies, Baglioni and colleagues[71] found that patients with insomnia, compared to good sleeper controls,

slept less (approximately 23 minutes), need longer to fall asleep (approximately 6 minutes) and had more awakenings (approximately 6) per night. Further, insomnia patients seemed to spend less time in slow-wave sleep and rapid eye movement (REM) sleep. However, the differences in sleep continuity were not large and did not reflect the subjectively estimated differences. Since there is a discrepancy between the subjective sleep complaint and objectively measured sleep through polysomnography, more fine-grained approaches such as spectral analysis of EEG sleep, the assessment of event-related potentials (ERP) prior to and during sleep and the analysis of micro-arousals and the cyclic alternating pattern (CAP) have generated significant interest.[66,72] For example, spectral analysis studies have shown that patients with insomnia have increased power in fast EEG frequencies during sleep.[73–77] These fast frequencies have been hypothesized to play a role in cortical processing of sensory information. Thus, the findings so far support the cortical hyperactivity hypothesis. Only few of the ERP studies that have been conducted so far suggest an increased sensitivity to auditory stimuli during wake and sleep onset in patients with insomnia.[66] Moreover, an increased frequency of micro-arousals during REM sleep was observed in patients with insomnia in comparison to healthy sleepers.[72,78] This "REM sleep instability" may contribute to the experience of disrupted and nonrestorative sleep and may play an important role in the pathophysiology of insomnia.[45,78] Consistent with the hyperarousal model, an increased CAP rate—a non-REM sleep EEG marker of unstable sleep and poor sleep quality—has been found in insomnia patients.[79,80] Altogether, findings of these fine-grained approaches might reflect a mixed or hybrid sleep–wake state[68] contributing to the sleep state misperception found in insomnia patients.

Evidence for the hyperarousal concept also comes from studies measuring autonomous and neuroendocrine variables and parameters of the immune system as well as from neuroimaging studies.[66] For instance, an elevated heart rate, altered heart rate variability,[81,82] and an increased basal metabolic rate[83] have been found in insomnia patients. Furthermore, some researchers found an increased cortisol secretion[84,85] while others did not find differences between insomnia patients and healthy controls.[86,87] A fluorodeoxyglucose positron emission tomography (FDG-PET) study by Nofzinger and colleagues[88] also provides evidence for the hyperarousal model. They observed an increased global cerebral glucose metabolism in parts of the arousal system, the emotion-regulating system and the cognitive system during sleep and wake in insomnia patients compared to good sleeper controls. With respect to the transition from wakefulness to sleep, insomnia patients also showed a significantly smaller decline of activity in wake-promoting regions. These results were replicated in a recent FDG-PET study by the same research group[89] using a larger sample size. In a review about the neurobiology of chronic insomnia, Riemann and colleagues[68] summarized findings of brain imaging studies (daytime and sleep investigations) identifying important brain areas that may be involved in the pathophysiology of insomnia. These areas include the hippocampus, the amygdala, the thalamus, the caudate head, the anterior cingulate cortex, and the frontal cortex. In a proton magnetic resonance spectroscopy study, Winkelman and colleagues[90] found reduced levels of γ-aminobutyric acid (GABA), the most important inhibitory neurotransmitter in the central nervous system, in patients with insomnia. This finding may account for difficulties in initiating and maintaining sleep.

Although substantial support for the idea that hyperarousal processes play a decisive role in the pathophysiology of insomnia has been delivered, it is important to note that all studies were cross-sectional, so no conclusions about cause–effect relationships can be drawn. Thus, it is still unclear whether hyperarousal leads to insomnia, or vice versa, or whether there is a bidirectional relationship. Moreover, there is partially conflicting evidence, and many studies drew findings based on rather small samples. Further research using larger sample sizes and longitudinal designs is needed.[66]

FURTHER APPROACHES

Circadian Factors

With respect to the development and maintenance of insomnia, circadian factors may also be relevant in a subgroup of individuals. For instance, in shift workers or blind patients the sleep–wake pattern and the circadian phase is desynchronized, which can lead to sleep initiation and sleep maintenance difficulties. Adolescents and young adults may also be affected by sleep-onset insomnia due to a circadian phase delay, whereas a phase advance may be associated with early awakening in elderly people.[15] If circadian factors are primarily causative, the problem would rather be classified as circadian rhythm sleep wake disorder instead of ID. Hence, this should be considered in the process of differential diagnosis.

Animal Models

In recent years, increasing efforts were dedicated to modelling insomnia in rodents.[91] Using a cage-exchange paradigm, Cano and colleagues[92] investigated the pattern of Fos expression to identify activated brain areas. Fos is a transcription factor that can be used as a marker of neuronal activity.[93] The authors transferred a male rat from his home cage to a cage that was previously occupied by another male rat. Since rats are very territorial, the cage exchange and the exposure to the odor of the other rat produced stress, leading to sleep disturbances. During this period of disturbed sleep, the authors found increased Fos in the cerebral cortex, limbic system, and parts of the arousal and autonomic systems. Interestingly, they observed a simultaneous activation of sleep-inducing brain areas probably driven by circadian and homeostatic pressure. The simultaneous activation of sleep-inducing and wake-promoting brain regions reflects a hybrid sleep–wake state that may result in instability of the flip-flop switch of sleep–wake regulation as suggested by Saper and colleagues.[69] It also suggests that circumscribed brain areas can independently be in different states of sleep and wakefulness[68] at the same time. This hybrid sleep–wake state may bear similarities to human insomnia characterized by fast EEG frequencies and micro-arousals. For instance, patients with insomnia subjectively experience daytime sleepiness and at the same time are unable to fall asleep when they intend to do so. Additionally, insomnia patients often show a misperception of sleep. Research in this area is still at an early age and future research may help to shed light on the neurobiology of insomnia as well as to foster the development of new pharmacological treatments for insomnia. However, the potential benefits of animal experimentation should be carefully weighed against ethical considerations.

Epigenetics

Epigenetics refer to the study of molecular or cellular alterations in response to environmental factors that influence gene expression but do not change the gene sequence. Epigenetic changes have the potential to influence physiology and behavior. Hence, epigenetic modifications provide an explanation of how stressful life events cause changes in the adult brain structure and function and, in a further step, may affect behavior. Epigenetic mechanisms have also been suggested to be involved in the development and perpetuation of insomnia.[24] It has been argued that stressful life events may have the capability to alter the activity of stress-regulatory systems and that this effect might be mediated by epigenetic mechanisms at the molecular level. It is hypothesized that this epigenetic change could evoke long-term alterations in brain structures such as the hippocampus, which is a particularly plastic and vulnerable brain region with respect to stress.[24,68] It can be hypothesized that the beneficial effects of cognitive behavioral treatment as well as pharmacological treatment for insomnia are explained through epigenetic mechanisms.[24] For example, a psychotherapy-epigenetic study investigating patients with panic disorder found epigenetic changes (reversibility of monoamine oxidase A hypomethylation) as a correlate of response to cognitive behavior therapy.[94] More detailed information on the role of epigenetics in insomnia can be found in a review by Palagini and colleagues.[24]

Metacognition

Ong and colleagues[95] presented a metacognitive model of insomnia that is based on the cognitive models. Metacognition refers to the awareness of one's own cognitive activity or, in other words, "thinking about thinking." The authors differentiate between primary and secondary arousal, and both are seen as key factors in the pathophysiology of ID. Primary arousal refers to cognitive activity concerning the inability to sleep (e.g., beliefs about daytime consequences of sleep loss), and secondary arousal refers to the way one relates to his or her thoughts about sleep (e.g., emotional valence, degree of attachment to these thoughts). The model suggests the use of mindfulness and acceptance-based approaches to reduce secondary arousal, which, in turn, is hypothesized to reduce primary arousal. Metacognitive therapies for insomnia seek to increase the awareness of the cognitive and physical states associated with insomnia. Patients learn to shift mental processes, promoting an adaptive stance between own thoughts and their appraisal. The aim of such techniques is to reduce secondary arousal and therefore prevent the perpetuation of negative emotions.[95]

Research on mindfulness and acceptance-based therapies for insomnia is still in its infancy and randomized controlled trials (RCT) are lacking. In one RCT, Gross and colleagues[96] compared mindfulness-based stress reduction with eszopiclone in insomnia patients. Both groups showed significant improvements on actigraphy-measured SOL, subjectively estimated SOL, total sleep time, and sleep efficiency, and no significant intergroup differences were found. Further research is needed to test the efficacy of metacognitive therapies for insomnia to identify treatment mechanisms and to compare mindfulness and acceptance-based therapies to other approaches such as cognitive behavioral therapy for insomnia (CBT-I) as well as their combination.

Misperception of Sleep

As previously mentioned, a discrepancy between objectively measured and subjectively estimated sleep has been noted in insomnia patients. It is not uncommon that patients with insomnia overestimate their SOL and underestimate their total sleep time. Researchers still are puzzled over this robust finding which nevertheless is not universal among insomnia patients.[97] Although the misperception of sleep is not a pathophysiologic model of insomnia per se, Harvey and Tang[97] suggest that the tendency to misperceive sleep might be a mechanism that may contribute to the development and maintenance of insomnia. Thus, insomnia outcomes may improve by reversing patients' misperceptions about their sleep as a part of a multicomponent treatment for insomnia. In a review, Harvey and Tang[97] outline and critically evaluate 13 possible explanations for the misperception of sleep. Finally, the authors propose an integrative model based on the best empirical evidence. The model involves seven processes that may contribute to the misperception of sleep. First, contextual factors (e.g., darkness, clock checking) provide a fertile ground for misperception. Next, worry, selective attention, and a cortical arousal, together with a fault in neuronal circuitry, lead to chronic activation of the arousal system. Due to this arousal state, more transient awakenings occur, and physiological sleep is often perceived as wakefulness. Taken together, this may lead to a misperception of sleep. Other possible explanations for the misperception of sleep that have been mentioned in this chapter may be added to parts of this model; for example, the REM instability hypothesis[78] could be part of "transient awakenings." Future research should aim at further explaining the discrepancy between objective and subjective sleep parameters in insomnia.

CONCLUSION AND FUTURE DIRECTIONS

Although insomnia is a highly prevalent disorder and a major public health burden, the underlying mechanisms of the development and perpetuation of the disorder are still not fully understood. There are several models that may explain the pathophysiology of insomnia—the exact interplay between genetic, behavioral, cognitive, emotional, and neurobiological factors, however, is still a matter of debate.[2] Most models are explicitly or implicitly based on the original version of the 3P model by Spielman et al.[10] describing the interaction of predisposing, precipitating, and perpetuating factors. While psychological perspectives emphasize the role of dysfunctional sleep-related cognitions and a selective attention toward sleep-related stimuli, neurobiological perspectives particularly emphasize the physiological alterations such as hyperactivity of arousal-promoting systems and/or a hypoactivity of sleep-promoting systems in the brain. Most of the models presented herein are not mutually exclusive[29] but rather complement each other (see Figure 8.1). Neurobiological and psychological processes are highly interdependent and interrelated.[66] Moreover, since insomnia is a very complex and heterogeneous disorder, there might probably be different causal mechanisms.[98] To improve the treatment of insomnia, Riemann and colleagues[12,15,68] promote a psycho-neurobiological approach to integrate psychological and neurobiological knowledge in the understanding of the pathophysiology of chronic insomnia. Due to limitations of the current research including small sample sizes, correlational designs, and the need for replication for numerous findings, it is not possible to draw final conclusions on the pathophysiology of insomnia, and therefore future research is needed. Since epigenetics, animal models, and metacognition are relatively new approaches in the field of insomnia, they might be interesting and promising topics for future research. CBT-I is the first-line treatment for chronic insomnia.[12,15] However, many patients retain sleep disturbances after CBT-I and up to 25% don't show any treatment response.[99] Further investigating the pathophysiology may help to identify underlying mechanisms of the development and perpetuation of insomnia and in a next step, to improve therapy.

KEY CLINICAL PEARLS

- Individual predisposing, precipitating, and perpetuating factors contributing to the development and maintenance of ID should be assessed to guide treatment decisions.
- Several etiological models have been proposed highlighting genetic, psychological, and neurobiological factors. Thus, interventions from multiple disciplines such as psychotherapy, pharmacotherapy, and noninvasive brain stimulation may be appropriate for the treatment of insomnia.
- The models described in this chapter shed light into how insomnia develops and becomes chronic. Thus, it provides a framework for future research and may help to understand why insomnia presents as it does and how different treatments may work.

SELF-ASSESSMENT QUESTIONS

1. Which of the following components does not belong to the Harvey model?
   a. Excessive cognitive activity
   b. Safety behaviors
   c. Sleep effort
   d. Monitoring sleep-related threats

Answer: c

2. Which of the following options is a central tenet of the A-I-E model by Espie and colleagues?[36]
   a. Sleep-interfering process
   b. Automaticity
   c. Metacognition
   d. Classical conditioning

Answer: b

3. Which is not a common alternative name for the 3P model?
   a. Spielman model
   b. Three-factor model
   c. Behavioral model
   d. Cognitive model

Answer: d

4. Which answer is not true for the hyperarousal model?
   a. The hyperarousal model posits that only physiological factors play a role in the development and perpetuation of insomnia.
   b. The hyperarousal model is based on the 3P model.
   c. Conditioned arousal expressed in terms of somatic, cognitive and cortical activation is a perpetuating factor of the disorder.
   d. The hyperarousal model posits a heightened arousal in the cognitive, emotional and

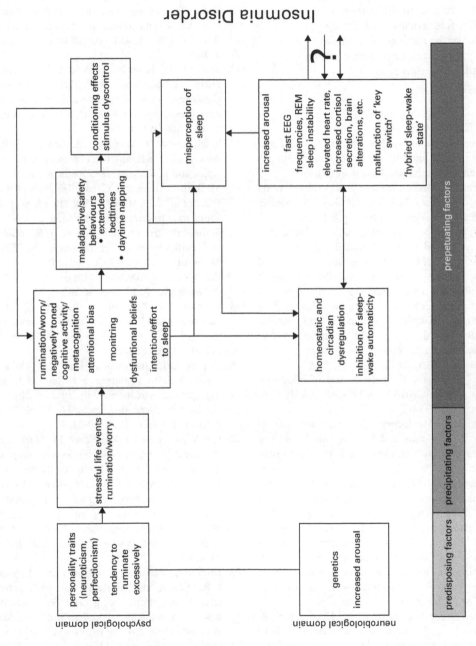

FIGURE 8.1. Predisposing, precipitating, and perpetuating factors for insomnia disorder.

physiological domains during night time
and daytime in patients with insomnia.

Answer: a

5. **Which factor may contribute to the misperception of sleep?**
   a. REM sleep instability
   b. A hybrid sleep–wake state
   c. Fast frequencies in EEG sleep
   d. All of the mentioned factors are
      hypothesized to contribute to the
      misperception of sleep.

Answer: d

REFERENCES

1. American Psychiatric Association. *Diagnostic and Statistical Manual of Mental Disorders.* 5th ed. American Psychiatric Association; 2013.
2. Morin CM, Drake CL, Harvey AG, et al. Insomnia disorder. *Nat Rev Dis Primer.* September 2015;1:15026. doi:10.1038/nrdp.2015.26.
3. Roth T, Coulouvrat C, Hajak G, et al. Prevalence and perceived health associated with insomnia based on DSM-IV-TR; International Statistical Classification of Diseases and Related Health Problems, Tenth Revision; and Research Diagnostic Criteria/International Classification of Sleep Disorders, Second Edition criteria: results from the America Insomnia Survey. *Biol Psychiatry.* 2011;69(6):592–600. doi:10.1016/j.biopsych.2010.10.023.
4. Léger D, Bayon V. Societal costs of insomnia. *Sleep Med Rev.* 2010;14(6):379–389. doi:10.1016/j.smrv.2010.01.003.
5. Katz DA, McHorney CA. The relationship between insomnia and health-related quality of life in patients with chronic illness. *J Fam Pract.* 2002;51(3):229–235.
6. Wickwire EM, Shaya FT, Scharf SM. Health economics of insomnia treatments: the return on investment for a good night's sleep. *Sleep Med Rev.* 2016;30:72–82. doi:10.1016/j.smrv.2015.11.004.
7. Sofi F, Cesari F, Casini A, Macchi C, Abbate R, Gensini GF. Insomnia and risk of cardiovascular disease: a meta-analysis. *Eur J Prev Cardiol.* 2014;21(1):57–64. doi:10.1177/2047487312460020.
8. Spiegelhalder K, Johann A, Hertenstein E, Baglioni C, Riemann D. Die Prävention körperlicher Erkrankungen durch eine Behandlung von Insomnien. *Somnologie—Schlafforschung Schlafmed.* 2015;19(2):93–97. doi:10.1007/s11818-015-0003-y.
9. Baglioni C, Battagliese G, Feige B, et al. Insomnia as a predictor of depression: a meta-analytic evaluation of longitudinal epidemiological studies. *J Affect Disord.* 2011;135(1-3):10–19. doi:10.1016/j.jad.2011.01.011.
10. Spielman AJ, Caruso LS, Glovinsky PB. A behavioral perspective on insomnia treatment. *Psychiatr Clin North Am.* 1987;10(4):541–553.
11. Ellis JG, Gehrman P, Espie CA, Riemann D, Perlis ML. Acute insomnia: current conceptualizations and future directions. *Sleep Med Rev.* 2012;16(1):5–14. doi:10.1016/j.smrv.2011.02.002.
12. Riemann D, Baum E, Cohrs S, et al. S3-Leitlinie Nicht erholsamer Schlaf/SchlafstörungenS3 Guidelines on non-restorative sleep/sleep disorders. *Somnologie.* 2017;21(1):2–44. doi:10.1007/s11818-016-0097-x.
13. Spielman, A. J, Yang, C. M, Glovinsky, P. B. Assessment techniques for insomnia in principles and practice of sleep medicine. In: Kryger M, Roth T, Dement WC, eds. *The Principles and Practice of Sleep Medicine.* Vol 5th ed. St. Louis: Saunders, Elsevier; 2011:1632–1656.
14. Perlis ML, Smith MT, Pigeon WR. Etiology and pathophysiology of insomnia. In: Kryger M, Roth T, Dement WC, eds. *Principles and Practice of Sleep Medicine.* (4th ed., pp. 714–725). Philadelphia, PA: Elsevier/Saunders; 2005.
15. Riemann D, Baglioni C, Bassetti C, et al. European guideline for the diagnosis and treatment of insomnia. *J Sleep Res.* 26(6):675–700. doi:10.1111/jsr.12594.
16. Harvey C-J, Gehrman P, Espie CA. Who is predisposed to insomnia: a review of familial aggregation, stress-reactivity, personality and coping style. *Sleep Med Rev.* 2014;18(3):237–247. doi:10.1016/j.smrv.2013.11.004.
17. Heath AC, Kendler KS, Eaves LJ, Martin NG. Evidence for genetic influences on sleep disturbance and sleep pattern in twins. *Sleep.* 1990;13(4):318–335. doi:10.1093/sleep/13.4.318.
18. Watson NF, Goldberg J, Arguelles L, Buchwald D. Genetic and environmental influences on insomnia, daytime sleepiness, and obesity in twins. *Sleep.* 2006;29(5):645–649. doi:10.1093/sleep/29.5.645.
19. Hublin C, Partinen M, Koskenvuo M, Kaprio J. heritability and mortality risk of insomnia-related symptoms: a genetic epidemiologic study in a population-based twin cohort. *Sleep.* 2011;34(7):957–964. doi:10.5665/SLEEP.1136.
20. Drake CL, Friedman NP, Wright KP, Roth T. Sleep reactivity and insomnia: genetic and environmental influences. *Sleep.* 2011;34(9):1179–1188. doi:10.5665/SLEEP.1234.
21. Deuschle M, Schredl M, Schilling C, et al. Association between a serotonin transporter

length polymorphism and primary insomnia. *Sleep*. 2010;33(3):343.

22. Buhr A, Bianchi MT, Baur R, et al. Functional characterization of the new human GABAA receptor mutation β3(R192H). *Hum Genet*. 2002;111(2):154–160. doi:10.1007/s00439-002-0766-7.

23. Serretti A, Benedetti F, Mandelli L, et al. Genetic dissection of psychopathological symptoms: insomnia in mood disorders and CLOCK gene polymorphism. *Am J Med Genet*. 2003;121B(1):35–38. doi:10.1002/ajmg.b.20053.

24. Palagini L, Biber K, Riemann D. The genetics of insomnia: evidence for epigenetic mechanisms? *Sleep Med Rev*. 2014;18(3):225–235. doi:10.1016/j.smrv.2013.05.002.

25. Bastien CH, Vallieres A, Morin CM. Precipitating factors of insomnia. *Behav Sleep Med*. June 2010. doi:10.1207/s15402010bsm0201_5.

26. Jansson-Fröjmark M, Lundqvist D, Lundqvist N, Linton SJ. Psychosocial work stressors for insomnia: a prospective study on 50–60-year-old adults in the working population. *Int J Behav Med*. 2007;14(4):222–228.

27. Morin CM, Rodrigue S, Ivers H. Role of stress, arousal, and coping skills in primary insomnia: *Psychosom Med*. 2003;65(2):259–267. doi:10.1097/01.PSY.0000030391.09558.A3.

28. Schwartz DR, Carney CE. Mediators of cognitive-behavioral therapy for insomnia: a review of randomized controlled trials and secondary analysis studies. *Clin Psychol Rev*. 2012;32(7):664–675. doi:10.1016/j.cpr.2012.06.006.

29. Perlis ML, Ellis JG, Kloss JD, Riemann DW. Etiology and pathophysiology of insomnia. In: *Principles and practice of sleep medicine*. New York: Elsevier; 2017:769–784. doi:10.1016/B978-0-323-24288-2.00082-9.

30. Bootzin RR. Stimulus control treatment for Insomnia. *Proceedings of the APA 80th Annual Convention*.1972;395–396.

31. Bootzin RR, Perlis ML. Stimulus control therapy. In: Perlis M, Aloia M, Kuhn B, eds. *Behavioral Treatments for Sleep Disorders: A Comprehensive Primer of Behavioral Sleep Medicine Interventions*. Amsterdam: Academic; 2011:21–30. doi:10.1016/B978-0-12-381522-4.00002-X.

32. Turner RM, Ascher LM. Controlled comparison of progressive relaxation, stimulus control, and paradoxical intention therapies for insomnia. *J Consult Clin Psychol*. 1979;47(3):500–508. doi:10.1037/0022-006X.47.3.500.

33. Engle-Friedman M, Bootzin RR, Hazlewood L, Tsao C. An evaluation of behavioral treatments for insomnia in the older adult. *J Clin Psychol*. 1992;48(1):77–90. doi:10.1002/1097-4679(199201)48:1<77::AID-JCLP2270480112>3.0.CO;2-J.

34. Lundh L-G, Broman J-E. Insomnia as an interaction between sleep-interfering and sleep-interpreting processes. *J Psychosom Res*. 2000;49(5):299–310. doi:10.1016/S0022-3999(00)00150-1.

35. Harvey A. A cognitive model of insomnia. *Behav Res Ther*. 2002;40(8):869–893. doi:10.1016/S0005-7967(01)00061-4.

36. Espie CA, Broomfield NM, MacMahon KMA, Macphee LM, Taylor LM. The attention–intention–effort pathway in the development of psychophysiologic insomnia: a theoretical review. *Sleep Med Rev*. 2006;10(4):215–245. doi:10.1016/j.smrv.2006.03.002.

37. Morin CM, Stone J, Trinkle D, Mercer J, Remsberg S. Dysfunctional beliefs and attitudes about sleep among older adults with and without insomnia complaints. *Psychol Aging*. 1993;8(3):463–467. doi:10.1037/0882-7974.8.3.463.

38. Carney CE, Edinger JD, Morin CM, et al. Examining maladaptive beliefs about sleep across insomnia patient groups. *J Psychosom Res*. 2010;68(1):57–65. doi:10.1016/j.jpsychores.2009.08.007.

39. Harvey AG. Pre-sleep cognitive activity: a comparison of sleep onset insomniacs and good sleepers. *Br J Clin Psychol*. 2000;39(3):275–286. doi:10.1348/014466500163284.

40. Kuisk LA, Bertelson AD, Walsh JK. Presleep cognitive hyperarousal and affect as factors in objective and subjective insomnia. *Percept Mot Skills*. August 2016. doi:10.2466/pms.1989.69.3f.1219.

41. Wicklow A, Espie CA. Intrusive thoughts and their relationship to actigraphic measurement of sleep: towards a cognitive model of insomnia. *Behav Res Ther*. 2000;38(7):679–693. doi:10.1016/S0005-7967(99)00136-9.

42. Mercer JD, Bootzin RR, Lack LC. Insomniacs' perception of wake instead of sleep. *Sleep*. 2002;25(5):559–566. doi:10.1093/sleep/25.5.559.

43. Mendelson WB, James SP, Garnett D, Sack DA, Rosenthal NE. A psychophysiological study of insomnia. *Psychiatry Res*. 1986;19(4):267–284. doi:10.1016/0165-1781(86)90120-4.

44. Means MK, Edinger JD, Glenn DM, Fins AI. Accuracy of sleep perceptions among insomnia sufferers and normal sleepers. *Sleep Med*. 2003;4(4):285–296. doi:10.1016/S1389-9457(03)00057-1.

45. Feige B, Al-Shajlawi A, Nissen C, et al. Does REM sleep contribute to subjective wake time in primary insomnia? A comparison of polysomnographic and subjective sleep in 100 patients.

J Sleep Res. 2008;17(2):180–190. doi:10.1111/j.1365-2869.2008.00651.x.

46. Harvey AG. Identifying safety behaviors in insomnia. *J Nerv Ment Dis.* 2002;190(1):16–21.

47. Woodley J, Smith S. Safety behaviors and dysfunctional beliefs about sleep: Testing a cognitive model of the maintenance of insomnia. *J Psychosom Res.* 2006;60(6):551–557. doi:10.1016/j.jpsychores.2006.03.002.

48. Jansson M, Linton SJ. Psychological mechanisms in the maintenance of insomnia: arousal, distress, and sleep-related beliefs. *Behav Res Ther.* 2007;45(3):511–521. doi:10.1016/j.brat.2006.04.003.

49. Borbély AA. A two process model of sleep regulation. *Hum Neurobiol.* 1982;1(3):195–204.

50. Semler CN, Harvey AG. An investigation of monitoring for sleep-related threat in primary insomnia. *Behav Res Ther.* 2004;42(12):1403–1420. doi:10.1016/j.brat.2003.09.003.

51. Semler CN, Harvey AG. Monitoring for sleep-related threat: a pilot study of the Sleep Associated Monitoring Index (SAMI). *Psychosom Med.* 2004;66(2):242–250. doi:10.1097/01.PSY.0000114870.50968.90.

52. Tang NKY, Anne Schmidt D, Harvey AG. Sleeping with the enemy: clock monitoring in the maintenance of insomnia. *J Behav Ther Exp Psychiatry.* 2007;38(1):40–55. doi:10.1016/j.jbtep.2005.07.004.

53. Woods H, Marchetti LM, Biello SM, Espie CA. The clock as a focus of selective attention in those with primary insomnia: an experimental study using a modified Posner paradigm. *Behav Res Ther.* 2009;47(3):231–236. doi:10.1016/j.brat.2008.12.009.

54. Taylor LM, Espie CA, White CA. Attentional bias in people with acute versus persistent insomnia secondary to cancer. *Behav Sleep Med.* 2003;1(4):200–212. doi:10.1207/S15402010BSM0104_3.

55. Jones BT, Macphee LM, Broomfield NM, Jones BC, Espie CA. Sleep-related attentional bias in good, moderate, and poor (primary insomnia) sleepers. *J Abnorm Psychol.* 2005;114(2):249–258. doi:10.1037/0021-843X.114.2.249.

56. Marchetti LM, Biello SM, Broomfield NM, Macmahon KMA, Espie CA. Who is pre-occupied with sleep? A comparison of attention bias in people with psychophysiological insomnia, delayed sleep phase syndrome and good sleepers using the induced change blindness paradigm. *J Sleep Res.* 2006;15(2):212–221. doi:10.1111/j.1365-2869.2006.00510.x.

57. MacMahon KMA, Broomfield NM, Espie CA. Attention bias for sleep-related stimuli in primary insomnia and delayed sleep phase syndrome using the dot-probe task. *Sleep.* 2006;29(11):1420–1427. doi:10.1093/sleep/29.11.1420.

58. Bonnet MH, Arand DL. The consequences of a week of insomnia. *Sleep.* 1996;19(6):453–461. doi:10.1093/sleep/19.6.453.

59. Bonnet MH, Arand DL. Activity, arousal, and the MSLT in patients with insomnia. *Sleep.* 2000;23(2):205–212.

60. Espie CA, Lindsay WR, Brooks DN, Hood EM, Turvey T. A controlled comparative investigation of psychological treatments for chronic sleep-onset insomnia. *Behav Res Ther.* 1989;27(1):79–88. doi:10.1016/0005-7967(89)90123-X.

61. Espie CA, Morin CM. Insomnia: a clinical guide to assessment and treatment [References]. University of Glasgow; 2003. http://eprints.gla.ac.uk/22313/.

62. Broomfield NM, Espie CA. Initial insomnia and paradoxical intention: an experimental investigation of putative mechanisms using subjective and actigraphic measurement of sleep. *Behav Cogn Psychother.* 2003;31(3):313–324. doi:10.1017/S1352465803003060.

63. Ansfield ME, Wegner DM, Bowser R. Ironic effects of sleep urgency. *Behav Res Ther.* 1996;34(7):523–531. doi:10.1016/0005-7967(96)00031-9.

64. Broomfield NM, Espie CA. Towards a valid, reliable measure of sleep effort. *J Sleep Res.* 2005;14(4):401–407. doi:10.1111/j.1365-2869.2005.00481.x.

65. Kohn L, Espie CA. Sensitivity and specificity of measures of the insomnia experience: a comparative study of psychophysiologic insomnia, insomnia associated with mental disorder and good sleepers. *Sleep.* 2005;28(1):104–112. doi:10.1093/sleep/28.1.104.

66. Riemann D, Spiegelhalder K, Feige B, et al. The hyperarousal model of insomnia: a review of the concept and its evidence. *Sleep Med Rev.* 2010;14(1):19–31. doi:10.1016/j.smrv.2009.04.002.

67. Perlis ML, Giles DE, Mendelson WB, Bootzin RR, Wyatt JK. Psychophysiological insomnia: the behavioural model and a neurocognitive perspective. *J Sleep Res.* 1997;6(3):179–188. doi:10.1046/j.1365-2869.1997.00045.x.

68. Riemann D, Nissen C, Palagini L, Otte A, Perlis ML, Spiegelhalder K. The neurobiology, investigation, and treatment of chronic insomnia. *Lancet Neurol.* 2015;14(5):547–558. doi:10.1016/S1474-4422(15)00021-6.

69. Saper CB, Scammell TE, Lu J. Hypothalamic regulation of sleep and circadian rhythms. *Nature.* 2005;437(7063):1257–1263.

70. Perlis, M. L, Pigeon, W. R., Drummond, S. P. The neurobiology of insomnia. *Neurobiol Dis.* 2006.

71. Baglioni C, Regen W, Teghen A, et al. Sleep changes in the disorder of insomnia: a meta-analysis of polysomnographic studies. *Sleep Med Rev.* 2014;18(3):195–213. doi:10.1016/j.smrv.2013.04.001.

72. Feige B, Baglioni C, Spiegelhalder K, Hirscher V, Nissen C, Riemann D. The microstructure of sleep in primary insomnia: an overview and extension. *Int J Psychophysiol.* 2013;89(2):171–180. doi:10.1016/j.ijpsycho.2013.04.002.

73. Merica H, Blois R, Gaillard J-M. Spectral characteristics of sleep EEG in chronic insomnia. *Eur J Neurosci.* 1998;10(5):1826–1834. doi:10.1046/j.1460-9568.1998.00189.x.

74. Perlis ML, Kehr EL, Smith MT, Andrews PJ, Orff H, Giles DE. Temporal and stagewise distribution of high frequency EEG activity in patients with primary and secondary insomnia and in good sleeper controls. *J Sleep Res.* 2001;10(2):93–104. doi:10.1046/j.1365-2869.2001.00247.x.

75. Krystal AD, Edinger JD, Wohlgemuth WK, Marsh GR. NREM Sleep EEG frequency spectral correlates of sleep complaints in primary insomnia subtypes. *Sleep.* 2002;25(6):626–636. doi:10.1093/sleep/25.6.626.

76. Israel B, Buysse DJ, Krafty RT, Begley A, Miewald J, Hall M. Short-term stability of sleep and heart rate variability in good sleepers and patients with insomnia: for some measures, one night is enough. *Sleep.* 2012;35(9):1285–1291. doi:10.5665/sleep.2088.

77. Spiegelhalder K, Regen W, Feige B, et al. Increased EEG sigma and beta power during NREM sleep in primary insomnia. *Biol Psychol.* 2012;91(3):329–333. doi:10.1016/j.biopsycho.2012.08.009.

78. Riemann D, Spiegelhalder K, Nissen C, Hirscher V, Baglioni C, Feige B. REM sleep instability: a new pathway for insomnia? *Pharmacopsychiatry.* 2012;45(05):167–176. doi:10.1055/s-0031-1299721.

79. Chouvarda I, Mendez MO, Rosso V, et al. CAP sleep in insomnia: New methodological aspects for sleep microstructure analysis. *Conf Proc IEEE Eng Med Biol Soc.* 2011;2011:1495–1498. doi:10.1109/IEMBS.2011.6090341.

80. Chouvarda I, Mendez MO, Rosso V, et al. Cyclic alternating patterns in normal sleep and insomnia: structure and content differences. *IEEE Trans Neural Syst Rehabil Eng.* 2012;20(5):642–652. doi:10.1109/TNSRE.2012.2208984.

81. Bonnet MH, Arand DL. Heart rate variability in insomniacs and matched normal sleepers: *Psychosom Med.* 1998;60(5):610–615. doi:10.1097/00006842-199809000-00017.

82. Farina B, Dittoni S, Colicchio S, et al. Heart rate and heart rate variability modification in chronic insomnia patients. *Behav Sleep Med.* 2014;12(4):290–306. doi:10.1080/15402002.2013.801346.

83. Bonnet MH, Arand DL. 24-hour metabolic rate in insomniacs and matched normal sleepers. *Sleep.* 1995;18(7):581–588. doi:10.1093/sleep/18.7.581.

84. Xia L, Chen G-H, Li Z-H, Jiang S, Shen J. Alterations in hypothalamus-pituitary-adrenal/thyroid axes and gonadotropin-releasing hormone in the patients with primary insomnia: a clinical research. Wolfe A, ed. *PLoS ONE.* 2013;8(8):e71065. doi:10.1371/journal.pone.0071065.

85. Seelig E, Keller U, Klarhöfer M, et al. Neuroendocrine regulation and metabolism of glucose and lipids in primary chronic insomnia: a prospective case-control study. *PLOS ONE.* 2013;8(4):e61780. doi:10.1371/journal.pone.0061780.

86. Riemann D, Klein T, Rodenbeck A, et al. Nocturnal cortisol and melatonin secretion in primary insomnia. *Psychiatry Res.* 2002;113(1-2):17–27. doi:10.1016/S0165-1781(02)00249-4.

87. Varkevisser M, Dongen V, P.a H, Kerkhof GA. Physiologic indexes in chronic insomnia during a constant routine: evidence for general hyperarousal? *Sleep.* 2005;28(12):1588–1596. doi:10.1093/sleep/28.12.1588.

88. Nofzinger EA, Buysse DJ, Germain A, Price JC, Miewald JM, Kupfer DJ. Functional neuroimaging evidence for hyperarousal in insomnia. *Am J Psychiatry.* 2004;161(11):2126–2128.

89. Kay DB, Karim HT, Soehner AM, et al. Subjective–objective sleep discrepancy is associated with alterations in regional glucose metabolism in patients with insomnia and good sleeper controls. *Sleep.* 2017;40(11). doi:10.1093/sleep/zsx155.

90. Winkelman JW, Buxton OM, Jensen JE, et al. Reduced brain GABA in primary insomnia: preliminary data from 4T proton magnetic resonance spectroscopy (1H-MRS). *Sleep.* 2008;31(11):1499–1506. doi:10.1093/sleep/31.11.1499.

91. Revel FG, Gottowik J, Gatti S, Wettstein JG, Moreau J-L. Rodent models of insomnia: a review of experimental procedures that induce sleep disturbances. *Neurosci Biobehav Rev.* 2009;33(6):874–899. doi:10.1016/j.neubiorev.2009.03.002.

92. Cano G, Mochizuki T, Saper CB. Neural circuitry of stress-induced insomnia in rats. *J Neurosci.* 2008;28(40):10167–10184. doi:10.1523/JNEUROSCI.1809-08.2008.

93. Sagar SM, Sharp FR, Curran T. Expression of c-fos protein in brain: metabolic mapping at the cellular level. *Sci Sci.* 1988;240(4857):1328–1331.

94. Ziegler C, Richter J, Mahr M, et al. MAOA gene hypomethylation in panic disorder—reversibility of

an epigenetic risk pattern by psychotherapy. *Transl Psychiatry*. 2016;6(4):e773. doi:10.1038/tp.2016.41.

95. Ong JC, Ulmer CS, Manber R. Improving sleep with mindfulness and acceptance: A metacognitive model of insomnia. *Behav Res Ther*. 2012;50(11):651–660. doi:10.1016/j.brat.2012.08.001.

96. Gross CR, Kreitzer MJ, Reilly-Spong M, et al. Mindfulness-based stress reduction versus pharmacotherapy for chronic primary insomnia: a randomized controlled clinical trial. *EXPLORE J Sci Heal*. 2011;7(2):76–87. doi:10.1016/j.explore.2010.12.003.

97. Harvey AG, Tang NKY. (Mis)perception of sleep in insomnia: a puzzle and a resolution. *Psychol Bull*. 2012;138(1):77–101. doi:10.1037/a0025730.

98. Bonnet MH, Burton GG, Arand DL. Physiological and medical findings in insomnia: implications for diagnosis and care. *Sleep Med Rev*. 2014;18(2):111–122. doi:10.1016/j.smrv.2013.02.003.

99. Harvey AG, Tang NKY: Cognitive behaviour therapy for primary insomnia: can we rest yet? Sleep Med Rev 2003 Jun;7:237–262.

9

Pharmacological Management of Insomnia

KARL DOGHRAMJI

INTRODUCTION

In this chapter, we will review essential characteristics of the pharmacological agents utilized in the management of insomnia. The clinical conditions and settings that lead to the decision to utilize a hypnotic agent are discussed elsewhere in this book.

A variety of substances have been utilized throughout history for the purpose of inducing sleep. In recent history, chloral hydrate was one of the first agents to be formally utilized to treat insomnia. Despite its rapid onset of action, it was soon noted to have a number of troublesome side effects, limiting its usefulness. These included daytime hangover, light-headedness, malaise, and ataxia as well as the rapid development of tolerance, usually within 5 weeks of use. Rapid discontinuation following chronic use was associated with a withdrawal syndrome characterized by delirium, seizures, and death. Its narrow therapeutic index was particularly troublesome, with overdoses resulting in severe respiratory depression, hepatic damage, hypotension, coma, and death. The more recently introduced barbiturates, although safer, tended to produce generalized depression of the central nervous system (CNS), ranging from mild sedation to general anesthesia, and were associated with rapid development of tolerance, noted within a few days of administration. Also common were rebound effects after rapid discontinuation, including a rebound of rapid eye movement (REM) sleep, associated with increased frequency and intensity of dreaming and nightmares. Barbiturates were also noted to be associated with residual sedation (hangover) and psychological dependence. Barbiturate overdoses, especially those involving alcohol, led to some fatalities.[1] Owing largely to these negative effects, chloral hydrate and the barbiturates are now rarely used for the management of insomnia. More recently introduced agents have a more favorable clinical profile relative to side effects and have largely displaced chloral hydrate and the barbiturates as sedative-hypnotic agents. Categories of prescription medications commonly used for this purpose are listed in Table 9.1. The clinical effects of hypnotic agents such as latency of onset, duration of action, and the predilection for daytime carryover effects are determined by multiple pharmacokinetic properties, including rate of absorption, extent of distribution, and elimination half-life. The most commonly utilized clinical efficacy variables for hypnotic agents are sleep latency (SL), a measure of the time spent in falling asleep after going to bed; wake after sleep onset (WASO), which is the total time spent awake after falling asleep, a measure of sleep discontinuity during the course of the night; and total sleep time (TST), a measure of the duration of sleep.

Although numerous hypnotic agents are available, an important determinant of the choice of the agent is the nature of the patient's specific insomnia complaint. For patients having difficulty falling asleep, the ideal medication would reach peak plasma concentrations rapidly, thus producing a rapid onset of action. For patients who have difficulty with sleep maintenance (i.e., multiple nocturnal awakenings or early morning awakening), the ideal medication would allow for mid-nocturnal administration, following middle-of-the-night (MOTN) awakening, and have a rapid onset of action, as well as a rapid elimination rate to prevent carry-over effects following morning awakening. Alternatively, the ideal medication for sleep maintenance would be taken just prior to bedtime and have a sufficiently long elimination half-life to ensure sleep maintenance during the problem period, yet have no residual effects following morning awakening. Finally, for patients having difficulties with both sleep initiation and sleep maintenance, the ideal medication would provide rapid onset of action and a sufficiently lengthy duration of action to prevent MOTN awakenings or result in rapid return to sleep if awakening does happen, yet have no residual effects.

- FDA-approved hypnotic agents
  - Benzodiazepine receptor agonists:
    - Benzodiazepines
    - Nonbenzodiazepines
  - Melatonin receptor agonists
  - H_1-receptor antagonists
  - Orexin receptor antagonists
- Agents not FDA-approved for insomnia
  - Sedating antidepressants
  - Anticonvulsants
  - Antipsychotics

FDA-APPROVED HYPNOTICS

Benzodiazepine Receptor Agonists

All agents in this class bind to benzodiazepine recognition site of the γ-aminobutyric acid type A (GABA$_A$) receptor complex and augment the effects of GABA. GABA is the most abundant inhibitory neurotransmitter in the CNS and is thought to mediate a wide variety of clinical effects, including anxiety, cognition, vigilance, memory, and learning, among others.[2] GABA is also the major neurotransmitter in brain structures thought to be critical for the generation of sleep, such as the ventrolateral preoptic nucleus of the hypothalamus.

GABA$_A$ receptors are widely distributed in the CNS, including the cortex, basal ganglia, and cerebellum. These receptors contain not only the GABA receptor itself but also a benzodiazepine recognition site and a chloride ion channel. GABA$_A$ receptors are composed of five subunits (α, β, γ, ε, and ρ). Most GABA$_A$ receptors are composed of 2α, 2β, and 1γ subunits. The benzodiazepine receptor agonists (BzRAs) bind to the benzodiazepine recognition site, located at the interface of α and γ subunits. Each of these subunits exists in multiple forms and different combinations of these forms may yield different pharmacologic properties, although this connection has not been firmly established.

Benzodiazepines act with comparable affinity at all GABA$_A$ receptors containing αβ, αγ-2, and any of 4α subunits (α1, α2, α3, or α5). They do not interact with receptor subtypes containing the α4 or α6 subunit. The newer hypnotic agents, such as zaleplon, zolpidem, and eszopiclone, bind more avidly to benzodiazepine receptors containing α1 subunit. These agents are collectively referred to

as selective BzRAs (sBzRAs).[3] In animal models, GABA$_A$ receptors with α1 subunits are thought to mediate the sedative, amnestic, and anticonvulsant effects, whereas those containing α2 subunits are more important for anxiolytic effects.[4] However, the connection between subunit composition and clinical effects in humans has not been firmly established.

The BzRAs are listed in Table 9.2 and Table 9.3.[5-7] Newer hypnotics with novel mechanisms are listed in Table 9.4. The first group represents agents that have a benzodiazepine molecular structure. The second group represents agents that are non-benzodiazepines in structure and are also referred to as sBzRAs. Plasma concentrations of available BzRA hypnotics follow a skewed pattern. In general, their plasma concentrations peak rapidly; therefore, with the possible exception of temazepam,[8] all are effective in reducing SL and are suitable for patients who complain of difficulty in falling asleep upon retiring (Table 9.5).

As a group, the older BzRAs are also effective in increasing TST and in maintaining sleep (i.e., reducing WASO).[9] However, these effects have not been well demonstrated with all of these agents.[10] Nevertheless, they are well suited for patients who complain that they awaken repeatedly during the course of the night or who cannot sleep for adequate periods of time. However, largely owing to their longer elimination half-lives, which result in plasma concentrations that persist into waking periods, the older BzRAs also have a tendency to produce daytime carryover effects, described in greater detail in the following discussion.[11-13]

Following the development of the first sBzRA, oral zolpidem, many of its newer formulations have been subsequently developed. These feature drug delivery via the oral mucosa by administration in the sublingual route, an area of the oral cavity that is more permeable than the cheek and palatal areas. Sublingual administration is useful when rapid onset of action is desired. The portion of drug absorbed through the sublingual blood vessels bypasses the hepatic first-pass metabolic processes and is protected from degradation by the low pH environment and digestive enzymes of the middle gastrointestinal tract. Similarly, sublingual sprays (ZolpiMist) improve the time to reach maximum plasma concentration as compared to oral zolpidem.

A sublingual formulation of zolpidem (Edluar) has been developed for the short-term treatment of insomnia characterized by difficulties with sleep initiation. Possibly owing to its

TABLE 9.2. BENZODIAZEPINE RECEPTOR AGONISTS: THE BENZODIAZEPINES

Generic (Trade) Name	Dose Range[a] (mg)	Onset of Action	Half-Life (h)	Active Metabolites	Indications and Usage
Estazolam (Prosom)	1–2	Rapid	10–24	No	Short-term management of insomnia characterized by difficulty in falling asleep, frequent nocturnal awakenings, and/or early morning awakenings
Flurazepam (Dalmane)	15–30	Rapid	47–100	Yes	Treatment of insomnia characterized by difficulty in falling asleep, frequent nocturnal awakenings, and/or early morning awakening
Quazepam (Doral)	7.5–15	Rapid	39–73	Yes	Treatment of insomnia characterized by difficulty falling asleep, frequent nocturnal awakenings, and/or early morning awakenings
Temazepam (Restoril)	7.5–30	Slow	3.5–18.4	No	Short-term treatment of insomnia (generally 7 to 10 days)
Triazolam (Halcion)	0.125–0.25	Rapid	1.5–5.5	No	Short-term treatment of insomnia (generally 7 to 10 days)

[a]Normal adult dose. Dose may require individualization.

rapid absorption, Edluar appears to provide an earlier onset of action than oral zolpidem and may be suitable for patients who still find SL to be too long following administration of traditional oral zolpidem.[14-16]

A lower-dose sublingual formulation of zolpidem (Intermezzo) was formulated specifically for the treatment of patients with insomnia characterized by difficulty returning to sleep following MOTN awakenings. This formulation has a rapid onset of action, and short duration of action, which is suitable for patients who wake up in the MOTN, with at least 4 hours of bedtime remaining.[16,17]

Zolpidem ER (Ambien CR), an extended-release formulation of zolpidem, consists of a coated two-layer tablet: one layer releases drug content immediately and another allows a slower release of additional drug content, thus providing extended plasma concentrations beyond 3 hours after administration.

All of the newer sBzRAs also increase TST; however, in the case of zaleplon, this feature is limited to the highest dose of 20 mg. With respect to effects on sleep discontinuity, eszopiclone also diminishes WASO and, therefore, enhances sleep continuity throughout the course of the night.[18,19] This feature may be due to its longer elimination

half-life (6 hours) when compared with the other sBzRAs. Zolpidem ER also enhances sleep continuity (decreases WASO), an effect that has been demonstrated in controlled trials. These effects have been noted for the first 7 hours following administration during the first 2 nights and for the first 5 hours following administration after 2 weeks of treatment.[7] This clearly distinguishes it from zolpidem.

Most common adverse effects of BzRA hypnotic medications (Table 9.6) are somnolence, headache, nausea, fatigue, hypokinesia, dizziness, and abnormal coordination. Severe sedation, nervousness, lethargy, dry mouth, diarrhea, and coma, probably indicative of drug intolerance or overdosage, have been reported. Similarly, the most commonly reported adverse events of sBzRAs include headache, nausea, fatigue, drowsiness, dizziness, diarrhea, and drugged feeling. These occur variably in each of the medications (refer to individual product inserts for detailed information on each medication).

All of the BzRAs are regarded as Schedule IV agents by the US Drug Enforcement Administration (DEA) and carry the risk of abuse liability. They should, therefore, be used with special caution in individuals with a prior history of alcohol and substance abuse. The benzodiazepine

TABLE 9.3. SELECTIVE BENZODIAZEPINE RECEPTOR AGONISTS: THE NON-BENZODIAZEPINES

Generic (Trade) Name	Dose Range[a] (mg)	Onset of Action	Half-Life (h)	Active Metabolites	Indications and Usage
Eszopiclone (Lunesta)	Men and women: Initial dose 1 mg, may be increased to max of 3 mg; elderly and patients with severe hepatic impairment, or taking potent CYP3A4 inhibitors: 2 mg	Rapid	6	No	Treatment of insomnia
Zaleplon (Sonata CIV)	Low weight: 5 Nonelderly adults: 10 Elderly/hepatic insufficiency: 5	Rapid	1	No	Short-term treatment of insomnia
Zolpidem (Ambien)	Women: 5 Men: 5–10 Geriatric/hepatic impairment: 5	Rapid	2.5–2.6	No	Short-term treatment of insomnia characterized by difficulties with sleep initiation
Zolpidem ER (Ambien CR)	Women: 6.25 Men: 6.25–12.5 Geriatric/hepatic impairment: 6.25	Rapid	2.8	No	Treatment of insomnia characterized by difficulties with sleep onset and/or sleep maintenance (as measured by wake time after sleep onset)
Zolpidem oral spray (Zolpimist)	Women: 5 Men: 5-10 Geriatric/hepatic impairment: 5	Rapid	2.5–3.1	No	Short-term treatment of insomnia characterized by difficulties with sleep initiation
Zolpidem SL (Edluar)[b]	Women: 5 Men: 5–10 Geriatric/hepatic impairment: 5	Rapid	2.65–2.85	No	Short-term treatment of insomnia characterized by difficulties with sleep initiation
Zolpidem SL (Intermezzo)[b]	Women: 1.75 Men: 3.5 Geriatric/hepatic impairment: 1.75	Rapid	1.4–3.6	No	Treatment of insomnia when a middle-of-the-night awakening is followed by difficulty returning to sleep

[a]Normal initial adult dose. Dose may require individualization.
[b]Sublingual tablet.

TABLE 9.4. OTHER HYPNOTICS

Generic (Trade) Name	Dose Range[a] (mg)	Onset of Action (T_{max})	Half-Life (h)	Metabolite (active?)	Indications and Usage
Doxepin (Silenor)	3 mg (elderly)		15.3	Nordoxepin (no)	Treatment of insomnia characterized by difficulties with sleep maintenance
	6 mg (adults)	Slow (3.5 hours)			
Ramelteon (Rozerem)	8	Rapid (45 minutes)	1–2.6	M-II (Yes)	Treatment of insomnia characterized by difficulty with sleep onset
Suvorexant (Belsomra)	5–20 mg	Rapid (2 hours)	12	Hydroxy-suvorexant (no)	Treatment of insomnia characterized by difficulties with sleep onset and/or sleep maintenance

hypnotics (BzRAs) are all unsafe to use in pregnancy, as they have a pregnancy safety category X, while all the sBzRAs are pregnancy category C, (no adequate and well-controlled studies exist in humans) with the exception of zolpidem, which is in category B; therefore, their benefits for usage in pregnancy must be weighed against their risks. None of these medications are indicated for pediatric usage nor for lactating mothers.[59]

Hypnotics introduced for clinical use over the past decade have had novel mechanisms, not involving the GABA receptor. These are listed in Table 9.4.

Melatonin Receptor Agonists

The central processes governing sleep and wakefulness are thought to be strongly influenced by two major CNS drives, named circadian and homeostatic. During the course of a typical day, sleep-producing homeostatic drive (sleep debt or sleep pressure) accumulates and intensifies in force as the day progresses. This is opposed by circadian wake-promoting drive, which is thought to be primarily mediated by the suprachiasmatic nucleus (SCN) of the anterior hypothalamus and which also intensifies as the day progresses. These circadian wakefulness drive counteracts the homeostatic drive, thus resulting in the maintenance of wakefulness and normal daytime functioning. Localized to the SCN are melatonin receptors, sites at which endogenous melatonin binds and affects the neuronal output of the SCN.[20]

There are two subtypes of such receptors, MT_1 and MT_2, and these are G–protein-coupled receptors.[21] Activation of MT_1 receptors inhibit the neuronal firing rate in the SCN, thus tipping the scale in the direction of the homeostatic

sleep-promoting drive, allowing sleep to occur. MT_2 receptor activation may play a role in readjustment of circadian rhythms.

Ramelteon (Rozerem) is a hypnotic agent that acts at MT_1 and MT_2 receptors with high selectivity and, presumably owing to its activity at the MT_1 receptors, is thought to mute the wakefulness force of the SCN, thus allowing the homeostatic drive to dominate, resulting in sleep. It has virtually no binding capacity to MT_3 receptors located in numerous locations outside the CNS.[22] Ramelteon is indicated for the treatment of insomnia characterized by difficulty with sleep onset. Ramelteon does not affect WASO or number of awakenings following sleep onset. The most common adverse events that are associated with ramelteon

TABLE 9.5. EFFECTS OF RECENTLY INTRODUCED HYPNOTIC AGENTS ON SELECTED SLEEP VARIABLES

Medication	Decrease Sleep Latency	Decrease WASO
Zaleplon	Yes	No
Zolpidem	Yes	No
Zolpidem ER	Yes	Yes
Zolpidem oral spray	Yes	No
Zolpidem sublingual	Yes	No
Eszopiclone	Yes	Yes
Ramelteon	Yes	No
Low-dose doxepin	No	Yes
Suvorexant	Yes	Yes

Abbreviation: WASO, wake after sleep onset.

TABLE 9.6. SELECTED ADVERSE EFFECTS OF HYPNOTIC AGENTS

Benzodiazepine receptor agonists

Daytime sedation, psychomotor and cognitive impairment (depending on dose and half-life)

Rebound insomnia

Respiratory depression in vulnerable populations

DEA Schedule IV

Melatonin receptor agonist

Headache, somnolence, fatigue, dizziness

Not recommended for use with fluvoxamine due to CYP 1A2 interaction

H1 receptor antagonist

Somnolence/sedation

Nausea

Upper respiratory tract infection

Orexin receptor antagonist

Somnolence

Risk of impaired alertness and motor coordination, including impaired driving; increases with dose

Contraindicated in narcolepsy

DEA Schedule IV

Abbreviation: DEA, Drug Enforcement Administration.

include somnolence, fatigue, and dizziness. It is not recommended for use with fluvoxamine due to a CYP1A2 interaction. A mild transitory elevation in prolactin levels has been noted in a small number of females, and a mild decrease in testosterone values has been noted in elderly males, yet the clinical relevance of these changes remains unclear. Possibly owing to its lack of activity at the GABA receptor, ramelteon does not demonstrate respiratory depression in mild to moderate chronic obstructive pulmonary disease and mild to moderate sleep apnea.[23] Ramelteon has an US Food and Drug Administration (FDA) pregnancy safety category C and is not scheduled by the DEA as a controlled substance. Its usage is not indicated in pediatric population nor in lactating mothers.

H₁-Receptor Antagonist

Low-dosage (3 mg and 6 mg) formulations of the tricyclic antidepressant doxepin (Silenor) are approved for the treatment of insomnia characterized by frequent or early morning awakenings and an inability to return to sleep. Although the mechanism of action of doxepin for treating insomnia remains unknown, ascending histaminic neurons are thought to be involved in the initiation and maintenance of wakefulness and the blockade of the H_1 receptor likely plays a role in reducing wakefulness, thereby allowing sleep to occur. Compared with other tricyclic antidepressants, doxepin's binding potency for H_1 receptor is approximately 100 times higher than its binding potency for serotonin and norepinephrine receptors. Thus, at low doses, doxepin acts as a highly selective H_1 antagonist and has minimal activity as an anticholinergic, adrenergic, and serotonergic agent, thus freeing it from some of the adverse events associated with these receptors.[24]

Doxepin is a pregnancy category C drug. It is not scheduled as a controlled substance by the DEA and thus may be of special value in patients with a history of substance abuse. It is not indicated for pediatric use nor for lactating mothers. Doxepin is contraindicated in patients with severe urinary retention and narrow angle glaucoma and in those who have used monoamine oxidase inhibitors (MAOIs) within the previous 2 weeks.

Orexin Receptor Antagonists

The neuropeptide hypocretin/orexin plays an important role as a stabilizer and maintainer of wakefulness by minimizing unplanned transitions to the sleep state through reinforcement of the wake-promoting signaling in the brain. Orexin deficiency results in narcolepsy in many species, suggesting that this system is particularly important for maintenance of wakefulness, although not necessarily its initiation.[20,25] Orexin peptides bind with different affinities to the two orexin receptors, OX1R and OX2R, to induce downstream wake signaling.[26]

Suvorexant (Belsomra) is the first dual orexin-antagonist to be approved for the treatment of insomnia. As an antagonist at both orexin receptors, it is thought to diminish wakefulness drive thus allowing sleep to occur. It is indicated for the treatment of insomnia characterized by difficulties with sleep onset and/or sleep maintenance. Suvorexant peak concentrations occur at a median T_{max} of 2 hours (range 30 minutes to 6 hours) under fasted conditions. Steady-state is achieved 3 days after ingestion. The mean $t_{1/2}$ is approximately 12 hours. The efficacy and safety of suvorexant has been established at doses of 10 mg to 20 mg in elderly and nonelderly adult patients. It safety has also been established in mild to moderate obstructive sleep apnea (OSA).[27]

Suvorexant is a DEA schedule IV medication and is a controlled substance. It is in pregnancy category C, and its use in not indicated in pediatric population nor in nursing mothers. It is contraindicated in patients with narcolepsy.

Under development is the dual orexin receptor antagonist lemborexant. A New Drug Application was submitted to FDA for insomnia disorder in January, 2019.[28] Controlled study in insomnia disorder demonstrated improvement in SL and continuity, and a phase 2 study is under way for irregular sleep–wake rhythm disorder and mild to moderate Alzheimer's dementia.[29]

OTHER CLINICAL CONSIDERATIONS IN USE OF HYPNOTIC AGENTS

Long-Term Use

The chronic nature of some patients' insomnia may necessitate longer treatment. The report of a recent National Institute of Health State of the Science Conference[30] expressed concern regarding the mismatch between the potentially lifelong nature of insomnia and the duration of clinical trials.

The main concerns in long-term use are tolerance, a decrement in clinical efficacy following repeated use, and rebound insomnia, which is an escalation of insomnia beyond baseline severity levels following abrupt discontinuation. The latter must be distinguished from a return of symptoms after discontinuation of the medication. Studies of the repeated administration of BzRA hypnotic agents for 2 to 5 weeks suggest that rebound phenomena following withdrawal are more pronounced following the administration of higher doses of BzRA hypnotics and following administration of the benzodiazepine agents that have a short elimination half-life, such as triazolam, than the longer-elimination half-life benzodiazepines and some of the newer sBzRAs.[31] They are less likely following the administration of long-acting drugs because of the gradual decline in their plasma concentration following discontinuation. Mild and transient withdrawal effects, generally lasting 1 day, have been noted with zolpidem.

Long-term use while utilizing a placebo control condition has been evaluated for zolpidem, zolpidem ER, ramelteon, and eszopiclone. In a study, utilizing intermittent treatment with zolpidem over the course of 3 months, clinical gains were sustained, and there was no evidence of subjective rebound insomnia on nights when the medication was not taken.[32] The long-term usage of zolpidem ER was evaluated in a 6-month, placebo-controlled study.[33] At every time point, zolpidem ER demonstrated sustained efficacy in TST, WASO, and

SL. No rebound insomnia was observed during the first 3 nights after discontinuation, and there were sustained improvements in morning sleepiness and ability to concentrate with zolpidem ER compared with placebo. Nightly eszopiclone at 3 mg for 6 months in a placebo-controlled design revealed no evidence of tolerance during the entire 6-month course; sustained improvement was noted in, among other measures, SL, WASO, and TST. There was also no evidence of rebound insomnia after rapid discontinuation in a subset of patients who received treatment for an additional 6 months in an open-label fashion.[18,34] In a 6-month randomized, placebo-controlled sleep laboratory study over the 6 months of treatment, ramelteon consistently reduced latency to persistent sleep compared with baseline and with placebo with significant decreases observed at week 1 and months 1, 3, 5, and 6. There were no significant next-morning residual effects during treatment and no withdrawal symptoms or rebound insomnia after discontinuation of ramelteon treatment.[35] In a 3-month clinical trial, a 3-mg dose of doxepin given nightly was shown to produce significant improvement in SL without evidence of next-day residual sedation.[36]

Despite favorable long-term findings, clinical wisdom suggests that hypnotics should be utilized for short periods of time as much as possible, and patients should be periodically evaluated during longer-term use. Withdrawal symptoms can occur in this class of compounds, and patients should be carefully monitored following abrupt discontinuation, especially in the case of agents with shorter half-lives. Even with medications prone to have these effects, the risk of rebound insomnia and withdrawal symptoms can be minimized by utilizing the lowest effective dose and by gradually tapering the dose downward over time for discontinuation.

As-Needed and Middle-of-the-Night Use

As-needed use of a hypnotic agent is generally recommended by clinicians, and preferred by patients, as a means of diminishing reliance on hypnotic agents and possibly minimizing the development of tolerance and dose escalation over time. Insomnia occurs on an intermittent basis in nearly half of all insomniacs seen in a primary care office[37] and the ability to predict its occurrence prior to onset would be of great benefit in implementing as-needed use. Unfortunately, being able to predict the occurrence of insomnia is typically not possible until it is too late to take a hypnotic in many patients. This is especially the case in insomnia characterized by mid-nocturnal awakenings, since MOTN administration following awakenings, especially in the case of the longer half-life medications, would introduce the possibility of next-day residual effects. Zaleplon, which has a short half-life of 1 hour, has been shown to be effective in assisting patients in falling back to sleep if administered after MOTN awakenings, although it is not specifically indicated for this usage by the FDA.[38] If utilized in this fashion, the patient should be advised to remain in bed for a minimum of 4 hours after taking the medication to avoid daytime sedation. The low-dose sublingual formulation of zolpidem (Intermezzo) is indicated for MOTN use.

Safety

The main adverse effects of all of the hypnotic agents are summarized in Table 9.6. Table 9.7 outlines certain populations that are vulnerable to the use of hypnotic medication. Hypnotics should be used with caution in individuals with respiratory depression (e.g., chronic obstructive pulmonary disease, OSA), in the elderly, and in those with hepatic disease, those with multiple medical conditions, and those who are taking other medications that have CNS-depressant properties. They should not be used in pregnant women. Individuals who must awaken during the course of the drug's active period should not take these medications.

All sedative-hypnotic medications include language concerning the potential for complex sleep-related behaviors, which may include sleep driving, defined as driving while not fully awake after ingestion of a sedative-hypnotic product,

---

TABLE 9.7. VULNERABLE POPULATIONS IN THE USE OF HYPNOTIC AGENTS

- Respiratory compromise (e.g., chronic obstructive pulmonary disease, obstructive sleep apnea)
- Elderly
- Women
- History of substance use disorders
- Pregnancy
- Multiple medication users (sedation mainly)
- Hepatic impairment
- Depression
- Pediatric patients: not indicated

---

with no memory of the event. The concern was triggered by anecdotal postmarketing reports of such events with some hypnotic agents. In the case of sleep driving, at least some of the episodes were associated with concomitant ingestion of alcohol and other sedating substances.[39] It is important, therefore, to advise patients who are receiving hypnotic agents to refrain from the use of alcohol and similar substances.

Lower doses are also recommended for women of various zolpidem preparations including Ambien, Ambien CR, Edluar, and Zolpimist due to the finding of high drug levels in the blood of some women the day following administration due to the slower rate of clearance of zolpidem. This may, in turn, impair activities that require alertness during the day, such as driving. In the case of eszopiclone, due to the observation of next day impairment at higher doses in some patients irrespective of gender, recommendations include a starting dose of 1 mg at bedtime with the potential for an increase in dose, if clinically indicated, to a maximum of 3 mg.

Dependence, Abuse, and Other Precautions

Dependence (addiction) and abuse (an exaggerated desire to obtain the medication in increasing amounts to the exclusion of all other activities)[1] continue to be significant concerns for physicians. A review the relative abuse liability of 19 hypnotic agents[40] regarded abuse liability as a function of both the likelihood that a drug will be abused (used for nonmedical reasons) and the liability of abuse (i.e., the untoward or toxic effects of using the drug nonmedically) and suggested that abuse liability of hypnotics is highest for the barbiturate and barbiturate-like medications, intermediate for the BzRAs, low for trazodone, and not present for ramelteon. Relative abuse liabilities for newer hypnotics were not assessed in this study. Since the risk of abuse or problematic use of hypnotic drugs appears to be more likely in patients with histories of drug or alcohol abuse or dependence, hypnotics that carry a DEA schedule should be used with caution or not used at all in patients with such backgrounds. Other groups at risk for the development of problematic hypnotic use include the elderly and patients with chronic pain.[1] In contrast to BzRAs and suvorexant, doxepin and ramelteon are not associated with abuse potential, nor do they appear to produce physical dependence. Nevertheless, patients should be monitored for signs of drug abuse, and observed carefully.

General guidelines for prescribing hypnotic medications, listing factors that should be taken into consideration, are presented in Table 9.8.

FDA-UNAPPROVED PRESCRIPTION AGENTS FOR INSOMNIA

Agents in this class are used as hypnotics but not indicated for this use by the FDA. Factors favoring their use include low abuse liability, availability of wide dose ranges, and, in some cases, low cost. Although these agents may have been studied for their effects on sleep in other conditions complicated by insomnia, only information relative to primary insomnia will be reviewed here.

Sedating Antidepressants

These agents are prescribed extensively[41] despite limited data on their safety and efficacy in insomnia. For insomnia, they are typically utilized at doses that are subtherapeutic for the treatment of depression or anxiety disorders.

Trazodone is a heterocyclic antidepressant that has an elimination half-life of 5 to 12 hours. It has received little scientific attention as a sleep aid in primary insomnia,[42] and the few available studies suggest the possibility of early development of tolerance, following 2 weeks of administration at a dosage of 50 mg. Doxepin (antidepressant dose) is a tricyclic antidepressant. At doses of 25 mg to 50 mg, it was the subject of a controlled study in 47 subjects with primary insomnia for 4 weeks; it demonstrated an improvement in TST but not in

---

TABLE 9.8. SELECTED GUIDELINES FOR HYPNOTIC USE

- Perform a comprehensive evaluation and provide specific treatment of insomnia comorbidities
- Caution in patients with respiratory and hepatic impairment, substance use disorders, or who are already taking sedatives; avoid alcohol
- Use lowest effective dose, lower dose in elderly (and in women for certain compounds)
- Take at bedtime (or MOTN for zolpidem SL low dose)
- 7–8 hours in bed (or minimum of 4 hours for zolpidem SL low dose and Zaleplon when used for MOTN insomnia)
- Efficacy may be improved on empty stomach
- Gradual dose reduction for discontinuation
- Periodic follow-up visits during chronic use

Abbreviations: MOTN, middle-of-the-night.

SL.[43] Withdrawal insomnia was evident following abrupt discontinuation. Mirtazapine is a newer antidepressant with an elimination half-life of 20 to 40 hours.[1] Although mirtazapine has been shown to improve symptoms of insomnia associated with major depressive disorder, there are no published reports on its use in primary insomnia patients. Therefore, despite their potential advantages, the paucity of available data regarding the effects of antidepressants on sleep and wakefulness in insomnia limits the use of these agents as first-line treatments for insomnia.

Atypical Antipsychotics

Several sedating antipsychotics (e.g., quetiapine and olanzapine) are occasionally used alone for the treatment of insomnia, even though they are not approved for this use. Nevertheless, studies demonstrating the usefulness for the management of insomnia are scant and suffer from methodological drawbacks. A recent literature review of the published studies and case reports in which quetiapine was used specifically for the treatment of insomnia as the primary endpoint concluded that while it has moderate sedative properties and was reported to provide improvements in several subjective and objective sleep parameters,[44] it, as well as other antipsychotics, can have adverse effects, such as periodic limb movements, akathisia, metabolic complications, and weight gain.[45] Therefore, although the use of antipsychotics for various psychiatric disorders that feature insomnia may be appropriate for the treatment of the primary psychiatric condition, their use in the treatment of primary insomnia cannot be wholeheartedly recommended.[30]

NONPRESCRIPTION AGENTS

Non-prescription agents commonly used for insomnia are summarized in Table 9.9.[46]

Antihistamines

The primary active ingredients in over-the-counter sleep aids are first-generation H1 antihistamines diphenhydramine and doxylamine, which produce mild to moderate sedation and may improve SL and continuity for some individuals. Diphenhydramine, the most commonly used agent, is well absorbed and is widely distributed throughout the body, including the CNS.[1] However, these antihistamines are also associated with morning grogginess since they may have long durations of action. In the case of diphenhydramine, peak serum concentration

TABLE 9.9 NONPRESCRIPTION AGENTS COMMONLY USED TO TREAT INSOMNIA

Histamine-1 Receptor Antagonists
- Diphenhydramine hydrochloride
- Diphenhydramine citrate
- Doxylamine succinate

Herbs
- Passionflower
- Valerian
- Jamaican dogwood
- Hops
- California poppy
- Chamomile
- Lemon balm
- St. John's wort
- Kava kava
- Wild lettuce
- Scullcap
- Patrinia root

Vitamins and Supplements
- Calcium
- Vitamin A
- Nicotinamide
- Magnesium
- Vitamin B12
- Tryptophans

is at 2 to 4 hours and the elimination half-life can be as long as 8 hours. Other potential side effects include delirium (especially in vulnerable individuals such as the elderly), urinary retention, constipation, dry mouth, blurry vision, orthostasis, CNS depression, paradoxical excitement, and tachycardia.[47,48] In addition, problems with chronic use, such as the development of tolerance to sedative-hypnotic actions and weight gain are possible, although not well studied.

Dietary Supplements and Herbal Agents

Although their use is not regulated by the FDA, dietary supplements and herbal remedies also enjoy extensive use for sleep disorders owing to their widespread availability, lack of prescription requirements, relatively low cost, and the widespread belief that they are safe and have a relatively low abuse risk.

Melatonin is a neurohormone secreted by the pineal gland that plays a major role in regulating circadian rhythms. Following administration of exogenous melatonin as a dietary supplement, it

is rapidly absorbed, with peak levels occurring in <30 minutes. It has an elimination half-life of 40 to 50 minutes. Oral doses of 1 to 5 mg result in serum melatonin concentrations that are 10 to 100 times higher than the usual nighttime peak within 1 hour after ingestion, followed by a decline to baseline values in 4 to 8 hours.[49] Although studies for insomnia suffer from a variety of methodological limitations, a recent meta-analysis indicated that melatonin has modest but significant effects in some sleep variable. The analysis revealed a decrease in SL of 7.06 minutes and an increase in TST of 8.25 minutes and an improvement of subjective sleep quality.[50] The effects did not appear to dissipate with continued melatonin use. Therefore, the absolute benefit of melatonin compared to placebo is smaller than other pharmacological treatments for insomnia.

Questions have been raised regarding purity and composition of melatonin preparations. In addition, owing to the widespread distribution of melatonin receptors throughout the body, it may have various negative clinical effects. One study revealed, for example, that acute melatonin administration in normal volunteers impaired glucose tolerance in both the morning and evening.[51] Therefore, caution should be exercised with the use of melatonin, especially for prolonged periods of time.

Valerian extract, derived from the root of *Valeriana officinalis*, a perennial that grows wildly in temperate areas of the Americas and Europe, has long been advocated and used for promoting sleep.[52] Valerian is used as a sedative and anxiolytic and is commonly available as an aqueous, alcohol, or dilute alcohol extract. However, the extraction method can strongly influence the presumed active components in any formulation. These components include sesquiterpenes (volatile oil components that account for valerian's unpleasant odor), valepotriates, and amino acids (such as GABA and glutamine).[46] However, its soporific mechanism of action is unknown. The typical dose is 400 to 900 mg of *V officinalis* root, 30 to 60 minutes before bedtime. Nevertheless, the available data are based on studies with inconsistent and flawed methodologies, often yielding mixed and contradictory results. Side effects are thought to be generally mild, consisting mostly of gastrointestinal irritation and headaches. There have also been case reports of hepatotoxicity in persons taking herbal products containing valerian.[53]

L-tryptophan is an essential amino acid that is a biochemical precursor to serotonin and is thought to function by increasing serotonin in certain brain cells, thus inducing sleep. It has been reported to reduce SL by increasing subjective "sleepiness" and also decreasing waking time.[46] Systematic evidence supporting the use of L-tryptophan, an endogenous amino acid available in a variety of dietary supplements, in the treatment of insomnia is very limited and based on studies in small numbers of patients.[30] In 1989, L-tryptophan was associated with cases of eosinophilic myalgia syndrome, attributed to contamination linked with bacterial fermentation methods used in processing. Consequently, L-tryptophan was recalled in the United States and is now only available by prescription.

5-hydroxytryptophan (5-HTP) is an intermediate metabolite of L-tryptophan in the serotonin pathway and is currently being used as a sleep aid, to treat depression, and as a weight loss tool. *Kava kava*, derived from the root of a plant endogenous to the western Pacific (*P methysticum*), has long been used as a hypnotic and anxiolytic. However, there have been few clinical trials of kava kava.[53] Reports of serious hepatotoxicity with this preparation have resulted in it being banned in many countries. There are two types of *chamomile* plants used in herbal preparations: German chamomile (*Matricaria recutita*), used for restlessness and insomnia, and Roman chamomile (*Chamaemelum nobile*), used orally for a variety of digestive, menstrual, and nasal-oral mucosal symptoms and topically for eczema, wounds, and inflammation. The sedative effects of German chamomile may be due to the avonoid, apigenin, that binds to benzodiazepine receptors in the brain, although its mechanism is unknown. When used orally as highly concentrated tea, chamomile can induce vomiting. Chamomile has been used traditionally as a sedative, and studies have observed few significant differences in the effects of chamomile on sleep architecture when compared to placebo, such as changes in TST, sleep efficiency, SL, WASO, sleep quality, and number of awakenings.[54]

In summary, nonprescription agents are widely utilized for the management of sleep disturbances. However, these treatments suffer from a number of drawbacks, including their lack of strict regulation by the FDA, the paucity of studies of their efficacy and side effects, the lack of definitive data regarding optimal dosages, the unknown potential for interactions with other medications, and questions regarding the purity of preparations.

SELECTION OF A HYPNOTIC AGENT

The clinical approach to the patient with insomnia is beyond the scope of this chapter. However, a variety of parameters are useful to obtain during the clinical interview, which can guide the clinician in choosing the proper hypnotic; for a thorough discussion of this topic, see Chapter 6 of this volume. Some of the considerations in selecting a hypnotic are listed in Table 9.10.

CONCLUSIONS

A variety of agents, spanning multiple receptor profiles, are now available for the treatment of insomnia. A thorough clinical evaluation should always precede pharmacological intervention, so that comorbid conditions can be addressed, whose management may well dissipate the complaint of insomnia. Direct treatment of the condition can also be accomplished with nonpharmacological techniques such as cognitive-behavioral therapy, which has a number advantages over pharmacotherapy that are discussed elsewhere in this textbook. If pharmacology is selected, it is optimal to tailor the agent to the patient's clinical characteristics as much as possible. Systematic follow-up with attention to sustained efficacy and safety is essential.

FUTURE DIRECTIONS

Lemborexant, like suvorexant, is a dual orexin receptor antagonist, being developed for the treatment of insomnia. A New Drug Application was submitted for lemborexant in January 2019, based on the

---

TABLE 9.10 SELECTED CONSIDERATIONS IN CHOICE OF HYPNOTIC AGENT

- Initiation or maintenance insomnia
  - Initiation: Zaleplon, zolpidem, ramelteon
  - Maintenance: Doxepin low dose, zolpidem SL MOTN
  - Initiation and maintenance: Zolpidem ER, eszopiclone, suvorexant
- Respiratory compromise; safety in mild to moderate OSA/COPD
  - Ramelteon, suvorexant
- Abuse potential
  - Lowest: Ramelteon, doxepin
- Prior failure of selected medication
- Patient preference

Abbreviations: COPD, chronic obstructive pulmonary disease; MOTN, middle of the night; OSA, obstructive sleep apnea.

results of two pivotal phase 3 clinical studies; the first was a head-to-head comparison with zolpidem ER and objectively assessed sleep parameters, and the second was a 12-month subjective assessment compared to placebo.[55] Recently published data indicate that it has no clinically meaningful effect on driving performance in healthy adults and elderly during the next day following bedtime administration.[56] In addition, although it diminishes the time to fall asleep after nocturnal awakenings on par with zolpidem, it does not appear to be associated with as much body sway during nocturnal awakenings.[57]

A variety of other pharmaceutical products are under development, whose mechanisms largely fall in the categories already discussed, including benzodiazepine and melatonin receptor agonists and orexin and histamine receptor antagonists. The future may also clarify the potential role of cannabinoid receptor agonists, which are increasingly being utilized for the management of pain, anxiety, and other conditions.[58]

CLINICAL PEARLS

- Obtain the profile of the patient's sleep patterns prior to direct treatment of insomnia.
- Ask about nonprescription agents that the patient may be taking.
- Select the pharmacological agent that best suits the patient's clinical profile.
- Use evidence-based information to guide you in the choice of hypnotic agents.

SELF-ASSESSMENT QUESTIONS

1. A patient complains of insomnia; although he has no difficulty in falling asleep, he wakes up repeatedly after sleep onset. Which of these agents is the most specific treatment for his condition?
    a. Zolpidem
    b. Ramelteon
    c. Zaleplon
    d. Suvorexant
    e. Doxepin

Answer: e

2. Which of the following hypnotic agents is not scheduled by the US Drug Enforcement Agency?
    a. Ramelteon
    b. Zolpidem
    c. Suvorexant
    d. Triazolam
    e. None of the above

Answer: a

3. Which of the following hypnotic agents does not modulate the activity of the GABA receptor?
    a. Flurazepam
    b. Eszopiclone
    c. Suvorexant
    d. Zaleplon
    e. Zolpidem

Answer: c

4. Suvorexant, an FDA-approved medication for insomnia, is a dual antagonist of which of the following receptors?
    a. Serotonin
    b. Orexin
    c. Dopamine
    d. Histamine
    e. Norepinephrine

Answer: b

5. Which of the following over-the-counter agents for insomnia has been associated with serious hepatotoxicity?
    a. Kava Kava
    b. Melatonin
    c. Chamomile
    d. 5-hydroxytryptophan (5-HTP)
    e. None of the above

Answer: e

REFERENCES

1. Laurence LB, ed. *Goodman & Gilman's the pharmacological basis of therapeutics.* 11th ed. New York, NY: The McGraw-Hill Companies; 2006.
2. Sieghart W, Sperk G. Subunit composition, distribution and function of GABA(A) receptor subtypes. *Curr Top Med Chem.* 2002;2(8):795–816.
3. Mendelson WB, Roth T, Cassella J, et al. The treatment of chronic insomnia: Drug indications, chronic use and abuse liability: summary of a 2001 new clinical drug evaluation unit meeting symposium. *Sleep Med Rev.* 2004;8(1):7–17. doi:10.1016/S1087-0792(03)00042-X [doi].
4. Möhler H, Fritschy JM, Rudolph U. A new benzodiazepine pharmacology. *J Pharmacol Exp Ther.* 2002;300(1):2–8.
5. Sateia MJ, Buysse DJ, Krystal AD, Neubauer DN, Heald JL. Clinical practice guideline for the pharmacologic treatment of chronic insomnia in adults: an American academy of sleep medicine clinical practice guideline. *J Clin Sleep Med.* 2017;13(2):307–349.
6. Wilt TJ, MacDonald R, Brasure M, et al. Pharmacologic treatment of insomnia disorder: an evidence report for a clinical practice guideline by the American college of physicians. *Ann*

Intern Med. 2016;165(2):103–112. doi:10.7326/M15-1781.

7. US Food and Drug Administration. Drugs@FDA: FDA approved drug products. https://www.accessdata.fda.gov/scripts/cder/daf/. Updated 2019.

8. Heel RC, Brogden RN, Speight TM, Avery GS. Temazepam: a review of its pharmacological properties and therapeutic efficacy as an hypnotic. *Drugs.* 1981;21(5):321–340. doi:10.2165/00003495-198121050-00001.

9. Greenblatt DJ. Pharmacology of benzodiazepine hypnotics. *J Clin Psychiatry.* 1992;53 Suppl:7–13.

10. Rosenberg RP. Sleep maintenance insomnia: strengths and weaknesses of current pharmacologic therapies. *Ann Clin Psychiatry.* 2006;18(1):49–56. doi:10.1080/10401230500464711.

11. Greenblatt DJ, Harmatz JS, von Moltke LL, et al. Comparative kinetics and dynamics of zaleplon, zolpidem, and placebo. *Clin Pharmacol Ther.* 1998;64(5):553–561. doi:10.1016/S0009-9236(98)90139-4.

12. Greenblatt DJ, Divoll M, Harmatz JS, MacLaughlin DS, Shader RI. Kinetics and clinical effects of flurazepam in young and elderly noninsomniacs. *Clin Pharmacol Ther.* 1981;30(4):475–486.

13. Roth T, Roehrs TA. A review of the safety profiles of benzodiazepine hypnotics. *J Clin Psychiatry.* 1991;52(Suppl):38–41.

14. Staner C, Joly F, Jacquot N, et al. Sublingual zolpidem in early onset of sleep compared to oral zolpidem: polysomnographic study in patients with primary insomnia. *Curr Med Res Opin.* 2010;26(6):1423–1431. doi:10.1185/03007991003788225.

15. Staner L, Eriksson M, Cornette F, et al. Sublingual zolpidem is more effective than oral zolpidem in initiating early onset of sleep in the post-nap model of transient insomnia: a polysomnographic study. *Sleep Med.* 2009;10(6):616–620. doi:10.1016/j.sleep.2008.06.008.

16. Roth T, Hull SG, Lankford DA, Rosenberg R, Scharf MB. Low-dose sublingual zolpidem tartrate is associated with dose-related improvement in sleep onset and duration in insomnia characterized by middle-of-the-night (MOTN) awakenings. *Sleep.* 2008;31(9):1277–1284.

17. Roth T, Krystal A, Steinberg FJ, Singh NN, Moline M. Novel sublingual low-dose zolpidem tablet reduces latency to sleep onset following spontaneous middle-of-the-night awakening in insomnia in a randomized, double-blind, placebo-controlled, outpatient study. *Sleep.* 2013;36(2):189–196. doi:10.5665/sleep.2370.

18. Krystal AD, Walsh JK, Laska E, et al. Sustained efficacy of eszopiclone over 6 months of nightly treatment: results of a randomized, double-blind, placebo-controlled study in adults with chronic insomnia. *Sleep.* 2003;26(7):793–799.

19. Rosenberg R, Caron J, Roth T, Amato D. An assessment of the efficacy and safety of eszopiclone in the treatment of transient insomnia in healthy adults. *Sleep Med.* 2005;6(1):15–22. doi:10.1016/j.sleep.2004.09.001.

20. Saper CB, Chou TC, Scammell TE. The sleep switch: hypothalamic control of sleep and wakefulness. *Trends Neurosci.* 2001;24(12):726–731.

21. Dubocovich ML, Rivera-Bermudez MA, Gerdin MJ, Masana MI. Molecular pharmacology, regulation and function of mammalian melatonin receptors. *Front Biosci.* 2003;8:1093.

22. Roth T, Stubbs C, Walsh JK. Ramelteon (TAK-375), a selective MT1/MT2-receptor agonist, reduces latency to persistent sleep in a model of transient insomnia related to a novel sleep environment. *Sleep.* 2005;28(3):303–307.

23. Kryger M, Roth T, Wang-Weigand S, Zhang J. The effects of ramelteon on respiration during sleep in subjects with moderate to severe chronic obstructive pulmonary disease. *Sleep Breathing.* 2009;13(1):79–84.

24. Markov D, Doghramji K. Doxepin for insomnia. *Current Psychiatry.* 2010;9(10):67–77.

25. Andlauer O, Moore H,4th, Hong SC, et al. Predictors of hypocretin (orexin) deficiency in narcolepsy without cataplexy. *Sleep.* 2012;35(9):55F.

26. Mignot E, Taheri S, Nishino S. Sleeping with the hypothalamus: emerging therapeutic targets for sleep disorders. *Nat Neurosci.* 2002;5(Suppl):1071–1075. doi:10.1038/nn944.

27. Sun H, Palcza J, Card D, et al. Effects of suvorexant, an orexin receptor antagonist, on respiration during sleep in patients with obstructive sleep apnea. *J Clin Sleep Med.* 2016;12(1):9–17. doi:10.5664/jcsm.5382.

28. Vision a New drug application for insomnia disorder treatment lemborexant submitted in the united states. http://eisai.mediaroom.com/2019-01-15-New-Drug-Application-for-Insomnia-Disorder-Treatment-Lemborexant-Submitted-in-the-United-States. Updated 2014.

29. Murphy P, Moline M, Mayleben D, et al. Lemborexant, a dual orexin receptor antagonist (DORA) for the treatment of insomnia disorder: results from a Bayesian, adaptive, randomized, double-blind, placebo-controlled study. *J Clin Sleep Med.* 2017;13(11):1289–1299. doi:10.5664/jcsm.6800.

30. National Institutes of Health. National Institutes of Health State of the Science Conference statement on manifestations and management of chronic insomnia in adults, June 13–15, 2005. *Sleep*. 2005;28(9):1049–1057.

31. Soldatos CR, Dikeos DG, Whitehead A. Tolerance and rebound insomnia with rapidly eliminated hypnotics: a meta-analysis of sleep laboratory studies. *Int Clin Psychopharmacol*. 1999;14(5):287–303.

32. Perlis ML, McCall WV, Krystal AD, Walsh JK. Long-term, non-nightly administration of zolpidem in the treatment of patients with primary insomnia. *J Clin Psychiatry*. 2004;65(8):1128–1137.

33. Krystal AD, Erman M, Zammit GK, Soubrane C, Roth T; ZOLONG Study Group. Long-term efficacy and safety of zolpidem extended-release 12.5 mg, administered 3 to 7 nights per week for 24 weeks, in patients with chronic primary insomnia: a 6-month, randomized, double-blind, placebo-controlled, parallel-group, multicenter study. *Sleep*. 2008;31(1):79–90.

34. Walsh JK, Krystal AD, Amato DA, et al. Nightly treatment of primary insomnia with eszopiclone for six months: effect on sleep, quality of life, and work limitations. *Sleep*. 2007;30(8):959–968.

35. Mayer G, Wang-Weigand S, Roth-Schechter B, Lehmann R, Staner C, Partinen M. Efficacy and safety of 6-month nightly ramelteon administration in adults with chronic primary insomnia. *Sleep*. 2009;32(3):351–360.

36. Krystal AD, Durrence HH, Scharf M, et al. Efficacy and safety of doxepin 1 mg and 3 mg in a 12-week sleep laboratory and outpatient trial of elderly subjects with chronic primary insomnia. *Sleep*. 2010;33(11):1553–1561.

37. Shochat T, Umphress J, Israel AG, Ancoli-Israel S. Insomnia in primary care patients. *Sleep*. 1999;22(Suppl 2):359.

38. Zammit GK, Corser B, Doghramji K, et al. Sleep and residual sedation after administration of zaleplon, zolpidem, and placebo during experimental middle-of-the-night awakening. *J Clin Sleep Med*. 2006;2(4):417–423.

39. Southworth MR, Kortepeter C, Hughes A. Nonbenzodiazepine hypnotic use and cases of "sleep driving." *Ann Intern Med*. 2008;148(6):486–487.

40. Griffiths RR, Johnson MW. Relative abuse liability of hypnotic drugs: a conceptual framework and algorithm for differentiating among compounds. *J Clin Psychiatry*. 2005;66(Suppl 9):31–41.

41. Walsh JK. Drugs used to treat insomnia in 2002: regulatory-based rather than evidence-based medicine. *Sleep*. 2004;27(8):1441–1442.

42. James SP, Mendelson WB. The use of trazodone as a hypnotic: a critical review. *J Clin Psychiatry*. 2004;65(6):752–755.

43. Hajak G, Rodenbeck A, Voderholzer U, et al. Doxepin in the treatment of primary insomnia: a placebo-controlled, double-blind, polysomnographic study. *J Clin Psychiatry*. 2001;62(6):453–463.

44. Wine JN, Sanda C, Caballero J. Effects of quetiapine on sleep in nonpsychiatric and psychiatric conditions. *Ann Pharmacother*. 2009;43(4):707–713. doi:10.1345/aph.1L320.

45. Richelson E. Receptor pharmacology of neuroleptics: Relation to clinical effects. *J Clin Psychiatry*. 1999;60(Suppl 10):5–14.

46. Meolie AL, Rosen C, Kristo D, et al. Oral nonprescription treatment for insomnia: an evaluation of products with limited evidence. *J Clin Sleep Med*. 2005;1(2):173–187.

47. Agostini JV, Leo-Summers LS, Inouye SK. Cognitive and other adverse effects of diphenhydramine use in hospitalized older patients. *Arch Intern Med*. 2001;161(17):2091–2097.

48. Basu R, Dodge H, Stoehr GP, Ganguli M. Sedative-hypnotic use of diphenhydramine in a rural, older adult, community-based cohort: effects on cognition. *Am J Geriatr Psychiatry*. 2003;11(2):205–213.

49. Hardeland R. New approaches in the management of insomnia: weighing the advantages of prolonged-release melatonin and synthetic melatoninergic agonists. *Neuropsychiatric disease and treatment*. 2009;5:341–354. doi:10.2147/NDT.S4234.

50. Ferracioli-Oda E, Qawasmi A, Bloch MH. Meta-analysis: melatonin for the treatment of primary sleep disorders. *PLoS One*. 2013;8(5):e63773.

51. Rubio-Sastre P, Scheer, Frank A J L, Gómez-Abellán P, Madrid JA, Garaulet M. Acute melatonin administration in humans impairs glucose tolerance in both the morning and evening. *Sleep*. 2014;37(10):1715–1719. doi:10.5665/sleep.4088.

52. Bent S, Padula A, Moore D, Patterson M, Mehling W. Valerian for sleep: a systematic review and meta-analysis. *Am J Med*. 2006;119(12):1005–1012. doi:10.1016/j.amjmed.2006.02.026.

53. Wheatley D. Medicinal plants for insomnia: a review of their pharmacology, efficacy and tolerability. *J Psychopharmacol (Oxford)*. 2005;19(4):414–421. doi:10.1177/0269881105053309.

54. Zick SM, Wright BD, Sen A, Arndt JT. Preliminary examination of the efficacy and safety of a standardized chamomile extract for chronic primary insomnia: a randomized placebo-controlled pilot

study. *BMC Complement Altern Med.* 2011;11:78. doi:10.1186/1472-6882-11-78.

55. New Drug Application for Insomnia Disorder Treatment Lemborexant Submitted in the United States [press release]. Stamford, CT: Eisai; 2019. http://eisai.mediaroom.com/2019-01-15-New-Drug-Application-for-Insomnia-Disorder-Treatment-Lemborexant-Submitted-in-the-United-States.

56. Vermeeren A, Jongen S, Murphy M, et al. *Sleep.* 2018;1–5

57. Murphy P, Kumar D, Zammit G, et al. Auditor awakening threshold to evaluate ability to awaken after administration of Lemborexant versus Zolpidem. *Sleep.* 2018;41:A156–A157.

58. Babson KA, Scottile J, Morabito D. Cannabis, cannabinoids, and sleep: a review of the literature. *Curr Psychiatry Rep.* (2017) 19: 23. doi:10.1007/s11920-017-0775-9

59. Armstrong C. ACOG guidelines on psychiatric medication use during pregnancy and lactation. *Am Fam Physician.* 2008 Sep 15;78(6):772–778

10

Insomnia—Behavioral Treatments

SHEILA N. GARLAND, IVAN VARGAS, MICHAEL A. GRANDNER, AND MICHAEL L. PERLIS

INTRODUCTION

The fifth edition of the *Diagnostic and Statistical Manual for Mental Disorders* removed the primary and secondary qualifiers for insomnia and reclassified it as *insomnia disorder* [1]. The impetus for this change in classification is related to a variety of factors including multiple demonstrations that insomnia disorder: (a) appears to have a unique etiology and pathophysiology [2]; (b) occurs *prior to* and represents a *risk factor for* new onset and recurrence of multiple psychiatric disorders [3]; (c) often persists following the successful treatment of the comorbid disorder(s) [4]; and (d) treatment may serve to augment standard treatment outcomes for other disorders (e.g., major depression) [5]. These findings challenged the utility of classifying insomnia as either a disorder or a symptom (i.e., primary vs. secondary insomnia) with the clear implication being that insomnia should be a target for treatment, in addition to the concurrent psychiatric disorder(s).

THEORETICAL PERSPECTIVES ON THE ETIOLOGY OF INSOMNIA

Behavioral Model

As originally described by Bootzin [6], stimulus control therapy is based on the behavioral principle that one stimulus may elicit a variety of responses, depending on the conditioning history. In the instance where one stimulus is always paired with a single behavior, there is a high probability that the stimulus will yield only one response. In the instance with a complex conditioning history, where a stimulus is paired with a variety of behaviors, there is a low probability that the stimulus will elicit only one response. In individuals with insomnia, the normal cues associated with sleep (e.g., bed, bedroom, bedtime, etc.) are frequently paired with behaviors other than sleep (e.g., reading, working, watching TV, on social media, planning, worrying, etc.). These practices set the stage for stimulus dyscontrol, that is, reduced probability that sleep-related stimuli will elicit the desired response of sleepiness and sleep.

Spielman 3P Model

Since its inception, the 3P model (predisposing, precipitating, and perpetuating) has gained wide acceptance among insomnia treatment providers and researchers [7]. Predisposing and precipitating factors explain insomnia development, whereas perpetuating factors explain the mechanisms by which insomnia can become chronic.

Predisposing factors increase the underlying vulnerability to develop insomnia and are comprised of biological features, such as age and sex, and psychological traits, such as the tendency to worry [8, 9]. A predisposition to insomnia, however, requires a sufficiently stressful precipitant, or combination of precipitants, before it may be expressed. Precipitating factors are thought to be acute occurrences of a stress-related trigger [10]. Perpetuating factors refer to the behaviors that an individual engages in while attempting to manage a sleep difficulty, which in turn actually contribute to the persistence of insomnia. Examples include going to bed earlier, "trying" harder to sleep, napping during the day, engaging in activities other than sleep while in bed, and delaying the time that an individual takes to get out of bed.

These are referred to as "sleep extension" behaviors. While enacted to attempt to recover lost sleep, they result in a mismatch between sleep opportunity (i.e., amount of time a person allows for sleep or time in bed [TIB]) and sleep ability (i.e., amount of time a person actually sleeps). For example, if the person's sleep ability is 7 hours, and they are in bed for 10 hours, they will "necessarily" have 3 hours of wakefulness over the course of the night).

Neurocognitive Model of Insomnia

The neurocognitive model extends the behavioral models of insomnia by suggesting that the repeated pairing of sleep-related stimuli with insomnia-related wakefulness leads to conditioned cortical hyperarousal. While hyperarousal is widely considered the underlying factor that gives rise to insomnia [11], the neurocognitive model proposes that hyperarousal is not a unitary construct and that there are several forms of hyperarousal which may be more or less relevant to how the disorder is expressed over time.

This model suggests that hyperarousal may be construed in at least three dimensions (somatic, cognitive, and cortical arousal) and that it is cortical hyperarousal (which may be indicated by increases in high frequency electroencephalography activity [beta/gamma activity between 16 and 45 Hz]) that is of primary relevance for chronic insomnia [12]. Heightened cortical arousal is hypothesized to allow for increased levels of sensory and information processing at and around sleep onset and during nonrapid eye movement (NREM) sleep and/or for the attenuation of the normal mesograde amnesia that occurs in association with sleep. These latter phenomena are hypothesized to increase the probability of difficulties falling and staying asleep and to contribute to subjective feelings of having not slept despite objective evidence that sleep occurred (sleep-state misperception) [13].

Cognitive Model of Insomnia

The cognitive model of insomnia suggests that individuals with insomnia have negatively toned cognitive activity throughout the day and before bed, which leads to an overall increase in anxiety and distress [14]. This initiates a process by which the individual begins to bias their attention toward monitoring of perceived internal (e.g., body sensations for signs of fatigue) and external (e.g., the alarm clock) sleep-related threats that might indicate to a person that they did (or will) not receive enough sleep. The detection of a sleep-related threat might validate the need to monitor and reinforce the need for worry and concern. This is problematic because selective attention and monitoring produces cognitive arousal, which creates additional physical sensations while also increasing the probability of detecting meaningless cues that would otherwise remain unnoticed. These processes work together to create an exaggerated perception of the deficit in sleep and its potentially negative impact on daytime performance.

Individuals with insomnia also tend to hold erroneous beliefs about the impact of sleep disruption and the utility of worry while also engaging in counterproductive safety behaviors, such as canceling appointments or taking a nap during the day. The cognitive model highlights the importance of targeting specific cognitive maintaining factors (i.e., attentional bias) and eliminating the use of safety behaviors in the successful treatment of insomnia.

Psychobiological Inhibition Model

The psychobiological inhibition model suggests that difficulty with sleep initiation and maintenance is caused by the failure to inhibit wakefulness [15], as opposed to the conditioned hyperarousal [12]. Failure to inhibit wakefulness is thought to occur from an activation of a cognitive *attention–intention–effort* pathway. When a person experiences difficulty sleeping, their *attention* shifts toward the process of sleep, something that is typically an automatic and passive event. This shift in attention prevents the normal disengagement from wakefulness and changes sleep to a purposive or *intentional* activity. When an individual experiences difficulty sleeping, they demonstrate active *effort* to sleep, which further impairs the inhibition of wakefulness.

ASSESSMENT AND MEASUREMENT

An understanding of the previously described theoretical models is necessary and invaluable to ensure an appropriate diagnosis and inform the treatment process. A recent clinical guideline outlines the best practices for the assessment and diagnosis of insomnia, which is summarized and tailored to the treatment of patients with comorbid psychiatric conditions described in the following discussion [16]. The assessment process typically begins with a semistructured clinical interview intended to identify predisposing, precipitating, and perpetuating factors while at the same time paying attention to possible comorbidities and differential diagnostic possibilities that may better explain the patient's difficulty.

Clinical Interview

A semistructured clinical interview should cover the following content areas:

1. *Characterization of the primary insomnia complaint*: It is helpful to have the patient describe the event or events that they

believe to have *precipitated* their insomnia. From here, one can easily assess the nature of the difficulty (i.e., difficulty falling asleep, staying asleep, or waking up too early); the frequency and duration of the problem; the success, or lack thereof, of any previous attempts at treatment; and whether adequate opportunity is available for sleep.

2. *Typical sleep–wake pattern*: A characterization of a typical sleep–wake schedule can be accomplished by asking the patient to report on the following: What time do they typically go to bed at night and wake up in the morning? What time do they actually fall asleep and wake up? How many times do they tend to wake up at night and how long do these awakenings last? What activities do they engage in when they are awake at night (e.g., checking social media, lying in bed, trying harder to sleep)? Does their routine change on weekends, when they are working different shifts, or with mood changes? This information is particularly beneficial to identify conditions that may incorrectly be identified as insomnia (e.g., delayed or advanced sleep phase syndrome) or to assess the contribution of psychiatric conditions to the presenting problem, as in the case of depressive disorder with seasonal pattern or bipolar disorder.

3. *Individual and family history*: This section is useful to identify factors that might predispose an individual to experience insomnia. The research is beginning to confirm what clinicians have long suspected: that there is a genetic predisposition to experience insomnia [17]. Patients will often report that one or more of their immediate family members have past or present experience with insomnia. It is also useful to query the presence of temperament or personality factors that are commonly observed in patients with insomnia, such as anxious, sensitive, or reactive temperament, perfectionistic tendencies, and/or behavioral rigidity.

4. *Behavioral, cognitive, and environmental presleep conditions*: This section includes an examination of what activities the individual engages in before bed and

these are likely to be consistent with the comorbid psychiatric condition(s). For example, patients may use distraction to cope with uncomfortable feelings and unwanted thoughts by watching television, working on the computer, or keeping busy with other tasks. They may also attempt to eliminate their negative emotionality by going to bed earlier and trying harder to "force" sleep. Patients with trauma and stress-related disorders are likely to pay close attention to what their sleep environment is like (e.g., Is it safe and free of noise?). Similarly, other patients with anxiety or obsessive-compulsive disorders may have strict rules about sleep routines and conditions that must be "just so" for sleep to occur (e.g., certain sounds or absolute silence). Lastly, regardless of the psychiatric condition, it is prudent to assess how the patient feels before bed. For example, do they feel anxious and worry about the future? Are they ruminating about past events and/or perceived failures? Are they fearful and/or hypervigilant? Close attention to the behavioral, cognitive and environmental presleep conditions will identify relevant *perpetuating* factors and potential targets of behavioral and/or cognitive remediation techniques.

5. *Perceived impact of insomnia, next day function, and compensatory behaviors*: Patients may report difficulty concentrating or paying attention, sleepiness and/or fatigue, affective disturbances, or worsening of comorbid physical or psychiatric conditions. They may also engage in, or discontinue, activities to try and cope with their daytime dysfunction. This may include daytime napping, stimulant use (e.g., caffeine), and canceling physical activity or social engagements. The perpetuating behaviors, while intended to help them cope, actually promote (i.e., *perpetuate*) the persistence of the insomnia and can be modified or eliminated to reduce their contribution to the insomnia disorder.

6. *The presence of other sleep disorders*: There are a number of other sleep disorders that may account for (or exacerbate) the presenting insomnia symptoms or represent an additional

comorbidity to be considered. Increased prevalence of obstructive sleep apnea [18], hypersomnolence disorder [19], restless legs syndrome [20], parasomnias [21], nightmare disorder [22], and narcolepsy [23] have all been demonstrated in patients with psychiatric disorders. To assess for these disorders, especially for clinicians less familiar with the signs and symptoms of the various intrinsic sleep disorders, it is recommended that a screening questionnaire be used. While many such instruments exist [24], only two are considered brief: the Global Sleep Assessment Questionnaire (GSAQ) [25] and the Sleep Disorders Symptom Checklist-25 (SDS-CL-25) [26]—and only one is both brief and comprehensive (the SDS-CL-25 [26]). If the patient presents with symptoms suggestive of one or more of these disorders, a sleep study (nocturnal polysomnogram) may be warranted.

7. *Medical and psychiatric history*: Comorbidity is the norm and not the exception in the case of insomnia. A number of medical and psychiatric conditions, along with their treatments, can contribute to and complicate insomnia [27]. Symptoms of these disorders (e.g., pain) will need to be considered when planning treatment. A thorough review of medications (both prescribed and over the counter) is necessary to identify any potential substances that may be contributing to insomnia. Commonly used antidepressant, antipsychotic, and stimulant medications are known to affect sleep [27, 28]. Attention should be paid to whether these are taken in the morning or evening depending on whether they impair or promote sleep. Anxiolytic medications are often used as hypnotic/sedative agents to reduce presleep arousal, but these are not recommended as a long-term solution for reasons of tolerance, dependence, and the potential for other negative outcomes [28, 29].

Measurement Instruments
Use of a prospective sleep diary is critical at (a) the time of assessment to properly evaluate the sleep wake pattern and the treatment plan and (b) throughout treatment to titrate recommendations

and evaluate treatment response. A standard sleep diary has been developed and is recommended for use [30]; however, should alternate versions be used they should include, at minimum, information on time to bed and wake time (which provide information on TIB), sleep latency (SL), frequency of nightly awakenings, wake after sleep onset (WASO), total sleep time (TST), early morning awakenings, subjective assessments of sleep quality, nap frequency and duration, fatigue ratings, stimulant consumption, and medication usage.

Information on TIB and TST is used to calculate sleep efficiency (SE) percentage, which is the TST, divided by the TIB, multiplied by 100. It is recommended that patients complete 2 weeks of sleep diaries before initiating treatment to allow for a stable evaluation of baseline sleep patterns. Additional tools may include the Insomnia Severity Index (ISI) [31], the Dysfunctional Beliefs and Attitudes about Sleep (DBAS-16) scale [32], and the Epworth Sleepiness Scale [33]. It is worthwhile to consider including other measures related to the comorbid psychiatric condition(s) (e.g., depression, anxiety, mania, etc.) to monitor the parallel effects of cognitive behavioral therapy for insomnia (CBT-I) on those symptoms. In the absence of another possible comorbid sleep disorder, the diagnosis of insomnia does not require the use of laboratory-based assessments (i.e., polysomnography) or ambulatory assessment (i.e., actigraphy).

COGNITIVE BEHAVIORAL THERAPY FOR INSOMNIA
The recognition that individuals with insomnia exhibit cognitive, physiological, and cortical hyperarousal; demonstrate particular cognitive patterns and attentional biases; strongly endorse problematic sleep-related beliefs; and engage in maladaptive sleep-related behaviors has led to the development of a treatment designed to address these inter-related components. CBT-I combines principles from stimulus control therapy and sleep restriction therapy with formal cognitive restructuring to target arousal, dysfunctional behaviors, and maladaptive thoughts, beliefs, and attitudes.

CBT-I traditionally requires 4 to 8 sessions with once a week face-to-face meetings with the clinical provider [34]. Patients with comorbid psychiatric conditions may require more sessions than this depending on motivation and how well the comorbid condition is managed. Sessions range from 30 to 90 minutes depending on the stage of treatment and the degree of patient compliance. Intake sessions are usually 60 to 90 minutes in duration. During the first session, the clinical history is obtained, and the patient is instructed in the use of sleep diaries. No intervention is provided during the first week as it is used to collect the baseline sleep wake data that will guide treatment for the remainder of therapy.

The primary interventions (stimulus control and sleep restriction) are deployed over the course of the next one to two 60-minute sessions [34]. Once these treatments are delivered, the patient enters into a phase of treatment where TST is upwardly titrated over the course of the next two to five visits. These follow-up sessions require about 30 minutes unless additional interventions are being integrated into the treatment program or extra effort is required to gain the patient compliance.

Stimulus Control

Stimulus dyscontrol refers to the tendency to engage in behaviors other than sleep in the bedroom thereby weakening the association between the sleep environment (stimulus) and the physiologic state of sleep (response) [35]. Stimulus control targets the conditioned arousal associated with insomnia that is caused by the failure to establish discriminative stimuli for sleep or the presence of sleep incompatible stimuli, such as reading or watching television in bed. Lying awake in bed while trying to sleep further strengthens the association between the bed and wakefulness, while falling asleep in places other than your bed, such as the couch, strengthens the association between sleep and nonsleeping environments. [36]

Stimulus Control Instructions

1. Lie down to sleep only when sleepy.
2. Avoid using the bed for activities other than sleep or intimacy.
3. Get out of bed if unable to sleep within 15 to 20 minutes and return to bed only when sleepy.
4. Repeat this pattern throughout the night as necessary.
5. Set an alarm and get up at the same time every day.
6. Avoid napping throughout the day.

Sleep Restriction

When Arthur Spielman first described sleep restriction in 1987, he challenged the typical and seemingly logical goal of most individuals with insomnia:

spend more TIB to get more sleep (i.e., sleep extension) [37]. Sleep extension refers to the tendency to increase TIB in an effort to recover lost sleep, which ultimately results in the mismatch between sleep opportunity and sleep ability. The aim of sleep restriction is not necessarily to "restrict" sleep, but to limit the patient's TIB (sleep opportunity) to the time that they are actually asleep (sleep ability). The first objective in sleep restriction is to determine a morning wake-up time that can be closely adhered to on a daily basis. The individual then determines their "sleep window" based on their current sleep ability as recorded in their sleep diary (during the 2-week baseline phase). Their current sleep ability is then subtracted from their wake-up time to determine their bedtime. For example, if a patient has a 6-hour sleep ability and needs to get up at 7:00 AM every morning, their designated bedtime would be 1:00 AM.

Sleep restriction has the following important objectives: (a) it reduces the increased arousal caused by an individual's effort to force sleep by keeping them out of bed until they are really sleepy, and (b) it reduces the time to fall asleep and time spent awake during the night by consolidating sleep into longer and more restorative sections. Once the individual is able to maintain an SE of 85% or greater, the sleep window is expanded in 15 to 30 minute intervals until no further gains are produced.

Sleep Restriction Instructions

1. Using a sleep diary, calculate mean TST for the baseline period (e.g., 1–2 weeks). This will become the client's prescribed TIB or sleep window.
2. Establish a fixed wake up time that the client will adhere to 7 days per week.
3. Set bedtime to approximate the mean TST to achieve a >85% SE (TST/TIB × 100%) over 7 days. Do not restrict the TIB to less than 5 hours.
4. Make weekly adjustments: (a) for SE (TST/TIB × 100%) >85% to 90% over 7 days, TIB can be increased by 15 to 30 minutes; (b) for SE <80%, TIB can be further decreased by 15 to 30 minutes.
5. Repeat TIB adjustment every 7 days until the individual sleep need is met or SE begins to decrease.

Cognitive Restructuring

Given the research on the influence of negative sleep beliefs, attentional biases and presleep cognitions, cognitive restructuring is increasingly being recognized as an important component of a comprehensive insomnia treatment [38]. According to the principles behind cognitive therapy, events are not inherently good or bad, rather it is how we appraise or interpret these events that determines their valence. The primary goal of cognitive therapy in insomnia treatment is to identify problematic thoughts that may contribute to the development of or reinforce behaviors that produce presleep arousal, examine these thoughts for accuracy, and, if necessary, modify them to be more rational and/or realistic.

The therapist initially helps the patient identify dysfunctional sleep cognitions and the resulting emotional reactions using thought records. The patient is instructed to describe the situation that produced the thought, the content of the thought, the emotional reaction, and its intensity in detail. These beliefs are then evaluated with cognitive restructuring techniques including, but not limited to, reappraisal, reattribution, decatastrophizing, attention shifting, and hypothesis testing. [39] The patient is then able to apply their revised or alternate thought to the situation and note the impact on the intensity of the emotion. Although psycho-education may serve the goal of delivering information, the use of these cognitive therapy techniques allows the person to realize that their beliefs may not be wholly accurate through a process of guided discovery. Once learned, the patient can continue to use cognitive therapy techniques to better manage their problematic sleep beliefs and cognitive responses.

Potential Adjunctive Treatments

The following are not recommended as stand-alone treatments but can be incorporated as necessary to address specific patient characteristics, needs, and/or preferences.

Sleep Hygiene Education

Sleep hygiene education addresses a variety of behaviors that may influence sleep quality and quantity. The intervention most often involves providing the patient with a handout and then reviewing the items and the rationales for them. Sleep hygiene education is most helpful when tailored to a behavioral analysis of the patient's sleep wake behaviors.

Sleep Hygiene Instructions

1. Keep a regular schedule. Regular times for sleeping, meals, medications, chores, and other activities help keep the inner body clock running smoothly.
2. Take time to unwind before bed. Begin rituals to promote relaxation each night before bed. This can include such things as a warm bath, light snack, or a few minutes of reading.
3. Exercise regularly. Schedule exercise times so that they do not occur within 3 hours of intended bedtime. Exercise makes it easier to initiate sleep and deepen sleep.
4. Make sure your bedroom is comfortable and free from light and noise. A comfortable, noise-free sleep environment will reduce the likelihood that you will wake up during the night. Noise that does not awaken you may still disturb the quality of your sleep.
5. Eat regular meals and do not go to bed hungry. Hunger may disturb sleep. A light snack at bedtime may help sleep but avoid greasy or "heavy" foods.
6. Cut down on all caffeine products. Caffeinated beverages and foods (coffee, tea, cola, chocolate) can cause difficulty falling asleep, awakenings during the night, and shallow sleep. Even caffeine early in the day can disrupt nighttime sleep.
7. Avoid alcohol, especially in the evening. Although alcohol helps tense people fall asleep more easily, it causes awakenings later in the night.
8. Avoid excessive liquids in the evening. Reducing liquid intake will minimize the need for nighttime trips to the bathroom.
9. Smoking may disturb sleep. Nicotine is a stimulant. Try not to smoke during the night when you have trouble sleeping.
10. Avoid naps. Avoid taking naps if you can. If you must take a nap, try to keep it short (20 minutes or less) and at least 6 hours prior to your desired bedtime.

Relaxation Therapy

The rationale for including relaxation therapy in a comprehensive nonpharmacological treatment program follows logically from research demonstrating that individuals with insomnia report higher levels of both daytime and nighttime cognitive and physiological arousal. Relaxation therapy is thought to improve sleep by reducing sympathetic nervous system activity and facilitating physiological and mental calmness [39]. Progressive muscle relaxation and imagery are among the most commonly included therapies but there is little evidence to suggest differential effectiveness between those and a range of other techniques [40].

Mindfulness Meditation

The practice of mindfulness meditation, defined as intentionally bringing awareness to present moment thoughts or sensations with an attitude of acceptance, patience, openness, curiosity, and kindness [41], has been suggested to reduce patterns of rumination [42], presleep arousal [43], and attention bias [44]. Trials comparing mindfulness-based interventions to CBT-I, or combining the two, suggest that CBT-I produces more immediate effects on sleep but that incorporating mindfulness techniques may enhance the durability of these effects [45, 46] and may be a useful ancillary treatment to CBT-I because it may serve as a major strategy for relapse prevention [47].

CONTEMPORARY ISSUES WITH THE CLINICAL DELIVERY OF CBT-I

Concurrent Use of Sleep Medications

In 2016, the American College of Physicians (ACP), the professional organization that represents internal medicine, released a position statement entitled, "Management of Chronic Insomnia Disorder in Adults: A Clinical Practice Guideline from the American College of Physicians" [48]. This document represents the results of a systematic review of the literature between 2004 and 2015 and states two recommendations:

1. All adult patients receive CBT-I as the initial treatment for chronic insomnia disorder.
2. Clinicians should use a shared decision-making approach, including a discussion of the benefits, harms, and costs of short-term use of medications, to decide whether to add pharmacological therapy in adults with chronic insomnia disorder in whom CBT-I alone was unsuccessful.

Thus, the official position of the ACP is that not only is CBT-I recommended as the first-line therapy of choice, but that pharmacotherapy is only recommended in cases where its use is short-term, and/or in combination with behavioral treatment,

and/or after discussion with patients regarding the limitations of this approach.

The endorsement of CBT-I over pharmacotherapy for insomnia is further supported by a position statement by the American Academy of Sleep Medicine (AASM), the organization that represents sleep physicians. This document focused exclusively on pharmacotherapy, reviewing the available literature on prescription and over-the-counter insomnia treatments (behavioral approaches were not evaluated) [49]. This statement evaluated a wide range of potential insomnia treatment options. According to this guideline: no pharmacological agent was rated as being supported by more than "weak" evidence, no pharmacological agent was recommended as superior to any other approach, and no over-the-counter approaches were recommended for insomnia treatment. This is consistent with the ACP guideline that considered pharmacological treatment only in combination with CBT-I or if CBT-I fails and only after discussion of the limitations of medications.

It was previously believed that sleep-promoting medication needed to be tapered prior to the initiation of treatment with CBT-I; however, recent research has demonstrated that it may be preferred to taper medication after treatment with CBT-I. In a direct comparison of 6 weekly sessions of CBT-I, with or without nightly hypnotic medication (10 mg zolpidem), in 160 patients with chronic insomnia, the group that received the combined CBT-I plus medication, followed by a medication taper, had slightly better results than the groups that received CBT-I alone or CBT-I with medication on a PRN basis in the extended 6 month follow-up phase [50]. The improvements were maintained at 6, 12, and 24 month follow-up assessments. [51, 52] Attention should be paid to individuals who experience withdrawal symptoms, increased psychological distress, and lower self-efficacy during medication tapering, as these are significant predictors of failure to discontinue hypnotic medication use [53].

Limitations and Side Effects of CBT-I

One of the main benefits identified of CBT-I is its low side effect profile compared to pharmacological interventions, but recent efforts have acknowledged that patients can still experience side effects of treatment. The side effects of CBT-I are most commonly associated with sleep restriction and tend to be minimal and short-lasting (2–3 weeks in duration). The side effects typically reported are mild and include daytime sleepiness and increased emotionality, but if not appropriately planned for and mitigated, these side effects can lead to other more potentially serious consequences (e.g., falling asleep behind the wheel of a car). Treatment providers are obligated to make patients aware of the potential for these side effects to occur and collaboratively plan to reduce the likelihood for unintended effects of treatment. This mitigation plan may include such things as making alternate transportation arrangements to avoid operating motor vehicles, making family members and coworkers aware in advance that the individual may be more irritable or emotional than usual. Having a prespecified plan in place beforehand can make the individual better able to cope with such effects if or when they occur.

While not restricted to CBT-I, the most apparent limitation is the need for qualified providers. There is a substantial disparity between evidence and practice in the case of treating insomnia. In a survey of providers who self-identified as having experience providing CBT-I, there were four states with no behavioral sleep medicine providers. Of the 167 U.S. cities with a population of > 150,000, 105 cities have no behavioral sleep medicine providers [54]. Even if this value did not capture all practitioners, the number would still be well below the number needed to treat the burden of insomnia. Espie [55] and Manber [56] advocate for a model that would see other healthcare providers, such as social workers, nurses, and master's level practitioners [57] provide CBT-I in straight-forward cases of insomnia, reserving the cases that are complicated by other physical or psychological comorbidities cases to doctoral trained providers. Graduate training programs represent an ideal place to provide training in CBT-I. At present, medical residents in North America receive at most 3 hours of sleep education. [58] This varies considerably with some programs offering comprehensive training and others offering none. Skill development in treating insomnia, the most common sleep disorder, is likely to enhance practice opportunities and interprofessional collaborations.

Alternate Delivery Models of CBT-I

To address the access limitation of CBT-I, increased attention has been paid to the development and evaluation of self-help [56], mobile [59], and online [60] CBT-I interventions. One of the key advantages of such alternate treatment models is that they can allow for people who might typically struggle with access (i.e., individuals in rural and remote locations) to benefit from treatment. While there is evidence that these programs can produce clinically meaningful improvements in insomnia [61], they are not likely to completely replace the need for qualified providers. A study by Lancee et al. [62] compared online CBT-I to face-to-face CBT-I and found that while the online treatment group showed clinically significant improvement, face-to-face treatment produced larger reductions in insomnia severity and improvements in secondary mood outcomes. The choice of when to use online treatment versus face-to-face interventions is likely to be different for each person and based on a number of considerations including patient preference, provider availability, and insurance coverage, among others. At present, the evidence suggests that for straightforward cases of insomnia, alternate delivery models of CBT-I or treatment with a master's level provider may be appropriate, but that doctoral level providers are still required to manage the complications that can arise when insomnia coexists with other medical and/or psychiatric disorders.

EVIDENCE FOR OVERALL USE OF CBT-I IN PATIENTS WITH PSYCHIATRIC DISORDERS

CBT-I, with or without relaxation therapy, is recommended by the AASM and the ACP [48]. Several systematic reviews and meta-analyses have validated the robust effect of CBT-I on a number of sleep outcomes regardless of delivery format [63–67]. With the growing recognition that individuals with psychiatric conditions more often than not have symptoms of insomnia [68], Wu and colleagues [69] conducted a meta-analysis of 37 randomized controlled studies on the impact of CBT-I not only on perceived insomnia severity and sleep continuity measures but also on the symptoms of the comorbid disorder in an overall sample of 2,189 participants. Of these studies, 10 were conducted in patients with comorbid psychiatric conditions, 26 with medical comorbidities, and 1 with a mixed sample. The psychiatric conditions included were substance use disorders, depressive disorders, and posttraumatic stress disorder. While patients with psychiatric and medical conditions improved equally on symptoms of insomnia, a larger effect of CBT-I was found for reducing symptoms of the comorbid psychiatric conditions ($g = 0.76$) than symptoms of medical comorbidities ($g = 0.20$). This suggests that psychiatric symptoms may be more responsive to CBT-I than those associated with a medical condition. Consistent with findings of other studies, the sleep improvements were maintained for 3 to 12 months after completing treatment.

Not surprisingly, the treatment of insomnia comorbid with psychiatric disorders requires more therapeutic skill and experience to effectively manage both disorders, but when employed appropriately, the cognitive and behavioral techniques employed in CBT-I map nicely onto cognitive-behavioral therapy for other psychiatric disorders. For example, setting a consistent wake-up time and engaging in morning and afternoon activities can be seen as forms of behavioral activation; avoiding triggers for rumination by staying out of the bed until very sleepy breaks conditioned ways of thinking; and challenging dysfunctional beliefs using cognitive restructuring can work equally well for sleep-related and depressive thoughts. Reviews suggest that CBT-I can be used effectively for insomnia that occurs comorbid with depression, anxiety, posttraumatic stress disorder, bipolar disorder, and psychotic conditions but that some modifications may be required. The potential modifications required for each condition have been described in detail elsewhere [70].

DELIVERING CBT-I IN A PATIENT WITH COMORBID DEPRESSION: A CASE EXAMPLE

We demonstrate use of these techniques using the case example of Eric, a 26-year-old man of Southeast Asian descent. He was referred by his psychiatrist for the treatment of chronic insomnia comorbid with recurrent major depressive disorder. In our first meeting, we focused on getting a complete sleep, medical, and psychiatric history to inform the treatment strategies that would be employed in the following weeks.

Session 1
Presenting Problem

Eric reported that his difficulty with sleep was, at the time, his biggest barrier to resuming normal functioning. His nightly routine consisted of being on the computer until 10:30 PM, having a shower, and reading in the kitchen until about 1:30 AM until he began to feel sleepy. He would then go up to his bedroom to initiate sleep but found that his mind turned on, and he began to think about things. Eric estimated that it would take him, on average, 90 minutes to fall asleep.

When Eric couldn't fall asleep, he would search the Internet on his phone while in bed. Once asleep, he was able to remain asleep for most of the night unless noise in the house woke him up. If awakened during the night, he would only be able to fall back asleep about half of the time. Eric woke up in the morning because of the light coming into his bedroom at around 10:30 AM but would not get out of bed until around noon. He estimated that he was currently getting 8 hours of sleep but he was not happy about sleeping so late into the day. Eric reports difficulty with sleep at least 5 days per week and stated that his routine on weekends was the same as on weekdays. He felt like his sleep quality was okay but was unhappy with how long it took him to get going in the morning. He denied drinking caffeine late into the day and did not engage in any formal exercise. He reported that his biggest current stressor was his uncertainty with work.

Relevant Sleep and Psychiatric History

Eric's difficulty with sleep began when he was in his third year of his undergraduate degree in economics, and it coincided with his first major depressive episode. Eric reported that he was always a good student but that he found it difficult to keep this up. With the encouragement of his parents, he had planned on going into business school because of his aptitude for numbers, but he stated that it was never really his passion. Eric reported that he was working too much and felt burned out. He had lost interest in his studies and began to find it hard to get up in the morning. The pressure to perform academically also led him to stop going out with friends. He struggled to complete his degree (e.g., failing some classes along the way) but ultimately graduated.

After graduating from college, Eric held various entry-level jobs but struggled to remain engaged. That year he also attempted suicide by overdosing on sleeping pills. He was hospitalized for 2 weeks and released into the care of a psychiatrist and was started on medication, which resulted in a moderate symptom improvement in his mood, but his insomnia remained unchanged. The next year, Eric began working approximately 50 hours per week as a delivery driver, which required him to get up at 5:00 AM. When he was lying in bed awake at night, Eric began worrying about the impact that the insomnia would have on his ability to function the next day, and he would get frustrated and angry. He estimated that he was getting 3 to 4 hours of sleep per night. He would try to make up for this on weekends, but he never really felt like he could recover from the week. After 4 months working at this job, Eric noticed that his depression was getting worse and he was getting more and more frustrated about not being able to sleep. Later that year, he injured his back at work and walked off the job. Eric described this time as very difficult for him. He was living off his savings and collecting unemployment insurance. At this time, he reported that he also thought of committing suicide but ultimately decided to check himself into the hospital. He reported thoughts of suicide but did not endorse immediate intent.

Eric had tried a number of prescription medications to help manage his depression and insomnia including escitalopram (Lexapro) and mirtazapine (Remeron), but these left him feeling groggy in the morning and into the day. He tried one other hypnotic but could not recall what it was called. His psychiatrist ultimately suggested that he take Benadryl to help him sleep, but this also impacted his daytime function. He was maintained on citalopram (Celexa) for 4 months but discontinued this because he felt it was not really helping his mood and was making his sleep worse. He tried taking melatonin at the suggestion of his mother but stated that this was also not helpful. At the time of Session 1, Eric was not on any prescribed or over-the-counter medication for sleep or depression. He reported that he did not believe that he would respond to medication and did not want to endure the side effects of something that is not going to work.

Relevant Social and Medical History

Eric is the oldest child of parents that emigrated from Thailand. He currently lives with his parents and brother. His father owns a restaurant, and his mother is a bookkeeper. His younger brother is 14 years old and in high school. Eric reports that his brother has been diagnosed with some sort of anxiety disorder but is not sure what kind. Eric also reports that his mother may have had postpartum depression as he remembers having to take care of his infant younger brother when his mother could not get out of bed. Eric does not report significant current or previous romantic relationships and has little social support. He stated that he is trying to learn how to meditate because he heard that it might help his mood and insomnia. He is currently taking metformin for type 2 diabetes and states that his blood sugars still vary between 6 and 8 mmol/L. He is also taking Celebrex daily

for an old knee injury. His daily routine consists of helping transport his brother and attending various medical appointments.

Baseline Symptom Measurement

Eric completed the ISI [31], a brief 7-item measure designed to assess the severity of sleep-onset and sleep maintenance difficulties, satisfaction with current sleep pattern, interference with daily functioning, impairment attributed to the sleep problem, and degree of distress elicited. Respondents are asked to rate the current (i.e., last 2 weeks) severity of their insomnia problems on a 5-point scale (0 = none; 4 = very severe). A total score is calculated by summing scores for all 7 items with a total score that ranges from zero to 28, with higher scores indicating more severe symptoms of insomnia. Optimal cut-off scores include: zero to 7 (no clinically significant insomnia), 8 to 14 (subthreshold insomnia), 15 to 21 (presence of clinically significant insomnia; moderate severity), and 22 to 28 (presence of clinically significant insomnia; severe). Eric's score on the ISI was 23, indicating clinically significant insomnia.

Eric also filled out the Hospital Anxiety and Depression Scale (HADS) [71], a 14-item, self-rated instrument for anxiety (7 items) and depression (7 items) symptoms in the past week. Established cutoffs are zero to 7, not significant; 8 to 10, subclinical; and 11 to 21, clinically significant depression/anxiety. Eric's score was 14 on the depression subscale and 8 on the anxiety subscale, indicating clinically significant depression and subclinical levels of anxiety.

Impression and Treatment Plan

Eric was diagnosed with chronic insomnia comorbid with major depressive disorder. He has a significant family history of anxiety and depression and may have a predisposition to internalizing disorders, which is likely exacerbated by self-imposed and familial performance demands. Based on his self-report, the precipitating event for the development of his insomnia and his major depressive episode was stress caused by academic performance demands. Perpetuating factors related to his insomnia include the following: (a) a conditioned association between his bed and worrying, which produces heightened cognitive arousal while he lays awake in bed; (b) a circadian phase shift caused by a lack of a daily routine and reason to get out of bed in the morning; (c) engaging in arousal producing activities in the bedroom environment (TV, computer, phone, etc.); and (d) inadequately managed major depressive disorder. Eric was recommended to keep all other appointments with his psychiatrist. Eric was provided with sleep diaries and instructed on how to use these to monitor his sleep over the next two weeks.

Session 2

The mismatch between sleep ability and sleep opportunity was discussed. The 3P model of insomnia was reviewed and personalized. Sleep restriction and stimulus control were introduced. Based on TST from the previous week, Eric's sleep ability was estimated at approximately 7 hours, but he is spending close to 10 hours in bed. On average, he wakes up for the day at 10:38 AM but waits until 11:55 AM to get up for the day. One of his goals is to shift his sleep phase earlier. He agreed to a sleep window of 3:00 AM to 10:00 AM. A 90-minute buffer zone was implemented prior to his designated bedtime to allow for cognitive and physiological de-arousal. During this time, Eric was instructed to eliminate his use of backlit devices and engage in activities that were pleasant and relaxing while being sedentary and in dim light. Eric was encouraged to use his seasonal affective disorder (SAD) light for 30 minutes upon awakening to help with mood and promote an earlier circadian entrainment.

Session 3

Eric struggled with implementing the changes from last week. He was able to wake up at 10:00 AM on 3 days but remained in bed for 1 to 2 hours before starting his day. He reports that he gets headaches and pains if he gets out of bed right away and did not have time to use his SAD light because he laid in bed so long. It was suggested that if Eric was not feeling well, he should still get out of bed in the morning and go to another comfortable spot. Eric was not able to eliminate the use of backlit devices during his buffer zone. He stated that one of the reasons he stays up so late and distracts himself is to avoid being alone with his thoughts. We discussed getting a notebook and devoting 30 minutes to processing his thoughts earlier in the evening. He identified several dysfunctional beliefs about himself and his standards for himself such as "I am a failure," "I am a disappointment to my family," and "I will never amount to anything." Eric was introduced to the cognitive behavioral model of depression, and techniques to identify and challenge automatic thoughts were discussed. There was no significant change in his sleep pattern and his target sleep window remained at 3:00 AM to 10:00 AM.

Session 4

Eric continued to struggle with implementing the CBT-I recommendations. He requested additional rationale for why these were necessary. His own goals were reviewed, including shifting his sleep phase. Eric was also told that he was free to change his mind about treating his insomnia. Eric reported that he and his father got into an argument a couple weeks ago and that he intends to move out on his own. Eric was tearful when describing the conflictual relationship with his father and his feelings of inadequacy. There is a great deal of ambivalence toward change, and in many ways Eric rebels against his father's wishes but also wants to please him and be rewarded with his approval. Part of the discussion today centered on Eric's belief that self-worth comes from achievement, and because he hasn't reached the goals he and his parents set, he is not worthy. Cognitive restructuring techniques were practiced, and Eric decided that he would like to continue to try to implement the CBT-I techniques. His target sleep window remained unchanged at 3:00 AM to 10:00 AM.

Session 5

Eric appeared to be in a lower mood today and did not bring his sleep diary to session. He reported that he has noticed mood change over the past few weeks and has been more tearful. He attributes this to a belief that he is responsible for all of the problems in his life and for making bad choices. He feels that because the antidepressant medication was not working that a flaw in his character is responsible for his depression. Eric was challenged on that belief and is amenable to trying medication again. He agreed to make an appointment with his psychiatrist to discuss medication management. Eric admitted to increased suicidal ideation but assured me that he was not a risk to himself at this time and if things change, he would seek medical assistance. Eric's score on the ISI was mostly unchanged at 24, however, his score of 14 on the depression subscale of the HADS had increased to 17, providing additional support for the need to intervene on his depression. His score on the anxiety subscale remained subclinical at 10.

Session 6

Eric cancelled his previous two sessions because of illness and a scheduling conflict but remained in contact; however, this meant that it had been 3 weeks since his last session. Eric reported that he met with his psychiatrist 4 days after our last meeting and was prescribed Effexor (venlafaxine), which he began taking immediately. He reported that the Effexor has resulted in improved mood and made him less emotionally reactive. He is taking the medication in the evening but does not feel like it has made a significant change either way on his sleep. We also discussed Eric's value of caring for his family above everything else and how this requires him to take care of his own mental and physical health. Eric felt like this was a turning point as it provided him with the motivation to address his insomnia and depression to make other significant life changes like employment. We reviewed the principles of sleep restriction and stimulus control. Eric agreed to resume completing the sleep diary and recommitted to the original target sleep window of 3:00 AM to 10:00 AM.

Session 7

Eric had clear improvements in his sleep onset latency and time spent awake during the night. His SE increased to 91%. He made arrangements to attend appointments and help his father with the restaurant in the morning, which required him to get out of bed for the day at the desired time. Eric regularly used his SAD light for 30 minutes in the morning. He also set an alarm to cut off his electronic use 90 minutes before his desired bedtime to help with cognitive disengagement and relaxation. He began going for walks in the afternoon to help with mood and alertness. On the one night that he struggled to fall asleep, he recognized that he was ruminating and blaming himself for past events. He was able to challenge these thoughts using the cognitive restructuring techniques he was introduced to in Session #4. Sleep hygiene recommendations were reviewed. Based on the success of the week, Eric felt like he would be able to move his sleep window back by 30 minutes. Because his SE was greater than 90%, an additional 30 minutes was added to his sleep window (2:00 AM–9:30 AM). Eric's score on the ISI decreased to 11, placing him in the subclinical range. This was driven mostly by the impact of his sleep on daytime functioning. His score on the depression subscale of the HADS dropped to 9 (subclinical range), and the anxiety subscale was no longer significant at 5.

Session 8

Eric was very happy with the progress that he made this week. He was falling asleep within 15 minutes and only woke up once to use the washroom but then fell right back asleep. His SE was 94%. He noted that his relationship with his family has improved as they have appreciated his increased involvement. Eric stated that he is feeling much better about himself. The effectiveness of the medication challenged his belief that he was "unfixable" and a character flaw was responsible for his depression. Eric reinitiated his mindfulness meditation practice and signed up for a weekend "retreat." Although he did not feel that it helped him fall or stay asleep, Eric felt that the meditation helped him manage his depressive thoughts during the day so they weren't so powerful at night. He started to investigate options to complete coursework required for him to become a chartered professional accountant. His sleep window was increased by 30 minutes and moved back 30 minutes (1:00 AM–9:00 AM).

Session 9

Eric continued to make progress, despite having one night where he was unable to keep his regular schedule because he needed to pick up his brother from the airport at 3:00 AM. His SE for the previous week was 92%. Eric felt that the 8-hour window allowed for an adequate amount of sleep but still wanted to start his day earlier to be more in line with his family and prepare to resume his education and employment. His target sleep window was set at 12:30 AM to 8:30 AM.

Session 10

In the last session, we reviewed relapse prevention strategies, drawing on Eric's established knowledge of the cognitive behavioral model of insomnia and the sleep restriction and stimulus control techniques. He feels confident to continue shifting his sleep phase back over the next couple weeks until he meets his target of 11:00 PM to 7:00 AM. Given his treatment gains and consistent use of CBT-I skills, we agreed to shift the focus of treatment to the individual and interpersonal factors contributing to his depression. Eric's final score on the ISI was 6, and his score on the depression and anxiety subscales of the HADS were 7 and 4, respectively. His sleep diary summary variables are presented in Figure 10.1.

Treatment Summary

Eric's case demonstrates the delivery of CBT-I in a patient with moderate to severe comorbid depression, a behaviorally induced delayed sleep phase, and extended terminal wakefulness. In the beginning, Eric's depression was being monitored but was untreated. He was unwilling to consider medication management because of culturally shaped beliefs about the nature of his depression.

	Baseline	Week 2	Week 3	Week 4–5	Week 6
SOL	15	14	16	No data	12
WASO	67	19	38		15
TST	7.01 hrs	5.89 hrs	5.96 hrs		6.34 hrs
TIB	9.24 hrs	8.19 hrs	8.00 hrs		7.00 hrs
SE	76%	72%	75%		91%

	Week 7	Week 8	Week 9
SOL	10	8	9
WASO	7	12	11
TST	7.05 hrs	7.34 hrs	7.28 hrs
TIB	7.50 hrs	8.00 hrs	8.00 hrs
SE	94%	92%	91%

FIGURE 10.1. Sleep diary data summary.

His cultural and family background needed to be incorporated when addressing the cognitive distortions related to his depression and his motivation for change. In the beginning, the severity of his depression negatively influenced his ability to participate in cognitive-behavioral therapy for his insomnia and depression. It was when his mood worsened to the point of considering suicide that he was willing to work with his psychiatrist to find an appropriate medication to allow him to engage in therapy. Because of the bidirectional relationship of depression and insomnia, effective treatment more often than not requires equal attention to both of the presenting concerns.

It is important not to view challenges to adherence as therapeutic failures but to identify opportunities to remove barriers and capitalize on willingness to change. Finding the motivation to engage in behavior change is essential as the "why" is a necessary precursor to the "how." Eric's need to care for himself so that he had ability to care for his family became his sense of purpose. This allowed him to more fully engage in therapy and he began to make progress addressing the behaviors and thoughts that were maintaining his insomnia and depression. Although there was a break in the middle of treatment, it did not ultimately impact treatment outcome for his insomnia. Once his insomnia was effectively addressed, the focus of treatment shifted to more thoroughly addressing the factors that contributed to his depressive disorder.

CONCLUSIONS
Insomnia and psychiatric disorders are highly comorbid, but the treatment of the psychiatric condition alone is often insufficient to resolve the insomnia. As such, it is essential that all

professionals working with people with psychiatric conditions be well versed in how to employ CBT-I, the treatment with the strongest efficacy and effectiveness for insomnia. It is our hope that this chapter will increase awareness of the application of CBT-I within the context of psychiatric disorders, which will lead to expanded use of this effective therapy and a reduction of the overall burden of insomnia worldwide.

FUTURE DIRECTIONS
There can be no question that change in standard clinical practice is something that takes time, but significant progress has been made. These advances have included the classification of a cluster of symptoms as a disorder, the evaluation of targeted treatments, and (perhaps the most important) the dissemination of this information so that new practices may be implemented. At present, all that remains is that the treatment that is recommended as first line practice, that is CBT-I, be adopted and available widely [51]. It is our hope that this chapter represents a step toward this goal. Finally, while the present chapter has focused on the assessment and treatment of insomnia within the context of psychiatric illness, it should be acknowledged that insomnia also appears to be a risk factor for multiple medical disorders and that the treatment of insomnia may also serve to reduce medical morbidity. For example, experiencing sleep difficulties at least 3 nights per week is associated with an 18% increased likelihood of obesity, an 18% increased likelihood of diabetes, and a 59% increased likelihood of coronary artery disease [72]. This set of parallel findings may also have relevance to the management of psychiatric disorders to the extent that better management of medical illness is likely to promote better mental health.

KEY CLINICAL PEARLS

1. Insomnia represents a risk factor for new onset and recurrence of multiple psychiatric disorders and often persists following the successful treatment of the comorbid disorder(s).
2. An understanding of the theoretical models of insomnia is necessary for proper assessment and treatment.
3. Appropriate assessment includes a semistructured interview, prospective sleep diaries, and validated measurements.
4. CBT-I is the treatment with the strongest efficacy and effectiveness for insomnia.
5. The treatment of insomnia comorbid with psychiatric disorders may require more therapeutic skill and experience to effectively manage both disorders.
6. Alternative delivery models of CBT-I may be used to increase access.
7. Professionals working with people with psychiatric conditions should be well versed in CBT-I to enhance recovery of mental health.

SELF-ASSESSMENT QUESTIONS

1. Going to bed earlier and trying harder to sleep are considered which of the following?
   a. Predisposing factors
   b. Precipitating factors
   c. Perpetuating factors
   d. All of the above

Answer: c

2. While evidence suggests that insomnia may have a number of roles in the development and maintenance of depression, previous research mostly strongly supports insomnia's role as a ____ _____ factor to depression.
   a. predisposing
   b. precipitating
   c. perpetuating
   d. prodromal

Answer: a

3. A patient's sleep opportunity (i.e., TIB) can be extended in 15-30 min increments if they have achieved a sleep efficiency of
   a. ≥80%.
   b. ≥85%.
   c. ≥90%.
   d. ≥95%.

Answer: b

4. What are the two primary components of Cognitive Behavioral Therapy for Insomnia?
   a. Stimulus control and cognitive restructuring
   b. Stimulus control and sleep restriction
   c. Stimulus control and sleep hygiene education
   d. Relaxation training and sleep compression

Answer: b

5. Stimulus control targets the tendency to engage in behaviors other than sleep in the bedroom thereby weakening the association between the bedroom environment and sleep. What behavioral principle is this related to?
   a. Reinforcement
   b. Bias
   c. Entrainment
   d. Conditioning

Answer: d

REFERENCES

1. American Psychiatric Association. *Diagnostic and statistical manual of mental disorders*. 5th ed. Washington, DC: American Psychiatric Association; 2013.
2. Riemann, D., et al., *The neurobiology, investigation, and treatment of chronic insomnia*. Lancet Neurol, 2015. **14**(5): p. 547–558.
3. Pigeon, W.R., T.M. Bishop, and K.M. Krueger, *Insomnia as a precipitating factor in new onset mental illness: a systematic review of recent findings*. Curr Psychiatry Rep, 2017. **19**(8): p. 44.
4. Soehner, A.M., K.A. Kaplan, and A.G. Harvey, *Insomnia comorbid to severe psychiatric illness*. Sleep Med Clin, 2013. **8**(3): p. 361–371.
5. Dolsen, M.R., L.D. Asarnow, and A.G. Harvey, *Insomnia as a transdiagnostic process in psychiatric disorders*. Curr Psychiatry Rep, 2014. **16**(9): p. 471.
6. Sloan, E.P., et al., *The nuts and bolts of behavioral therapy for insomnia*. J Psychosom Res, 1993. **37**(Suppl 1): p. 19–37.
7. Spielman, A.J., L.S. Caruso, and P.B. Glovinsky, *A behavioral perspective on insomnia treatment*. Psychiatr Clin North Am, 1987. **10**(4): p. 541–553.
8. Singareddy, R., et al., *Risk factors for incident chronic insomnia: a general population prospective study*. Sleep Med, 2012. **13**(4): p. 346–353.
9. van de Laar, M., et al., *The role of personality traits in insomnia*. Sleep Med Rev, 2010. **14**(1): p. 61–8.
10. Drake, C.L., V. Pillai, and T. Roth, *Stress and sleep reactivity: a prospective investigation of the*

stress-diathesis model of insomnia. Sleep, 2014. **37**(8): p. 1295–1304.

11. Riemann, D., et al., *The hyperarousal model of insomnia: a review of the concept and its evidence.* Sleep Med Rev, 2010. **14**(1): p. 19–31.

12. Perlis, M.L., et al., *Psychophysiological insomnia: the behavioural model and a neurocognitive perspective.* J Sleep Res, 1997. **6**(3): p. 179–188.

13. Bastien, C.H., et al., *Insomnia and sleep misperception.* Pathol Biol (Paris), 2014. **62**(5): p. 241–251.

14. Harvey, A.G., *A cognitive model of insomnia.* Behav Res Ther, 2002. **40**(8): p. 869–893.

15. Espie, C.A., et al., *The attention-intention-effort pathway in the development of psychophysiologic insomnia: a theoretical review.* Sleep Med Rev, 2006. **10**(4): p. 215–245.

16. Schutte-Rodin, S., et al., *Clinical guideline for the evaluation and management of chronic insomnia in adults.* J Clin Sleep Med, 2008. **4**(5): p. 487–504.

17. Hammerschlag, A.R., et al., *Genome-wide association analysis of insomnia complaints identifies risk genes and genetic overlap with psychiatric and metabolic traits.* Nat Genet, 2017. **49**(11): p. 1584–1592.

18. Gupta, M.A. and F.C. Simpson, *Obstructive sleep apnea and psychiatric disorders: a systematic review.* J Clin Sleep Med, 2015. **11**(2): p. 165–175.

19. Barateau, L., et al., *Hypersomnolence, hypersomnia, and mood disorders.* Curr Psychiatry Rep, 2017. **19**(2): p. 13.

20. Mackie, S. and J.W. Winkelman, *Restless legs syndrome and psychiatric disorders.* Sleep Med Clin, 2015. **10**(3): p. 351–357, xv.

21. Waters, F., U. Moretto, and T.T. Dang-Vu, *Psychiatric illness and parasomnias: a systematic review.* Curr Psychiatry Rep, 2017. **19**(7): p. 37.

22. van Schagen, A., et al., *Nightmare disorder, psychopathology levels, and coping in a diverse psychiatric sample.* J Clin Psychol, 2017. **73**(1): p. 65–75.

23. Ruoff, C.M., et al., *High rates of psychiatric comorbidity in narcolepsy: findings from the Burden of Narcolepsy Disease (BOND) study of 9,312 patients in the United States.* J Clin Psychiatry, 2017. **78**(2): p. 171–176.

24. Klingman, K.J., C.R. Jungquist, and M.L. Perlis, *Questionnaires that screen for multiple sleep disorders.* Sleep Med Rev, 2017. **32**: p. 37–44.

25. Roth, T., et al., *A new questionnaire to detect sleep disorders.* Sleep Med, 2002. **3**(2): p. 99–108.

26. J. Klingman, K., C. R. Jungquist, and M. L. Perlis, *Introducing the Sleep Disorders Symptom Checklist-25: a primary care friendly and comprehensive screener for sleep disorders.* Sleep Med Res, 2017. **8**(1): p. 17–25.

27. Doufas, A.G., et al., *Insomnia from drug treatments: evidence from meta-analyses of randomized trials and concordance with prescribing information.* Mayo Clin Proc, 2017. **92**(1): p. 72–87.

28. McCall, W.V., et al., *Hypnotic medications and suicide: risk, mechanisms, mitigation, and the FDA.* Am J Psychiatry, 2017. **174**(1): p. 18–25.

29. Mallon, L., J.E. Broman, and J. Hetta, *Is usage of hypnotics associated with mortality?* Sleep Med, 2009. **10**(3): p. 279–286.

30. Carney, C.E., et al., *The consensus sleep diary: standardizing prospective sleep self-monitoring.* Sleep, 2012. **35**(2): p. 287–302.

31. Bastien, C.H., A. Vallieres, and C.M. Morin, *Validation of the insomnia severity index as an outcome measure for insomnia research.* Sleep Med, 2001. **2**(4): p. 297–307.

32. Morin, C.M., A. Vallieres, and H. Ivers, *Dysfunctional beliefs and attitudes about sleep (DBAS): validation of a brief version (DBAS-16).* Sleep, 2007. **30**(11): p. 1547–1554.

33. Johns, M.W., *Reliability and factor analysis of the Epworth Sleepiness Scale.* Sleep, 1992. **15**(4): p. 376–381.

34. Perlis, M.J., C.; Smith, M.; Posner, D.;, *Cognitive behavioral treatment of insomnia: A session by session guide.* New York: Springer-Verlag; 2005.

35. Bootzin, R.R.P., M.L.;, *Stimulus Control.* In: Perlis M, Aloia M, Kuhn B.,eds. *Behavioral treatments for sleep disorders.* Amsterdam: Elsevier; 2011, p. 21–30.

36. Perlis, M.L., et al., *Cognitive-behavioral therapy for insomnia.* In: .Attarian P, Schuman C, eds. *Clinical Handbook of Insomnia.* Humana Press: New York; 2010: p. 281.

37. Spielman, A.J., P. Saskin, and M.J. Thorpy, *Treatment of chronic insomnia by restriction of time in bed.* Sleep, 1987. **10**(1): p. 45–56.

38. Espie, C.A., *Understanding insomnia through cognitive modelling.* Sleep Med, 2007. **8**(Suppl 4): p. S3–S8.

39. Morin, C.M. and C. Espie, *Insomnia: A clinical guide to assessment and treatment.* New York, NY: Springer; 2004.

40. Chesson, A.L., Jr., et al., *Practice parameters for the nonpharmacologic treatment of chronic insomnia: an American Academy of Sleep Medicine report. Standards of Practice Committee of the American Academy of Sleep Medicine.* Sleep, 1999. **22**(8): p. 1128–1133.

41. Carlson, L.E., *Mindfulness-based interventions for physical conditions: a narrative review evaluating levels of evidence.* ISRN Psychiatry, 2012. **2012**: p. 651583.

42. Carney, C.E., et al., *Distinguishing rumination from worry in clinical insomnia.* Behav Res Ther, 2010. **48**(6): p. 540–546.

43. Ong, J.C., C.S. Ulmer, and R. Manber, *Improving sleep with mindfulness and acceptance: a metacognitive model of insomnia.* Behav Res Ther, 2012. **50**(11): p. 651–660.

44. Larouche, M., et al., *Kind attention and nonjudgment in mindfulness-based cognitive therapy*

applied to the treatment of insomnia: state of knowledge. Pathol Biol (Paris), 2014. **62**(5): p. 284–291.

45. Garland, S.N., et al., *Mindfulness-based stress reduction compared with cognitive behavioral therapy for the treatment of insomnia comorbid with cancer: a randomized, partially blinded, noninferiority trial.* J Clin Oncol, 2014. **32**(5): p. 449–457.

46. Ong, J.C., et al., *A randomized controlled trial of mindfulness meditation for chronic insomnia.* Sleep, 2014. **37**(9): p. 1553–1563.

47. Gong, H., et al., *Mindfulness meditation for insomnia: a meta-analysis of randomized controlled trials.* J Psychosom Res, 2016. **89**: p. 1–6.

48. Qaseem, A., et al., *Management of chronic insomnia disorder in adults: a clinical practice guideline from the American College of Physicians.* Ann Intern Med, 2016. **165**(2): p. 125–133.

49. Sateia, M.J., et al., *Clinical practice guideline for the pharmacologic treatment of chronic insomnia in adults: an American Academy of Sleep Medicine clinical practice guideline.* J Clin Sleep Med, 2017. **13**(2): p. 307–349.

50. Morin, C.M., et al., *Cognitive behavioral therapy, singly and combined with medication, for persistent insomnia: a randomized controlled trial.* JAMA, 2009. **301**(19): p. 2005–2015.

51. Beaulieu-Bonneau, S., et al., *Long-term maintenance of therapeutic gains associated with cognitive-behavioral therapy for insomnia delivered alone or combined with zolpidem.* Sleep, 2017. **40**(3): p. 1–6.

52. Morin, C.M., et al., *Cognitive-behavior therapy singly and combined with medication for persistent insomnia: Impact on psychological and daytime functioning.* Behav Res Ther, 2016. **87**: p. 109–116.

53. Belleville, G. and C.M. Morin, *Hypnotic discontinuation in chronic insomnia: impact of psychological distress, readiness to change, and self-efficacy.* Health Psychol, 2008. **27**(2): p. 239–248.

54. Thomas, A., et al., *Where are the behavioral sleep medicine providers and where are they needed? A geographic assessment.* Behav Sleep Med, 2016. **14**(6): p. 687–698.

55. Espie, C.A., *"Stepped care": a health technology solution for delivering cognitive behavioral therapy as a first line insomnia treatment.* Sleep, 2009. **32**(12): p. 1549–1558.

56. Manber, R., N.S. Simpson, and R.R. Bootzin, *A step toward stepped care: delivery of CBT-I with reduced clinician time.* Sleep Med Rev, 2015. **19**: p. 3–5.

57. Fields, B.G., et al., *Master's-level practitioners as cognitive behavioral therapy for insomnia providers: an underutilized resource.* J Clin Sleep Med, 2013. **9**(10): p. 1093–1096.

58. Mindell, J.A., et al., *Sleep education in medical school curriculum: a glimpse across countries.* Sleep Med, 2011. **12**(9): p. 928–931.

59. Kuhn, E., et al., *CBT-I Coach: a description and clinician perceptions of a mobile app for cognitive behavioral therapy for insomnia.* J Clin Sleep Med, 2016. **12**(4): p. 597–606.

60. Elison, S., et al., *Feasibility of a UK community-based, eTherapy mental health service in Greater Manchester: repeated-measures and between-groups study of "Living Life to the Full Interactive," "Sleepio" and "Breaking Free Online" at 'Self Help Services'.* BMJ Open, 2017. **7**(7): p. e016392.

61. Ritterband, L.M., et al., *Effect of a Web-based cognitive behavior therapy for insomnia intervention with 1-year follow-up: a randomized clinical trial.* JAMA Psychiatry, 2017. **74**(1): p. 68–75.

62. Lancee, J., et al., *Guided online or face-to-face cognitive behavioral treatment for insomnia: a randomized wait-list controlled trial.* Sleep, 2016. **39**(1): p. 183–191.

63. Irwin, M.R., J.C. Cole, and P.M. Nicassio, *Comparative meta-analysis of behavioral interventions for insomnia and their efficacy in middle-aged adults and in older adults 55+ years of age.* Health Psychol, 2006. **25**(1): p. 3–14.

64. Zachariae, R., et al., *Efficacy of Internet-delivered cognitive-behavioral therapy for insomnia: a systematic review and meta-analysis of randomized controlled trials.* Sleep Med Rev, 2016. **30**: p. 1–10.

65. Cheng, S.K. and J. Dizon, *Computerised cognitive behavioural therapy for insomnia: a systematic review and meta-analysis.* Psychother Psychosom, 2012. **81**(4): p. 206–216.

66. Trauer, J.M., et al., *Cognitive behavioral therapy for chronic insomnia: a systematic review and meta-analysis.* Ann Intern Med, 2015. **163**(3): p. 191–204.

67. Koffel, E.A., J.B. Koffel, and P.R. Gehrman, *A meta-analysis of group cognitive behavioral therapy for insomnia.* Sleep Med Rev, 2015. **19**: p. 6–16.

68. Seow, L.S.E., et al., *Evaluating DSM-5 insomnia disorder and the treatment of sleep problems in a psychiatric population.* J Clin Sleep Med, 2018. **14**(2): p. 237–244.

69. Wu, J.Q., et al., *Cognitive behavioral therapy for insomnia comorbid with psychiatric and medical conditions: a meta-analysis.* JAMA Intern Med, 2015. **175**(9): p. 1461–1472.

70. Garland, S.N., et al., *Treating insomnia in patients with comorbid psychiatric disorders: a focused review.* Canadian Psychology/Psychologie canadienne, 2018. **59**(2): p. 176–186.

71. Bjelland, I., et al., *The validity of the Hospital Anxiety and Depression Scale: an updated literature review.* J Psychosom Res, 2002. **52**(2): p. 69–77.

72. Grandner, M.A., et al., *Sleep disturbance is associated with cardiovascular and metabolic disorders.* J Sleep Res, 2012. **21**(4): p. 427–433.

11

Hypersomnolence Disorders

SULAIMAN ALHIFZI, NEVIN ZAKI, ALJOHARA S. ALMENEESIER, AND AHMED S. BAHAMMAM

INTRODUCTION

The terms *hypersomnolence* and *hypersomnia* are commonly used interchangeably despite the different operational definition of each. Hypersomnia has been defined as long sleep time across multiple published studies.[1–4] *The Diagnostic and Statistical Manual of Mental Disorders* (fifth edition; DSM-5)[5] uses the term *hypersomnia* as a symptom, such as in the criteria of major depressive disorder (MDD) "with atypical features" specifier and define it as either an extended period of nighttime sleep or daytime napping that totals at least 10 hours of sleep per day (or at least 2 hours more than when not depressed). The DSM-5 uses the term *hypersomnolence* more broadly to define a core feature of hypersomnolence disorder that include recurrent periods of sleep or lapses into sleep within the same day, prolonged main sleep episode duration (to more than 9 hours without restoration) or difficulty sustaining wakefulness occurring at least 3 months with excessive sleepiness occurring at least 3 times per week despite at least 7 hours of sleep during a main sleep period. Additionally, these symptoms are not attributable to disturbed nighttime sleep, circadian rhythm disorder, other sleep disorders, drug abuse or medication, or mental and medical disorders.

On the other hand, ICSD-3[6] refers to hypersomnia to define specific disorders like idiopathic hypersomnia (IH) but uses the term *hypersomnolence* to more broadly define the symptom of excessive sleepiness which is somewhat similar to DSM-5. According to ICSD-3, hypersomnolence is the (i) inability to stay awake and alert during the major waking episodes of the day, resulting in periods of irrepressible need for sleep or unintended lapses into drowsiness or sleep; (ii) excessive sleepiness that associated with large increases in total daily amount of sleep without any genuine feeling of restoration; or (iii) excessive sleepiness that can be alleviated temporarily by naps but

reoccurs. The ICSD-3 also states that in young children excessive sleepiness may manifest as excessively long night sleep or with a recurrence of previously discontinued daytime napping, or present differently such as inattentiveness, emotional lability, hyperactive behavior, or decreased performance at school. Table 11.1 summarizes the differences in terminology and classification between the DSM-5 and the ICSD-3.

The ICSD-3 has a broad category of central disorders of hypersomnolence with hypersomnolence or excessive sleepiness as a core symptom. This category includes narcolepsy type 1 (NT1) and type 2 (NT2), IH, and Kleine–Levin syndrome (KLS), in addition to hypersomnia associated with or due to various environmental, sleep deprivation, or medical/psychiatric causes. Hypersomnolence presents a great challenge to practicing physicians as it can be difficult to differentiate between sleepiness and fatigue, which are symptoms loosely reported by the general population and patients with psychiatric disorders.[7] Fatigue is best characterized as difficulty in initiating or sustaining voluntary activities in absence of irrepressible need to sleep.

This chapter examines hypersomnolence as a symptom and hypersomnia disorders, with emphasis on clinical features and treatment strategies. In addition, it discusses the current understanding of the relationships between hypersomnolence and psychiatric disorders.

PREVALENCE OF HYPERSOMNOLENCE

Long sleep duration in humans may be considered a normal variant. Long sleep duration (more than 9 hours per 24 hours) was estimated to be 8.4% in a cross-sectional study with a sample of 19,136 adults aged 18 years or older in 15 states in the United States.[8] In the same study, individuals with a mood disorder were noted to be 3 to 12 times

TABLE 11.1. DIAGNOSTIC CLASSIFICATION OF HYPERSOMNOLENCE
DISORDERS IN ICSD-3 VERSUS DSM-V

	ICSD-3	DSM-V
Disorders characterized by hypersomnolence	• Narcolepsy type 1 • Narcolepsy type 2 • Idiopathic hypersomnia • Klein–Levin syndrome • Insufficient sleep syndrome • Hypersomnia due to a medical disorder • Hypersomnia associated with a psychiatric disorder • Hypersomnia due to a medication or substance	• Hypersomnolence disorder • Narcolepsy

Abbreviations: DSM-V, *Diagnostic and Statistical Manual of Mental Disorders* (fifth edition; DSM-V)[5]; ICSD-3, *International Classification of Sleep Disorders* (third edition; ICSD-3)[6].

more likely to suffer from an excessive quantity of sleep, defined in the study as a subjective estimate of long sleep duration, and an increased frequency and duration of napping. Another study including 15,929 individuals representative of the adult general population residing in 15 states in the United States,[9] used specific criteria to determine the prevalence of excessive sleepiness in the study population. The first criterion in the study was a report of excessive sleepiness with recurrent episodes of an irrepressible need to sleep, recurrent naps, prolonged main sleep episode (>9 hours a day), or unusual difficulty being fully awake. The second criterion was the frequency of symptoms, which was set at 3 or more days per week for the past 3 months despite adequate main sleep period duration. The third criterion was distress or impairment in cognitive, social, occupational, or other areas of functioning. Approximately, 16% of the study population had at least one symptom in the first criterion. When the second criterion was added, specifying the frequency of symptoms, the prevalence dropped to 4.7%. And when the third criterion was added, specifying distress or impairment, the prevalence was noted to be 2.6%. Drowsiness results in a variety of neurocognitive impairments, such as reduced reaction time, decreased attention, and impaired decision-making skills.[10] The Centers for Disease Control and Prevention reported that drowsy drivers were responsible for nearly 72,000 accidents, 44,000 injuries, and 800 deaths in 2013.[6] Additionally, data obtained around the world support hypersomnolence and sleep disorders as important causes of industrial accidents.[11]

The neurobiology of sleepiness is a complex area that is yet to be fully understood. Several neurotransmitters have been implicated in the biological regulation of sleep and wakefulness. In narcolepsy, there is a loss of neurons that produce hypocretin (HRT) neuropeptides.[6] HRT neuropeptides activate the histaminergic system via HRT receptor 2, which implicates decreased histaminergic function in excessive daytime sleepiness (EDS) seen in patients with narcolepsy.[2] The monoamine system is also involved in the regulation of sleep and wakefulness.[3] Loss of adrenergic neurons and dopaminergic dysfunction have both been associated with hypersomnia disorders.[12,13] Dysregulation in the monoamine system is also implicated in the pathophysiology of psychiatric disorders,[14] which may partly explain the complex relationship between hypersomnolence and psychiatric disorders.

ASSESSMENT OF HYPERSOMNOLENCE

Clinical Interview and History Taking

Hypersomnolence is associated with some behavioral signs including yawning, ptosis, reduced behavioral activity, lapses in attention, and head nodding; which can be elicited during clinical interviewing. Furthermore, history taking can help thoroughly understand subjective complaints of the patient including sleep propensity during activities like driving for extended periods, reading, watching television, talking on the phone, interacting with friends, and completing desk work and identify other underlying sleep-related and medical/psychiatric causes of hypersomnolence that should be excluded before diagnosing a patient with a central disorder of hypersomnolence. At times, the central hypersomnolence disorders could be complicated by other coexisting sleep disorders like sleep-related breathing and movement disorders and circadian rhythm sleep-wake disorders, which themselves tend to produce hypersomnolence by disrupting sleep or curtailing sleep duration. Please see respective chapters on these sleep disorders for a more thorough review. Multiple medical conditions that can potentially cause sleepiness (directly and/or via use of medications to treat them) including but not limited to myotonic dystrophy, stroke, tumors and sarcoidosis affecting hypothalamus or midbrain, Parkinson disease, Alzheimer's disease, multiple sclerosis, hypothyroidism, encephalopathy/delirium, nutritional deficiencies (iron, vitamin B12, vitamin D), fibromyalgia, chronic obstructive pulmonary disease, migraines, congestive heart failure, cancer, and traumatic brain injury can coexist with central disorders of hypersomnolence.[15] Similarly, psychiatric disorders with sleepiness inducing potential (directly and/or due to use of psychotropics) such as MDD, bipolar disorder (BD), posttraumatic stress disorder (PTSD), obsessive-compulsive disorder, eating disorder, schizophrenia, attention deficit-hyperactivity disorder (ADHD), and most anxiety disorders especially social anxiety disorder can complicate central disorders of hypersomnolence with varying rates of comorbidity that is higher than general population.[15,40] A comprehensive review of medication/substance use either prescribed or nonprescribed such as illicit drug use, and behavioral/lifestyle factors that may lead to insufficient sleep syndrome (ISS) is very important part of hypersomnolence evaluation.[16] Compensatory behaviors and mechanisms to overcome hypersomnolence should also be taken into consideration, such as excess caffeine intake especially since compensatory behaviors can potentially worsen hypersomnolence; for example, caffeine use in the evening can cause sleep disturbance at night and add to pre-existing hypersomnolence the next day.

Questionnaires

Hypersomnolence or EDS, which is a requirement for diagnosing disorders of hypersomnolence, is a subjective, self-reported complaint. Several self-administered questionnaires have been created for the assessment of EDS. One of the most commonly used questionnaires for the evaluation of EDS is the Epworth Sleepiness Scale (ESS).[17] It is a self-administered questionnaire that provides a measurement of the subject's general level of daytime sleepiness. It measures sleep propensity in eight situations of daily living during the month before answering the questionnaire. The ESS has been validated in clinical populations, showing a 74% sensitivity and 50% specificity relative to the multiple sleep latency test (MSLT).[18] A score greater than 10 (maximum score is 24) is suggestive of pathological daytime sleepiness requiring further assessment to delineate the underlying cause of hypersomnolence.[19] The Stanford Sleepiness and the Karolinska Sleepiness scales are only used for a momentary assessment of sleepiness.[18,20,21] Another common questionnaire is the Pittsburgh Sleep Quality Index (PSQI),[22] which is a self-administered questionnaire with 19 items. It measures subjective sleep quality in the last month, a global score and seven component scores. The PSQI has been shown to have test–retest reliability.[23]

A sleep diary, which is a record of the individual's sleep and wake times with other related information, better characterizes the sleep/wake pattern over several weekday and weekend timetables. This tool may be helpful to precisely quantify the regularity of sleep/wake habits and to rule out poor sleep hygiene and circadian rhythm sleep disorders.[24]

Polysomnography and Multiple Sleep Latency Test (MSLT)

Polysomnography is a diagnostic test that uses multiple parameters to aid in the assessment and diagnosis of sleep disorders and other sleep-related conditions that could potentially lead to EDS. The MSLT measures physiological sleep tendency under standardized conditions; it is based on predicting the degree of sleepiness as reflected by sleep latency. The MSLT objectively measures the tendency of a subject to fall asleep during the daytime. It measures the time from the start of a daytime nap period to the first signs of sleep (sleep latency) in four to five naps; the mean of these times is referred to as the mean sleep latency.[25] If a subject falls asleep during a nap, the recording continues for 15 min after sleep onset. If rapid eye movement (REM) occurs during within these 15 minutes, it is recorded as sleep onset REM period (SOREMP).

Adult healthy subjects have a sleep latency of 10 to 20 minutes.[26] On the other hand, a mean sleep latency of less than 8 minutes is considered pathological and indicative of EDS.[25,27] SOREMP in two or more naps is suggestive of narcolepsy in the right clinical setting; however, sleep deprivation and major depression are other possible causes of SOREMP. Several factors may affect performance and interpretation of MSLT results in patients who suffer from psychiatric illnesses or in patients who take psychotropic medications that should be taken into consideration when performing MSLT. First, several psychiatric disorders disrupt sleep continuity and affect sleep architecture[28]; second, psychotropic medications may affect sleep architecture and MSLT readings[28]; and third, an agitated or severely anxious patient may not be compliant with the instructions of MSLT (e.g., may use benzodiazepine before the nap trial which can confound the sleep onset latency) or have confounded result due to anxiety (inability of sleep during the test due to anxiety). If MSLT is clinically indicated to determine underlying cause of hypersomnolence, the finding of one or no SOREMPs on MSLT conducted in presence of a REM-suppressing psychotropic medication as an invalid result should be part of the discussion with the patient prior to conducting MSLT. With importance of holding REM-suppressing psychotropic medications for 2 weeks (6 weeks for fluoxetine) prior to performing MSLT, a psychiatrist must be consulted while collaborating with the patient to assess the safety of stopping/ tapering the psychotropic medication and check if it is feasible to implement an alternative management plan like psychotherapy or watching the patient closely during the time he or she is off psychotropic medication (usually an antidepressant). Similarly, stimulant and stimulant-like medications should be ideally stopped 2 weeks before the MSLT, and during these 2 weeks, the patient should be strongly recommended to avoid long-distance driving (or any driving if actively sleepy) and activities requiring sustained alertness. The stimulant and other psychotropic medications held prior to MSLT can be resumed on the day after the MSLT.

Maintenance of wakefulness test (MWT) is an objective test that evaluates one's ability to stay awake.[29] This test requires the subject to lie in bed or sit in a chair in a darkened room and try to remain awake. The latency to sleep onset indirectly measures one's ability to sustain wakefulness. The test has not been standardized yet; there are 20-minute and 40-minute versions, and the subject either sits in a chair or lies down in

bed. The reliability of the MWT has not been established either. The rationale for the MWT is that, clinically, the critical issue for sleepy patients is how long they can maintain wakefulness. The MWT assumes that a set of events can be evaluated in the laboratory that will reflect an individual's ability to stay awake during daily activities. However, such an assumption might not be accurate because the environment, motivation, circadian phase, and any competing drive states (e.g., sleep deprivation, sedating medications that patient did not use during MWT and so forth) can affect an individual's tendency to remain awake.[30] The MSLT, on the other hand, addresses the question of the individual's tendency to fall asleep in the absence of external alerting factors under conditions standardized by the American Academy of Sleep Medicine (AASM).

Actigraphy

Actigraphy is a procedural measurement of limb movement activity by a wearable device that has a built-in accelerometer that detects movements. It has been validated for measuring sleep patterns and sleep duration.[31] The AASM guidelines suggest assessing sleep/wake schedules and adequacy of sleep duration leading up to the MSLT before conducting an MSLT.[31] However, there is no consensus guideline about whether actigraphy, sleep diaries, or both should be used. Wrist actigraphy is certainly a more objective measurement of sleep patterns.

Actigraphy can be useful in situations where long-term monitoring is warranted, or when a measure of sleep in subjects' natural environment is needed. In addition, actigraphy can be helpful in assessing sleep patterns before polysomnography, evaluating ISS and circadian rhythm sleep–wake disorders, and assessing treatment outcomes in patients with hypersomnolence or EDS. However, actigraphy should not substitute a structured clinical interview and the multiparameter polysomnography.[32,33]

CENTRAL DISORDERS OF HYPERSOMNOLENCE

In the ICSD-3,[6] central disorders of hypersomnolence were divided into four main types: NT1, NT2, IH, and KLS. Other central disorders of hypersomnolence in the ICSD-3 include hypersomnia due to a medical disorder, hypersomnia due to a medication or substance, hypersomnia associated with a psychiatric disorder, and ISS. On the other hand, in the DSM-5,[5] under the category of sleep/wake disorders, hypersomnolence disorder was newly introduced. It is defined as self-reported excessive sleepiness at least three times per week for at least 3 months, accompanied by significant distress or dysfunction and not being secondary or better explained by another disorder.

Narcolepsy

Narcolepsy is a chronic neurological disorder characterized by irresistible attacks of sleep with or without symptoms of REM sleep intrusion like cataplexy, sleep paralysis and hypnagogic/hypnopompic hallucinations, and fragmented nocturnal sleep. In the ICSD-3, narcolepsy is divided into two types, NT1 and NT2.

Narcolepsy Type 1

NT1 is characterized by cataplexy. Cataplexy is a sudden transient episode of loss of muscle tone accompanied by full consciousness.[6] Cataplexy is triggered by strong, generally positive emotions such as laughter, joking, or excitement although emotions like anger and grief have also been implicated. It can evolve over seconds, may render the subject at risk of injury from sudden falls, and usually last from seconds to a few minutes.[34] The prevalence of NT1 has been reported to range between 25 and 50 per 100,000 people.[35]

According to the ICSD-3,[6] the diagnostic criteria for NT1 are as follows:

A. The patient has daily periods of an irrepressible need to sleep or daytime lapses into sleep occurring for at least 3 months;
B. The presence of one or both of the following:
    1. Cataplexy (as defined under "Essential features") and a mean sleep latency of ≤8 min and two or more sleep-onset REM periods (SOREMPs) on an MSLT performed according to standard techniques. A SOREMP (within 15 min of sleep onset) on the preceding nocturnal polysomnogram may replace one of the SOREMPs on the MSLT;
    2. Cerebrospinal fluid (CSF) HRT-1 concentration, measured by immunoreactivity, is either ≤110 pg mL or <1/3 of mean values obtained in normal subjects with the same standardized assay.

For diagnosing NT2, the following criteria must be met:

A. The patient has daily periods of an irrepressible need to sleep or daytime lapses into sleep occurring for at least 3 months;
B. A mean sleep latency of ≤8 min and two or more sleep-onset REM periods (SOREMPs) are found on MSLT performed according to standard techniques; a SOREM period (within 15 min of sleep onset) on the preceding nocturnal polysomnogram may replace one of the SOREMPs on the MSLT;
C. Cataplexy is absent;
D. Either CSF HRT-1 concentration has not been measured or CSF HRT-1 concentration measured by immunoreactivity is either >110 pg mL or >1/3 of mean values obtained in normal subjects with the same standardized assay; and
E. The hypersomnolence and/or MSLT findings are not explained more clearly by other causes such as insufficient sleep, obstructive sleep apnea (OSA), delayed sleep phase disorder or the effect of medication or substances or their withdrawal.

Additionally, a diagnosis of NT1 can be more accurately made with CSF concentration of HRT-1 equal to or less than 110 pg/ml, with or without the presence of cataplexy. However, this diagnostic testing is not freely available. Mayo Clinic in Rochester, Minnesota in United States offer this testing.

Hypocretin/Orexin System in NT1

HRT (orexin) is a neuropeptide involved in the regulation of arousal and sleep states. It has been established that HRT signaling deficiency in the hypothalamus is causative towards NT1.[6] The cells that produce HRT-1 in the lateral hypothalamus are selectively destroyed possibly via T-cell mediated autoimmune attack in genetically susceptible individuals carrying one or more alleles of HLA DQB1*0602.[36–38]

Psychiatric Comorbidities of Narcolepsy: Schizophrenia, ADHD, and Depression

The psychiatric illnesses are commonly comorbid to narcolepsy.[15] In a large, systematic, US population–based analysis of medical comorbidities associated with narcolepsy,[39] the high prevalence of psychiatric illnesses was replicated. Another study showed similar commonality of psychiatric disorders in patients with narcolepsy. Hence, it is important for a sleep physician to pay attention to psychiatric disorders for comprehensive management of patients with narcolepsy especially since psychiatric disorders can complicate the symptom of hypersomnolence directly as in atypical major depression and bipolar depression or indirectly via use of psychotropic medications to treat them (e.g., sedating antidepressants for depression, benzodiazepines for anxiety, mood stabilizers/neuroleptics for BD, etc.). Conversely, it is important for psychiatrists not formally trained in sleep medicine to understand that narcolepsy could be a coexisting condition in their patients with hypersomnolence as a prominent symptom especially if it persists despite resolution of other psychiatric symptoms and predated the use of potentially sedating psychotropic medications. Mental health comorbidities in patients with narcolepsy may be related to chronic disabling nature of narcolepsy (psychological basis) or perhaps common psychopathologic mechanisms between narcolepsy and mental illnesses (biological basis).[40] The axons of HRT neurons in the lateral hypothalamus project widely throughout the cortex in variable densities. HRT and dopamine (DA) have significant overlap, particularly in the basal forebrain, thalamic paraventricular nucleus, and prefrontal cortex[41] with similar overlapping circuits for HRT and other monoamines, such as serotonin and norepinephrine. The dopaminergic activity within the mesolimbic circuitry is regulated by HRT neurotransmission. HRT has also been shown to have direct excitatory effects on serotonergic neurons, especially in the dorsal raphe nucleus. Similarly, there is a direct excitatory effect on the noradrenergic neurotransmission in Locus ceruleus, with HRT-1 neurons having five times the excitatory effect compared to HRT-2 neurons.

Schizophrenia and narcolepsy have significant overlap in clinical presentation including early age of onset (adolescence), hallucinations, and sleep fragmentation, which can potentially lead to misdiagnosis or missed diagnosis (if both co-occur in same patient). Use of sedating antipsychotics in schizophrenia magnifies this overlap by causing hypersomnolence that is a core symptom of narcolepsy. Sansa et al.[42] highlighted several possible reasons behind overlap between narcolepsy and schizophrenia. The authors suggested that stimulant therapy might precipitate hallucinations, although this is an infrequent side effect even in patients treated with high doses of stimulants over a prolonged time period. Another explanation was that some symptoms of narcolepsy, especially hypnagogic and hypnopompic hallucinations, can be misdiagnosed as an active psychotic state of schizophrenia although there is clear difference between multisensory hallucinations of narcolepsy happening at sleep–wake interface and predominantly auditory hallucinations (occurring during full wakefulness) commonly accompanied by delusions in schizophrenia. Finally, Sansa et al. suggested coexistence of narcolepsy and schizophrenia in the same patient due to shared underlying pathophysiologic basis or simply by chance.

In children with narcolepsy, ADHD symptoms were twofold higher compared to children without narcolepsy.[43] Narcolepsy can cause ADHD-like symptoms, and ADHD, especially the inattentive subtype, can resemble narcolepsy. Despite this, there is no strong overlap in the diagnostic criteria between ADHD and narcolepsy, making it appear that they are easily distinguishable from one another; however, the truth of the matter is that they might be commonly comorbid, and there is blurring of clinical features with potential for missed diagnosis and misdiagnosis (toward ADHD), respectively. The stimulant medication use is common to both ADHD and narcolepsy, and use of stimulant medication intended for ADHD can potentially mask comorbid narcolepsy. The mental fogginess due to hypersomnolence in narcolepsy could mimic inattentiveness of ADHD. The hyperactivity as a compensatory response to hypersomnolence may mimic hyperactivity of ADHD. The HRT deficiency as a common underpinning for both ADHD and narcolepsy has been ruled out.[43] The core symptoms of sleepiness and fragmented sleep are likely responsible for commonality of ADHD like symptoms in narcolepsy similar to other sleep disorders with symptoms of sleepiness and fragmented sleep like sleep apnea rather than primary ADHD unless there is coexistence of primary ADHD and narcolepsy.

The comorbidity between depression and narcolepsy is complex. The hypersomnolence may be a risk factor for depression. Conversely, depression could contribute to hypersomnolence in narcolepsy. A large observational study of patients with narcolepsy with and without cataplexy and IH indicated that majority of the patients had varying degrees of depressive symptoms, and depressed patients had higher ESS scores than nondepressed patients. Denton et al.[44] found high prevalence of depression in patients being formally evaluated with MSLT for hypersomnolence and a weak but significant correlation between subjective (and not objective) measures of sleepiness and depression. This correlation, together with the higher ESS scores in patients with depression, raises the possibility that depression contributes to the subjective sleepiness in narcolepsy and that treatment of depression may improve subjective sleepiness. There may be both psychological and biological bases for high depression and narcolepsy comorbidity. Depression could certainly be the result of chronic and disabling nature of narcolepsy. In addition, a shared pathophysiology related to HRT deficiency has been suggested.

Management of Narcolepsy

The treatment of narcolepsy comprises of behavioral modifications, patient education, treatment of comorbid disorders that can contribute to sleepiness (e.g., continuous positive airway pressure for OSA, sleep extension for ISS, iron replacement for iron deficiency, etc.), and multimodal pharmacological therapies.

Behavioral modifications include strategically scheduled naps during the daytime and adopting good sleep hygiene principles. Strategically timed naps between 15 to 20 minutes in duration two to three times a day (e.g., at lunch time) can be helpful. Good sleep hygiene includes consistent sleep–wake schedules, avoidance of caffeine in the evening, avoidance of heavy meals within 2 hours of bedtime, and avoidance of alcohol in the evening. Both sleep hygiene and strategic napping can improve symptom control in narcolepsy. Patient education includes counseling regarding high-risk activities avoidance, such as driving and operating heavy machinery when sleepy.[45] In addition, career counseling is an important component of the management plan. Patients and their employers must be educated about jobs that patients with narcolepsy should avoid including shift work, on-call schedules, driving, and tasks requiring sustained attention for long hours without breaks, especially under monotonous conditions. The employer can always help by especially accommodating 15- to 20-minute naps two to

three times during the daytime. Besides, certain drugs are best avoided in patients with narcolepsy. These include the ones which can worsen daytime sleepiness include benzodiazepines, opiates, antipsychotics, and alcohol or ones that can worsen cataplexy like prazosin.

Pharmacological therapies aim to manage the primary symptoms of narcolepsy, which include EDS, disturbed night-time sleep, and cataplexy. Modafinil and its dextro-enantiomer armodafinil are wakefulness promoting agents. They are both effective in the treatment of EDS in narcolepsy.[32,46] Modafinil has not been shown to bind to or inhibit any receptors or enzymes of known neurotransmitters.[47] The studies have demonstrated that modafinil binds to the DA transporter (DAT) and inhibits dopamine (DA) reuptake, which has been associated with increased extracellular DA levels in the striatum in rats and dog brain.[47,48] Interestingly, it has been shown that DAT knockout mice were completely unresponsive to the wake-promoting effects of modafinil,[47] which supports the role of DAT in mediating the wake-promoting effects of modafinil. Amphetamines and methylphenidate are psychostimulant medications that act by altering neurotransmission of monoamine neurotransmitters in the brain.[49] They have been conventionally used in the treatment of EDS in narcolepsy.[50] However, due to the higher potential for addiction and serious side effects, they are not considered first-line agents for treatment of EDS in narcolepsy but can be used as adjunctive treatments with modafinil and armodafinil when the latter are only partially effective.[49,50] Amphetamines and methylphenidate can also be used in place of modafinil/armodafinil when the latter are not effective.

Solriamfetol was added to the armamentarium of wakefulness promoting agents on March 21, 2019, after it received US Food and Drug Administration (FDA) approval as the first and only dual-acting DA and norepinephrine reuptake inhibitor for treatment of EDS in adults with narcolepsy and OSA. This approval was based on data from the Treatment of Obstructive sleep apnea and Narcolepsy Excessive Sleepiness (TONES) phase 3 clinical trial program, which consisted of four studies evaluating approximately 900 adults. The drug will be recommended as once-daily treatment with doses of 75 mg and 150 mg for patients with narcolepsy and doses of 37.5 mg, 75 mg, and 150 mg for patients with OSA.

$GABA_A$ receptor modulators like clarithromycin and flumazenil have been studied for treatment of hypersomnolence based on CSF finding of potentiation of GABAA receptors in some individuals with hypersomnolence. Clarithromycin 500 mg twice a day for 5 weeks significantly reduced daytime sleepiness with a 4-point reduction in ESS in 20 hypersomnolent patients, 4 of whom had NT2, when compared to the placebo group. In a study of 153 patients treated with flumazenil transdermal cream and/or sublingual flumazenil titrated up to 12 mg four times daily showed symptomatic reduction in sleepiness in 62.8% of patients with treatment refractory hypersomnia, with mean reduction of ESS by 4.7±4.7. Patients in this study either had previously used or were using wake-promoting drugs. The positive response was seen mostly in females with sleep inertia. The scientific evidence on efficacy and safety of clarithromycin and flumazenil is too limited at this time to recommend their use for narcolepsy that is refractory to standard treatments.

Sodium oxybate is effective in treating cataplexy, EDS, and nocturnal sleep fragmentation.[51] It is the sodium salt of gamma-hydroxybutyrate (GHB). Sodium oxybate is $GABA_B$ receptor agonist, but its mechanism of action in narcolepsy is not fully understood.[51] Sodium oxybate is the only drug approved by FDA for the treatment of cataplexy in adult patients with narcolepsy. The FDA approval was obtained in 2002. Sodium oxybate attained approval by the European Medicines Agency (EMA) in 2005 for the treatment of narcolepsy with cataplexy. In 2005, the FDA also approved it for treatment of EDS in patients with narcolepsy with or without cataplexy.[52] Sodium oxybate is not approved for the treatment of other narcolepsy symptoms, such as nocturnal sleep fragmentation, sleep paralysis, or hypnagogic hallucinations.[51] It is administered orally after mixing with water. It is rapidly absorbed and eliminated with a mean elimination half-life of 30 to 60 minutes, and its duration of action is 2 to 4 hours.[53] Typically, an initial dose of 4.5 g is administered divided into two equivalent doses; the first at bedtime and the second approximately 2.5 to 4 hours later.[51] The patient is recommended not to drive within 6 hours of the second nightly dose. The dose is gradually increased on a weekly basis by 1.5 g per night until symptoms are controlled, side effects appear, or the maximum nightly dose of 9.0 g is achieved.[51] The typical dose for adults is 6 to 9 g per night. Doses higher than 9 g per night have not been studied and should not be administered.[51]

It must be noted that sodium oxybate overdose has been known to cause apnea, hypopnea, or respiratory failure. A decrease in respiratory rate occurs, accompanied by a compensatory increase in tidal volume, allowing minute volume to be maintained until doses approach lethality. The concomitant ingestion of alcohol typically alters the concentration–effect relationship, leading to respiratory depression without the compensatory increase in tidal volume, thereby potentiating the respiratory depressant effect of sodium oxybate.[54] Similarly, concomitant use of benzodiazepines and opioids increases risk for respiratory depression due to which these drugs are contraindicated for use along with sodium oxybate.

Additionally, there is debate over the use of sodium oxybate in patients with narcolepsy who also suffer from OSA. The matter is complicated as we know that the Apnea–Hypopnea Index (AHI) during sleep is elevated in many patients who suffer from narcolepsy.[55] About 31% of narcolepsy patients show an AH of >5.[56] and 24.8% show an AHI of >10.[57] In 1986, Chokroverty[58] warned about this common link, suggesting a neural dysfunction in those areas of the brain where respiratory and sleep–waking systems are interrelated, such as the nucleus tractus solitarius and ponto-medullary reticular formation. There is evidence on worsening of pre-existing obstructive sleep after starting sodium oxybate, which indicates that clinical monitoring for breathing related parameters is crucial in patients placed on sodium oxybate therapy.[59] A 2-week study compared sodium oxybate therapy to placebo with polysomnography at baseline and day 14. The study demonstrated that short-term use of sodium oxybate at 4.5 g/night dose did not worsen obstructive or central respiratory event count or oxygen saturation status.[60] Another study of 42 patients with mild to moderate OSA patients administered sodium oxybate at a dose of 9 g/night showed 7% incidence of clinically significant increase in central apneas and oxygen desaturations but without worsening in obstructive respiratory events.[61] It has been suggested that effect of sodium oxybate on sleep-disordered breathing is dose dependent.[62] Nevertheless, further studies are needed to assess this effect.

The psychiatric complications including parasomnia (sleepwalking), mood swings, depression, and anxiety have been reported in patients taking sodium oxybate.[63] Therefore, caution is recommended prior to initiating sodium oxybate in patients with psychiatric comorbidities. In these cases, appropriate psychiatric assessment is recommended.[51] Patients should be particularly screened for suicidality before initiating treatment with sodium oxybate since suicidal attempts and suicides have been reported. Perhaps this risk is higher in patients with history of depression and suicidality. Symptoms of psychosis like paranoia, agitation, confusion, and hallucinations are potential and infrequent side effects of sodium oxybate.[51] Therefore, the use of sodium oxybate is best avoided in patients with comorbid narcolepsy and psychosis. The monitoring for emergence or exacerbation of psychotic symptoms after the initiation and dose escalation should be undertaken.[64]

Antidepressant medications including selective serotonin reuptake inhibitors (SSRIs) like fluoxetine, tricyclic antidepressants (TCAs) like protriptyline and clomipramine, serotonin and norepinephrine reuptake inhibitors (SNRIs) like venlafaxine and selective norepinephrine reuptake inhibitors (NRIs) like atomoxetine and reboxetine have been used in the treatment of cataplexy, hypnogogic hallucinations, and sleep paralysis.[32] Antidepressants' effect on reducing cataplexy has been commonly referred to as an anticataplectic effect.[32] However, none of the antidepressants have been FDA approved for treatment of cataplexy.

In the AASM practice parameters for the treatment of narcolepsy and other hypersomnias of central origin,[32] TCAs, SSRIs, and venlafaxine were noted as probably effective treatment options for cataplexy. These medications were also recommended as options in the treatment of sleep paralysis and hypnogogic hallucinations. In addition, reboxetine (NRI), which is not available in the United States, was in the guidelines for the treatment of cataplexy. Table 11.2 presents a summary of the common drugs in use to treat narcolepsy and cataplexy.[49,65,66]

Tips for Managing EDS in Patients with Narcolepsy and Comorbid Psychiatric Disorders

The potential link of narcolepsy with psychiatric disorders makes both the diagnosis and management of narcolepsy more complex especially since medications used to manage narcolepsy can influence the comorbid psychiatric conditions. According to Barateau et al,[65] dopaminergic stimulants and sodium oxybate may worsen psychiatric symptoms (particularly anxiety, depression, or psychosis).

The optimal management of depression and psychotic symptoms is not easy in patients with narcolepsy. For patients with coexisting narcolepsy and psychotic disorder (a rare, but very serious comorbid association), pitolisant may be more appropriate for treating hypersomnolence than dopaminergic agents (modafinil, methylphenidate, and amphetamines). Pitolisant is an inverse agonist/antagonist at the H3 receptor. H3 receptor is an auto-receptor that suppresses histamine neuronal firing and inhibits synthesis and release of histamine. Hence, pitolisant works by increasing histaminergic tone in the wakefulness-promoting system of the brain.[67] Pitolisant was approved in United States in August, 2019 for EDS in narcolepsy. It is approved in European Union for both EDS and cataplexy.

Reported side effects of pitolisant include gastrointestinal pain, increased appetite, weight gain, headache, insomnia, and anxiety.[68] Pitolisant is taken as a single morning dose, starting at 4.5 to 9 mg. The dose can be increased to 18 mg in week 2 up to maximum dose of 36 mg in week 3 except if there is renal or moderate hepatic impairment where maximum dose should not exceed 18 mg once daily. Pitolisant is contraindicated if there is severe hepatic impairment. It may reduce efficacy of oral contraceptives; thus, alternative methods of contraception should be recommended. Concomitant administration of antidepressants like fluoxetine, paroxetine and bupropion which are potent CYP2D6 inhibitors can result in higher pitolisant exposure.

In absence of coexisting psychotic disorder, dopaminergic agents are preferred for treatment of EDS in narcolepsy. However, dopaminergic treatment can be complicated by treatment emergent psychosis especially when doses higher than maximum recommended are utilized. This complication may respond to dose reduction or necessitate cessation of the offending dopaminergic agent altogether. Psychosis is generally short lived but may persist beyond 1 month after drug cessation in some individuals. It is a clinical judgment to consider antipsychotic in such cases versus wait and watch. Although any antipsychotic medication can potentially address the treatment emergent persistent psychosis, aripiprazole might be particularly useful because of its unique mechanism of action as a DA D2 receptor partial agonist, serotonin 5-hydroxytryptamine 2A (5-HT1A) receptor partial agonist, and serotonin 5-HT2A receptor antagonist. Recent evidence suggests that activation of postsynaptic DA (D1 or D2) receptors increases wakefulness, and selective stimulation of DA D2 autoreceptors or blockade of DA D1 or D2 receptors produces

TABLE 11.2. SUMMARY OF THE COMMON DRUGS USED TO TREAT EXCESSIVE SLEEPINESS AND CATAPLEXY IN PATIENTS WITH NARCOLEPSY

Drug	Mechanism(s) of Action	Dosage and Preparations	Practical Considerations
Traditional psychostimulants: (Second-line treatment of EDS)	1. Inhibit dopamine and norepinephrine reuptake into presynaptic neuron leading to increase in dopamine and norepinephrine concentrations in neuronal synapse. 2. Increase dopamine and norepinephrine release into extra-neuronal space 3. Stimulation of adrenergic receptors	▲ Methylphenidate Start with 5 mg in the morning and 5 mg in the afternoon (second dose to be avoided within 6 to 8 hours of bedtime); increase by 5–10 mg weekly to control symptoms, then switch to either ER or SR 10–30 mg, and use IR as add-on at 10–30 mg at noon for pm sleepiness if necessary ▲ Amphetamines -Dextro-amphetamine [start with immediate release formulation at 5 mg twice or three times daily at 4–6 hour intervals (no dose within 6–8 hours of bedtime), increase by 5–10 mg at weekly intervals up to 30 mg twice daily as necessary to get optimal wake promotion, and then switch to equivalent dose of sustained release formulation once stable dosing is achieved. For example, 10–30 mg of sustained release in the morning plus as needed 10–30 mg of immediate release as add-on for pm sleepiness] - Mixed amphetamine salts (start with immediate release at 5 mg twice daily (second dose should not be within 6–8 hours of bedtime) with weekly increment of 10 mg up to 30 mg twice per day as necessary to get optimal wake promotion, and once stable dosing is achieved switch to equivalent dose of extended release once daily with or without immediate release as necessary for pm sleepiness. For example, switch to equivalent dose of extended release formulation at 10–30 mg in the morning plus 10–30 mg of immediate release if needed as add-on for pm sleepiness)	Adverse effects: are dose dependent; include psychosis, anorexia, addiction, increase in systolic BP, arrhythmias, sudden death, lowered threshold for seizures; patients should be carefully informed about these risks Monitoring: BP, pulse, weight, abuse

(continued)

TABLE 11.2. CONTINUED

Drug	Mechanism(s) of Action	Dosage and Preparations	Practical Considerations
Modafinil (First line treatment of EDS)	Inhibition of dopamine reuptake by binding to dopamine transporter	Starting dose is 200 mg in am; increase to 400 mg either as single dose in the morning or split dosing—200 mg in the morning and 200 mg at noon). Usual dose: 200 mg twice daily. Maximum dose: usually 400 mg/d although doses up to 600 mg/day have been used	Modafinil is a reversible inhibitor of the drug-metabolizing enzyme CYP2C19; therefore, co-administration of modafinil with drugs such as diazepam and phenytoin, which are largely eliminated via that pathway, may increase their circulating levels. In addition, the levels of CYP2D6 substrates such as tricyclic antidepressants and selective serotonin reuptake inhibitors, which have ancillary routes of elimination through CYP2C19, may be increased by co-administration of modafinil. Dose adjustments may be necessary for patients being treated with these and similar medications. The effectiveness of steroidal contraceptives may be reduced when used with modafinil and for 1 month after discontinuation of therapy. Safety and effectiveness in pediatric patients, below age of 17 years have not been established. Serious skin rashes, including erythema multiforme major and Stevens–Johnson syndrome have been associated with modafinil use in pediatric patients.
Armodafinil (First line treatment of EDS)	R enantiomer of modafinil with longer duration of action compared to modafinil; mechanism of action is same as modafinil	Usual dose is 150–250 mg given as single morning dose	Indication: First line treatment of EDS. FDA category C; should not be used during pregnancy and lactation. Side effects: Headache, rhinitis, nervousness, nausea, dizziness, diarrhea, rare severe skin rash (Stevens–Johnson syndrome). Caution about increased risk of pregnancy when using steroidal contraceptives and for 1 month after discontinuation of therapy. Alternate means of contraception is recommended.
Solriamfetol (will likely become first line treatment of EDS)	dual-acting dopamine and norepinephrine reuptake inhibitor	75–150 mg given as single morning dose	Recently approved by FDA for treatment of EDS in narcolepsy and OSA.

Drug	Mechanism	Dosing	Notes
Pitolisant	Inverse agonist of the histamine H3 receptor	Available as 4.5 mg and 18 mg tablets. Start at 9 mg/day and increase weekly by 9 mg. Usual dose 18–36 mg	It improves EDS and attention, and reduces cataplexy frequency by 60%. Side effects: Insomnia headache, nausea, anxiety, irritability, vertigo, depression, tremor, tiredness, dyspepsia. Serious but rare side effects are abnormal loss of weight and spontaneous abortion. Supratherapeutic doses led to slight prolongation of QTc interval. It may lower efficacy of oral contraceptives due to which alternate means of contraception should be done. Not recommended during pregnancy unless benefit exceeded the risk. The drug is approved in European Union for treatment of both EDS and cataplexy in narcolepsy. The US FDA approved it for treatment of EDS in narcolepsy in August, 2019.
Sodium oxybate (First line treatment for EDS and cataplexy; off-label use for nocturnal sleep disturbance in narcolepsy)	Sodium salt of γ-hydroxybutyric acid (GHB) that acts as putative neurotransmitter and neuromodulator at the GABA-B receptor.	Start at 4.5 g/night split into two doses (2.25 g initially and 2.25 g 2.5–4 hours later). Increase by 1.5 g/night at weekly intervals. Usual dose range: 6–9 g/night for adolescents and adults.	FDA category C. Not recommended during pregnancy and breast-feeding. Side effects: Nausea, weight loss, headache, confusion, enuresis, sleep walking; sedation; memory impairment. Single pharmacy source (Xyrem REMS program) and regular follow-up (q 3 months) with provider. Patient education (i) Store securely out of reach of children/pets. (ii) Prepare both doses before bedtime. Take first dose at least 2 hours after eating; dilute each dose in 60 mL of water. Take doses while lying in bed (likely to fall asleep within 5–15 minutes or may be dizzy). (iii) Remain in bed after both doses. May need to set alarm for second dose. (iv) Allow 6 hours after dose 2 before doing activities requiring alertness. (v) No alcohol or other sedative hypnotics or opioids while on sodium oxybate and inform about risk of respiratory depression. (vi) Caution on operating dangerous machinery for at least 6 hours after taking 2nd dose. (vii) Report to provider any symptoms of depression, anhedonia, significant appetite and weight change, psychomotor agitation or retardation, fatigue, suicidal ideation. (viii) Higher risk of sleep walking, incontinence at night. (ix) Caution regarding high salt load. (x) Fine-tune timing and dose of medication—may need to either split into three doses, or delay first dose if no sleep onset difficulties but current dose insufficient to maintain entire night's sleep.

TABLE 11.2. CONTINUED

Drug	Mechanism(s) of Action	Dosage and Preparations	Practical Considerations
Antidepressants medications (second line treatment of cataplexy)	Blockade of norepinephrine and serotonin reuptake, suppression of REM sleep	▲ SNRI -venlafaxine immediate release (start at 37.5 mg b.i.d., increase by 75 mg weekly to usual target dose of 75–100 mg b.i.d.) or venlafaxine extended release (start at 37.5 mg in the morning, increase to 75 mg in a week, and then in 75 mg increment after a week to 150 mg in the morning; usual dose is 75–150 mg in the morning) ▲ SSRIs -fluoxetine (start 20 mg in the morning, titrate by 20 mg weekly increments as necessary to maximum dose of 80 mg in the morning) -sertraline (start 50 mg in the morning, titrate by 50 mg weekly increments as necessary to maximum dose of 200 mg in the morning) ▲ TCAs -Clomipramine (start at 25 mg at bedtime with 25 mg weekly increments as necessary to usual target dose of 75–125 mg at bedtime; maximum dose is 250 mg at bedtime) -Protriptyline (start at 5 mg three times daily; titrate by 5 mg weekly increments as indicated to maximum dose of 10 mg 3 times daily) ▲ Selective norepinephrine reuptake inhibitor -Atomoxetine (start at 40 mg daily, increase to 80 mg daily in a week, and then after 1 week to the maximum of 100 mg daily as necessary	FDA category C; prescribe only if expected benefits outweigh risks. Caution regarding nursing as it is excreted in breast milk. Side effects: Nausea, dizziness, sexual dysfunction, dry mouth, headache, blood pressure increase, insomnia, anxiety, headache, and loss of appetite. Very effective for cataplexy but has short T1/2 so extended formulation is preferred. Has slight stimulant effect; FDA category C; not recommended during pregnancy and lactation. Side effects: Nausea is most common, headache, dry mouth, less sexual dysfunction (erectile and ejaculation problems) than other SSRIs, diarrhea, weight gain FDA category C. Prescribe to pregnant women only if expected benefits outweigh risks. Caution in nursing. Side effects: Nausea, sexual dysfunction, weight gain, diarrhea, headache FDA category C; prescribe to pregnant women only if expected benefits outweigh risks; not for use during nursing. Side Effects: Dry mouth, constipation, sweating, dizziness, weight gain, orthostatic hypotension. Protriptyline is not recommended for use in pregnant/nursing women and children. Side effects: Dry mouth, constipation, urinary retention Serious adverse effects (TCAs): Dangerous in overdose with cardiotoxicity, including heart block, arrhythmias, and sudden death; also higher risk of myocardial infarction; higher risk for seizures; caution against coadministration with and within 14 days of use of MAO inhibitors. Alcohol should be avoided with TCAs.

Caution with SSRI coadministration and when switching between TCAs and SSRIs (fluoxetine, sertraline, paroxetine, fluvoxamine); sufficient time must elapse before starting therapy when switching from fluoxetine (at least 5 weeks may be necessary).

Sudden discontinuation is not advised since rebound cataplexy can happen.

FDA category C. Prescribe to pregnant women only if expected benefits outweigh risks to fetus. Avoid atomoxetine during breast-feeding.

Side effects: Nausea, dry mouth, headache, increased BP and HR, erectile dysfunction; liver dysfunction

Abbreviations: BP, blood pressure; EDS, excessive daytime sleepiness; ER, extended release; FDA, US Food and Drug Administration; HR, heart rate; MAO, monoamine oxydase; NDA, New Drug Application; IR, immediate release; OSA, obstructive sleep apnea; SNRI, serotonin and norepinephrine reuptake inhibitors; SR, sustained release; SSRI, selective serotonin reuptake inhibitors; TCA, tricyclic antidepressants.

sedation.[69,70] Activation of serotonergic 5-HT1A receptors leads to increased DA release in the ventral tegmental area (VTA), which may also result in increased wakefulness; however, effects of serotonergic 5-HT2A receptor activation are unclear.

Dopaminergic agents are preferred for treatment of narcolepsy in patients with comorbid unipolar depression especially since these agents could also serve as augmenting strategies for depression. While these agents could also be used if there is comorbid bipolar depression, their use is tricky in such cases since treatment emergent mania has been reported. However, modafinil and armodafinil have significantly lower risk of precipitating mania compared to methylphenidate and amphetamines.

Idiopathic Hypersomnia (IH)

IH is another sleep disorder characterized by EDS as a core symptom. In the ICSD-2,[71] IH was divided into two disorders, one with prolonged sleep duration and the other without it. However, the two disorders were considered as a single entity in the ICSD-3, where IH can be diagnosed with or without the presence of prolonged sleep duration.[6] IH is a diagnosis of exclusion, which means that other more common causes of EDS need to be ruled out first before arriving at this diagnosis based on polysomnographic investigation.

In the ICSD-3, as with NT1 and NT2, the diagnostic criteria of IH include daily periods of an irrepressible need to sleep or daytime lapses into sleep for at least 3 months. However, in IH, cataplexy is absent, and an MSLT shows less than two SOREM periods or no SOREM periods if the REM latency on the preceding polysomnogram was less than or equal to 15 minutes.[6] Additional criteria include either a mean sleep latency (during MSLT) of equal to or less than 8 minutes, or polysomnographically measured (performed after correcting chronic sleep deprivation) total sleep time of more than or equal to 660 minutes in a 24-hour period. Objective measurement of total sleep duration can alternatively be done by wrist actigraphy averaged over minimum of 7 days of unrestricted sleep accompanied by a sleep log during this period.

Modafinil has been noted to improve EDS in IH in two recent randomized, double-blind, placebo-controlled studies; one of these studies indicated significant improvement in both subjective and objective measures of sleepiness,[72] while the other study indicated significant improvement in subjective EDS with modafinil therapy in IH patients.[73] Pitolisant and sodium oxybate have also been shown to be effective in patients with IH.[74,75]

Kleine–Levin Syndrome (KLS)

KLS is recurrent hypersomnia characterized by relapsing–remitting episodes of hypersomnolence and hypersomnia (increased sleep duration) associated with cognitive, behavioral (disinhibited sexual behavior), and psychiatric (anorexia or hyperphagia, depression, anxiety, hallucinations, delusions) disturbances. The episodes usually last from 1 to several weeks with median of 10 days, with 1- to 12-month-long period of normalcy between episodes.[76] The prevalence of KLS is approximately two cases per million in Western populations.[77] The diagnosis is often delayed or missed, with many patients getting treated for psychiatric conditions for prolonged period before a definitive diagnosis is made.[76]

KLS has a putative genetic component to its etiology (first-degree relatives have an 800 to 4,000-fold increased risk of developing KLS; multiplex families including affected monozygotic twins have been described implicating organic pathology, but the exact etiology and pathophysiology remain uncertain.[78,79]

Diagnosis of KLS

According to ICSD-3, criteria A to E must be met for diagnosis of KLS[6]:

A. The patient experiences at least two recurrent episodes of excessive sleepiness and increased sleep duration, each persisting for two days to five weeks.
B. Episodes usually recur more than once a year and at least once every 18 months.
C. The patient has normal alertness, cognitive function, behavior, and mood between episodes.
D. The patient must demonstrate at least one of the following during episodes:
   1. Cognitive dysfunction.
   2. Altered perception.
   3. Eating disorder (anorexia or hyperphagia).
   4. Disinhibited behavior (such as hypersexuality).
E. The hypersomnolence and related symptoms are not better explained by another sleep disorder, other medical, neurologic, or psychiatric disorder (especially BD), or use of drugs or medications.

To date, there are no specific diagnostic markers of KLS.[80] However, several biochemical parameters have been measured in both serum and CSF of individuals with KLS. In two recent studies,[81,82] low CSF levels of HRT-1 were found suggesting recurrent functional alterations of the hypothalamus as underlying etiology of EDS in some individuals with KLS. The thalamic and frontotemporal cortical regions of the brain have also been implicated.[83] Electroencephalography has demonstrated nonspecific diffuse slowing of background activity along with bursts of bisynchronous, generalized, moderate- to high-voltage waves in KLS patients during an episode.[83] Polysomnography might be useful in the diagnosis of KLS. However, data are limited.[84]

Brain imaging studies (magnetic resonance imaging, computed tomography) are mostly normal, although functional brain imaging (with single-photon emission computed tomography, for instance) has revealed a spectrum of perfusion pathway and metabolic changes in the brains of KLS patients.[85]

Psychiatric Comorbidity

During an episode of hypersomnia in KLS, patients might exhibit low mood, with around 15% of cases reported to have suicidal ideation.[86] A few cases have been reported to become hypomanic towards the end of a KLS episode.[87,88] Mood symptoms in KLS appear to be transient and in most cases are limited to the duration of a KLS episode.

Management of KLS

No medication has been found to be significantly and consistently efficacious in the treatment of KLS during an episode or interepisodically (to prevent recurrence). The best modality for KLS is supportive and symptomatic management. For example, mood and anxiety symptoms should be monitored and treated accordingly.[89]

A Cochrane review done in 2009,[90] with an update in 2016,[91] found no randomized, placebo-controlled trials of pharmacological treatments for KLS. Lithium has been used to control KLS. Mayer[92] proposed that the pharmacologic mechanisms of lithium in KLS are multifold. Lithium induces slow-wave sleep and reduces REM sleep, may improve memory consolidation in sleep-deprived animals, enhances neuroplasticity, and has effects on the period gene *PER*, thus strengthening the period of the circadian sleep–wake cycle. By depletion of free myo-inositol concentrations, it can alter cell signaling; by inhibiting glycogen synthase kinase 3, it influences insulin receptor signaling, immunity and inflammation responses, neurotransmission, and memory function.[92] Inflammation may be a cause of KLS, and memory dysfunction is one of the residual

symptoms of KLS.[78] Gabapentin, carbamazepine, and valproate are some other options primarily for relapse prevention while amphetamines and amantadine could be used for treatment of EDS during an episode.

INSUFFICIENT SLEEP SYNDROME (ISS)

ISS is characterized by failure to meet the minimum sleep duration requirement necessary to maintain adequate wakefulness and alertness.

The ICSD-3[6] criteria for the diagnosis of ISS include daily periods of an irrepressible need to sleep or daytime lapses into sleep for 3 months, with a duration of sleep shorter than expected for age being present for at least 3 months. When patients with ISS extend their sleep duration, symptoms resolve. In case of prepubertal children, lack of sleep might present as behavioral abnormalities attributable to sleepiness.

PSYCHIATRIC DISORDERS AND HYPERSOMNOLENCE

The relationship between psychiatric disorders and hypersomnolence is complex and not yet well understood. Three models of association between psychiatric disorders and sleep disorders were conceptualized by Honda[93] to facilitate its understanding. The first model regards hypersomnolence as symptom of psychiatric disorders. The second model identifies psychiatric disorders and hypersomnolence having independent mechanisms that have bidirectional influence on one another. The third model suggests that hypersomnolence and psychiatric disorders share common pathophysiological mechanisms, indicating that various psychiatric symptoms may be regarded as distinct phenotypes of sleep/wake dysregulation.

ROLE OF HYPOCRETIN/OREXIN IN PSYCHIATRIC DISORDERS

HRT/orexin is involved in the regulation of a variety of behavioral and physiological processes, including sleep and metabolism.[94] There are two types of HRT neuropeptides: HRT-1 (orexin A) and HRT-2 (orexin B). The neurons that secrete HRT have widespread projections to mono-aminergic (serotonin, norepinephrine, and DA) neuronal network. Studies have indicated presence of feedback loop between dorsal raphe and hypothalamus where HRT stimulates serotonin neurotransmission from dorsal raphe nucleus while serotonin exerts an inhibitory influence on HRT secretion from perifornical-lateral hypothalamic area.

The preclinical studies in mice models of depression have suggested the role of HRT in pathophysiology of depression. In mice exposed to unpredictable chronic mild stress (UCMS), HRT antagonist almorexant normalized hypothalamic–pituitary–adrenal axis activity and imparted antidepressant effect. Additionally, in mice subjected to UCMS, fluoxetine was noted to reverse HRT neuronal activation in dorsomedial and perifornical hypothalamic areas with concomitant reversal of depressive behaviors. On the other hand, escitalopram was shown to have no such effect on depressive behaviors or HRT activated neurons in mice representing the "genetic" model of depression, perhaps mimicking treatment resistance seen in clinically depressed humans exposed to relatively low levels of stress but with heightened stress responsiveness due to predisposing genetic makeup.

Clinical studies have observed dysregulation of HRT signaling in MDD that may explain sleep–wake cycle dysfunction, which constitutes a core symptom of MDD. However, clinical studies have revealed conflicting results. For example, a study reported reduced diurnal variations of HRT-1 in depressed patients, which is consistent with sleep/wake dysregulation in MDD, and noted that sertraline but not bupropion slightly decreased cerebrospinal fluid HRT-1 indicating a serotoninergic influence on HRT tone. On the other hand, other studies have observed decreased CSF levels of HRT in MDD patients at times of attempted suicide; followed by an increase in CSF HRT levels accompanied by clinical improvement in depression 1 year after the suicidal attempt.[95-97] Perhaps, more clinical studies (with different antidepressants within the same and different class, and different depressive subtypes) are needed since data on HRT and depression are equivocal. The equivocality is probably reflective of what we see in clinical practice that different antidepressants have different clinical responses in different individuals with different depressive subtypes. The depressed population is a nonhomogenous group of people with mental illness, and antidepressants are nonhomogenous groups of drugs.

It is likely that HRT may have a role in patients with schizophrenia. Sansa and coworkers[42] reported that patients with schizophrenia showed a positive correlation with human leukocyte antigen (HLA) DQB1*0602 . Narcolepsy has a strong association with the HLA DQB1 *0602. This is suggestive of role of HRT neurotransmission in the development of schizophrenia.

The subnuclei of the basolateral and central amygdala, the prefrontal cortex, and the paraventricular thalamic nucleus are regions known to be involved in the development of anxiety symptoms, and they all are part of the HRT system in the brain. Studies have shown an increase in the release of HRT in the amygdala and high HRT levels in the cerebrospinal fluid of patients with panic disorder, suggesting that high hypocretinergic tone is contributory toward panic anxiety.[98]

HYPERSOMNOLENCE AND PSYCHIATRIC DISORDERS

Major Depressive Disorder

The frequency of hypersomnolence in MDD varies across studies; this may be attributed to the different definitions of hypersomnolence. The definition of hypersomnolence includes EDS, long duration of sleep, impaired vigilance during major wakeful period, or sleep inertia.[99] A recent study examined the longitudinal association between hypersomnolence and depression.[100] In this study, subjective EDS or hypersomnolence was demonstrated to have a longitudinal relationship with the development of depression, and this is consistent with previous studies.[101,102] The hypersomnolence associated with MDD with atypical features specifier has been shown to be associated with a more severe and disabling course of illness.[104] Hypersomnolence, when seen as a symptom of MDD, may be an indication of treatment-resistant depression.[104] Patients may continue to suffer from hypersomnolence despite being considered in remission from an episode of MDD.[105]

A systematic evaluation of sleep propensity measured by MSLT in patients with hypersomnolence associated with psychiatric disorders (mostly mood disorders) noted that (a) patients with hypersomnolence associated with psychiatric disorders have mean sleep latency on the MSLT that are mostly comparable to normative values and (b) mean sleep latency below 8 minutes (which is the cutoff point defining pathologic sleepiness), is seen in just one-fourth of the patients with psychiatric disorders reporting subjective hypersomnolence. The prevalence of MSLT measured pathological sleepiness in hypersomnolent psychiatric patients is similar to prevalence in general population, which raises multiple questions (a) if mean sleep latency of 8 minutes is an appropriate cutoff for assessing objective hypersomnolence or pathological sleepiness in patients with psychiatric disorders; (b) if subjective hypersomnolence in psychiatric patients more commonly involves other facets of sleepiness such as excessive sleep duration, excessive sleep inertia, or the reduced ability to maintain vigilance that MSLT does not quantify; or (c) if hypersomnolence reported by psychiatric patients is actually "clinophilia" (French word for "love for bed") where they do spend excessive time in bed but are not necessarily sleeping. SOREMPs have also been described in patients with MDD. All this issues indicate that MSLT has many limitations as an objective test that could segregate hypersomnia associated with psychiatric disorder from central hypersomnias. A later study tried to provide answers by demonstrating that patients with major depression and comorbid hypersomnolence do have increased sleep duration relative to healthy sleepers, as well as similar objective sleep efficiency as measured by naturalistic actigraphic recordings followed by ad libitum polysomnography (without prescribed wake time) in 22 patients with MDD and comorbid hypersomnolence against age- and sex-matched healthy sleeper controls.

Bipolar Disorder (BD)

In the DSM-5, BDs have criteria for the diagnosis of manic or hypomanic episodes. A patient in a manic or hypomanic state commonly reports decreased need for sleep, characterized by feeling rested after fewer hours of sleep than usual. However, patients with BD more commonly present with a major depressive episode during the course of their illness; this is commonly referred to as bipolar depression, a state in which they may have insomnia or hypersomnolence. Hypersomnolence appears to be highly prevalent in bipolar depression, with a prevalence ranging from 38% to 78% across studies.[106] It was also shown that hypersomnolence occurred in 25% of BD patients during periods of partial or full remission, which was subsequently associated with recurrence of depressive episodes.[106] Hypersomnolence in the interepisodic periods of BD is a predictor of relapse and a determinant of future depressive severity.[106]

Table 11.3 highlights various putative mechanisms underlying occurrence of hypersomnolence in the setting of mood disorders and management strategies based on the presumed mechanism(s) as suggested by Lopez at al.[99]

Attention Deficit Hyperactivity Disorder (ADHD)

ADHD is a developmental disorder characterized by a persistent pattern of inattention with or without accompanying hyperactivity or impulsivity,[5] with predisposing genetic etiology and a heritability of approximately 75%.[107] A study explored the possibility of diagnostic confusion between central disorders of hypersomnolence and the adult form of ADHD.[108] A high percentage of symptom overlap was found, with a correlation between inattention scores and EDS score in the ESS, raising the possibility of misdiagnosis. A recent study proposed that ADHD may be a variant of NT2. The investigators reported that hypersomnia patients with ADHD tend to show shorter REM latencies and tend to fulfill NT2 diagnostic criteria in the absence of the DQB1*0602 allele.[109]

CONCLUSIONS

Central disorders of hypersomnolence are sleep disorders with EDS as a core symptom. They are primarily classified to include narcolepsy and IH. Hypersomnolence is an area of sleep medicine with a growing body of literature, leading to advancement in its understanding and management. Hypersomnolence and hypersomnia have been used interchangeably in literature, which has made it difficult to study and analyze the association between hypersomnolence and psychiatric disorders. There is a need for universal terminology to further understand the complicated but probable relationship between hypersomnolence and psychiatric disorders. This area of sleep medicine may hold a key to understanding nonhomogeneity of psychiatric intradisorder phenotypes and responses to currently available psychotropic treatments.

FUTURE DIRECTIONS

Potential approaches to hypocretin (HRT) in the brain for narcolepsy include intranasal administration of HRT peptides, developing small molecule HRT receptor agonists, HRT neuronal transplantation, transforming HRT stem cells into hypothalamic neurons, and HRT gene therapy. Besides these, immunotherapy to prevent HRT neuronal death is a potential future treatment approach.[110] It has been shown that partial agonists at trace amine-associated receptor 1 (TAAR1) promote wakefulness in mice and rats.[111] Recently, Black et al.[112] assessed the beneficial effects of TAAR1 agonist in two mouse models of narcolepsy and demonstrated that TAAR1 agonism is a promising potential new therapeutic pathway for narcolepsy with cataplexy, probably involving the suppression of rapid eye movement sleep.[112]

TABLE 11.3. PUTATIVE MECHANISMS AND STRATEGIES FOR MANAGEMENT OF HYPERSOMNOLENCE ASSOCIATED WITH MOOD DISORDERS

Putative Mechanisms	Potential Management Strategies
1. Disturbance in monoamine activity as a common pathway to both depression and hypersomnolence	-Choose first line antidepressant which has preferential stimulant profile for use in morning and preferential sedative profile for night time use, and emphasize correct timing of medication to the patient e.g. fluoxetine, venlafaxine, duloxetine, reboxetine, nortriptyline, bupropion for morning use; amitriptyline, clomipramine, mirtazapine, trazodone, paroxetine and agomelatine for night time use. Switch timing of medications if some individuals get opposite to the intended effect (e.g. fluoxetine caused sedation instead of activation when given in the morning)
2. Sedation induced by psychotropic medications and comorbid substance abuse	-Lower the dose of sedating psychotropic drugs while monitoring for return of depressive symptoms -Switch to shorter acting medications -Switch timing of medication from morning to evening if there is clear relationship with daytime sedation -Switch to antidepressant (in major depressive disorder) or mood stabilizer (in bipolar disorder) with lesser risk of causing hypersomnolence -Treat substance use disorders simultaneously to the mood disorder
3. Disturbance of sleep architecture (e.g. poor sleep continuity, reduced slow wave sleep)	-Can use lowest possible dose (to avoid increase in daytime hypersomnolence as side effect) of certain agents to enhance sleep continuity and possibly slow wave sleep like trazodone, mirtazapine, gabapentin and pregabalin.
4. Coexisting sleep disorder(s)	-Screen for obstructive sleep apnea with STOP-Bang or Berlin questionnaire and screen for central disorders of hypersomnolence (as described in the content of chapter), and collaborate with sleep physician to pursue formal investigations like actigraphy, PSG, and MSLT.
5. Coexisting medical disorder(s)	-Perform review of other body systems followed by focused physical exam -Check basic labs as clinically indicated (e.g. CBC, CMP, vitamin-D, vitamin-B12, fasting iron profile, TSH, etc.) -Refer to primary care provider or appropriate specialists for management of untreated medical disorders that could potentially cause hypersomnolence e.g. referral to pulmonology for possible chronic obstructive pulmonary disease (chronic smoker reporting shortness of breath on review of systems, noted to have wheezing on lung auscultation, with low normal SpO2 during office visit, and high recent serum bicarbonate)
6. Circadian rhythm issues (e.g., delayed sleep phase is commonly seen in bipolar disorder and seasonal affective disorder; this can cause sleepiness in first hours of the day if sleep is curtailed due to awakening prior to their delayed spontaneous wake up time)	-Recommend good sleep hygiene (reduce exposure to artificial light in evening hours, avoid using stimulating substances like caffeine close to bedtime, avoid prolonged and multiple naps) -Consider chronotherapeutic interventions (e.g. morning bright light therapy can advance sleep phase while also improving depression in seasonal affective and bipolar disorders; strategically timed melatonin is another approach to advance the sleep phase)
7. Persistent hypersomnolence of uncertain cause (after managing above)	-Can consider off-label use of psychostimulants with careful monitoring (e.g. theoretically increased risk of emergent manic symptoms in patients with bipolar disorder but no clear evidence of such risk with optimal mood stabilizer on board) -Future potential for drugs like Pitolisant which can help both hypersomnolence and potentially even depression (preclinical data on potential antidepressant benefit)

Adapted from Lopez et al.[99]

KEY CLINICAL PEARLS

- Narcolepsy is an autoimmune disorder with loss of hypocretin-producing neurons as an underlying pathology.
- Hypocretin is a neuropeptide involved in the regulation of arousal and sleep states, and is deficient in patients with NT1
- Per ICSD-3, narcolepsy has two subtypes: NT1 (with cataplexy and/or hypocretin deficiency) and NT2 (without cataplexy and hypocretin deficiency); both types share same MSLT criteria.
- PSG followed by MSLT is the gold standard for the diagnosis of narcolepsy.
- There is a high prevalence of psychiatric illnesses in patients with narcolepsy, and there may be common underlying pathophysiological mechanisms between narcolepsy and psychiatric disorders.
- Comprehensive management of narcolepsy includes behavioral modifications, education, pharmacological treatments, and management of comorbid conditions.
- Strategic naps of 15 to 20 minutes two or three times daily are recommended to improve alertness, functionality and safety.
- Modafinil and armodafinil are FDA-approved wakefulness-promoting agents for treatment of EDS in narcolepsy.
- Amphetamines and methylphenidate are stimulants used as second-line agents in treating EDS either as replacement of modafinil/armodafinil when these are ineffective or as add-on agents when wake promotion from modafinil/armodafinil monotherapy is not robust.
- Sodium oxybate is FDA-approved for treatment of cataplexy and EDS in patients with narcolepsy.
- Antidepressants such as SSRIs and SNRIs can be effective in the management of cataplexy and other REM intrusion symptoms like sleep paralysis and hypnagogic/hypnopompic hallucinations.
- While EDS is a core symptom of both narcolepsy and idiopathic hypersomnia (IH) with pathological sleep latency (less than or equal to 8 minutes) during MSLT, a diagnosis of narcolepsy requires minimum of two SOREMP during PSG and MSLT (taken together) while IH is diagnosed when there is one SOREMP during PSG and MSLT (taken together) after other more common causes of sleepiness are excluded.

- Modafinil, sodium oxybate, and pitolisant are potential treatment options for EDS in IH.
- Kleine–Levin syndrome (KLS) is a sleep disorder characterized by recurrent episodes of excessive sleepiness lasting 2 days to 5 weeks.
- Cognitive dysfunction, altered perception, anorexia or hyperphagia, and hypersexuality are present in patients with KLS during the episode of hypersomnolence and hypersomnia.
- No medication has been found to be significantly effective in the treatment of KLS but lithium can be used due to positive effect on EDS and ancillary behavioral symptoms along with efficacy for relapse prevention.
- Hypocretin is involved in the regulation of a variety of behavioral and physiological processes and may play a role in the pathophysiology of multitude of psychiatric conditions, including MDD, anxiety and schizophrenia.

ACKNOWLEDGMENTS

The preparation of this manuscript was supported by a grant from the Strategic Technologies Program of the National Plan for Sciences and Technology and Innovation in the Kingdom of Saudi Arabia (08-MED511-02).

SELF-ASSESSMENT QUESTIONS

1. A 16-year-old male presents to your clinic for the first time describing recent recurrent episodes of "sleeping all the time." The patient describes the episodes as severe to the degree that he only wakes up to eat and go to the bathroom. Further history showed cognitive dysfunction during an episode and complete remission between episodes. What is the most likely diagnosis?
   a. Obstructive sleep apnea/hypopnea syndrome
   b. Narcolepsy
   c. Kleine–Levin syndrome
   d. Idiopathic hypersomnia

Answer: c

2. Which of the following medications is approved by the FDA to treat cataplexy and excessive daytime sleepiness?
   a. Modafinil
   b. Venlafaxine
   c. Sodium oxybate
   d. Methylphenidate

Answer: c

3. Idiopathic hypersomnia can be differentiated from narcolepsy by which of the following?
   a. The presence of excessive daytime sleepiness
   b. The presence of cataplexy
   c. The absence of sleep onset REM periods in multiple sleep latency test
   d. Low CSF hypocretin concentration

Answer: c

4. Which of the following statements BEST DESCRIBE the findings in multiple sleep latency test (MSLT) of patients with a major depressive disorder (MDD)?
   a. Mean sleep latency values of ≤ 8 minutes may be present in one-fourth of patients with MDD.
   b. MSLT is a useful tool to differentiate between central disorders of hypersomnolence and hypersomnolence in MDD.
   c. More than three-quarters of patients with MDD will have abnormal MSLT values.
   d. MSLT can be used as an objective diagnostic tool of MDD.

Answer: a

5. Which of the following statements BEST DESCRIBE the relationship between hypersomnolence and bipolar disorder (BD)?
   a. Hypersomnolence rarely occurs in patients with BD.
   b. Presence of hypersomnolence is associated with subsequent depressive episodes in BD.
   c. Hypersomnolence occurs solely during depressive episodes in BD.
   d. Hypersomnolence is one of the criteria to diagnose a manic episode in BD.

Answer: b

REFERENCES

1. Soehner AM, Kaplan KA, Harvey AG. Prevalence and clinical correlates of co-occurring insomnia and hypersomnia symptoms in depression. *J Affect Disord*. 2014;167:93–97.
2. Parker G, Malhi G, Hadzi-Pavlovic D, Parker K. Sleeping in? The impact of age and depressive sub-type on hypersomnia. *J Affect Disord*. 2006;90(1):73–76.
3. Williamson DE, Birmaher B, Brent DA, Balach L, Dahl RE, Ryan ND. Atypical symptoms of depression in a sample of depressed child and adolescent outpatients. *J Am Acad Child Adolesc Psychiatry*. 2000;39(10):1253–1259.
4. Tam EM, Lam RW, Robertson HA, Stewart JN, Yatham LN, Zis AP. Atypical depressive symptoms in seasonal and non-seasonal mood disorders. *J Affect Disord*. 1997;44(1):39–44.
5. American Psychiatric Association., American Psychiatric Association. DSM-5 Task Force. *Diagnostic and statistical manual of mental disorders: DSM-5*. 5th ed. Washington, DC: American Psychiatric Association; 2013.
6. American Academy of Sleep Medicine. *International classification of sleep disorders*. 3rd ed. Darien, IL.: American Academy of Sleep Medicine; 2014.
7. BaHammam AS. Hypersomnolence. *Sleep Med Clin*. 2017;12(3):xvii.
8. Ohayon MM, Reynolds CF, 3rd, Dauvilliers Y. Excessive sleep duration and quality of life. *Ann Neurol*. 2013;73(6):785–794.
9. Ohayon MM, Dauvilliers Y, Reynolds CF, 3rd. Operational definitions and algorithms for excessive sleepiness in the general population: implications for DSM-5 nosology. *Arch Gen Psychiatry*. 2012;69(1):71–79.
10. Drowsy driving—19 states and the District of Columbia, 2009–2010. *MMWR Morb Mortal Wkly Rep*. 2013;61(51-52):1033–1037.
11. Gupta R, Pandi-Perumal SR, Almeneessier AS, BaHammam AS. Hypersomnolence and Traffic Safety. *Sleep Med Clin*. 2017;12(3):489–499.
12. Kanbayashi T, Kodama T, Kondo H, et al. CSF histamine contents in narcolepsy, idiopathic hypersomnia and obstructive sleep apnea syndrome. *Sleep*. 2009;32(2):181–187.
13. Montplaisir J, de Champlain J, Young SN, et al. Narcolepsy and idiopthic hypersomnia: biogenic amines and related compounds in CSF. *Neurology*. 1982;32(11):1299–1302.
14. Kurian MA, Gissen P, Smith M, Heales SJR, Clayton PT. The monoamine neurotransmitter disorders: an expanding range of neurological syndromes. *The Lancet Neurology*. 2011;10(8):721–733.
15. Ohayon MM. Narcolepsy is complicated by high medical and psychiatric comorbidities: a comparison with the general population. *Sleep Med*. 2013;14(6):488–492.
16. Chattu VK, Sakhamuri S, Kumar R, Spence DW, BaHammam AS, Pandi-Perumal SR. Insufficient sleep syndrome: Is it time classify it as a major noncommunicable disease? *Sleep Sci*. 2018;11(2):in press.
17. Johns MW. A new method for measuring daytime sleepiness: the Epworth sleepiness scale. *Sleep*. 1991;14(6):540–545.
18. Hoddes E, Zarcone V, Smythe H, Phillips R, Dement WC. Quantification of sleepiness: a new approach. *Psychophysiology*. 1973;10(4):431–436.
19. Rosenthal LD, Dolan DC. The Epworth sleepiness scale in the identification of obstructive sleep apnea. *J Nerv Ment Dis*. 2008;196(5):429–431.

20. Akerstedt T, Gillberg M. Subjective and objective sleepiness in the active individual. *Int J Neurosci.* 1990;52(1-2):29–37.

21. Murray BJ. Subjective and Objective Assessment of Hypersomnolence. *Sleep Med Clin.* 2017;12(3):313–322.

22. Buysse DJ, Reynolds CF, 3rd, Monk TH, Berman SR, Kupfer DJ. The Pittsburgh Sleep Quality Index: a new instrument for psychiatric practice and research. *Psychiatry Res.* 1989;28(2):193–213.

23. Carpenter JS, Andrykowski MA. Psychometric evaluation of the Pittsburgh Sleep Quality Index. *J Psychosom Res.* 1998;45(1):5–13.

24. Barateau L, Lopez R, Franchi JA, Dauvilliers Y. Hypersomnolence, hypersomnia, and mood disorders. *Curr Psychiatry Rep.* 2017;19(2):13.

25. Sullivan SS, Kushida CA. Multiple sleep latency test and maintenance of wakefulness test. *Chest.* 2008;134(4):854–861.

26. Richardson GS, Carskadon MA, Orav EJ, Dement WC. Circadian variation of sleep tendency in elderly and young adult subjects. *Sleep.* 1982;5 Suppl 2:S82–S94.

27. Littner MR, Kushida C, Wise M, et al. Practice parameters for clinical use of the multiple sleep latency test and the maintenance of wakefulness test. *Sleep.* 2005;28(1):113–121.

28. Plante DT, Winkelman JW. Polysomnographic features of medical and psychiatric disorders and their treatments. *Sleep Med Clin.* 2009;4(3):407–419.

29. Mitler MM, Gujavarty KS, Browman CP. Maintenance of wakefulness test: a polysomnographic technique for evaluation treatment efficacy in patients with excessive somnolence. *Electroencephalogr Clin Neurophysiol.* 1982;53(6): 658–661.

30. Goldstein C, Chervin R. Maintenance of wakefulness test. In: Chokroverty S, ed. *Sleep disorders medicine.* New York, NY: Springer; 2017.

31. Morgenthaler T, Alessi C, Friedman L, et al. Practice parameters for the use of actigraphy in the assessment of sleep and sleep disorders: an update for 2007. *Sleep.* 2007;30(4): 519–529.

32. Morgenthaler TI, Kapur VK, Brown TM, et al. Practice parameters for the treatment of narcolepsy and other hypersomnias of central origin. *Sleep.* 2007;30(12):1705–1711.

33. Martin JL, Hakim AD. Wrist actigraphy. *Chest.* 2011;139(6):1514–1527.

34. Scammell TE. Narcolepsy. *N Engl J Med.* 2015;373(27):2654–2662.

35. Longstreth WT, Jr., Koepsell TD, Ton TG, Hendrickson AF, van Belle G. The epidemiology of narcolepsy. *Sleep.* 2007;30(1):13–26.

36. Matsuki K, Grumet FC, Lin X, et al. DQ (rather than DR) gene marks susceptibility to narcolepsy. *Lancet.* 1992;339(8800):1052.

37. Neely S, Rosenberg R, Spire JP, Antel J, Arnason BG. HLA antigens in narcolepsy. *Neurology.* 1987;37(12):1858–1860.

38. Rogers AE, Meehan J, Guilleminault C, Grumet FC, Mignot E. HLA DR15 (DR2) and DQB1*0602 typing studies in 188 narcoleptic patients with cataplexy. *Neurology.* 1997;48(6):1550–1556.

39. Black J, Reaven NL, Funk SE, et al. Medical comorbidity in narcolepsy: findings from the Burden of Narcolepsy Disease (BOND) study. *Sleep Med.* 2017;33:13–18.

40. Morse AM, Sanjeev K. Narcolepsy and psychiatric disorders: comorbidities or shared pathophysiology? *Med Sci (Basel).* 2018;6(1).

41. Deutch AY, Bubser M. The orexins/hypocretins and schizophrenia. *Schizophr Bull.* 2007;33(6):1277–1283.

42. Sansa G, Gavalda A, Gaig C, et al. Exploring the presence of narcolepsy in patients with schizophrenia. *BMC psychiatry.* 2016;16:177.

43. Lecendreux M, Lavault S, Lopez R, et al. Attention-deficit/hyperactivity disorder (ADHD) symptoms in pediatric narcolepsy: a cross-sectional study. *Sleep.* 2015;38(8):1285–1295.

44. Denton EJ, Barnes M, Churchward T, et al. Mood disorders are highly prevalent in patients investigated with a multiple sleep latency test. *Sleep Breath.* 2018;22(2):305–309.

45. Schneider L, Mignot E. Diagnosis and management of narcolepsy. *Semin Neurol.* 2017;37(4):446–460.

46. Ahmed I, Thorpy M. Clinical features, diagnosis and treatment of narcolepsy. *Clin Chest Med.* 2010;31(2):371–381.

47. Takenoshita S, Nishino S. Pharmacologic management of excessive daytime sleepiness. *Sleep Med Clin.* 2017;12(3):461–478.

48. Dopheide MM, Morgan RE, Rodvelt KR, Schachtman TR, Miller DK. Modafinil evokes striatal [(3)H]dopamine release and alters the subjective properties of stimulants. *Eur J Pharmacol.* 2007;568(1-3):112–123.

49. Thorpy MJ, Dauvilliers Y. Clinical and practical considerations in the pharmacologic management of narcolepsy. *Sleep Med.* 2015;16(1):9–18.

50. Billiard M. Narcolepsy: current treatment options and future approaches. *Neuropsychiatr Dis Treat.* 2008;4(3):557–566.

51. BaHammam AS, Neubauer DN, Pandi-Perumal SR. Sodium oxybate (xyrem®): a new and effective treatment for narcolepsy with cataplexy. In: Guglietta A, ed. *Drug Treatment of Sleep Disorders. Milestones in Drug Therapy.* Cham: Springer; 2015.

52. Zaharna M, Dimitriu A, Guilleminault C. Expert opinion on pharmacotherapy of narcolepsy. *Expert Opin Pharmacother.* 11(10):1633–1645.

53. Owen RT. Sodium oxybate: efficacy, safety and tolerability in the treatment of narcolepsy

with or without cataplexy. *Drugs Today (Barc)*. 2008;44(3):197–204.

54. Ortega-Albás J, Ortega-Gabás S, Carratalá S, Leal D. Sodium Oxybate and Respiration. *Dual Diagnosis: Open Access*. 2016;1(3).

55. BaHammam AS, Alenezi AM. Narcolepsy in Saudi Arabia. Demographic and clinical perspective of an under-recognized disorder. *Saudi Medical Journal*. 2006;27(9):1352–1357.

56. Pizza F, Tartarotti S, Poryazova R, Baumann CR, Bassetti CL. Sleep-disordered breathing and periodic limb movements in narcolepsy with cataplexy: a systematic analysis of 35 consecutive patients. *Eur Neurol*. 2013;70(1-2):22–26.

57. Sansa G, Iranzo A, Santamaria J. Obstructive sleep apnea in narcolepsy. *Sleep medicine*. 2010;11(1):93–95.

58. Chokroverty S. Sleep apnea in narcolepsy. *Sleep*. 1986;9(1):250–253.

59. Seeck-Hirschner M, Baier PC, von Freier A, Aldenhoff J, Goder R. Increase in sleep-related breathing disturbances after treatment with sodium oxybate in patients with narcolepsy and mild obstructive sleep apnea syndrome: two case reports. *Sleep Med*. 2009;10(1):154–155.

60. George CF, Feldman N, Zheng Y, et al. A 2-week, polysomnographic, safety study of sodium oxybate in obstructive sleep apnea syndrome. *Sleep Breath*. 2011;15(1):13–20.

61. George CF, Feldman N, Inhaber N, et al. A safety trial of sodium oxybate in patients with obstructive sleep apnea: Acute effects on sleep-disordered breathing. *Sleep Med*. 2010;11(1):38–42.

62. Mason M, Cates CJ, Smith I. Effects of opioid, hypnotic and sedating medications on sleep-disordered breathing in adults with obstructive sleep apnoea. *Cochrane Database Syst Rev*. 2015;(7):CD011090.

63. Russell IJ, Holman AJ, Swick TJ, Alvarez-Horine S, Wang YG, Guinta D. Sodium oxybate reduces pain, fatigue, and sleep disturbance and improves functionality in fibromyalgia: results from a 14-week, randomized, double-blind, placebo-controlled study. *Pain*. 2011;152(5):1007–1017.

64. Moturi S, Ivanenko A. Complex diagnostic and treatment issues in psychotic symptoms associated with narcolepsy. *Psychiatry (Edgmont)*. 2009;6(6):38–44.

65. Barateau L, Lopez R, Dauvilliers Y. Treatment Options for Narcolepsy. *CNS Drugs*. 2016;30(5):369–379.

66. Abad VC, Guilleminault C. New developments in the management of narcolepsy. *Nature and science of sleep*. 2017;9:39–57.

67. Calik MW. Update on the treatment of narcolepsy: clinical efficacy of pitolisant. *Nature and science of sleep*. 2017;9:127–133.

68. Leu-Semenescu S, Nittur N, Golmard JL, Arnulf I. Effects of pitolisant, a histamine H3 inverse agonist, in drug-resistant idiopathic and

symptomatic hypersomnia: a chart review. *Sleep Med*. 2014;15(6):681–687.

69. Hawkins RD. Possible contributions of a novel form of synaptic plasticity in Aplysia to reward, memory, and their dysfunctions in mammalian brain. *Learn Mem*. 2013;20(10):580–591.

70. Monti JM, Jantos H. The roles of dopamine and serotonin, and of their receptors, in regulating sleep and waking. *Progress in brain research*. 2008;172:625–646.

71. Diagnostic Classification Steering Committee. *International Classification of Sleep Disorders: Diagnostic and Coding Manual—2*. Westchester: American Academy of Sleep Medicine; 2005.

72. Philip P, Chaufton C, Taillard J, et al. Modafinil improves real driving performance in patients with hypersomnia: a randomized double-blind placebo-controlled crossover clinical trial. *Sleep*. 2014;37(3):483–487.

73. Mayer G, Benes H, Young P, Bitterlich M, Rodenbeck A. Modafinil in the treatment of idiopathic hypersomnia without long sleep time—a randomized, double-blind, placebo-controlled study. *Journal of sleep research*. 2015;24(1):74–81.

74. Dauvilliers Y, Bassetti C, Lammers GJ, et al. Pitolisant versus placebo or modafinil in patients with narcolepsy: a double-blind, randomised trial. *The Lancet Neurology*. 2013;12(11):1068–1075.

75. Leu-Semenescu S, Louis P, Arnulf I. Benefits and risk of sodium oxybate in idiopathic hypersomnia versus narcolepsy type 1: a chart review. *Sleep medicine*. 2016;17:38–44.

76. Arnulf I. Kleine-Levin Syndrome. *Sleep Med Clin*. 2015;10(2):151–161.

77. Lavault S, Golmard JL, Groos E, et al. Kleine-Levin syndrome in 120 patients: differential diagnosis and long episodes. *Ann Neurol*. 2015;77(3):529–540.

78. Al Suwayri SM, BaHammam AS. The "Known Unknowns" of Kleine-Levin Syndrome: A Review and Future Prospects. *Sleep Med Clin*. 2017;12(3):345–358.

79. BaHammam AS, GadElRab MO, Owais SM, Alswat K, Hamam KD. Clinical characteristics and HLA typing of a family with Kleine-Levin syndrome. *Sleep Med*. 2008;9(5):575–578.

80. Dauvilliers Y, Lopez R. Time to find a biomarker in Kleine-Levin Syndrome. *Sleep Med*. 2016;21:177.

81. Wang JY, Han F, Dong SX, et al. Cerebrospinal Fluid Orexin A Levels and Autonomic Function in Kleine-Levin Syndrome. *Sleep*. 2016;39(4):855–860.

82. Lopez R, Barateau L, Chenini S, Dauvilliers Y. Preliminary results on CSF biomarkers for hypothalamic dysfunction in Kleine-Levin syndrome. *Sleep Med*. 2015;16(1):194–196.

83. Papacostas SS, Hadjivasilis V. The Kleine-Levin syndrome. Report of a case and review of the literature. *Eur Psychiatry*. 2000;15(4):231–235.

84. Al Shareef SM, Almeneessier AS, Hammad O, Smith RM, BaHammam AS. The sleep architecture of Saudi Arabian patients with Kleine-Levin syndrome. *Saudi Med J*. 2018;39(1):38–44.

85. Hong SB. Neuroimaging of Narcolepsy and Kleine-Levin Syndrome. *Sleep Med Clin*. 2017;12(3):359–368.

86. Arnulf I, Zeitzer JM, File J, Farber N, Mignot E. Kleine-Levin syndrome: a systematic review of 186 cases in the literature. *Brain*. 2005;128(Pt 12):2763–2776.

87. Reynolds CF, 3rd, Black RS, Coble P, Holzer B, Kupfer DJ. Similarities in EEG sleep findings for Kleine-Levin syndrome and unipolar depression. *Am J Psychiatry*. 1980;137(1):116–118.

88. Goldberg MA. The treatment of Kleine-Levin syndrome with lithium. *Can J Psychiatry*. 1983;28(6):491–493.

89. Miglis MG, Guilleminault C. Kleine-Levin syndrome: a review. *Nature and science of sleep*. 2014;6:19–26.

90. Oliveira MM, Conti C, Saconato H, Fernandes do Prado G. Pharmacological treatment for Kleine-Levin Syndrome. *Cochrane Database Syst Rev*. 2009(2):CD006685.

91. de Oliveira MM, Conti C, Prado GF. Pharmacological treatment for Kleine-Levin syndrome. *Cochrane Database Syst Rev*. 2016(5): CD006685.

92. Mayer G. Lithium treatment of Kleine-Levin syndrome An advance for a disorder of hypersomnolence. In: AAN Enterprises; 2015.

93. Honda M. Psychiatry and hypersomnia: remaining research area in sleep medicine. *Sleep and Biological Rhythms*. 2017;15(3):187–188.

94. Adamantidis A, de Lecea L. The hypocretins as sensors for metabolism and arousal. *J Physiol*. 2009;587(1):33–40.

95. Brundin L, Bjorkqvist M, Petersen A, Traskman-Bendz L. Reduced orexin levels in the cerebrospinal fluid of suicidal patients with major depressive disorder. *Eur Neuropsychopharmacol*. 2007;17(9):573–579.

96. Brundin L, Bjorkqvist M, Traskman-Bendz L, Petersen A. Increased orexin levels in the cerebrospinal fluid the first year after a suicide attempt. *J Affect Disord*. 2009;113(1-2): 179–182.

97. Brundin L, Petersen A, Bjorkqvist M, Traskman-Bendz L. Orexin and psychiatric symptoms in suicide attempters. *J Affect Disord*. 2007;100(1-3):259–263.

98. Johnson PL, Truitt W, Fitz SD, et al. A key role for orexin in panic anxiety. *Nature medicine*. 2010;16(1):111–115.

99. Lopez R, Barateau L, Evangelista E, Dauvilliers Y. Depression and Hypersomnia: A Complex Association. *Sleep Med Clin*. 2017;12(3):395–405.

100. Plante DT, Finn LA, Hagen EW, Mignot E, Peppard PE. Longitudinal associations of hypersomnolence and depression in the Wisconsin Sleep Cohort Study. *J Affect Disord*. 2017;207:197–202.

101. Fernandez-Mendoza J, Vgontzas AN, Kritikou I, Calhoun SL, Liao D, Bixler EO. Natural history of excessive daytime sleepiness: role of obesity, weight loss, depression, and sleep propensity. *Sleep*. 2015;38(3):351–360.

102. Jaussent I, Bouyer J, Ancelin ML, et al. Insomnia and daytime sleepiness are risk factors for depressive symptoms in the elderly. *Sleep*. 2011;34(8): 1103–1110.

103. Matza LS, Revicki DA, Davidson JR, Stewart JW. Depression with atypical features in the National Comorbidity Survey: classification, description, and consequences. *Arch Gen Psychiatry*. 2003;60(8):817–826.

104. Iovieno N, van Nieuwenhuizen A, Clain A, Baer L, Nierenberg AA. Residual symptoms after remission of major depressive disorder with fluoxetine and risk of relapse. *Depress Anxiety*. 2011;28(2):137–144.

105. Zimmerman M, McGlinchey JB, Posternak MA, Friedman M, Boerescu D, Attiullah N. Differences between minimally depressed patients who do and do not consider themselves to be in remission. *J Clin Psychiatry*. 2005;66(9):1134–1138.

106. Kaplan KA, Gruber J, Eidelman P, Talbot LS, Harvey AG. Hypersomnia in inter-episode bipolar disorder: does it have prognostic significance? *J Affect Disord*. 2011;132(3):438–444.

107. Sadock BJ, Sadock VA, Ruiz P. *Kaplan and Sadock's Synopsis of Psychiatry: Behavioral Sciences/Clinical Psychiatry*. Wolters Kluwer Health; 2014.

108. Oosterloo M, Lammers GJ, Overeem S, de Noord I, Kooij JJ. Possible confusion between primary hypersomnia and adult attention-deficit/hyperactivity disorder. *Psychiatry Res*. 2006;143(2-3):293–297.

109. Ito W, Honda M, Ueno T, Nobumasa K. Hypersomnia with ADHD: a possible subtype of narcolepsy type 2. *Sleep Biol Rhythms* 2017;(ahead of print): https://doi.org/10.1007/s41105-41017-40139-41101.

110. Takenoshita S, Sakai N, Chiba Y, Matsumura M, Yamaguchi M, Nishino S. An overview of hypocretin based therapy in narcolepsy. *Expert Opin Investig Drugs*. 2018;27(4):389–406.

111. Schwartz MD, Black SW, Fisher SP, et al. Trace amine-associated receptor 1 regulates wakefulness and eeg spectral composition. *Neuropsychopharmacology*. 2017;42(6):1305–1314.

112. Black SW, Schwartz MD, Chen TM, Hoener MC, Kilduff TS. Trace amine-associated receptor 1 agonists as narcolepsy therapeutics. *Biol Psychiatry*. 2017;82(9):623–633.

12

Parasomnias

JESSICA JUNG AND ERIK K. ST. LOUIS

INTRODUCTION

Parasomnias are undesirable and abnormal movements, behaviors, emotions, perceptions, and dreams occurring during or immediately surrounding sleep. The parasomnias are categorized as nonrapid eye movement (NREM) sleep parasomnias, rapid eye movement (REM) sleep parasomnias, and other parasomnias. This chapter will provide an overview to the epidemiology, clinical characteristics, differential diagnosis, diagnostic approach, and treatment of common parasomnias encountered in clinical practice.

The range of NREM, REM, and other parasomnias as categorized by the *Diagnostic and Statistical Manual of Mental Disorders* (fifth edition; DSM-5) and, where appropriate, the *International Classification of Sleep Disorders* (third edition; ICSD-3)[1] is shown in Table 12.1, which serves as an outline for each of the major disorders within each category discussed within this chapter. A brief broader consideration of other common nocturnal events that must also be considered in the differential diagnoses and clinical approach to patients presenting with possible parasomnias or spells related to sleep will be presented following a detailed discussion of each of the parasomnias. Sleep-related eating disorder (SRED) is also covered in Chapter 30 of this volume on sleep and eating disorders.

NONRAPID EYE MOVEMENT SLEEP-RELATED PARASOMNIAS

NREM parasomnias are a group of disorders resulting from abnormal arousal from NREM sleep. NREM parasomnias are seen most commonly in children and adolescents but may continue through or develop in adulthood. Disorders of arousal are defined as (a) recurrent incomplete arousals from sleep, occurring especially during the first third of the sleep, (b) absent or inappropriate response to external stimuli (e.g.,

intervention or redirection) during the episodes, (c) limited or absent dream imagery, (d) partial or complete amnesia involving the events, and (e) absence of other sleep, psychiatric, or medical conditions or medication/substance use that may explain the symptoms.[1] The ICSD-3 classifies NREM parasomnias to consist of disorders of arousal, including confusional arousals, sleepwalking, sleep terrors, and SRED.[1] Although these disorders are distinguished by their distinct clinical phenotypic features, they share key characteristics involving the pathophysiology of impaired arousal from NREM sleep, common triggers of sleep fragmentation and/or preceding sleep deprivation, inappropriate or disruptive behaviors arising from sleep, and complete or partial amnesia for the events. The following subheadings of this section of this chapter will review the clinical features, epidemiology, pathophysiology, diagnostic evaluation, and treatment of NREM parasomnias.

CLINICAL FEATURES AND EPIDEMIOLOGY

Confusional Arousals (Elpenor Syndrome)

Individuals with confusional arousals have episodes of sudden awakening, followed by confusion or disorientation that may be accompanied by confused behaviors and excessive motor activity. Mumbling or vocalization is often heard. During these episodes, the individual typically remains in bed. If ambulation is present, the episodes are considered instead to be sleepwalking and not confusional arousals. These episodes usually last for several minutes. During this period, patients do not respond appropriately to external stimuli and have complete or partial amnesia for the events. Typically, autonomic features such as tachycardia, tachypnea, mydriasis, and diaphoresis are absent.[1] The ICSD-3 diagnostic criteria for confusional arousals are as follows[1]:

TABLE 12.1. PARASOMNIAS AS CATEGORIZED BY THE INTERNATIONAL CLASSIFICATION OF SLEEP DISORDERS (THIRD EDITION)

Nonrapid eye movement (NREM) sleep-related parasomnias
    Confusional arousals
    Sleepwalking (somnambulism)
    Sleep Terrors
    Sleep-related eating disorder
Rapid eye movement (REM) sleep-related parasomnias
    Recurrent isolated sleep paralysis
    Nightmare disorder
    REM sleep behavior disorder
Other parasomnias
    Exploding head syndrome
    Sleep-related hallucinations
    Sleep enuresis
    Parasomnia due to a medical disorder
    Parasomnia due to a medication or substance use
    Parasomnia, unspecified
Isolated symptoms
    Sleep talking (somniloquy)

This table delineates the common categories of parasomnias specified within the ICSD-3, including the NREM sleep-related, REM sleep-related, and others categories of parasomnia disorders, and directly parallels the outline of the discussion of each disorder within this chapter.

1. The episodes meet the general NREM disorders of arousal diagnostic criteria.
2. The events are characterized by mental confusion or confusional behavior while the patient remains in bed.
3. Ambulation out of bed or terror is absent.

The prevalence of confusional arousals in the pediatric population is estimated to be as high as 17%[2] but decreases with age, and adult prevalence is between 4% to 15%.[3,4] Comorbid psychiatric disorders are present in a high proportion of individuals with confusional arousals. In a cross-sectional study of over 19,000 individuals from the United States, 37.4% of patients with confusional arousals had mental health disorders, most commonly bipolar and panic disorders, as well as major depressive, dysthymic, and generalized anxiety disorders; however, agoraphobia, obsessive-compulsive disorder, and social anxiety disorder were not significantly associated with confusional arousals.[4]

Sleepwalking (Somnambulism)

Sleepwalking is a disorder of arousal associated with ambulation. Ambulatory behavior can be simple walking and wandering but also can be complex motor activity, such as an attempt to escape one's house, driving, or urination in an inappropriate place such as the closet. Similar to confusional arousals, individuals with sleepwalking are either partially or completely unresponsive to external stimuli, including efforts toward redirection. Unintentional injuries or violence can occur during sleepwalking. In adults with childhood- and adult-onset sleepwalking, injuries were seen in 33% to 45%, and violent behaviors were observed in 29% to 44%.[5] The ICSD-3 diagnostic criteria for sleepwalking are[1]:

1. The events meet the general diagnostic criteria for NREM disorders of arousal.
2. The episodes of arousal are associated with ambulation or other out-of-bed complex behaviors.

The prevalence of sleepwalking over the lifetime is estimated to be 7% to 22%.[6,7] The prevalence of sleep walking in childhood is around 29%, with the peak prevalence at age of 10 years.[8] Sleepwalking occurs more frequently in individuals with a positive family history. The prevalence of sleepwalking was 23% in children who had parents without a history of sleepwalking, 47% in children who had one parent with a history of sleepwalking, and 62% in children in whom both parents had a history of sleepwalking.[8] As in confusional arousals, there are maturational influences, and sleepwalking prevalence declines to only about 2% in adulthood.[6] Data are conflicting with regards to an association between psychiatric comorbidities and sleepwalking in adults. In a study of psychiatric outpatients, sleepwalking was observed in 9%, which is higher than the general adult population.[9] Increased odds of sleepwalking were seen in individuals with alcohol abuse/dependence, major depressive disorder, or obsessive-compulsive disorder in an epidemiologic study of the US population.[10] However, no significant association with depression or anxiety was noted in a cohort of Canadian adults with sleepwalking.[11]

Sleep Terrors

Sleep terrors are characterized by abrupt arousals associated with terror, piercing screaming, and autonomic symptoms such as tachycardia, tachypnea, mydriasis, and diaphoresis. During the events, the patients cannot be consoled. Attempts to comfort the individuals can increase the risk of aggression. Violent behaviors are frequently seen in episodes of sleep terrors.[12] The individuals are generally amnestic to the events, although the episodes can distress the parents and bedpartners. The ICSD-3 defines sleep terrors as follows[1]:

1. The episodes meet the NREM disorders of arousal general criteria.
2. The events are characterized by abrupt terror, starting with a frightening scream and vocalization.
3. Intense fear and autonomic symptoms, including mydriasis, tachycardia, and diaphoresis are present.

The lifetime prevalence of sleep terrors is estimated to be 10%.[7] Sleep terrors occur in up to 56% of children.[8] Children with a history of sleep terrors between ages 1.5 and 3.5 years tend to develop sleepwalking after age 5 years, compared to the children without a history of sleep terrors in early childhood.[8] Although the prevalence decreases in adults, 4% to 5% of adults experience sleep terrors.[13] The association between sleep terrors and psychiatric disorders is not clear. In the UK population, comorbid mood and anxiety disorders were observed in 30% of those with sleep terrors.[3] In another study, however, the presence of sleep terrors was not significantly different between patients with and without psychiatric conditions, and treatment of the concurrent psychiatric disorders did not improve sleep terrors.[14,15]

Sleep-Related Eating Disorder (SRED)

SRED is characterized by compulsive eating behaviors associated with incomplete arousal from sleep. These behaviors are involuntary and unintentional. Individuals with SRED are completely or partially amnestic to the events. Oftentimes, these individuals binge on high-caloric food or consume inedible or bizarre objects. SRED can lead to potentially hazardous health consequences, including morning anorexia, weight gain, impaired glucose tolerance, injuries related to food preparation, or ingestion of toxic material. SRED is different from night eating syndrome, which instead is characterized by intentional excessive nocturnal eating of usual daytime food items close to bedtime or after awakening in the middle of the night. The ICSD-3 diagnostic criteria for SRED are as follows[1]:

1. The disorder is characterized by recurrent arousal associated with dysfunctional eating during the sleep period.
2. Inedible, toxic, or peculiar food consumption, injury or potential for injury associated with food seeking or cooking, and/or adverse health outcome associated with sleep-related eating are present.
3. Partial or complete amnesia about the events is present.
4. There is absence of another sleep disorder, psychiatric condition, medication, or substance use that serves as an alternative cause for the behaviors.

SRED is more common in women, similar to other eating disorders.[16] The overall frequency is about 0.5% in patients who are referred to a sleep clinic and is increased especially in college students and people with daytime eating disorders, depression, and dissociation.[9,17-19] The lifetime prevalence of SRED is thought to be 5%.[7] Sleepwalking is frequent in individuals with SRED. In the first two series of SRED published, about 70% of individuals had polysomnographic findings consistent with sleepwalking.[17,18] SRED is likely part of the continuum of sleepwalking, as ambulation out of bed after partial, incomplete arousal from NREM sleep precedes and overlaps with the sleep-related eating behavior.

Sexsomnia

Sexsomnia is another NREM sleep-related parasomnia, characterized by sexual acts such as masturbation, orgasm, fondling a bedpartner, attempted or actual sexual intercourse, or even sexual assault that may have legal consequences. Sleep deprivation, shift work, and certain medications (antidepressants, pramipexole treatment in Parkinson's disease [PD]) may be triggers, and it appears that rarely sleep-related epilepsy may be an alternative cause.

PATHOPHYSIOLOGY

The transition from NREM sleep to wakefulness is thought to be compromised in NREM parasomnias. NREM parasomnias most commonly occur out of N3 (slow wave) sleep, although they can be seen out of N2 (light NREM) sleep.[20] Most, although not all, NREM parasomnias occur in the first half of the night, especially the first third of the night, being maximal during N3 and consolidated N2 sleep stages. More frequently, NREM parasomnia episodes are noted in individuals with frequent arousals from slow-wave or N3 sleep.[21] Therefore, factors that disrupt sleep continuity and increase the threshold for complete awakening tend to predispose individuals to NREM parasomnias. Untreated sleep disorders, such as obstructive sleep apnea (OSA), periodic limb movement disorder (PLMD), and restless legs syndrome (RLS), as well as other conditions that can lead to sleep fragmentation such as pain, increase the propensity toward NREM parasomnias, especially in adults with de-novo or worsened frequency of NREM parasomnia behaviors. Hypnotics, especially non-benzodiazepine benzodiazepine receptor agonists such as zolpidem, as well as preceding sleep deprivation may also be associated with NREM parasomnias, as these influences increase the threshold for complete arousal and awakening from NREM sleep. In addition, several other medications, including selective serotonin reuptake inhibitors (SSRIs), amitriptyline, bupropion, antipsychotics, beta-blockers, fluoroquinolones, and montelukast, as well as alcohol and substance use, have been linked to NREM parasomnias.[22–24] Other medical conditions, including chronic pain, migraines, hyperthyroidism, head injury, encephalitis, and stroke, have been associated with NREM parasomnias as well.[1,25,26] Genetic and familial patterns have been described. Human leukocyte antigen (HLA) DQB1*05:01 and DQB1*04 alleles have been associated with various NREM parasomnias.[27,28] Autosomal dominant inheritance of sleepwalking with reduced penetrance at the genetic locus of chromosome 20q12-q13.12 has also been observed.[29]

CLINICAL EVALUATION AND DIAGNOSIS

Obtaining a detailed and comprehensive history of the nocturnal events from the patient, and collateral history from the parents or bed partner is the most important first step for diagnosing NREM parasomnias. Since NREM parasomnias most often occur during N3 or N2 sleep, they are most likely to have a history of being reported to occur during the first half of the night, especially during the first third of the night, which can be a helpful feature to distinguish these events from REM parasomnias, which are most apt to occur during the second half of the night where REM sleep occurs more compared to first half of the night.

If the details of the nocturnal events are not available or witnesses of the events are absent, overnight in-lab video polysomnography should be considered. In-lab polysomnography can also be helpful if the history is atypical or when there are concerns for other primary sleep disorders or nocturnal seizure activity.[30,31] Unlike seizures, the nocturnal episodes of NREM parasomnias are not stereotyped and occur less frequently. Given that these events occur intermittently, a typical nocturnal episode may not be captured during the overnight in-lab polysomnography. However, features suggestive of NREM instability, such as frequent arousals from NREM sleep, especially in N3 sleep, may be seen. In addition, polysomnography is helpful for excluding the presence of other comorbid sleep disorders that may increase the tendency for sleep fragmentation, such as OSA and PLMD. Addition of extended electroencephalography (EEG) and electromyography (EMG) channels is useful for monitoring epileptiform activity to rule out seizures and to evaluate muscle activity during REM sleep to exclude REM sleep behavior disorder (RBD), respectively.[30] Monitoring of the video-recording of nocturnal events and correlating with EEG changes can be helpful in identifying nonepileptic behavioral spells in some cases.

TREATMENT OF THE NREM PARASOMNIAS

The primary focus of NREM parasomnia management should be injury prevention. Modifying the sleep environment is the initial and most important step in preventing sleep-related injury. Potentially injurious objects, including nightstands, tables, and any sharp objects, need to be removed from the bedside, and firearms or other weapons should be removed from the bedroom and, whenever possible, kept in a locked cabinet or safe to prevent access of the weapon to the patient. Pads or cushions should be used for the sharp corners of bedroom furniture. The bed should be placed away from windows, and window locks and door alarms should be considered. The use of a sleeping bag can be considered to limit opportunities to leave the bed.

Factors that predispose individuals to increased arousals during sleep should be minimized and appropriately addressed. Sleep deprivation and an irregular sleep–wake schedule or swing shift work should be avoided. Use of hypnotics, especially zolpidem and other central nervous system depressants that have been shown to be associated with NREM parasomnias, should be avoided or minimized. Comorbid sleep disorders, such as OSA, RLS, and PLMD, should be adequately treated. In particular, diagnosis and treatment of comorbid OSA with nasal continuous positive airway pressure in adults or with tonsillectomy in children and some adolescents can be effective for reducing NREM parasomnia behavior frequency and severity.

In most pediatric confusional arousals and sleep terrors, reassuring and educating the parents and patient can be sufficient. If these nocturnal episodes are timed in a predictable manner, regular anticipatory awakenings, which involve waking up the children about 15 to 30 minutes before the habitual anticipated time of occurrence, can be effective.[32] Psychotherapy and hypnosis have been successfully used in NREM parasomnias.[32–34] One or two sessions of a mindfulness-based hypnosis approach with classic induction, progressive suggested relaxation, and guided imagination of a parasomnia-free night followed by nightly practice by patients can be effective. Individuals with comorbid anxiety are more likely to respond to hypnosis.[35]

Clonazepam is a typical first-line pharmacologic treatment option. In individuals with sleepwalking and sleep terrors, clonazepam, alprazolam, and other benzodiazepines were shown to completely or substantially control the symptoms in 86% of the patients over a mean duration of 3.5 years without significant escalation of the dose.[36] The average initial and final doses of clonazepam used in this study were 0.77 ± 0.46 mg and 1.10 ± 0.96 mg, respectively.[36] Several case reports also showed that antidepressants, including paroxetine, sertraline, and trazodone can be effective in treating sleep terrors and/or sleepwalking.[37–39] For treatment of SRED, in addition to clonazepam,[18] topiramate was beneficial in 68% of patients in a retrospective case series of 25 patients.[40] Low doses of pramipexole (0.18–0.36 mg) were also effective in a pilot randomized double-blind crossover study.[41] In addition, agomelatine, a melatonin receptor agonist, improved SRED in a patient with comorbid depression and panic disorder.[42]

REM SLEEP-RELATED PARASOMNIAS

The next section of this chapter discusses the range of REM parasomnias, which include nightmare disorder, recurrent isolated sleep paralysis, and RBD.

Nightmare Disorder

Dreaming may occur in any stage of sleep, although REM-sleep related dreams tend to be more vivid and have a deeper narrative structure. Nightmares are repetitive dreams that most often involve elaborate, vivid, and an unpleasant or threatening content or theme such as being physically attacked or chased, and while these could also occur during any sleep stage, REM sleep is the most frequent and representative of the type of dreaming seen in nightmares. Upon awakening following a nightmare, the dreamer can usually recall the unpleasant dream and is fully alert and coherent. Nightmares are common enough to be considered a normal variant in most people when they are singular or infrequent. However, in some individuals, nightmares evolve into a clinical disorder, and nightmare disorder is diagnosed (a) when there are repeated occurrences of extended, extremely dysphoric, and well-remembered dreams involving threats to survival, security, or physical integrity; (b) when on awakening from these dysphoric dreams the patient rapidly becomes alert and oriented; and (c) when the dream or sleep disturbance associated with the nightmare causes clinically significant distress, mood disturbance, sleep resistance, cognitive impairment, behavioral problems, daytime sleepiness or fatigue, impairment in work or educational roles, or in interpersonal or social functioning, including disruption to the sleep of the patient's family or caregiver.

Nightmare disorder has an estimated frequency of approximately 4% of the population.[1] Nightmare disorder may occur as a primary sleep disorder or accompany another sleep, medical, or psychiatric disorder such as narcolepsy, OSA syndrome, RBD, a mood disorder (i.e., depression, bipolar affective disorder), an anxiety or panic disorder, or posttraumatic stress disorder. Certain medications might precipitate nightmares and nightmare disorder, especially beta-blocking antihypertensive drugs, antidepressants, varenicline (Chantix), and alcohol and other substances (or their withdrawal).

Treatment for nightmare disorder is indicated when nightmares cause distress and/or impairment in sleep-related, social, school, or occupational functioning. Image rehearsal therapy, cognitive-behavioral therapies and hypnosis are all reasonable options. Of these, image rehearsal therapy involving "rewriting" the nightmare's theme and/or conclusions toward a more positive theme/conclusion while awake, practiced for 10 to 20 minutes daily following instruction in its conceptual basis, may be particularly effective. Nightmares associated with posttraumatic stress disorder may benefit from prazosin 1 to 10 mg nightly, although evidence for its success is mixed.[43]

RECURRENT ISOLATED SLEEP PARALYSIS

The presumed pathophysiology of recurrent isolated sleep paralysis involves an intrusion of normal, physiologic REM sleep muscle atonia into an awakening from sleep, generally lasting from a few seconds to 1 minute. An episode of sleep paralysis is characterized by complete paralysis and inability to move during wakefulness, typically during sleep–wake transitions. Sleep paralysis is considered to be hypnagogic when occurring during sleep onset and hypnopompic when occuring upon awakening from sleep. These episodes may also be associated with hypnagogic or hypnopompic hallucinatory experiences. Respiratory and eye muscles are typically unaffected. Treatment is generally not necessary beyond reassurance of the patient and education to avoid/treat factors that may trigger its occurrence such as sleep deprivation or comorbid OSA.

REM SLEEP BEHAVIOR DISORDER

RBD is a common parasomnia, with an estimated prevalence near 1% to 2%, that may lead to serious injury to patients or their bedpartners and has a strong association with alpha-synucleinopathy neurodegenerative disorders such as PD, dementia with Lewy bodies (DLB), or multiple system atrophy (MSA).[44] RBD is diagnosed when there is a clinical history of dream enactment behavior, accompanied by finding of loss of REM sleep-related atonia (aka, REM sleep without atonia [RSWA], an abnormally elevated muscle activity during REM sleep) during polysomnography, which is required for diagnosis.[1] Thematic content of dreams in RBD patients characteristically involve being chased or attacked by assailants or animal characters, with the dreamer feeling that they are defending themselves against the attackers. Dream enactment behaviors most often involve violent thrashing arm or leg movements, accompanied by screaming or shouting vocalizations during REM sleep. Polysomnography is necessary for determination of RSWA and making a diagnosis of RBD, and video during polysomnography enables visual review of any corresponding excessive complex motor behavior typical of dream enactment and auditory review of sleep-related vocalizations. Usually, there is accompanying excessive limb jerking during REM sleep. Comorbid OSA often occurs in patients with RBD, and rarely can lead to "pseudo-RBD," where respiratory resuscitative arousals during OSA mimic RBD episodes.

RBD has been very strongly associated with alpha-synucleinopathy neurodegeneration over the last several years, so much so that some experts are now beginning to shift terminology toward calling idiopathic RBD (without other overt associated neurological symptoms or signs of motor, cognitive, or autonomic disorders at presentation) instead as "isolated RBD," meaning that it can be considered as the first sign of an otherwise covert neurodegenerative disease that is already present in some (or maybe even most) older adults presenting with RBD symptoms. RBD appears in majority of older adults to actually be a prodrome of an underlying neurodegenerative disease, occurring long before the future development of overt and more devastating memory, motor, or autonomic disorders including mild cognitive impairment (MCI), DLB, PD, or MSA.[44-45] Older adult patients presenting with idiopathic/isolated RBD carry an approximate 50% to 70% (or higher) risk of developing MCI, DLB, PD, or MSA over the subsequent 10 to 20 years of longitudinal follow-up, annualized to approximately 6% per year following diagnosis.[45] The practical implication is that all patients with RBD merit careful longitudinal serial neurological follow-up annually to permit an accurate eventual diagnosis and prognosis for the patient and to enable early symptomatic therapy for any evolving cognitive, motor, or autonomic symptoms or signs that may otherwise deteriorate quality of life and functioning. RBD may signify a time window during which future neuroprotective therapies could be strategically administered to hopefully arrest or delay development of PD or DLB.[44]

RBD may also occur as a secondary disorder, and in older adults, the main secondary cause for RBD is also the alpha-synucleinopathy neurodegenerative disorders, in which initial cognitive, motor, or autonomic symptoms or signs exist prior to the onset of dream enactment behaviors. However, stroke is also suspected to be a cause in some older adults and in some younger adults, and multiple sclerosis can be an alternative etiology for RBD with lesions occurring in the brainstem REM atonia control regions. See Chapter 25 of this volume on neurocognitive disorders and the sections relating to RBD there for a complete discussion of these causes of secondary RBD.

RBD may have a broader spectrum of secondary nondegenerative etiologies in younger (i.e., <60 years old) adults, and evidence suggests that younger adults with RBD have more frequent psychiatric comorbidity and antidepressant use, autoimmune disorders, brain lesion pathology, and narcolepsy. RBD has been particularly strongly associated with antidepressant medication use especially SSRIs, but may also be associated with serotonin and norepinephrine reuptake inhibitors (SNRIs) and tricyclic antidepressants. A current, unresolved controversy is whether antidepressant-associated RBD may be reversible when anti-depressant medications are discontinued, and further longitudinal cohort studies will be necessary to resolve this uncertainty. RBD may rarely even occur in children and adolescents, where narcolepsy type 1 or neurodegenerative disorders of infancy or childhood may cause RSWA and dream enactment.[44] Stopping or changing antidepressants may improve RBD symptoms in some patients, and while there is no good evidence basis for good or poor choices of antidepressant treatment in the setting of RBD, many favor the use of bupropion rather than another SSRI, SNRI, or tricyclic antidepressant medication trial when a switch is considered. Additional longitudinal cohort studies following these younger adult patients are needed to determine if they too may harbor neurodegenerative pathology covertly.

The other main concern with RBD is injury potential for the patient or their bed partner. Injuries have been reported to occur in approximately 55% of RBD patients, and while most injuries are only of mild severity such as bruises or lacerations, about 11% may be serious, including subdural hematoma requiring surgical intervention and broken ribs.[44]

RBD treatment is important to reduce the risk of injury to patients and their bedpartners. Unfortunately, the evidence basis for any treatment for RBD remains quite thin. Bedroom safety counseling is much the same as recommended for NREM parasomnias (lower the bed mattress to the floor if/as possible, or place cushions or floor rugs near the bed to prevent fall related injuries, removing sharply cornered furniture or night tables from close proximity to the bed, considering use of a bed alarm if the patient has a history of leaving the bed, and removing or locking any firearms or weapons away from the bedroom environment). Melatonin 3 to 12 mg (average effective dosage 6 mg) and clonazepam 0.5 to 2.0 mg (average effective dosage 0.5 mg) have been the mainstays of pharmacotherapy for RBD and may have adverse effects of somnolence, dizziness, unsteadiness, or, rarely, sexual side effects such as decreased libido or erectile dysfunction, which are worse with clonazepam than melatonin. Beyond these, there are few effective options although donepezil or pramipexole may be tried, which are especially attractive options for patients who have already developed concurrent cognitive or motor parkinsonism impairments that may benefit symptomatically from these alternatives.

OVERLAP PARASOMNIA DISORDERS

Overlap parasomnia disorder is characterized by clinical features of both NREM and REM parasomnias, with features of one or more of the heterogeneous spectrum of NREM disorder of arousal such as sleepwalking or confusional arousals, occurring together with RBD. Overlap parasomnia may be a distinct disorder given that it often has a relatively younger age of onset with initial NREM parasomnia features, and later evolution of RBD features. Overlap parasomnia has also been associated with narcolepsy, multiple sclerosis, psychiatric disorders like posttraumatic stress disorder, and substance and alcohol abuse and withdrawal. Polysomnography typically shows sleep instability typical of NREM parasomnia together with RSWA typical for RBD.

Related to the overlap parasomnias, an even more extreme form of sleep state dissociation (known as status dissociatus) may occur in which not only are there combined features of NREM and REM sleep-related parasomnias, but the differentiation among sleep stages during polysomnography can become challenging even for sleep medicine experts. Several such disorders are symptomatic and occur either as secondary parasomnias in advanced neurodegenerative diseases or, in some patients, dissociated states may occur as a presenting manifestation of rare but increasingly recognized autoimmune encephalopathy syndromes.

In one of these entities that is associated with antibodies against IgLON5, a neuronal cell surface adhesion protein, both REM and NREM parasomnias may occur, as well as features of severe sleep architecture disturbance (although N2 architectural features of K complexes and sleep spindles may still be present), and sleep disordered breathing (OSA, sleep related hypoventilation, or even sleep stridor, which is usually seen in MSA), gait instability, movement disorders including choreiform movements, and symptoms or signs involving the brainstem. Undifferentiated or poorly differentiated NREM sleep is also seen.[46,47] Sleep disturbance noted in dipeptidyl-peptidase-like protein-6 (DPPX) potassium channel antibody autoimmune disorder is characterized by abnormalities in both NREM and REM sleep, and REM or NREM parasomnias may also occur in this entity.[48]

Status dissociatus is an extreme case of wake/sleep state dissociation where the boundaries of the wakefulness, NREM and REM sleep are blurred and recognizable sleep stages are absent.[49,50] Status dissociatus is observed in alcohol withdrawal, anti-*N*-methyl-D aspartate (NMDA) receptor antibody associated autoimmune encephalopathy, and alpha synucleinopathies such as advanced PD, DLB, or MSA.[51–53] Agrypnia excitata is an extreme variant of status dissociatus seen in association with fatal familial insomnia, Morvan syndrome, and delirium tremens[53] and is characterized by severe insomnia, loss of slow-wave sleep, reduced sleep spindles and K complexes, abnormal REM sleep with loss of muscle atonia and resultant dream enactment, and generalized motor and sympathetic hyperactivity related to thalamo-limbic dysfunction.[53,54] Oneiric stupor, a state of unresponsiveness with repetitive semipurposeful motor activity, is seen in agrypnia excitata.[55] Cases of agrypnia excitata and similar milder syndromic presentations have been described in association with LGI1 and CaspR2, and other voltage-gated potassium channel complex autoimmunity targets have been reported. Given the clinical heterogeneity that is possible in clinical characteristics across individuals, work-up for a possible autoimmune encephalopathy involving antibodies targeting VGKC, LGI1, CaspR2, DPPX, and IgLON5 should be considered in patients with complex sleep disturbances including NREM and/or REM parasomnias, and other subacute symptoms or signs of a broad range of neuropsychiatric disturbances including mood, cognition, motor, cerebellar, cranial nerve, or peripheral nerve disorders.

Careful clinical history with PSG evaluation, as well as other diagnostic work-up for a possible underlying etiology, is warranted. Management includes treating comorbid sleep disorders such as OSA or RLS and the optimization of sleep and environmental safety. Clonazepam is the most frequently used agent for these rare parasomnia disorders, although alprazolam, temazepam, carbamazepine, and melatonin use may also be considered. For autoimmune etiologies, immunotherapeutic agents such as steroids, intravenous immunoglobulin, and plasma exchange have been used in some cases of status dissociatus associated with autoimmune encephalopathy.

DIFFERENTIAL DIAGNOSIS OF NOCTURNAL EVENTS

Diagnosis of NREM parasomnias most often can be done confidently by a careful clinical history and examination. However, polysomnography is required for the diagnosis of clinically suspected RBD, for documenting confirmatory evidence of REM sleep atonia loss (aka, REM sleep without atonia). The American Academy of Sleep Medicine recommends performing polysomnography in the evaluation of parasomnias that are atypical or unusual in age of onset, duration, or behavioral characteristics, when they are potentially injurious, or if potentially epileptogenic activity needs to be excluded (which also requires appropriate adjunctive monitoring with full electroencephalography; i.e., 10–20 International Electrode Systems placements), and full electromyography montages with monitoring of all four limbs should be considered when RBD is a possibility.[56] Usually, a single night of video–EEG–polysomnography can provide a high diagnostic yield for sufficiently frequent nocturnal events or at least provide insight through documentation of RSWA to support a diagnosis of RBD or, alternatively, provide evidence for supportive interictal epileptiform discharges when sleep-related epilepsies may be in consideration (or lack of these, which gives further weight to NREM parasomnia diagnosis).

When captured during polysomnography, NREM parasomnia events most often involve an otherwise spontaneous arousal from NREM sleep, usually from N2 or N3 (slow-wave) sleep, although they sometimes may be triggered by a respiratory arousal associated with sleep apnea or possibly periodic limb movement associated arousals. Clinical manifestations may include nonstereotyped behavior with confusion, variable vocalization, or sleepwalking. The accompanying polysomnogram may show no change other than arousal, but occasionally shows a generalized or bifrontal dominant rhythmic slow-wave (delta or theta) EEG pattern lasting for several seconds or even minutes following the arousal. RBD is instead characterized by vocalization, variable complex motor behavior paralleling dream content consistent with dream enactment, and REM sleep atonia loss (REM sleep without atonia) as its neurophysiological hallmark seen in the chin and limb muscles during REM sleep.

Nocturnal events that must be discriminated from parasomnias include sleep-related epilepsies. The main distinction with these are that nocturnal seizures are typically highly stereotyped clinical events with features of vocalization and complex motor behaviors that most often involve oral, limb, or even proximal truncal automatisms. Nocturnal temporal lobe seizures have focal rhythmic activity, while frontal lobe seizures often show little EEG change before or during the seizure, and frequently if there are prominent movements, the EEG may be obscured by muscle and movement artifact; so the diagnosis of these frontal lobe seizure events instead relies chiefly upon observation of the typically stereotyped complex motor and vocal behaviors. Psychogenic nonepileptic spells (PNES) are frequently also confused with epilepsy or other nocturnal events including parasomnias. PNES closely resemble epileptic seizures but lack clinical and electrophysiologic features of true epilepsy and appear to have features of unresponsiveness, abnormal movements, and postictal behavioral alterations. In addition, PNES often show eye closure during the spell and often have bizarre voluntary appearing movements, including "yes-yes" head nodding or "no-no" head shaking, pelvic thrusting, or atypical nonanatomical movement spread such as clonic-type limb movements starting in a leg that then spread to the face or head, and then on to an arm, as compared to a "Jacksonian" seizure progression, which is more anatomic (i.e., face and head to arm, arm to leg). In distinction to true epileptic seizures, PNES lack stereotypy between different events and lack any epileptiform EEG discharges before or during the spells. However, expert review and diagnosis is needed since true epileptic seizures may sometimes share some of these atypical clinical characteristics and lack an EEG change, especially sleep-related focal frontal lobe epilepsies. Last and least probable, the possibility of presyncope or syncope, or a migrainous event (i.e., migraine equivalent, which may cause focal neurological symptoms in the absence of headache) needs to be considered in some cases, although these etiologies are rarely sleep-related specifically and more often have daytime spells and characteristic clinical features that provide sufficient information for diagnosis. If a single night of video–EEG–polysomnography fails to provide a diagnosis, patients with continued and sufficiently frequent undiagnosed nocturnal events should be referred for inpatient video–EEG monitoring in an epilepsy monitoring unit.

OTHER PARASOMNIAS

The category of other parasomnias are a spectrum of "leftovers," which do not map well to NREM or REM sleep-related parasomnias, including exploding head syndrome, sleep-related hallucinations, sleep enuresis, and parasomnias ascribed to medical disorders, medication or substance use, or unspecified etiologies. These entities will be described briefly here.

Exploding head syndrome is a distinctive yet rare phenomenon theorized to represent a very peculiar hypnogogic or hypnopompic hallucination or hypnic phenomena at sleep–wake transition. The patient describes an extremely loud explosive sound that is nonpainful and associated with a sudden awakening from sleep. Exploding head syndrome should not be confused with a "thunderclap" headache, characteristically associated with a severe and sudden headache that may arise from either wakefulness or sleep and that may frequently represent a neurological emergency resulting from aneurysmal subarachnoid hemorrhage. In contrast, while exploding head syndrome can be very upsetting to the patient, it is an invariably benign phenomenon for which the patient can simply be reassured.

Sleep-related hallucinations can be a normal variant associated with sleep paralysis but can also occur as a distinctive parasomnia in older adults characterized usually by complex formed hallucinations such as people or animals by the bedside visible upon awakening from sleep. The patient most often experiences these as nonfrightening, may have preserved insight into the false nature of their vision, and may realize that the hallucinatory vision is associated with another normal object in the room once they turn up the lights or replace their glasses to improve visual acuity (i.e., mistake a bathrobe in the closet as a standing person or animal). When these characteristic associated features are present, this entity has been called by the eponymous Charles Bonnet syndrome.[57] When sleep-related hallucinations occur de-novo in later life, especially if also associated with waking hallucinations, there should be a strong index of suspicion for prodromal Lewy body disease (since hallucinations can be an initial symptom expression of Lewy body disease similar to RBD), and neuropsychological testing and brain imaging should be considered for evaluation. Recent evidence has shown that many such patients with sleep-related hallucinations go on to develop DLB over longitudinal follow-up.[57] On the other hand, in earlier adulthood, other neuropsychiatric comorbidities in those with sleep-related hallucinations deserve consideration, including migraine, epilepsy, or comorbid anxiety disorders.

Sleep enuresis (aka bedwetting) is often a normal maturational variant that is outgrown after age 7 to 10 years and for which reassurance toward this eventuality can be offered. However, occasionally sleep enuresis persists into adolescence or even early adulthood or grows to become so socially problematic that evaluation and treatment become necessary. A family history of enuresis suggests genetically enriched sleep homeostatic drive (i.e., especially deep NREM sleep) as a contributing cause. Secondary enuresis, defined as when enuresis returns after a 6-month dry spell of maintaining bladder control with or without development of other urological symptoms (dysuria, hesitancy or urinary frequency, daytime urge incontinence), should prompt urological evaluation. Limiting fluid intake at night, avoidance of caffeine, and scheduled voiding may be sufficient treatments, but prescription moisture alarms (that awaken the patient when undergarments or bedclothes are wet) or prescribed desmopressin (ddAVP) or oxybutynin can also be considered if underlying causative urological disorders are appropriately excluded.

There is ample evidence to suggest that some parasomnia behaviors may be associated with medical disorders, medications, or substance/alcohol use/abuse or withdrawal. The implication here is that if the parasomnia is symptomatic and secondary to the underlying disorder and that disorder can be corrected or removed, the parasomnia behaviors may abate or improve significantly. Specific examples include zolpidem precipitating sleepwalking, which led the US Food and Drug Administration to recently issue a boxed warning for all the "Z" drug hypnotics, including eszopiclone and zaleplon, as possible precipitants of sleep-related amnestic behaviors that are typically NREM disorders of arousal, as well as sodium oxybate that may also precipitate sleepwalking and enuresis. The main culprits in precipitating RBD are the SSRI or SNRI antidepressant drugs. If parasomnias persist despite resolution of the apparently triggering disorder, further evaluation and consideration of primary sleep disorders and specific type of parasomnia presentation should be considered.

CONCLUSIONS

NREM parasomnias are a phenotypically heterogeneous group of disorders of arousal from NREM sleep, including confusional arousals, sleep terrors, and sleepwalking. The pathophysiology of these disorders is an incomplete or abortive arousal from NREM sleep, and these events can be potentially injurious. REM sleep parasomnias include recurrent isolated sleep paralysis, which typically requires no specific treatment other than reassurance; nightmare disorder for which dream image rehearsal therapy is helpful; and RBD, frequently a prodrome to, or occurring secondary to, alpha-synucleinopathy neurodegenerative disorders (i.e., PD, DLB) in older adults. RBD has also been linked with several other etiologies including antidepressant medications, autoimmunity, narcolepsy, and brain lesions in younger adults below the age of 60 years. The other parasomnia category includes a heterogeneous group of disorders that are linked neither to NREM nor REM sleep specifically, including exploding head syndrome sleep-related hallucinations, and sleep enuresis, as well as parasomnias associated with medical disorders, hypnotic medications, and substance/alcohol abuse or withdrawal.

The treatment approach to all parasomnias with injury potential should include counseling on bedroom safety with patients and any involved bedpartners or parents, with removal of potentially injurious objects from the bedside and moving any firearms or weapons out of the bedroom environment. For the NREM sleep-related parasomnias, factors that promote rebound slow-wave sleep, such as sleep deprivation, an irregular sleep wake schedule, or shift work, or that disturb sleep continuity leading to increased arousals should be corrected when possible, and in-lab polysomnography should be considered when there is a clinical suspicion for a comorbid primary sleep disorder such as OSA or PLMD that could be triggering or aggravating the parasomnia or sleep-related epilepsy is in question.

RBD requires polysomnography for diagnosis, to document REM sleep without atonia. Clonazepam has been the most used pharmacologic approach for both parasomnia types, whereas behavioral interventions such as anticipatory awakening or hypnosis may also be helpful therapies for the NREM parasomnias. Melatonin is also an option for RBD, but there is no evidence it is helpful for NREM parasomnia. When patients present with parasomnias accompanying unusual clinical syndromes of complex neuropsychiatric symptoms or signs, work-up for autoimmune encephalopathies should also be considered. Following RBD diagnosis, careful annual longitudinal monitoring for symptoms and signs of concurrent or future development of neurodegenerative disorders with overt cognitive, autonomic, and motor impairments is necessary.

FUTURE DIRECTIONS

The first-half century of parasomnias research has built a solid foundation for diagnostic recognition and categorization of these disorders. The basic pathophysiology of the parasomnias has also been elucidated, in that NREM parasomnias appear to predominantly be disorders of arousal from NREM sleep, while RBD results from REM sleep atonia loss (aka REM sleep without atonia). However, the causes and factors underlying isolated REM sleep paralysis and nightmare disorder remain largely opaque and enigmatic.

A vastly improved understanding of the neurobiology of both NREM and REM parasomnias will be necessary to inform more specific and evidence-based treatment strategies. Definition of genetic and other etiologic factors and the underlying pathophysiologic mechanisms remain a frontier for the parasomnias in general and NREM parasomnias in particular. While current evidence suggests that majority of older adults who develop RBD have or will develop an overt synucleinopathy, understanding Lewy body disease biology also remains poor; so neuroprotective therapy development to prevent Parkinsonism and dementia from developing will likely also require patience and long-term development strategies. Even before mechanistic insights, refinement of current recommended treatment strategies with a stronger evidence basis is sorely needed, as all current pharmacotherapy and behavioral strategies still largely rely on retrospective case series level evidence.

CASE VIGNETTE

A 55-year-old man is evaluated for new onset of complex behaviors and vocalization during sleep. For the last 6 months, he has begun to apparently act out his dreams, with nightmares characteristically involving a chase or attack theme. His wife provides collateral history that he frequently flails his arms or makes punching or kicking movements in the second half of the night. Initially infrequently occurring, the behaviors are now

occurring nightly, and an episode of his inadvertently punching his wife in the eye and blackening it, prompted medical evaluation in the sleep clinic. Additional specific questioning reveals that he has had little sense of smell or taste for the last 5 years and notes constipation for the last few years as well. He denies any history of a tremor, gait slowing, handwriting difficulties, drooling, or lightheadedness upon arising in the mornings. There are no subjective restless legs symptoms. He notes no appreciable daytime sleepiness with an Epworth Sleepiness Scale score of only 4. He sleeps soundly on a regular schedule, bedtime and rise time averaging 10 PM to 6 AM, without features of insomnia. He is receiving no medications.

His full neurological and general medical examinations were normal, without features of rigidity, bradykinesia, tremor, or postural instability present. A polysomnogram shows abundant REM sleep without atonia in the submentalis (chin) and all four limb EMG channels (flexor digitorum superficialis and anterior tibialis), without evidence for OSA. His periodic leg movement index during sleep was 80 per hour, but movement arousals were only 3 per hour.

He was diagnosed with idiopathic/isolated RBD and started on melatonin 3 mg, with instructions to titrate biweekly to 6 to 12 mg as needed and tolerated should violent parasomnia behaviors continue. He is worried, sharing that he read on the Internet several articles about the risk of this disease becoming a form of PD. He dug further into his family background and learned that his paternal uncle developed PD in his mid-60s, with eventual development of dementia and death at age 77.

At 3 months clinical follow-up, this patient's sleep behaviors were infrequent, perhaps occurring only once per month, on melatonin 6 mg nightly. He had no adverse effects of sleepiness, drowsiness, or dizziness with treatment. Serial annual neurological examinations remains normal for the next 3 years, but in year 4, he showed a subtle degree of cogwheel rigidity in his right arm on examination, a "soft sign" of parkinsonism, in the absence of resting tremor, postural instability, or bradykinesia.

Comment

This is a very typical clinical history, exam, and polysomnography findings for the diagnosis of idiopathic/isolated RBD. A personal history of other nonmotor or even motor features of parkinsonism may be seen at presentation and should be sought in the history and examination. A family history of another Lewy body disease is not uncommon. Symptomatic treatment for injury prevention with melatonin 3 to 12 mg or clonazepam 0.5 to 2.0 mg (with melatonin preferred in most elderly patients given equivalent efficacy and superior tolerability), and annual neurological history and examination in follow-up are indicated to monitor for evolving features of a Lewy body disorder (i.e., PD, DLB, or MSA). Prognostic counseling remains difficult, but current evidence suggests lifetime risk for phenoconversion is 70% or greater, with an approximate 6% per year risk following the diagnosis of RBD for developing PD or DLB.

KEY CLINICAL PEARLS

- Parasomnias are classified as NREM or REM sleep parasomnias.
- The NREM parasomnias are disorders of arousal in which an incomplete or abortive arousal from NREM sleep leads to abnormal cognitive and motor behaviors including confusional arousals, sleep terrors, sleep walking, and SREDs.
- The REM parasomnias include RBD, nightmare disorder, and recurrent isolated sleep paralysis.
- RBD is strongly associated with the alpha synucleinopathy neurodegenerative diseases, including PD, DLB, and MSA.
- The diagnostic workup for the parasomnias includes a through history and physical examination, and video polysomnography for RBD and selected cases of NREM parasomnia.
- Provoking causes of arousal from NREM sleep and important sleep comorbidities such as OSA and PLMD should be sought and treated appropriately to reduce the frequency and severity of parasomnia behaviors, especially for the NREM disorders of arousal.
- The NREM parasomnias and RBD may both be treated symptomatically with clonazepam 0.5 to 2 mg nightly (or other shorter acting benzodiazepines such as lorazepam or triazolam), and RBD also appears to benefit from melatonin 3 to 12 mg nightly.
- Nightmare disorder may benefit from dream image rehearsal therapy, hypnosis, and other behavioral strategies, discontinuation of any precipitating medications, and diagnosis and treatment of mental health comorbidities.

SELF-ASSESSMENT QUESTIONS

1. Which of the following clinical characteristics is a usual feature of NREM sleep-related parasomnia?
   a. Onset after age 60 years
   b. Highly stereotypic clinical behaviors
   c. Occurrence in first third of night
   d. Second half of night predominance

Answer: c

2. Which of the following is most commonly seen during polysomnography in patients with NREM sleep-related parasomnias?
   a. Prominent respiratory arousals during NREM sleep
   b. Spontaneous arousals and rhythmic EEG slow waves
   c. Periodic leg movements of sleep
   d. Periodic limb movement disorder

Answer: b

3. Which of the following is considered as a first-line treatment for NREM parasomnia?
   a. Antidepressants
   b. Beta-blockers
   c. Clonazepam
   d. Dilaudid

Answer: c

4. Which of the following has been most strongly associated with REM sleep behavior disorder in adults under age 60?
   a. Antidepressants
   b. Beta-blockers
   c. Clonazepam
   d. Dilaudid

Answer: a

5. Which of the following is considered as a first-line treatment for REM sleep behavior disorder?
   a. Memantine
   b. Melatonin
   c. Mimosa
   d. Methylphenidate

Answer: b

REFERENCES

1. American Academy of Sleep Medicine. *International Classification of Sleep Disorders*. 3rd ed. Darien, IL: American Academy of Sleep Medicine, 2014.

2. Laberge L, Tremblay RE, Vitaro F, Montplaisir J. Development of parasomnias from childhood to early adolescence. *Pediatrics.* 2000;106:67–74.

3. Ohayon MM, Guilleminault C, Priest RG. Night terrors, sleepwalking, and confusional arousals in the general population: their frequency and relationship to other sleep and mental disorders. *J Clin Psychiatry.* 1999;60:268–276.

4. Ohayon MM, Mahowald MW, Leger D. Are confusional arousals pathological? *Neurology.* 2014;83:834–841.

5. Bargiotas P, Arnet I, Frei M, Baumann CR, Schindler K, Bassetti CL. Demographic, clinical and polysomnographic characteristics of childhood- and adult-onset sleepwalking in adults. *Eur Neurol.* 2017;78:307–311.

6. Stallman HM, Kohler M. Prevalence of sleepwalking: a systematic review and meta-analysis. *PLoS One.* 2016;11:e0164769.

7. Bjorvatn B, Gronli J, Pallesen S. Prevalence of different parasomnias in the general population. *Sleep Med.* 2010;11:1031–1034.

8. Petit D, Pennestri MH, Paquet J, et al. Childhood sleepwalking and sleep terrors: a longitudinal study of prevalence and familial aggregation. *JAMA Pediatr.* 2015;169:653–658.

9. Lam SP, Fong SY, Ho CK, Yu MW, Wing YK. Parasomnia among psychiatric outpatients: a clinical, epidemiologic, cross-sectional study. *J Clin Psychiatry.* 2008;69:1374–1382.

10. Ohayon MM, Mahowald MW, Dauvilliers Y, Krystal AD, Leger D. Prevalence and comorbidity of nocturnal wandering in the U.S. adult general population. *Neurology.* 2012;78:1583–1589.

11. Labelle MA, Desautels A, Montplaisir J, Zadra A. Psychopathologic correlates of adult sleepwalking. *Sleep Med.* 2013;14:1348–1355.

12. Ohayon MM, Schenck CH. Violent behavior during sleep: prevalence, comorbidity and consequences. *Sleep Med.* 2010;11:941–946.

13. Crisp AH. The sleepwalking/night terrors syndrome in adults. *Postgrad Med J.* 1996;72:599–604.

14. Schenck CH, Milner DM, Hurwitz TD, Bundlie SR, Mahowald MW. A polysomnographic and clinical report on sleep-related injury in 100 adult patients. *Am J Psychiatry.* 1989;146:1166–1173.

15. Szelenberger W, Niemcewicz S, Dabrowska AJ. Sleepwalking and night terrors: psychopathological and psychophysiological correlates. *Int Rev Psychiatry.* 2005;17:263–270.

16. Inoue Y. Sleep-related eating disorder and its associated conditions. *Psychiatry Clin Neurosci.* 2015;69:309–320.

17. Schenck CH, Hurwitz TD, Bundlie SR, Mahowald MW. Sleep-related eating disorders: polysomnographic correlates of a heterogeneous syndrome distinct from daytime eating disorders. *Sleep.* 1991;14:419–431.

18. Schenck CH, Hurwitz TD, O'Connor KA, Mahowald MW. Additional categories of sleep-related eating disorders and the current status of treatment. *Sleep.* 1993;16:457–466.

19. Winkelman JW, Herzog DB, Fava M. The prevalence of sleep-related eating disorder in psychiatric and non-psychiatric populations. *Psychol Med.* 1999;29:1461–1466.

20. Gibbs SA, Proserpio P, Terzaghi M, Pigorini A, Sarasso S, Lo Russo G, Tassi L, Nobili L. Sleep-related epileptic behaviors and non-REM-related parasomnias: insights from stereo-EEG. *Sleep Med Rev.* 2016;25:4–20.

21. Buskova J, Pisko J, Pastorek L, Sonka K. The course and character of sleepwalking in adulthood: a clinical and polysomnographic study. *Behav Sleep Med.* 2015;13:169–177.

22. Pressman MR. Factors that predispose, prime and precipitate NREM parasomnias in adults: clinical and forensic implications. *Sleep Med Rev.* 2007;11:5–30; discussion 31–33.

23. Stallman HM, Kohler M, White J. Medication induced sleepwalking: a systematic review. *Sleep Med Rev.* 2018;37:105–113.

24. von Vigier RO, Vella S, Bianchetti MG. Agitated sleepwalking with fluoroquinolone therapy. *Pediatr Infect Dis J.* 1999;18:484–485.

25. Lopez R, Jaussent I, Dauvilliers Y. Pain in sleepwalking: a clinical enigma. *Sleep.* 2015;38:1693–1698.

26. Giuliano L, Fatuzzo D, Mainieri G, La Vignera S, Sofia V, Zappia M. Adult-onset sleepwalking secondary to hyperthyroidism: polygraphic evidence. *J Clin Sleep Med.* 2019;14(2):285–287.

27. Heidbreder A, Frauscher B, Mitterling T, Boentert M, Schirmacher A, Hörtnagl P, Schennach H, Massoth C, Happe S, Mayer G, Young P, Högl B. Not only sleepwalking but NREM parasomnia irrespective of the type is associated with HLA DQB1*05:01. *J Clin Sleep Med.* 2016;12:565–570.

28. Horvath A, Papp A, Szucs A. Progress in elucidating the pathophysiological basis of nonrapid eye movement parasomnias: not yet informing therapeutic strategies. *Nat Sci Sleep.* 2016;8:73–79.

29. Licis AK, Desruisseau DM, Yamada KA, Duntley SP, Gurnett CA. Novel genetic findings in an extended family pedigree with sleepwalking. *Neurology.* 2011;76:49–52.

30. Kushida CA, Littner MR, Morgenthaler T, et al. Practice parameters for the indications for polysomnography and related procedures: an update for 2005. *Sleep.* 2005;28:499–521.

31. Kotagal S, Nichols CD, Grigg-Damberger MM, et al. Non-respiratory indications for

polysomnography and related procedures in children: an evidence-based review. *Sleep.* 2012;35:1451–1466.

32. Hauri PJ, Silber MH, Boeve BF. The treatment of parasomnias with hypnosis: a 5-year follow-up study. J Clin Sleep Med 2007;3:369–373.

33. Galbiati A, Rinaldi F, Giora E, Ferini-Strambi L, Marelli S. Behavioural and cognitive-behavioural treatments of parasomnias. *Behav Neurol.* 2015;2015:786928.

34. Hurwitz TD, Mahowald MW, Schenck CH, Schluter JL, Bundlie SR. A retrospective outcome study and review of hypnosis as treatment of adults with sleepwalking and sleep terror. *J Nerv Ment Dis.* 1991;179:228–233.

35. Larsen V, Sandness DJ, Richardson J, Boeve BF, Silber MH, St. Louis EK. Clinical characteristics and treatment outcomes of patients treated with hypnosis for parasomnias [Abstract]. *Sleep.* 2016;39(Suppl):A237.

36. Schenck CH, Mahowald MW. Long-term, nightly benzodiazepine treatment of injurious parasomnias and other disorders of disrupted nocturnal sleep in 170 adults. *Am J Med.* 1996;100:333–337.

37. Lillywhite AR, Wilson SJ, Nutt DJ. Successful treatment of night terrors and somnambulism with paroxetine. *Br J Psychiatry.* 1994;164:551–554.

38. Wilson SJ, Lillywhite AR, Potokar JP, Bell CJ, Nutt DJ. Adult night terrors and paroxetine. *Lancet.* 1997;350:185.

39. Balon R. Sleep terror disorder and insomnia treated with trazodone: a case report. *Ann Clin Psychiatry.* 1994;6:161–163.

40. Winkelman JW. Efficacy and tolerability of open-label topiramate in the treatment of sleep-related eating disorder: a retrospective case series. *J Clin Psychiatry.* 2006;67:1729–1734.

41. Provini F, Albani F, Vetrugno R, Vignatelli L, Lombardi C, Plazzi G, Montagna P. A pilot double-blind placebo-controlled trial of low-dose pramipexole in sleep-related eating disorder. *Eur J Neurol.* 2005;12:432–436.

42. Zapp AA, Fischer EC, Deuschle M. The effect of agomelatine and melatonin on sleep-related eating: a case report. *J Med Case Rep.* 2017;11:275.

43. Morgenthaler TI, Auerbach S, Casey KR, et al. Position paper for the treatment of nightmare disorder in adults: an American Academy of Sleep Medicine position paper. *J Clin Sleep Med.* 2018;14(6):1041–1055.

44. St. Louis EK, Boeve BF. REM sleep behavior disorder: diagnosis, clinical implications, and future directions. *Mayo Clin Proc.* 2017;92(11):1723–1736.

45. Postuma RB, Iranzo A, Hu M, et al. Risk and predictors of dementia and parkinsonism in idiopathic REM sleep behaviour disorder: a multicentre study. *Brain.* 2019;142(3):744–759.

46. Gaig C, Graus F, Compta Y, et al. Clinical manifestations of the anti-IgLON5 disease. *Neurology.* 2017;88:1736–1743.

47. Sabater L, Gaig C, Gelpi E, et al. A novel non-rapid-eye movement and rapid-eye-movement parasomnia with sleep breathing disorder associated with antibodies to IgLON5: a case series, characterisation of the antigen, and post-mortem study. *Lancet Neurol.* 2014;13:575–586.

48. Tobin WO, Lennon VA, Komorowski L, et al. DPPX potassium channel antibody: frequency, clinical accompaniments, and outcomes in 20 patients. *Neurology.* 2014;83:1797–1803.

49. Mahowald MW, Schenck CH. Status dissociatus: a perspective on states of being. *Sleep.* 1991;14:69–79.

50. Antelmi E, Ferri R, Iranzo A, et al. From state dissociation to status dissociatus. *Sleep Med Rev.* 2016;28:5–17.

51. Stamelou M, Plazzi G, Lugaresi E, Edwards MJ, Bhatia KP. The distinct movement disorder in anti-NMDA receptor encephalitis may be related to Status Dissociatus: a hypothesis. *Mov Disord.* 2012;27:1360–1363.

52. Vetrugno R, Alessandria M, D'Angelo R, et al. Status dissociatus evolving from REM sleep behaviour disorder in multiple system atrophy. *Sleep Med.* 2009;10:247–252.

53. Montagna P, Lugaresi E. Agrypnia excitata: a generalized overactivity syndrome and a useful concept in the neurophysiopathology of sleep. *Clin Neurophysiol.* 2002;113:552–560.

54. Lugaresi E, Provini F. Agrypnia excitata: clinical features and pathophysiological implications. *Sleep Med Rev.* 2001;5:313–322.

55. Guaraldi P, Calandra-Buonaura G, Terlizzi R, et al. Oneiric stupor: the peculiar behaviour of agrypnia excitata. *Sleep Med.* 2011;12 Suppl 2:S64–S67.

56. Kushida CA, Littner MR, Morgenthaler T, et al. Practice parameters for the indications for polysomnography and related procedures: an update for 2005. *Sleep.* 2005; 28:499–521.

57. Lapid MI, Burton MC, Chang MT, Rummans TA, Cha SS, Leavitt JA, Boeve BF. Clinical phenomenology and mortality in Charles Bonnet syndrome. *J Geriatr Psychiatry Neurol.* 2013;26(1):3–9.

13

Circadian Rhythm Sleep Disorders

GREGORY M. BROWN, SEITHIKURIPPU R. PANDI-PERUMAL,
AND DANIEL P. CARDINALI

INTRODUCTION

Circadian rhythm sleep disorders (CRSDs) are characterized by disturbances in sleep and wakefulness resulting from a misalignment between the timing of the body's intrinsic circadian clock with environmental light/day and social activity cycles. The key objectives of this chapter are to review the clinical features, pathophysiology, and treatment of CRSDs with circadian rhythm adjustment techniques, including light therapy and melatonin, and to discuss their relationship with psychiatric disorders.

Circadian rhythms exist in almost all body and brain functions including neurochemical and hormonal processes.[1,2] Moreover, circadian rhythms permit the organism to prepare for anticipated circadian events. As an example, before daily waking, there are rises in plasma cortisol, sympathetic tone, and body temperature that prepare the organism for postural change and increased activities that are associated with wakefulness.

The two-process model of sleep regulation which is currently widely accepted is conceptually useful.[3] The model postulates that a homeostatic process (Process S), which is a pressure for sleep, interacts with a process controlled by the circadian pacemaker (Process C), with the resulting time-courses derived from both physiological and behavioral variables.

The individuals with CRSDs may go to sleep (as in delayed sleep–wake phase syndrome [DSPD]) or wake up (as in advanced sleep–wake phase syndrome [ASPD]) at their intrinsic time while simultaneously meeting their social obligations. This can result in a significant reduction in sleep duration due to earlier wake up than the circadian rhythm determined wake up time in DSPD and later bedtime than the circadian rhythm determined bedtime in ASPD. Adequate duration of sleep is necessary to restore energy and repair DNA damage.[4,5] Major industrial, air, and train accidents have been attributed to the decrement in alertness

due to cognitive impairment caused by sleep loss in a CRSD (see Chapter 5). Improper entrainment of the body clock due to factors such as nocturnal light exposure, unusual timing of food, irregular sleep/wake schedules and traveling between different time zones have been linked to numerous disorders including diabetes,[6] obesity,[7] metabolic syndrome,[8] cancer,[9] and cardiovascular disease.[10,11]

Disturbances in circadian rhythms are found in many patients with psychiatric disorders including bipolar disorder, major depressive disorder and schizophrenia.[12–17] The close relationship between the circadian rhythm and psychiatric disorders has led to the notion that chronobiologic treatment of the rhythm disturbances could be a helpful strategy in treating psychiatric disorders.

DIAGNOSTIC CLASSIFICATION

The fifth edition of the *Diagnostic and Statistical Manual* (DSM-5) of the American Psychiatric Association lists five disorders under the heading CRSDs: delayed sleep phase type, advanced sleep phase type, irregular sleep–wake type, non-24-hour sleep–wake type (N24), and shift work type (night).[18] Missing from this list is jet lag disorder, a disorder listed in the third edition of the *International Classification of Sleep Disorders*, a diagnostic manual widely used by sleep physicians in their clinical practice.[19] The diagnostic criteria used in these two manuals are similar.

Diagnostic criteria for CRSDs as listed in the DSM-5 are

- A persistent or recurrent pattern of sleep disruption that is primarily due to an alteration of the circadian system or to a misalignment between the endogenous circadian rhythm and the sleep-wake schedule required by an individual's physical environment or social or professional schedule.

- Sleep disruption that leads to excessive sleepiness, insomnia, or both.
- The sleep disturbance causes clinically significant distress or impairment in social, occupational, and other important areas of functioning.[18,20]

CIRCADIAN RHYTHMS: BASIC PHYSIOLOGY

Circadian rhythm regulation is reviewed in Chapter 4. Briefly, the mechanisms regulating body clocks exist in majority of the cells in the body, and most tissues are capable of independent cycling.[1,21,22] The suprachiasmatic nuclei (SCN) in the anterior hypothalamus contains the master circadian (close to 24 hours) clock that coordinates all of these body clocks along with the sleep–wake cycle through a combination of neural and hormonal links.[23–25]

Because the SCN produces a daily rhythm that is close to 24 hours, the SCN rhythm needs regular synchronization to optimize adaptation to the external environment of daily activity.[26] Light provides this synchronization to the SCN, and this process is known as entrainment. Light input is via the retinohypothalamic tract, which originates in a tiny group of intrinsically photosensitive retinal ganglion cells (IPRGCs) that are only sensitive to blue light and contain the photopigment melanopsin.[27–29] IPRGCs do not send visual information but provide a signal of the presence of light to cue the SCN rhythm to the light cycle and also to send an alerting signal to other brain areas.

The pineal gland synthesizes melatonin that acts as a major circadian rhythm signal. The pineal gland is under the control of the SCN via a complex indirect multisynaptic pathway that projects to the superior cervical ganglia which then sends postganglionic fibers to the pineal gland.[30] Although many tissues synthesize melatonin, virtually all circulating hormone comes from the pineal gland.[31] Melatonin is a highly lipophilic and pleotropic hormone that readily penetrates tissues. Once produced, melatonin is immediately released into the CSF and blood stream.

Melatonin can be readily measured in blood, saliva, or urine to provide a profile of its secretion. Melatonin levels typically begin to rise shortly before the onset of darkness, continue rising for about six hours, and then fall. It is virtually nonexistent in blood during the daytime. The melatonin profile is used as an index of the bodies' circadian phase, commonly by measurements obtained by sampling saliva or blood melatonin levels under dim light conditions during the expected rise time (dim light melatonin onset [DLMO]).[30]

There are numerous targets for melatonin.[31] These include two G protein-linked membrane receptors (MT_1 and MT_2) that subserve rhythm regulation widely in the brain and body as well as in the SCN itself where they provide a feedback loop. There is a third receptor G protein-coupled receptor 50 (GPR50), sharing 45% of the amino acid sequence with MT_1 and MT_2, but does not bind melatonin. While GPR50 has no effect on MT2 function, GPR50 prevents MT_1 from binding melatonin. Certain polymorphisms of the GPR50 gene in Scottish females has been associated with increased risk of developing bipolar affective disorder and major depressive disorder.[32]

DIAGNOSTIC TOOLS

Prior to diagnostic procedures, it is important to assess the degree of variability of the patient's sleep–wake schedule on workdays versus work free days, which can cause variability in the light/dark schedule that may go beyond correction by the circadian system if it is large. The variability in exposure to artificial light in the evenings and in the schedule on work free days should be minimized to less than three hours per week to prevent errors due to such schedule changes.[33]

Current diagnostic guidelines from the American Academy of Sleep Medicine recommend obtaining sleep logs for at least 7 and preferably 14 days, along with actigraphy monitoring for assessment of patients with a suspected CRSD.[34] Actigraphs are devices generally worn on the wrist (although they can also be placed on the ankle or trunk) to record movement over a period of time. Collected data are downloaded to a computer for display and analysis of activity/inactivity that, in turn, can be further analyzed to estimate wake/sleep.[35] Actigraphy should be performed in unrestricted conditions so the sleep–wake pattern represent patient's native rhythm rather than one imposed by societal demands.

Although not commonly used in clinical settings, the DLMO is currently the best single marker of circadian rhythms in humans.[36] It can assist both with diagnosis and with timing of circadian-based treatments. It has been shown that home kits can be used successfully for this purpose.[36] It is unfortunate that most clinics do not yet have the DLMO. It has been slow to be widely accepted despite strong recommendations. This is possibly because of the inconvenience and expense of repeated melatonin measurements or simply because of inertia.[37] To test for the DLMO, seven hourly samples of saliva or serum are collected for melatonin assay beginning at

5 PM under dim light conditions (10–30 lux).[38] Alternatively, the timing of sampling may bracket the individual's habitual bedtime.[39,40] The time at which melatonin levels in serum rise above 10 pg/ml (3 pg/ml in saliva) is usually defined as the individual's DLMO.[38] In the absence of DLMO testing or as a supplement, circadian questionnaires can be used that document daily profiles including sleep.[41] One such questionnaire is the Morningness–Eveningness Questionnaire (MEQ) that generates a chronotype score. Chronotype is basically an individual's preference to be a night owl or early bird or neutral type. Another one is the Munich ChronoType Questionnaire (MCTQ).[42] There is a good but not perfect agreement between these three measures (DLMO, MEQ, and MCTQ). Furthermore, in the absence of formal testing for the DLMO, the DLMO could be estimated to occur on average 2.5 hours before habitual or natural bedtime.[33]

TREATMENTS

The predominant treatments that can remove misalignment between bodily circadian rhythms and

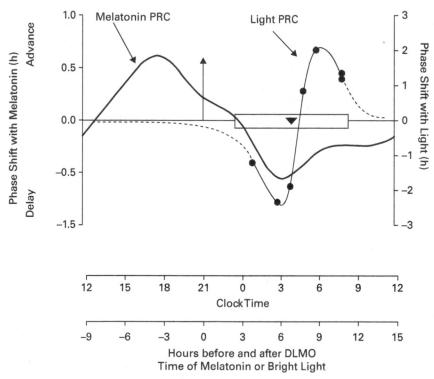

FIGURE 13.1. The light PRC was generated from seven subjects who free-ran through about 3 days (73.5 hours) of an ultradian LD cycle (2.5 hours wake in dim light <100 lux alternating with 1.5 hours sleep in dark; Eastman and Burgess, unpublished data). Subjects lived on the ultradian schedule on two different occasions, once with bright light pulses, about 3,500 lux, for 2 hours at the same time each day, and once without bright light pulses, counterbalanced. Phase shifts of the midpoint of the melatonin rhythm collected in dim light (<5 lux) before and after the 3 days were plotted against the time of the light pulse relative to each subject's baseline dim light melatonin onset (DLMO) and corrected for the free run when the bright light was not applied. Upward arrow: average baseline DLMO, rectangle: average baseline sleep schedule, triangle: estimated time of body temperature minimum (DLMO+ 7 hours). The solid line is a smoothed curve fit to the 7 points. The melatonin phase response curve was calculated from the data of Lewy et al. (1998). Subjects ($n = 6$), living at home, took 0.5 mg melatonin at the same time each day for 4 days. Phase shifts of the DLMO were plotted against the time of melatonin administration relative to each subject's baseline DLMO. A smoothed curve was fit to the data after averaging the 70 data points into 3-hour bins. Figure from Revell and Eastman, Journal of Biological Rhythms, Vol. 20(4), 2005, pp 353–365, © 2005 Sage Publications, Reprinted by Permission of SAGE Publications, Inc.

the external environment are light and melatonin. Hence, light and melatonin are called chronobiotics. Both light and melatonin affect circadian rhythms in a unique fashion known as a phase response curve (PRC). The phasing conditions for both bright light and melatonin treatments have been well worked out based on these PRCs.[33,43]

When administered in the evening, light produces phase delays while when administered in the morning, it causes phase advances.[44] In contrast, melatonin treatment acts on the MT_1 and MT_2 receptors in the SCN to produce a PRC that is the inverse of PRC for light, being about 12 hours out of phase with light.[43,45] A detailed PRC for melatonin (3 mg) established that the maximum advance portion peaks about five hours before DLMO; the maximum delay portion is about 11 hours after DLMO, which is shortly after habitual awakening and a dead zone is in the first half of usual sleep.[46]

Light therapy is typically given via a light box administered for 30 to 60 minutes per day with the patient seated close to the light so that the intensity is approximately 10,000 lux.[33] The timing of bright light treatment (BLT) is derived from use of the DLMO.[43] In the absence of DLMO information, habitual sleep and wake times may be used.[33] Light in the evening prior to habitual bedtime and for a few hours thereafter will cause a phase delay; in contrast, light exposure within 3 hours before habitual wake up time as well as for several more hours afterwards will cause a phase advance. The switch from phase delays to phase advance on average is about three hours before habitual wake up time.

Because of inconvenience of light treatment leading to reduced adherence, alternatives are being examined, including a light visor with a light above the eye (myluminette.com) and a device similar to glasses with a light below the eye (Retimer.com).[36] As lightweight wearable devices, they are far more convenient and are likely to be more acceptable. Early studies using blue light to cause phase changes have also been done.[47,48] In addition, other studies have provided preliminary

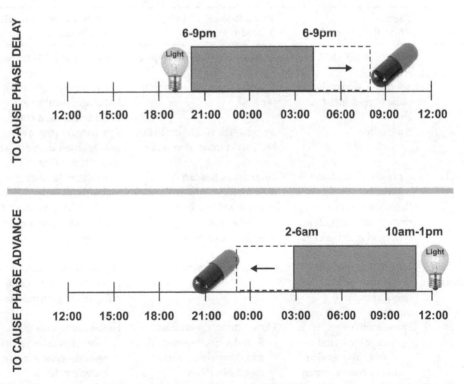

FIGURE 13.2. Times for scheduling the phase resetting agents, bright light and melatonin, are based on their phase response curves (PRCs). The PRCs for bright light and low-dose melatonin (see text and Figure 13.1) provide the best times to schedule these phase-resetting agents, according to clinical experience as well as by the time provided by the dim light melatonin onset (DLMO) if it is available in a given patient. The crossover times between advance and delay zones for the bright light PRC are around 6 to 8 hours before and 4 hours after the DLMO. Timing for melatonin is about 12 hours out of phase with bright light. Examples are shown in the figure.

evidence that flashes of light may be effective in phase resetting.[49,50] One or more of these alternative approaches may eventually be adopted as standard treatment(s).

BLT can be associated with side effects including headaches, eye strain, nausea, and agitation, which often disappear over time.[51,52] A rare but serious side effect is the development of mania in some patients with bipolar illness who overexpose to bright light.[51,52] A recent review of 10 studies concluded that BLT can be effective for bipolar patients when given between noon and 2 PM, potentially treating phase delays and thus preventing relapse as well as being unlikely to precipitate mania.[53] Potential contraindications are migraine precipitated by light, existing eye disease and use of phototoxic medication.[33]

With the discovery that blue light is the most active wavelength of the visible light spectrum with regards to the light's circadian phase effects, blue blocking glasses have recently been explored

as therapeutic tools that can impede both the alerting effect and the melatonin suppression caused by evening light.[54,55]

Melatonin and other melatonergic drugs have minimal side effects in most people (see Table 13.1 and 13.2).[36] With a short half-life of about 45 minutes, doses of 3 mg or less of oral melatonin produce a short-lived pulse that is not sedating and is ideal as a cue. With such small doses, morning drowsiness is very rare, probably occurring only in slow metabolizers. Higher doses can yield such a prolonged effect that may not provide a pulse. Doses from 0.3 to 1 mg of melatonin attain "physiological" melatonin blood levels and when administered prior to sleep onset reduce sleep latency and increase sleep efficiency in healthy human subjects.[56] However, in most studies, higher amounts of melatonin (2–6 mg) have been given to obtain similar effects (probably unnecessarily high).[57] Doses of 0.02 mg and 0.3 mg can synchronize circadian rhythms in blind

TABLE 13.1 CHARACTERISTICS OF DIFFERENT FORMULATIONS OF MELATONIN

Type	Regular (immediate release)	Timed Release (Circadin®)	Over the Counter (Regular and Timed Release)
Class	Agonist at MT_1/MT_2 receptors	Agonist at MT_1/MT_2 receptors	Agonist at MT_1/MT_2 receptors
Action	Short half-life produces a pulse to reset melatonin rhythm	Mimics nocturnal melatonin profiles	If content too high or low, may last longer than normal or fail to achieve desired effect
Dose	3 mg or less	2 mg tablet 1 to 2 hours before bedtime in those 55 years or over	5 or 10 mg, variable as not regulated except those submitted to FDA
Side effects	Drowsiness, headache, nightmares	Drowsiness, headache, nightmares	Drowsiness, headache, nightmares
Uses	Resetting circadian rhythm may help sleep onset and maintenance,	Helps sleep onset and maintenance in the aged who have decreased nocturnal melatonin	May help with insomnia and sleep onset depending on type and actual dose
Contra-indications	Hepatic impairment, pregnancy, breastfeeding, safety in children unknown	Hepatic impairment	Hepatic impairment, pregnancy, breast feeding, safety in children unknown
Interactions	Fluvoxamine, cimetidine 5- and 8- methoxypsoralen and estrogens increase melatonin levels Possible warfarin interaction	Fluvoxamine, cimetidine, 5- and 8- methoxypsoralen and estrogens increase melatonin levels Possible warfarin interaction	Fluvoxamine, cimetidine, 5- and 8-methoxypsoralen and estrogens increase melatonin levels Possible warfarin interaction
Source(s) of information	Burgess and Emens 2016, Herxheimer et al 2002	Burgess and Emens 2016, EMA assessment	Burgess and Emens 2016

EMA = European Medicines Agency; FDA = US Food and Drug Administration.

TABLE 13.2 COMPARISON OF MELATONERGIC DRUGS

Drug	Agomelatine (Valdoxan®)	Ramelteon (Rozerem®)	Tasimelteon (Hetlioz®)
Class	Agonist at MT_1/MT_2 receptors antagonist at 5HT2C receptors	Agonist at MT_1/MT_2 receptors	Agonist at MT_1/MT_2 receptors
Action	Acts on sleep and anhedonia within one week and may work for years	Decreases sleep onset latency and increases sleep time	Resets circadian rhythms to synchronize sleep–wake cycle
Dose	25 to 50 mg at bedtime with precautionary liver function tests repeated regularly	8 mg 30 minutes prior to bedtime, take without food	20 mg at bedtime; effect may take weeks or months
Side Effects	Increased transaminase, rarely hepatitis, liver failure, rare angioedema	Mild nausea and dizziness, behavioral changes rare respiratory depression	Headache nightmares high amino-transferase infection of urinary tract or upper respiratory tract
Uses	Major depressive disorder generalized anxiety disorder if no history of bipolar disorder	Insomnia especially with sleep onset	Non-24-hour sleep–wake Disorder
Contra-indications	Hepatic impairment pregnancy, breast feeding, safety in those under 18 unknown	Hepatic impairment in those over 75; those over 65 may have greater side effects	Use in pregnancy only if essential; safety in children unknown
Interactions	Increased by fluvoxamine, ciprofloxacin and estrogens; rifampicin decreases levels	Increased by fluvoxamine, ketoconazole, doxepin and donepezil, rifampin decreases ramelteon	Strong CYP1A2 inhibitors and CYP3A4 inducers
Source(s) of information	EMA assessment report	FDA prescribing information	FDA prescribing information

EMA = European Medicines Agency; FDA = US Food and Drug Administration.

individuals.[58] Melatonin sold as a natural health product, claiming 3 to 10 mg doses of melatonin, may have a highly variable content of melatonin with some products also containing serotonin.[59] Some suppliers participate in a USP-verified program establishing the purity and dosage of their products.[33,36]

Circadin® (Neurim Pharmaceuticals), a prolonged release 2 mg melatonin formulation that mimics the natural nocturnal profile of melatonin has been certified by the European Medicines Agency as monotherapy for the short-term treatment of primary insomnia characterized by poor quality of sleep in patients aged 55 or over.

Rozerem (Ramelteon©, Takeda Pharmaceuticals), a MT_1 and MT_2 receptor agonist with long acting melatonergic action, is certified by the US Food and Drug Administration (FDA) for the treatment of insomnia characterized by difficulty with sleep onset.

Agomelatine (Valdoxan©, Melitor©, Thymanax©; Servier Pharmaceuticals), a MT_1 and MT_2 receptor agonist with long-acting melatonergic action combined with 5-HT2C antagonism, is approved by the European Medicines Agency for treatment of major depressive disorder (MDD). The melatonergic function is intended to improve sleep patterns, whereas the serotonergic antagonism is supposed to cause release of norepinephrine and dopamine to improve mood. Because it may cause hepatic impairment, it is necessary to check hepatic function before initiating treatment, and at intervals during treatment.[60] It is contraindicated in those with pre-existing hepatic disease and must be discontinued if it develops.

Tasimelteon (Hetlioz©; Vanda Pharmaceuticals), a short-acting MT$_1$ and MT$_2$ agonist that, like melatonin, provides a short lived melatonergic pulse, is approved by the FDA for treatment of non-24 hour sleep–wake disorder (N24) in the totally blind.[61]

The Clinical Practice Guidelines (CPGs) of the American Academy of Sleep Medicine for the treatment of intrinsic circadian rhythm sleep–wake disorders were published in 2015,[37] and then an updated review was published.[36] Evidence for treatments was generally weak, and there is a clear need for more clinical trials.[36]

DELAYED SLEEP PHASE DISORDER (DSPD)

In DSPD, there is a pattern of delayed sleep onset and awakening times with an inability to fall asleep and to wake up at a desired or conventionally acceptable earlier time. Habitual sleep and wake times are between two and six hours later than the normal or socially desired ones. Those with DSPD have difficulty falling asleep as well as difficulty waking up, so that when awakened at an earlier time than their spontaneous awakening, they are tired; when allowed to sleep until spontaneous awakening, they may exhibit normal sleep quality and duration for age.[18] When consistent awakening as socially necessary is coupled with a late bedtime, it can lead to short sleep time resulting in impaired cognitive function, excessive daytime sleepiness, irritable mood and reduced quality of life, and potentially reduce life prospects.[62,63] DSPD can masquerade as insomnia disorder. The main differences between these conditions are (i) patients with insomnia disorder are unable to fall asleep at their usual bedtimes commonly due to ruminative thinking while patients with DSPD just don't feel sleepy until later times like 2 AM to 6 AM; (ii) patients with insomnia disorder find it difficult to initiate sleep whenever they go to bed while patients with DSPD have no problem initiating sleep at a later bedtime; and (iii) patients with insomnia disorder start feeling sleepy outside of bed (when their internal circadian alertness signal goes down) but get a second wind when they lay down in bed. In contrast, when DSPD patients naturally start feeling sleepy, they do not get a second wind when they go to bed unless there is a comorbid insomnia disorder, which can certainly happen in some cases. Similarly, excessive daytime sleepiness experienced by patients with DSPD due to imposed early morning awakening, and resultant sleep deprivation may be mislabeled as hypersomnia disorder and result in unnecessary use of psychostimulants, which may further delay their circadian rhythm.[64] Therefore, it is vitally important to distinguish insomnia and hypersomnia disorders (primary and comorbid) from delayed sleep phase syndrome.

DSPD, the most common CRSD, has an estimated prevalence between 0.2% and 10% of the population.[65] There is a significant variability in prevalence between clinical samples, with those presenting with insomnia symptoms having highest prevalence rates (7%–16%)[19,62] while, in contrast, survey studies in the general population report much lower prevalence estimates (below 1.5%) likely because no strict diagnostic criteria can be applied as is done in clinical populations and also because only the more severe cases present to the clinic.[66,67] Survey prevalence rates in the adolescent population tend to be higher (see following discussion); however, these studies also lack strict diagnostic criteria.[68-71]

The DSM-5 identifies two subtypes of DSPD—a familial type and one that overlaps with N24.[18] There are several possible explanations regarding the etiology of nonfamilial DSPD, including alterations in circadian rhythm regulation along with behavioral, cognitive, personality, and emotional factors.[72]

The long-known familial type of the disorder has been thought to be due to genetic factors with a variety of theories on the cause.[72] A missense variation in the clock gene PER3 has been reported to be a risk factor[73] and was substantiated in some studies,[74,75] but in other studies, some probands were unaffected.[76-78] Recently, a mutation of the CRY1 gene (CRY1 D11 variant) was identified in a number of patients who display circadian rhythm abnormalities consistent with an intrinsic delayed circadian rhythm including a DLMO delayed about 5.5 hours with a subset reporting fragmented sleep.[79]

An important external cause of delayed sleep phase is environmental light, the predominant cue for circadian rhythms. Our modern society uses artificial light extensively, extending daytime into the evening with a resultant change in sleep–wake patterns.[80-82] Moreover, television, e-readers, computers, and smartphones are frequently used late into the evening.[54,83] Adolescents and young adults who are especially frequent users of smartphones and e-readers have a higher prevalence in population survey studies of DSPD.[54,69,84] This practice has become so widespread, especially among youth that it has been labeled as "cell phone addiction"[85] with consequences like sleep phase delay and sleep deprivation.

For the diagnosis of DSPD, a detailed history, sleep logs, and/or actigraphy are recommended for at least seven days (preferably 14 days). Salivary DLMO and morningness/eveningness questionnaires can provide supplementary information.

Treatment of DSPD focuses on advancing the delayed rhythm.[34,36] The CPGs weak recommendation for treating adults, children, and adolescents is with strategically timed melatonin and post awakening light therapy combined with behavioral treatments. In adults, low doses of melatonin given 2 to 5 hours before DLMO have been used successfully to cause phase advance.[86,87] The treatment with bright light could also be attempted in adults with DSPD for which various protocols have been proposed. One such protocol is for the patient to use BLT at his or her spontaneous wake up time for 30 minutes for two days and then begin advancing BLT and wake up time by 30 minutes daily until desired wake-up timing is achieved. After desired wake-up timing is achieved, BLT can be discontinued with enforcement of desired wake-up time on daily basis. If there is relapse of delayed sleep phase after discontinuing BLT, the BLT can be reintroduced and used in the same way as the first time.[88]

ADVANCED SLEEP PHASE DISORDER (ASPD)

ASPD is characterized by preferentially advanced sleep onset and wake up times as compared to socially conventional times. Those with ASPD typically report average sleep onset at 6 to 9 PM with a wake up time of 2 to 5 AM. As with DSPD, if they sleep during preferred times, the quality and duration of sleep are normal for age.[19] There is a familial subtype of this condition described in the DSM-5.[18,89]

Prevalence estimates of ASPD are lower than those of DSPD.[66,67] In a survey of 10,000 adult Norwegians, no cases were identified using questionnaires based in the 10th edition of the *International Classification of Sleep Disorders* while 0.17% of that population had DSPD.[66] In a survey of 9,100 adults in New Zealand using the MCTQ supplemented with additional information, prevalence estimates of ASPD were 0.25% to 7.13% while those for DSPD were 1.51% to 8.90% depending on the definition used.[67]

Several familial groups have been identified but to date only two different mutations have been implicated. The first mutation identified was in the phosphorylation site for PER2[89,90]; another is a missense mutation in the CK1 delta gene, which alters phosphorylation activity.[91,92]

Both alterations decrease phosphorylation, which stabilizes PER2 so that transcription–translation increases, resulting in a shortened circadian period. There are several other familial groups with ASPD that have no known genetic cause.

For establishing the diagnosis of ASPD, it is recommended that sleep logs and/or actigraphy be done for at least seven days. In addition, salivary DLMO and morningness/eveningness questionnaires can be helpful in supporting the diagnosis of ASPD but are not recommended to establish the diagnosis

The CPGs treatment recommendation is for evening bright light therapy (at least 5000 lux for 2 hours; e.g. 7–9 PM) in adults with ASPD with the objective of delaying the circadian phase.[37] There is limited evidence to support the use of melatonin or melatonergic analogs in treatment of ASPD.[93]

NON-24 HOUR SLEEP–WAKE RHYTHM DISORDER

Diagnosis of N24 is based primarily on a history of symptoms of insomnia or excessive sleepiness related to abnormal synchronization between the 24-hour light–dark cycle and the endogenous circadian rhythm.[18] Individuals typically present with periods of insomnia, excessive sleepiness, or both, which alternate with short asymptomatic periods. In N24, the intrinsic sleep–wake cycle is not entrained/synchronized with the extrinsic light–dark cycle. This results in progressive delay in sleep–wake pattern each day as the native circadian rhythm usually has a period longer than 24 hours. The symptoms emerge when the intrinsic circadian period fall out of alignment with the external 24-hour light/dark cycle.

Originally diagnosed in those with no light perception, it is now also reported in some individuals with normal vision. Blind individuals with N24 presumably fail to receive the appropriate retinal signals to the SCN.[25,29] In a study of absolutely blind women aged 50.8 ± 13.4 years, the majority showed abnormally phased (24%) or not entrained (39%) urinary 6-suphatoxymelatonin patterns while the minority (37%) were normally entrained.[94] In contrast, the majority of those with some degree of light perception were normally entrained (69%). The underlying cause of N24 in the sighted individuals is uncertain, whether it is due to decreased or absent sensitivity of the appropriate signals or possibly a longer circadian rhythm[34]; although lengthened circadian rhythm due to a mutated *CRY1* gene in familial delayed sleep disorder revealed no probands with N24.[79]

Again, the recommendation for diagnosis is a sleep log and/ or actigraphy for at least seven days (up to 14 days). Sequential measurement of phase markers (e.g. urinary 6-sulphatoxymelatonin) or DLMO can be helpful.[34]

The CPGs recommendation is to use strategically timed melatonin for treatment of N24.[37] However, the drug Hetlioz® (tasimelteon) was approved for treatment of N24 by the FDA in late 2013.[61,95] Unlike melatonin, it is available as a prescription drug, and therefore its quality is tightly regulated, although it is much more expensive. However, it should be noted that melatonin, an over-the-counter drug, has been repeatedly reported to be effective for treatment of N24.[96–101] To our knowledge, no head-to-head comparison of tasimelteon and melatonin has yet been published. Timed light exposure may be an option in sighted individuals with N24 based on anecdotal evidence.[39]

IRREGULAR SLEEP–WAKE DISORDER

The DSM-5 diagnosis of CRSD, irregular sleep–wake type is based on symptoms of insomnia at night (during the usual sleep period) and excessive sleepiness (with multiple napping intervals) during the day. This type is characterized by a lack of discernible sleep–wake circadian rhythm. There is no major sleep period, and sleep is fragmented into at least three periods during the 24-hour period.[18,20]

The prevalence is unknown, but it is more common in later life. It can be due to a problem in the central pacemaker or interference with the normal melatonin signaling pathway.[34] It may accompany disorders such as Alzheimer's disease, Parkinson's disease, Huntington's disease, traumatic brain injury, and neurodevelopmental disorders in children. Another possible cause is decreased exposure to external cues like light (e.g. in those with aging-related visual disorders like cataracts), which, combined with limited structured activities, may decrease the rhythmic stimulation necessary to counteract the circadian irregularity.[102] There may also be a genetic component in some, as a small subset of those with a variation in clock gene CRY1, usually associated with DSPD, were affected with fragmented sleep at night and napping during the daytime.[79]

Diagnostic markers are sleep history and sleep diaries (completed by caregivers) as well as actigraphy. The major recommended treatments for this disorder are melatonin in the evening and regular exposure to morning light and to social activities.[36]

SHIFT WORK DISORDER

As with other CRSDs, shift work issues arise from societal demands.[103] Diagnosis is primarily based on a history of the individual working outside of the normal 8 AM to 6 PM daytime window on a regularly scheduled (i.e., non-overtime) basis.[18] Symptoms of excessive sleepiness at work and impaired sleep at home on a persistent basis are prominent. Diagnosis requires the presence of both of these symptoms. Moreover, when switched to a normal daytime work schedule, symptoms usually disappear. Shift work is common with reports ranging from 15% to 25% of workers in various countries.[104]

Shift work may be of various types including permanent night shifts, early morning shifts, afternoon–evening shifts, and rotating shifts (rapid or slow; slow shift is >4 days per shift). Shift work also includes split shifts or irregular shifts, which are unpredictable.

Diagnosis is usually based on history. However, as in other types of CRSDS, actigraphy and sleep logs can be helpful. The Karolinska Sleepiness Scale may also be useful in providing a means of assessing the severity of sleepiness in shift work disorder.[105,106] It is a subjective 9-point sleepiness scale, with 1 being "very alert," 5 being "neither alert nor sleepy," and 9 being "very sleepy." Those affected with shift work disorder may have a shortened sleep duration, shorter sleep latency on the multiple sleep latency test, react more to novel stimuli, and have reduced brain responses to auditory stimuli.[107,108]

There are major differences in individual susceptibility. The causes of these differences have been the subject of a recent review.[34] Shift work disorder susceptibility is related to age, sex, and chronotype.[34] A genetic basis for susceptibility has been shown in some night shift workers. Those with a PER3 gene length polymorphism are more likely to be sleepy, and a common genetic variation near the MT_1 gene is linked to job-related exhaustion in shift workers.[109]

Shift workers are liable to have various disorders related to difficulties in daily functioning. They are more likely to use alcohol in excess, and have substance abuse and depression.[110] Shift work can make relationships with family and friends more difficult.[100] Marital problems may also arise leading to divorce.[111]

There is a higher risk of near-crash driving incidents following a night shift.[112] There is also a reported higher incidence of excessive sleepiness and poor daytime sleep quality in nighttime bus drivers.[113] Relationship between shift work and both sickness and absence due to work-related accidents has been reported.[114,115] Shift workers have a higher risk of a host of physical disorders including diabetes, obesity, cardiovascular disease, and cancer.[6,7,9,116–118] A recent study demonstrated that the shift workers, with lower levels of circulating melatonin during night work as compared with night sleep, excreted significantly lower levels of 8-hydroxydeoxyguanosine in urine during night work relative to night sleep, which may reflect decreased oxidative DNA damage repair.[4]

Given that the need for shift work will not disappear in our society, the underlying mechanisms of the altered sleep patterns in shift workers need urgent and continuing investigations to determine the best strategies to combat the problem.[119]

Treatment of problems related to shift work ideally should be circadian-based (i.e., making use of sleep hygiene) and cuing by light or melatonergic agents. Because of the large variety of shift work schedules, it is necessary to tailor the treatment approach individually (based on shift work type and chronotype[120]). It is recommended that the hours dedicated to sleep should be regular, adequate, and allow time to wind down and wake up spontaneously or naturally. It is also important to have sleep environment that is dark and quiet so that it is conducive to sleep. Bright light in the first part of the work shift can help to immediately produce alertness and eventually shift the circadian system.[33,121–124] Melatonin given before daytime sleep (after the night shift) is helpful to improve sleep quality and phase shift the circadian rhythm.[123,125,126]

The systematic studies of shift work schedules and strategies to mitigate health problems associated with shift work disorder are urgently needed to determine the best practices.[7] For now, a combination of forward-rotating shifts (day-evening–night) with adequate recovery periods (>11 hours) can be recommended.[7]

The key features of CRSDs described above are illustrated in Table 13.3.

CHRONOBIOLOGY AND PSYCHIATRIC DISORDERS

As noted in the introduction, disturbances in circadian rhythms are found in many patients with psychiatric disorders like bipolar disorder, MDD, and schizophrenia.[12–17] They are often assumed to be the result of the underlying psychiatric disorder. However, it is also possible that altered circadian rhythms in brain function actually disturb the mental processes to produce psychiatric symptoms.[127–130] It has been amply documented that the

brain mechanisms that underlie the neural substrate of sleep and circadian rhythm regulation overlap with those of psychiatric disorders.[12,131] Alterations in circadian rhythms may be due to the environmental or behavioral factors or due to changes in the endogenous circadian clock system itself.[74,80,89] Whether or not the psychiatric illness in a given individual is due to the disturbed rhythm, it is certain that a desynchronized circadian rhythm could aggravate psychiatric symptoms in that particular individual.[132] Based on this concept, a chronobiologic approach, using timed melatonin or light, could always be useful to normalize sleep/circadian rhythm as a complementary treatment.[131,133]

There are several theories regarding the association of mood and circadian rhythm disorders.[133] The social zeitgeber theory of depression proposed that susceptible individuals experience severe circadian rhythm and sleep disturbances when social rhythms are disrupted by factors like life stressors which result in emergence of a depressive episode.[134] Because in this theory disruption of circadian rhythms is responsible for the onset of a major depressive episode, the enhancement of circadian zeitgebers or time giving cues by a highly regular environment would potentially be a corrective strategy.[135] Differing circadian rhythm based theories have been proposed. The first such model was the internal coincidence model developed by Wehr and Wirz-Justice in 1980.[136] This model asserts that the phase angle difference between the SCN and the sleep–wake cycle is depressogenic. In other words, the model asserts that sleep can prompt depression when it is not synchronized (or coincident) with a critically relevant circadian phase.[136,137] An S-deficiency hypothesis was proposed in 1987.[138] As an extension of the two-process theory of sleep regulation, this hypothesis attributed the changes in sleep in depression to the deficiency of Process S (sleep pressure or drive) and proposed that the abnormally low level of Process S is normalized by prolonged waking and that this normalization is the basis for the antidepressant effect of sleep deprivation. The phase-shift hypotheses of depression proposed that mood disturbances result from a phase advance or delay of the central pacemaker and related circadian rhythms that regulate temperature, cortisol, melatonin, and REM sleep relative to other circadian rhythms, and with a marked phase-shift relative to the sleep-wake rhythm.[139] None of these models have been definitively established.

A variety of abnormalities in clock and related genes have been reported in depressive disorders. Polymorphisms of *PER3*, *CRY1*, *CLOCK*, *NPAS2*,

TABLE 13.3 KEY FEATURES OF CRSDs

CRSD	Key clinical features	Diagnosis	Treatment
Delayed sleep phase type	Delayed sleep onset and awakening with inability to fall asleep and wake up at conventional times; possible "cell phone addiction" in young	Sleep logs or actigraphy for 7–14 days Elective: salivary DLMO, morningness/eveningness questionnaires	Advance the delayed rhythm: Low dose melatonin (≤3mg), taken 5 hour before habitual bedtime; bright light (5,000 lux) on waking for 30 minutes to 2 hours
Advanced sleep phase type	Advanced sleep onset and wake times as compared to conventional times	Sleep logs or actigraphy for 7 to 14 days Elective. salivary DLMO, Morningness/eveningness questionnaires	Delay the rhythm: bright light (5,000 lux) in the evening for 2 hours; theoretically, extra-low-dose melatonin (≤0.5 mg) taken when fully awake should safely help but as yet no published studies exist
Non-24-h sleep-wake type	Insomnia or excessive sleepiness based on abnormal synchronization of 24-hour light–dark cycle and endogenous circadian rhythm.	Sleep logs or actigraphy for 14 or more days Elective: sequential salivary DLMO or urinary aMT6s	Entrainment: Blind: melatonin (0.5) mg before habitual bedtime Sighted: Bright light on waking, regulated sleep schedule, melatonin (0.5) mg before habitual bedtime
Irregular sleep–wake type	Symptoms of insomnia at night during usual sleep times and excessive sleepiness during the day. No discernable sleep-wake rhythm	Clinical history and sleep diary (by caregiver if necessary) Elective: actigraphy	Consolidate nighttime sleep using daytime bright light, structured activity and melatonin (0.5) mg before habitual bedtime
Shift work type (nighttime shift)	History of working outside of normal daytime window on a regularly scheduled basis	Clinical history and sleep diary Elective actigraphy	Synchronize body rhythm to shift using sleep hygiene, bright light periodically at work (as necessary); in morning avoid bright light and take melatonin (0.5 mg) prior to sleep time. During day: for sleepinesss day use modafinil or armodafinil, caffeine, bright light, and naps For insomnia, use melatonin (0.5 mg)

DLMO = dim light melatonin onset.

and *SIRT1* genes have been reported to be associated with MDD.[140–145] In postmortem studies, *PER1*, *PER2*, *PER3*, *BMAL1*, *NR1D1*, *DBP*, *DEC1*, and *DEC2* genes were reported to be altered in MDD brains.[146] In seasonal depression, mutations have been reported in *PER2*, *CRY2*, *BMAL1*, and *NPAS2* genes.[147–151] In bipolar disorder, polymorphisms have been reported in *PER3*, *CRY2*, *BMAL1*, *BMAL2*, *CLOCK*, *DBP*, *TIM*, *CSNK1ε*, and *NR1D1* (*REV-ERBα; EAR1*) genes. However, several other studies have not revealed similar findings in these disorders.[152] Despite no precise knowledge of causality, it remains well established that there is a relationship of circadian rhythm abnormalities with depressive disorders.

POTENTIAL FOR CHRONOTHERAPY IN DEPRESSIVE DISORDERS

A recent review of the relationship between sleep and clocks in affective disorders concludes that sleep disturbances are ubiquitous, not specific to the disorder, but that specific manipulations may have powerful clinical effects.[153] The various treatments used to alter timing of the body clock as previously described, especially light therapy, have been used extensively and found to be helpful in stabilizing the sleep–wake cycle and relieving some symptoms in seasonal and nonseasonal depressive disorders, as well as other disorders like eating disorders, attention deficit/hyperactivity disorder, and so forth.[53] Morning BLT was shown to be a viable (and perhaps safer) alternative to antidepressants for treatment of depression during pregnancy in a randomized controlled trial.[154] BLT could accelerate treatment response to antidepressants in patients with MDD and could be instituted at the start of antidepressant therapy. In other cases, BLT could be added as adjunctive treatment when there is partial or delayed response to an antidepressant.[155] For bipolar disorder, a recent review suggests that BLT given between noon and 2 PM may be highly effective and that this mid-day timing reduces the risk of inducing mania.[53] To recapitulate from the previous discussion on CRSDs, blue light acts on a tiny group of uniquely photosensitive ganglion cells that send melanopsin containing fibers to the SCN, helping regulate rhythms, and to other brain areas that may also improve alertness.

Sleep deprivation treatment (often 36 hours of wakefulness from 7 AM until 7 PM the following day) when given alone causes a rapid antidepressant response (within 24 to 48 hours) in 50% to 80% of depressed patients.[156] Relapse is often prevented by combination with effective mood stabilizers/antidepressants or with BLT combined with sleep phase advance. Success rates are equivalent to the most effective psychiatric treatments.[156–158] Bipolar depression and unipolar depression can both respond to this type of protocol. The patient should be advised not to drive or engage in tasks requiring sustained attention and alertness during the period of prolonged sleep deprivation. Careful assessment for mixed states is advised when a patient with bipolar disorder presents with depression prior to recommending BLT or sleep deprivation since such treatments can potentially cause switch from depression predominant mixed state to mania predominant mixed state or even pure mania.[158]

Although treatment of manic episodes relies heavily on antipsychotic and mood stabilizing agents, they are slow to act.[159] Recently, a pilot study reported that blue blocking glasses worn from 6 PM to 8 AM for seven days added to treatment as usual were a highly effective add-on

treatment yielding results as early as one day and definitive improvement within three days.[160] This is an exciting first report, which requires corroboration. However, it is suggestive of the potential of chronotherapy as a tool that can be added to the armamentarium of psychiatric disorder management.

CONCLUSION
CRSDs represent alterations in a fundamental body system that can have far-reaching effects. It merits reiterating that all CRSDs can lead to compromised sleep and that sleep is essential for restoration of several body and brain reserves.[4,7] With respect to psychiatric disorders, it is clear that dysregulation of body clocks can aggravate psychiatric symptoms. Because CRSDs can lead to a wide variety of psychiatric and sleep-related symptoms, the further development of effective treatments is urgently needed.

FUTURE DIRECTIONS
Knowledge of the processes underlying the circadian system and of the mechanisms in which the circadian system affects virtually all the body systems is proceeding rapidly. Hence, this review is only a snapshot of this dynamic section of the healthcare field. Current practice guidelines need continuous revision to take into account new information, such as the recent availability of the prescription melatonergic drug, tasimelteon, in the United States and other countries, novel BLT delivery methods, and so forth. Moreover, the discovery that blue light is the most effective part of the white light as a visual cue to the circadian system needs to be evaluated further to determine its potential utility along with blue blocking glasses.

Most current strategies only allow gradual phase shifts in circadian rhythms. However, there are hints of new possibilities. For instance, it has been shown that the nuclear receptors (REV-ERBα and REV-ERBβ), the key regulators of the molecular clock, can be successfully targeted in animals with small molecular ligands.[161] Another finding is that heme is the natural ligand of REV-ERBα and REV-ERBβ.[162] These agents may have potential for treatment of circadian disorders.

KEY CLINICAL PEARLS
- Insomnia or hypersomnia disorders may be diagnosed in patients with MDD or bipolar disorder instead of DSPD. Thorough history-taking, sleep log, and, if possible,

actigraphy are helpful in making the right connection between the sleep symptom and underlying disorder. The correct diagnosis is essential to help guide treatment since chronotherapy may be correct treatment instead of hypnotic or stimulant that may otherwise be given for insomnia or hypersomnia, respectively.

- Young adults with DSPD, commonly with comorbid cell phone addiction, frequently stay up late at night but wake up prior to their natural/spontaneous wake-up time to meet societal demands. This results in suboptimal sleep duration leading to complaints of poor concentration and reduced alertness at school or work. Chronobiologic treatments like melatonin and BLT can be helpful in such cases. Use of blue blocking glasses in the evening can also be useful.
- Morning BLT is the treatment of choice for seasonal affective disorder.[163–165] Mid-day BLT is recommended for bipolar depression due to reduced risk of manic precipitation.

CASE-BASED ILLUSTRATION

A 22-year-old female adult presented with complaints of difficulty in advancing bedtime to meet school and work schedule and poor school performance but without any somatic or psychiatric symptoms. She completed the MEQ to which this question was added: "If you consider yourself to be an 'evening' type, does your habitual sleep schedule cause you problems at work or school? If yes, is this problem 'mild,' 'moderate,' 'marked,' 'severe,' or 'disabling.'" She replied moderate. Her habitual bedtime of 1:34 AM and wake time of 9:26 AM were confirmed by screening questionnaires and a one-week sleep diary. As a university student, she attempted to avoid all morning classes. Her score was seven on the Pittsburgh Sleep Quality Index,[166] and she used no medication known to affect sleep (e.g., hypnotics, anxiolytics, antidepressants, neuroleptics, stimulants), melatonin secretion (beta-blockers, nonsteroidal anti-inflammatory drugs), or light sensitivity (some antibiotics). However, she used a cell phone incessantly, right up to the time she went to bed. Circadian phase as estimated with salivary DLMO was 11:23 PM. Diagnosis was DSPD with a contributing factor of excessive evening cell phone usage. Treatment was instituted with melatonin 3 mg at 9:30 PM daily, use of blue blocking glasses from 9:30 PM until bedtime, a recommendation to

cease cell phone use at that time, and light therapy or exposure to outdoor light immediately on waking. The patient responded well to treatment over the next two weeks.

SELF-ASSESSMENT QUESTIONS

1. Which of the following disorders usually respond to bright light therapy? (Select all that apply.)
   a. Irregular sleep–wake phase disorder
   b. Advanced sleep–wake phase disorder
   c. Non-24-hour sleep–wake rhythm disorder
   d. Seasonal affective disorder
   e. Shift work disorder

Answers: a yes, b yes, c no, d yes, e yes.

2. Which of the following disorders often display sleep loss and exhaustion? (Select all that apply.)
   a. Insomnia
   b. Shift work disorder
   c. Non-24-hour sleep–wake rhythm disorder
   d. Major depressive disorder
   e. Delayed sleep–wake disorder

Answers: a yes, b yes, c yes, d yes, e, yes

3. Which of the following interact with melatonin receptors exclusively? (Select all that apply.)
   a. Circadin®
   b. Agomelatine
   c. Rozerem
   d. Melatonin
   e. Tasimelteon

Answers: a yes, b no, c yes, d yes, e yes

REFERENCES

1. Dibner C, Schibler U, Albrecht U. The mammalian circadian timing system: organization and coordination of central and peripheral clocks. *Annu Rev Physiol.* 2010;72:517–549. doi:10.1146/annurev-physiol-021909-135821.
2. Schmidt C, Collette F, Cajochen C, Peigneux P. A time to think: circadian rhythms in human cognition. *Cog Neuropsychol.* 2007;24(7):755–789. doi:10.1080/02643290701754158.
3. Borbély AA, Daan S, Wirz-Justice A, Deboer T. The two-process model of sleep regulation: a reappraisal. *J Sleep Res.* 2016;25(2):131–143. doi:10.1111/jsr.12371.
4. Bhatti P, Mirick DK, Randolph TW, et al. Oxidative DNA damage during sleep periods among nightshift workers. *Occup Environ Med.* 2016;73(8):537–544. doi:10.1136/oemed-2016-103629.

5. Skuladottir GV, Nilsson EK, Mwinyi J, Schiöth HB. One-night sleep deprivation induces changes in the DNA methylation and serum activity indices of stearoyl-CoA desaturase in young healthy men. *Lipids Health Dis.* 2016;15(1):137. doi:10.1186/s12944-016-0309-1.

6. Karthikeyan R, Marimuthu G, Spence DW, et al. Should we listen to our clock to prevent type 2 diabetes mellitus? *Diabetes Res Clin Pract.* 2014;106(2):182–190. doi:10.1016/j.diabres.2014.07.029.

7. Kecklund G, Axelsson J. Health consequences of shift work and insufficient sleep. *BMJ.* 2016:i5210. doi:10.1136/bmj.i5210.

8. Karlsson B. Commentary: metabolic syndrome as a result of shift work exposure? *Int J Epidemiol.* 2009;38:854–855.

9. Haus EL, Smolensky MH. Shift work and cancer risk: potential mechanistic roles of circadian disruption, light at night, and sleep deprivation. *Sleep Med Rev.* 2013;17(4):273–284. doi:10.1016/j.smrv.2012.08.003.

10. Pandi-Perumal SR, BaHammam AS, Ojike NI, et al. Melatonin and human cardiovascular disease. *J Cardiovasc Pharmacol Ther.* 2017;22(2):122–132. doi:10.1177/1074248416660622.

11. Touitou Y, Reinberg A, Touitou D. Association between light at night, melatonin secretion, sleep deprivation, and the internal clock: Health impacts and mechanisms of circadian disruption. *Life Sci.* 2017;173. doi:10.1016/j.lfs.2017.02.008.

12. Jones SG, Benca RM. Circadian disruption in psychiatric disorders. *Sleep Med Clin.* 2015;10(4):481–493. doi:10.1016/j.jsmc.2015.07.004.

13. Byrne EM, Heath AC, Madden PAF, et al. Testing the role of circadian genes in conferring risk for psychiatric disorders. *Am J Med Genet Part B Neuropsychiatr Genet.* 2014;165(3):254–260. doi:10.1002/ajmg.b.32230.

14. Nechita F, Pirlog M-C, Chiriţă AL. Circadian malfunctions in depression—neurobiological and psychosocial approaches [Review]. *Rom J Morphol Embryol.* 2015;56(3):949–955.

15. McClung CA. How might circadian rhythms control mood? Let me count the ways . . . *Biol Psychiatry.* 2013;74(4):242–249. doi:10.1016/j.biopsych.2013.02.019.

16. Jagannath A, Peirson SN, Foster RG. Sleep and circadian rhythm disruption in neuropsychiatric illness. *Curr Opin Neurobiol.* 2013;23(5):888–894. doi:10.1016/j.conb.2013.03.008; 10.1016/j.conb.2013.03.008.

17. Wulff K, Dijk DJ, Middleton B, Foster RG, Joyce EM. Sleep and circadian rhythm disruption in schizophrenia. *Br J Psychiatry.* 2012;200(4):308–316. doi:10.1192/bjp.bp.111.096321.

18. American Psychiatric Association. *Diagnostic and Statistical Manual of Mental Disorders.* 5th ed. Washington, DC: American Psychiatric Association; 2013.

19. American Academy of Sleep Medicine. *The International Classification of Sleep Disorders.* 3rd ed. Darien, IL: American Academy of Sleep Medicine; 2014.

20. Reynolds CF 3rd, O'Hara R. DSM-5 sleep–wake disorders classification: overview for use in clinical practice. *Am J Psychiatry.* 2013;170(10):1099–1101. doi:10.1176/appi.ajp.2013.13010058.

21. DeBruyne JP, Weaver DR, Reppert SM. Peripheral circadian oscillators require CLOCK. *Curr Biol.* 2007;17:R538–R539.

22. Reddy AB, Wong GK, O'Neill J, Maywood ES, Hastings MH. Circadian clocks: neural and peripheral pacemakers that impact upon the cell division cycle. *Mutat Res.* 2005;574(0027-5107;0027-5107;1-2):76–91.

23. Hastings MH, Brancaccio M, Maywood ES. Circadian pacemaking in cells and circuits of the suprachiasmatic nucleus. *J Neuroendocrinol.* 2014;26(1):2–10. doi:10.1111/jne.12125.

24. Sollars PJ, Pickard GE. The neurobiology of circadian rhythms. *Psychiatr Clin North Am.* 2015;38(4):645–665. doi:10.1016/j.psc.2015.07.003.

25. Saper CB, Lowell BB. The hypothalamus. *Curr Biol.* 2014;24(23):R1111–R1116. doi:10.1016/j.cub.2014.10.023.

26. Golombek DA, Rosenstein RE. Physiology of circadian entrainment. *Physiol Rev.* 2010;90(3):1063–1102. doi:10.1152/physrev.00009.2009.

27. Berson DM. Phototransduction in ganglion-cell photoreceptors. *Pflügers Arch—Eur J Physiol.* 2007;454(5):849–855. doi:10.1007/s00424-007-0242-2.

28. David C. Klein, Robert Y. Moore and Steven M. Reppert. The suprachiasmatic nucleus and the circadian timing system. *Prog Mol Biol Transl Sci.* 2013;119:1–28. doi:10.1016/B978-0-12-396971-2.00001-4.

29. Hannibal J, Christiansen, AT; Heegaard S, Fahrenkrug J, Kiilgaard J. Melanopsin containing human retinal ganglion cells: subtypes, distribution, and intraretinal connectivity. *J Comp Neurol.* 2017;525(8):1934.1961. doi:10.1002/cne.24181.

30. Lewy AJ, Sack RL. The dim light melatonin onset as a marker for circadian phase position. *Chronobiol Int.* 1989;6(1):93–102.

31. Hardeland R. Melatonin: signaling mechanisms of a pleiotropic agent. *Biofactors.* 2009;35(2):183–192. doi:10.1002/biof.23; 10.1002/biof.23.

32. Khan MZ, He L, Zhuang X. The emerging role of GPR50 receptor in brain. *Biomed Pharmacother.* 2016;78:121–128. doi:10.1016/j.biopha.2016.01.003.

33. Emens JS, Burgess HJ. Effect of light and melatonin and other melatonin receptor agonists on human circadian physiology. *Sleep Med Clin.* 2015;10(4). doi:10.1016/j.jsmc.2015.08.001.

34. Abbott SM, Reid KJ, Zee PC. Circadian rhythm sleep–wake disorders. *Psychiatr Clin North Am.* 2015;38(4):805–823. doi:10.1016/j.psc.2015.07.012.

35. Ancoli-Israel S, Cole R, Alessi C, Chambers M, Moorcroft W, Pollak CP. The role of actigraphy in the study of sleep and circadian rhythms. *Sleep.* 2003;26(3):342–392. doi:10.1093/sleep/26.3.342.

36. Burgess HJ, Emens JS. Circadian-based therapies for circadian rhythm sleep-wake disorders. *Curr Sleep Med Reports.* 2016;2:158–165. doi:10.1007/s40675-016-0052-1.

37. Auger RR, Burgess HJ, Emens JS, Deriy L V, Thomas SM, Sharkey KM. Clinical practice guideline for the treatment of intrinsic circadian rhythm sleep–wake disorders. *J Clin Sleep Med.* 2015;11(10):1199–1236. doi:10.5664/jcsm.5100.

38. Lewy AJ. Melatonin and human chronobiology. *Cold Spring Harb Symp Quant Biol.* 2007;72:623–636. doi:10.1101/sqb.2007.72.055.

39. Molina TA, Burgess HJ. Calculating the dim light melatonin onset: the impact of threshold and sampling rate. *Chronobiol Int.* 2011;28(8):714–718. doi:10.3109/07420528.2011.597531.

40. Baker EK, Richdale AL, Hazi A, Prendergast LA. Assessing the dim light melatonin onset in adults with autism spectrum disorder and no comorbid intellectual disability. *J Autism Dev Disord.* 2017;47(7):2120–2137. doi:10.1007/s10803-017-3122-4.

41. Kantermann T, Sung H, Burgess HJ. Comparing the Morningness–Eveningness Questionnaire and Munich ChronoType Questionnaire to the Dim Light Melatonin Onset. *J Biol Rhythms.* 2015;30(5):449–453. doi:10.1177/0748730415597520.

42. Roenneberg T, Wirz-justice A, Merrow M. Life between clocks : daily temporal patterns of human chronotypes. *J Biol Rhythms.* 2003;18(1):80–90. doi:10.1177/0748730402239679.

43. Skene DJ. Optimization of light and melatonin to phase-shift human circadian rhythms. *J Neuroendocrinol.* 2003;15(4):438–441.

44. Boulos Z, Campbell SS, Lewy AJ, Terman M, Dijk DJ, Eastman CI. Light treatment for sleep disorders: consensus report. VII: jet lag [Review]. *J Biol Rhythms.* 1995;10(2):167–176.

45. Lewy AJ, Bauer VK, Ahmed S, et al. The human phase response curve (PRC) to melatonin is about 12 hours out of phase with the PRC to light. *Chronobiol Int.* 1998;15(0742-0528; 1):71–83.

46. Burgess HJ, Revell VL, Eastman CI. A three pulse phase response curve to three milligrams of melatonin in humans. *J Physiol.* 2008;586(0022-3751; 2):639–647.

47. Ackermann K, Sletten TL, Revell VL, Archer SN, Skene DJ. Blue-light phase shifts PER3 gene expression in human leukocytes. *Chronobiol Int.* 2009;26(4):769–779. doi:10.1080/07420520902929045.

48. Figueiro MG, Plitnick B, Rea MS. The effects of chronotype, sleep schedule and light/dark pattern exposures on circadian phase. *Sleep Med.* 2014;15(12):1554–1564. doi:10.1016/j.sleep.2014.07.009.

49. Zeitzer JM, Fisicaro RA, Ruby NF, Heller HC. Millisecond flashes of light phase delay the human circadian clock during sleep. *J Biol Rhythms.* 2014;29(5):370–376. doi:10.1177/0748730414546532.

50. Zeitzer JM, Ruby NF, Fisicaro RA, Heller HC. Response of the human circadian system to millisecond flashes of light. *PLoS One.* 2011;6(7):1–5. doi:10.1371/journal.pone.0022078.

51. Pail G, Huf W, Pjrek E, et al. Bright-light therapy in the treatment of mood disorders. *Neuropsychobiology.* 2011;64(3):152.162.

52. Terman M, Terman J. Light therapy for seasonal and nonseasonal depression: efficacy, protocol, safety, and side effects. *CNS Spectr.* 2005;10(8):647–663.

53. Nasr S, Elmaadawi A, Patel R. Bright light therapy for bipolar depression. *Curr Psychiatr.* 2018;17(11):28–32.

54. van der Lely S, Frey S, Garbazza C, et al. Blue blocker glasses as a countermeasure for alerting effects of evening light-emitting diode screen exposure in male teenagers. *J Adolesc Heal.* 2015;56(1):113–119. doi:10.1016/j.jadohealth.2014.08.002.

55. Sasseville A, Hébert M. Using blue-green light at night and blue-blockers during the day to improves adaptation to night work: a pilot study. *Prog Neuro-Psychopharmacol Biol Psychiatr.* 2010;34(7):1236–1242. doi:10.1016/j.pnpbp.2010.06.027.

56. Dollins N, Zhdanova I V, Wurtman RJ, Lynch HJ, Deng MH. Effect of inducing nocturnal serum melatonin concentrations in daytime on sleep, mood, body temperature, and performance. *Proc Natl Acad Sci USA.* 1994;91(5):1824–1828.

57. Buscemi N, Vandermeer B, Hooton N, et al. Efficacy and safety of exogenous melatonin for secondary sleep disorders and sleep disorders accompanying sleep restriction: meta-analysis. *BMJ.* 2006;332(1468-5833; 7538):385–393.

58. Lewy AJ, Emens JS, Lefler BJ, Yuhas K, Jackman AR. Melatonin entrains free-running blind people according to a physiological dose-response curve. *Chronobiol Int.* 2005;22(6):1093–1106.

59. Erland LAE, Saxena PK. Melatonin natural health products and supplements: presence of serotonin and significant variability of melatonin content. *J Clin Sleep Med.* 2017;13(2):275–281. doi:10.5664/jcsm.6462.

60. Montastruc F, Scotto S, Vaz IR, et al. Hepatotoxicity related to agomelatine and other new antidepressants: a case/noncase approach with information from the Portuguese, French, Spanish, and Italian pharmacovigilance systems. *J Clin Psychopharmacol.* 2014;34(3):327–330. doi:10.1097/JCP.0000000000000094.

61. Dhillon S, Clarke M. Tasimelteon: first global approval. *Drugs.* 2014;74(4):505–511. doi:10.1007/s40265-014-0200-1.

62. van Maanen A, Dewald-Kaufmann JF, Smits MG, Oort FJ, Meijer AM. Chronic sleep reduction in adolescents with delayed sleep phase disorder and effects of melatonin treatment. *Sleep Biol Rhythms.* 2013;11(2):99–104. doi:10.1111/sbr.12010.

63. Solheim B, Langsrud K, Kallestad H, Olsen A, Bjorvatn B, Sand T. Difficult morning awakening from rapid eye movement sleep and impaired cognitive function in delayed sleep phase disorder patients. *Sleep Med.* 2014;15(10):1264–1268. doi:10.1016/j.sleep.2014.05.024.

64. Snitselaar MA, Smits MG, van der Heijden KB, Spijker J. Sleep and circadian rhythmicity in adult ADHD and the effect of stimulants: a review of the current literature. *J Atten Disord.* 2017;21(1):14–26. doi:10.1177/1087054713479663.

65. Zee PC, Attarian H, Videnovic A. Circadian rhythm abnormalities. *Continuum.* 2013;19(1 Sleep Disorders):132–147. doi:10.1212/01.CON.0000427209.21177.aa.

66. Schrader H, Bovim G, Sand T. The prevalence of delayed and advanced sleep phase syndromes. *J Sleep Res.* 1993;2:51–55.

67. Paine S-J, Fink J, Gander PH, Warman GR. Identifying advanced and delayed sleep phase disorders in the general population: a national survey of New Zealand adults. *Chronobiol Int.* 2014;31(5):627–636. doi:10.3109/07420528.2014.885036.

68. Thorpy MJ, Korman E, Spielman AJ, Glovinsky PB. Delayed sleep phase syndrome in adolescents. *J Adolesc Heal Care.* 1988;9(1):22–27.

69. Sivertsen B, Pallesen S, Stormark KM, Bøe T, Lundervold AJ, Hysing M. Delayed sleep phase syndrome in adolescents: prevalence and correlates in a large population based study. *BMC Public Health.* 2013;13(1). doi:10.1186/1471-2458-13-1163.

70. Saxvig IW, Pallesen S, Wilhelmsen-Langeland A, Molde H, Bjorvatn B. Prevalence and correlates of delayed sleep phase in high school students. *Sleep Med.* 2012;13(2):193–199. doi:10.1016/j.sleep.2011.10.024.

71. Lovato N, Gradisar M, Short M, Dohnt H, Micic G. Delayed sleep phase disorder in an Australian school-based sample of adolescents. *J Clin Sleep Med.* 2013;9(9):939–944. doi:10.5664/jcsm.2998.

72. Micic G, Lovato N, Gradisar M, Ferguson SA, Burgess HJ, Lack LC. The etiology of delayed sleep phase disorder. *Sleep Med Rev.* 2016;27:29–38. doi:10.1016/j.smrv.2015.06.004.

73. Ebisawa T, Uchiyama M, Kajimura N, et al. Association of structural polymorphisms in the human period3 gene with delayed sleep phase syndrome. *EMBO Rep.* 2001;2(1469-221; 4):342–346.

74. Archer SN, Robilliard DL, Skene DJ, et al. A length polymorphism in the circadian clock gene Per3 is linked to delayed sleep phase syndrome and extreme diurnal preference. *Sleep.* 2003;26(0161-8105; 4):413–415.

75. Hida A, Kitamura S, Katayose Y, et al. Screening of clock gene polymorphisms demonstrates association of a PER3 polymorphism with morningness-eveningness preference and circadian rhythm sleep disorder. *Sci Rep.* 2014;4:6309. doi:10.1038/srep06309.

76. Kripke DF, Klimecki WT, Nievergelt CM, et al. Circadian polymorphisms in night owls, in bipolars, and in non-24-hour sleep cycles. *Psychiatry Investig.* 2014;11(4):345–362. doi:10.4306/pi.2014.11.4.345.

77. Osland TM, Bjorvatn BR, Steen VM, Pallesen S. Association study of a variable-number tandem repeat polymorphism in the clock gene PERIOD3

and chronotype in Norwegian university students. *Chronobiol Int.* 2011;28(9):764–770. doi:10.3109/07420528.2011.607375.

78. Pereira DS, Tufik S, Louzada FM, et al. Association of the length polymorphism in the human Per3 gene with the delayed sleep-phase syndrome: does latitude have an influence upon it? *Sleep.* 2005;28(0161-8105; 1):29–32.

79. Patke A, Murphy PJ, Onat OE, et al. Mutation of the human circadian clock gene CRY1 in familial delayed sleep phase disorder. *Cell.* 2017;169(2):203–215.e13. doi:10.1016/j.cell.2017.03.027.

80. Ohayon MM, Milesi C. Artificial outdoor nighttime lights associate with altered sleep behavior in the American general population. *Sleep.* 2016;39(6):1311–1320. doi:10.5665/sleep.5860.

81. Haim A, Zubidat AE. Artificial light at night: melatonin as a mediator between the environment and epigenome. *Philos Trans R Soc B Biol Sci.* 2015. doi:10.1098/rstb.2014.0121.

82. Smolensky MH, Sackett-Lundeen LL, Portaluppi F. Nocturnal light pollution and underexposure to daytime sunlight: complementary mechanisms of circadian disruption and related diseases. *Chronobiol Int.* 2015. doi:10.3109/07420528.2015.1072002.

83. Chang A-M, Aeschbach D, Duffy JF, Czeisler CA. Evening use of light-emitting eReaders negatively affects sleep, circadian timing, and next-morning alertness. *Proc Natl Acad Sci.* 2014;112(4). doi:10.1073/pnas.1418490112.

84. Hysing M, Pallesen S, Stormark KM, Jakobsen R, Lundervold AJ, Sivertsen B. Sleep and use of electronic devices in adolescence: results from a large population-based study. *BMJ Open.* 2015;5(1):e006748–e006748. doi:10.1136/bmjopen-2014-006748.

85. Gutiérrez JDS, de Fonseca FR, Rubio G. Cell-phone addiction: a review. *Front Psychiatry.* 2016;7:175. doi:10.3389/fpsyt.2016.00175.

86. Saxvig IW, Wilhelmsen-Langeland A, Pallesen S, Vedaa Ø, Nordhus I-H, Bjorvatn B. A randomized controlled trial with bright light and melatonin for delayed sleep phase disorder: effects on subjective and objective sleep. *Chronobiol Int.* 2014;31(1):72–86.

87. Nagtegaal JE, Kerkhof GA, Smits MG, Swart AC, van der Meer YG. Delayed sleep phase syndrome: a placebo-controlled cross-over study on the effects of melatonin administered five hours before the individual dim light

melatonin onset. *J Sleep Res.* 1998;7(0962-1105; 2):135–143.

88. Gradisar M, Dohnt H, Gardner G, etc. A randomized controlled trial of cognitive-behavior therapy plus bright light therapy for adolescent delayed sleep phase disorder. *Sleep.* 2011;34(12):1671–1680. doi:10.5665/sleep.1432.

89. Ptáček LJ, Jones CR, Campbell SS, et al. Familial advanced sleep-phase syndrome: a short-period circadian rhythm variant in humans. *Nat Med.* 1999;5(1078-8956; 9):1062–1065. doi:10.1038/12502.

90. Toh KL, Jones CR, He Y, et al. An hPer2 phosphorylation site mutation in familial advanced sleep phase syndrome. *Science (80-).* 2001;291(0036-8075; 5506):1040–1043. doi:10.1126/science.1057499.

91. Shanware NP, Hutchinson JA, Kim SH, Zhan L, Bowler MJ, Tibbetts RS. Casein kinase 1-dependent phosphorylation of familial advanced sleep phase syndrome-associated residues controls PERIOD 2 stability. *J Biol Chem.* 2011;286(14):12766–12774. doi:10.1074/jbc.M111.224014.

92. Xu Y, Padiath QS, Shapiro RE, et al. Functional consequences of a CKIdelta mutation causing familial advanced sleep phase syndrome. *Nature.* 2005;434(1476-4687; 7033):640–644.

93. Zee PC. Melatonin for the treatment of advanced sleep phase disorder. *Sleep.* 2008;31(7):923; author reply 925.

94. Flynn-Evans EE, Tabandeh H, Skene DJ, Lockley SW. Circadian rhythm disorders and melatonin production in 127 blind women with and without light perception. *J Biol Rhythms.* 2014;29(3):215–224.

95. Traynor K. Tasimelteon approved for circadian disorder in blind adults. *Am J Heal Pharm.* 2014;71(5):350–350. doi:10.2146/news140017.

96. Folkard S, Arendt J, Aldhous M, Kennett H. Melatonin stabilises sleep onset time in a blind man without entrainment of cortisol or temperature rhythms. *Neurosci Lett.* 1990;113(2):193–198.

97. Aldhous ME, Arendt J. Radioimmunoassay for 6-sulphatoxymelatonin in urine using an iodinated tracer. *Ann Clin Biochem.* 1988;25:298–303.

98. Tzischinsky O, Dagan Y, Lavie P. The effects of melatonin on the timing of sleep in patients with delayed sleep phase syndrome. In: Touitou Y, Arendt J, Pevet P, eds. *Melatonin and the Pineal Gland: From Basic Science to Clinical Application.*

Amsterdam, The Netherlands: Excerpta Medica; 1993:351–354.

99. Rosenthal NE, Sack DA, Jacobsen FM, Skwerer RG, Wehr TA. Seasonal affective disorder and light: past, present and future. *Clin Neuropharmacol*. 1986;9(Suppl 4):193–195.

100. Sack RL, Brandes RW, Kendall AR, Lewy AJ. Entrainment of free-running circadian rhythms by melatonin in blind people. *N Engl J Med*. 2000;343(15):1070–1077.

101. Lewy AJ, Emens JS, Sack RL, Hasler BP, Bernert RA. Low, but not high, doses of melatonin entrained a free-running blind person with a long circadian period. *Chronobiol Int 19 649-58*. 2002;19(3):649–658.

102. Zee PC, Vitiello MV. Circadian rhythm sleep disorder: irregular sleep wake rhythm type. *Sleep Med Clin*. 2009;4(2):213–218.

103. Stevens RG. Circadian disruption and health: Shift work as a harbinger of the toll taken by electric lighting. *Chronobiol Int*. 2016;33(6):589–594. doi:10.3109/07420528.2016.1167732.

104. Wickwire EM, Geiger-Brown J, Scharf SM, Drake CL. Shift work and shift work sleep disorder: clinical and organizational perspectives. *Chest*. 2017;151(5):1156–1172. doi:10.1016/j.chest.2016.12.007.

105. Akerstedt T. Sleep loss and fatigue in shift work and SWD. *Sleep Med Clin*. 2009;4(2):257–271. doi:10.1016/j.jsmc.2009.03.001.Sleep.

106. Wright KP, Bogan RK, Wyatt JK. Shift work and the assessment and management of shift work disorder (SWD). *Sleep Med Rev*. 2013;17(1):41–54. doi:10.1016/j.smrv.2012.02.002.

107. Gumenyuk V, Howard R, Roth T, Korzyukov O, Drake CL. Sleep loss, circadian mismatch, and abnormalities in reorienting of attention in night workers with shift work disorder. *Sleep*. 2014;37(3):545–556. doi:10.5665/sleep.3494.

108. Gumenyuk V, Belcher R, Drake CL, Roth T. Differential sleep, sleepiness, and neurophysiology in the insomnia phenotypes of shift work disorder. *Sleep*. 2015;38(1):119–126. doi:10.5665/sleep.4336.

109. Sulkava S, Ollila H, Alasaari J, et al. Common genetic variation near melatonin receptor 1A gene linked to job-related exhaustion in shift workers. *Sleep*. 2017;40(1). doi:10.1093/sleep/zsw011.

110. Drake CL, Roehrs T, Richardson G, Walsh JK, Roth T. Shift work sleep disorder: prevalence

and consequences beyond that of symptomatic day workers. *Sleep*. 2004;27(8):1453–1462.

111. White L, Keith B. The effect of shift work on the quality and stability of marital relations. *J Marriage Fam*. 1990;52(2):453–462. doi:10.2307/353039.

112. Lee ML, Howard ME, Horrey WJ, et al. High risk of near-crash driving events following nightshift work. *Proc Natl Acad Sci*. 2016;113(1):176–181. doi:10.1073/pnas.1510383112.

113. Krishnaswamy UM, Chhabria MS, Rao A. Excessive sleepiness, sleep hygiene, and coping strategies among night bus drivers: A cross-sectional study. *Indian J Occup Environ Med*. 2016;20(2):84–87. doi:10.4103/0019-5278.197526.

114. Alali H, Braeckman L, van Hecke T, de Clercq B, Janssens H, Wahab MA. Relationship between non-standard work arrangements and work-related accident absence in Belgium. *J Occup Health*. 2017;59(2):177–186. doi:10.1539/joh.16-0119-OA.

115. Drongelen A Van, Boot CRL, Hlobil H, Beek AJ Van Der, Smid T. Cumulative exposure to shift work and sickness absence: associations in a five-year historic cohort. *BMC Public Health*. 2017;17(67):1–12. doi:10.1186/s12889-016-3906-z.

116. Jankowiak S, Backé E, Liebers F, et al. Current and cumulative night shift work and subclinical atherosclerosis: results of the Gutenberg Health Study. *Int Arch Occup Environ Health*. 2016;89(8):1169–1182. doi:10.1007/s00420-016-1150-6.

117. Copertaro A, Bracci M, Barbaresi M, Santarelli L. Assessment of cardiovascular risk in shift healthcare workers. *Eur J Cardiovasc Prev Rehabil*. 2008;15(2):224–229.

118. Costa G, Haus E, Stevens R. Shift work and cancer—Considerations on rationale, mechanisms, and epidemiology. *Scand J Work Environ Heal*. 2010;36(2):163–179. doi:10.5271/sjweh.2899.

119. Neil-Sztramko SE, Pahwa M, Demers PA, Gotay CC. Health-related interventions among night shift workers: a critical review of the literature. *Scand J Work Environ Heal*. 2014;40(6):543–556. doi:10.5271/sjweh.3445.

120. Vetter C, Fischer D, Matera JL, Roenneberg T. Aligning work and circadian time in shift workers improves sleep and reduces circadian disruption. *Curr Biol*. 2015;25(7). doi:10.1016/j.cub.2015.01.064.

121. Boudreau P, Dumont GA, Boivin DB. Circadian adaptation to night shift work influences sleep,

performance, mood and the autonomic modulation
of the heart. *PLoS One.* 2013;8(7):e70813. doi:10.
1371/journal.pone.0070813; 10.1371/journal.
pone.0070813.

122. Burgess HJ, Sharkey KM, Eastman CI. Bright
light, dark and melatonin can promote circadian
adaptation in night shift workers. *Sleep MedRev.*
2002;6(5):407–420.

123. Crowley SJ, Lee C, Tseng CY, Fogg LF, Eastman
CI. Combinations of bright light, scheduled
dark, sunglasses, and melatonin to facilitate circadian entrainment to night shift work. *J Biol
Rhythms.* 2003;18(6):513–523. doi:10.1177/
0748730403258422.

124. Smith MR, Fogg LF, Eastman CI. A compromise circadian phase position for permanent
night work improves mood, fatigue, and performance. *Sleep.* 2009;32(0161-8105; 0161-8105;
11):1481–1489.

125. Sharkey KM, Eastman CI. Melatonin phase
shifts human circadian rhythms in a placebo-controlled simulated night-work study.
Am J Physiol Regul Integr Comp Physiol.
2002;282(2):R454–R463.

126. Smith MR, Lee C, Crowley SJ, Fogg LF,
Eastman CI. Morning melatonin has
limited benefit as a soporific for daytime sleep after night work. *Chronobiol
Int.* 2005;22(5):873–888. doi:10.1080/
09636410500292861.

127. Reid KJ, Abbott SM. Jet lag and shift work disorder. *Sleep Med Clin.* 2017;10(4):523–535.
doi:10.1016/j.jsmc.2015.08.006.

128. Coderre TJ, Abbott F V, Melzack R. Effects of
peripheral antisympathetic treatments in the
tail-flick, formalin and autotomy tests. *Pain.*
1984;18:13–23.

129. Alloy LB, Nusslock R, Boland EM. The development and course of bipolar spectrum disorders: an integrated reward and circadian
rhythm dysregulation model. *Annu Rev
Clin Psychol.* 2015;11:213–250. doi:10.1146/
annurev-clinpsy-032814-112902.

130. Karatsoreos IN. Links between circadian
rhythms and psychiatric disease. *Front
Behav Neurosci.* 2014;8:162. doi:10.3389/
fnbeh.2014.00162.

131. Wulff K, Gatti S, Wettstein JG, Foster RG.
Sleep and circadian rhythm disruption in
psychiatric and neurodegenerative disease.
Nat Rev. 2010;11(8):589–599. doi:10.1038/
nrn2868.

132. Barandas R, Landgraf D, McCarthy MJ, Welsh
DK. Circadian clocks as modulators of metabolic comorbidity in psychiatric disorders. *Curr
Psychiatry Rep.* 2015;17(12):98. doi:10.1007/
s11920-015-0637-2.

133. Zaki NFW, Spence DW, BaHammam
AS, Pandi-Perumal SR, Cardinali DP,
Brown GM. Chronobiological theories of
mood disorder. *Eur Arch Psychiatry Clin
Neurosci.* 2018;268(2):107–118. doi:10.1007/
s00406-017-0835-5.

134. Ehlers CL, Frank E, Kupfer DJ. Social zeitgebers
and biological rhythms: a unified approach to
understanding the etiology of depression. *Arch
Gen Psychiatry.* 1988;45:948–952.

135. Monk TH. Enhancing circadian zeitgebers.
Sleep. 2010;33(4):421–422.

136. Wehr TA, Wirz-Justice A. Internal coincidence model for sleep deprivation and
depression. In: Koella WP, ed. *Sleep.* Basel,
Switzerland: Karger; 1980:26–33.

137. Borbely AA, Wirz-Justice A. Sleep, sleep deprivation and depression: a hypothesis derived from
a model of sleep regulation. *Hum Neurobiol.*
1982;1(3):205–210.

138. Borbély AA. The S-deficiency hypothesis
of depression and the two-process model
of sleep regulation. *Pharmacopsychiatry.*
1987;20(1):23–29.

139. Germain A, Kupfer DJ. Circadian rhythm disturbances in depression. *Hum Psychopharmacol
Clin Exp.* 2008;23:571–585.

140. Melhuish Beaupre L, Brown GM, Kennedy JL.
Circadian genes in major depressive disorder. *World J Biol Psychiatry.* 2018. doi:10.1080/
15622975.2018.1500028. [Epub ahead of
print]

141. Hua P, Liu W, Chen D, et al. Cry1 and Tef gene
polymorphisms are associated with major
depressive disorder in the Chinese population.
J Affect Disord. 2014;157:100–103. doi:10.1016/
j.jad.2013.11.019.

142. Shi SQ, White MJ, Borsetti HM, et al. Molecular
analyses of circadian gene variants reveal sex-
dependent links between depression and clocks.
Transl Psychiatry. 2016;6(3):e748. doi:10.1038/
tp.2016.9.

143. Soria V, Martínez-Amorós E, Escaramís G,
et al. Differential association of circadian
genes with mood disorders: CRY1 and NPAS2
are associated with unipolar major depression
and CLOCK and VIP with bipolar disorder.

Neuropsychopharmacology. 2010;35(6):1279–1289. doi:10.1038/npp.2009.230.

144. Soria V, Martinez-Amoros E, Escaramis G, et al. Resequencing and association analysis of arylalkylamine N-acetyltransferase (AANAT) gene and its contribution to major depression susceptibility. *J Pineal Res.* 2010;49(1):35–44. doi:10.1111/j.1600-079X.2010.00763.x.

145. Kishi T, Yoshimura R, Kitajima T, et al. SIRT1 gene is associated with major depressive disorder in the Japanese population. *J Affect Disord.* 2010;126(1-2):167–173. doi:10.1016/j.jad.2010.04.003.

146. Li JZ, Bunney BG, Meng F, Hagenauer MH, Walsh DM, Vawter MP. Circadian patterns of gene expression in the human brain and disruption in major depressive disorder. *PNAS.* 2013;110(24):9950–9955. doi:10.1073/pnas.1305814110.

147. Partonen T, Treutlein J, Alpman A, et al. Three circadian clock genes Per2, Arntl, and Npas2 contribute to winter depression. *Ann Med.* 2007;39(3):229–238.

148. Johansson C, Smedh C, Partonen T, et al. Seasonal affective disorder and serotonin-related polymorphisms. *Neurobiol Dis.* 2001;8(2):351–357.

149. Lavebratt C, Sjöholm LK, Partonen T, Schalling M, Forsell Y. PER2 variation is associated with depression vulnerability. *Am J Med Genet Part B Neuropsychiatr Genet.* 2010;153(2):570–581. doi:10.1002/ajmg.b.31021.

150. Lavebratt C, Sjöholm LK, Soronen P, et al. CRY2 is associated with depression. *PLoS One.* 2010;5(2 e9407):1–8.

151. Rajendran B, Janakarajan VN. Circadian clock gene aryl hydrocarbon receptor nuclear translocator-like polymorphisms are associated with seasonal affective disorder: an Indian family study. *Indian J Psychiatry.* 2016;58(1):57–60.

152. Brown GM, McIntyre RS, Rosenblat J, Hardeland R. Depressive disorders: processes leading to neurogeneration and potential novel treatments. *Prog Neuro-Psychopharmacol Biol Psychiatr.* 2018;80(1):189–204. doi:10.1016/j.pnpbp.2017.04.023.

153. Wirz-Justice A, Benedetti F. Perspectives in affective disorders: clocks and sleep. *Eur J Neurosci.* 2019;51(1):346–365. doi:10.1111/ejn.14362.

154. 4. Wirz-Justice A, Bader A, Frisch U, et al. A randomized, double-blind, placebo-controlled study of light therapy for antepartum depression. *J Clin Psychiatry.* 2011;72(7):986-93. doi:10.4088/JCP.10m06188blu.

155. Wirz-Justice A, Benedetti F, Terman M. *Chronotherapeutics for Affective Disorders.* Rev. 2nd ed. Basel, Switzerland: Karger; 2013.

156. Dallaspezia S, Suzuki M, Benedetti F. Chronobiological therapy for mood disorders. *Curr Psychiatry Rep.* 2015;17(12):95. doi:10.1007/s11920-015-0633-6.

157. Bunney BG, Bunney WE. Rapid-acting antidepressant strategies: mechanisms of action. *Int J Neuropsychopharmacol.* 2012;15(5):695–713. doi:10.1017/S1461145711000927.

158. Goodwin FK, Jamison K. Fundamentals of treatment, medical treatment of hypomania, mania, and mixed states. In: Goodwin FK, ed. *Manic-Depressive Illness.* 2nd ed. New York, NY: Oxford University Press; 2007:699–744.

159. Henriksen TE, Skrede S, Fasmer OB, et al. Blue-blocking glasses as additive treatment for mania: A randomized placebo-controlled trial. *Bipolar Disord.* 2016;18(3):221–232. doi:10.1111/bdi.12390.

160. Johnsson A. Influence of lithium ions on human circadian rhythms. *Z Naturforsch.* 1980;35c:503–507.

161. Amador A, Huitron-Resendiz S, Roberts AJ, Kamenecka TM, Solt LA, Burris TPB. Pharmacological targeting the REV-ERBs in sleep/wake regulation. *PLoS One.* 2016;11(9):1–16. doi:10.1371/journal.ponc.0162452.

162. Raghuram S, Stayrook KR, Huang P, et al. Identification of heme as the ligand for the orphan nuclear receptors REV-ERBα and REV-ERBβ. *Nat Strut Mol Biol.* 2007;14(12):1207–1213. doi:10.1038/nsmb1344. Identification.

163. Rastad C, Ulfberg J, Lindberg P. Improvement in fatigue, sleepiness, and health-related quality of life with bright light treatment in persons with seasonal affective disorder and subsyndromal SAD. *Depress Res Treat.* 2011;2011:543906. doi:10.1155/2011/543906.

164. Gordijn MCM, Mannetje D 't, Meesters Y. The effects of blue-enriched light treatment compared to standard light treatment in

Seasonal Affective Disorder. *J Affect Disord.* 2012;136(1–2):72–80.

165. Brown GM, Pandi-Perumal SR, Trakht I, Cardinali DP. The role of melatonin in seasonal affective disorder. In: Partonen T, Pandi-Perumal SR, eds. *Seasonal Affective Disorder Practice and Research.* Vol 2. New York, NY: Oxford University Press; 2010:149–162.

166. Buysse DJ, Reynolds CF 3rd, Monk TH, Berman SR, Kupfer DJ. The Pittsburgh Sleep Quality Index: a new instrument for psychiatric practice and research. *Psychiatry Res.* 1989;28(2):193–213.

14

Sleep-Related Movement Disorders

RAVI GUPTA

INTRODUCTION

Abnormal movements are seen across a wide range of sleep disorders. However, they vary in complexity and duration as well as their relation to sleep-wake stages. For example, abnormal movements are observed in patients with sleepwalking, restless legs syndrome (RLS), and those with nocturnal frontal lobe epilepsy. Within the scope of this chapter, we will focus on RLS, which is included under broad diagnostic category of "sleep-related movement disorders," with special emphasis on its pathophysiology, clinical assessment and management.[1] Besides RLS, other diagnoses in this category include periodic limb movement disorder (PLMD), sleep-related bruxism, sleep-related leg cramps (SRLCs), sleep-related rhythmic movement disorder (RMD), benign sleep myoclonus of infancy, propriospinal myoclonus, and sleep-related movement disorders caused by medical conditions or medication/substance use. While the *International Classification of Sleep Disorders* (third edition; ICSD-3)[1] includes these multiple conditions under the rubric of "Sleep Related Movement Disorders," the *Diagnostic and Statistical Manual* (fifth edition; DSM-5) describes only RLS in this category.[2]

RESTLESS LEGS SYNDROME (RLS)

RLS is a sensorimotor disorder characterized by an intense urge to move legs, which may or may not be associated with uncomfortable sensations in legs.[1] The symptoms follow a circadian pattern, at least early in the course of disease, with daily onset of symptoms in the latter part of the day. Rest or periods of inactivity may lead to initiation or exacerbation of RLS symptoms. Lastly, the movement or stretching of legs brings relief of varying magnitude ranging from slight improvement to complete relief. The symptoms tend to reappear when movement/stretching is halted. For clinical diagnosis of RLS, symptoms must interfere with

sleep, cause distress or adversely affect functioning during the day, and all the diagnostic features (as above) have to be present.[1,2] The International RLS Study Group (IRLSLSG) describes interference with functioning as a clinical specifier.[3]

There are some differences among diagnostic criteria proposed by IRLSLSG,[3] American Psychiatric Association (DSM-5),[2] and American Academy of Sleep Medicine (AASM; ICSD-3).[1] DSM-5 had added a frequency and duration criteria where symptoms must be present for at least 3 nights per week for at least 3 months.[2] On the other hand, IRLSSG provides specifiers such as "chronic persistent" where symptoms when not treated would occur at least 2 nights per week during past 1 year and "chronic intermittent" where symptoms when not treated, are less frequent over the past year but there are at least 5 episodes during lifetime.[3] Lastly, ICSD-3[1] does not describe any frequency or duration criteria.

A number of medical and neurological conditions that mimic RLS should be ruled out before making a definitive diagnosis of RLS. These conditions include leg cramps, discomfort from keeping limb in the same position for a long period, varicose veins, limb edema, leg muscle pain, joint pain, and habitual foot tapping (see Table 14.1).[1,3] Symptoms of peripheral neuropathy may also mimic symptoms of RLS. However, peripheral neuropathy can be differentiated from RLS based upon history and physical examination. Patients with peripheral neuropathy generally report pins and needles or burning type of sensation in their legs. These types of sensations are typically absent in RLS. History and physical examination are usually helpful to confirm RLS, although laboratory investigations are recommended with particular emphasis on evaluating for underlying iron deficiency that has been shown to precipitate restless leg symptoms in a high percentage of individuals, with suppression of these symptoms noted after repletion of iron stores. Differentiating features

TABLE 14.1. CONDITIONS THAT MIMIC RESTLESS LEG SYNDROME

Conditions	How to Differentiate
Leg Cramps	Patients often complain of "knot" in the muscle of calves or feet. The symptoms tend to come on at night and are relieved with stretching or walking. However, leg cramps are usually associated with severe pain and abnormal posturing of the affected limb, not seen in RLS. Also, known as "Charley horse". Unlike dysesthesias seen in RLS patients, it is not associated with "urge to move." Most often unilateral with localized symptoms with sudden onset.
Positional discomfort	Movement of the limb only once (i.e., change of posture brings relief in symptoms). On the other hand, patients with RLS have to continue moving the limb(s) to relieve the uncomfortable sensation. Circadian pattern is lacking in positional discomfort.
Varicose veins	Examination of limb shows prominent veins and other signs of venous stasis like skin discoloration. Varicose veins may cause achy or heavy feeling, burning, throbbing in lower legs with worsening of discomfort after sitting or standing for a long time. "Urge to move" is usually not reported, and discomfort is relieved by resting or massage.
Myalgia	Movement generally worsens the pain. Pain also worsens after prolonged physical activity. There is no "urge to move" or circadian pattern.
Arthralgia	Pain is localized to joints and worsens with movement. Circadian pattern and "urge to move" are not present.
Habitual foot tapping	This is usually seen during periods of anxiety or boredom with no sensory symptoms or "urge to move". No circadian pattern. Tapping does not cause distress or sleep disturbances.
Peripheral neuropathy	Sensations felt superficially rather than deep inside the muscles as in RLS. There is burning or pins and needles type of sensation, which is not reported by patients with RLS. Nocturnal worsening (circadian pattern) can be seen but sensory symptoms are not relieved by movement and there is no "urge to move."
Akathisia	This is inner sense of restlessness accompanied by an intense desire to move, which is usually generalized but may be more predominant in legs and simulate RLS. However, akathisia does not cause unpleasant sensory symptoms and there is less relief from movement and circadian variance compared with RLS.
Peripheral vascular disease	The pain worsens with activity and improves with rest, which is exact opposite to RLS. In addition, there is no "urge to move" or circadian pattern.

Abbreviation: RLS, restless leg syndrome.

between various RLS mimics are depicted in Table 14.1.[4]

Clinicians are advised to consider variations in clinical presentations of patients with RLS. First, although it has been named as restless *legs* syndrome, approximately quarter to half of the patients with RLS have symptoms in their arms.[1] Because of this reason, IRLSSG suggested that it should be termed as restless legs syndrome/ Willis Ekbom disease (RLS/WED) instead of RLS, a nomenclature that is retained in the ICD-3.[1] In some atypical cases, symptoms have been reported in arms only or in other body parts such

as face and trunk.[3,5] Burning mouth syndrome and restless sensations in genital area have also been described as rare clinical variants of RLS.[6] However, the scientific evidence available for these variants is merely anecdotal. Besides, these variants have some diagnostic limitations; for example, urge to move the legs was not seen in all of the reported cases and improvement by movement was difficult to establish as body parts other than legs were involved.[6] Second, using the term "legs" does not mean that symptoms should be present in both legs as in a sizable number of patients, RLS symptoms are seen just in one leg.[3] Clinical presentation of patients with unilateral symptoms is similar to those with bilateral symptoms except that these patients may not have significant family history of RLS.[7] Unilateral RLS symptoms may present as a manifestation of subcortical stroke in contralateral hemisphere.[7] Technically, this condition would be included under sleep-related movement disorder due to a medical disorder. Third, the description of quality of uncomfortable sensations tends to differ among different ethnic populations. For example, in the Western population, sensations may be described as uncomfortable, painful, "need to stretch," creepy, crawling, buzzing, itching sensations.[1,8] Among Asians, "tingling," "tickling," "just restlessness," "just pain" or "stretching sensations in calves" are commonly reported sensations.[3,9] Children may describe RLS symptoms as "ants or spiders in legs" or "legs want to stretch."[10]

Thus, a clinician needs to be aware of the choice of various phrases/words used for description of RLS sensations. Finally, careful questioning is required to assess relief in symptoms with the activity. For correct assessment, patients should be questioned whether they feel "any relief while the activity continues" as symptoms are bound to recur after discontinuation of activity even for a brief period of time.[3] Most of the patients report that "moving legs in bed" or "keep walking" relieve their symptoms. In severe cases of RLS, circadian variation may be lost. However, late night or morning periods are often symptom free even in these cases.[3] Symptoms of RLS have multiple dimensions, and each of these require careful consideration during history taking and examination to make an accurate clinical diagnosis.[3] Where diagnostic clarity is lacking, certain supportive features can be helpful in confirming the diagnosis. Four supportive features of RLS—periodic limb movements during sleep (PLMS), response to dopaminergic therapy, family history of RLS, and lack of profound daytime sleepiness—have been described in literature.[3,11] PLMS are seen not only in RLS, but also in various other sleep disorders (like REM behavior disorder, untreated obstructive sleep apnea (OSA), and narcolepsy), medical/neurologic/psychiatric disorders (like Parkinson's disease, uremia, post-traumatic stress disorder) and even in healthy individuals.[1,3,12] Thus, PLMS have high sensitivity but lack specificity for RLS. PLMS represents underlying biology of the disease and PLMS index (movements/hour) is a good indicator of RLS severity.[3] For the diagnosis of RLS, PLMS

are considered important, especially when PLMS occurs with an intensity or pattern that is not explained by factors including age, medications, and comorbid medical conditions known to cause or worsen PLMS.[3] On the contrary, periodic leg movements during wakefulness, as observed in the suggested immobilization test (SIT), have greater sensitivity and specificity for RLS, especially when this information is combined with subjective report of discomfort in legs or urge to move legs.[3]

Nearly three-fourths of the RLS patients show good response to dopaminergic therapy.[3] If the patient does not show *any* improvement in symptoms with dopaminergic therapy, the diagnosis should be revisited. However, nonresponse to dopaminergic therapy does not necessarily rule out diagnosis of RLS.

Most of the patients with RLS have a positive family history, which is supportive of the diagnosis of RLS.[3] Finally, lack of excessive daytime sleepiness is a supporting feature of RLS that may seem counterintuitive. Symptoms of RLS are disruptive to sleep and can lead to reduction in total sleep time. Despite chronic partial sleep deprivation, even patients with moderate to severe RLS often do not complain of daytime sleepiness in a magnitude that would be expected with the amount of sleep loss.[3] The complaint of excessive daytime sleepiness in a patient with RLS should alert the clinician to look for other comorbid conditions that can cause daytime somnolence, for example, insufficient sleep syndrome, central disorders of hypersomnolence, OSA, and hypersomnia due to a medication or substance, to name a few.[3]

Diagnosis of RLS in Special Populations

Diagnostic criteria are similar for the pediatric population and requires the description of symptoms in child's own words, depending upon the level of cognitive development.[13] Proxy report of symptoms by parents or caregivers are not sufficient for the diagnosis of RLS among children.[13] In addition, research diagnostic criteria for "possible" and "probable RLS" have been proposed for pediatric population to stimulate further research.[13] "Probable RLS" indicates presence of all criteria for RLS except circadian variation and "possible RLS" depicts a child with observable behavior showing restlessness in legs at rest but without subjective report of an urge to move legs, and the affected child must fulfil all other criteria for RLS.[13]

Since diagnosis of RLS is purely clinical, patients who cannot communicate well and those who are cognitively impaired are two challenging populations when it comes to diagnosing RLS. To date, no definitive methods are available to establish the diagnosis of RLS in these populations but behavioral observations along with evidence of PLMS and response to dopaminergic therapy may be considered to support diagnosis of RLS although this approach remains to be confirmed.[3]

Epidemiology

RLS has been found to be more prevalent among European and North American population as compared to Asian and African populations.[1,14,15] The prevalence estimates are 1.9% to 4.6% in European and North American general adult populations. In addition, European and North American populations demonstrate an age-related increase in RLS prevalence, while Asian populations do not. In most of the studies, RLS has been noted to be about twice higher in women than in men.[14] Studies using a single question have reported prevalence of RLS to range between 9% to 15% in the adult population.[14] When symptoms were assessed using IRLSLSG criteria, the prevalence of RLS ranged between 5% to 15%.[1,14] Besides diagnostic method, prevalence is also affected by clinical definition used in an individual study as there is a wide variation in the frequency of occurrence of symptoms criterion used between individual studies. Upon inclusion of "criterion for frequency of RLS symptoms," a drop in prevalence was observed across studies. Prevalence dropped by 40%, 50%, and 80% when frequency of symptoms was set to at least once a week, at least 2 nights a week, and almost nightly symptoms, respectively.[14] This suggests that most of the patients do not experience symptoms of RLS on nightly basis. The ethnicity also influences prevalence of RLS. Among Asians, a Japanese study reported RLS prevalence of 5%, and nearly 2% prevalence has been reported in India, which is lower than that reported among whites.[14,16,17] African population seems to have lowest prevalence of 0.01%.[15] In addition, geographical factors also appear to influence prevalence of RLS with increasing prevalence toward greater northern latitude as a function of distance from equator.[15]

In children, prevalence varies between 2% to 4%.[1] RLS has been found to be more frequent among elderly population across different studies.[14] Higher prevalence among females after the age of 35 years has been reported across studies;

however, in younger population, gender difference was not observed.[1,3,14] Gender predisposition for the RLS among females is thought to be related to the pregnancy and parity as prevalence comparable to men has been found in nulliparous women.[3] Thus, multiple factors including environment, geography, race, gender, age, pregnancy, parity and diagnostic criteria appear to influence the prevalence of RLS.

Predisposing Factors

Certain people have biological predisposition to have RLS while extrinsic factors precipitate the symptoms. Common predisposing and precipitating factors are mentioned in Table 14.2. Biological predisposition is evident from family studies showing higher prevalence of RLS in twins and first-degree relatives of patients with RLS.[3] Among twins, monozygotic twins are at higher concordance for RLS.[1,18] Certain genes like BTBD-9, MEIS1, MAP2K5/LNXCOR, and PTPRD have been shown to increase predisposition, although

TABLE 14.2. PREDISPOSING AND PRECIPITATING FACTORS FOR RESTLESS LEG SYNDROME

Medical conditions	Iron deficiency anemia
	Chronic renal failure
	Prolonged immobilization
	Pregnancy
Medications	Antipsychotics
	Anti-histaminics
	Antidepressants
	Antiemetics like metoclopramide
	Opioid withdrawal
Family history	Positive family history for RLS
Possible factors with preliminary or insufficient evidence	Systemic hypertension
	Diabetes mellitus
	Migraine
	Parkinson's disease
	fibromyalgia
	Multiple sclerosis
	Stroke
	Chronic obstructive pulmonary disease
	Narcolepsy
	Spinocerebellar ataxia

Abbreviation: RLS, restless leg syndrome.

each of them have a small effect.[1,18] In addition, genetics of RLS does not follow Mendelian pattern (i.e., linkage with single disease-causing gene), and expression of RLS symptoms has been found to be dependent upon environmental/epigenetic factors.[18]

Certain medical conditions (also mentioned in Table 14.2) can precipitate RLS. The patients who develop RLS symptoms in their fourth decade or later have higher likelihood of having underlying medical disorders precipitating the symptoms of RLS.[11] Among these medical conditions, higher prevalence of RLS has been reported among subjects with liver cirrhosis.[19,20] Although chronic kidney disease is a known risk factor for the RLS, some reports question this association.[21] A study reported a possibility that muscle ischemia, leg cramps, neuropathy, neurogenic claudication, and unspecified leg discomfort in patients with chronic kidney disease might be mistaken for RLS in absence of comprehensive neurological examination.[21] Additionally, nicotine use and opiate withdrawal syndrome have been associated with RLS symptoms in a sizeable

TABLE 14.3. INITIAL PHARMACOTHERAPY (EXCEPT IRON) OF RESTLESS LEG SYNDROME

Drug	Dose	Common Adverse Effects
Dopaminergic medications[45]		
Levodopa	100–300 mg/day (use only for intermittent RLS)	Nausea, vomiting, postural hypotension, impulse control disorders
Nonergot derived Dopamine agonists		
Pramipexole immediate release	0.125 mg starting dose with increments by 0.125 mg every 2–3 nights up to maximum of 0.75 mg; to be given 2–3 hours before bedtime	Nausea, somnolence, nasopharyngitis, augmentation
Ropinirole immediate release	0.25 mg starting dose with increments by 0.25 mg every 2–3 nights up to maximum dose of 4 mg; to be given 1–3 hours before bedtime	Nausea, vomiting, headache, dizziness, Somnolence
Rotigotine transdermal patch	Start at 1 mg per 24 hour patch and assess weekly for increment by 1 mg/ weekly up to maximum of 4 mg per 24 hour	Nausea, headache, nasopharyngitis, backache, application site reactions; use with caution in liver disease
Alpha-2-delta ligands		
Gabapentin enacarbil	600 mg at 5 PM	Dizziness, somnolence, suicidal thoughts (rare); dose adjustment is advised in renal disease
Gabapentin	300–600 mg 2 hours before RLS symptoms onset	Sedation, dizziness, vision changes, suicidal thoughts (rare); dose adjustment is advised in renal disease
Pregabalin	50–75 mg starting dose given 1–3 hours before bedtime and assess weekly for dose titration by 50–75 mg/week to maximum of 300 mg	Unsteadiness, daytime sleepiness, suicidal thoughts (rare); dose adjustment is advised in renal disease

number of patients.[22-27] Interestingly, nicotine has been reported both as exacerbating as well as alleviating factor for RLS.[22-24]

Available data suggest that antidepressants can precipitate or aggravate RLS/PLMS, although these studies had methodological limitations, and conclusions could not be reached.[28] Among antidepressants, mirtazapine has strong evidence on induction or aggravation of RLS and PLMS while bupropion has been found to reduce symptoms of RLS, at least in short term.[28,29] Antipsychotic medications have been found to induce RLS in female subjects with tryptophan hydroxylase geneVal81Met polymorphism, but no association has been found with D1, D2, D3, and D4 receptor polymorphisms.[30,31] Recently, higher prevalence of RLS and PLMS were reported among subjects living at high altitudes.[32-34]

Differentiation between "causative" and "precipitating" factors is worth a little discussion. It is possible that certain conditions do not *cause* RLS but *precipitate* this condition in people with genetic predisposition thereby bringing the dichotomy of primary and secondary RLS in question.[35] In short, recent evidence indicates that RLS could be considered as a complex disorder where genetic factors interact with environmental factors to precipitate symptoms.[35] Of note, the DSM-5 criteria no longer differentiate between primary and secondary RLS.

Course of RLS

RLS has variable course ranging from relapsing remitting to gradually progressive disease. Based on the frequency of symptoms, IRLSLSG has proposed course specifiers: chronic persistent RLS and intermittent RLS for *untreated* cases.[3] Intermittent RLS represents a condition where symptoms would occur less than two times a week during the past 1 year and the patient has at least five episodes of RLS during their lifetime. However, IRLSLSG criteria do not define "episode" or "event" in terms of duration and interval between two episodes to be considered as two separate episodes/events.[3] On the other hand, chronic persistent RLS represents a condition where symptoms would occur on two or more nights a week during the past year. Cut-off of 2 nights per week is based upon the data related to disease burden as reported in REST study.[36] However, these specifiers do not apply to situations where a known precipitating factor such as pregnancy or a medication seems to result in RLS symptoms.[3]

Pathophysiology

Despite extensive research, pathophysiology of RLS is still an enigma.[11,37] Most of the hypotheses seem to have been derived from observational studies where the treatment of this condition has been traced back to uncover underlying pathophysiological processes.[38] However, cerebrospinal fluid (CSF) studies, functional neuroimaging, and animal models have also contributed to understanding of pathophysiology of RLS.[35]

Genetic Factors

As already discussed, RLS should be seen as a complex disease where genetic factors interact with epigenetic factors to manifest symptoms. Genome-wide studies have shown association of RLS with five genes: *MEIS1, BTBD9, PTPRD, MAP2k/SKOR1,* and *TOX3/BC034767*.[39] These genes have been found to be associated with periodic limb movements, which are considered as motor signature of RLS.[39] In addition, *BTBD9* has been found to be associated with reduced iron stores, a common finding in patients with RLS.[39] *MEIS1* has also been found to influence some aspects of iron metabolism.[18] However, genome-wide association studies had some methodological limitations. First, the number of subjects included in these studies were inadequate to really uncover this complex disorder[11]; second, less frequent variants were not included[11]; and third, these studies were conducted in the United States and Canada, and it is uncertain whether results can be extrapolated to other populations across the globe.

Iron Metabolism

Before exploring the role of iron in RLS, some discussion regarding normal iron metabolism is required. Iron is a critical element for human body functioning. Most cells use iron as a cofactor for fundamental biochemical activities, such as oxygen transport, energy metabolism, and DNA synthesis.[41] Iron metabolism is a tightly regulated body process, which depends upon iron concentration as well as presence of oxygen. Iron is absorbed through duodenum through divalent metal transporters (DMT-1) present on the apical membrane of duodenal cells after conversion into ferrous form (Fe^{+2}). From the duodenal cells, it gets secreted into blood plasma where it binds with apo-transferrin to form transferrin. Transferrin then delivers the iron to body cells via process of endocytosis occurring after binding with transferrin receptors (TfR1). Internalized iron is transported to mitochondria to integrate into metallo-proteins while excess iron goes back to cytoplasm where it combines with apo-ferritin in ferrous state (Fe^{+2}), converts into ferric state (Fe^{+3}) and form ferritin.[40] Ferritin is found in most tissues as a cytoplasmic protein and consists of light (L) and heavy (H) chains or subunits. Ferritin is secreted in small amounts into the serum where it functions as an iron carrier. Serum ferritin is also an indirect marker of the total amount of iron stored in the body due to which serum ferritin is used as a diagnostic test for iron-deficiency anemia. Ferritin serves to store iron in a nontoxic form and to transport it to areas in the body where it is required. Free iron is toxic to cells as it can catalyze formation of free radicals from reactive oxygen species like peroxide via Fenton reaction.

The expression of TfR1 and apo-ferritin is regulated at post-transcriptional level depending upon the availability of iron. This molecular mechanism involves iron-regulatory proteins 1 and 2 (IRP1 and IRP2) and their binding with iron-response elements (IRE) present on the mRNA of these proteins. During iron deficiency, IRPs bind with IREs to increase and block translations of TfR1 mRNA and apo-ferritin mRNA, respectively. These actions increase the mobilization of iron and reduce its cellular storage.[40]

Iron metabolism is also linked with hypoxia through hypoxia inducible factors (HIFs), which become active in response to hypoxia and iron deficiency.[42] HIFs have multiple effects that include increase in erythropoietin production, iron absorption, and utilization, as well as changes in the bone marrow to increase erythropoiesis.[42] The HIF system has two transcription factors— HIF-1 alpha and HIF-2 alpha—whose activation or deactivation is pivotal to the activity of this system. Under normal conditions, these proteins continuously get inactive (due to hydroxylation) owing to binding of oxygen, iron, and alpha-ketoglutarate with proline hydroxylase domain 2 (PHD-2). Thus, HIF system responds not only to hypoxia, but also to iron deficiency and to the reduction of alpha-ketoglutarate resulting from anaerobic respiration. Of note, alpha-ketoglutarate is an intermediate in Krebs cycle, which is an aerobic metabolic cellular process, being heavily dependent on oxygen. Under hypoxic conditions, HIF-1 alpha and HIF-2 alpha form dimers upon combining with HIF-1 beta, thereby resulting in activation of HIF system or pathway. The activation of HIF pathway then leads to increase in bioavailable iron by increasing iron absorption (via increased DMT-1) and iron transport (via increased translation of transferrin receptor TfR1 mRNA) and by reducing iron storage (via reduced translation of apo-ferritin mRNA).[38]

Iron deficiency is a well-defined environmental factor implicated in causation of RLS. This deficiency in patients with RLS was first described in the groundbreaking studies by Ekbom and Norlander in 1945 and 1953, respectively. Peripheral iron studies have shown inconsistent results among patients with RLS. However, studies that assessed iron status in the central nervous system (CNS) have shown the association between iron and RLS. Low CNS iron status as evident from increased CSF transferrin, and low CSF ferritin has been shown in patients with RLS.[38] Other CSF studies have shown that patients with RLS have lower levels of CSF prohepcidin, which furthers the biological evidence of a low CNS iron status in RLS. Overall, these studies support the alteration in brain iron homeostasis in RLS patients and that peripheral iron stores (as determined by serum values) do not always reflect the state of iron homeostasis in the brain. A higher serum concentration of soluble transferrin receptor, possibly indicating early iron deficiency, has also been shown in patients with RLS. Brain autopsy studies tend to confirm these findings. Connor et al. showed a dramatic decrease in iron and ferritin heavy chains, and an increase in transferrin staining in the substantia nigra of RLS brains compared to controls. Later studies also showed reduced iron content both inside as well as outside the neuronal cells, especially in the nigro-striatal area of the brain.[38,39] However, findings related to ferritin light chains were contradictory, showing either no change or a reduction compared to controls.[38] Even within a cell, iron has been found to have a differential distribution in patients with RLS. For example, sequestration of iron has been found in mitochondria with reduced iron in cytoplasm in cells of choroid plexus.[39] Similarly, increased mitochondrial ferritin reflecting increased mitochondrial iron status has been found in the cells of substantia nigra. Iron pathophysiology is also supported by the fact that allelic variants of BDBT9 genomic region implicated in RLS are either associated with decreased peripheral iron stores (reduced serum ferritin) or greater decreases in peripheral iron stores with blood donations.[39]

Overall, the available data point toward decreased acquisition of iron by cells in the brain and low brain iron despite normal peripheral iron as the best-established neurobiological abnormality in RLS. This brain iron deficiency is regional and localized to certain areas like substantia nigra, choroid plexus, red nucleus, and thalamus, and in some of these areas, like substantia nigra and choroid plexus, the available iron is preferentially located in mitochondria at the expense of cytoplasmic iron. The regional brain deficiency of iron likely results from failure to provide optimal iron transport across blood–brain barrier exacerbated by regional failure to provide iron to critical brain areas like substantia nigra and sequestration of available iron preferentially in mitochondria versus cytoplasm. The role of iron in pathophysiology of RLS is further emphasized by the fact that iron supplementation has been found to improve/alleviate symptoms in many RLS patients.[43] This brain-specific alteration in iron homeostasis is also considered a putative cause of dopamine abnormalities seen in RLS.

Molecular mechanisms of iron metabolism support the role of iron in causation of RLS symptoms. Iron regulatory proteins (IRPs) bind to the IREs on mRNA of various proteins that take part in iron metabolism. IRPs are present in two forms, IRP-1 and IRP-2, both having similar biological functions.[38] During iron deficiency, binding of IRP-1 to IRE reduces translation of ferritin-mRNA and increases translation of transferrin mRNA.[38] These effects are manifested by reduced iron storage and increment in iron transportation in the body. In addition, IREs are also present in DMT-1 mRNA. DMT-1 is present in duodenum, and it helps in absorption of iron. Thus, IRPs help in mobilization of iron during iron deficiency. However, in such conditions, certain areas of brain (e.g., neuro-melanin cells of substantia nigra) show paradoxical response characterized by reduced IRP-1 activity leading to impaired transport of iron across brain.[39]

It may be perplexing to understand the mechanisms that explain iron deficiency in brain leading to RLS symptoms. Iron deficiency can lead to two outcomes: (a) activation of hypoxia inducible pathway and (b) loss of myelin. IRP is also present on mRNA of proteins involved in hypoxia inducible pathway (HIF), especially HIF-2 alpha. Activation of HIFs occurs in hypoxic conditions, as iron is important for oxygen transport (see the following discussion).[39] In addition, iron is an important co-factor, along with tetra-hydrobiopterin for the synthesis of dopamine through tyrosine–hydroxylase pathway.[38] Hence, iron deficiency appears to negatively influence dopaminergic neurotransmission involving tyrosine hydroxylase pathway.[38] Increased HIF-1 alpha in substantia nigra tissue and increased HIF-2 alpha in cortical microvasculature have been reported among subjects with RLS, suggesting a role of HIF pathway in RLS.[44]

Dopamine

Considering the efficacy of dopaminergic drugs in treatment of RLS, it may be considered as a hypo-dopaminergic state. Contrary to these expectations, an increase in dopamine content and increased production has been reported across different studies.[39] CSF studies of patients with RLS have shown increased concentration of 3-O-methyl-dopa along with increased homovanillic acid and increased tetra-hydro-biopterin, suggesting increased presynaptic synthesis of dopamine.[38] In addition, reduction in postsynaptic D2 receptor density and fluoro-DOPA uptake in striatal regions has been reported.[39] Lastly, reduced membrane bound dopamine transporters (DAT) have been found in patients with RLS.[39] Together, the evidence suggests an increased availability of synaptic dopamine in striatal regions along with downregulation of postsynaptic D2 receptors.

Interestingly, dopamine concentration in brain follows a circadian pattern with increasing availability in the morning and reduction by the evening. This circadian variation explains evening onset of RLS symptoms in predisposed individuals due to a state of functional dopamine deficiency (reduced postsynaptic D2 receptors due to downregulation from high synaptic dopamine during morning hours along with reduced synaptic dopamine during evening hours) in striatal regions during evening and night.[39] This model also explains the phenomenon of augmentation related to use of dopamine agonists for treatment of RLS. Augmentation is seen after long-term dopaminergic therapy and is characterized by overall increase in RLS symptom severity with increasing doses of dopaminergic medication, including earlier onset of symptoms, increased intensity of symptoms, shorter duration of drug action, or topographic spread of symptoms to other body parts, including the trunk and arms. A small dose of dopaminergic agent in the evening intends to correct the relative evening decline in dopamine, but this could mean adding fuel to the fire. The treatment with dopaminergic agent can lead to increasing the downregulation beyond that is already occurring with the disease, thus making the underlying RLS worse and augmenting the symptoms. The eventual adjustment to the treatment leads to a need for adding even more stimulation and higher doses to be effective. This initially looks like tolerance to the medication, but in this situation, tolerance is essentially a worsening of the underlying pathology or augmentation.[39]

There is emerging experimental and clinical evidence implicating hyperglutamatergic and hypoadenosinergic states in the brain resulting from brain iron deficiency in pathophysiology of RLS. The hypoadenosinergic state may explain enhanced arousal state at night in patients with RLS despite relative dopamine deficiency at night.

Diagnostic Assessment in Patients with RLS

RLS is a clinical diagnosis to be suspected in patients who complain of an urge to move the legs when lying in bed or sitting down during evening hours. The diagnosis is made by clinical history and does not require additional testing, except for an assessment of iron stores in all patients (see previous discussion) and blood urea nitrogen and creatinine if uremia is suspected. Any other potentially contributing or aggravating factors like medications should be identified.

Diagnostic criteria for RLS published by IRLSSG are based on five key clinical features of the disorder, all of which are required for the diagnosis:

1. An urge to move the legs, usually accompanied or caused by uncomfortable and unpleasant sensations in the legs. Sometimes the urge to move is present without the uncomfortable sensations, and sometimes the arms or other body parts are involved in addition to the legs.
2. The urge to move or unpleasant sensations begin or worsen during periods of rest or inactivity such as lying or sitting.
3. The urge to move or unpleasant sensations are partially or totally relieved by movement, such as walking or stretching, at least as long as the activity continues.
4. The urge to move or unpleasant sensations are worse in the evening or night than during the day, or only occur in the evening or night. When symptoms are severe, the worsening at night may not be noticeable but must have been previously present.

5. Symptoms are not solely accounted for by another medical or behavioral condition, such as leg cramps or habitual foot tapping (see Table 14.2).

Diagnostic criteria for RLS in ICSD-3 are similar to those of the IRLSSG and also contain a requirement that symptoms cause concern, distress, sleep disturbance, or impairment in functioning.[1] Neither a minimum frequency nor duration of events is part of the current diagnostic criteria. The clinical distress associated with RLS symptoms tends to increase when symptoms are present at least 3 days per week.

A single diagnostic question, "When you try to relax in the evening or sleep at night, do you ever have unpleasant, restless feelings in your legs that can be relieved by walking or movement?" was shown to have good predictive power for diagnosis of RLS. Screening questionnaires without involving clinical interview can overdiagnose RLS. A polysomnographic evaluation is not required for the diagnosis of RLS. It is usually reserved for patients in whom the diagnosis is in doubt, in cases where PLMS are suspected to be severe and result in arousals, or if comorbid other sleep disorders, such as sleep apnea, are suspected based on clinical assessment.

Occasionally, symptoms of RLS are difficult to distinguish from those of a neuropathy especially since neuropathic symptoms are worse during evening/nighttime hours. However, in neuropathy, sensations are felt superficially rather than deep inside the muscles as in RLS. There is burning or pins and needles type of sensation in neuropathy, which is not reported by patients with RLS. The sensory symptoms in neuropathy are not relieved by movement, and there is generally no "urge to move." If it continues to remain uncertain if presenting symptoms are due to RLS or neuropathy, nerve conduction studies and electromyogram can be considered.

RLS and Psychiatric Disorders

RLS is common among patients with psychiatric disorders, especially those with depression.[47] Nearly one-third of subjects with depression report RLS. However, it appears unrelated to age, duration of depressive disorder, or number of depressive episodes.[48] RLS increases the risk for depression by two- to fourfolds.[49] Patients with RLS commonly have personality traits of high harm avoidance and low self-directedness, which may also contribute to depression.[50] The self-directedness is an ability to regulate and adapt behavior to the demands of a situation to achieve personally chosen goals and values. Mounting evidences suggest that RLS-associated sleep disturbance contributes to depression, with prevalence of depression increasing with worsening severity of RLS.[49,51] Furthermore, a study showed that the subjects with mild RLS are not more likely to be depressed compared to individuals of the same age and education who do not have RLS.[52] A multicenter, randomized, placebo-controlled study showed significant improvement in depression in patients with moderate to severe idiopathic RLS and at least mild depressive symptoms with ropinirole, a dopaminergic agent commonly used to treat RLS.[53] This study suggested that that mild to moderate depressive symptoms should not be treated with antidepressant medication before sufficient therapy for moderate to severe RLS especially when coupled with evidence that depression emerged after onset of RLS in a given individual and since some antidepressants can potentially aggravate RLS symptoms. The authors of this study proposed that antidepressant medications are suitable options if depressive symptoms persist after RLS symptoms are ameliorated. Of note, most antidepressants are thought to precipitate or worsen RLS, but scientific evidence indicates that this association is likely overrated, except for mirtazapine.[28,54]

Among children, RLS has been found to be associated with attention deficit-hyperactivity disorder (ADHD; 25%), depressive disorders (nearly 30%), and anxiety (11%).[55] Relationship between RLS and ADHD in children seems to have neurobiological basis. Among children with ADHD, the parents with RLS have significantly higher prevalence of psychiatric disorders than parents without RLS.[56]

Management of RLS
Both pharmacological and nonpharmacological strategies have been described for management of RLS. However, the evidence is insufficient to assess effect of nonpharmacological strategies.[57] Among nonpharmacological strategies, cognitive-behavior therapy (CBT), mindfulness techniques, and stress-reducing strategies have been found to be effective. Exercise therapy and leg compression devices have also been reported to be effective in small trials.[57] The avoidance of alcohol, caffeine, and nicotine is also effective as these substances are known to exacerbate RLS.[58] There are no data to recommend use of other sleep hygiene

practices to treat RLS. CBT for insomnia (CBT-I) has been found to be beneficial for RLS in patients with comorbid insomnia.[58] Exercise prior to bedtime may be effective in management of RLS in some individuals.[58] Exercise seems to make sense considering the fact that RLS symptoms tend to increase with prolonged inactivity and to be alleviated with physical activity. However, some other individuals report exacerbation of RLS symptoms with exercise. Overall (besides CBT-I), the suggested nonpharmacological strategies include maintaining a healthy weight and diet, getting moderate exercise, using support groups, and taking a hot bath, cold shower, and/or brief walk before bedtime. With the exception of exercise for RLS (for which randomized controlled trials exist), all of these suggested strategies are based on nothing more than just anecdotal evidence.

Pharmacotherapy Therapy of RLS
The pharmacological treatment of RLS is divided into three phases: initial therapy, long-term therapy, and prevention and management of augmentation.

Initial Therapy
The initial pharmacotherapy of RLS (except iron) is summarized in Table 14.3.

Iron Replacement
Oral iron replacement therapy is advised for treatment of patients with RLS who have "fasting" serum ferritin at or below 75 microgram/L.[43] The iron can be replaced orally with ferrous sulphate 325 mg given twice daily along with vitamin C 100 mg twice daily. This strategy has been shown in research studies to be effective in controlling RLS symptoms commensurate with increase in serum ferritin levels.[43] Another approach to replace iron orally could involve administration of ferrous sulfate 325 mg tablet (containing 65 mg of elemental iron), 1 to 2 tablets along with 200 mg vitamin C given every other day since there is increasing evidence suggesting that alternate-day dosing (taking the iron every other day rather than every day) may result in better iron absorption than daily dosing. The findings from a study of the response of 54 iron-deficient women (without evidence of anemia) to daily oral iron suggest that giving multiple doses per day could actually cause a paradoxical decrease in iron absorption. These iron deficient women (ferritin ≤20 ng/mL) were given various doses of oral iron that contained a traceable isotope to track absorption. Iron absorption

was best when dosing was restricted to lower doses and less frequent administration (40 to 80 mg of iron no more than once a day). Higher or more frequent doses of iron raised circulating hepcidin levels. Hepcidin is the key iron-regulating peptide that inhibits intestinal iron absorption . Ferrous sulphate is also available in liquid forms for those who cannot swallow tablets. These forms include oral elixir (containing 44 mg elemental iron per 5 mL) and oral solution (containing 15 mg elemental iron per 1 mL).

The addition of vitamin C enhances absorption of iron from the gut. It also enhances cellular iron uptake by reducing ferric form of iron to ferrous form of iron, and regulates iron-responsive element binding proteins and HIF systems involved in iron metabolism.[43] Vitamin C· also modulates iron metabolism by stimulating ferritin synthesis, inhibiting lysosomal ferritin degradation, and decreasing cellular iron efflux.

The iron supplementation frequently causes gastrointestinal side effects (especially when taken on an empty stomach) including nausea, vomiting, heartburn, epigastric pain/discomfort, metallic taste, flatulence, and either constipation or diarrhea. Other side effects include itching and black/green or tarry stools that stain clothing or cause anxiety about bleeding. These side effects could lower compliance to oral iron. The occurrence of these side effects can be potentially reduced by taking iron supplement after meal even though iron absorption is better on an empty stomach. Other strategies to reduce occurrence of side effects include avoidance of liquid iron supplements because they can stain the teeth, taking iron supplement with a full cup of water to make sure it does not get stuck in the esophagus, not lying down (to reduce risk of reflux) for 30 to 60 minutes after taking iron supplement, and increasing fiber and water intake (to manage constipation). Next, if the person poorly tolerates one formulation of iron supplementation, another formulation (with lower amount of elemental iron) could be tried. One such example of alternative formulation (with elemental iron content and dosing) is ferrous gluconate (325 mg tablet containing 38 mg elemental iron per tablet; 1 tablet daily). The extended-release iron formulations like iron protein succinylate or ferrous glycine sulfate are better tolerated by not releasing large quantities of elemental iron into the stomach. However, these preparations cannot be whole-heartedly recommended as these are poorly absorbed due to iron released too far distally in the intestinal tract;

in some cases, the intact tablets are excreted in stool. Finally, another option is switching to IV iron, which eliminates all of the gastrointestinal side effects of iron that are due to direct effects of iron on the intestinal mucosa. Patient can be referred to the hematologist for consideration of IV iron infusion. If the patient switches to IV iron, oral iron should be discontinued. Overall, IV iron therapy is preferred over oral iron therapy in patients with malabsorption syndromes, complete intolerance to oral iron preparations, moderate to severe symptoms despite a trial of oral iron, or the need for a more rapid response due to severity of symptoms.

Monitoring is critical in patients on oral iron replacement. A fasting iron panel should be obtained after 3 months of initiating therapy, and then every 3 to 6 months until the serum ferritin level is >75 mcg/L and iron saturation is greater than 20%. Monitoring is important to avoid the rare but serious complication of iron overload in patients with hemochromatosis genes. Iron therapy can be discontinued when target values are reached if an ongoing cause for iron deficiency has not been established. The etiologic evaluation of iron deficiency is beyond the scope of this chapter. The patient can be referred to his primary care provider to evaluate for underlying causes of iron deficiency.

In patients who do not respond to nonpharmacologic treatment and correction of iron deficiency, pharmacologic treatment with a dopamine agonist or an alpha-2-delta calcium channel ligand can be considered. Table 14.6 summarizes the doses, mechanism of action and side effects of the commonly used medications for management of RLS. Among these, pramipexole, ropinirole, rotigotine, and gabapentin enacarbil are approved by US Food and Drug Administration (FDA) for the treatment of RLS.[59]

Dopaminergic Medications

The dopaminergic medications used in treatment of RLS include levodopa and nonergot dopamine receptor D3 agonists like pramipexole, ropinirole, and rotigotine. These medications should be cautiously used at the lowest possible dose as their use may lead to dopamine dysregulation syndrome, end of dose effect, and augmentation of RLS symptoms.[57] The patients with dopamine dysregulation syndrome may exhibit an addictive pattern of dopamine replacement therapy use and/or behavioral disturbances including punding and impulse control disorders such as pathologic gambling, compulsive shopping, compulsive eating, and hypersexuality.[60,61] Dopamine dysregulation syndrome has higher prevalence in patients with Parkinson's disease likely due to use of higher doses of dopamine agonists compared to patients with RLS. The male gender increases the risk.[61] Management includes reduction of dopaminergic medication dose or elimination altogether. Another potentially useful strategy is switching from short-acting dopaminergic agent to extended release dopaminergic agent like rotigotine transdermal patch, which provide continuous drug delivery with a stable plasma concentration over 24 hours, although dopamine dysregulation syndrome has also been described with rotigotine transdermal patch. The addition of valproate has also been found useful in some cases.[60,61] The end of dose rebound phenomenon occurs in up to 35% of RLS patients and refers to the reappearance of symptoms in the early morning, the time at which the medication concentration is falling. Hence, it is more common with drugs with a shorter half-life such as levodopa and less frequent when longer-acting dopamine agonists such as ropinirole or pramipexole are given early evening.[45] Delaying the timing of dopaminergic medication in the evening or giving half of the dose of medication at usual time followed by remaining dose a few hours later may prove to be beneficial in addressing end of dose rebound phenomenon. The end of dose rebound may look like augmentation. Similar to augmentation, the symptoms of rebound are worse compared to baseline, but there is no spread of symptoms to the arms, nor a worsening with increased dose, or conversely no improvement with decreased dose as seen in augmentation, which is described in detail in the following discussion.

Among all the dopaminergic drugs, levodopa has the highest potential for causing augmentation and early morning end of dose rebound.[57] However, levodopa is a good medication choice for patients who require intermittent therapy for infrequent RLS symptoms.[57] Pramipexole and ropinirole are less likely to induce augmentation compared to levodopa.[57] Finally, another dopaminergic medication rotigotine, which is available as a transdermal patch for treatment of RLS has minimum chances of rebound and augmentation out of all the dopaminergic agents known to treat RLS.[57] It was withdrawn from US market because of crystallization of drug in 2008 to be reintroduced in 2012.[62]

Alpha-2-Delta Ligands

Three medications in this category are available for the treatment of RLS: gabapentin, gabapentin enacarbil, and pregabalin.[57] Among these medications, gabapentin enacarbil has the most robust available evidence.[57] These medications have potential to cause sedation and anxiolysis. Both gabapentin and pregabalin are used off-label for the treatment of various anxiety disorders. Pregabalin is currently approved for the treatment of generalized anxiety disorder by the European Medicines Agency, but not by the FDA. Hence, these medications may be particularly useful in RLS patients with comorbid insomnia and/or anxiety. Since these medications also possess analgesic property, these are preferred over dopamine agonists for use in RLS patients with comorbid peripheral neuropathy or other pain conditions. These medications are also preferred in patients with history of impulse control disorder or addiction associated with use of dopamine agonists. All of these medications are excreted unchanged by kidney. Hence, these medications should be used with caution in patients with kidney disease.

The alpha-2-delta ligands are now considered first-line medications in the treatment of RLS since these do not cause iatrogenic worsening or augmentation of RLS with long-term treatment. However, for patients with very severe RLS, comorbid depression, obesity, or metabolic syndrome, a dopamine agonist is preferred as initial therapy.

Opioids

Medications including oxycodone, methadone, and tramadol have been used for management of RLS. These medications have been found to be effective for management of treatment refractory RLS and usually do not lead to augmentation.[57] Given the risks, however, including opiate-induced central sleep apnea and addictive potential, these medications are best reserved for nonresponders or patients with augmentation that is nonresponsive to alpha-delta ligands.[57] Their use is described in detail in the following discussion.

Benzodiazepines

The evidence is scarce for the use of benzodiazepines to treat RLS.[57] Clonazepam is the best-studied benzodiazepine for RLS. Due to long half-life, clonazepam has potential to cause adverse effects like nocturnal unsteadiness, drowsiness, or cognitive impairment in the morning. Clonazepam can also lead to exacerbation of sleep apnea if comorbidly seen in patients with RLS. In addition, long-term maintenance treatment with clonazepam is limited by tolerance in many patients. Because of these drawbacks, use of clonazepam at 0.5 to 2 mg dose for RLS should be reserved to patients that require only intermittent therapy or as an add-on agent in patients with refractory symptoms. Benzodiazepine receptor agonists such as zolpidem should be avoided due to high prevalence of complex sleep-related behaviors like sleepwalking associated with their use in the setting of RLS.

Long-Term Therapy for RLS

As previously discussed, medications (except iron) used for treatment of RLS may lose efficacy or cause serious adverse effects over time. Based on extensive literature review, the IRLSSG task force suggested that dopamine D3 agonists pramipexole, ropinirole, and rotigotine have been found to be effective for up to 6 months in uncontrolled studies for the treatment of RLS.[63] On the other hand, pregabalin has been reported to be effective for 1 year in uncontrolled studies for the treatment of RLS.[63] Since RLS tends to have a fluctuating course, reduction of dose or drug holidays can be planned during long-term therapy.[45]

Prevention and Management of Augmentation

Two decades ago, the main issue was spreading awareness among physicians to improve recognition and treatment of patients with clinical significant restless leg symptoms with levodopa. However, soon it became clear that symptoms of RLS worsened profoundly over time in majority of patients with persistent use of levodopa. This gave rise to longer-acting dopaminergic agents like ropinirole, pramipexole, and rotigotine, which were approved for RLS between 2004 and 2008 due to clinical trials showing robust clinical efficacy for short-term treatment of RLS. Over time, it became apparent that augmentation developed in many patients on these agents, being least common among patients on rotigotine. Currently, the main issue is management of RLS over the long term and preventing augmentation and managing augmentation if it were to develop. Augmentation definitely hinders long-term treatment of RLS with dopaminergic agents with incidence rate of augmentation being 8% per year in patients on these medications.[45]

The emergence of augmentation in a patient with RLS who has taken dopaminergic medication for at least 6 months[45] can be suspected when a patient reports advancement in time of onset of RLS symptoms compared to time of onset of RLS symptoms prior to starting dopaminergic medication. This is usually accompanied by requirement for higher medication dosages to suppress RLS symptoms. The overall worsening of RLS symptoms in either severity and/or extension to other body parts (e.g., arms) points toward augmentation.[45] The worsening of RLS symptoms with dosage increase after initial suppression and reduction in symptom severity with dosage reduction further support emergence of augmentation in a given individual.[45] However, an astute clinician would also carefully evaluate for other conditions that may mimic augmentation (Table 14.4).

To prevent the augmentation, alpha-2-delta ligands may be started as the first-line therapy, if not contraindicated for other reasons.[45] If

TABLE 14.4. CONDITIONS MIMICKING AUGMENTATION OF RESTLESS LEG SYNDROME/WILLIS–EKBOM DISEASE

Conditions	Clinical Features
End of dose rebound	Symptoms emerge during early morning hours. There is no spread to areas other than legs, worsening with increased dose or improvement with decreased dose.
Tolerance to drugs	There is breakthrough symptomatology seen at night related to loss of efficacy of drug over time. There is no topographic spread of symptoms, worsening compared to baseline, earlier onset of symptoms, worsening with increased dose or improvement with decreased dose.
Natural progression of disease	This is very similar clinical scenario to augmentation with worsening of symptoms compared to baseline, earlier onset of symptoms, spread to areas other than legs and breakthrough at night but unlike augmentation, there is no worsening with increased dose or improvement with decreased dose.
Exacerbating factors	Same as "natural progression of disease"

dopaminergic medications are preferred over alpha-2-delta ligands based in patient profile, the lowest effective dose should be used.

If augmentation develops during the course of RLS treatment with dopaminergic medication, one should begin management of augmentation with modification/correction of extrinsic exacerbating factors such as low iron stores (serum ferritin below 75 mcg/ml and/or transferrin saturation below 17%) and medications like antidepressants, antipsychotics, and antihistaminics.[45] Augmentation severity can range from mild to severe that can be measured using augmentation severity rating scale.[46] If augmentation prompts the dopaminergic medication dose increase, the switch to a nondopaminergic agent is probably a better approach than increasing the dose of dopaminergic medication especially in cases of severe augmentation.[45] However, in mild augmentation, splitting or advancing the current dose of dopaminergic medication and, if these measures fail, increasing the dose (while still keeping it at or below maximum approved daily dose) of dopaminergic medication are other options.[45] If all of these measures fail in cases of mild augmentation, a switch to another class of drugs is recommended. This switch can be done abruptly or gradual cross-titration method can be used, depending upon clinical severity of RLS symptoms.[45] For management of severe augmentation symptoms, it is recommended that initial short-acting dopaminergic agent be substituted with a long-acting dopaminergic agent like rotigotine or be switched to an alpha-2-delta ligand either abruptly or in a gradual cross titration fashion.[45] Some experts have suggested a 10-day wash-out with no medication on board to evaluate if treatment is even necessary before considering switch to a different class of medications. This approach makes sense but can result in severe RLS symptoms and marked sleep reduction during the wash-out period. If all of these approaches fail or if patient has severe relentless symptoms, opioid therapy should be considered for management of RLS.[45] One could start short-acting oxycodone and consider switching after 1 week to long-acting oxycodone to prevent end-of-dose rebound of RLS symptoms that could happen with use of short-acting oxycodone. The Centers for Disease Control and Prevention advises against starting long-acting opioid for chronic pain in opioid-naïve individuals until a short-acting opioid has been trialed for minimum of 1 week, which makes it reasonable to start with short-acting opioid in patients with severe augmentation as well. The typical starting dose is 5 mg and can go up to 30 mg. Methadone is another option with starting dose of 2.5 mg and going up to 20 mg. Similarly, controlled-release morphine (7.5 mg to 45 mg) and hydrocodone (10 mg to 45 mg) are other options. Both hydrocodone and oxycodone are available as immediate and extended release formulations.

The factors that may aggravate RLS symptoms or result in augmentation include iron deficiency, poor medication adherence, sleep deprivation, lifestyle changes (e.g., sedentary lifestyle), appearance of physiological or pathological conditions known to trigger or exacerbate RLS (pregnancy, renal insufficiency, other sleep disorders particularly sleep-disordered breathing), and medications such as antihistamines (like diphenhydramine and doxylamine found in over-the-counter sleep aids), dopamine-receptor blocking agents like antipsychotic medications, antiemetics like metoclopramide, and serotonergic antidepressants. The prevalence of these factors should be evaluated as a part of comprehensive assessment in a given individual and addressed accordingly.

PERIODIC LIMB MOVEMENT DISORDER (PLMD)

Many patients complain of chronic nonrefreshing sleep or daytime fatigue and their clinical history is not indicative of common sleep disorders. In such cases, objective investigation with in-lab polysomnography (PSG) may reveal excessive PLMS. These movements are usually associated with autonomic and/or cortical arousals or frank awakenings with resultant sleep maintenance or middle insomnia (Figure 14.3). The AASM suggests that a diagnosis of PLMD can be made if PLMS index on a PSG is higher than the normative values (i.e., >5 hours in children and >15 hours in adults).[1] PLMD cannot be diagnosed in the absence of sleep disturbance or daytime fatigue even if PLMS index is elevated above normative values. However, in such cases, the presence of PLMS should be acknowledged as elevated PLMS count that may be clinically correlated to other sleep disorders like sleep apnea, narcolepsy, REM behaviors disorder and RLS. That being said, PLMD is characterized by excessive PLMS with significant sleep disturbance or daytime fatigue in absence of other sleep disorders that could explain these symptoms and cause excessive PLMS including sleep apnea, RLS, narcolepsy, and REM sleep behavior disorder (RBD). PLMD is a rare condition and a diagnosis of exclusion.

A variant of PLMD mimicking RBD has been described with patients kicking, punching, gesticulating, falling out of bed, assaulting the bed partner, and talking or shouting during sleep with or without unpleasant dreams. The PSG in these patients indicated that such behaviors occurred during arousals immediately following PLMS during NREM or REM sleep and responded to dopaminergic therapy.[64]

PLMS has significant overlap with RLS in terms of pathophysiology.[1,65] At present, standard guidelines for treatment of PLMD do not exist. However, medications used for RLS management such as dopamine agonists and alpha-2-delta ligands can be considered for treatment of PLMD.[57,64]

SLEEP-RELATED LEG CRAMPS (SRLCs)

SRLCs are characterized by painful, involuntary, sudden, and intense contractions of leg muscles or muscle groups (calves, thighs, feet) lasting for few seconds to several minutes with an average of 9 minutes (thigh cramps tend to be longest) in adults and 1.7 minutes in children and adolescents.[1] SRLCs are known by many different colloquial names such as "Charlie horses," "leg stitches," "leg or foot spasms," or "knots." SRLC usually resolve spontaneously, but most of them are followed by painful discomfort due to soreness in the muscle that may persist from 30 minutes to several hours. SRLC occur during time in bed, arising either from sleep or wakefulness.[1] SRLC can cause a brief arousal or frank awakening from sleep. Patients with SRLC can have one or two episodes per night, several times a week. These can usually be relieved by local massage, application of heat, movement of the affected limb, or dorsiflexing the foot to relieve the spasm. SRLC can occur in all age groups, but their frequency increases with aging. SRLC may be idiopathic or secondary to a medical disorder or use of medications such as long-acting beta blockers, IV iron sucrose, statins, oral contraceptives, and diuretics.[1,66] Electrolyte imbalance, diabetes mellitus, peripheral vascular disease, hemodialysis, neuromuscular disorders like amyotrophic lateral sclerosis, prolonged standing at work, excessive exercise, dehydration, and cirrhosis are some predisposing and precipitating factors for SRLC.[1] Clinicians need to differentiate SRLC from dystonia that is characterized by simultaneous contraction of both agonist and antagonist muscles, while during SRLC, antagonist and agonist muscles do not contract at the same time. In addition, dystonia unlike SRLC do not respond to stretching of the affected muscle or muscle group.

Management

The first step in management involves treating the underlying condition and withdrawing the medicines suspected of causing nocturnal leg cramps (NLCs). The next step is educating the patient about nonpharmacologic management strategies aiming at prevention of cramping.

Nonpharmacologic Treatments

These include drinking six to eight glasses of water daily to prevent dehydration, stretching the calves regularly throughout the day and at night, riding a stationary bicycle for a few minutes before bedtime, keeping blankets loose at the foot of the bed, doing aquatic exercises to help stretch and condition the muscles, and wearing proper fitting shoes. For an acute attack, helpful strategies include walking on or jiggling the affected leg and then elevating it, straightening the leg, flexing the foot toward the knee, and grabbing the toes and pulling them toward the knee, taking hot shower or warm bath, or applying ice massage to the cramped muscle. Stretching has been shown to be the most effective strategy for acutely aborting the attack but various studies investigating its effectiveness for prophylaxis have yielded mixed results. However, a recent randomized controlled trial in the Netherlands showed that nightly stretching of calf and hamstring muscles before going to sleep can reduce the frequency and severity of nocturnal leg cramps in adults older than 55 years. Other measures like raising the head of the bed, raising feet on pillows, lying in prone position with the feet hanging over the end of the bed, ice cold massage, and warm bath do not have more than just anecdotal evidence. Overall, the evidence for nonpharmacological strategies for management of NLCs is very limited.

Pharmacologic Treatments

Various medications have been studied for the treatment of NLCs and include quinine, magnesium, calcium channel blockers, naftidrofuryl, orphenadrine, vitamin E, vitamin B complex, antiepileptics, lidocaine, and botulinum toxin. For dosing recommendations, refer to a nice review by Monderer et al.[67]

SLEEP-RELATED BRUXISM

This condition is usually reported by bed-partners who would hear significant teeth grinding sounds produced by their co-sleeper (i.e., the patient during their periods of sleep). These sounds are usually loud enough to interfere with bed partner's sleep. Patients may present with complaints of fatigue or pain in temporalis-masseters in the morning (that improves as day progresses), temporal headaches, tooth pain, and arousals from sleep due to locking of jaws.[1,68] There may be signs of tooth wear. Sleep-related bruxism may be idiopathic or may occur in association with use of psychotropic medications like selective serotonin reuptake inhibitors, venlafaxine, methylphenidate, atomoxetine, lithium, haloperidol, and chlorpromazine and medical conditions such as RBD, Parkinson's disease, psychiatric disorders like anxiety and depression, RLS, and particularly OSA.[1] Caffeine and alcohol intake are also associated with sleep-related bruxism. It is more frequent among children. In some children, it has been associated with ADHD.[1] The prevalence of bruxism seems to lessen with aging. The estimated prevalence is 17% in children and 8% in middle-aged adults, whereas it drops down to 3% in elderly individuals. The exact pathophysiology of bruxism is unknown. Polysomnography shows rhythmic masticatory muscle activity.[68] This activity is either tonic (isolated sustained contraction) or phasic (series of repetitive activity). It should be differentiated from other conditions that may produce muscle activity involving jaw and facial muscles such as seizures or oromandibular myoclonus occurring during sleep.[1] Management of sleep-related bruxism is focused on prevention of teeth damage, reduction of sounds produced, lessening of muscle discomfort, and minimizing damage to temporo-mandibular joint.[69] Teeth guards are prescribed in severe cases of sleep related bruxism. Caffeine, nicotine, and alcohol use should be eliminated or minimized. Any other potentially contributing or aggravating factors like medications should be identified and removed as feasible. Underlying contributing medical/psychiatric/sleep disorders like OSA should be treated. Other therapeutic measures including medications have not been systematically analyzed for treatment of sleep related bruxism althoughbenzodiazepines, clonidine, anticonvulsants, beta-blockers, dopamine agents, antidepressants, muscle relaxants, local injections of botulinum toxin, and other drugs have been tested in the treatment of sleep related bruxism.

SLEEP-RELATED RHYTHMIC MOVEMENT DISORDER

Patients with SRRMD show rhythmic, repetitive, and stereotyped movements that involve large muscle groups occurring during sleep or drowsy state. There is significant impact on daytime function or interference with normal sleep due to these movements. If adequate precautions are not taken, such patients may also sustain bodily injuries.[1] RMD is common during childhood and may present in various forms like body rocking, head banging, side to side head rolling, body rolling, or banging of legs.[1] Atypical cases where hand was used to bang on the head have also been reported.[70] Although the disorder is self-limiting and improves with age, in some cases it may persist during adolescence.[71] RMD has been reported in association with RLS, OSA, narcolepsy, and RBD.[1] Pathophysiology of RMD is poorly understood. However, resolution of symptoms has been reported with positive airway pressure therapy in patients with OSA and with clonazepam in other patients.[70–72] Stereotypic movement disorder (SMD), a DSM-V disorder seen in children with autism spectrum disorder may be mistaken for RMD but can be distinguished by lack of sleep-related prominence of movements in SMD.

BENIGN SLEEP MYOCLONUS OF INFANCY

This condition is characterized by repetitive myoclonic twitches that may involve a part or whole of the body and usually seen during sleep among infants under 6 months of age. There is disappearance of movements upon awakening. This condition is benign with the affected infant often showing normal neurological examination.[1] The pathophysiology of Benign sleep myoclonus of infancy (BSMI) is poorly understood. BSMI can be confused with myoclonic seizures that could result in unnecessary investigation. The absence of movements in BSMI during wakefulness is the single most important distinguishing feature.

PROPRIO-SPINAL MYOCLONUS AT SLEEP ONSET

Proprio-spinal myoclonus (PSM) is characterized by sudden myoclonic jerks occurring during transition from wakefulness to sleep. These jerks usually start in abdominal, neck, and truncal muscles with subsequent rostral and caudal spread. These episodes occur with varying frequency ranging from an isolated incident to recurrent events. The jerks disappear upon mental activation or with onset of stable sleep and remain absent during various sleep stages. These jerks/movements can lead to significant sleep initiation difficulty. PSM may be divided into three categories based upon the etiopathogenesis: idiopathic, functional, and secondary.[73] These three categories can be differentiated based upon electromyography (EMG) findings.[73] Secondary cases often have structural lesions in the spinal cord.[73] PSM has not been reported among children and is primarily seen in adults. PSM should be differentiated from hypnic jerks, phasic REM twitches, fragmentary myoclonus, epileptic myoclonus, and PLMS.[1] Various kinds of pharmacological as well as nonpharmacological treatments have been tested with varying efficacies for management of PSM.[73]

CONCLUSIONS

In conclusion, SRMDs represent a cluster of conditions characterized by simple and repetitive movements during/around sleep that interfere with sleep and functioning during wakefulness. At present, our understanding regarding pathophysiology of SRMDs is limited. RLS is the most common prototypical SRMD seen in psychiatric practice and, if left untreated, may produce symptoms akin to ADHD, somatic symptom disorders, fibromyalgia, insomnia, and depression. The patients should be clinically screened for RLS, especially if they report sleep initiation difficulties. If patient has moderate to severe RLS, one should consider treating RLS before considering psychotropic treatment of the comorbid psychiatric condition especially if the psychiatric condition is not severe and could await full management of RLS to see if psychiatric condition would abate with treatment of RLS, thereby preventing unnecessary treatment with psychotropic medication, which has the potential to worsen RLS.

KEY CLINICAL PEARLS

1. RLS, a prototypical sleep-related movement disorder is commonly seen in patients with psychiatric disorders.
2. RLS is a genetically moderated sensorimotor circadian disorder related to regional brain iron deficiency stemming from faulty iron acquisition by brain leading to hyperdopaminergic, hyperglutamatergic, and hypoadenosinergic states in the brain.
3. RLS can result in difficulty with sleep initiation that could be mistaken for insomnia in patients with psychiatric

disorders, thereby leading to treatment like sedating antidepressants and antipsychotics with potential of worsening RLS and possibly even the psychiatric disorder.
4. Comprehensive history, which includes probing for sleep-related movement disorders, particularly RLS is important in patients with depression and comorbid sleep initiation problem since treatment of RLS if found could lead to resolution of depression without need for separate antidepressant therapy.
5. Initial treatment includes non-pharmacologic strategies, and oral or IV iron replacement (advised for patients with RLS who have serum ferritin at or below 75 mcg/L).
6. Alpha-2-delta ligands and dopaminergic agents are treatments options for persistent RLS (i.e., if RLS is nonresponsive to iron replacement (if indicated) and nonpharmacologic strategies.
7. Dopamine D3 agonists are no longer considered first line pharmacotherapy for treatment of persistent RLS since they are commonly associated with augmentation/worsening of RLS symptoms over time but can considered as first line (instead of alpha-2-delta ligands) in select cases (very severe RLS, comorbid depression, obesity, or metabolic syndrome).
8. Opioids can be considered for refractory cases of RLS and augmentation due to dopaminergic therapy.

CASE VIGNETTE

A 63-year-old man presented with complaints of depressed mood, poor focus, low appetite, and fatigue during the day worsening over the past 3 months. Further evaluation revealed significant sleep initiation difficulty due to active mind. Past psychiatric history was significant for chronic depression with failed multiple antidepressant trials. Family history was noncontributory. Due to symptoms of low mood with fatigue, poor focus, low appetite, and sleep-onset insomnia indicative of underlying depressive disorder, he was started on mirtazapine 15 mg nightly. During follow up visit 4 weeks later, he reported worsening in his sleep initiation difficulty while depressed mood lifted to some extent. Upon further assessment, he was noted to have emergence of RLS on nightly basis due to mirtazapine that interfered with sleep initiation. At this time, he denied having active mind as a major contributor to his sleep initiation difficulty as it did prior to initiation of mirtazapine. He was reluctant about discontinuing mirtazapine due to overall mood benefit and past history of multiple failed antidepressants. Fasting iron profile was obtained. His serum ferritin was noted to be quite low at 4.3 microgram/L with transferrin saturation of 10%, highly indicative of iron deficiency. Due to ferritin being extremely low, he was referred to hematology for consideration of IV iron infusion since oral iron supplementation would be expected to correct iron deficiency over the course of several months. He received ferric carboxymaltose (Injectafer) 750 mg intravenously as per protocol, 2 doses 1 week apart with rather quick subsidence of his restless leg symptoms. His iron panel was rechecked 6 weeks after second dose with ferritin now at 87 and transferrin saturation at 34%. He also underwent upper and lower gastrointestinal endoscopic studies to find out source of blood (iron) loss, which were unremarkable. Poor iron stores were attributed to previous history of frequent blood donations. Hematology recommended annual check-ups from that point on or earlier as clinically indicated. During a psychiatric clinical follow-up 1 month after IV iron infusion, he indicated complete resolution of RLS symptoms and actually felt that his mood improved remarkably after IV iron infusion. His energy also increased remarkably. Mirtazapine was continued at this point with no further symptoms of restless legs over the next 6-month period.

Case Discussion

As previously noted, iron deficiency can predispose an individual to having RLS symptoms, while antidepressant medications like mirtazapine can act as precipitating agents. Iron replacement can simply correct the predisposition, alleviate restless leg symptoms, and allow continuation of the precipitating agent without further consequence. In addition, iron is known to function in the enzymatic reactions involved in production of neurotransmitters like serotonin, norepinephrine, and epinephrine, while concurrently augmenting their binding to their respective receptors in the frontal cortex. This might explain marked improvement in mood after iron replacement with IV iron infusion in this individual considering these neurotransmitters are involved in mood regulation. This case also highlights an importance of obtaining thorough sleep history as sleep initiation difficulty on mirtazapine could

have been easily dismissed as simple worsening in the problem that existed even before initiation of mirtazapine, and resulted in increase in dose of mirtazapine from 15 to 30 mg without looking for underlying iron deficiency, potentially making the problem worse and even resulting in nonadherence to mirtazapine due to perceived side effect from mirtazapine.

SELF-ASSESSMENT QUESTIONS

1. RLS mimics include all of the following conditions *except*
   a. ADHD.
   b. anxiety.
   c. leg edema.
   d. depression.

Answer: d

2. To assess severity of RLS, following may be used in clinical practice:
   a. International RLS Severity Rating Scale.
   b. suggested immobilization test.
   c. periodic limb movement during sleep index.
   d. algesiometer.

Answer: a

3. Mild RLS in patients with serum ferritin of 40 microgram/L is best managed by
   a. levodopa.
   b. ropinirole.
   c. oral iron therapy.
   d. rotigotine transdermal patch.

Answer: c

4. Daytime symptoms of RLS may mimic
   a. anxiety
   b. depression
   c. alcohol withdrawal
   d. psychosis

Answer: a

5. Patients with morning headache should be screened for
   a. propriospinal myoclonus at sleep onset.
   b. RLS.
   c. sleep-related bruxism.
   d. sleep-related leg cramps

Answer: c

REFERENCES

1. American Academy of Sleep Medicine. *International Classification of Sleep Disorders.*

3rd ed. Darian, IL: American Academy of Sleep Medicine; 2014.

2. American Psychiatric Association. *Diagnostic and Statistical Manual of Mental Disorders.* 5th ed. Arlington, VA: American Psychiatric Association; 2013.

3. Allen RP, Picchietti DL, Garcia-Borreguero D, et al. Restless legs syndrome/Willis–Ekbom disease diagnostic criteria: updated International Restless Legs Syndrome Study Group (IRLSSG) consensus criteria—history, rationale, description, and significance. *Sleep Med.* 2014;15(8):860–873. doi:10.1016/j.sleep.2014.03.025.

4. Jones R, Cavanna AE. The neurobiology and treatment of restless legs syndrome. *Behav Neurol.* 2013;26(4):283–292. doi:10.3233/BEN-2012-120271.

5. Gupta R, Lahan V, Goel D. Restlessness in right upper limb as sole presentation of restless legs syndrome. *J Neurosci Rural Pract.* 2013;4(1):78–80. doi:10.4103/0976-3147.105625.

6. Turrini A, Raggi A, Calandra-Buonaura G, Martinelli P, Ferri R, Provini F. Not only limbs in atypical restless legs syndrome. *Sleep Med Rev.* 2018;38:50–55. doi:10.1016/J.SMRV.2017.03.007.

7. Shukla G, Gupta A, Pandey RM, et al. What features differentiate unilateral from bilateral restless legs syndrome? A comparative observational study of 195 patients. *Sleep Med.* 2014;15(6):714–719. doi:10.1016/j.sleep.2014.01.025.

8. Cotter PE, O'Keeffe ST. Restless leg syndrome: is it a real problem? *Ther Clin Risk Manag.* 2006;2(4):465–475.

9. Gupta R, Ahmad S, Dhar M, Goel D, Lahan V. Clinical presentation of restless legs syndrome: does the gender matter? *Sleep Biol Rhythms.* 2014;12(3). doi:10.1111/sbr.12059.

10. de Weerd A, Aricò I, Silvestri R. Presenting symptoms in pediatric restless legs syndrome patients. *J Clin Sleep Med.* 2013;9(10):1077–1080. doi:10.5664/jcsm.3086.

11. Garcia-Borreguero D, Cano-Pumarega I. New concepts in the management of restless legs syndrome. *BMJ.* 2017;356:j104. doi:10.1136/bmj.j104.

12. Vertrugno R, Montagna P. Periodic limb movements: diagnosis and clinical associations. *Pract Neurol.* 2009:23–27.

13. Picchietti DL, Bruni O, de Weerd A, et al. Pediatric restless legs syndrome diagnostic criteria: an update by the International Restless Legs Syndrome Study Group. *Sleep Med.* 2013;14(12):1253–1259. doi:10.1016/j.sleep.2013.08.778.

14. Ohayon MM, O'Hara R, Vitiello M V. Epidemiology of restless legs syndrome: a synthesis of the literature. *Sleep Med Rev.* 2012;16(4):283–295. doi:10.1016/j.smrv.2011.05.002.

15. Koo BB. Restless legs syndrome: relationship between prevalence and latitude. *Sleep Breath.* 2012;16(4):1237–1245. doi:10.1007/s11325-011-0640-8.

16. Gupta R, Ulfberg J, Allen RP, Goel D. High prevalence of restless legs syndrome/Willis Ekbom Disease (RLS/WED) among people living at high altitude in the Indian Himalaya. *Sleep Med.* 2017;35:7–11. doi:10.1016/j.sleep.2017.02.031.

17. Rangarajan S, Rangarajan S, D'Souza GA. Restless legs syndrome in an Indian urban population. *Sleep Med.* 2007;9(1):88–93. doi:10.1016/j.sleep.2006.11.004.

18. Winkelmann J, Schormair B, Xiong L, Dion PA, Rye DB, Rouleau GA. Genetics of restless legs syndrome. *Sleep Med.* 2017;31:18–22. doi:10.1016/j.sleep.2016.10.012.

19. Franco RA, Ashwathnarayan R, Deshpandee A, et al. The high prevalence of restless legs syndrome symptoms in liver disease in an academic-based hepatology practice. *J Clin Sleep Med.* 2008;4(1):45–49.

20. Anderson K, Jones DEJ, Wilton K, Newton JL. Restless leg syndrome is a treatable cause of sleep disturbance and fatigue in primary biliary cirrhosis. *Liver Int.* 2013;33(2):239–243. doi:10.1111/liv.12035.

21. Calviño J, Cigarrán S, Lopez LM, Martinez A, Sobrido M-J. Restless legs syndrome in non-dialysis renal patients: is it really that common? *J Clin Sleep Med.* 2015;11(1):57–60.

22. Lahan V, Ahmad S, Gupta R. RLS relieved by tobacco chewing: paradoxical role of nicotine. *Neurol Sci.* 2012;33(5):1209–1210. doi:10.1007/s10072-011-0882-z.

23. Lavigne GJ, Lobbezoo F, Rompre PH, Nielsen TA, Montplaisir J, Lavigne G. Smoking and sleep cigarette smoking as a risk factor or an exacerbating factor for restless legs syndrome and sleep bruxism. *Sleep.* 20(4):290–293.

24. Oksenberg A. Alleviation of severe restless legs syndrome (RLS) symptoms by cigarette smoking. *J Clin Sleep Med.* 2010;6(5):489–490.

25. Gupta R, Ali R, Ray R. Willis–Ekbom disease/restless legs syndrome in patients with opioid withdrawal. *Sleep Med.* 2018;45:39–43. doi:10.1016/j.sleep.2017.09.028.

26. Högl B, Lohner H, Mikus G, Huff H. Acute and painful exacerbation of RLS and PLM induced by opioid interaction—withdrawal syndrome. *Sleep Med.* 2017;36:186–187. doi:10.1016/j.sleep.2017.05.010.

27. Freye E, Levy J. Acute abstinence syndrome following abrupt cessation of long-term use of

tramadol (Ultram): a case study. *Eur J Pain.* 2000;4(3):307–311. doi:10.1053/eujp.2000.0187.

28. Kolla BP, Mansukhani MP, Bostwick JM. The influence of antidepressants on restless legs syndrome and periodic limb movements: a systematic review. *Sleep Med Rev.* 2018;38:131–140. doi:10.1016/j.smrv.2017.06.002.

29. Vishwakarma K, Kalra J, Gupta R, Sharma M, Sharma T. A double-blind, randomized, controlled trial to compare the efficacy and tolerability of fixed doses of ropinirole, bupropion, and iron in treatment of restless legs syndrome (Willis–Ekbom disease). *Ann Indian Acad Neurol.* 2016;19(4):472–477. doi:10.4103/0972-2327.194424.

30. Cho C-H, Kang S-G, Choi J-E, Park Y-M, Lee H-J, Kim L. Association between antipsychotics-induced restless legs syndrome and tyrosine hydroxylase gene polymorphism. *Psychiatry Investig.* 2009;6(3):211–215. doi:10.4306/pi.2009.6.3.211.

31. Kang S-G, Lee H-J, Choi J-E, et al. Association study between antipsychotics- induced restless legs syndrome and polymorphisms of dopamine D1, D2, D3, and D4 receptor genes in schizophrenia. *Neuropsychobiology.* 2008;57(1-2):49–54. doi:10.1159/000129667.

32. Vizcarra-Escobar D, Mendiola-Yamasato A, Risco-Rocca J, et al. Is restless legs syndrome associated with chronic mountain sickness? *Sleep Med.* 2015;16(8):976–980. doi:10.1016/j.sleep.2015.03.013.

33. Gupta R, Ulfberg J, Allen RP, Goel D. High prevalence of restless legs syndrome/Willis Ekbom Disease (RLS/WED) among people living at high altitude in the Indian Himalaya. *Sleep Med.* 2017;35:7–11. doi:10.1016/j.sleep.2017.02.031.

34. Stefani A, Heidbreder A, Hackner H, Burtscher M, Högl B. Influence of high altitude on periodic leg movements during sleep in individuals with restless legs syndrome and healthy controls: A pilot study. *Sleep Med.* 2017;29:88–89. doi:10.1016/J.SLEEP.2016.06.037.

35. Trenkwalder C, Allen R, Högl B, Paulus W, Winkelmann J. Restless legs syndrome associated with major diseases: a systematic review and new concept. *Neurology.* 2016;86(14):1336–1343. doi:10.1212/WNL.0000000000002542.

36. Allen RP, Walters AS, Montplaisir J, et al. Restless legs syndrome prevalence and impact. *Arch Intern Med.* 2005;165(11):1286. doi:10.1001/archinte.165.11.1286.

37. Daubian-Nosé P, Frank MK, Esteves AM. Sleep disorders: a review of the interface between restless legs syndrome and iron metabolism.

Sleep Sci (São Paulo, Brazil). 2014;7(4):234–237. doi:10.1016/j.slsci.2014.10.002.

38. Earley CJ, Connor J, Garcia-Borreguero D, et al. Altered brain iron homeostasis and dopaminergic function in restless legs syndrome (Willis–Ekbom disease). *Sleep Med.* 2014;15(11):1288–1301. doi:10.1016/j.sleep.2014.05.009.

39. Allen RP. Restless leg syndrome/Willis–Ekbom disease pathophysiology. *Sleep Med Clin.* 2015;10(3):207–214, xi. doi:10.1016/j.jsmc.2015.05.022.

40. Wang J, Pantopoulos K. Regulation of cellular iron metabolism. *Biochem J.* 2011;434(3):365–381. doi:10.1042/BJ20101825.

41. Sammarco MC, Ditch S, Banerjee A, Grabczyk E. Ferritin L and H subunits are differentially regulated on a post-transcriptional level. *J Biol Chem.* 2008;283(8):4578–4587. doi:10.1074/jbc.M703456200.

42. Haase VH. Hypoxic regulation of erythropoiesis and iron metabolism. *Am J Physiol Physiol.* 2010;299(1):F1–F13. doi:10.1152/ajprenal.00174.2010.

43. Allen RP, Picchietti DL, Auerbach M, et al. Evidence-based and consensus clinical practice guidelines for the iron treatment of restless legs syndrome/Willis–Ekbom disease in adults and children: an IRLSSG task force report. *Sleep Med.* 2018;41:27–44. doi:10.1016/J.SLEEP.2017.11.1126.

44. Patton SM, Ponnuru P, Snyder AM, Podskalny GD, Connor JR. Hypoxia-inducible factor pathway activation in restless legs syndrome patients. *Eur J Neurol.* 2011;18(11):1329–1335. doi:10.1111/j.1468-1331.2011.03397.x.

45. Garcia-Borreguero D, Silber MH, Winkelman JW, et al. Guidelines for the first-line treatment of restless legs syndrome/Willis–Ekbom disease, prevention and treatment of dopaminergic augmentation: a combined task force of the IRLSSG, EURLSSG, and the RLS Foundation. *Sleep Med.* 2016;21:1–11. doi:10.1016/j.sleep.2016.01.017.

46. García-Borreguero D, Kohnen R, Högl B, et al. Validation of the Augmentation Severity Rating Scale (ASRS): a multicentric, prospective study with levodopa on restless legs syndrome. *Sleep Med.* 2007;8(5):455–463. doi:10.1016/j.sleep.2007.03.023.

47. Becker PM, Sharon D. Mood disorders in restless legs syndrome (Willis–Ekbom disease). *J Clin Psychiatry.* 2014;75(7):e679–e694. doi:10.4088/JCP.13r08692.

48. Gupta R, Lahan V, Goel D. Prevalence of restless leg syndrome in subjects with depressive

disorder. *Indian J Psychiatry.* 2013;55(1):70–73. doi:10.4103/0019-5545.105515.

49. Hornyak M. Depressive disorders in restless legs syndrome: epidemiology, pathophysiology and management. *CNS Drugs.* 2010;24(2):89–98. doi:10.2165/11317500-000000000-00000.

50. Altunayoglu Cakmak V, Gazioglu S, Can Usta N, et al. Evaluation of temperament and character features as risk factors for depressive symptoms in patients with restless legs syndrome. *J Clin Neurol.* 2014;10(4):320–327. doi:10.3988/jcn.2014.10.4.320.

51. Hornyak M, Kopasz M, Berger M, Riemann D, Voderholzer U. Impact of sleep-related complaints on depressive symptoms in patients with restless legs syndrome. *J Clin Psychiatry.* 2005;66(9):1139–1145.

52. Driver-Dunckley E, Connor D, Hentz J, et al. No evidence for cognitive dysfunction or depression in patients with mild restless legs syndrome. *Mov Disord.* 2009;24(12):1840–1842. doi:10.1002/mds.22701.

53. Benes H, Mattern W, Peglau I, et al. Ropinirole improves depressive symptoms and restless legs syndrome severity in RLS patients: a multicentre, randomized, placebo-controlled study. *J Neurol.* 2011;258(6):1046–1054. doi:10.1007/s00415-010-5879-7.

54. Brown LK, Dedrick DL, Doggett JW, Guido PS. Antidepressant medication use and restless legs syndrome in patients presenting with insomnia. *Sleep Med.* 2005;6(5):443–450. doi:10.1016/j.sleep.2005.03.005.

55. Pullen SJ, Wall CA, Angstman ER, Munitz GE, Kotagal S. Psychiatric comorbidity in children and adolescents with restless legs syndrome: a retrospective study. *J Clin Sleep Med.* 2011;7(6):587–596. doi:10.5664/jcsm.1456.

56. Steinlechner S, Brüggemann N, Sobottka V, et al. Restless legs syndrome as a possible predictor for psychiatric disorders in parents of children with ADHD. *Eur Arch Psychiatry Clin Neurosci.* 2011;261(4):285–291. doi:10.1007/s00406-010-0140-z.

57. Aurora RN, Kristo DA, Bista SR, et al. The treatment of restless legs syndrome and periodic limb movement disorder in adults—an update for 2012: practice parameters with an evidence-based systematic review and meta-analyses: an American Academy of Sleep Medicine Clinical Practice Guideline. *Sleep.* 2012;35(8):1039–1062. doi:10.5665/sleep.1988.

58. Pigeon WR, Yurcheshen M. Behavioral sleep medicine interventions for restless legs syndrome and periodic limb movement disorder. *Sleep Med Clin.* 2009;4(4):487–494. doi:10.1016/j.jsmc.2009.07.008.

59. Comella CL. Treatment of restless legs syndrome. *Neurotherapeutics.* 2014;11(1):177–187. doi:10.1007/s13311-013-0247-9.

60. O'Sullivan SS, Evans AH, Lees AJ. Dopamine Dysregulation Syndrome. *CNS Drugs.* 2009;23(2):157–170. doi:10.2165/00023210-200923020-00005.

61. Warren N, O'Gorman C, Lehn A, Siskind D. Dopamine dysregulation syndrome in Parkinson's disease: a systematic review of published cases. *J Neurol Neurosurg Psychiatry.* 2017;88(12):1060–1064. doi:10.1136/jnnp-2017-315985.

62. Nakaki T. Drugs that affect autonomic functions or the extrapyramidal system. *Side Eff Drugs Annu.* 2014;36:179–202. doi:10.1016/B978-0-444-63407-8.00013-7.

63. Garcia-Borreguero D, Kohnen R, Silber MH, et al. The long-term treatment of restless legs syndrome/Willis–Ekbom disease: evidence-based guidelines and clinical consensus best practice guidance: a report from the International Restless Legs Syndrome Study Group. *Sleep Med.* 2013;14(7):675–684. doi:10.1016/j.sleep.2013.05.016.

64. Gaig C, Iranzo A, Pujol M, Perez H, Santamaria J. Periodic limb movements during sleep mimicking REM sleep behavior disorder: a new form of periodic limb movement disorder. *Sleep.* 2017;40(3). doi:10.1093/sleep/zsw063.

65. Haba-Rubio J, Marti-Soler H, Marques-Vidal P, et al. Prevalence and determinants of periodic limb movements in the general population. *Ann Neurol.* 2016;79(3):464–474. doi:10.1002/ana.24593.

66. Brown TM. Sleep-related leg cramps. *Sleep Med Clin.* 2015;10(3):385–392. doi:10.1016/j.jsmc.2015.05.002.

67. Monderer RS, Wu WP, Thorpy MJ. Nocturnal leg cramps. Curr Neurol Neurosci Rep. 2010;10(1):53–59. doi:10.1007/s11910-009-0079-5.

68. Das S, Gupta R, Dhyani M, Goel D. Headache secondary to sleep-related bruxism: A case with polysomnographic findings. *J Neurosci Rural Pract.* 2015;6(2):248–251. doi:10.4103/0976-3147.150293.

69. Guo H, Wang T, Li X, Ma Q, Niu X, Qiu J. What sleep behaviors are associated with bruxism in children? A systematic review and meta-analysis. *Sleep Breath.* 2017;21(4):1013–1023. doi:10.1007/s11325-017-1496-3.

70. Yeh S-B, Schenck CH. Atypical headbanging presentation of idiopathic sleep related rhythmic movement disorder: three cases with video-polysomnographic

documentation. *J Clin Sleep Med*. 2012;8(4):403–411. doi:10.5664/jcsm. 2034.

71. Gupta R, Goel D, Dhyani M, Mittal M. Head banging persisting during adolescence: A case with polysomnographic findings. *J Neurosci Rural Pract*. 2014;5(4):405–408. doi:10.4103/0976-3147.140004.

72. Gharagozlou P, Seyffert M, Santos R, Chokroverty S. Rhythmic movement disorder associated with respiratory arousals and improved by CPAP titration in a patient with restless legs syndrome and sleep apnea. *Sleep Med*. 2009;10(4):501–503. doi:10.1016/j.sleep.2009.03.003.

73. van der Salm SMA, Erro R, Cordivari C, et al. Propriospinal myoclonus: clinical reappraisal and review of literature. *Neurology*. 2014;83(20):1862–1870. doi:10.1212/WNL.0000000000000982.

15

Breathing-Related Sleep Disorders

AHMED S. BAHAMMAM, SULAIMAN ALHIFZI, AND SALIH ALEISSI

INTRODUCTION

Breathing-related sleep disorders (BRSDs) are common in psychiatric patients with more than one-third of psychiatric patients suffering from a BRSD in their lifetime.[1] The relationship between psychiatric disorders and BRSDs is bidirectional, as both disorders share common features including risk factors, symptoms, disease course, and outcomes. For example, obstructive sleep apnea (OSA) and depressive disorders share symptoms such as fatigue, sleepiness, decreased concentration, and insomnia. In addition, both conditions have insidious courses that delay presentation and diagnosis, which can lead to worsened outcomes.[1,2] Both BRSDs and psychiatric disorders worsen cardiovascular morbidity and mortality,[3] as they share common risk factors including, but not limited to, obesity, metabolic syndrome, and inflammation.[4]

BRSDs worsen cardiovascular morbidity in the psychiatric patients and also contribute to other comorbidities such as cognitive decline and dementia thereby influencing psychosocial functioning and quality of life.[5,6] In some psychiatric disorders, like posttraumatic stress disorder (PTSD), sleep disturbance is a cardinal manifestation. The patients with PTSD frequently wake during sleep with complaints of insomnia, nightmares, and nocturnal symptoms of comorbid OSA.[7] The positive airway pressure (PAP) treatment of concomitant OSA is known to improve not just the nightmares but also global PSTD symptomatology although adherence to PAP therapy can pose a substantial challenge.[7-9]

BRSDs could present initially or be misinterpreted as a psychiatric condition, thus leading to difficulties in its diagnosis and management.[10] Therefore, the aim of the current chapter is to enable early recognition of BRSDs for optimal clinical outcomes in psychiatric patients. According to the *International Classification of Sleep Disorders*, (third edition; ICSD-3),[11] in addition to isolated symptoms and normal variants like snoring and catathrenia, BRSDs can be classified into four major groups as follows: OSA, central sleep apnea (CSA) disorders, sleep-related hypoventilation (SRH) disorders, and sleep-related hypoxemic disorders.[11] We review the first three BRSD groups and their association with psychiatric disorders in the present chapter.

OBSTRUCTIVE SLEEP APNEA (OSA)

OSA, which is a systemic disorder, is considered as a syndrome with constellation of symptoms.[12] Additionally, it is a chronic stressor, with affected patients usually presenting after failure of their adaptive mechanisms. The obstruction of the upper airway can occur during sleep in two main forms: recurrent complete (apnea) or partial collapse (hypopnea) of the upper airway. Then, there is another form of respiratory event characterized by increasing respiratory effort for 10 seconds or longer, leading to an arousal from sleep but one that does not fulfill the criteria for a hypopnea or apnea. This is known as respiratory effort–related arousal (RERA) for which the American Academy of Sleep Medicine (AASM) recommends esophageal manometry for measurement that is uncomfortable for patients and impractical to use at most sleep centers.

Assessment and Diagnosis of OSA

It is usually helpful to have the patient's bed partner or a family member present during the interview because they may be able to give additional information about the patient's symptomatology while asleep. Snoring is a common feature of OSA. It is associated with a sensitivity of 80% to 90% for the diagnosis of OSA, although its specificity is below 50%.[13] History should also cover other features for OSA including witnessed apneas, gasping/choking episodes during sleep, total sleep amount, nocturia, morning headaches, night sweats, sleep fragmentation/sleep maintenance insomnia, reduced daytime energy and alertness, and decreased concentration and memory. These symptoms may be reported during the evaluation of another complaint, detected during health maintenance screening, or reported during preoperative screening or as a part of the comprehensive evaluation of patients at high risk for OSA. Evaluation should include a history of medical conditions that commonly occur with OSA, such as hypertension, chronic obstructive pulmonary disease, stroke, ischemic heart disease, cor pulmonale, and motor vehicle accidents. Sleep history for patients suspected to have OSA should include evaluation of excessive daytime sleepiness (EDS) that cannot be explained by other medical and psychiatric conditions or use of medications, although there may be multiple concomitant reasons for EDS. Epworth Sleepiness Scale (ESS) is a commonly used questionnaire to evaluate EDS in patients with suspected OSA.[14]

The common physical exam findings in OSA patients include obesity (body mass index [BMI] >30 kg/m^2) and a crowded oropharyngeal airway. Anatomical features like retrognathia, micrognathia, lateral peritonsillar narrowing, macroglossia, scalloped tongue, tonsillar hypertrophy, an elongated or enlarged uvula, a high arched or narrow palate, nasal septal deviation, and nasal polyps can lead to the narrowing of the upper airway thus increasing the risk of OSA. Furthermore, a large neck (along with waist circumference) has a stronger correlation with OSA than general obesity and is highly predictive of OSA in men and women who have a neck size greater than 17 and 16 inches, respectively. Patients should also be evaluated for complications of OSA including elevated blood pressure, signs of pulmonary hypertension or cor pulmonale, and cardiac dysrhythmias.

Diagnostic Testing

Objective confirmation of OSA is always necessary.[13] Patients with suspected OSA usually undergo an attended, overnight, in-laboratory polysomnography (PSG), which is the gold standard diagnostic test for OSA (i.e., a type 1 diagnostic sleep study). If patients who are subsequently diagnosed with OSA plan on initiating PAP therapy to treat their OSA, another study may be conducted to determine the fixed PAP pressure setting that would optimally control their OSA in all different sleep stages and sleep positions. Split-night attended, in-laboratory PSG is another approved diagnostic test, where the first half of the night is used to diagnose OSA, and PAP is applied in the second half, as indicated.[15] Figure 15.1 shows a hypnogram of a patient with OSA who underwent a split-night sleep study.

Out-of-center sleep testing (OCST) or home sleep apnea testing (HSAT), which are unattended

sleep studies performed at patient's home can be considered for (a) patients without comorbidities (significant cardiorespiratory disease, potential respiratory muscle weakness due to neuromuscular condition, awake hypoventilation or suspicion of sleep related hypoventilation, chronic opioid medication use, history of stroke or severe insomnia) that would preclude the use of unattended sleep studies and (b) patients who have a high likelihood of moderate or severe OSA.[16,17] Most OCST devices record airflow, respiratory effort, and blood oxygenation (Type 3 sleep studies). Some OCST devices measure peripheral arterial tonometry.[16,17]

Diagnostic Criteria

In addition to the frequency of respiratory events (i.e., number of apneas, hypopneas, and RERAs per hour of sleep during a PSG or per hour of monitoring time during a OCST), the diagnosis of OSA may depend on the presence of symptoms (daytime sleepiness; unrefreshing sleep; fatigue; insomnia; unintentional sleep episodes during wakefulness; awakening with breath holding, gasping, or choking; and bed partner' report of loud snoring, breathing interruptions, or both during the patient's sleep) and/or comorbid conditions (hypertension, mood disorder, cognitive dysfunction, coronary artery disease, stroke, congestive heart failure (HF), atrial fibrillation, or type 2 diabetes mellitus). The Apnea Hypopnea Index (AHI) is the number of apneas and hypopneas per hour of sleep recorded on PSG. Respiratory disturbance index is the number of apneas, hypopneas, and RERAs per hour of sleep recorded on PSG. The scoring of RERAs is optional since these are not easy to score, and Medicare, along with most insurances in United States, do not regard them as scorable respiratory event for diagnosis of OSA. The Respiratory Event Index (REI) is analogue of AHI on OCST. REI is defined as number of apneas and hypopnea per hour of monitoring time (instead of sleep time) since sleep is not scored on OCST due to lack of encephalographic (EEG) sleep recording capability on OCST. Per AASM guidelines, follow-up PSG is recommended if REI is less than 5 on OCST.[17] Table 15.1 provides the diagnostic criteria for OSA in adults.

Patients who meet criteria for the diagnosis of OSA are classified into mild, moderate, or severe disease on the basis of symptoms and the AHI/ REI as follows[18]:

  Mild: Patients with an AHI/REI between 5 and 14 with concomitant symptoms and/ or comorbidities

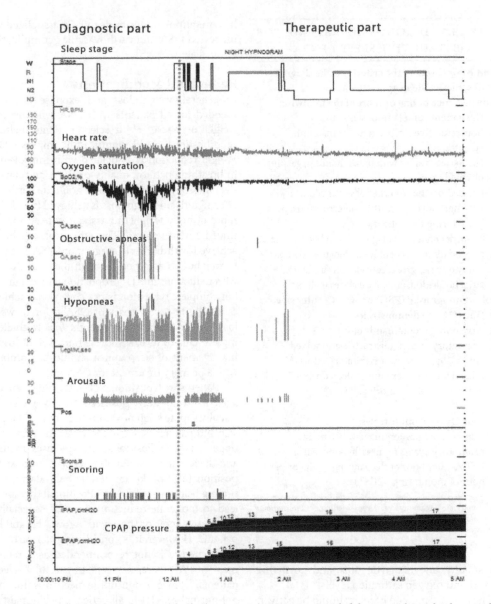

FIGURE 15.1. A hypnogram of a patient with obstructive sleep apnea, recorded during a split-night sleep study. The first part of the study, which was diagnostic, shows a high number of apneas and hypopneas associated with significant desaturation and arousals. The patient's sleep remained at stages N1 and N2 alone. The second part of the study focused on the therapeutic use of continuous positive pressure airway therapy (CPAP). Optimal CPAP pressure eliminated apneas and hypopneas and maintained oxygen saturation at >90%. The patient's sleep progressed into stages N3 and REM sleep.

Moderate: Patients with an AHI/REI between 15 and 29 with or without concomitant symptoms

Severe: Patients with an AHI/REI greater than 30 with or without concomitant symptoms

Management of Obstructive Sleep Apnea

OSA is a chronic disease with multiple comorbidities that requires a long-term, multidisciplinary approach. Management of OSA starts with patient education and an emphasis on goals to improve

TABLE 15.1. DIAGNOSTIC CRITERIA FOR OBSTRUCTIVE SLEEP APNEA

(A and B) or C satisfy the criteria for the diagnosis of obstructive sleep apnea (OSA)

A. The presence of one or more of the following:

1. The patient complains of sleepiness, nonrestorative sleep, fatigue, or insomnia symptoms.
2. The patient wakes with breath holding, gasping, or choking.
3. The bed partner or other observer reports habitual snoring, breathing interruptions, or both during the patient's sleep.
4. The patient has been diagnosed with hypertension, a mood disorder, cognitive dysfunction, coronary artery disease, stroke, congestive heart failure, atrial fibrillation, or type 2 diabetes mellitus.

B. Polysomnography (PSG) or out-of-center sleep testing (OCST) demonstrates:

Five or more predominantly obstructive respiratory events (obstructive and mixed apneas, hypopneas, or respiratory effort–related arousals per hour of sleep during a PSG or per hour of monitoring (OCST).

OR

C. PSG or OCST demonstrates:

Fifteen or more predominantly obstructive respiratory events (apneas, hypopneas, or RERAs) per hour of sleep during a PSG or per hour of monitoring (OCST)

From American Academy of Sleep Medicine. *International Classification of Sleep Disorders.* 3rd ed. Darien, IL: American Academy of Sleep Medicine, 2014.

sleep quality, alleviate symptoms, and normalize the AHI and oxygen saturation levels.

The patient and bed partner should be actively involved in making decisions about treatment options. PAP therapy is the first-line treatment for mild, moderate, and severe OSA. However, alternative therapies may be considered, based on the severity of the OSA and the patient's condition and preferences. Although there have been many published clinical practice guidelines for the management of OSA in adults, we will focus on the AASM guidelines in Chapter 19 of this volume.

Patient Education

Once the diagnosis of OSA is confirmed and its severity has been determined, it is important to educate patients about the risk factors, natural history, and consequences of OSA,[19] including the increased risk while operating motor vehicle or heavy equipment due to sleepiness associated with untreated OSA and cardiovascular complications of untreated OSA.[20]

Behavioral Modifications

In general, weight loss and exercise is recommended for all patients with OSA who are overweight or obese.[19,21] In select patients, behavior modifications could significantly improve OSA. Weight reduction is associated with improvement in breathing pattern, quality of sleep, and daytime sleepiness.[22] A follow-up PSG should be performed after significant weight loss is achieved (i.e., 10% or more of body weight) to assess the need for continued PAP therapy.[15] The effects of weight loss achieved with bariatric surgery on OSA is similar to weight loss achieved through diet and exercise, with reductions in AHI proportional to weight loss, but complete remission is not commonly achieved especially in severe cases of OSA prior to weight loss, and maintenance of weight loss is challenging.[23,24] Due to its low success rate, weight loss for management of sleep apnea should be combined with a primary treatment for OSA.[19,25]

Patients with positional OSA should be encouraged to avoid sleep positions that worsen OSA. Usually supine sleep positions tend to affect airway size and patency, since it decreases the area of the upper airway.[26] Positional therapy uses methods and devices that maintain patients in a nonsupine position (e.g., backpack, tennis ball, alarm, positioning belts and pillow).[19,25] Positional therapy can lead to moderate reductions in AHI especially in younger patients or those with a low AHI and lean patients. However, it is considered inferior to PAP and therefore is not recommended as a replacement of PAP therapy, except in carefully selected patients.[22] Since a nonsupine sleep position does not normalize AHI in all patients, positional therapy should be evaluated with PSG for optimal efficacy if prescribed as a primary therapy for OSA.[19]

All patients with untreated OSA should be advised to avoid alcohol, even during the day, because it can suppress the central nervous system, worsen OSA and sleepiness, and increase weight.[27] Moreover, sedatives, such benzodiazepines, should also be avoided or used carefully with close monitoring.[28]

Positive Airway Pressure (PAP) Therapy

PAP therapy maintains the patency of the upper airway during sleep by acting as a pneumatic splint. PAP can be delivered using the following modes: continuous PAP (CPAP), bilevel (BPAP), or auto-titrating PAP (APAP). PAP is applied through a nasal, or oro-nasal interface during sleep.[19,29] The AASM recommends offering PAP to all patients who have been diagnosed with OSA.[19]

The available modes of PAP are summarized as follows[19]:

- CPAP: It provides PAP at a fixed level throughout the respiratory cycle; it is often the initial therapy.
- BPAP: It provides inspiratory PAP (IPAP) and expiratory PAP (EPAP). The tidal volume is related to the difference between the IPAP and EPAP (pressure support) and the patient's effort. There is no proven advantage of using BPAP over CPAP for routine management of OSA.
- APAP: It increases or decreases the level of PAP in relation to signs indicating upper airway resistance changes, such as airflow changes, circuit pressure changes, or vibratory snore.
- Adaptive servo-ventilation (ASV) is a type of BPAP that dynamically adjusts pressure support and respiratory rate to stabilize the patient's breathing. The operation of ASV is different from that of CPAP. The expiratory pressure is set at the level of CPAP to eliminate obstructive apneas. The device provides a variable amount of inspiratory support (above the expiratory pressure) to eliminate hypopneas. In addition, a backup rate can be set at fixed or auto setting, which aborts any central apneas. With these settings, the device can effectively control both obstructive and CSA.[30]

PAP therapy improves symptoms of OSA, reduces the risk of traffic and workplace accidents, and reduces the risk of cardiovascular complications.[31,32]

CPAP is a safe mode of treatment, with generally minor side effects, like dryness of the upper airways and nose, local skin irritation (from mask), nasal congestion, eye irritation, aerophagia, sinusitis, and epistaxis. Nevertheless, suboptimal compliance, which is a major challenge with this therapy, is likely to reduce the potential benefits.[33] Previous studies demonstrated that patients with OSA on CPAP therapy use their CPAP, on average, 4.5 to 5.5 hours per night, with a compliance rate (an average of 4 hours a night for at least 70% of the nights) ranging from 30% to 85%.[34] Patient education and regular follow-up, especially during the first few weeks of therapy can help identify therapy-related side effects and troubles to enable early trouble-shooting and potentially improving long-term compliance.[35]

Alternative (Non-PAP) Therapies

Table 15.2 presents a summary of non-PAP therapies for OSA and the available evidence.[22,36,37]

Oral Appliances

Oral appliances (OAs) or mandibular advancement devices (MADs) are an effective treatment for a group of patients with mild or moderate OSA, particularly if they decline, do not respond to, or fail to adhere to PAP.[19,38] OAs may improve the patency of the upper airway during sleep by enlarging the upper airway and/or decreasing its collapsibility.[19] The OA covers the upper and lower teeth and push the mandible into an advanced position with respect to the resting position to increase the retro-lingual space. The modification of OA, known as tongue-retaining devices (TRDs), hold the tongue in a forward position with respect to the resting position without mandibular repositioning.[19] Studies have shown that OAs/MADs improve sleep apneas, subjective daytime sleepiness, and quality of life. There is emerging evidence that MADs might also have beneficial cardiovascular effects. In general, TRDs are not recommended; however, they can be used in select patients with mild to moderate OSA, when other therapeutic options have failed or are not possible.[22] A few studies show that TRDs result in reductions in sleep apneas; nevertheless, compliance might be a limitation.[22] The side effects of using MADs are generally minor. Excessive salivation and discomfort are the most common side effects. Persistent temporomandibular joint pain and changes in occlusion may necessitate the cessation of treatment.

Upper Airway Surgery

Upper airway surgical treatments, which are specifically tailored to the airway obstruction of individual patients, aim to modify airway anatomy through a variety of upper airway reconstructive or bypass procedures. Although surgery is not considered a first-line treatment for OSA, it could be the primary treatment in patients with mild OSA with severe obstructing anatomy, which is surgically correctible (e.g., tonsillar hypertrophy obstructing the pharyngeal airway). Nevertheless, surgery is reserved as a secondary approach for patients who fail to adequately respond or comply with PAP or OAs.[19,22]

TABLE 15.2. A SUMMARY OF NON-POSITIVE AIRWAY PRESSURE THERAPIES FOR OBSTRUCTIVE SLEEP APNEA AND THE AVAILABLE EVIDENCE

Treatment Modality	Evidence
Weight reduction	Current evidence shows that weight reduction results in improvement in breathing pattern, an increase in REM sleep and a decrease in daytime sleepiness. Most available studies have level 4 evidence
Positional therapy	Positional therapy may be useful in carefully selected patients with mild position-related OSA. However, long-term compliance is poor.
Mandibular advancement devices (MADs)	MADs can be used for the treatment of patients with mild to moderate OSA, and in patients who do not tolerate CPAP.
Tongue retaining devices (TRDs)	TRDs can be used in selected patients with mild to moderate OSA, when other therapeutic options have failed or are not possible.
Training of the upper airway muscles	This therapy could serve as an adjunct to other OSA treatments particularly in children. More research is needed.
Upper airway surgery • Tonsillectomy and/or adenoidectomy • Nasal surgery, including turbinectomy or straightening of the nasal septum • Uvulopalatopharyngoplasty or laser-assisted uvulopalatoplasty • Reduction of the tongue base • Hyoid suspension • Maxillo-mandibular advancement (MMA)	MMA is effective in selected group of patients; however, the benefits should be weighed against the risk of complications. Tonsillectomy and/or adenoidectomy are effective in children. There is no good evidence to support the use of the other modalities
Hypoglossal nerve stimulation or upper airway stimulation	Current data demonstrate significant reductions in AHI and oxygen saturation index, and improvement in subjective measures of sleepiness after device implantation in selected patients
Pharmacological therapy	No evidence of efficacy

Sources: Camacho M, Certal V, Abdullatif J, et al. Myofunctional therapy to treat obstructive sleep apnea: a systematic review and meta-analysis. *Sleep*. 2015;38(5):669–675; Halle TR, Oh MS, Collop NA, Quyyumi AA, Bliwise DL, Dedhia RC. Surgical treatment of OSA on Cardiovascular outcomes: a systematic review. *Chest*. 2017;152(6):1214–1229; and Randerath WJ, Verbraecken J, Andreas S, et al. Non-CPAP therapies in obstructive sleep apnoea. *Eur Respir J*. 2011;37(5):1000–1028.
Abbreviations:

There are a number of different surgical procedures that may be performed including the following[22,39]:

• Tonsillectomy and/or adenoidectomy.

• Nasal surgery, including turbinectomy or straightening of the nasal septum.
• Uvulopalatopharyngoplasty or laser-assisted uvulopalatoplasty; modern variants of this procedure sometimes use

radiofrequency waves to heat and remove tissue.

- Reduction of the tongue base, either with laser excision or radiofrequency ablation.
- Genioglossus advancement, in which a small portion of the lower jaw that attaches to the tongue is moved forward, to pull the tongue away from the back of the airway.
- Hyoid suspension, in which the hyoid bone in the neck, another attachment point for tongue muscles, is pulled forward in front of the larynx.
- Maxillo-mandibular advancement, which involves forward-fixing of the maxilla and mandible.

A recent systematic review of surgical treatment of OSA on cardiovascular outcomes indicated that examination of cardiovascular endpoints following surgical treatment of OSA is limited in the literature. The review stressed the need for larger, randomized, prospective trials with a more rigorous study design.[37]

Hypoglossal Nerve Stimulation or Upper Airway Stimulation Therapy

Recently, hypoglossal nerve stimulation (HGNS) using an implantable neurostimulator device was introduced as a novel strategy to treat patients with moderate to severe OSA. This modality of treatment was approved by the US Food and Drug Administration in April 2014, based on data demonstrating significant reductions in AHI and Oxygen Desaturation Index (ODI) and improvement in subjective measures of sleepiness after device implantation in selected patients.[40–42]

Guilleminault et al.[43] in 1978 were the first to attempt enhancing upper airway patency in humans using neurostimulation. Initial attempts with transcutaneous submental and intraoral electrical stimulation of the upper airway muscles had limited success. Subsequent intramuscular stimulation was associated with better results.[44] The first clinical trial treated 21 patients (AHI between 20 and 100 events per hour) with the new technique.[45] Follow-up after 6 months revealed a reduction of AHI of >50%.[45] A large multicenter 1-year phase 2–3 trial of 126 patients was completed in 2014 and reported significant clinical improvement with a reduction of 68% of the median AHI score and 70% of the ODI score.[46] A recent meta-analysis of 16 studies that included 381 patients revealed that at 6 months, the mean Sleep Apnea Quality of Life Index (SAQLI) improved by 3.1 (95% confidence interval [CI] 2.6–3.7). At 12

months, the mean AHI was reduced by 21.1 (95% CI 16.9–25.3), the mean ODI was reduced by 15.0 (95% CI 12.7–17.4), the mean ESS was reduced by 5.0 (95% CI 4.2–5.8), and the mean Functional Outcomes of Sleep Questionnaire (FOSQ) improved by 3.1 (95% CI 2.6–3.4).[47] In a prospective single-arm interventional trial of 21 patients with moderate to severe OSA who underwent HGNS treatment, the Beck Depression Inventory (BDI) score decreased after 3 months of treatment from 15.8 to 8.8, and at 6 month was 9.7 (*p* < 0.001).[45]

The HGNS system (Inspire, Maple Grove, MN, USA) comprises three components: (a) stimulation cuff electrode, (b) pleural pressure sensing lead, and (c) implantable pulse generator (IPG). The pleural pressure sensing lead senses the ventilatory efforts and then activates the IPG to stimulate the hypoglossal nerve.[48] Stimulation is delivered between end-expiration through the inspiratory period to diminish the risk of neuromuscular fatigue.[49]

Although HGNS is not as effective as CPAP therapy, it still has several advantages. The daily use of HGNS was 86% at 12 months and 84% at 18 months (based on self-report), which is significantly better than CPAP use.[50] Additionally, HGNS is a titratable therapy similar to CPAP and mandibular advancement devices, which is important in chronic diseases like OSA that may have a changing course due to age, weight changes, and emerging/worsening comorbid conditions.[48]

The overall reported rate of serious adverse effects is less than 2%.[46] Additionally, no serious IPG device-related infection that required explantation has been reported, and no permanent hypoglossal nerve damage has been reported.[46] Postoperative discomfort is not a prominent symptom in patients undergoing this procedure (compared to traditional tongue surgeries like tongue base suspension, tongue base reduction, and so forth).[49] Nevertheless, the following side effects have been reported: discomfort in the IPG site, tongue stiffness, tongue abrasion, transient ipsilateral tongue paresis, and postoperative swelling.[48] A recent meta-analysis showed that pain, tongue abrasion, and internal/external device malfunction are common adverse events.[47]

It is important to mention here that studies assessing HGNS had excluded patients with a BMI over 32 kg/m², which is a limitation of this procedure in terms of patient selection especially when there are so many patients with OSA who have BMI much higher than 32 kg/ m². Also, the fact that HGNS is a costly procedure is another limitation to utilize this procedure on a wider group of patients although this upfront cost may not be much higher than long-term costs of CPAP replacement parts over time as well as the persistent public health costs and increased psychiatric/cardiovascular disease burden in patients with untreated OSA due to CPAP intolerance.[49] The device interrogation in the office can provide feedback on hours of usage and stimulation settings like CPAP data download technology. In-office adjustments in voltage and electrode configuration can also be performed if patient is reporting persistent symptoms and/or intolerability. However, this therapy lacks capability to indicate objective efficacy unlike CPAP data download, and one has to mostly depend on improvement in symptoms to assess efficacy. The patient can certainly return to the sleep lab for overnight PSG with IPG turned on or chose to undergo OCST with IPG turned on to objectively prove efficacy. We usually follow this paradigm at our sleep center since it is critical to objectively prove resolution of sleep apnea to reduce long-term cardiovascular risk even when patient reports significant symptomatic improvement/resolution. The in-lab PSG is preferred as it also gives us opportunity to adjust the voltage and electrode configuration on the IPG to objectively ensure optimal treatment of their OSA.

Pharmacological Treatment

Currently, there is no evidence that pharmacological treatment helps patients with OSA. The therapeutic potentials of several pharmacological agents have been investigated for the management of OSA. This includes drugs that might act by stimulating respiratory drive, either directly (e.g., theophylline) or indirectly (e.g., acetazolamide). However, none of these agents were sufficiently effective to replace conventional therapies.[22,51] Medical cannabis is worth mentioning under pharmacological treatment section primarily due to small pilot or proof-of-concept studies suggesting that the synthetic medical cannabis extract dronabinol may improve respiratory stability and improve OSA by affecting serotonin neurotransmission in the airway. At least one US state announced that OSA will be added to the list of medical indications for the use of medical cannabis. There is a rapidly increasing number of patients getting medical cannabis for other conditions. We have encountered several patients inquiring into this as a non-PAP treatment alternative at our sleep center. The AASM recommends that medical cannabis and/or its synthetic extracts should not be used for the treatment of OSA due to unreliable delivery methods and insufficient evidence of treatment effectiveness, tolerability, and safety, that OSA should be excluded from the list of chronic medical conditions for state medical cannabis programs, and that patients with OSA should be advised to discuss their treatment options with a licensed medical provider at an accredited sleep facility.

Patients who continue to have EDS despite adequate conventional therapy, which is severe enough to warrant treatment, may benefit from adjunctive pharmacological therapy with agents like modafinil or armodafinil at standard doses.[19]

OSA and Psychiatric Disorders

The relationship between OSA and psychiatric disorders is bidirectional, where the presence of one disorder could worsen the other. For example, OSA is highly prevalent in psychiatric patients, especially those with depression,[52–53] anxiety,[54] and PTSD. Conversely, patients with OSA have a higher risk of developing psychiatric symptoms and comorbidities, in comparison to the general population.[55] Moreover, patients with OSA have a higher rate of mood disorders, anxiety disorders, PTSD, and psychotic disorders, compared with non-OSA patients.[52,56]

Although OSA encompasses the majority of BSRD, it is underdiagnosed,[57] which could be attributed to a lack of awareness about the disorder or its heterogeneous nature.[58] Therefore, OSA can be misdiagnosed as a psychiatric condition. Patients with OSA may suffer from the disorder for years before it is diagnosed, which could result in medical and mental disorders that can stem from untreated OSA via various pathophysiological mechanisms. For example, OSA results in intermittent hypoxia and sleep fragmentation, increased negative intrathoracic pressure, and poor sleep quality, which can lead to pathophysiological consequences including high sympathetic and depressed parasympathetic activity. This, in turn, can lead to acute intermittent changes in blood pressure and heart rate and changes in blood oxygen and carbon dioxide levels. It can also lead to pathological changes in cardiac structure and function. In addition, OSA can also result in dysfunction in metabolic and inflammatory processes,[59] impaired vascular endothelial function,[60] and activation of clotting pathways.[61] Together, these changes can increase incidence and progression of coronary heart disease, HF, stroke, and atrial fibrillation in patients with OSA.

OSA and Brain Function

Healthy sleep is vital for brain development and function. Sleep homeostasis and circadian rhythm work together for optimal sleep–wake cycle. During the entire night of sleep, there is cycling between nonrapid eye movement (NREM) and rapid eye movement (REM) stages of sleep. The sleep spindles, which define stage NREM N2 sleep, are important for the restoration of brain function.[62] REM sleep significantly increases during the second half of the night and is important for creativity and thinking.[63] Any disruption of sleep architecture could impair brain function and development.[64]

The natural history of OSA effects on brain function remains to be fully elucidated. The mechanisms like sleep fragmentation and hypoxemia are likely implicated in the pathogenesis of cognitive impairment in patients with OSA. In addition to the duration of the disease, brain function may also be affected by the severity of OSA, which is reflected by the AHI and the Desaturation Index, OSA comorbidities, OSA symptoms and systemic inflammation, levels of cerebral blood flow, hormonal imbalance, and genetic vulnerability.[12,65–67] Loss of wakefulness drive during sleep predisposes high-risk patients to recurrent pharyngeal obstruction, which leads to intermittent hypoxia and reoxygenation. This may lead to ischemic reperfusion and neuroinflammatory injuries.

Although, the brain tries to adapt to changes in oxygen levels via ischemia preconditioning, the bouts of desaturation that are too severe, frequent, or have a long duration can cause infarcts.[68] Further, not all areas of the brain will be resilient to changes in blood oxygen levels, even in young patients.[69] A wide range of brain areas are susceptible to OSA pathology; the prefrontal cortex, hippocampus, and amygdala are particularly worth mentioning because of their role in the regulation of cognition and emotion.[70]

The prefrontal regions of the cerebral cortex, the master of the "executive system," responsible for behavioral inhibition, attentive shifting, emotion and arousal self-regulation, working memory, and contextual memory are affected, to varying degrees, in patients with OSA.[71] Memory dysfunction and affective disorders are common in patients with OSA, which are attributed to hippocampal dysfunction.[69,72] In addition, levels of brain-derived neurotrophic factor (BDNF) have been found to be low in depression[69] and in OSA patients,[69] when compared to healthy subjects. Since BDNF is considered a key mediator of memory and cognition, its reduction is proposed

to be one of the causes of the cognitive impairment observed in OSAS.[69]

Intermittent hypoxia can affect the prefrontal cortex by disrupting restorative cellular processes.[73] Hypometabolism and slowing of neural activity may occur in patients with OSA, particularly if oxygen saturation (SpO_2) is less than 90%.[73] Although the effect of hypercapnia on cognition is not well studied, there is evidence that hypercapnia can affect cognition in patients with OSA through the reduction of cerebrovascular reactivity.[74] The ability of the brain to withstand variation in blood gases is an important factor that determines cognitive implications.[75]

Sleep fragmentation with the resultant changes in sleep architecture and sleep deprivation are known to have deleterious effects on brain function. Frequent arousals disturb sleep, which leads to EDS. Sleep fragmentation mainly affects attention and memory. Moreover, sleep deprivation induces neuroinflammation and prevents the restorative function of neural cells, which make them vulnerable to neurodegenerative disorders, like the early cognitive decline and dementia.[76]

Patients with OSA also have cognitive dysfunction, including visuospatial deficits. A recent meta-analysis demonstrates that visuospatial deficits were unique to patients with OSA, compared to those with chronic obstructive pulmonary disease (COPD) and insomnia. This suggests that mechanisms other than sleep disturbance and hypoxia/hypercapnia may also be implicated in specific cognitive deficits in OSA.[77] In fact, a study demonstrated that maze performance was significantly attenuated in patients with severe OSA, after a night of REM disruption, without changes to psychomotor vigilance.[78] These findings indicated a novel role for REM sleep in human spatial navigational memory. REM sleep is suppressed in a significant proportion of patients with severe OSA, which may affect visuospatial memory via REM sleep deprivation.[78]

Overall, adult patients with OSA usually suffer from attention and executive function impairment and memory problems, with varying severity.[79] Children with BRSD suffer from the same neurocognition dysfunctions, in addition to problems with their phonological behavior, which is essential for their development.[80] Current evidence suggests that the early recognition (preferably before the age of 5 years) and treatment of BRSD can improve the neurodevelopmental stages in children.[81] In fact, the longer the duration of nonrecognition of BRSD, the worse are the cognitive outcomes.[82]

Emotional behaviors are under direct control of amygdala, locus coeruleus, and prefrontal cortex.[70] Healthy sleep is a cornerstone for regulating the amygdalar response to various emotional stimuli. REM sleep, in terms of duration, circadian, and neurochemical changes, is important for the regulation of emotions.[70] The disturbance of slow-wave sleep (SWS) and REM sleep works as a nidus for evolving neurological and psychiatric disorders. Disturbance of SWS, sleep spindles, and REM sleep are common among patients with OSA.

Impact of OSA Treatment on Depression

Most studies that assessed the prevalence of depression among patients with OSA could not determine whether OSA preceded depression, or vice versa.[52] However, if a causal relationship exists between OSA and depression with OSA coming first, then depression would be expected to improve with effective OSA therapy. The previous studies that assessed depression in patients with OSA used clinical questionnaires for mood disorders, clinician assessments, or patients' self-reported symptoms to diagnose depression. The prevalence of depression among OSA patients was assessed in clinical settings and in community samples. Several questionnaires that have been utilized include BDI,[83] the Center for Epidemiological Studies Depression Scale (CES-D),[84] the Minnesota Multiphasic Personality Inventory (MMPI),[85] the Profile of Mood States (POMS), the Hospital Anxiety and Depression Scale (HADS),[86] the Patient Health Questionnaire (PHQ-9),[87] the Hamilton Rating Scale for Depression (HRSD), the Structured Interview Guide for the Hamilton Depression Rating Scale-Seasonal Affective Disorder Version-Self-Rating Version (SIGH-SAD-SR), the Symptom Checklist 90 (SCL-90),[88] the Mini International Neuropsychiatric Interview 6.0 (MINI),[89] and the Zung Depression Rating Scale (ZDRS).[90] It is important to note that among the previously mentioned instruments, only the CES-D and MINI were specifically designed to diagnose depression.[52] The remaining scales are designed to assess the severity of depression and are meant to be used after the clinical diagnosis of depression is established. Randomized clinical trials assessing the positive effects of CPAP treatment in patients with OSA have demonstrated a beneficial effect of therapy on several symptoms and comorbidities, including daytime sleepiness, quality of life, and blood pressure.[91,92] However, only a few studies have explored the effects of CPAP therapy on depression in patients with OSA.

Most observational studies assessing the effect of CPAP therapy on depression among patients with OSA demonstrated a reduction in depressive symptoms.[93–95] In addition, a 2006 Cochrane meta-analysis, which included data from five clinical trials comparing CPAP with placebo, showed that the pooled fixed effects significantly favored CPAP over placebo for depression. There was, however, no significant effect of CPAP treatment after the application of random effects modeling.[96]

A randomized controlled trial, using the Geriatric Depression Scale, reported no significant difference in the change in depression between the control and CPAP therapy arms.[97] Two subsequent short-term (i.e., 2 weeks of CPAP therapy) randomized controlled trials reported no mood improvement associated with CPAP.[98,99] However, most of the previously mentioned studies assessed the outcome of depressive symptoms after only 2 to 4 weeks of CPAP use. Intervention studies assessing the effect of antidepressant treatment, however, typically take 4 to 6 weeks, or longer, to show a significant response to treatment.[100] A subsequent study that included 17 patients with treatment-resistant depression and comorbid OSA revealed that 2 months of CPAP therapy resulted in significant reductions in depression scores.[101]

A more recent multicenter observational longitudinal study, which included 300 patients with OSA and depressive symptoms measured by the 13-item, self-rated Pichot depression scale (QD2A) ≥7 at diagnosis and during follow-up for at least 1 year, demonstrated a significant improvement in depression scores in response to CPAP therapy.[102] However, 42% of the patients displayed persistent depressive symptoms after 1 year of CPAP therapy. Persistence of depressive symptoms was independently associated with persistent EDS (odds ratio [OR] 2.72), comorbid cardiovascular disease (OR, 1.76), and female sex (OR 1.53).[102] The findings of this study corroborated with previous research demonstrating the association between persistent EDS and persistent depression in patients with OSA who were treated with CPAP.[101,103]

A recent systematic review and meta-analysis evaluated the efficacy of CPAP or MADs in treating depression in patients with OSA. CPAP treatment resulted in significant improvement in depression compared with control groups (Q statistic, $p < 0.001$; $I^2 = 71.3\%$, 95% CI 54%, 82%).[100] Additionally, treatment with a MAD was also significantly beneficial for depressive symptoms. Overall, it seems that depression may persist in some patients, despite good adherence with CPAP therapy. Current evidence indicates that patients with OSA with persistent daytime sleepiness, despite regular CPAP use, are at a higher risk for persistence of depression compared to OSA patients without daytime sleepiness. Perhaps, use of wake-promoting agents like modafinil and armodafinil can be considered in such cases to see if there is improvement in persistent daytime sleepiness with concomitant improvement in persistent depression.

Relationship between Depression and CPAP Adherence

In a questionnaire-based study that assessed self-reported adherence to CPAP therapy in 178 established CPAP users, depression was associated with lower CPAP use.[103] Another study that objectively assessed the adherence of 122 patients with OSA to CPAP therapy, 1 month after beginning CPAP treatment, reported no effect of depression on CPAP adherence.[104] A more recent multicenter observational longitudinal study, which followed 300 patients with OSA and depressive symptoms at diagnosis for at least 1 year, reported that the percentage of patients who used CPAP >4 hour/night was not different between patients with persistent depressive symptoms and those without persistent depressive symptoms (23.2% and 18.9%, respectively).[102] In another study, which was conducted on 240 CPAP-naïve OSA patients, depression significantly predicted fewer hours of auto-PAP use.[105] The majority of previous studies did not control for confounders, such as OSA symptoms (e.g., daytime sleepiness); comorbid conditions of both OSA and depression, like insomnia and anxiety; or use and compliance with antidepressant medications, which could all influence CPAP adherence.

A study assessing rates of CPAP adherence in a large sample of African American and white American military veterans, with and without comorbid mental health disorders, showed that mental health disorders (including mood disorders) influenced CPAP adherence in African Americans, but not in whites.[106] African Americans with a mental health diagnosis used CPAP fewer nights per week and for less time per night at 1 month and for less time per night at 3 months, compared with African Americans without mental health disorders.[106] Therefore, mental disorders may influence CPAP acceptance and adherence in ethnic minorities.

The Role of Psychiatrists in OSA Treatment

It is essential for the psychiatrists to acquire the knowledge and skills to recognize patients with OSA during the early stages of the disease and refer them to a sleep specialist for diagnosis. Additionally, psychiatrists should be familiar with available treatment modalities for OSA and potential mental and physical complications of untreated OSA. This knowledge will allow psychiatrists to facilitate management of this otherwise insidious comorbid condition, which, if left untreated, may prevent complete recovery from a psychiatric condition.

The lack of education in sleep medicine has resulted in a culture of physicians with limited knowledge of diagnosis and treatment of sleep disorders including OSA.[107–114] Therefore, collective efforts are required to educate psychiatrists about sleep disorders in general and OSA in particular, given the high prevalence of OSA among psychiatric patients.

CENTRAL SLEEP APNEA SYNDROMES

Introduction

CSA syndromes (CSASs) are a group of disorders, which are characterized by cessation of airflow due to the absence of respiratory effort. According to the ICSD-3,[11] CSASs can be classified as follows:

- CSA with Cheyne-Stokes breathing (CSB)
- Central apnea due to a medical disorder without CSB
- CSA due to high altitude periodic breathing
- CSA due to a medication or substance
- Primary CSA
- Primary CSA of infancy
- Primary CSA of prematurity
- Treatment-emergent CSA

As noted, CSASs can be primary or secondary. Also categorizing CSASs into hyperventilation-related and hypoventilation-related central apnea helps in planning its management. Hyperventilation-related CSASs include primary CSA, CSA associated with CSB, CSA due to a medical condition without CSB, and CSA due to high altitude periodic breathing. Hypoventilation-related central apnea includes CSA due to central nervous system diseases, central nervous system suppressing drugs or substances, neuromuscular disorders, or severe abnormalities in pulmonary mechanics.

The first step in managing symptomatic patients is the treatment of underlying cause or the precipitating factor.

Cheyne–Stokes Breathing

The AASM defines CSB as a breathing disorder in which there are cyclical fluctuations in breathing, with periods of central apneas or hypopneas

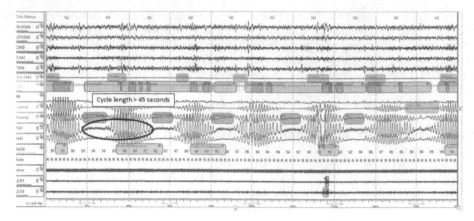

FIGURE 15.2. A zoomed epoch (5 minutes) of the breathing of a patient with Cheyne–Stokes, showing the typical cyclical breathing with crescendo–decrescendo pattern.

that alternate with periods of hyperpnoea in a gradual waxing and waning fashion (Figure 15.2). Although CSB is mostly seen in patients with HF, it has also been described in patients recovering from acute pulmonary edema, advanced renal failure, and central nervous system lesions like stroke.[115] Several clinical and epidemiological studies have shown that a large proportion of patients with left ventricular systolic dysfunction suffer from CSB or other sleep-related breathing disorders.[115]

The presence of CSB in patients with HF is associated with increased morbidity and mortality and impaired quality of life.[116] Those suffering from advanced HF, with an ejection fraction as low as 35% to 40%, are prone to develop pulmonary congestion and elevated pulmonary venous pressure, which results in the stimulation of pulmonary "J" receptors, eventually leading to hyperventilation at night and during the daytime.[115] Central apneas are triggered when the P_aCO_2 level falls below the apnea threshold due to hyperventilation. This cycle of hyperventilation and apnea happens during sleep to constitute CSB.

Diagnosis

CSB may present with nonspecific symptoms, such as poor sleep quality, daytime somnolence or insomnia, paroxysmal nocturnal dyspnea, and easy fatigability. Therefore, a high index of suspicion is required for patients with HF to prevent unjustified delays in diagnosis. In general, patients with HF and CSB tend usually to have a lower BMI than patients who have concomitant OSA.[117] Moreover, CSB is more common among male patients and patients with comorbid atrial fibrillation.[115] Table 15.3 outlines the AASM diagnostic criteria for CSB.[11]

TABLE 15.3. DIAGNOSTIC CRITERIA FOR CHEYNE–STOKES RESPIRATION

(A or B) + C + D satisfy the criteria:

A. The presence of one or more of the following:
1. Sleepiness
2. Difficulty initiating or maintaining sleep, frequent awakenings, or nonrestorative sleep
3. Awakening short of breath
4. Snoring
5. Witnessed apneas

B. The presence of atrial fibrillation/flutter, congestive heart failure, or a neurological disorder

C. PSG (during diagnostic or positive airway pressure titration) shows all the following:
1. Five or more central apneas and/or central hypopneas per hour of sleep
2. The total number of central apneas and/or central hypopneas is >50% of the total number of apneas and hypopneas.
3. The pattern of ventilation meets the criteria for Cheyne–Stokes breathing
4. The disorder is not better explained by another current sleep disorder, medication use (e.g., opioids), or substance use disorder.

D. The disorder is not better explained by another current sleep disorder, medication use (e.g., opioids), or substance use disorder.

From American Academy of Sleep Medicine. *International Classification of Sleep Disorders.* 3rd ed. Darien, IL: American Academy of Sleep Medicine, 2014.

Arterial blood gas (ABG) analysis while awake can be considered in the diagnosis of CSB. Patients with CSB usually have low or low-normal PaCO2.[118] Previous studies have demonstrated that the severity of underlying HF does not always correlate with the severity of CSB. Thus, other factors must be considered.[115] It is not uncommon to find that patients with HF have coexisting OSA and CSB.[115]

Overnight PSG typically shows crescendo–decrescendo breathing pattern (Figure 15.2), with periods of central apnea or hypopnea that alternate with periods of hyperpnea, that predominates during stages N1 and N2 of NREM sleep.

CSB among patients with HF has been linked to poor prognosis. Studies that assessed the systemic consequences of CSB in patients with HF found that laboratory markers indicative of enhanced sympathetic nervous system activity (e.g., plasma and urinary catecholamine levels) are elevated in such patients.[115,119]

Management of CSB

There is still no consensus regarding the best management for CSB in patients with HF. Optimizing cardiac function is the initial and most important step in the management of CSB. Medical management of HF does not only improve BRSDs, it is also the cornerstone for the management of a dysfunctional heart, thereby, increasing patient survival.[115]

Pharmacological Therapy

Several drugs have been used to treat patients with HF and CSB. Although these drugs frequently reduce BRSD, they may cause undesirable side effects and/or interactions with other drugs. The most commonly administered drugs are methylxanthines (theophylline), acetazolamide, and benzodiazepines. Unfortunately, all studies that assessed the effects of these medications were short-term and used small sample sizes.[115] Hence, there is limited knowledge of the long-term efficacy and safety profile of these medications. Theophylline appears to be associated with arrhythmia, which could have deleterious effects on a poorly functioning left ventricle. Currently, none of these drugs are recommended as a first-line approach to manage CSB of patients with HF.

Oxygen

The theory behind using oxygen supplementation is that it will offset the hypoxic ventilatory drive and, suppress periodic breathing. The AASM recommended nocturnal oxygen therapy as the treatment of CSA related to HF (Standard).[120]

Positive Airway Pressure (PAP) Support

A multicenter trial (i.e., CANPAP) was conducted to evaluate the efficacy of CPAP in reducing mortality and morbidity associated with CSB in patients with HF.[121] The study revealed that CPAP had positive effects on oxygen saturation, left ventricular ejection fraction (LVEF), and 6-minute walk distance and resulted in a 53% reduction in AHI. However, there were no significant differences in transplant-free survival, the rate of hospitalization, or quality of life. The study group advised against routine use of CPAP in patients with HF and CSB. However, in the subsequent post-hoc analysis of the study, it was reported that patients with residual AHI <15/hour on CPAP had improvement in both LVEF and heart transplant–free survival.[122] Therefore, the authors recommended continuing CPAP only if it significantly suppressed AHI.

ASV is a new mode of automated pressure support that performs breath-to-breath analysis and delivers ventilation accordingly to prevent hyperventilation that drives CSB. Numerous observational studies have demonstrated the beneficial effect of ASV in CSB in patients with HF.[123] However, long-term randomized controlled clinical trials are required to determine the long-term clinical efficacy and safety of these devices. The ResMed Company issued a serious safety concern in May 2015, after the preliminary primary data analysis from the SERVE-HF clinical trial came into the limelight.[124,125] The investigators of SERVE-HF clinical trial reported that patients with symptomatic chronic HF (CHF) and reduced LVEF (45% or below) using ASV for treatment of CSA related to CHF are at increased risk of cardiovascular mortality.[124] One of the speculations by SERVE-HF investigators was that central apneas are compensatory and protective in HF, and ASV can cause harm by eliminating this protective mechanism. This finding from SERVE-HF study resulted in AASM making an update to the recommendation regarding use of ASV for treatment of CSASs related to CHF in May 2016.[126] The recommendation stated that "ASV targeted to normalize the AHI should not be used for the treatment of CSB related to HF in adults with left ventricular ejection fraction (LVEF) ≤ 45% and moderate or severe CSA predominant, sleep-disordered breathing" (STANDARD level recommendation).[126] Again, this recommendation against the use of ASV is based on evidence of increased risk of death from cardiovascular causes in patients with CHF and a LVEF ≤45%. Nevertheless, ASV has been approved for the use in patients with CSB related to HF, with an ejection fraction >45% (OPTION level recommendation).[127] An ongoing trial, the ADVENT-HF study is expected to be completed in June 2020 with an intent to reassess this connection (between ASV and increased cardiovascular mortality if LVEF ≤45%) by using Respironics ASV in the study since SERVE-HF study studied the connection with ResMed ASV.[128] If similar results are not obtained with Respironics ASV, it may indicate that increase in cardiovascular mortality with ASV in SERVE-HF may be device-specific rather than representing an ASV class effect.

The CSA related to HF has been shown to increase mortality in patients with HF[129] although SERVE-HF study cast doubt on this by suggesting that mortality can increase with ASV treatment of CSA in HF patients. Among several pitfalls of SERVE-HF study,[130] poor adherence (average use of 3.7 hours/night) was thought to be one of the possible reasons for observation of excess cardiovascular mortality in patients who used ASV, since 3.7 hours of average usage is definitely not adequate in addressing CSA, especially since the recent study by Javaheri et al.[131] indicated that the burden of CSA (frequency, duration, and associated arousals) increases during late sleep hours in patients with HF with LVEF <40. The authors suggested that this increased burden of CSA in the later hours of sleep, which is normally when most subjects take the mask off and sleep for few hours without using the PAP device could have contributed to observation of excess mortality in SERVE-HF study and recommend full use of PAP therapy throughout sleep for full cardiovascular benefits.

Transvenous Phrenic Nerve Stimulation

Transvenous phrenic nerve stimulation (PNS) is a novel therapeutic approach for CSA that was approved by FDA in 2017, for treating moderate to severe CSA. The phrenic nerve descends down through the neck and the thoracic cavity and passes across the wall of the thoracic cavity in adjacency to several veins. This passage allows a transvenous electrode stimulation approach of the nerve, which is anatomically feasible and minimally invasive.[132]

In right thoracic cavity, the phrenic nerve passes near the right wall of the superior vena cava or the right brachiocephalic vein, and on the left side, it passes along the wall of the left pericardiophrenic vein in left thoracic cavity.[132] The stimulation electrode is usually placed within the brachiocephalic or in left pericardiophrenic vein using percutaneous routes.

Temporary, transvenous, unilateral PNS was reported to reduce central apnea events and

significantly improve important sleep parameters.[133,134] Subsequently, permanent transvenous PNS and stimulator implantation was developed.

A recent large multicenter long-term follow-up study that was conducted in Europe and the United States and included 151 patients with HF reported elimination of CSA events and elevation of oxygen saturation compared with no PNS.[135] Another recent randomized controlled trial (Remedē System Pivotal Trial) randomized 96 patients with HF.[136] Sleep parameters and quality of life improved from baseline at 6 and 12 months in the treatment group.[136] The 6-month rate of HF hospitalization was 4.7% in the treatment group and 17.0% in in the control group.[136]

The most common adverse events reported included interaction with concomitant devices, infection at the site of implant, swelling, and local tissue damage or pocket erosion. In nutshell, while this treatment modality may offer a novel approach to management of CSA, it is not currently included as one of the treatment options in AASM practice parameters for treatment of CSASs.[120]

Drug-Induced Central Sleep Apnea (CSA)

Drugs like narcotics, baclofen and sodium oxybate can cause CSA. However, the exact mechanisms and outcomes have not yet been elucidated.[137,138] Apart from its antialgesic effect, opioids also influence stress responses, appetite, thermoregulation, respiration, and sleep. Opioid-treated patients may suffer from CSA, OSA, irregular breathing, hypoxemia and hypercapnia during sleep, and fragmentation of sleep. During daytime, they may also have hypoventilation and hypercapnia. Combining benzodiazepines with opioids may worsen hypoventilation.[139] Opioids affects respiration during sleep by causing respiratory depression and decreasing central respiratory control sensitivity to hypercapnia and decreasing peripheral sensitivity to hypoxemia, which leads to unstable ventilation and recurrent CSA.[140] Irregular breathing with central apneas seen in patients on chronic opioid therapy is referred to as Biot's or ataxic respiration. Morphine equivalent doses were correlated with the prevalence of ataxic respiration with 92% of patients on morphine dose equivalent to ≥200 mg having ataxic respiration in study by Walker et al.[141] This dose dependence was so profound in this study that with each 100-mg morphine dose equivalent increase, the rate of central apneas was noted to increase by 29.2%.[141] Additionally, patients treated with opioids may be at risk of OSA due to the effects of opioids on upper airway muscles.[142] PAP therapy may be effective in improving CSA in patients who chronically use opioids. Sophisticated modes of PAP, such as ASV, are much more effective than conventional CPAP for the treatment of CSA in patients using opioids.[143]

SLEEP-RELATED HYPOVENTILATION DISORDERS

The most recent version of the ICSD-3 defined SRH disorders as insufficient ventilation during sleep leading to abnormally elevated $PaCO_2$ during sleep.[11]

SRH disorders include the following[11]:

- Obesity hypoventilation syndrome (OHS)
- Congenital central alveolar hypoventilation
- Late-onset central hypoventilation with hypothalamic dysfunction
- Idiopathic central alveolar hypoventilation
- SRH due to a medication or substance
- SRH due to a medical disorder

Awake hypoventilation is defined as P_aCO_2 $\geq$45 mmHg.[11] Since OHS is the most common form of sleep related hypoventilation in adults, we will discuss OHS in the present chapter.

Obesity Hypoventilation Syndrome (OHS)

OHS is also called hypercapnic sleep apnea or SRH associated with obesity.[11] Although it was previously known as Pickwickian syndrome, the use of this term is now discouraged.

OHS is a clinical diagnosis that requires the presence of the following criteria:[11]

A. Presence of hypoventilation during daytime wakefulness (P_aCO_2 $\geq$45 mmHg) as measured by arterial PCO_2, end-tidal PCO_2, or transcutaneous PCO_2.
B. Presence of obesity (BMI >30 kg/m^2).
C. Hypoventilation is not primarily due to lung parenchymal or airway disease, pulmonary vascular pathology, chest wall disorder (other than mass loading from obesity), medication use, neurologic disorder, muscle weakness, or a known congenital or idiopathic central alveolar hypoventilation syndrome.

Although arterial oxygen desaturation is common in patients with OHS, it is not a criterion for OHS diagnosis. It is important to note that OSA often coexists with OHS. In those cases, a diagnosis of both OSA and OHS should be made.

Assessment and Diagnosis

Since 90% of patients with OHS have coexisting OSA, the symptoms of patients with OHS are similar to those of patients with OSA.[144,145] These symptoms include EDS, snoring, choking during sleep, morning headaches, fatigue, mood disturbance, and impairments of memory or concentration.[145] However, when compared to patients with eucapnic OSA, those with OHS tend to complain more often of dyspnea and to present with right-sided HF.[144,145]

By definition, patients with OHS are obese, and most of them are morbidly obese (BMI $\geq$40 kg/m^2). At the time of presentation, most OHS patients exhibit signs of cor pulmonale (right-sided HF) or circulatory congestion, including plethora, scleral injection, peripheral edema, and a prominent pulmonic component of the second heart sound.[145,146]

OHS is diagnosed based on the exclusion of other conditions. Thus, diagnostic tests should be performed to distinguish OHS from other disorders, such as chronic pulmonary diseases, skeletal restriction, neuromuscular disorders, hypothyroidism, or pleural pathology, in which hypercapnia is a common finding.[11,145] Diagnostic tests include ABG analysis, pulmonary function tests (PFTs), chest imaging, electrocardiography (ECG), transthoracic echocardiogram, and PSG with CO_2 monitoring, as well as complete blood count and renal and hepatic profiles. ABG is an essential test as hypercapnia, while awake, is one of the diagnostic criteria. The ABG analysis usually reveals high P_aCO_2 and high bicarbonate levels, which reflect the chronic nature of the disease.

Serum bicarbonate level is a useful test in the evaluation of OHS. Mokhlesi et al.[147] demonstrated that among obese patients with OSA and normal renal function, serum bicarbonate level below 27 mEq/L had a 97% negative predictive value for excluding the diagnosis of OHS. In addition, abnormal resting pulse oximetry during wakefulness has been suggested as a clinical measure that should increase the suspicion for OHS among obese OSA patients.[147] Usually, individuals with OHS have BMI $\geq$40, although not all individuals with BMI $\geq$40 have OHS. However, BMI $\geq$40 in presence of recent serum bicarbonate $\geq$27 and/or abnormal resting pulse oximetry should raise suspicion for comorbid OHS in patients with suspected OSA. In such cases, PSG should be ordered with CO_2 monitoring to evaluate for both OSA and OHS.

PFTs are essential to exclude other causes of hypercapnia, such as chronic pulmonary diseases. Although the PFT can be normal, a mild-to-moderate restrictive pattern is common due to obesity.[147] ECG and transthoracic echocardiogram could show features of right heart strain, right ventricular hypertrophy, right atrial enlargement, and elevated pulmonary artery pressure.[145,146] Other laboratory testing should include a complete blood count and thyroid function test to exclude severe hypothyroidism and secondary erythrocytosis, respectively.[45,148,149]

PSG of patients with OHS may show sustained oxygen desaturation and hypercapnia during sleep, which is not related to obstructive apneas and hypopneas periods. Hypoventilation is usually more prominent during REM sleep compared to NREM sleep.[15] If end-tidal or transcutaneous CO_2 is monitored, it may also demonstrate an increase of more than 10 mmHg in P_aCO_2 level during sleep, compared with levels during wakefulness.[145] The AASM recommends scoring SRH during PSG if either one of the following occur: there is an increase in the arterial PCO_2 (or surrogate) to a value >55 mmHg for >10 minutes, or there is ≥10 mmHg increase in arterial PCO_2 (or surrogate) during sleep (in comparison to an awake supine value) to a value exceeding 50 mmHg for ≥10 minutes.[150]

Management of Obesity Hypoventilation Syndrome (OHS)

Given the multiple comorbidities associated with OHS, the management of patients with OHS requires a multidisciplinary approach, including different medical and surgical subspecialties. Affected patients often require the care of the following: internists and endocrinologists, regarding their diabetes mellitus, hypertension, hyperlipidemia, HF, and hypothyroidism therapy; a dietician, for weight reduction planning; a pulmonologist for respiratory failure management; and a surgeon, for potential bariatric surgery. Moreover, patients with OHS have higher rates of intensive care admissions than obese patients without hypoventilation for the management of acute on chronic respiratory failure episodes.[145]

Although there is no consensus for the management of OHS, treatment approaches are based on reversing the underlying pathophysiology of OHS, including the reversal of sleep-disordered breathing, weight reduction, and treatment of comorbid conditions.

Weight Loss

Significant weight loss is desirable in patients with OHS because it improves pulmonary physiology

and function, including the improvement of alveolar ventilation and nocturnal oxyhemoglobin saturation.[151] Furthermore, in patients with coexisting OSA, weight loss decreases the frequency of obstructive respiratory events.[152–154] All patients with OHS should pursue lifestyle modifications to lose weight. If lifestyle modifications are not sufficient, bariatric surgery should be considered. The benefits of weight loss appear to occur regardless of whether weight loss is due to lifestyle modification (i.e., diet or exercise) or surgery. However, it is important to realize that weight loss cannot be used as the sole initial treatment for OHS.[145]

Positive Airway Pressure Therapy

PAP therapy is the mainstay treatment for OHS. Since the majority of OHS patients have coexisting OSA, it is recommended to start therapy with CPAP. CPAP was effective in a group of patients with stable OHS, particularly those with severe OSA.[155,156] There are no clear guidelines on when to start or switch to BPAP; however, BPAP should be strongly considered for patients with OHS without OSA; those with OHS and coexisting OSA, where CPAP is insufficient and hypercapnia has persisted despite being on long-term CPAP; or those who fail to tolerate CPAP.[156] In addition, BPAP should be used for patients with OHS who experience acute-on-chronic respiratory failure.[156–158] Several studies have shown that treatment of OHS with PAP improves blood gases within 2 to 4 weeks. Therefore, early follow-up is important and should include repeat measurement of ABG with assessment of adherence to PAP.[155]

Volume-Targeted Pressure Support

Volume-targeted pressure support (VtPS) is a hybrid mode of ventilation that combines pressure support and volume-controlled modes of ventilation into one ventilation mode to ensure a more consistent tidal volume and, hence, minute volume ventilation.[158] Current evidence suggests a more consistent tidal volume is advantageous in lowering transcutaneous PCO_2 readings.[159] However, VtPS does not seem to provide further clinical benefits in terms of sleep quality and health-related quality of life.[159,160] Nevertheless, this does not preclude use of this mode of ventilatory support, especially in patients who fail fixed BPAP.

Oxygen Therapy

Oxygen therapy is needed if hypoxemia persists, despite the relief of upper airway obstruction and hypercapnia with PAP therapy, to prevent long-term consequences of hypoxemia on pulmonary vasculature and other vital organs. However, it is important to note that treatment with oxygen alone is inadequate and not recommended, since it does not reverse hypoventilation or airway obstruction on its own.[145,158]

Tracheostomy
Tracheostomy is rarely required and is generally reserved for patients who do not tolerate or adhere to PAP therapy or have difficulty in weaning themselves from invasive ventilation.[158]

Treatment of Comorbid Conditions and Complications
Untreated OHS is associated with a high mortality rate, reduced quality of life, and numerous comorbidities, including hypertension, pulmonary hypertension, right HF, angina, and acute hypercapnic respiratory failure.[115,158] Therefore, it is important to manage comorbid conditions that impair ventilation or reduce the ventilatory response to hypoxemia or hypercapnia, which are likely to worsen OHS, such as COPD and hypothyroidism. In addition, complications associated with OHS should be investigated and managed appropriately.

CONCLUSIONS
BRSDs are common and underrecognized disorders. The early recognition and treatment of OSA and BRSDs, in general, is crucial, given the associated substantial adverse medical and psychosocial consequences of untreated BRSDs. Although PAP therapy is still the gold-standard treatment, other therapies, such as OAs, have proven to be an effective treatment option. A multidisciplinary approach is the best treatment for these systemic disorders.

Current evidence indicates that depression is prevalent among patients with BRSD. Clinicians in general and psychiatrists, in particular, should be aware of this significant association and should aim at treating both of these conditions simultaneously for optimal outcomes. Simple and practical screening tools for depression can be applied in sleep disorder clinics to facilitate the evaluation of depression among patients with BRSD. Conversely, simple and practical tools like STOP-Bang questionnaire could be used in psychiatric clinics to evaluate for the likelihood for BRSD, especially OSA. Patients with persistent daytime sleepiness despite optimal CPAP use for OSA should be assessed for possible comorbid depression especially since persistent sleepiness has been linked to persistent depressive symptoms in patients with treated OSA although the direction of this link is uncertain.

FUTURE DIRECTIONS
Large-scale longitudinal studies are needed to establish the cause and effect relationship between BRSD and depression while controlling for possible confounders. Additionally, more research is needed to elucidate the effect of treatment of depression with antidepressants on PAP adherence in patients with BRSDs.

ACKNOWLEDGMENTS
The preparation of this manuscript was supported by a grant from the Strategic Technologies Program of the National Plan for Sciences and Technology and Innovation in the Kingdom of Saudi Arabia (08-MED511-02).

KEY CLINICAL PEARLS
- More than one-third of psychiatric patients suffer from BRSDs in their lifetime.
- The relationship between psychiatric disorders and BRSD is bidirectional.
- The presence of BRSD in a patient with psychiatric disorder(s) is associated with worsening course of both conditions.
- OSA is a systemic disorder, presenting with partial or complete obstruction of the upper airway.
- Assessment of OSA involves a comprehensive approach, taking into account the patient's physical, psychological, and social conditions.
- PSG is the gold standard diagnostic test for OSA although HSAT can be considered in select patients.
- Negative, inconclusive, or technically inadequate home sleep apnea testing should be followed with PSG to definitely rule out OSA.
- PAP therapy is the first-line treatment of OSA.
- OAs or MADs are effective for managing mild to moderate OSA.
- Surgery is usually reserved for patients that are unable to use or benefit from PAP therapy.
- Hypoglossal nerve stimulation is a novel and effective method of treating OSA.
- Medical cannabis is not recommended for treatment of OSA.
- Misinterpretation of OSA symptoms as psychiatric symptoms leads to a delay in diagnosis and treatment of OSA.
- OSA affects numerous brain functions, which, in turn, worsen psychiatric comorbidities.

- Depression may affect compliance with OSA management modalities,
- Treatment of OSA improves depression in many patients; however, comorbid EDS persisting despite treatment of OSA may lead to a persistence of depression in those patients.
- Psychiatrists could play a key role in detecting BRSDs among psychiatric patients.
- CSASs are a group of disorders that are characterized by airflow cessation due to the absence of respiratory effort.
- CSB is a breathing disorder presenting with cyclical fluctuations in breathing, is mostly associated with HF, and contributes to a poor prognosis in HF patients.
- Opioids can cause CSA in dose-dependent fashion for which ASV is more effective than conventional CPAP.
- Sleep related hypoventilation disorders are disorders characterized by insufficient ventilation during sleep leading to abnormally elevated $PaCO_2$ during sleep.
- OHS is highly comorbid with OSA; treatment with PAP, in addition to weight loss, can improve both conditions.

SELF-ASSESSMENT QUESTIONS

1. A 40-year-old male patient presents to the clinic with a hand injury; he is a heavy machine operator in a steel factory. The patient reported that he fell asleep while performing his task at his workplace; in fact, he claimed that he received warning many times of impending sleep during working hours. His body mass index is 39 kg/m^2, and apnea hypopnea index is 32. The initial management for this patient is weight reduction and
   a. nonsupine sleep position.
   b. CPAP therapy.
   c. tongue-retaining devices.
   d. laser-assisted uvulopalatoplasty.

Answer: b

2. A 38-year-old male patient presents to the clinic with 3 years history of low mood, interrupted sleep, and impairment of concentration. He was started on antidepressant treatment with no improvement. He is a smoker, drinks alcohol on social occasions, and his medications include fluoxetine and atenolol and metformin. The proper management of this patient is
   a. investigate for cardiovascular complications.
   b. investigate for sleep-related breathing disorders
   c. measure the brain-derived neurotrophic factor level.
   d. use another antidepressant medication.

Answer: b

3. A 52-year-old diabetic male patient presented to the clinic with daytime sleepiness, mood changes, and reduced concentration. Based on patient interview and investigation, he was diagnosed with depression and obstructive sleep apnea. You decide to start him on CPAP as the main treatment modality. The strategy that could most likely enhance adherence to CPAP therapy is
   a. prescribing a sleeping tablet.
   b. treatment of comorbid depression.
   c. prescribing a stimulant medication to be used in the daytime.
   d. using auto-titrating CPAP.

Answer: b

4. A 60-year-old male patient who was diagnosed with heart failure due to ischemic heart disease, presented to the clinic complaining of interrupted sleep at night, daytime somnolence and easy fatigability. He was diagnosed to have CSA with Cheyne–Stokes breathing. Further investigations are expected to reveal
   a. LV ejection fraction of 55% on echocardiogram.
   b. high or high-normal awake $PaCO_2$ level.
   c. low plasma and urinary catecholamine levels.
   d. crescendo–decrescendo breathing pattern on polysomnogram.

Answer: d

5. A 58-year-old female patient presented to the clinic complaining of shortness of breath, excessive daytime sleepiness, and fatigability. The husband has witnessed frequent choking attacks during sleep. Her examination reveals an obese woman with a body mass index of 42 kg/m^2, an arterial P_aCO_2 of 48 mmHg, and serum bicarbonate level of 29 mEq/L. The initial treatment of this patient after PSG reveals OSA and OHS is
   a. positive airway pressure therapy during sleep
   b. oxygen therapy
   c. tracheostomy
   d. weight loss

Answer: a

REFERENCES

1. Gupta MA, Simpson FC. Obstructive sleep apnea and psychiatric disorders: a systematic review. *J Clin Sleep Med*. 2015;11(2):165.
2. Haynes PL, Emert SE, Epstein D, Perkins S, Parthasarathy S, Wilcox J. The effect of sleep disorders, sedating medications, and depression on cognitive processing therapy outcomes: a fuzzy set qualitative comparative analysis. *J Traumatic Stress*. 2017;30(6):635–645.
3. Gilat H, Vinker S, Buda I, Soudry E, Shani M, Bachar G. Obstructive sleep apnea and cardiovascular comorbidities: a large epidemiologic study. *Medicine*. 2014;93(9):e45.
4. Katon W, Lin EH, Kroenke K. The association of depression and anxiety with medical symptom burden in patients with chronic medical illness. *Gen Hosp Psychiatry*. 2007;29(2):147–155.
5. Chang W-P, Liu M-E, Chang W-C, et al. Sleep apnea and the risk of dementia: a population-based 5-year follow-up study in Taiwan. *PloS One*. 2013;8(10):e78655.
6. Zhu X, Zhao Y. Sleep-disordered breathing and the risk of cognitive decline: a meta-analysis of 19,940 participants. *Sleep Breathing*. 2017;22(1):165–173.
7. Lettieri CJ, Collen JF, Williams SG. Challenges in the management of sleep apnea and PTSD: is the low arousal threshold an unrealized target? *J Clin Sleep Med*. 2017;13(6):845–846.
8. BaHammam AS, Al-Shimemeri SA, Salama RI, Sharif MM. Clinical and polysomnographic characteristics and response to continuous positive airway pressure therapy in obstructive sleep apnea patients with nightmares. *Sleep Med*. 2013;14(2):149–154.
9. Ullah MI, Campbell DG, Bhagat R, Lyons JA, Tamanna S. Improving PTSD symptoms and preventing progression of subclinical PTSD to an overt disorder by treating comorbid OSA with CPAP. *J Clin Sleep Med*. 2017;13(10):1191–1198.
10. Sweetman AM, Lack LC, Catcheside PG, et al. Developing a successful treatment for co-morbid insomnia and sleep apnoea. *Sleep Med Rev*. 2017;33:28–38.
11. American Academy of Sleep Medicine. *International Classification of Sleep Disorders*. 3rd ed. Darien, IL: American Academy of Sleep Medicine, 2014.
12. Kryger MH, Roth T, Dement WC. Principles and practice of sleep medicine. In: Elsevier; 2017.
13. Myers KA, Mrkobrada M, Simel DL. Does this patient have obstructive sleep apnea?: The Rational Clinical Examination systematic review. *JAMA*. 2013;310(7):731–741.
14. Johns MW. A new method for measuring daytime sleepiness: the Epworth sleepiness scale. *Sleep*. 1991;14(6):540–545.
15. Kushida CA, Littner MR, Morgenthaler T, et al. Practice parameters for the indications for polysomnography and related procedures: an update for 2005. *Sleep*. 2005;28(4):499–521.
16. Collop NA, Tracy SL, Kapur V, et al. Obstructive sleep apnea devices for out-of-center (OOC) testing: technology evaluation. *J Clin Sleep Med*. 2011;7(5):531–548.
17. Kapur VK, Auckley DH, Chowdhuri S, et al. Clinical practice guideline for diagnostic testing for adult obstructive sleep apnea: an American Academy of Sleep Medicine clinical practice guideline. *J Clin Sleep Med*. 2017;13(3):479–504.
18. Ruehland WR, Rochford PD, O'Donoghue FJ, Pierce RJ, Singh P, Thornton AT. The new AASM criteria for scoring hypopneas: impact on the apnea hypopnea index. *Sleep*. 2009;32(2):150–157.
19. Epstein LJ, Kristo D, Strollo PJ, Jr., et al. Clinical guideline for the evaluation, management and long-term care of obstructive sleep apnea in adults. *J Clin Sleep Med*. 2009;5(3):263–276.
20. Strohl KP, Brown DB, Collop N, et al. An official American Thoracic Society Clinical Practice Guideline: sleep apnea, sleepiness, and driving risk in noncommercial drivers. An update of a 1994 statement. *Am J Respir Crit Care Med*. 2013;187(11):1259–1266.
21. Epstein LJ, Kristo D, Strollo PJ, Jr., et al. Clinical guideline for the evaluation, management and long-term care of obstructive sleep apnea in adults. *J Clin Sleep Med*. 2009;5(3):263–276.
22. Randerath WJ, Verbraecken J, Andreas S, et al. Non-CPAP therapies in obstructive sleep apnoea. *Eur Respir J*. 2011;37(5):1000–1028.
23. Sutherland K, Kairaitis K, Yee BJ, Cistulli PA. From CPAP to tailored therapy for obstructive sleep Apnoea. *Multidiscip Respir Med*. 2018;13:44.
24. Dixon JB, Schachter LM, O'Brien PE, et al. Surgical vs conventional therapy for weight loss treatment of obstructive sleep apnea: a randomized controlled trial. *JAMA*. 2012;308(11):1142–149.
25. Morgenthaler TI, Kapen S, Lee-Chiong T, et al. Practice parameters for the medical therapy of obstructive sleep apnea. *Sleep*. 2006;29(8):1031–1035.
26. Pevernagie DA, Stanson AW, Sheedy PF, 2nd, Daniels BK, Shepard JW, Jr. Effects of body position on the upper airway of patients with obstructive sleep apnea. *Am J Respir Crit Care Med*. 1995;152(1):179–185.

27. Issa FG, Sullivan CE. Alcohol, snoring and sleep apnea. *J Neurol Neurosurg Psychiatry.* 1982;45(4):353–359.

28. Al-Jawder SE, Bahammam AS. Comorbid insomnia in sleep-related breathing disorders: an under-recognized association. *Sleep Breath.* 2012;16(2):295–304.

29. BaHammam AS, Singh T, George S, Acosta KL, Barataman K, Gacuan DE. Choosing the right interface for positive airway pressure therapy in patients with obstructive sleep apnea. *Sleep Breath.* 2017;21(3):569–575.

30. Javaheri S, Malik A, Smith J, Chung E. Adaptive pressure support servoventilation: a novel treatment for sleep apnea associated with use of opioids. *J Clin Sleep Med.* 2008;4(4):305–310.

31. Ou Q, Chen YC, Zhuo SQ, et al. Continuous Positive Airway Pressure Treatment Reduces Mortality in Elderly Patients with Moderate to Severe Obstructive Severe Sleep Apnea: A Cohort Study. *PloS One.* 2015;10(6):e0127775.

32. Campos-Rodriguez F, Martinez-Garcia MA, de la Cruz-Moron I, Almeida-Gonzalez C, Catalan-Serra P, Montserrat JM. Cardiovascular mortality in women with obstructive sleep apnea with or without continuous positive airway pressure treatment: a cohort study. *Ann Intern Med.* 2012;156(2):115–122.

33. Kryger MH, Berry RB, Massie CA. Long-term use of a nasal expiratory positive airway pressure (EPAP) device as a treatment for obstructive sleep apnea (OSA). *J Clin Sleep Med.* 2011;7(5):449–453B.

34. Barbe F, Duran-Cantolla J, Capote F, et al. Long-term effect of continuous positive airway pressure in hypertensive patients with sleep apnea. *Am J Respir Crit Care Med.* . 2010;181(7):718–726.

35. Wozniak DR, Lasserson TJ, Smith I. Educational, supportive and behavioural interventions to improve usage of continuous positive airway pressure machines in adults with obstructive sleep apnoea. *Cochrane Database Syst Rev.* 2014;1:CD007736.

36. Camacho M, Certal V, Abdullatif J, et al. Myofunctional therapy to treat obstructive sleep apnea: a systematic review and meta-analysis. *Sleep.* 2015;38(5):669–675.

37. Halle TR, Oh MS, Collop NA, Quyyumi AA, Bliwise DL, Dedhia RC. Surgical treatment of OSA on cardiovascular outcomes: a systematic review. *Chest.* 2017;152(6):1214–1229.

38. Kushida CA, Morgenthaler TI, Littner MR, et al. Practice parameters for the treatment of snoring and Obstructive Sleep Apnea with oral appliances: an update for 2005. *Sleep.* 2006;29(2):240–243.

39. Smith DF, Cohen AP, Ishman SL. Surgical management of OSA in adults. *Chest.* 2015;147(6):1681–1690.

40. Van de Heyning PH, Badr MS, Baskin JZ, et al. Implanted upper airway stimulation device for obstructive sleep apnea. *Laryngoscope.* 2012;122(7):1626–1633.

41. Strollo PJ, Jr., Soose RJ, Maurer JT, et al. Upper-airway stimulation for obstructive sleep apnea. *N Engl J Med.* 2014;370(2):139–149.

42. Woodson BT, Gillespie MB, Soose RJ, et al. Randomized controlled withdrawal study of upper airway stimulation on OSA: short- and long-term effect. *Otolaryngol Head Neck Surg.* 2014;151(5):880–887.

43. Guilleminault C, Hill MW, Simmons FB, Dement WC. Obstructive sleep apnea: electromyographic and fiberoptic studies. *Exp Neurol.* 1978;62(1):48–67.

44. Schwartz AR, Bennett ML, Smith PL, et al. Therapeutic electrical stimulation of the hypoglossal nerve in obstructive sleep apnea. *Arch Otolaryngol Head Neck Surg.* 2001;127(10):1216–1223.

45. Eastwood PR, Barnes M, Walsh JH, et al. Treating obstructive sleep apnea with hypoglossal nerve stimulation. *Sleep.* 2011;34(11):1479–1486.

46. Strollo PJ, Jr., Soose RJ, Maurer JT, et al. Upper-airway stimulation for obstructive sleep apnea. *N Engl J Med.* 2014;370(2):139–149.

47. Kompelli AR, Ni JS, Nguyen SA, Lentsch EJ, Neskey DM, Meyer TA. The outcomes of hypoglossal nerve stimulation in the management of OSA: A systematic review and meta-analysis. *World J Otorhinolaryngol Head Neck Surg.* 2019;5(1):41–48.

48. Hong SO, Chen YF, Jung J, Kwon YD, Liu SYC. Hypoglossal nerve stimulation for treatment of obstructive sleep apnea (OSA): a primer for oral and maxillofacial surgeons. *Maxillofac Plast Reconstr Surg.* 2017;39(1):27.

49. Dedhia RC, Strollo PJ, Soose RJ. Upper Airway Stimulation for Obstructive Sleep Apnea: Past, Present, and Future. *Sleep.* 2015;38(6):899–906.

50. Strollo PJ, Jr., Gillespie MB, Soose RJ, et al. Upper Airway Stimulation for Obstructive Sleep Apnea: Durability of the Treatment Effect at 18 Months. *Sleep.* 2015;38(10):1593–1598.

51. Mason M, Welsh EJ, Smith I. Drug therapy for obstructive sleep apnoea in adults. *Cochrane Database Syst Rev.* 2013;5:CD003002.

52. BaHammam AS, Kendzerska T, Gupta R, et al. Comorbid depression in obstructive sleep apnea: an under-recognized association. *Sleep Breath.* 2016;20(2):447–456.

53. Kendzerska T, Gershon AS, Hawker GA, Tomlinson GA, Leung RS. Obstructive sleep apnoea is not a risk factor for incident hospitalised depression: a historical cohort study. *Eur Respir J.* 2017;49(6):1601361.

54. Rezaeitalab F, Moharrari F, Saberi S, Asadpour H, Rezaeetalab F. The correlation of anxiety and depression with obstructive sleep apnea syndrome. *J Res Med Sci.* 2014;19(3):205–210.

55. Lu M-K, Tan H-P, Tsai I-N, Huang L-C, Liao X-M, Lin S-H. Sleep apnea is associated with an increased risk of mood disorders: a population-based cohort study. *Sleep Breath.* 2017;21(2):243–253.

56. Sharafkhaneh A, Giray N, Richardson P, Young T, Hirshkowitz M. Association of psychiatric disorders and sleep apnea in a large cohort. *Sleep.* 2005;28(11):1405–1411.

57. Young T, Skatrud J, Peppard PE. Risk factors for obstructive sleep apnea in adults. *JAMA.* 2004;291(16):2013–2016.

58. Zinchuk AV, Gentry MJ, Concato J, Yaggi HK. Phenotypes in obstructive sleep apnea: A definition, examples and evolution of approaches. *Sleep Med Rev.* 35:113–123. doi:10.1016/j.smrv.2016.10.002.

59. Kasasbeh E, Chi DS, Krishnaswamy G. Inflammatory aspects of sleep apnea and their cardiovascular consequences. *South Med J.* 2006;99(1):58–67.

60. Chung S, Yoon I-Y, Lee CH, Kim J-W. The association of nocturnal hypoxemia with arterial stiffness and endothelial dysfunction in male patients with obstructive sleep apnea syndrome. *Respiration.* 2010;79(5):363–369.

61. Mehra R, Xu F, Babineau DC, et al. Sleep-disordered breathing and prothrombotic biomarkers: cross-sectional results of the Cleveland Family Study. *Am J Respir Crit Care Med.* 2010;182(6):826–833.

62. Urakami Y, Ioannides AA, Kostopoulos GK. Sleep spindles—as a biomarker of brain function and plasticity. In: Ajeena IM, ed. *Advances in Clinical Neurophysiology.* London: Intech Open; 2012:73–108.

63. Landmann N, Kuhn M, Piosczyk H, et al. The reorganisation of memory during sleep. *Sleep Med Rev.* 2014;18(6):531–541.

64. D'Rozario AL, Cross NE, Vakulin A, et al. Quantitative electroencephalogram measures in adult obstructive sleep apnea: potential biomarkers of neurobehavioural functioning. *Sleep Med Rev.* 2016.

65. Rosenzweig I, Glasser M, Polsek D, Leschziner GD, Williams SC, Morrell MJ. Sleep apnoea and the brain: a complex relationship. *Lancet Resp Med.* 2015;3(5):404–414.

66. Alex RM, Mousavi ND, Zhang R, Gatchel RJ, Behbehani K. Obstructive sleep apnea: Brain hemodynamics, structure, and function. *J Appl Biobehav Res.* 2017;22(4):e12101.

67. Bucks RS, Olaithe M, Rosenzweig I, Morrell MJ. Reviewing the relationship between OSA and cognition: where do we go from here? *Respirology.* 2017;22(7):1253–1261.

68. Rosenzweig I, Kempton MJ, Crum WR, et al. Hippocampal hypertrophy and sleep apnea: a role for the ischemic preconditioning? *PloS One.* 2013;8(12):e83173.

69. Devita M, Montemurro S, Ramponi S, et al. Obstructive sleep apnea and its controversial effects on cognition. *J Clin Exp Neuropsychol.* 2017;39(7):659–669.

70. Goldstein AN, Walker MP. The role of sleep in emotional brain function. *Annu Rev Clin Psychol.* 2014;10:679–708.

71. Glasser M. Neuroanatomical correlates of cognitive dysfunction in obstructive sleep apnoea. *Am J Resp Crit Care Med.* 2013;187:A2319.

72. Gao H, Han Z, Huang S, et al. Intermittent hypoxia caused cognitive dysfunction relate to miRNAs dysregulation in hippocampus. *Behav Brain Res.* 2017;335:80–87.

73. Xia Y, Fu Y, Xu H, Guan J, Yi H, Yin S. Changes in cerebral metabolites in obstructive sleep apnea: a systemic review and meta-analysis. *Sci Rep.* 2016;6:28712.

74. Brugniaux JV, Foster GE, Beaudin AE. What role for hypercapnia in obstructive sleep apnea? *J Appl Physiol.* 2016;121(1):362.

75. Parrino L, Vaudano AE. The resilient brain and the guardians of sleep: New perspectives on old assumptions. *Sleep Med Rev.* 2018;39:98–107.

76. Elble R. Alzheimer disease and sleep. Neurobio Aging. 2016;39(Suppl 1):S3.

77. Olaithe M, Bucks RS, Hillman DR, Eastwood PR. Cognitive deficits in obstructive sleep apnea: insights from a meta-review and comparison with deficits observed in COPD, insomnia, and sleep deprivation. *Sleep Med Rev.* 2018;38:39–49. doi: 10.1016/j.smrv.2017.03.005.

78. Varga AW, Kishi A, Mantua J, et al. Apnea-induced rapid eye movement sleep disruption impairs human spatial navigational memory. *J Neuroscience.* 2014;34(44):14571–14577.

79. Olaithe M, Bucks RS. Executive dysfunction in OSA before and after treatment: a meta-analysis. *Sleep.* 2013;36(9):1297–1305.

80. Krysta K, Bratek A, Zawada K, Stepańczak R. Cognitive deficits in adults with obstructive sleep apnea compared to children and adolescents. *J Neural Transmission.* 2017;124(1):187–201.

81. Urquhart DS, Hill EA, Morley A. Sleep-disordered breathing in children. *Paed Child Health.* 2017;27(7):328–336

82. Quan SF, Chan CS, Dement WC, et al. The association between obstructive sleep apnea and neurocognitive performance—the Apnea Positive Pressure Long-term Efficacy Study (APPLES). *Sleep.* 2011;34(3):303–314.

83. Beck AT, Ward CH, Mendelson M, Mock J, Erbaugh J. An inventory for measuring depression. *Arch Gen Psychiatry*. 1961;4:561–571.

84. Weissman MM, Sholomskas D, Pottenger M, Prusoff BA, Locke BZ. Assessing depressive symptoms in five psychiatric populations: a validation study. *Am J Epidemiol*. 1977;106(3):203–214.

85. Gough HG. Diagnostic patterns on the Minnesota multiphasic personality inventory. *J Clin Psychol*. 1946;2:23–37.

86. Chandarana PC, Eals M, Steingart AB, Bellamy N, Allen S. The detection of psychiatric morbidity and associated factors in patients with rheumatoid arthritis. *Can J Psychiatry*. 1987;32(5):356–361.

87. Kroenke K, Spitzer RL, Williams JB. The PHQ-9: validity of a brief depression severity measure. *J Gen Intern Med*. 2001;16(9):606–613.

88. Derogatis LR, Lipman RS, Covi L. SCL-90: an outpatient psychiatric rating scale--preliminary report. *Psychopharmacol Bull*. 1973;9(1):13–28.

89. Sheehan DV, Lecrubier Y, Sheehan KH, et al. The Mini-International Neuropsychiatric Interview (M.I.N.I.): the development and validation of a structured diagnostic psychiatric interview for DSM-IV and ICD-10. *J Clin Psychiatry*. 1998;59(Suppl 20):22–33; quiz 34–57.

90. Zung WW. A Self-Rating Depression Scale. *Arch Gen Psychiatry*. 1965;12:63–70.

91. McDaid C, Griffin S, Weatherly H, et al. Continuous positive airway pressure devices for the treatment of obstructive sleep apnoea-hypopnoea syndrome: a systematic review and economic analysis. *Health Technol Assess*. 2009;13(4):iii–iv, xi–xiv, 1–119, 143–274.

92. Bazzano LA, Khan Z, Reynolds K, He J. Effect of nocturnal nasal continuous positive airway pressure on blood pressure in obstructive sleep apnea. *Hypertension*. 2007;50(2):417–423.

93. Schwartz DJ, Kohler WC, Karatinos G. Symptoms of depression in individuals with obstructive sleep apnea may be amenable to treatment with continuous positive airway pressure. *Chest*. 2005;128(3):1304–1309.

94. Kawahara S, Akashiba T, Akahoshi T, Horie T. Nasal CPAP improves the quality of life and lessens the depressive symptoms in patients with obstructive sleep apnea syndrome. *Intern Med*. 2005;44(5):422–427.

95. Diamanti C, Manali E, Ginieri-Coccossis M, et al. Depression, physical activity, energy consumption, and quality of life in OSA patients before and after CPAP treatment. *Sleep Breath*. 2013;17(4):1159–1168.

96. Giles TL, Lasserson TJ, Smith BH, White J, Wright J, Cates CJ. Continuous positive airways pressure for obstructive sleep apnoea in adults. *Cochrane Database Syst Rev*. 2006(3):CD001106.

97. Henke KG, Grady JJ, Kuna ST. Effect of nasal continuous positive airway pressure on neuropsychological function in sleep apnea-hypopnea syndrome. A randomized, placebo-controlled trial. *Am J Respir Crit Care Med*. 2001;163(4):911–917.

98. Haensel A, Norman D, Natarajan L, Bardwell WA, Ancoli-Israel S, Dimsdale JE. Effect of a 2 week CPAP treatment on mood states in patients with obstructive sleep apnea: a double-blind trial. *Sleep Breath*. 2007;11(4):239–244.

99. Bardwell WA, Norman D, Ancoli-Israel S, et al. Effects of 2-week nocturnal oxygen supplementation and continuous positive airway pressure treatment on psychological symptoms in patients with obstructive sleep apnea: a randomized placebo-controlled study. *Behav Sleep Med*. 2007;5(1):21–38.

100. Povitz M, Bolo CE, Heitman SJ, Tsai WH, Wang J, James MT. Effect of treatment of obstructive sleep apnea on depressive symptoms: systematic review and meta-analysis. *PLoS Med*. 2014;11(11):e1001762.

101. Habukawa M, Uchimura N, Kakuma T, et al. Effect of CPAP treatment on residual depressive symptoms in patients with major depression and coexisting sleep apnea: Contribution of daytime sleepiness to residual depressive symptoms. *Sleep Med*. 2010;11(6):552–557.

102. Gagnadoux F, Le Vaillant M, Goupil F, et al. Depressive symptoms before and after long-term CPAP therapy in patients with sleep apnea. *Chest*. 2014;145(5):1025–1031.

103. Kjelsberg FN, Ruud EA, Stavem K. Predictors of symptoms of anxiety and depression in obstructive sleep apnea. *Sleep Med*. 2005;6(4):341–346.

104. Poulet C, Veale D, Arnol N, Levy P, Pepin JL, Tyrrell J. Psychological variables as predictors of adherence to treatment by continuous positive airway pressure. *Sleep Med*. 2009;10(9):993–999.

105. Law M, Naughton M, Ho S, Roebuck T, Dabscheck E. Depression may reduce adherence during CPAP titration trial. *J Clin Sleep Med*. 2014;10(2):163–169.

106. Means MK, Ulmer CS, Edinger JD. Ethnic differences in continuous positive airway pressure (CPAP) adherence in veterans with and without psychiatric disorders. *Behav Sleep Med*. 2010;8(4):260–273.

107. Saleem AH, Al Rashed FA, Alkharboush GA, et al. Primary care physicians' knowledge of sleep medicine and barriers to transfer of patients with sleep disorders. A cross-sectional study. *Saudi Med J*. 2017;38(5):553–559.

108. Almohaya A, Qrmli A, Almagal N, et al. Sleep medicine education and knowledge among medical students in selected Saudi Medical Schools. *BMC Med Educ*. 2013;13:133.

109. Senthilvel E, Auckley D, Dasarathy J. Evaluation of sleep disorders in the primary care setting: history taking compared to questionnaires. *J Clin Sleep Med*. 2011;7(1):41–48.

110. Rosen RC, Zozula R, Jahn EG, Carson JL. Low rates of recognition of sleep disorders in primary care: comparison of a community-based versus clinical academic setting. *Sleep Med*. 2001;2(1):47–55.

111. Zozula R PB, Boehlecke B, Avidan A, Consens F, Dunagan D, Zee P, Rosen RC. The Medical Education in Sleep (MEDSleep) Survey. 2001;15(Suppl): S110.

112. Kovacic Z, Marendic M, Soljic M, Pecotic R, Kardum G, Dogas Z. Knowledge and attitude regarding sleep medicine of medical students and physicians in Split, Croatia. *Croatian Med J*. 2002;43(1):71–74.

113. Cherrez Ojeda I, Jeffe DB, Guerrero T, et al. Attitudes and knowledge about obstructive sleep apnea among Latin American primary care physicians. *Sleep Med*. 2013;14(10):973–977.

114. Papp KK, Penrod CE, Strohl KP. Knowledge and attitudes of primary care physicians toward sleep and sleep disorders. *Sleep Breath*. 2002;6(3):103–109.

115. AlDabal L, BaHammam AS. Cheyne-stokes respiration in patients with heart failure. *Lung*. 2010;188(1):5–14.

116. Carmona-Bernal C, Ruiz-Garcia A, Villa-Gil M, et al. Quality of life in patients with congestive heart failure and central sleep apnea. *Sleep Med*. 2008;9(6):646–651.

117. Sin DD, Fitzgerald F, Parker JD, Newton G, Floras JS, Bradley TD. Risk factors for central and obstructive sleep apnea in 450 men and women with congestive heart failure. *Am J Respir Crit Care Med*. 1999;160(4):1101–1106.

118. Xie A, Skatrud JB, Puleo DS, Rahko PS, Dempsey JA. Apnea-hypopnea threshold for CO2 in patients with congestive heart failure. *Am J Respir Crit Care Med*. 2002;165(9):1245–1250.

119. Carmona-Bernal C, Quintana-Gallego E, Villa-Gil M, Sanchez-Armengol A, Martinez-Martinez A, Capote F. Brain natriuretic peptide in patients with congestive heart failure and central sleep apnea. *Chest*. 2005;127(5):1667–1673.

120. Aurora RN, Chowdhuri S, Ramar K, et al. The treatment of central sleep apnea syndromes in adults: practice parameters with an evidence-based literature review and meta-analyses. *Sleep*. 2012;35(1):17–40.

121. Bradley TD, Logan AG, Kimoff RJ, et al. Continuous positive airway pressure for central sleep apnea and heart failure. *N Engl J Med*. 2005;353(19):2025–2033.

122. Arzt M, Floras JS, Logan AG, et al. Suppression of central sleep apnea by continuous positive airway pressure and transplant-free survival in heart failure: a post hoc analysis of the Canadian Continuous Positive Airway Pressure for Patients with Central Sleep Apnea and Heart Failure Trial (CANPAP). *Circulation*. 2007;115(25):3173–3180.

123. Javaheri S, Brown LK, Randerath WJ. Clinical applications of adaptive servoventilation devices: part 2. *Chest*. 2014;146(3):858–868.

124. ResMed. Important medical device warning. http://www.thoracic.org.au/imagesDB/wysiwyg/ServeHFDoctorLetter.pdf. 2015.

125. Cowie MR, Woehrle H, Wegscheider K, et al. Adaptive Servo-Ventilation for Central Sleep Apnea in Systolic Heart Failure. *N Engl J Med*. 2015;373(12):1095–1105.

126. Aurora RN, Bista SR, Casey KR, et al. Updated adaptive servo-ventilation recommendations for the 2012 AASM Guideline: "The treatment of central sleep apnea syndromes in adults: practice parameters with an evidence based literature review and meta-analyses." *J Clin Sleep Med*. 2016;12(5):757–761.

127. Perger E, Lyons OD, Inami T, et al. Predictors of 1-year compliance with adaptive servoventilation in patients with heart failure and sleep disordered breathing: preliminary data from the ADVENT-HF trial. *Eur Respir J*. 2019;53(2).

128. Effect of adaptive servo ventilation (ASV) on survival and hospital admissions in heart failure (ADVENT-HF) [clinical trial]. Identifier: NCT01128816National Library of Medicine (US). https://clinicaltrials.gov/ct2/show/NCT01128816. May 24, 2010.

129. Terziyski K, Draganova A. Central sleep apnea with Cheyne–Stokes breathing in heart failure—from research to clinical practice and beyond. *Adv Exp Med Biol*. 2018;1067:327–351.

130. Javaheri S, Brown LK, Randerath W, Khayat R. SERVE-HF: more questions than answers. *Chest*. 2016;149(4):900–904.

131. Javaheri S, McKane SW, Cameron N, Germany RE, Malhotra A. In patients with heart failure the burden of central sleep apnea increases in the late sleep hours. *Sleep*. 2019;42(1). doi:10.1093/sleep/zsy195.

132. Ding N, Zhang X. Transvenous phrenic nerve stimulation, a novel therapeutic approach for central sleep apnea. *J Thorac Dis*. 2018;10(3):2005–2010.

133. Zhang XL, Ding N, Wang H, et al. Transvenous phrenic nerve stimulation in patients with Cheyne-Stokes respiration and congestive heart failure: a safety and proof-of-concept study. *Chest.* 2012;142(4):927–934.

134. Ponikowski P, Javaheri S, Michalkiewicz D, et al. Transvenous phrenic nerve stimulation for the treatment of central sleep apnoea in heart failure. *Eur Heart J.* 2012;33(7):889–894.

135. Costanzo MR, Ponikowski P, Javaheri S, et al. Transvenous neurostimulation for central sleep apnoea: a randomised controlled trial. *Lancet.* 2016;388(10048):974–982.

136. Costanzo MR, Ponikowski P, Coats A, et al. Phrenic nerve stimulation to treat patients with central sleep apnoea and heart failure. *Eur J Heart Fail.* 2018;20(12):1746–1754.

137. Correa D, Farney RJ, Chung F, Prasad A, Lam D, Wong J. Chronic opioid use and central sleep apnea: a review of the prevalence, mechanisms, and perioperative considerations. *Anesthesia Analgesia.* 2015;120(6):1273–1285.

138. Frase L, Schupp J, Sorichter S, Randelshofer W, Riemann D, Nissen C. Sodium oxybate-induced central sleep apneas. *Sleep Med.* 2013;14(9):922–924.

139. Hassamal S, Miotto K, Wang T, Saxon AJ. A narrative review: the effects of opioids on sleep disordered breathing in chronic pain patients and methadone maintained patients. *Am J Addict.* 2016;25(6):452–465.

140. Weil JV, McCullough RE, Kline J, Sodal IE. Diminished ventilatory response to hypoxia and hypercapnia after morphine in normal man. *N Engl J Med.* 1975;292(21):1103–1106.

141. Walker JM, Farney RJ, Rhondeau SM, et al. Chronic opioid use is a risk factor for the development of central sleep apnea and ataxic breathing. *J Clin Sleep Med.* 2007;3(5):455–461.

142. Ehsan Z, Mahmoud M, Shott SR, Amin RS, Ishman SL. The effects of anesthesia and opioids on the upper airway: A systematic review. *Laryngoscope.* 2016;126(1):270–284.

143. Wang D, Teichtahl H. Opioids, sleep architecture and sleep-disordered breathing. *Sleep Med Rev.* 2007;11(1):35–46.

144. Qasrawi SO, BaHammam AS. NIV in type 2 (Hypercapnic) acute respiratory failure. In: Esquinas A, Lemyze M, eds. *Mechanical Ventilation in the Critically Ill Obese Patient.* Cham, Switzerland: Springer; 2018:229–238.

145. Al Dabal L, Bahammam AS. Obesity hypoventilation syndrome. *Ann Thorac Med.* 2009;4(2):41–49.

146. Almeneessier AS, Nashwan SZ, Al-Shamiri MQ, Pandi-Perumal SR, BaHammam AS. The prevalence of pulmonary hypertension in patients with obesity hypoventilation syndrome: a prospective observational study. *J Thorac Dis.* 2017;9(3):779–788.

147. BaHammam AS. Prevalence, clinical characteristics, and predictors of obesity hypoventilation syndrome in a large sample of Saudi patients with obstructive sleep apnea. *Saudi Med J.* 2015;36(2):181–189.

148. Bahammam SA, Sharif MM, Jammah AA, Bahammam AS. Prevalence of thyroid disease in patients with obstructive sleep apnea. *Respir Med.* 2011;105(11):1755–1760.

149. BaHammam AS, Pandi-Perumal SR, Piper A, et al. Gender differences in patients with obesity hypoventilation syndrome. *J Sleep Res.* 2016;25(4):445–453.

150. Berry RB, Brooks R, Gamaldo C, et al. AASM Scoring Manual Updates for 2017 (Version 2.4). *J Clin Sleep Med.* 2017;13(5):665–666.

151. Aaron SD, Fergusson D, Dent R, Chen Y, Vandemheen KL, Dales RE. Effect of weight reduction on respiratory function and airway reactivity in obese women. *Chest.* 2004;125(6):2046–2052.

152. Guardiano SA, Scott JA, Ware JC, Schechner SA. The long-term results of gastric bypass on indexes of sleep apnea. *Chest.* 2003;124(4):1615–1619.

153. Harman EM, Wynne JW, Block AJ. The effect of weight loss on sleep-disordered breathing and oxygen desaturation in morbidly obese men. *Chest.* 1982;82(3):291–294.

154. Nguyen NT, Hinojosa MW, Smith BR, Gray J, Varela E. Improvement of restrictive and obstructive pulmonary mechanics following laparoscopic bariatric surgery. *Surg Endosc.* 2009;23(4):808–812.

155. Mokhlesi B. Obesity hypoventilation syndrome: a state-of-the-art review. *Respir Care.* 2010;55(10):1347–1362; discussion 1345–1363.

156. Piper AJ, BaHammam AS, Javaheri S. Obesity hypoventilation syndrome: choosing the appropriate treatment of a heterogeneous disorder. *Sleep Med Clin.* 2017;12(4):587–596.

157. BaHammam A. Acute ventilatory failure complicating obesity hypoventilation: update on a "critical care syndrome." *Curr Opin Pulm Med.* 2010;16(6):543–551.

158. Bahammam AS, Al-Jawder SE. Managing acute respiratory decompensation in the morbidly obese. *Respirology.* 2012;17(5):759–771.

159. Storre JH, Seuthe B, Fiechter R, et al. Average volume-assured pressure support in obesity hypoventilation: A randomized crossover trial. *Chest.* 2006;130(3):815–821.

160. Murphy PB, Davidson C, Hind MD, et al. Volume targeted versus pressure support non-invasive ventilation in patients with super obesity and chronic respiratory failure: a randomised controlled trial. *Thorax.* 2012;67(8):727–734.

16

Pediatric Sleep–Wake Disorders

REBECCA MARSHALL, KYLE P. JOHNSON, AND ANNA IVANENKO

INTRODUCTION

For accurate assessment of sleep disturbances in infancy, childhood and adolescence, it is vital to understand the normal sleep changes that occur during these developmental stages. While sleep needs vary by individual, in general, following are the sleep duration recommendations for typically developing children during different developmental stages[1]:

- Newborns (0–3 months): 14–17 hours
- Infants (4–11 months): 12–15 hours
- Toddlers (1–2 years): 11–14 hours
- Preschoolers (3–5 years): 10–13 hours
- School-age children (6–13 years): 9–11 hours
- Teenagers (14–17 years): 8–10 hours

In the first few weeks of life, newborns sleep approximately two thirds of the time; sleeping and waking times are spread throughout a 24-hour period, and are mostly influenced by hunger and satiety.[2] As infants begin to respond to light/dark and environmental cues, they begin to develop a circadian rhythm, which leads to increased sleep at night and increased periods of wakefulness during the day. Sleep consolidates between 6 and 9 months of age, with most infants sleeping approximately 10 to 12 hours at night, with two or three daytime naps.[3] By one year, infants have fewer nighttime awakenings and generally take two naps a day.[4] Importantly, developmental changes such as motor development during the first year may have a significant impact on sleep.[5]

During the toddler and preschool period, sleep continues to consolidate. On average, toddlers sleep from 11 to 14 hours daily, and preschoolers sleep 10 to 13 hours daily; children who spend more time napping during the day tend to sleep less at night. Daytime sleep decreases during this time: approximately 92% of 3-year-olds take one nap per day, with many children discontinuing napping between ages 4 and 5.[6] Night awakenings commonly occur during these years; as per parent report, 10% of children wake at least once per night, and 50% wake at least 1 night per week. While various factors influence night awakenings, a child's ability to return to sleep without parental help predicts the degree to which night awakenings persist.[7]

School-aged children generally sleep about 10 hours per night and wake spontaneously.[8] Predictably, older school-aged children tend to sleep less than younger school-aged children. Children in sixth grade go to sleep more than an hour later than second-grade children, resulting in total sleep time of 457 to 465 minutes in sixth-grade children versus 513 to 520 minutes in second-grade children.[9] Notably, older school-aged children report more morning sleepiness, and parents report that they are more likely to fall asleep unintentionally as compared to younger children.[10]

In adolescence, average sleep time decreases to 7.5 to 8 hours by age 16.[11] This decrease reflects a shift in sleep–wake patterns that begins in puberty and corresponds to later bedtimes and earlier rise times.[12,13] Although environmental factors such as school times and homework are believed to affect adolescents' sleep habits, biological processes regulating sleep and wakefulness may also influence sleep patterns during this period.[14] Teenagers often build up a "sleep debt" during the week, resulting in longer sleep periods on the weekend and proving disruptive to both the circadian rhythm and homeostatic sleep pressure.[15] Common sleep disturbances in adolescence include insufficient sleep, difficulty initiating and maintaining sleep, and/or a delayed circadian phase.[16]

Throughout the developmental phases of childhood and adolescence, parents can help children develop healthy sleep habits. Maintaining a consistent sleep schedule, choosing an age-appropriate bedtime and establishing a consistent, sleep-promoting bedtime routine are important elements in developing good sleep habits that will extend into adulthood. While sleep is a critical aspect of development and well-being, sleep disruption among children is common, with approximately 25% of children experiencing some type of sleep disturbance during childhood. Problems range from short-term difficulties to primary sleep disorders such as obstructive sleep apnea (OSA). Some research suggests that this estimate of prevalence is consistent across different cultures.[17]

Among children with psychiatric disorders, numerous studies have demonstrated high rates of sleep initiation and maintenance insomnia, restless sleep, nocturnal fears, nightmares, and daytime sleepiness.[18] This prevalence represents a complex association which appears to be bidirectional[19] as early sleep problems are known to predict later childhood psychiatric symptom severity and functional impairment.[20,21] Throughout childhood and adolescence, there are strong associations between sleep problems and various mental health symptoms and disorders. A recent study of preschoolers estimated an overall rate of sleep disorders of 19.2%, and the sleep disorders appeared to be particularly related to symptoms of anxiety disorders.[22] Among 6-year-old children, 13% with sleeping difficulties were found to have clinically elevated anxiety and depression scores, compared to 3% without sleep disturbances. At age 11, the percentage of children with anxiety and depressive symptoms increased to 29% and 4%, respectively.[23] Among adolescents, sleep problems are associated with higher rates of depression, anxiety, low self-esteem, excessive worry, and irritability, as well as increased risk of substance use.[24-28] Adolescents with insomnia also have increased rates of suicidal ideation and suicide attempts compared to adolescents without insomnia.[29]

In addition to evidence that sleep disturbances and disorders have an impact on the mental health of children and adolescents, there is also evidence that treating sleep disorders has a positive impact on psychiatric outcomes. For example, there is substantial evidence that treatment of obstructive sleep disordered breathing improves cognitive, behavioral, and academic outcomes in children and adolescents.[30] This chapter will provide an overview of pediatric sleep disorders. Specifically, the chapter will review the

comorbidity and treatment of sleep disturbances associated with the common psychiatric disorders in children and adolescents. Next, the chapter will review the clinical features and management of the most common pediatric sleep disorders including insomnia disorder, parasomnia disorders, narcolepsy and hypersomnolence disorders, restless legs syndrome (RLS), and periodic limb movement disorder (PLMD), OSA, and circadian rhythm sleep–wake disorders.

CLINICAL APPROACH TO CHILDHOOD SLEEP DISORDERS

Given the ubiquity of sleep complaints in children and adolescents suffering with psychiatric conditions, it is prudent to include sleep- and alertness-related questions in any initial assessment. This query could be made part of the clinical history obtained orally or by means of written intake materials. Fortunately, the questions to be asked are informed by research. Owen and colleagues developed the BEARS to assist pediatric residents in assessing for sleep disorders in busy outpatient practices.[31] BEARS is a mnemonic with B standing for bedtime issues, E for excessive daytime sleepiness, A for night awakenings, R for regularity and duration of sleep, and S for snoring. When the BEARS was incorporated into the medical chart, the frequency of sleep being mentioned in the impression and plan doubled.[29]

Subjective questionnaires have an important role in screening specific sleep disorders in children and adolescents. The Pediatric Sleep Questionnaire (PSQ) developed by Chervin for clinical research can be used to screen pediatric sleep problems, particularly breathing-related disorders and sleepiness.[32] It is a reliable measure validated by polysomnography (PSG). The Children's Sleep Habits Questionnaire (CSHQ) by Owens is another useful screening instrument for school-aged children.[33] The CSHQ gives both a total score and eight subscale scores, reflecting the important sleep domains of the major behavioral and medical sleep disorders in this age group. The Sleep Disorders Inventory for Students (SDIS) is a validated parent-reported screening inventory for children ages 2 through 10 years (SDIS-C), and adolescents, ages 11 through 18 years (SDIS-A).[34] The Epworth Sleepiness Scale (ESS) screens for the subjective propensity to fall asleep in several, common daytime situations and has been modified for use in children and adolescents.[35] Chronotype (morningness or eveningness preference) can be evaluated as well with the morningness–eveningness scale for children.[36]

Sleep diaries are an inexpensive, efficient means of collecting data on sleep and wake times prospectively. Typically, patients are sent home with diaries to complete over at least 2 weeks. On a return visit, the diaries are analyzed with special attention paid to total sleep time and sleep–wake schedule. Sleep diaries are particularly useful in assessing for insufficient sleep, the primary cause of daytime sleepiness in adolescents, and circadian rhythm disorders such as delayed sleep phase syndrome. It must be noted that data collected are subjective and prone to recall bias.

If initial screening is positive for sleep and alertness concerns, a more detailed sleep history should be undertaken including questions regarding sleep schedule and environment, unusual behaviors during sleep and sleep-related breathing problems. The clinician should also assess daytime alertness by questioning the patient, parents, and possibly collateral sources such as teachers. It is important to obtain a family sleep history since several sleep disorders run in families such as sleepwalking and RLS. Since sleep problems can be due to underlying, unrecognized medical problems, a focused medical history taking is also recommended. The differential diagnoses of the most common pediatric sleep disorder, insomnia, is listed in Table 16.1.

A tailored physical exam is also needed especially as it relates to risk factors for OSA. These risk factors include but are not limited to micrognathia (small jaw), enlarged tonsils, deviated nasal septum and abnormal palate and uvula. Weight and height measurements are important for assessing obesity, which is a major risk factor for OSA. Laboratory tests should be ordered on a case-by-case basis, depending on the condition suspected. OSA is common in patients with hypothyroidism; so thyroid function testing is indicated in patients with concomitant symptoms and/or signs of suggestive hypothyroidism. Given the association between iron deficiency and RLS, obtaining fasting iron indices, particularly ferritin levels, in patients with a clinical history consistent with RLS is appropriate. Drug screening should be considered in adolescents with excessive daytime sleepiness.

A sleep specialist may also order an overnight PSG. The PSG is considered the "gold standard" procedure for studying sleep and involves electroencephalogram (EEG), electro-oculogram, and chin electromyogram recordings while simultaneously measuring airflow, respiratory and abdominal effort, oxygen saturation, end tidal CO_2 ($ETCO_2$), heart rate and rhythm, and limb muscle activity. PSG requires a child to spend a night in the sleep

TABLE 16.1. DIFFERENTIAL DIAGNOSES FOR PEDIATRIC INSOMNIA

Medical	Substances/ Medications
Allergies/eczema	Alcohol
Asthma	Antiepileptic drugs
Gastroesophageal reflux disease	Antidepressants
Migraine headaches	Antipsychotics
Neuromuscular disorders	Lithium
Arnold–Chiari malformation	Stimulants
	Opioids
Chronic renal failure	Hypnotic agents
Seizure disorders	Corticosteroids
Ear infections	Caffeine
Diabetes mellitus	Nicotine
Pain syndromes	Theophylline
Iron deficiency anemia	
Hyperthyroidism	
Hypothyroidism	

Psychiatric	Psychosocial
Anxiety disorders	Abuse
Mood disorders	Chaotic home life
Disruptive behavior disorders	TV/computer in bedroom
Posttraumatic stress disorder	Parental sleep disorder
Pervasive developmental disorder	Inappropriate sleep-onset associations
Psychotic disorders	Marital conflict
Substance use disorders	New infant in home
Reactive attachment disorder	
Obsessive compulsive disorder	

laboratory accompanied by a parent or caregiver. A sleep technician is present during an in-lab PSG allowing timely attention to any technical challenges. Although home sleep apnea testing is commonly used in assessing adults at substantial risk for OSA, in-lab PSG remains preferable for children and adolescents.[37] A PSG is most often ordered when assessing for breathing-related sleep disorders but is also useful when assessing for PLMD, parasomnias, and nocturnal seizures.

The multiple sleep latency test (MSLT) is a series of four or five naps conducted at 2-hour intervals that begins 2 hours after the final morning awakening following nocturnal PSG. The MSLT is used to assess daytime sleepiness and propensity to enter rapid eye movement (REM) sleep when sleep occurs. The MSLT is most commonly used to assess a patient for potential narcolepsy. The maintenance of wakefulness test

(MWT) is similar to the MSLT but the patient is asked to remain awake while sleep latency in measured. This test has not been validated in children and therefore is rarely used in the pediatric setting. A pediatric sleep specialist has the ability to collect objective data on sleep and wakefulness. One tool available is actigraphy. An actigraph is a watch-like device worn on a patient's wrist for prolonged period of time. The actigraph measures movement, which algorithmically correlates with sleep and wakefulness. Actigraphy has particular utility when assessing for circadian rhythm disorders such as delayed sleep phase syndrome.[38]

Referral to a pediatric sleep specialist is warranted when underlying sleep disrupters such as sleep apnea or periodic limb movements are suspected. Consultation with a pediatric sleep specialist is also indicated for the evaluation and management of children with excessive daytime sleepiness, RLS, parasomnia disorders, or treatment-refractory insomnia.

Treatment plans addressing sleep problems in children and adolescents should include attention to sleep hygiene. Sleep hygiene refers to healthy sleep practices, which include avoiding caffeine close to bedtime, avoiding electronics for 1 to 2 hours before bedtime, implementing a calming bedtime routine, maintaining consistent bedtime and wake time schedules, sleeping in a dark, cool and quiet room, and adopting healthy daytime habits such as regular exercise. Behavioral treatments may be useful for children with insomnia (see Table 16.2). These approaches vary depending on the age of the child but

TABLE 16.2. BEHAVIORAL INTERVENTIONS FOR TREATING PEDIATRIC INSOMNIA

Intervention	Method
Sleep education	Educate parents and child regarding purpose of sleep, sleep needs and patterns for different age groups, and impact of inadequate sleep on daytime behavior and functioning
Sleep hygiene	Educate the child and parent regarding sleep-promoting behaviors prior to bedtime; eliminate environmental stimulation
Positive bedtime routine	Establish relaxing, low stress interactions between a parent and a child before lights-out; consider use of a transitional object
Unmodified extinction	Instructing parents to consistently ignore a child's disruptive behavior at bedtime
Graduated extinction	Gradual reduction of parental presence in the bedroom or of parental attention to inappropriate bedtime behaviors; can be combined with periodic "check-ins"
Extinction with parental presence	The parent remains in the child's bedroom while ignoring disruptive behavior at bedtime
Scheduled awakenings	Establish a pre-treatment pattern of nocturnal awakenings; then instruct parents to awaken the child 15–20 minutes prior to the anticipated awakenings followed by usual response to nocturnal awakening like feeding to aid return to sleep. Although beneficial for middle of the night insomnia with predictable pattern of nocturnal awakenings, this strategy is most helpful for parasomnias such as sleepwalking and sleep terrors.
Relaxation training	Identify symptoms associated with increased somatic and cognitive tension. Teach progressive muscle relaxation, guided imagery, and deep diaphragmatic (belly) breathing.

generally include establishing a consistent routine, removing overly stimulating activities prior to bedtime, eliminating unhealthy coping strategies (i.e., parents staying in room while child falls asleep; using the TV to fall asleep), and avoiding giving attention to bedtime-delaying behavior. The clinician and caregivers should collaborate to develop a specific behavioral plan, which includes the goal (i.e., falling asleep without parents in the room), and specific steps and timeline to accomplish that goal.

While clinicians are often asked for medications to be used as sleep aids, it should be noted that there are no medications currently approved by the US Food and Drug Administration (FDA) for treating any sleep disorders in children under 18 years of age. The majority of sleep disturbances in children and adolescents can be managed with behavioral treatments, as previously described. However, in some cases, pharmacologic intervention may be appropriate for management of the child or adolescent with significant difficulties in initiating or maintaining sleep. Medications should be used with clear expectations and goals; for example, with a goal of reducing sleep onset latency from 2 hours to 30 minutes. The treatment should be for the shortest possible duration and at the lowest possible dose for efficacy.

The medications commonly used as sleep-aids in pediatric setting include antihistaminic agents, melatonin, trazodone, zolpidem, and alpha agonists. However, it is important to note that there are no FDA approved medicines for pediatric insomnia; therefore, all medicines are used "off-label." See Table 16.3 for more specific information regarding medication treatments for pediatric insomnia. In addition, medication recommendations are provided in the following sections on specific sleep disorders.

SLEEP AND PSYCHIATRIC DISORDERS IN CHILDREN AND ADOLESCENTS

The research evidence increasingly supports the concept of a bidirectional relationship between sleep disturbances and psychiatric disorders. The sleep disturbance can result from a psychiatric disorder while sleep disturbance can contribute toward development of a psychiatric disorder.[39–41] In this section, we present a review of assessment and management of sleep disturbance associated with common psychiatric disorders in children and adolescents.

Sleep Disturbances in Depressive Disorders
Prevalence and Clinical Characteristics

Major depressive disorder (MDD) is typically characterized by depressed mood and/or loss of interest in previously enjoyable activities, along with other symptoms like decreased energy, prominent feelings of guilt or worthlessness, appetite change, and sleep disturbance.[42] In children, depression may present with irritability rather than depressed mood, as well as behavior changes and failure to achieve normal weight targets.[43] Prevalence in childhood has been estimated at 1% to 2 %[44]; in adolescence, prevalence is approximately 8%[45] with a lifetime prevalence of approximately 12%.[46]

Children and adolescents with MDD commonly express subjective sleep complaints including delayed sleep onset, nighttime awakenings, early morning awakenings, and daytime sleepiness.[47] In a large community study ($n = 1,710$), 88.6% of those meeting criteria for MDD reported sleep disturbances.[48] Among depressed children, insomnia is more common than hypersomnia.[49] As with many psychiatric disorders, there is likely a bidirectional relationship between sleep disturbances and depression.[50] A study of 3,134 youth 11 to 17 years of age found that baseline insomnia increased the risk of developing MDD by two- to threefold; reciprocally, MDD at baseline increased the risk of subsequent insomnia by two- to threefold.[51] Not only are adolescents' subjective sleep complaints linked with a higher severity of depression; sleep disturbance has also been associated with increased suicidality in this population.[52]

Neurobiology

While the neurobiological basis of MDD and sleep disturbance in adolescents is not well understood, both have been linked with abnormal neuronal connectivity. In adolescent MDD, research points to abnormal connectivity within the circuits mediating emotion processing,[53] in particular the subgenual region of the anterior cingulate cortex.[54–56] There is also evidence that sleep problems in youth affect brain structure and function. Sleep duration has been positively correlated with bilateral hippocampal grey matter volume as well as grey matter volume in the right dorsolateral prefrontal cortex.[57] Other research points to sleep deprivation changing adolescents' brain activity during task performance,[58] and sleep parameters being associated with changes in brain activity patterns, especially in the pre-frontal cortex and

TABLE 16.3. MEDICATIONS USED FOR PEDIATRIC SLEEP DISORDERS (PARTICULARLY INSOMNIA)

Drug	Mechanism of Action	Dose Range to Consider in Children	Safety Profile	Effects on Sleep	Uses in children*
Clonazepam	GABA-agonist	0.125 mg to 0.5 mg	Strong abuse potential	Suppresses SWS, reduces frequency of arousals	Partial arousals (sleepwalking, night terror, REM sleep behavior disorder)
Clonidine	Alpha-2 agonist	0.025 mg to 0.2 mg; increase by 0.05 mg increments	Narrow therapeutic index; dry mouth, bradycardia, hypotension; hypertension following abrupt discontinuation	Decreases SOL	Sleep onset and maintenance disturbances; ADHD
Guanfacine	Alpha-2 agonist	0.5 mg to 2 mg	Narrow therapeutic index; dry mouth, bradycardia, hypotension; hypertension following abrupt discontinuation; less sedating that clonidine	Decreases SOL	Sleep onset and maintenance disturbances; ADHD
Diphenhydramine	H1 agonist	12.5 mg to 50 mg	In overdose may cause hallucinations, seizures, agitation	Reduces SOL; improves sleep continuity in children	Mild sedative effect; high level of parental acceptance
Trazadone	5-HT serotonin agonist and reuptake inhibitor; blocks histamine receptors	12.5 mg to 100 mg	orthostatic hypotension, dizziness, priapism (rare)	Increases SWS, reduces SOL	Insomnia with comorbid depression and anxiety disorders
Mirtazapine	5-HT2, 5-HT3 antagonist, muscarinic antagonist, H1 receptor antagonist	3.75 mg to 15 mg	Increased appetite, weight gain, dry mouth	Reduces SOL, increases sleep duration	At low doses in cases of insomnia with co-morbid depression

Melatonin	Melatonin receptor agonist	0.3 mg to 6 mg	Not well defined	Decreases SOL	Shown to be effective in insomnia with comorbid autism spectrum disorder, developmental disabilities, ADHD, blindness, neurological impairments
Zolpidem	Non-benzodiazepine, benzodiazepine receptor agonist	2.5 mg to 10 mg	Complex sleep-related behaviors, retrograde amnesia, headaches, dizziness, residual sedation; has abuse potential	Decreases SOL, little to no effect on sleep architecture	At a dose of 0.25 mg/kg (max 10 mg) failed to reduce latency to persistent sleep in children and adolescents with insomnia associated with ADHD
Eszopiclone	Non-benzodiazepine, benzodiazepine receptor agonist	1 mg to 3 mg	Complex sleep-related behaviors, retrograde amnesia, headaches, dizziness, residual sedation; has abuse potential	Decreases SOL and WASO, little to no effect on sleep architecture	At doses up to 3 mg was generally well tolerated by pediatric patients, but failed to reduce latency to persistent sleep in children ages 6 to 17 years with ADHD-associated insomnia

*Not approved for these uses by the US Food and Drug Administration.
Abbreviations: SWS, slow wave sleep; SOL, sleep onset latency; ADHD, attention deficit-hyperactivity disorder; WASO, wake after sleep onset

the striatum.[59-61] In sum, there is some support for the combined effect of sleep disturbance and depression on affective and cognitive control networks; however, further research is needed to better understand these mechanisms.

Objective Findings

While PSG studies in adults with MDD consistently show prolonged sleep latency, fragmented sleep, disinhibited REM sleep, and decreased slow-wave sleep (SWS),[62] PSG studies in adolescents with depression are less consistent. Some studies have found similar features to those seen in adult depression, but to a lesser degree, and some studies have not revealed any differences between depressed adolescents and healthy controls.[63,64]

Treatments

Treating depression when combined with sleep disturbances in children and adolescents is often more difficult than treating depression or sleep disturbance alone. Therapeutic approaches to sleep disruption associated with MDD include pharmacological, circadian rhythm-based, cognitive-behavioral, and relaxation training–based interventions.

In a study including 309 youth, the authors found that insomnia was associated with higher depression severity. Additionally, this study found that adolescents with insomnia who were treated with fluoxetine were less likely to respond than those without insomnia. In contrast and interestingly, this same study showed that children with insomnia treated with fluoxetine were more likely to respond than those without insomnia. This suggests that adolescents with insomnia may need additional interventions targeting sleep.[65] Another study found that depressed adolescents receiving medication for sleep problems, particularly trazodone, were less likely to respond to depression treatment than those without sleep medication. This finding suggests that sleep medications are not particularly helpful in improving depression outcomes in youth with comorbid insomnia, although this suggestion may apply to trazodone alone.[66]

The sleep abnormalities may impair adolescents' response to cognitive-behavioral therapy (CBT) targeting depression, likely through increased hypothalamic–pituitary–adrenocortical (HPA) activity, which is thought to predict poor depression treatment response.[67,68] Furthermore, in depressed youth, decreased sleep efficiency and delayed sleep onset has been found to predict depression recurrence following treatment.[69] A CBT protocol for insomnia (CBT-I) targeted specifically at youth was shown to improve sleep; however, this did not target depressed youth.[70] There are efforts to develop joint treatment approaches using sleep-specific treatment strategies in conjunction with depression-specific treatment strategies, including insomnia-focused CBT for youth.[71] Further research on how different types of sleep disturbance respond to different types of treatment for depression is needed.

Recently, there has been interest in the positive effects of bright light therapy (monotherapy and add-on treatment) for unipolar adolescent depression, with finding that bright light therapy also improves sleep.[72] Other treatments include a personalized chronobiologic therapeutic intervention for those with both sleep and circadian rhythm disturbances, which involves intensive 2-week evaluation of depression and both subjective and objective measurements of sleep, followed by tailored behavioral and potentially pharmacologic strategies to improve sleep.[73]

Sleep Disturbances in Anxiety Disorders

Prevalence and Clinical Characteristics

Anxiety disorders comprise the largest class of psychiatric disorders among children and adolescents. Reported prevalence rates vary widely. However, the prevalence rate is probably between 15% to 25% among children and adolescents.[74] Anxiety disorders listed in the *Diagnostic and Statistical Manual* (fifth edition; DSM-5) include generalized anxiety disorder (GAD), social anxiety disorder, specific phobia, panic disorder, agoraphobia, separation anxiety disorder, selective mutism, and unspecified anxiety disorder. Obsessive-compulsive disorder (OCD), previously categorized as an anxiety disorder, is now included in a distinct category of OCD and related disorders in the DSM-5. Anxiety disorders typically present with excessive worry, fear or panic, avoidance, and marked distress; they are associated with significant academic, social, and family impairments.[75] Untreated anxiety disorders may contribute to later other mental comorbidities, physical comorbidities, substance misuse, suicidality, and reduced quality of life.[76-78]

The most frequent disorders among children and adolescents are separation anxiety disorder with prevalence estimates of 2.8% and 8%, respectively[79-81] and specific and social phobias with rates of approximately 10% and 7%, respectively.[82] Agoraphobia and panic disorder in childhood have low prevalence compared to adolescence (i.e., 1% or lower in children vs. 2%–3% for panic disorder and 3%–4% for agoraphobia in adolescents).[83] GAD appears to present later with on average, affecting approximately 1% of children and 3% of adolescents.[84]

Studies suggest that 80% to 90% of anxious youth have at least one sleep problem.[85] The most common problems reported are sleep initiation difficulty, nighttime awakenings, nightmares, and bedtime resistance.[86] More specifically, 94% of children with GAD may have sleep problems including nightmares and daytime sleepiness.[87] Up to 97% of children with separation anxiety disorder identify having one or more sleep problem; these include insomnia, reluctance or refusal to sleep alone, and nightmares.[88] Parents of children with separation anxiety disorder report higher rates of parasomnias (including sleepwalking, bedwetting and night terrors) than parents of children with other anxiety disorders. Finally, in a study of 66 pediatric patients with OCD, 92% experienced at least one type of sleep problem, with 27% of the sample reporting five or more sleep related problems. The most common parent-reported problems were "overtired" and "has trouble sleeping" although the exact nature of the sleep trouble was not specified. Furthermore, the greater severity of OCD symptoms was associated with lesser sleep.[89] A recent study of 435 children and adolescents shows that sleep may mediate link between childhood anxiety and irritability.[90]

Neurobiology

Research points to various shared neurobiological mechanisms for sleep, anxiety and depressive disorders. Genetic variations in 5-HT and dopamine pathways appear to contribute to anxiety, depression, and sleep dysregulation; interactions between these pathways can be traced to circadian function. Other mechanisms include alterations in corticolimbic and mesolimbic brain circuits, cortisol reactivity to stress, and inflammatory cytokine dysregulation.[91] The number of shared pathways in multiple biological systems that have been implicated in anxiety, mood, and sleep disorders underscores both the complicated nature of these disorders as well as the need for further research on a systemic basis.[92]

Objective Findings

Different studies using PSG support the presence of disrupted sleep among anxious youth. A small study (*n* = 9) of adolescents with OCD compared with healthy controls found that adolescents with OCD took twice as long as control adolescents to initiate sleep.[93] Children with GAD without comorbid mood disorders showed significantly increased sleep onset latency and reduced latency to REM sleep compared to controls. Marginal differences in the form of reduced sleep efficiency and increased total REM sleep were also found in the GAD group.[94]

Treatments

While there is convincing data regarding treatment of anxiety disorders in children and adolescents, there is limited research regarding the effect of treatments for anxiety on co-occurring sleep problems. Treatment of anxiety disorders with concomitant sleep disorders can be complicated. However, there is research suggesting that treating youth for anxiety disorders can have a beneficial effect on sleep related problems. For example, a large study (*n* = 128) examined sleep problems among youth with GAD, separation anxiety disorder, and social anxiety disorder. The frequency of eight subjective sleep-related problems was examined in relation to age, gender, type of anxiety disorder, anxiety severity, and functional impairment. When treated with fluvoxamine, significantly greater reductions in sleep related problems were found among children treated with fluvoxamine compared to placebo.[95] One study reported general decreases in "sleep disturbance" among children with GAD after CBT for anxiety, although reductions in specific sleep related problems were not examined.[96]

Sleep Disturbances in Posttraumatic Stress Disorder and Trauma
Prevalence and Clinical Characteristics

A 2009 national survey of 4,503 youth aged 1 month through 17 years found that 58% of the children and adolescents had experienced or witnessed at least one of five aggregate traumatic events (assaults and bullying, sexual victimization, maltreatment by a caregiver, property victimization, or witnessing victimization) in the prior year. Furthermore, 48% had more than 1 of 50 possible specific traumatic exposures (direct or indirect/witnessed), 15% had 6 or more, and 5% had 10 or more specific traumatic exposures.[97] Of the youth who experience or witness trauma, approximately 0.5% to 5% tend to develop posttraumatic stress disorder (PTSD).[98,99] PTSD symptoms relate to an exposure to, or threat of, death, serious injury, or sexual violence, either toward self or others, or learning of a close friend or relative who experienced an actual or threatened accidental or violent death. This traumatic event is re-experienced through symptoms such as intrusive memories or nightmares or marked physiological reactivity following reminders of the trauma; elicits persistent attempts to avoid reminders of the trauma; leads to negative alterations in cognition and mood; and causes significant distress or impairment. For children under 6, symptoms may be expressed through play and may manifest in a variety of behaviors such as aggression, tantrums, withdrawal, or sleep problems.

For children with PTSD, the common sleep disruptions are difficulty falling asleep, difficulty maintaining sleep, and parasomnias such as nightmares and bedwetting.[100] In one study including 147 females, childhood sexual abuse remained associated with significant sleep disturbances 10 years after disclosure.[101] Children who have been abused show prolonged sleep latency, decreased sleep efficiency, and higher levels of nocturnal activity compared to both depressed and nonabused children.[102] A study of 9,582 adolescents found that those exposed to childhood adversity had almost two times the risk of insomnia compared to their nonexposed peers. The effects of adversity appeared to differ by type. Exposure to interpersonal violence conferred the largest risk for insomnia symptoms. There was a dose–response relationship between the number of specific types of adversities reported by the child and risk for insomnia, such that each additional exposure to a different type of adversity was associated with an elevated risk for insomnia as compared to those unexposed to adversity.[103]

Neurobiology

In adults, the neurobiology of PTSD has been extensively researched; it appears that PTSD is associated with volumetric reductions in the hippocampus and anterior cingulate cortex as well as with functional dysregulation in the amygdala and medical prefrontal cortex.[104] There are few investigations relating to sleep disturbances in PTSD, with only a few showing that during REM sleep, PTSD is associated with a hypermetabolism in the brain stem, limbic regions, and basal ganglia.[105,106] It is not well understood whether or how these mechanisms differ in children.

Objective Findings

There are currently no published studies in which PSG has been performed on children with PTSD. Actigraphic measurements suggest that children who have experienced physical abuse appear to have greater fragmentation of sleep and poorer overall sleep quality[107] and that children with PTSD have higher sleep onset latencies and increased nocturnal activity compared to depressed and control groups.[108]

Treatments

There are currently no FDA-approved medications for either PTSD or insomnia in children. A 2010 review concluded that current research does not support the use of selective serotonin reuptake inhibitors as first-line treatments for PTSD in children and adolescents and that there is limited evidence that the brief use of antiadrenergic agents, second-generation antipsychotics, and various mood stabilizers may attenuate some PTSD symptoms in youth.[109] Alpha-2 adrenoreceptor agonists such as clonidine and guanfacine and an alpha-1 adrenoreceptor antagonist prazosin have been used to decrease hyperarousal and decrease nightmares in youth with PTSD, with some promising case reports and early research.[110-114] Side effects of these medications include dizziness, nausea, hypotension, and rebound hypertension if stopped abruptly. CBTs, such as trauma-focused CBT, are first-line treatments for children and adolescents who have experienced trauma. However, the impact of these therapies on trauma-specific sleep disturbances is not well established.[115]

Sleep Disturbance in Bipolar Disorder
Prevalence and Clinical Characteristics

While there has been controversy over the past two decades regarding the core characteristics, diagnosis, and prevalence of pediatric bipolar disorder, several studies and a recent meta-analysis have supported that bipolar spectrum disorder does occur in youth, at a rate of approximately 2.1% of the population aged 7 to 21 years.[116] The spectrum of bipolar disorders includes bipolar I disorder, bipolar II disorder, cyclothymic disorder, unspecified bipolar and related disorders, and other specified bipolar and related disorders. Bipolar disorder is characterized by periods of mania, hypomania, depression, or mixed mood states that interfere with daily functioning.

By both parent and child report, in a study including 133 children aged 8 to 11 years with early-onset bipolar disorder, 96.2% experienced sleep disturbances, which were linked to manic, depressive, or other comorbid psychiatric symptoms, most frequently separation anxiety.[117] The common sleep problems included insomnia, daytime sleepiness, parasomnias, night awakenings, bedtime resistance, anxiety, and sleep-disordered breathing. Diurnal variations of mood have been described in youth with bipolar disorder with evening acceleration of mood and energy and delayed sleep onset with difficulty waking up in the morning. A study indicated that nearly 30% children with bipolar disorder can exhibit elevated mood during the day with switching into depression overnight.[118]

Neurobiology
Current pathophysiologic models of bipolar disorder suggest the role of abnormalities in the emotional control brain network, which regulates emotion and attention. The emotional control brain network is comprised of ventrolateral and ventromedial prefrontal networks, which modulate the limbic system, specifically the amygdala, in conjunction with subcortical nuclei, such as the thalamus and striatum.[119] Theories regarding the interplay of neurobiological abnormalities in bipolar disorder and sleep disturbances are not well supported, but include the presence of variants in the genes or gene products responsible for the expression of the primary circadian clock.[120]

The relationship between sleep and bipolar disorder is complex. While sleep problems may be conceptualized as symptom of bipolar disorder, these may also contribute to relapse of a mood episode in pediatric bipolar disorder (e.g., sleep deprivation leading to onset of hypomania or mania).[121] Children with bipolar disorder have significantly higher rates of sleep difficulties from an early age.[122] Addressing the sleep problems related to bipolar disorder are critical since resultant sleep insufficiency during mood episodes can contribute to a number of adverse outcomes associated with bipolar disorder, such as obesity, substance use, risk-taking, and suicidality.[123]

Objective Findings
Using PSG,[124] there is some indication that objective sleep abnormalities may distinguish bipolar from unipolar trajectories in adolescence, with specifically increased stage one sleep and decreased stage four sleep with preserved REM sleep profile in bipolar illness and REM sleep abnormalities (reduced REM latency, higher REM density, and increased overall REM sleep) in unipolar depression.[125]

Treatments
There are no FDA-approved medications for treatment of sleep disturbance in pediatric bipolar disorder. A study of 4- to 6-year-old children with bipolar disorder found that an 8-week trial of monotherapy with olanzapine or risperidone equally improved sleep, in addition to manic symptoms.[126] Another study including adolescents (13–17 years) found that olanzapine compared to placebo resulted in greater reduction in decreased need for sleep as well as manic symptoms.[127]

Sleep Disturbances in Schizophrenia Spectrum Disorders
Prevalence and Clinical Characteristics
Schizophrenia in subjects younger than 13 years is rare, with prevalence estimated at 1 in 10,000.[128] Early-onset schizophrenia in youth between 13 and 17 years old is estimated to have a prevalence of about 1 to 2 in 1,000.[129] Schizophrenia is characterized primarily by psychotic symptoms such as hallucinations, delusions, disorganized behavior, and negative symptoms such as flat affect, alogia, and lack of motivation. It is likely that schizophrenia is not a single disease entity but rather a group of disorders resulting in similar clinical symptomatology. Sleep is of particular importance in schizophrenia, since abnormal brain connectivity and plasticity are thought to be core pathological features of the disorder; both are reflected in EEG.[130] Insomnia is a common complaint of patients with schizophrenia.[131] There is evidence that sleep disturbances are present prior to onset of psychosis, in prodromal phases in youth with schizophrenia, with sleep disturbance severity correlated to symptom severity.[132-134]

Neurobiology
Many biological abnormalities have been identified in schizophrenia, many of which may be involved in sleep dysfunction as well.[135] These include abnormalities in neurotransmitter pathways, gray and white matter structures, and cortical circuits that are involved in both sleep and brain plasticity.[136-139] In particular, the dysfunction of thalamic circuitry is thought to play a central role in pathogenesis of electrographic sleep disturbance of reduced spindle activity in schizophrenia.[140] Neurotransmitter systems implicated in the pathogenesis of schizophrenia include dopamine, gamma-aminobutyric acid (GABA), acetylcholine, glutamate, and neuromodulators

such as melatonin and orexin. As sleep–wake regulation occurs through complex interactions of neurotransmitters throughout the brain, abnormalities in these systems in schizophrenia are likely to be tied to sleep dysfunction in a patient with schizophrenia.[141]

Objective Findings

While there are no PSG studies in youth with schizophrenia, studies in adults have shown that patients with schizophrenia exhibit increased sleep latency, reduced sleep efficiency and total sleep time, whole-night deficits in slow and fast spindles, reduced REM latency and density, and disturbed non-REM sleep architecture.[142,143]

Treatments

Antipsychotics are the first-line medications used to treat schizophrenia. These medications comprise of typical (first-generation) and atypical (second-generation) antipsychotics. As discussed earlier in this chapter, there are no FDA-approved medications for treatment of insomnia in children. However, many antipsychotics are highly sedating and may be used jointly to treat schizophrenia as well as comorbid insomnia. Side effects of second-generation antipsychotics include weight gain and associated metabolic adverse effects, hypotension, sedation, anticholinergic symptoms, hyperprolactinemia, extrapyramidal symptoms, cardiac effects like QTc prolongation, myocarditis and cardiomyopathy, cataracts, and sexual dysfunction.

While there is no current evidence regarding the treatment of sleep disturbance on treatment outcomes in schizophrenia and related disorders in children and adolescents, there are some promising studies in adults. A recent study of adults with sleep apnea and schizophrenia found that treating sleep apnea improved cognition; however, this has not been replicated in youth.[144] Also in adults, a recent meta-analysis of Z-drugs alpidem and eszopiclone for schizophrenia did not show significant improvement in symptoms of schizophrenia, but those treated with eszopiclone showed improvement compared to placebo in Insomnia Severity Index scores.[145]

PRIMARY SLEEP DISORDERS IN CHILDREN AND ADOLESCENTS

This section will review the prevalence, clinical characteristics, diagnosis, and treatment of primary sleep disorders in children and adolescents.

Primary sleep disorders covered in this section include insomnia disorder, parasomnias, narcolepsy, and other hypersomnolence disorders, RLS and PLMD, OSA, and circadian rhythm sleep–wake disorders.

Insomnia Disorder
Prevalence and Clinical Characteristics

Insomnia, the most common sleep disorder presenting to pediatric healthcare providers, can be conceptualized as a set of symptoms with varying etiologies. There are two main categories of pediatric insomnia: behavioral insomnia of childhood (BIC) and psychophysiological insomnia. BIC is the most common behavioral sleep disorder of young children. It is mostly seen in children before age 5 years. Overall, 20% to 30% of children are reported to have significant bedtime problems or nocturnal awakenings.[146–148] Approximately 25% to 50% of children from 6 months through toddler-age continue to awaken during the night, while 10% to 15% of toddlers demonstrate bedtime resistance. Difficulties falling asleep and nocturnal awakenings are reported in 15% to 30% of preschoolers.[149,150] BIC is further categorized into sleep-onset association type (SOA), limit setting type (LST), and combined type.

BIC-SOA involves trouble initiating sleep at bedtime and frequent extended nighttime awakenings, requiring the caregiver to help the child initiate sleep or return to sleep. Diagnostic criteria include (a) prolonged sleep onset time that requires particular conditions, (b) demanding sleep-onset conditions, (c) significant delay of sleep onset in absence of those conditions, and (d) caregiver intervention is required to return the child to sleep after night awakenings.[151] Generally, this diagnosis is not made before the age of 6 months. Various intrinsic and extrinsic factors contribute to this disorder. These include parental behaviors around sleep initiation for the child; parental mental health issues such as anxiety or depression, medical conditions such as reflux or illness, temperament, and other factors such as schedule transitions or the child reaching new developmental milestones. In addition, child's own underlying anxiety or fears may be implicated (e.g., fear of sleeping alone, being in the dark, or having nightmares) that may result in demand of having parent in the bedroom. Importantly, cultural factors must also be taken into consideration as such factors play a prominent role in the development as well as the interpretation of sleep-onset association type insomnia.

BIC-LST involves behaviors at bedtime such as refusal to go to bed, verbal opposition, and multiple demands before going to bed. Diagnostic criteria include (a) trouble initiating or maintaining sleep, (b) stalling or refusing to go to sleep at bedtime or after nocturnal awakenings, and (c) lack of or insufficient limits set by caregiver regarding bedtime and sleep behaviors.[152] BIC-LST presents most commonly in children who are preschool-age and older. It often develops as a result of a caregiver not consistently reinforcing bedtime rules and schedules. Various intrinsic and extrinsic factors may also contribute and these include developmental issues such as developing imaginations, separation anxiety, and opposition. Medical issues such as asthma or anxiety and familial factors such as parenting style and temperament may contribute as well.

BIC-combined type presents as both bedtime resistance as well as frequent night awakenings, usually related to lack of clear rules and limits at bedtime, often resulting in the need for sleep associations for child to be able to return to sleep.

Psychophysiological insomnia is typically experienced by older children and adolescents. The rate of psychophysiological insomnia in 13- to 16-year-old youth is estimated at around 11%. Up to 35% of adolescents report insomnia at least several times a month.[153] Psychophysiological insomnia is characterized by difficulty with sleep onset and /or sleep maintenance. It results from a combination of learned negative sleep associations and heightened physiologic arousal, leading to a complaint of sleeplessness. Psychophysiological insomnia is associated with excessive worry about sleep and potential daytime consequences of decreased sleep. It may be caused by a combination of genetic predisposition, mental health difficulties, stress, or other external factors and perpetuating factors such as sleep habits, substance use including caffeine, and maladaptive thought patterns about sleep.

Diagnosis

The diagnosis of insomnia is based on a detailed clinical history from both the child and the parent or caregiver that includes assessment of current sleep patterns, usual sleep duration, and sleep–wake schedule. Enquiry should be done regarding the sleeping environment, bedtime routines, and parental behaviors around bedtime.

Medical evaluation should be conducted to rule out underlying medical reasons causing insomnia. Screening questionnaires for insomnia such as the CSHQ, Adolescent Sleep Hygiene Scale, and Children's Report of Sleep Patterns may be helpful as well. Clinicians may ask youth or parents to maintain a sleep diary for two consecutive weeks, which includes bedtime, estimated sleep onset time, timings of awakenings during the night, wake up time, and naps. Finally, actigraphy can provide an objective assessment of sleep–wake parameters, although results are most useful in conjunction with accompanying sleep diaries.

Treatment

Behavioral approaches are the mainstay of insomnia treatment. Numerous studies and reviews have found that behavioral therapies are effective and produce sustained improvements in insomnia.[154–156] In addition, behavioral interventions do not appear to lead to any short- or long-term negative effects on children or their caregivers.[157,158] See Table 16.2 for details on the behavioral approaches for insomnia management in younger children. The psychophysiologic insomnia of older children and adolescents is best addressed with CBT-I, which is covered in detail elsewhere in this book.

In the United States, there are no FDA-approved drugs to treat insomnia in children. Use of melatonin in both children with typical development and with autism spectrum disorder has been shown to have minimal side effects and to result in improvement in sleep onset.[159–161] Typical dosing of melatonin is 1 to 5 mg given 30 to 45 minutes before lights out.

Parasomnias
Prevalence and Clinical Features

Parasomnias occur more frequently in childhood than in adolescence or adulthood. The prevalence of parasomnias peaks at 34% between ages 1 and 5 years, with a prevalence of 10% by age 7.[162] However, up to 84% of children between ages 2.5 and 6 years may experience a parasomnia at least once.[163] More specifically, childhood prevalence estimates for parasomnias include sleep terrors (1%–6%), sleepwalking (up to 17% with a peak at 8–12 years), and confusional arousals (up to 17%).[164] Parasomnias have been more commonly reported in children with epilepsy, attention deficit-hyperactivity disorder (ADHD), or developmental coordination disorders than in community controls.[165–167]

Parasomnias are defined as undesirable physical events or experiences that occur during entry into sleep, during sleep, or during arousal from sleep. According to the International Classification of Sleep Disorders (third edition), parasomnias fall into three categories: (a) non-REM (NREM) sleep-related parasomnias, (b) REM parasomnias, and (c) other parasomnias.[168] In the DSM-5, parasomnias are categorized as NREM sleep arousal disorders (sleepwalking and sleep terror types), nightmare disorder (formerly known as dream anxiety disorder), and REM sleep behavior disorder (RBD).[169]

NREM-related parasomnias consist of sleepwalking, confusional arousals, and sleep terrors. These parasomnia behaviors occur most often during SWS, or stage N3 of NREM sleep, and therefore tend to occur within a few hours after sleep onset, when SWS is most prominent. NREM parasomnia episodes are characterized by abnormal transition between SWS and wakefulness, which leads to a prolonged state between deep sleep and wakefulness in children. Episodes usually last from a few minutes to 30 minutes, although they may last a few hours. The child may appear agitated or disoriented, resist comforting, and appear confused and disoriented if awakened. Amnesia regarding the episode is common. Although these events might be triggered by stress, in most cases, they do not reflect a primary underlying psychological problem. Triggers for parasomnias include sleep deprivation, alcohol consumption, withdrawal of drugs that suppress SWS such as benzodiazepines, and environmental stimuli that induce arousals during SWS.

Diagnosis

Diagnosis of parasomnias is made by detailed clinical history, including video recordings of the episodes if available. Overnight PSG is usually not necessary for diagnosis. PSG with video-monitoring is indicated for children with parasomnias who have a high likelihood of having OSA. Another reason to consider a sleep study is when limb movements in the night are suspected and the criteria for RLS is not met. In this situation, a sleep study is needed to confirm the diagnosis of PLMD.[170] An underlying seizure disorder should be considered, as well as other potential disorders including medical disorders such as syncope, breath holding, migraines, or transient ischemic attacks. Evaluation by PSG as well as further medical workup is indicated in cases where the underlying etiology is unclear.

Treatment

The management of parasomnias should include reassurance and education of the family, as in most instances the parasomnia behaviors tend to resolve. The family should be counseled regarding safety measures, if indicated, such as placing a mattress on the bedroom floor, using a gate on the bedroom door, locking outside doors and windows, and installing alarm systems. In addition, attempts should be made to identify triggers and exacerbating factors for the parasomnia behaviors. Scheduled awakening is one behavioral technique, which has been shown to have immediate and long-term benefits for sleepwalking or sleep terrors.[171] Scheduled awakenings are most likely to be effective if episodes occur nightly. Parents should be coached to wake the child 15 to 30 minutes before the time that episodes typically occur. After a scheduled awakening, the child needs to open his or her eyes and at least mumble a response before being allowed to return to sleep. This should continue for 2 to 4 weeks. In particularly severe cases, medications that suppress SWS, such as benzodiazepines, may be used; tricyclic antidepressants may also be effective.[172] In our clinical experience, doses of clonazepam in the 0.125 mg to 0.5 mg range are effective in treating the parasomnias. One can also consider doxepin in the 5 to 10 mg dose range for school-aged or older children. A medication should be trialed for 3 to 4 weeks with an attempt to withdraw the medication if symptoms have resolved.

Narcolepsy and Other Hypersomnolence Disorders
Prevalence and Clinical Characteristics

Narcolepsy is a lifelong disorder that most commonly begins in the first or second decade or in the early 20s. Approximately one-third of patients become symptomatic prior to 15 years of age, and up to 5% of cases begin before the age of 5.[173] With increased awareness of narcolepsy in children, there seems to be a trend toward increasing recognition of this disorder in the first decade of life. There are few population-based estimates of the incidence and prevalence of narcolepsy in children. One European study estimated a pooled incidence rate of 0.83 per 100,000 person-years in children aged 5 to 19 years.[174] The overall prevalence of narcolepsy in Western countries has been estimated at 20 to 50 cases per 100,000.[175] The disruption of orexin neurotransmission has been implicated in pathogenesis of narcolepsy.

While the exact cause remains uncertain in most cases of narcolepsy, hypothalamic glioma, craniopharyngioma, sarcoidosis, head injury, and genetic syndromes like Prader–Willi syndrome or Niemann–Pick disease type C have been implicated as secondary causes of orexin disturbance leading to narcolepsy in children. Finally, H1N1 influenza vaccine and streptococcal infections have also been suggested as putative underlying etiologic factors.

The classic tetrad of excessive daytime sleepiness, cataplexy (emotion triggered muscle weakness), hypnagogic/hypnopompic hallucinations (vivid dreams at sleep onset/offset), and sleep paralysis (momentary inability to move, breathe or scream during sleep–wake transitions) is often not recognizable in the early stages of the disorder and may gradually appear over time; this may contribute to delays in diagnosis.[176] Cataplexy has been reported in up to 80% of children with early-onset narcolepsy[177] and typically involves oculo-bucco-facial muscles.[178] Neurobehavioral symptoms are frequently reported in children and adolescents with narcolepsy. Depression and anxiety disorders are among the most common neuropsychiatric comorbidities of narcolepsy.[179,180] Aggressive behavior, attentional difficulties, social and emotional distress, and decreased school performance are often noted in pediatric patients with narcolepsy.[181]

Diagnosis

Validated scales for subjective assessment of daytime sleepiness in children, including Pediatric Daytime Sleepiness Scale (PDSS) and a modified version of the ESS, can be used to assess the severity of daytime somnolence and to monitor clinical response to treatment.[182,183] The diagnosis of narcolepsy requires sleep laboratory evaluation to include overnight PSG followed by daytime MSLT to demonstrate pathological sleepiness (mean sleep onset latency of <8 minutes) and at least two sleep-onset REM (SOREM) periods during 4 to 5 nap opportunities.

Idiopathic hypersomnia (IH) is characterized by excessive daytime sleepiness with nonrefreshing sleep. Patients with IH may share other symptoms that are common in narcolepsy like sleep attacks, sleep paralysis, or hypnogogic hallucinations. Absence of cataplexy and fewer than two SOREM periods on the MSLT differentiates IH from narcolepsy.

Kleine–Levin syndrome is characterized by reoccurring episodes of severe hypersomnolence associated with psychiatric and behavioral disturbances that last from 2.5 days to up to 80 days. Between the episodes, the patient resumes normal level of alertness and behavioral and emotional function. Usual onset is during late adolescence with a median course of illness of 14 years.

Treatment

Management for excessive daytime sleepiness associated with narcolepsy and IH is similar and include both behavioral interventions and pharmacological treatment. Disabling symptoms of cataplexy and excessive daytime sleepiness almost always require pharmacotherapy. Parents and their children should receive education on lifestyle modifications and good sleep habits. Maintaining good sleep hygiene with a regular sleep–wake schedule and adequate amount of nocturnal sleep are essential parts of management of excessive daytime sleepiness. Scheduled naps, lasting 25 to 30 minutes, during school hours and after school may reduce daytime drowsiness and increase alertness. Staying physically active and doing regular daily exercises are also recommended to enhance alertness.

School accommodations may need to be implemented to promote optimal learning and help manage daytime sleepiness in the school setting. Clinicians should be encouraged to advocate for daily scheduled naps, preferential seating in front of the classroom, more frequent breaks, extended time for long tests or exams. Adolescent patients should be instructed to avoid alcohol and recreational substances and cautioned against driving or operating machinery during periods of daytime sleepiness. Patients with cataplexy may need to be cautioned about risks associated with swimming or climbing if these activities trigger cataplexy attacks. Additional education and support groups are available through nonprofit organizations such as the Narcolepsy Network and Wake-Up Narcolepsy for patients, families, and professionals.

Pharmacological treatment is required in nearly all cases of narcolepsy and IH with the goal of reducing sleepiness and improving daytime alertness. Currently, there is only one medicine approved for the treatment of excessive daytime sleepiness in the pediatric population. This medicine, sodium oxybate, has FDA approval to treat the daytime sleepiness and cataplexy associated with narcolepsy in children 7 to 17 years old. Pharmacological treatment should be individualized given patient's symptom severity, age, medical and psychiatric co-morbidities, possible side effects, and risks of drug abuse, misuse, and diversion. Treatment of daytime sleepiness also includes wake-promoting medications like modafinil and armodafinil.[184,185] Psychostimulants such as methylphenidate or dextroamphetamine can be used alone or in combination with modafinil or armodafinil in treating excessive sleepiness in children.[186-188] A recent retrospective study showed the long-term use of modafinil and armodafinil to be effective and well tolerated in treatment of pediatric patients with narcolepsy, even when co-administered with other psychiatric medications.[189] Modafinil dose for children and adolescents ranges from 50 to 400 mg/day while armodafinil can be used between 25 to 250 mg/day.

Sodium oxybate is indicated for narcolepsy with cataplexy in adults and was recently approved by the FDA for pediatric use. Studies demonstrate sodium oxybate to effectively treat excessive daytime sleepiness and cataplexy in children and adolescents.[190-193] A retrospective study showed that up to 82% of children treated with sodium oxybate reported improvement in daytime sleepiness and cataplexy, and majority of the patients experienced improvement in sleep continuity and sleep quality.[194] Results from a recent double-blind, placebo-controlled multicenter study in pediatric subjects with narcolepsy supported the efficacy and safety of sodium oxybate for the treatment of cataplexy and excessive daytime sleepiness consistent with previously published findings.[195] Pharmacological treatment of cataplexy in pediatric patients may also be accomplished by use of tricyclic antidepressants (clomipramine, imipramine, protriptyline); mixed action antidepressants, like venlafaxine; or selective serotonin reuptake inhibitors like fluoxetine, sertraline, and citalopram. Patients should be carefully monitored for side effects including increased suicidal ideation.[196,197]

Restless Legs Syndrome and Periodic Limb Movement Disorder
Prevalence and Clinical Characteristics
RLS is a common sensorimotor disorder characterized by urge to move the legs, usually accompanied by uncomfortable sensations in the legs happening in sitting/lying position exclusively/predominantly in evening or night with transient relief in the symptoms with movement. RLS has an estimated prevalence of 2% to 4% in the pediatric population, depending on the studied sample.[198,199] Incidence rates of RLS in children are similar to adults ranging from 0.8% to 1.7%.[200]

The PLMD is characterized by sleep disturbance resulting from repetitive limb jerking during sleep that is not better explained by another condition or medication or substance use. The prevalence of PLMD in children is less well understood. RLS can be diagnosed based on subjective reports alone, not requiring a PSG. However, a PSG is required to make the diagnosis of PLMD with a periodic limb movement index of >5/hour considered as significant in children.

Pediatric patients frequently report symptoms of RLS differently from adults, which makes the diagnosis of RLS in children more challenging. There have been new diagnostic criteria of RLS established for children and adolescents.[201] Children commonly use different words to describe sensations associated with RLS like "want to move," "got to kick," "bugs," "ants," "tingling," "wiggly," "itchy," "pain," and "hurts."[202-204] It is important to consider use of different descriptors of sensory experience associated with RLS when interviewing children, especially of a younger age.

There is a high degree of association between RLS and neuropsychiatric conditions. ADHD, depression, and anxiety occur more frequently in children with RLS. In some clinical samples, almost 25% of children with RLS fulfilled diagnostic criteria for ADHD while 12 to 35% of individuals with ADHD had symptoms of RLS or PLMD.[205-207] Almost two-thirds of patients evaluated at a pediatric sleep center were found to have psychiatric disorders.[208] The most common psychiatric disorders noted among children with RLS were ADHD, mood disorders, anxiety disorders, and disruptive behavioral disorders.

Treatment
Nonpharmacological interventions for RLS and PLMD include establishing healthy sleep habits such as maintaining consistent sleep–wake schedule, avoiding sleep loss, reducing caffeine intake, eliminating tobacco and alcohol, and avoiding stimulating activities close to bedtime. Physical exercise is beneficial and should be encouraged by the parents. Leg massage may help on the nights when RLS symptoms are more severe and bothersome.

Effectiveness of iron supplementation is supported by both pediatric case reports and several clinical trials of oral iron in children with RLS or PLMD.[209] Pharmacological intervention with oral iron supplementation is usually recommended if the child's serum ferritin level is below 50 mcg/L, although it could be considered even when serum ferritin is in 50 to 75 mcg/L range. For youth 12 years and older, ferrous sulphate is suggested with 65 mg of elemental iron per tablet, one to two tablets once daily. For children younger than 12 years, ferrous sulfate is suggested with 3 mg/kg/day (no more than 130 mg per day) of elemental iron once daily. Vitamin C should be consumed while milk products should be avoided along with iron supplementation to improve absorption of iron. Intravenous iron supplementation is an alternative with serum ferritin less than 50 mcg/L when oral iron is either ineffective in improving ferritin level or oral iron absorption is hindered for some reason. The treatment goal is to achieve target serum ferritin levels between 50 and 100 mg mcg/L.[210] Serum ferritin level should be monitored every 3 to 4 months.

There are no FDA approved medications for pediatric RLS and PLMD. Gabapentin is approved by the FDA as an anticonvulsant for pediatric use and has been shown to be effective in reducing sensory symptoms of RLS in children and adolescents.[211] Dopamine agonists like pramipexole and ropinirole are approved treatments for adults with some published evidence of their effectiveness for pediatric RLS and PLMD.[212–214] A small double-blind, placebo-controlled study of carbidopa/L-DOPA CR demonstrated that it is a safe and effective treatment for RLS but not comorbid ADHD in children.[215] There are no published clinical trials of pramipexole or ropinirole in pediatric patients with RLS with the exception of few case reports. However, due to potential serious adverse effects like augmentation and impulse control problems, dopamine agonists should be reserved for more severe cases of RLS with careful monitoring for these side effects.

Other medications, with sedating properties, have shown to be effective in alleviating difficulty falling asleep associated with RLS. These include clonidine, melatonin, and low doses of benzodiazepines such as clonazepam. Since RLS commonly presents with other comorbidities like ADHD, depression, and anxiety, recognition of psychiatric disorders in children is important while making a treatment selection for RLS. Several classes of medications used to treat psychiatric disorders in pediatric patients like antidepressants, psychostimulants, and antipsychotics may aggravate symptoms of RLS leading to worsening of sleep-related complaints.

Obstructive Sleep Apnea
Prevalence and Clinical Characteristics
The pediatric mental health practitioner should maintain a level of suspicion for OSA since it is relatively common and can mimic or exacerbate neuropsychiatric symptoms and behaviors. OSA is relatively easy to screen and awareness of its risk factors (see Table 16.4) can prompt referral for additional assessment for this condition. OSA occurs in approximately 1% to 6% of youth with higher rates in African Americans and children belonging to families of lower socioeconomic status.[216,217] Adeno-tonsillar hypertrophy is a well-recognized risk factor for pediatric OSA. The second most common predisposing factor for pediatric OSA is obesity.[218] Conditions that impact the size or function of the upper airway are also known risk factors for OSA. Examples include cerebral palsy, muscular dystrophy, achondroplasia, Prader–Willi syndrome, and craniofacial anomalies such as micrognathia and midface hypoplasia.[219] It is estimated that upwards of 60% of patients with Down syndrome have OSA with this population being more likely to have severe OSA.[220] This high prevalence of OSA has led experts to advocate for screening sleep studies in all young children with Down syndrome.[221]

The most common symptoms of OSA include habitual snoring, witnessed apneas, and mouth breathing during sleep. Associated symptoms include excessive sweating in sleep, enuresis, nonrestorative sleep, and daytime fatigue. ADHD-type symptoms are common in younger children

---

TABLE 16.4. SYMPTOMS AND SIGNS OF PEDIATRIC OBSTRUCTIVE SLEEP APNEA

Nightly or near-nightly snoring

Sweating excessively while sleeping

Arousing from sleep with a gasp

Witnessed pauses in breathing especially when followed by a snort

ADHD-type symptoms and behaviors during the day

Sleep enuresis

Enlarged tonsils

Midface hypoplasia

Retrognathia and micrognathia

Chronic rhinorrhea suggesting enlarged adenoids

Obesity

Enlarged neck circumference

with OSA, since preadolescents tend to manifest the consequences of sleep disruption/deprivation as compensatory hyperactive behaviors rather than subjective or objective sleepiness. Numerous research studies demonstrate the comorbidity between OSA and ADHD with several of them showing resolution of ADHD when OSA is treated with adenotonsillectomy.[222,223]

A targeted physical exam can highlight risk factors for OSA including tonsillar hypertrophy, obesity, enlarged neck circumference, and a high-arched hard palate. This exam can be conducted briefly by a physician, nurse practitioner, or physician assistant specializing in mental health care with little investment in equipment beyond a light source, weight scale, height scale, and measuring tape. It is important to note that even "small" tonsils may cause upper airway obstruction during sleep. Visualization of the adenoids requires nasal endoscopy or lateral neck radiography.

Diagnosis

When pediatric OSA is suspected, the patient should be referred for further diagnostic sleep assessment. OSA cannot be definitively diagnosed without an overnight PSG study, but there are not enough pediatric sleep laboratory beds to serve the assessment needs. Therefore, many patients undergo adenotonsillectomy without a presurgery sleep study. Otolaryngology surgeons engage risk stratification to determine which pediatric patients can go straight to surgery versus those needing a prior sleep study to determine whether surgery is indicated. Screening instruments have been developed to aid in the risk stratification process although there remain concerns regarding their validity.[224–226] In general, pediatric patients with symptoms of OSA, in absence of tonsillar hypertrophy, should undergo a sleep study prior to consideration of surgery as should patients with medical complexity. The Apnea–Hypopnea Index (AHI) is used to determine severity of OSA. The AHI represents the number of apneas and hypopneas per hour of sleep. In general, mild pediatric OSA is defined by AHI of 2 to 5, moderate pediatric OSA by AHI of 6 to 15, and severe pediatric OSA by AHI of greater than 15. Patients with severe OSA diagnosed by sleep study should also undergo a postsurgical sleep study as should patients with risk factors for persistent OSA (i.e., obese patients and those with Down syndrome). If OSA symptoms persist in mild to moderate cases, a postsurgical PSG should be performed.

Treatment

Adenotonsillectomy is the first-line treatment for management of pediatric OSA. Continuous or bilevel positive airway pressure (CPAP or BIPAP, respectively) is another effective treatment for pediatric OSA, typically used in patients who have already undergone surgery but have persistent OSA or in those where the surgery is contraindicated. Pediatric patients requiring CPAP or BIPAP are typically managed in a sleep clinic. In a minority of cases, adenotonsillectomy and positive airway pressure are not effective or not tolerated. In such cases, particularly if the OSA is severe, additional surgical procedures including maxillomandibular advancement and uvulopalatopharyngoplasty can be considered. Tracheotomy may even be necessary when the OSA is life-threatening. When the OSA is mild, more conservative treatments can be considered such as weight loss or sleeping nonsupine.

Circadian Rhythm Sleep–Wake Disorders
Prevalence and Clinical Characteristics

Circadian rhythm sleep–wake disorders are characterized by a persistent or recurrent pattern of sleep disruption related to an alteration in the circadian system or a misalignment between the endogenous circadian rhythm and the sleep–wake schedule imposed by the society.[227] Although rare, structural or molecular alterations in the circadian system can occur due to congenital anomalies, trauma, or genetics. Circadian rhythm sleep–wake disorders are more typically due to misalignment with sleep occurring at the "wrong" time due to societal demands.

The most common type of circadian rhythm sleep–wake disorder afflicting youth is the delayed sleep phase type (also known as delayed sleep–wake phase disorder). Although children can be affected by this condition, adolescents are at particular risk for this circadian rhythm disturbance given their propensity to delay their sleep–wake preference.[228] It is estimated that approximately 8% of adolescents meet criteria for this condition.[229] Adolescents with a delayed sleep phase type of circadian rhythm sleep–wake disorder present with insomnia and excessive sleepiness during wakeful periods due to sleep insufficiency resulting from awakening prior to spontaneous wake-up time. The excessive sleepiness is most problematic in the morning hours. The sleep insufficiency often causes academic impairment, depressed mood and affective instability, attentional deficits, and family conflict.

Less common types of circadian rhythm sleep–wake disorders impacting youth include non-24-hour sleep–wake type and irregular sleep–wake type. The non-24-hour type occurs primarily in patients who are totally blind and therefore do not receive the light signal, which is necessary to set the biological clock. A relative absence of a circadian pattern to the sleep–wake cycle characterizes the irregular sleep–wake type.[230] These patients end up taking multiple long naps over the course of a 24-hour period rather than consolidating sleep in to a longer nighttime sleep episode. This mode of existence is problematic when attempting to attend school, hold a job, or have a social life. In healthy youth, the condition may be the result of very poor sleep hygiene including little to no daily structure. The irregular sleep–wake type is more commonly associated with neurological impairments such as intellectual disability.

Diagnosis
A circadian rhythm sleep–wake disorder diagnosis is made by taking a careful history and collecting sleep–wake data prospectively with use of sleep log and, ideally, actigraphy for 7 to 14 days.

Treatment
The treatment of delayed sleep–wake phase disorder include family and child education, improving sleep hygiene (minimizing or eliminating caffeine, nicotine, and alcohol, avoiding daytime naps, refraining from engaging in stimulating activity for at least 2 hours prior to the desired sleep onset time), and the gradual advancement of the sleep–wake schedule. Exposure to bright light (5,000–10,000 lux) upon awakening in the morning will induce phase advancement (make sleep-onset and wake times earlier) over several days. Use of blue light can induce more dramatic phase shifts often with lesser exposure time.[231] Melatonin administered in small doses (0.25 to 0.33 mg) 5 hours before lights out can assist with phase advancement as can melatonin in larger, pharmacologic doses (1–5 mg) given 30 to 60 minutes before lights out.[232] Youth with more severe delayed sleep–wake phase disorder can be treated by progressively delaying their sleep–wake schedule, typically in 3-hour increments, until the desired sleep–wake schedule is reached. This progressive delaying of the sleep–wake schedule is known as chronotherapy and requires the youth to miss daytime activities for several days.

CONCLUSIONS
While sleep disturbances are common in all children and adolescents, they are particularly prevalent in youth with neuropsychiatric conditions. These sleep disturbances can be caused by primary psychiatric disorders or be manifestation of primary sleep disorders. The sleep disturbances due to primary sleep disorders can often result in symptoms and behaviors that may suggest presence of an underlying psychiatric condition. These symptoms include inattention, poor impulse control, academic impairment, mood changes, fatigue, and excessive daytime sleepiness. It is important for the pediatric clinician to assess the youth, presenting with sleep and psychiatric symptomatology, for presence of comorbid primary sleep disorders. Consultation with a sleep physician for further evaluation and treatment is recommended if a primary sleep disorder is suspected.

FUTURE DIRECTIONS
There is a lot yet to be understood regarding the bidirectional relationship between sleep and psychiatric illness in youth. Sleep problems often manifest in infancy and toddlerhood, much before the onset of anxiety disorders and mood disorders. Are these measurable sleep problems markers for future development of psychiatric illnesses? If so, does intervening early to treat sleep problems like insomnia decrease the likelihood of developing an anxiety disorder or mood disorder later? Prospective, long-term research could answer these questions.

KEY CLINICAL PEARLS
- Sleep deprivation and disruption in young children can cause daytime neurocognitive symptoms and disruptive behaviors suggestive of ADHD.
- Children with ADHD and ADHD-type symptoms and behaviors have high likelihood of comorbid OSA and RLS.
- The most common cause of daytime sleepiness in teenagers is insufficient sleep.
- There are no FDA approved medicines to treat pediatric insomnia.
- The most common type of circadian rhythm sleep–wake disorder in youth is the delayed sleep phase type.
- Reassurance and education of the family is the primary treatment of parasomnias.

SELF-ASSESSMENT QUESTIONS

1. What is a first line intervention for insomnia in children and adolescents?
   a. Melatonin
   b. Diphenhydramine
   c. Clonidine
   d. Cognitive behavioral therapy for insomnia)

Answer: d

2. What is the first line treatment for obstructive sleep apnea in children?
   a. Adenotonsillectomy
   b. Bariatric surgery
   c. CPAP therapy
   d. Nasal steroids

Answer: a

3. Restless legs disorder is frequently seen in children with the following psychiatric disorder?
   a. Anxiety
   b. Depression
   c. ADHD
   d. Learning disability

Answer: c

4. Which symptom is not associated with narcolepsy?
   a. Cataplexy
   b. Sleep paralysis
   c. Catatonia
   d. Hypnagogic hallucinations

Answer: c

5. Sleepwalking is usually associated with the following sleep stage?
   a. Stage N1
   b. Stage N2
   c. Stage N3
   d. REM sleep

Answer: c

CLINICAL VIGNETTE: CASE OF AN ADOLESCENT WITH CIRCADIAN RHYTHM SLEEP–WAKE DISORDER, DELAYED SLEEP PHASE TYPE COMORBID WITH DEPRESSION

Clinical Presentation

Jim is a 15-year-old adolescent male who presents with a primary concern of difficulty falling asleep and "feeling exhausted all the time."

Parents report that they noticed a change in his sleeping pattern during his freshman year of high school. He has been going to bed at around 11 PM but will not be able to fall asleep until 3 AM. During summer break he was waking up between 12 PM and 2 PM. Since he returned back to school in the fall, he has not been able to get up on time and has been missing class. Jim reports poor sleep hygiene with use of electronics, eating in bed, and an inconsistent bedtime. He reports feeling tired and unmotivated, lacking interest in social and academic activities. His parents noticed that he has been more isolative and withdrawn and no longer interested in athletics or going out with friends. Jim described himself as being tired and sleepy during the morning hours, having trouble focusing on schoolwork, especially before lunch and usually having more energy during the evening. On the weekends, he still falls asleep at around 3 AM and wakes up by 2 PM. He admits feeling increasingly irritable, "overly sensitive," having difficulty concentrating, and having a negative outlook on life.

Management

For 2 weeks, Jim kept a sleep diary while wearing a wrist actigraph. This prospective data collection confirmed the diagnosis of circadian rhythm sleep–wake disorder, delayed sleep phase type. The psychiatric interview was consistent with the diagnosis of MDD. Jim was referred for individual psychotherapy to address his depressive symptoms and an antidepressant medication trial was initiated.

A number of treatment modalities were utilized to address his circadian rhythm sleep–wake disorder. Patient education regarding sleep was provided including ways to improve sleep habits and patterns (sleep hygiene). It was decided to gradually advance (make earlier) his sleep–wake schedule. This was accomplished by having him go to bed and wake up 30 minutes earlier every three days until the desired sleep–wake schedule of 10 PM to 7 AM was reached. Advancing his sleep–wake schedule was facilitated with well-timed, morning bright light exposure and evening melatonin administration. Bright light therapy (10,000 lux) was delivered via a light box for 30 minutes immediately upon awakening. A physiologic dose of melatonin (0.3 mg) was given 5 hours before lights out and advanced by 30 minutes every 3 days. Once his ideal lights out time was reached (10 PM), he was taking melatonin at 5 PM.

Recommendations for sleep hygiene included maintaining regular and consistent sleep and wake times 7 days a week, use of bed for sleep only, not allowing the use of electronic devices in bed (bedroom), avoiding caffeinated beverages within 6 hours of bedtime, avoiding rigorous exercise 2 hours before bedtime, and avoiding heavy meals at night.

REFERENCES
1. National Sleep Foundation. National Sleep Foundation guidelines. https://www.sleep-foundation.org/press-release/national-sleep-foundation-recommends-new-sleep-times. February 2, 2015.
2. Mindell JA, Owens JA. A clinical guide to pediatric sleep: diagnosis and management of sleep problems. Philadelphia: Lippincott Williams & Wilkins; 2003.
3. Anders TF, Halpern LF, Hua, J. Sleeping through the night: a developmental perspective. *Pediatrics.* 1992;90:554–560.
4. So, K., Adamson TM, Horne RS. The use of actigraphy for assessment of the development of sleep/wake patterns in infants during the first 12 months of life. *J Sleep Res.* 2007;16:181–187. http://dx.doi.org/10.1111/j.1365-2869.2007.00582.x.
5. Scher A. Crawling in and out of sleep. *Infant Child Dev.* 2005;14:491–500. http://dx.doi.org/10.1002/icd.427.
6. Meltzer, LJ, Crabtree VM. *Pediatric Sleep problems: A Clinician's Guide to Behavioral Interventions.* Washington, DC: American Psychological Association; 2015.
7. Touchette E, Petit D, Trembley RE, et al. Factors associated with fragmented sleep at night across early childhood. *Arch Pediatr Adolesc Med.* 2005;159:242–249.
8. Owens JA, Spirito A, McGuinn M. The Children's Sleep Habits Questionnaire (CSHQ): psychometric properties of a survey instrument for school-aged children. *Sleep.* 2000;23:1–9.
9. Crabtree VM, Dayyat E, Molfese D, et al. Objective quantification of sleep duration in healthy children [abstract supplement]. *Sleep.* 2007;30:A74.
10. Sadeh A, Raviv A, Gruber R. Sleep patterns and sleep disruptions in school-age children. *Dev Psychol.* 2000;36:291–301.
11. Wolfson AR, Carskadon MA, Acebo C, et al. Evidence for the validity of a sleep habits survey for adolescents. *Sleep.* 2003;26:213–216.
12. Carskadon MA, Acebo C. Regulation of sleepiness in adolescents: update, insights, and speculation. *Sleep.* 2002;25:606–614.
13. Wolfson AR, Carskadon MA. Sleep schedules and daytime functioning in adolescents. *Child Dev.* 1998;69:875–887.
14. Carskadon MA, Acebo C, Jenni OG. Regulation of adolescent sleep: implications for behavior. *Ann N Y Acad Sci.* 2004;1021:276–291.
15. Crowley SJ, Acebo C, Carskadon MA. Sleep, circadian rhythms, and delayed phase in adolescence. *Sleep Med.* 2007;8:602–612. doi:10.1016/j.sleep.2006.12.002.
16. Meltzer, LJ, Crabtree VM. Pediatric sleep problems: A clinician's guide to behavioral interventions. Washington, DC: American Psychological Association; 2015.
17. Liu X, Liu L, Owens JA, et al. Sleep patterns and sleep problems among schoolchildren in the United States and China. *Pediatrics.* 2005;115:241–249.
18. Ramtekkar U, Ivanenko A. Sleep in children with psychiatric disorders. *Semin Pediatr Neurol.* 2015;22:148–155.
19. Ivanenko A, Crabtree VM, Gozal D. Sleep in children with psychiatric disorders. *Pediatr Clin North Am.* 2004;51:51–68.
20. Liu X, Buysse DJ, Gentzler AL, et al. InsominaInsomnia and hypersomnia associated with depressive phenomenology and comorbidity in childhood depression. *Sleep.* 2007;30:83–90.
21. Liu X, Hubbard JA, Fabes RA, et al. Sleep disturbances and correlates of children with autism spectrum disorders. *Child Psychiatry Hum Dev.* 2006;37:179–191.
22. Steinsbekk, S.k Berg-Nielsen, TS., Wichstrom L. Sleep disorders in preschoolers: prevalence and comorbidity with psychiatric symptoms. *J Dev Behav Pediatr.* 2013;34(9):633–641.
23. Johnson EO, Chilcoat HD, Breslau N. Trouble sleeping and anxiety/depression in childhood. *Psychiatry Res.* 2000;94:93–102.
24. Price VA, Coates TJ, Thoresen CE, et al. Prevalence and correlates of poor sleep among adolescents. *Am J Dis Child.* 1978;132:583–586.
25. Kirmil-Gray K, Eagleston JR, Gibson E, et al. Sleep disturbance in adolescents: sleep quality, sleep habits, beliefs about sleep, and daytime functioning. *J Youth Adol.* 1984;13:375–384.
26. Morrison DN, MCGee R, Stanton WR. Sleep problems in adolescence. *J Am Acad Child Adolesc Psychiatry.* 1992;31:94–99.
27. Manni R, Ratti MT, Marchioni E, et al. Poor sleep in adolescents: a study of 869 17 year-old Italian secondary school students. *J Sleep Res.* 1997;6:44–49.
28. Saarenpaa-Heikkila O, Laippala P, Koivikko M. Subjective daytime sleepiness and its predictors in Finnish adolescents in an interview study. *Acta Paediatr.* 2001;90:552–557.
29. Roane BM, Taylor DJ. Adolescent insomnia as a risk factor for early adult depression and substance abuse. *Sleep.* 2008;31(10):1351–1356.

30. Trosman I, Trosman SJ. Cognitive and behavioral consequences of sleep disordered breathing in children. *Med Sci.* 2017;5:30. doi:10.3390/medsci5040030.

31. Owens JA, Dalzell V. Use of the "Bears" sleep screening tool in a pediatric residents' continuity clinic: a pilot study. *Sleep Med.* 2005; 6(1):63–69.

32. Chervin RD, Hedger K, Dillon JE, Pituch KJ. Pediatric Sleep Questionnaire (PSQ): validity and reliability of scales for sleep-disordered breathing, snoring, sleepiness, and behavioral problems. *Sleep Med.* 2000;1:21–32.

33. Owens JA, Spirito A, McGuinn M. The Children's Sleep Habits Questionnaire (CSHQ): psychometric properties of a survey instrument for school-aged children. *Sleep.* 2000;23(8):1043–1051.

34. Luginbuehl M, Bradley-Klug KL, Ferron J, Anderson WM, Bendadis SR. Pediatric sleep disorders: validation of the Sleep Disorders Inventory for Students. *School Psych Rev.* 2008;37(3):409–431.

35. Drake C, Nickel C, Burduvali E, Roth T, Jefferson C, Badia P. The Pediatric Daytime Sleepiness Scale (PDSS): sleep habits and school outcomes in middle-school children. *Sleep.* 2003;26(4):455–458.

36. Carskadon MA, Vieira C, Acebo C. Association between puberty and delayed phase preference. *Sleep.* 1993;16(3):258–262.

37. Tan H, Kheirandish-Gozal L, Gozal D. Pediatric home sleep apnea testing: slowly getting there! *Chest.* 2015;148(6):1382–1395.

38. Morgenthaler T, Alessi C, Friedman L, et al. Practice parameters for the use of actigraphy in the assessment of sleep and sleep disorders: an update for 2007. *Sleep.* 2007;30(4):519–529.

39. Sadeh A, Gruber R, Raviv A. Sleep, neurobehavioral functioning, and behavior problems in school-age children. *Child Dev.*2003;72(3):405–417. doi:10.1111/1467-8624.00414.

40. Cousins JC et al. The Bidirectional Association Between Daytime Affect and Nighttime Sleep in Youth With Anxiety and Depression. *J Pediatr Psychol.* 2011;36(9):969–979.

41. Dahl RE, Lewis DS. Pathways to adolescent health: sleep regulation and behavior. *J Adol Health.* 2001;31:175–184.

42. American Psychiatric Association. *Diagnostic and Statistical Manual of Mental Disorders.* 5th ed. Washington, DC: American Psychiatric Association; 2013.

43. Ibid.

44. Birmaher B, Birmaher B, Brent D, et al. Practice parameter for the assessment and treatment of children and adolescents with depressive disorders. *J Am Acad Child Adolesc Psychiatry.* 2007;46:1503–1526.

45. Ibid.

46. Merikangas KR, He J-P, Burstein M, et al. Lifetime prevalence of mental disorders in US adolescents: results from the national comorbidity survey replication – Adolescent supplement (NCS-A). *J Am Acad Child Adolesc Psychiatry.* 2010;49(10):980–989.

47. Ivanenko A, CrabtreeVM, O'Brien LM, et al. Sleep complaints and psychiatric symptoms in children evaluated at a pediatric mental health clinic. *J Clin Sleep Med.* 2006;2:42–48.

48. Roberts RE, Lewinsohn PM, Weeley JR. Symptoms of DSM-III-R major depression in adolescence: evidence from an epidemiological survey. *J Am Acad Child Adolesc Psychiatry.* 1995;34:1608–1617.

49. Roberts RE, Lewinsohn PM, Seeley JR. Symptoms of DSM-III-R major depression in adolescence: Evidence from an epidemiological survey. *J Am Acad Child Adolesc Psychiatry.* 1995;34:1608–1617.

50. Liu X, Buysse DJ, Gentzler AL, et al. Insomnia and hypersomnia associated with depressive phenomenology and comorbidity in childhood depression. *Sleep.* 2007;30:83–90.

51. Roberts RE, Duong HT. depression and insomnia among adolescents: a prospective perspective. *J Affect Disord.* 2013;148:66–71.

52. Goldstein TR, Bridge JA, Brent DA. Sleep disturbance preceding completed suicide in adolescents. *J Consult Clin Psychol.* 2008;76:84–91.

53. Cullen KR, Gee DG, Klimes-Dougan B, et al. A preliminary study of functional connectivity in comorbid adolescent depression. *Neurosci Lett.* 2009;460:227–231.

54. Connolly CG, Wu J, Ho TC, et al. Resting-state functional connectivity of subgenual anterior cingulate cortex in depressed adolescents. *Biol Psychiatry.* 2013;74:898–907.

55. Davey CG, Harrison BJ, Yucel M, Allen NB. Regionally specific alterations in functional connectivity of the anterior cingulate cortex in major depressive disorder. *Psychol Med.* 2012;42:2071–2081.

56. Ho TC, Yang G, et al. Functional connectivity of negative emotional processing in adolescent depression. *J Affect Disord.* 2014;155:65–74.

57. Taki Y, Hashizume H, Thyreau B, et al. Sleep duration during weekdays affects hippocampal gray matter volume in healthy children. *NeuroImage.* 2012;60:471–475.

58. Beebe DW, Difrancesco MW, Tlustos SJ, McNally KA, Holland SK. Preliminary fMRI findings in experimentally sleep-restricted adolescents engaged in a working memory task. *Behav Brain Funct.* 2009;5:9.

59. Holm SM, Forbes EE, Ryan ND, Phillips ML, Tarr JA, Dahl, RE. Reward-related brain function and sleep in pre/early pubertal and mid/late pubertal adolescents. *J Adolesc Health*. 2009;45:326–334.

60. Hasler BP, Dahl RE, Holm SM, Jakubcak JL, Ryan ND, Silk JS, Phillips ML, Forbes EE. Weekend-weekday advances in sleep timing are associated with altered reward-related brain function in healthy adolescents. *Biol Psychol*. 2012;91:334–341.

61. Telzer EH, Fuligni AJ, Lieberman MD, Galvan A. The effects of poor quality sleep on brain function and risk taking in adolescence. *NeuroImage*. 2013;71:275–283.

62. Steiger A, Kimura M. Wake and sleep EEG provide biomarkers in depression. *J Psychiatr Res*. 2010;44:242–252.

63. Dahl RE, Ryan ND, Matty MK, et al. Sleep onset abnormalities in depressed adolescents. *Biol Psychiatry*. 1996;39:400–410.

64. Rao U, Dahl RE, Ryan ND, et al. The relationship between longitudinal clinical course and sleep and cortisol changes in adolescent depression. *Biol Psychiatry*. 1996;40:474–484.

65. Emslie GJ, Kennard BD, Mayes TL, et al. Insomnia moderates outcome of serotonin-selective reuptake inhibitor treatment in depressed youth. *J Child Adolesc Psychopharmacol*. 2012;22:21–28.

66. Shamseddeen W, Clarke G, Keller MB, et al. Adjunctive sleep medications and depression outcome in the treatment of serotonin-selective reuptake inhibitor resistant depression in adolescents study. *J Child Adolesc Psychopharmacol*. 2012;22:29–36.

67. Ising M, Horstmann S, Kloiber S, et al. Combined dexamethasone/corticotropin releasing hormone test predicts treatment response in major depression: A potential biomarker? *Biol Psychiatry*. 2007;62(1)47–54[PubMed].

68. Brouwer JP, Appelhof BC, van Rossum EF, et al. Prediction of treatment response by HPA-axis and glucocorticoid receptor polymorphisms in major depression. *Psychoneuroendocrinology*. 2006;31:1154–1163.

69. Emslie GJ, Armitage R, Weinberg WA, et al. Sleep polysomnography as a predictor of recurrence in children and adolescents with major depressive disorder. *Int J Neuropsychopharmacol*. 2001;4:159–168.

70. De Bruin, EJ, Bögels SM, Oort FJ, Meijer AM. Efficacy of cognitive behavioral therapy for insomnia in adolescents: a randomized controlled trial with internet therapy, group therapy and a waiting list condition. *Sleep*. 2015;38(12):1913–1926.

71. Clarke G, Harvey AG. The complex role of sleep in adolescent depression. *Child Adolesc Psychiatr Clin N Am*. 2012;21:385–400.

72. Bogen S, Legenbauer T, Bogen T, et al. Morning light therapy for juvenile depression and severe mood dysregulation: study protocol for a randomized controlled trial. *Trials*. 2013;14:178.

73. Hickie, I.B, Naismith SL, Robillard R, Scott EM, Hermens DF. Manipulating the sleep-wake cycle and circadian rhythms to improve clinical management of major depression. *BMC Med*. 2013;11:79.

74. Beesdo K, Knappe S, Pine DS. Anxiety and anxiety disorders in children and adolescents: developmental issues and implications for DSM-V. *Psychiatr Clin North Am*. 2009;32(3):483–524.

75. Langley AK, Bergman RL, McCracken J, Piacentini JC. Impairment in childhood anxiety disorders: preliminary examination of the Child Anxiety Impact Scale-Parent Version. *J Child Adolesc Psychopharmacol*. 2004;14:105–114.

76. Comer JS, Blanco C, Grant B, et al. Health-related quality of life across the anxiety disorders: results from the national epidemiologic survey on alcohol and related conditions. *J Clin Psychiatry*. 2011;72:43–50.

77. Lopez B, Turner RJ, Saavedra LM. Anxiety and risk for substance dependence among late adolescents/young adults. *J Anxiety Disord*. 2005;19(3):275–294.

78. Weissman MM, Bland RC, Canino GJ, et al. Prevalence of suicide ideation and suicide attempts in nine countries. *Psychol Med*. 1999;29:9–17.

79. Pine DS, Cohen P, Gurley D, Brook J, Ma Y. The risk for early-adulthood anxiety and depressive disorders in adolescents with anxiety and depressive disorders. *Arch Gen Psychiatry*. 1998;55(1): 56–64.

80. Bowen RC, Offord DR, Boyle MH. The prevalence of overanxious disorder and separation anxiety disorder: results from the Ontario Child Health Study. *J Am Acad Child Adolesc Psychiatry*. 1990;29(5):753–758.

81. Bolton D, Eley TC, O'Connor TG, et al. Prevalence and genetic and environmental influences on anxiety disorders in 6-year-old twins. *Psychol Med*. 2006;36(3):335–344.

82. Beesdo K, Knappe S, Pine DS. Anxiety and anxiety disorders in children and adolescents: developmental issues and implications for DSM-V. *Psychiatr Clin North Am*. 2009;32(3):483–524.

83. Ibid.

84. Gale CK, Millichamp J. Generalised anxiety disorder in children and adolescents. *BMJ Clin Evid*. 2016;1002.

85. Chase R, Pincus D. Sleep-related problems in children and adolescents with anxiety disorders. *Behav Sleep Med*. 2011;9:224–236.

86. Alfano CA, Pina AA, Zerr AA, et al. Pre-sleep arousal and sleep problems of anxiety-disordered youth. *Child Psychiatry Hum Dev*. 2010;41(2):156–167.

87. Alfano CA, Beidel DC, Turner SM, et al. Preliminary evidence for sleep complaints among children referred for anxiety. *Sleep Med.* 2006;7(6):467–473.

88. Alfano CA, Ginsberg GA, Kingery JN. Sleep-related problems among children and adolescents with anxiety disorders. *J Am Acad Child Adolesc Psychiatry.* 2007;46:224–232.

89. Storch EA, Murphy TK, Lack CW, et al. Sleep-related problems in pediatric obsessive-compulsive disorder. *J Anxiety Disord.* 2008;22(5):877–885.

90. Poznanski B, Cornacchio D, Coxe S, et al. The link between anxiety severity and irritability among anxious youth: evaluating the mediating role of sleep problems. *Child Psychiatry Hum Dev.* 2018;49:352–359. doi:10.1007/s10578-017-0769-1.

91. Uhde TW, Cortese BM, Vedeniapin A. Anxiety and sleep problems: emerging concepts and theoretical treatment implications. *Curr Psychiatry Rep.* 2009;11(4):269–276.

92. Blake MJ, Trinder JA, Allen NB. Mechanisms underlying the association between insomnia, anxiety, and depression in adolescence: Implications for behavioral sleep interventions. *Clin Psychology Rev.* 2018;63:25–40.

93. Rapoport J, Elkins R, Langer DH, et al. Childhood obsessive-compulsive disorder. *Am J Psychiatry.* 1981;138:1545–1554.

94. Alfano C, Reynolds K, Scott N, Dahl R, Mellman T. Polysomnographic sleep patterns of non-depressed, non-medicated children with generalized anxiety disorder. *J Affect Disord.* 2013;147:379–384.

95. Alfano CA, Ginsberg GA, Kingery JN. Sleep-related problems among children and adolescents with anxiety disorders. *J Am Acad Child Adolesc Psychiatry.* 2007;46:224–232.

96. Kendall PC, Pimentel SS. On the physiological symptom constellation in youth with Generalized Anxiety Disorder (GAD). *J Anxiety Disord.* 2003;17(2):211–221.

97. Finkelhor D, Turner HA, Shattuck A, Hamby SL. Violence, crime and abuse exposure in a national sample of children and youth: An update. *JAMA Pediatr.* 2013;167(7):614–621. doi:10.1001/jamapediatrics.2013.42.

98. Merikangas KR, He JP, Burstein M, et al. Lifetime prevalence of mental disorders in U.S. adolescents: results from the National Comorbidity Survey Replication--Adolescent Supplement (NCS-A). *J Am Acad Child Adolesc Psychiatry.* 2010;49(10):980–989.

99. Copeland WE, Keeler G, Angold A, Costello EJ. Traumatic events and posttraumatic stress in childhood. *Arch Gen Psychiatry.* 2007;64(5):577–584.

100. Chorney DB, Detweiler MF, Morris TL, Kuhn BR. The interplay of sleep disturbance, anxiety and depression in children. *J Pediatr Psychol.* 2008;33(4): 339–348.

101. Noll JG, Trickett PK, Susman EJ, Putnam FW. Sleep disturbances and childhood sexual abuse. *J Pediatr Psychol.* 2006;31(5):469–480.

102. Glod CA, Teicher MH, Hartman CR, Harakal T. Increased nocturnal activity and impaired sleep maintenance in abused children. *J Am Acad Child Adolesc Psychiatry.* 1997;36:1236–1243.

103. Wang Y, Raffeld MR, Slopen N, Hale L, Dunn EC. Childhood adversity and insomnia in adolescence. *Sleep Med.* 2016;21:12–18.

104. Nardo D, Högberg G, Jonsson C, et al. Neurobiology of sleep disturbances in PTSD patients and traumatized controls: MRI and SPECT findings. *Front Psychiatry.* 2015;6(13):134. doi:10.3389/fpsyt.2015.00134.

105. Ebdlahad S, Nofzinger EA, James JA, et al. Comparing neural correlates of REM sleep in posttraumatic stress disorder and depression: a neuroimaging study. *Psychiatry Res.* 2013;214:422–428. doi:10.1016/j.pscychresns.2013.09.007.

106. Germain A, James J, Insana S, et al. A window into the invisible wound of war: functional neuroimaging of REM sleep in returning combat veterans with PTSD. *Psychiatry Res.* 2013;211:176–179. doi:10.1016/j.pscychresns.2012.05.007.

107. Sadeh A, McGuire JP, Sachs H, et al. Sleep and psychological characteristics of children on a psychiatric inpatient unit. *J Am Acad Child Adolesc Psychiatry.* 1995;34(6):813–819.

108. Glod CA, Teicher MH, Hartman CR, Harakal T. Increased nocturnal activity and impaired sleep maintenance in abused children. *J Am Acad Child Adolesc Psychiatry.* 1997;36(9):1236–1243.

109. Strawn JR, Keeshin BR, DelBello MP, Geracioti TD, Putnam FW. Psychopharmacologic treatment of posttraumatic stress disorder in children and adolescents: a review. *J Clin Psychiatry.* 2010;71(7):932–941. doi:10.4088/JCP.09r05446blu.

110. Donnelly CL. Pharmacologic treatment approaches for children and adolescents with posttraumatic stress disorder. *Child Adolesc Psychiatr Clin N Am.* 2003;12:251–269. doi:10.1016/S1056-4993(02)00102-5.

111. Harmon RJ, Riggs PD. Clonidine for posttraumatic stress disorder in preschool children. *J Am Acad Child Adolesc Psychiatry.* 1996;35:1247–1249. doi: 10.1097/00004583-199609000-00022.

112. Horrigan JP, Barnhill LJ. The suppression of nightmares with guanfacine. *J Clin Psychiatry.* 1996;57:371

113. Sallee FR, Lyne A, Wigal T, McGough JJ. Long-term safety and efficacy of guanfacine extended release in children and adolescents with attention-deficit/hyperactivity disorder. *J Child Adolesc Psychopharmacol.* 2009;19:215–226. doi: 10.1089/cap.2008.0080

114. Keeshin BR, Ding Q, Presson AP, Berkowitz SJ, Strawn JR. Use of prazosin for pediatric PTSD-associated nightmares and sleep disturbances: a retrospective chart review. *Neurol Ther.* 2017;6(2):247–257.

115. Keeshin BR, Strawn JR. Psychological and pharmacologic treatment of youth with posttraumatic stress disorder: an evidence-based review. *Child Adolesc Psychiatr Clin N Am.* 2014;23:399–411. doi:10.1016/j.chc.2013.12.002.

116. Goldstein BI, Birmaher B, Carlson GA, et al. The international society for bipolar disorders task force report on pediatric bipolar disorder: knowledge to date and directions for future research. *Bipolar Disord.* 2017;19:524–543.

117. Lofthouse N, Fristad M, Splaingard M, et al. Parent and child reports of sleep problems associated with early-onset bipolar spectrum disorders. *J Fam Psychol.* 2007;2191:114–123.

118. Staton D, Volness LJ, Beatty WW. Diagnosis and classification of pediatric bipolar disorder. *J Affect Disord.* 2008;105(1-3):205–212.

119. Goldstein BI, Birmaher B, Carlson GA, et al. The international society for bipolar disorders task force report on pediatric bipolar disorder: Knowledge to date and directions for future research. *Bipolar Disord.* 2017;19:524–543.

120. Staton, D. The impairment of pediatric bipolar sleep: Hypotheses regarding a core defect and phenotype-specific sleep disturbances. *J Affect Disord.* 2008;108(3):199–206.

121. Harvey AG. The adverse consequences of sleep disturbance in pediatric bipolar disorder: Implications for intervention. *Child Adolesc Psychiatric Clin N Am.* 2009;18(2):321–338.

122. Geller B, Zimerman B, Williams M, et al. DSM0IV mania symptoms in a prepubertal and early adolescent bipolar phenotype compared to attention-deficit hyperactive and normal controls. *J Child Adolesc Psychopharmacol.* 2002;12:11–25.

123. Harvey AG. The adverse consequences of sleep disturbance in pediatric bipolar disorder: Implications for intervention. *Child Adolesc Psychiatric Clin N Am.* 2009;18(2):321–338.

124. Harvey AG. The adverse consequences of sleep disturbance in pediatric bipolar disorder: Implications for intervention. *Child Adolesc Psychiatric Clin N Am.* 2009;18(2):321–338.

125. Dahl RE, Puig-Antich J, Ryan ND, et al. EEG sleep in adolescents with major depression: the role of suicidality and inpatient status. *J Affective Disorders.* 1990;19:63–75.

126. Biederman J, Mick E, Hammerness P, et al. Open-label, 8-week trial of olanzapine and risperidone for the treatment of bipolar disorder in preschool-age children. *Biol Psychiatry.* 2005;58(7):589–594.

127. Tohen M, Kryzhanovskaya L, Carlson G, et al. Olanzapine versus placebo in the treatment of adolescents with bipolar mania. *Am J Psychiatry.* 2007;164(10):1547–1556.

128. McClennan J. Sadock BJ, Sadock VA. Early onset schizophrenia. In: Sadock BJ, Sadock VA, eds. Comprehensive Textbook of Psychiatry. 8th ed. Vol. 2. Philadelphia: Lippincott Williams & Wilkins; 2005:3257–3261.

129. Hafner H, Nowotny B. Epidemiology of early-onset schizophrenia. *Eur Arch Psychiatry Clin Neurosci.* 1995;245:80–92.

130. Stephan KE, Baldeweg T, Friston KJ. Synaptic plasticity and dysconnection in schizophrenia. *Biol Psychiatry.* 2006;59(10):929–939. doi:10.1016/j.biopsych.2005.10.005.

131. Keshavan MD, Montrose DM, Miewald JM, Jindal RD. Sleep correlates of cognition in early course psychotic disorders. *Schizophr Res.* 2011;131:231–234.

132. Lunsford-Avery, JR, Orr J, Gupta T, Pelletier-Baldelli A, Dean DJ. Sleep dysfunction and thalamic abnormalities in adolescents at ultra high-risk of psychosis. *Schizophrenia Res.* 2013;151(1-3):148–153.

133. Lee YJ, et al. The relationship between psychotic-like experiences and sleep disturbances in adolescents. *Sleep Med.* 2012;13:1021–1027

134. Mattai AA, Tossell J, Greenstein DK, et al. Sleep disturbances in childhood-onset schizophrenia. *Schizophr Res.* 2006;86(1–3):123–129.

135. MacDonald AW, Schulz SC. What we know: findings that every theory of schizophrenia should explain. *Schizophr Bull.* 2009;35(3):493–508. doi:10.1093/schbul/sbp017.

136. Stephan KE, Friston KJ, Frith CD. Dysconnection in schizophrenia: from abnormal synaptic plasticity to failures of self-monitoring. *Schizophr Bull.* 2009;35(3):509–527. doi:10.1093/schbul/sbn176.

137. Howes OD, Kapur S. The dopamine hypothesis of schizophrenia: version III—the final common pathway. *Schizophr Bull.* 2009;35(3):549–562. doi:10.1093/schbul/sbp006

138. Olney JW, Newcomer JW, Farber NB. NMDA receptor hypofunction model of schizophrenia. *J Psychiatric Res.* 1999;33(6):523–533. doi: 10.1016/S0022-3956(99)00029-1

139. Kim Y, Zerwas S, Trace SE, Sullivan PF. Schizophrenia genetics: where next? *Schizophr*

Bull. 2011;37(3):456–463. doi:10.1093/schbul/sbr031.

140. Gilmour G, Dix S, Fellini L, et al. NMDA receptors, cognition and schizophrenia—testing the validity of the NMDA receptor hypofunction hypothesis. *Neuropharmacology.* 2012;62(3):1401–1412. doi:10.1016/j.neuropharm.2011.03.015.

141. Sprecher KE, Ferrarelli F, Benca RM. Sleep and plasticity in schizophrenia. In: Meerlo P, Benca R., Abel T eds., Sleep, Neuronal Plasticity and Brain Function: Current Topics in Behavioral Neurosciences. Vol 25. Berlin: Springer; 2015.

142. Monti JS, BaHammam AS, Pandi-Perumal SR, et al. Sleep and circadian rhythm dysregulation in schizophrenia. *Prog Neuropsychopharmacology Biol Psychiatry.* 2013;43:209–216.

143. Chouinard S, Poulin J, Stip E, et al. Sleep in untreated patients with schizophrenia: a meta-analysis. *Schizophr Bull.* 2004;30:957–967.

144. Myles H, Myles N, Coetzer CLC, et al. Cognition in schizophrenia improves with treatment of severe obstructive sleep apnoea: A pilot study. *Schizophrenia Res Cogn.* 2018;15:14–20. doi:10.1016/j.scog.2018.09.001.

145. Kishi T, Inada K, Matsui Y, Iwata N. Z-drug for schizophrenia: a systematic review and meta-analysis. *Psychiatry Res.* 2017;256:365–370. doi:10.1016/j.psychres.2017.06.063.

146. Goodlin-Jones BL, Burnham MM, Gaylor EE, et al. Night waking, sleep–wake organization, and self-soothing in the first year of life. *J Dev Behav Pediatr.* 2001;22:226–233.

147. Mindell JA, Meltzer LJ, Carskadon MA, et al. Developmental aspects of sleep hygiene: Findings from the 2004 National Sleep Foundation Sleep in America Poll. *Sleep Med.* 2009;10:771–779.

148. Burnham MM, Goodlin-Jones BL, Gaylor EE, et al. Nighttime sleep–wake patterns and self-soothing from birth to one year of age: a longitudinal intervention study. *J Child Psychol Psychiatry.* 2002;43:713–725.

149. Mindell JA, Meltzer LJ, Carskadon MA, et al. Developmental aspects of sleep hygiene: findings from the 2004 National Sleep Foundation Sleep in America Poll. *Sleep Med.* 2009;10:771–779.

150. Kerr S, Jowett S. Sleep problems in pre-school children: a review of the literature. *Child Care Health Dev.* 1994;20:379–391.

151. American Academy of Sleep Medicine. International Classification of Sleep Disorders: Diagnostic and Coding Manual. 2nd ed. Westchester, IL: American Academy of Sleep Medicine, 2005.

152. Ibid.

153. Johnson EO, Roth T, Schultz L, et al. Epidemiology of DSM-IV insomnia in adolescence: lifetime prevalence, chronicity, and an emergent gender difference. *Pediatrics.* 2006;117:e247–e256.

154. Mindell JA. Empirically supported treatments in pediatric psychology: bedtime refusal and night wakings in young children. *J Pediatr Psychol.* 1999;24:465–481.

155. Kuhn BR, Elliott AJ. Treatment efficacy in behavioral pediatric sleep medicine. *J Psychosom Res.* 2003;54:587–597.

156. Mindell JA, Kuhn B, Lewin DS, et al. Behavioral treatment of bedtime problems. *Sleep.* 2006;29(10):1263–1267.

157. Price AM, Wake M, Ukoumunne OC, Hiscock H. Five-year follow-up of harms and benefits of behavioral infant sleep intervention: randomized trial. *Pediatrics.* 2012;130:643–651.

158. Gradisar M, Jackson K, Spurrier NJ, et al. Behavioral interventions for infant sleep problems: a randomized controlled trial. *Pediatrics.* 2016;137:e20151486.

159. Rossignol DA, Frye RE. Melatonin in autism spectrum disorders: A systematic review and meta-analysis. *Dev Med Child Neurol.*2011;53:783–792.

160. Cortesi F, Giannotti F, Sebastiani T, Panunzi S, Valente D. Controlled-release melatonin, singly and combined with cognitive behavioural therapy, for persistent insomnia in children with autism spectrum disorders: A randomized placebo-controlled trial. *J Sleep Res.* 2012; 21:700–709

161. van Geijlswijk IM, Mol RH, Egberts TC, Smits MG. Evaluation of sleep, puberty and mental health in children with long-term melatonin treatment for chronic idiopathic childhood sleep onset insomnia. *Psychopharmacology.* 2011;216:111–120.

162. Petit D, Pennestri MH, Paquet J, et al. Childhood sleepwalking and sleep terrors: a longitudinal study of prevalence and familial aggregation. *JAMA Pediatr.* 2015;169:653–658.

163. Petit D, Touchette E, Tremblay RE, Boivin M, Montplaisir J. Dyssomnias and parasomnias in early childhood. *Pediatrics.* 2007;119:e1016–e1025.

164. AASAM 2014.

165. Ekinci O, Isik U, Gunes S, Ekinci N. Understanding sleep problems in children with epilepsy: associations with quality of life, attention-deficit hyperactivity disorder and maternal emotional symptoms. *Seizure.* 2016;40:108–113.

166. Rodopman-Arman A, Perdahli-Fis N, Ekinci O, Berkem M. Sleep habits, parasomnias and associated behaviors in school children

with attention deficit hyperactivity disorder (ADHD). *Turk J Pediatr.* 2011;53:397–403.

167. Barnett AL, Wiggs L. Sleep behaviour in children with developmental co-ordination disorder. *Child Care Health Dev.* 2012;38:403–411.

168. ASAM 3rd edition.

169. American Psychiatric Association. *Diagnostic and Statistical Manual of Mental Disorders.* 5th ed. Washington, DC: American Psychiatric Association, 2013.

170. Kotogal S, Nichols CD, Grigg-Damberger MM, et al. Non-respiratory indications for polysomnography and related procedures in children: an evidence-based review. *Sleep.* 2012;35(11):1451–1466. doi:10.5665/sleep.2188.

171. Frank NC, Spirito A, Stark L, Owens-Stively J. The use of scheduled awakenings to eliminate childhood sleepwalking. *J Pediatr Psychol.* 1997;22:345–353.

172. Attarian H, Zhu L. Treatment options for disorders of arousal: a case series. *Int J Neurosci.* 2013;123(9):623–625.

173. Challamel MJ, Mazzola ME, Nevsimalova S, et al. Narcolepsy in children. *Sleep.* 1994;8(Suppl):S17–S20.

174. Wijnans L, Lecomte C, de Vries C, et al. The incidence of narcolepsy in Europe: before, during, and after the influenza A(H1N1)pdm09 pandemic and vaccination campaigns. *Vaccine.* 2013;31(8):1246–1254.

175. Longstreth WT Jr, Koepsell TD, Ton TG, et al. The epidemiology of narcolepsy. *Sleep.* 2007;30:13–26.

176. Maski K, Steinhart E, Williams D, et al. Listening to the patient voice in narcolepsy: diagnostic delay, disease burden, and treatment efficacy. *J Clin Sleep Med.* 2017;13:419–425.

177. Challamel MJ, Mazzola ME, Nevsimalova S, et al. Narcolepsy in children. *Sleep.* 1994;8(Suppl):S17–S20.

178. Serra L, Montagna P, Mignot E, et al. Cataplexy features in childhood narcolepsy. *Mov Disord.* 2008; 23(6):858–865.

179. Stores G, Montgomery P, Wiggs L. The psychosocial problems of children with narcolepsy and those with excessive daytime sleepiness of uncertain origin. *Pediatrics.* 2006;118:e1116.

180. Maski K, Steinhart E, Williams D, et al. Listening to the patient voice in narcolepsy: diagnostic delay, disease burden, and treatment efficacy. *J Clin Sleep Med.* 2017;13:419–425.

181. Avis KT, Shen J, Weaver P, Schwebel DC. Psychosocial characteristics of children with central disorders of hypersomnolence versus matched healthy children. *J Clin Sleep Med.* 2015;11:1281–1288.

182. Drake C, Nickel C, Burduvali E, et al. The pediatric daytime sleepiness scale (PDSS): sleep habits and school outcomes in middle-school children. *Sleep.* 2003;26:455–458.

183. Lee J, Na G, Joo EY, Lee M, Lee J. Clinical and polysomnographic characteristics of excessive daytime sleepiness in children. *Sleep Breath.* 2017;21(4):967–974.

184. Aran A, Einen M, Lin L, et al. Clinical and therapeutic aspects of childhood narcolepsy-cataplexy: a retrospective study of 51 children. *Sleep.* 2010;33:1457–1464.

185. Lecendreux M, Bruni O, Franco P, et al. Clinical experience suggests that modafinil is an effective and safe treatment for paediatric narcolepsy. *J Sleep Res.* 2012; 21:481–483.

186. Babiker MO, Prasad M. Narcolepsy in children: a diagnostic and management approach. *Pediatr Neurol.* 2015;52:557–565.

187. Aran A, Einen M, Lin L, et al. Clinical and therapeutic aspects of childhood narcolepsy-cataplexy: a retrospective study of 51 children. *Sleep.* 2010; 33:1457.

188. Lecendreux M. Pharmacological management of narcolepsy and cataplexy in pediatric patients. *Paediatr Drugs.* 2014;16:363–372.

189. Ivanenko A., Kek L., Grosrenaud J. Long-term use of modafinil and armodafinil in pediatric patients with narcolepsy. *Sleep.* 2017;40(Abstract Suppl):A354–A355.

190. Aran A, Einen M, Lin L, et al. Clinical and therapeutic aspects of childhood narcolepsy-cataplexy: a retrospective study of 51 children. *Sleep.* 2010;33:1457–1464.

191. Murali H, Kotagal S. Off-label treatment of severe childhood narcolepsy-cataplexy with sodium oxybate. *Sleep.* 2006;29:1025–1029.

192. Lecendreux M. Pharmacological management of narcolepsy and cataplexy in pediatric patients. *Paediatr Drugs.* 2014;16:363.

193. Vendrame M, Havaligi N, Matadeen-Ali C, et al. Narcolepsy in children: a single-center clinical experience. *Pediatr Neurol.* 2008;38(5):314–320.

194. Lecendreux M, Poli F, Oudiette D, et al. Tolerance and efficacy of sodium oxybate in childhood narcolepsy with cataplexy: a retrospective study. *Sleep.* 2012;35:709–711.

195. Plazzi G, Ruoff C, Lecendreux M, et al. A double-blind, placebo-controlled, randomized-withdrawal, multicenter study on the efficacy and safety of sodium oxybate in pediatric subjects with narcolepsy with cataplexy. *Sleep.* 2017;40(Abstract Suppl) A239.

196. Møller LR, Østergaard JR. Treatment with venlafaxine in six cases of children with narcolepsy and with cataplexy and hypnagogic

hallucinations. *J Child Adolesc Psychopharmacol.* 2009;19:197–201.

197. Ratkiewicz M, Splaingard M. Treatment of cataplexy in a three-year-old using venlafaxine. *J Clin Sleep Med.* 2013;9:1341–1342.

198. Picchietti D, Allen RP, Walters AS, et al. Restless legs syndrome: prevalence and impact in children and adolescents—the Peds REST study. *Pediatrics.* 2007;120:253–266.

199. Sander HH, Eckeli AL, Costa Passos AD, et al. Prevalence and quality of life and sleep in children and adolescents with restless legs syndrome/Willis-Ekbom disease. *Sleep Med.* 2017;30:204–209.

200. Goodwin J, Vasquez MM, Quan SF. Prevalence of restless legs syndrome among adolescent children in the Tucson Children's Assessment if Sleep Apnea Study (TUCASA). *Sleep.* 2012;34:A268.

201. Picchietti DL, Bruni O, de Weerd A, et al. Pediatric restless legs syndrome diagnostic criteria: an update by the International Restless Legs Syndrome Study Group. *Sleep Med.* 2013;14:1253–1259.

202. Picchietti DL, Arbuckle RA, Abetz L, et al. Pediatric restless legs syndrome: analysis of symptom descriptions and drawings. *J Child Neurol.* 2011;26:1365–1376.

203. Arbuckle R, Abetz L, Durmer JS, et al. Development of the Pediatric Restless Legs Syndrome Severity Scale (P-RLS-SS): a patient-reported outcome measure of pediatric RLS symptoms and impact. *Sleep Med.* 2010; 11:897.

204. de Weerd A, Aricò I, Silvestri R. Presenting symptoms in pediatric restless legs syndrome patients. *J Clin Sleep Med.* 2013;9:1077–1080.

205. Picchietti D, Allen RP, Walters AS, et al. Restless legs syndrome: prevalence and impact in children and adolescents—the Peds REST study. *Pediatrics.* 2007;120:253–266.

206. Cortese S, Konofal E, Lecendreux M, et al. Restless legs syndrome and attention deficit/hyperactivity disorder: a review of the literature. *Sleep.* 2005;28:1007–1013.

207. Silvestri R, Gagliano A, Arico I, et al. Sleep disorders in children with ADHD recorded overnight by video-polysomnography. *Sleep Med.* 2009;10:1132–1138.

208. Pullen SJ, Wall CA, Angstman ER, et al. Psychiatric comorbidity in children and adolescents with restless legs syndrome: a retrospective study. *J Clin Sleep Med.* 2011;7:587–596.

209. Picchietti MA, Picchietti DL. Advances in pediatric restless legs syndrome: Iron, genetics, diagnosis and treatment. *Sleep Med.* 2010;11:643–651.

210. Durmer JS. Restless legs syndrome, periodic leg movements and periodic limb movement disorder. In: Sheldon SH, Ferber R, Kryger MH, Gozal D, eds. Principles and Practice of Pediatric Sleep Medicine. 2nd ed, Amsterdam: Elsevier; 2014:337–350.

211. Frenette E. Restless legs syndrome in children: A review and update on pharmacological options. *Curr Pharm Des.* 2011;17:1436–1442.

212. Konofal E, Arnulf I, Lecendreux M, Mouren MC. Ropinirole in a child with attention-deficit hyperactivity disorder and restless legs syndrome. *Pediatr Neurol.* 2005;32:350–351.

213. Walters AS, Mandelbaum DE, Lewin DS, et al. Dopaminergic therapy in children with restless legs/periodic limb movements in sleep and ADHD: dopaminergic therapy study group. *Pediatr Neurol.* 2000;22:182–186.

214. Cortese S, Konofal E, Lecendreux M. Effectiveness of ropinirole for RLS and depressive symptoms in an 11-year-old girl. *Sleep Med.* 2009;10:259–261.

215. England SJ, Picchietti DL, Couvadelli BV, et al. L-dopa improves restless legs syndrome and periodic limb movements in sleep but not attention-deficit-hyperactivity disorder in a double-blind trial in children. *Sleep Med.* 2011;12:471–477.

216. Garetz SL. Behavior, cognition, and quality of life after adenotonsillectomy for pediatric sleep-disordered breathing: summary of the literature. *Otolaryngol Head Neck Surg.* 2008;138(1 Suppl):S19–S26. doi:10.1016/j.otohns.2007.06.738.

217. Marcus CL, Brooks LJ, Draper KA, et al. American Academy of Pediatrics. Diagnosis and management of childhood obstructive sleep apnea syndrome. *Pediatrics.* 2012;130(3):e714–e755.

218. Verhulst SL, Schrauwen N, Haentjens D, et al. Sleep-disordered breathing in overweight and obese children and adolescents: prevalence, characteristics and the role of fat distribution. *Arch Dis Child.* 2007;92(3):205–208.

219. Aurora RN, Zak RS, Karippot A, et al. Practice parameters for the respiratory indications for polysomnography in children. *Sleep.* 2011;34(3):379–388.

220. Dudoignon B, Amaddeo A, Frapin A, et al. Obstructive sleep apnea in Down syndrome: benefits of surgery and noninvasive respiratory support. *Am J Med Genet.* 2017;173A:2074–2080.

221. Shott S. Down syndrome: common otolaryngologic manifestations. *Am J Med Genet.* 2006;142C:131–140.

222. Youssef NA, Ege M, Angly SS, Strauss JL, Marx CE. Is obstructive sleep apnea associated with ADHD? *Ann Clin Psychiatry.* 2011;23(3):213–224.

223. Aksu H, Günel C, Özgür BG, Toka A, Başak S. Effects of adenoidectomy/adenotonsillectomy

on ADHD symptoms and behavioral problems in children. *Int J Pediatr Otorhinolaryngol.* 2015;79(7):1030–1033.

224. Constantin E, Tewfik TL, Brouillette RT. Can the OSA-18 Quality-of-Life questionnaire detect obstructive sleep apnea in children? *Pediatrics.* 2010;125(1):e162–e168.

225. Borgstrom A, Nerfeldt P, Friberg D. Questionnaire OSA-18 has poor validity compared to polysomnography in pediatric obstructive sleep apnea. *Int J Pediatr Otorhinolaryngol.* 2013;77(11):1864–1868.

226. Chervin RD, Weatherly RA, Garetz SL, et al. Pediatric sleep questionnaire: prediction of sleep apnea and outcomes. *Arch Otolaryngol Head Neck Surg.* 2007;133(3):216–222.

227. American Psychiatric Association. *Diagnostic and Statistical Manual of Mental Disorders.* 5th ed. Washington, DC: American Psychiatric Association; 2013.

228. Carskadon MA. Patterns of sleep and sleepiness in adolescents. *Pediatrician.* 1990;17(1): 80–90.

229. Saxvig IW, Pallesen S, Wilhelmsen-Langeland A, Molde H, Bjorvatn B. Prevalence and correlates of delayed sleep phase in high school students. *Sleep Med.* 2012;13(2):193–199.

230. Sack RL, Auckley D, Auger R, et al. Circadian rhythm sleep disorders: part II, advanced sleep phase disorder, delayed sleep phase disorder, free-running disorder, and irregular sleep–wake rhythm. *Sleep.* 2007;30(11):1484–1501.

231. Revell VL, Molina TA, Eastman CI. Human phase response curve to intermittent blue light using a commercially available device. *J Physiol.* 2012;590(19):4859–4868.

232. Mundey K, Benloucif S, Harsanyi K, Dubocovich ML, Zee PC. Phase-dependent treatment of delayed sleep phase syndrome with melatonin. *Sleep.* 2005;28(10):1271–1278.

PART 3 ————————————

Sleep and Psychiatric Disorders

17

Depressive Disorders

AMIT CHOPRA, RAMYA BACHU, AND MICHAEL J. PETERSON

INTRODUCTION

Depressive disorders are the most prevalent mood disorders affecting 8% to 17% of the population worldwide [1–3]. In the United States alone, it is estimated that 20 million individuals experience a major depressive episode each year. Depression is one of the leading causes of disability and the fourth leading contributor to the global burden of disease. By 2020, depression is projected to be the first leading contributor to global burden of disease for all ages and both genders. Approximately one-third of patients in a major depressive episodes are refractory to medication and psychotherapeutic treatments [4], and presence of untreated severe depression is a major risk factor for death by suicide [5].

Approximately 90% of patients with depression report sleep disturbances [6, 7], which can persist even during periods of remission from depression [8]. When compared to patients with depression without sleep disturbance, those with associated sleep disturbances have more severe depressive symptoms and lower rates of treatment response or remission [9]. Of note, patients with depression who experience sleep disturbances including early morning awakening are also more likely to have suicidal ideation than those without such disturbances. Moreover, persistent insomnia following the acute phase of depression treatment poses a significant risk for relapse of depression. According to a study by Reynolds et al. [10], two-thirds of patients with persistent insomnia at the end of depression treatment with nortriptyline and interpersonal psychotherapy relapsed within one year after switching to placebo. Conversely, 90% of the patients with good sleep at the end of the acute treatment of depression remained well during the first year, even after discontinuing antidepressant medications and interpersonal psychotherapy.

Based on epidemiological data, insomnia is not only considered a symptom of depression but

also a risk factor for onset of depression [11–14]. Ford and Kamerow [15] noted that patients with persistent insomnia are at a substantially higher risk of developing new-onset major depressive disorder (MDD) than those with resolution of insomnia or no insomnia complaints. The study results suggested that concurrent depression was present in 14% of the insomnia patients as compared to less than 1% in those without insomnia. During prospective follow-up, the authors noted a significantly higher risk of developing major depression in patients with persistent insomnia (odds ratio [OR] 39.8) as compared to those whose insomnia had resolved (OR 1.6). Therefore, presence of insomnia should prompt clinicians to inquire about depression, and vice versa.

Sleep disturbances not only precede or manifest during acute episodes of depression but can persist in patients who have remitted from depression. Residual sleep-related disturbances, including insomnia, fatigue, and nightmares, can persist despite optimal antidepressant treatment in up to 20% to 60% of patients with depression. Presence of residual sleep symptoms is an established risk factor for relapse of major depression and suicide. The residual sleep disturbances in remitted patients correlate with impaired quality of life and suicidal ideation according to a 4-year prospective follow-up study [16]. Interestingly, the residual sleep symptoms may not be predicted by baseline clinical characteristics of MDD including the severity and duration of index episode of depression. These findings suggest, among other possibilities, that sleep dysfunction may be a comorbid and independent pathophysiological entity rather than merely a manifestation of depression with coexistence of these two entities stemming from dysfunction in the common neurological substrates involved in both mood and sleep regulation [16].

The *Diagnostic and Statistical Manual of Mental Disorders* (fifth edition; DSM-5) classification of depressive disorders includes MDD, persistent depressive disorder, disruptive mood dysregulation disorder, premenstrual dysphoric disorder, substance/medication-induced depressive disorder, depressive disorder due to another medical condition, other specified depressive disorder, and unspecified depressive disorder. A bidirectional link exists between sleep disturbances and depressive disorders based on the epidemiological data and shared common underlying neurobiological mechanisms. There is a greater need to understand the origins and treatment of sleep disturbances in depression to develop preventative strategies and optimize treatment outcomes in patients with depressive disorders.

This chapter illustrates the current understanding of the neurobiological mechanisms, sleep architectural changes, and treatment strategies for the commonly prevalent sleep disturbances in depressive disorders with a particular focus on MDD. This chapter also includes sections on sleep therapies as treatment of major depression and effects of somatic therapies, used for management of treatment refractory depression, on sleep outcomes. A separate section focusing on the association of sleep disorders and suicide has been included in this chapter. Sleep disturbance

in depressive episodes associated with bipolar and related disorders has been covered in detail in Chapter 18 of this volume.

NEUROBIOLOGY

Sleep dysfunction in depression can be attributed to common underlying neurobiological mechanisms including neurotransmitter deficits, over-activity of the hypothalamic–pituitary–adrenal (HPA) axis, circadian rhythm abnormalities, impairment of brain plasticity-related gene cascades, and common neural substrates (see Figure 17.1).

Neurotransmitters

Normal sleep architecture is comprised of alternating cycles of nonrapid eye movement (NREM) and rapid eye movement (REM) sleep. NREM sleep is further divided in to three stages: N1, N2, and N3 (slow-wave sleep [SWS]). REM sleep initiation is associated with surge in cholinergic activity along with a decrease in serotonergic and noradrenergic activity [17] whereas REM sleep cessation is associated with an increase in serotonergic activity and a decrease in cholinergic activity. Depression is characterized by sleep architectural changes that include reduced SWS

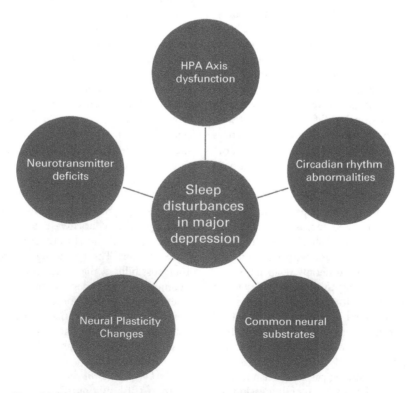

FIGURE 17.1. Neurobiology of sleep disturbances in major depression.

and increased REM propensity characterized by reduced REM latency, increased proportion of REM sleep, and increased REM density (increased number of eye movements per minute) [18]. A state of REM disinhibition has been attributed to monoamine–cholinergic imbalance in depression. Antidepressants that increase serotonergic and/or noradrenergic neurotransmission tend to cause REM suppression with resultant increased REM latency and decreased REM density, thus reversing many of the sleep architectural changes seen in depression [19, 20].

In addition to reduced monoaminergic transmission in depression, more recent studies have investigated role of other neurotransmitter classes. In particular, there has been an emphasis on the role of glutamate, a major excitatory neurotransmitter involved in neuroplasticity, pathophysiology, and treatment of major depression. Glutamate signaling also plays an important role in regulation of NREM and REM sleep. Excitatory glutamate transmission is crucial for the generation of thalamo-cortical slow oscillations of NREM sleep. Glutamate also regulates REM sleep onset due to its interaction with cholinergic neurons by increasing the activity of reticular activating system [17]. Several groups have identified decreased glutamate in the prefrontal cortex in unipolar depression and subsequent normalization following successful treatment with electroconvulsive therapy (ECT) [21–23]. N-methyl-D-aspartate (NMDA) receptors have highest affinity for glutamate, and ketamine, an NMDA receptor antagonist, has been shown to have rapid and potent antidepressant effects in patients with treatment refractory depression, including a reduction of suicidal ideation in these patients [24].

Circadian Rhythms

Human sleep is regulated mainly by two processes: homeostatic (increasing drive to sleep with prolonged wakefulness, or sleep pressure) and circadian (diurnal timing of sleep). Both processes can be disrupted in depression, with some aspects of insomnia and/or hypersomnia related to the homeostatic disruption (e.g., excessive napping during day), which can affect sleep onset latency (SOL) at night. Depression is also characterized by irregularities in the most obvious circadian rhythm in humans, the sleep–wake cycle [25]. In a subgroup of patients with depression, a dysregulation in diurnal rhythmicity affecting sleep, mood, temperature and hormone secretion has been noted [26]. Dysregulation of circadian rhythms

has been correlated with severity of depression [27], and normal rhythms are frequently restored upon improvement in depression symptoms [28].

A core set of CLOCK genes (*BMAL1, CLOCK, PER3, CRY*) plays a central role in generating virtually all the circadian rhythms in the body. Patients with depression, who also have CLOCK gene abnormalities (C/C variant), have been noted to have lifetime insomnia, higher recurrence of insomnia, and worse insomnia during antidepressant treatment [29]. Other gene polymorphisms include the monoamine-oxidase A gene and the promoter of the serotonin transporter gene; both of these genes are regulated by circadian rhythms and have been associated with both insomnia and major depression [30].

Treatments that aim to correct circadian timing, such as sleep deprivation, bright light, and pharmacological therapy, have been shown to alleviate depressive symptoms, which further substantiates the role of circadian dysfunction in depression pathophysiology. Agomelatine, a melatonergic antidepressant with an innovative mode of action (MT1/MT2 receptor agonist and 5-HT2c antagonist), has been noted to be an effective treatment of MDDs [29].

Hypothalamic-Pituitary-Adrenal (HPA) Axis

Dysregulation of the HPA axis has long been associated with depressive disorders and is considered by some investigators to be the final common pathway for development of mood disorders. Stress activates the HPA axis and is also often associated with onset of depressive episodes. During a major depressive episode, about 50% of patients will have excessive activity of the HPA axis, characterized by hypercortisolemia, elevated levels of corticotrophin-releasing hormone (CRH), and/or an abnormal response on the dexamethasone suppression test (DST) [31].

Elevated CRH has been implicated in the causation of depression. Both stress and depression are associated with the activation of CRH neurons and increased CRH mRNA in the paraventricular nucleus. Antidepressant treatments have been shown to normalize the elevated levels of CRH [32], and CRH1 receptor antagonists have also been noted to have antidepressant action [33]. Overactivity of the HPA axis has been linked to hyperarousal of the nervous system leading to reduced SWS and total sleep time (TST) [34]. CRH also affects sleep in a pattern similar to the sleep disturbances in depression by reducing

NREM cycles, suppressing slow-wave activity (SWA) and potentially increasing REM sleep. Conversely, CRH1 receptor antagonist (R121919) has been associated with increased SWS and improved sleep efficiency (SE) in patients with depression [35].

Neural Plasticity

Brain-derived neurotrophic factor (BDNF), a neurotrophin that influences neuronal development, survival, maintenance, and plasticity, has been implicated in the pathophysiology of depression. Serum levels of BDNF have been found to be lower in individuals with depression as compared to control subjects and low BDNF levels correlate with greater severity of depression, global volumetric loss in the cerebral cortex, and higher risk of relapse of depressive episodes [36, 37]. BDNF levels are also influenced by monoamines and the HPA axis [38], and evidence suggests that chronic antidepressant treatment is associated with an increase in hippocampal BDNF levels [31]. Furthermore, increases in BDNF have been associated with increased NREM sleep and SWA during sleep [39].

Sleep plays a pivotal role in the maintenance of normal biological functions. As compared to controls with no sleep disturbances, subjects with insomnia have been noted to exhibit significantly decreased serum BDNF levels according to a study by Giese and colleagues [40]. The authors reported insomnia to be a mediator of the association between perceived stress and serum BDNF levels. Sleep, particularly SWS, is needed for expression of genes related to downscaling of neural synapses [41], and this process could be affected by sleep alterations caused by sleep or mood disorders or both. Ketamine, a rapid-acting treatment for depression, has been shown to concomitantly increase serum BDNF and SWA, both markers of neural plasticity, in patients with major depression [42].

Neural Substrates

Based on neuroimaging studies, various brain regions have been implicated in the shared pathophysiology of sleep and depression. Major depression involves dysfunction of multiple brain structures including prefrontal cortex, hippocampus, nucleus accumbens, and amygdala [31]. Ventromedial prefrontal cortex (VmPFC) may be a critical area for regulating both depression and sleep as it has been suggested to be an important site for REM sleep abnormalities and depressive behaviors. VmPFC lesions have been correlated with increased sleep fragmentation and shortened REM latency in rodent models, similar to sleep architectural changes in patients with depression [43].

Patients with depression exhibit higher brain activity in several cortical and subcortical structures, especially frontal cortex, during wake–NREM transition. Major depression is associated with wake and REM sleep hypermetabolism in the limbic and paralimbic areas (amygdala and medial prefrontal cortex) and basal ganglia structures (caudate nucleus, putamen, and globus pallidus) [44]. Altered functioning of these neural structures can potentially explain cognitive, attention, emotional, and sleep dysregulation (reduced SWS, increased REM sleep) in depression. Lateral habenula (LHb), a brain structure that controls monoaminergic activity and REM sleep, negatively regulates the monoaminergic systems in the central nervous system and inhibits the firing activity of serotonergic and dopaminergic neurons. Hyperactivation of habenula has been implicated in both depression and sleep dysfunction [45].

Intrinsic functional connectivity studies suggest that several large-scale brain networks including the default mode network, the frontoparietal and dorsal attention network, and the salience network are potential neural substrates in MDD [46, 47]. The salience network, which mainly involves the amygdala, the anterior insula, and the dorsal anterior cingulate cortex, plays an important role in both insomnia and MDD [48, 49]. Increased salience activity has been reported in patients with depression with co-occurring insomnia (n = 24) as compared to patients with depression without significant insomnia (n = 37) and healthy controls (n = 51) [50].

CLINICAL APPROACH

This section includes assessment of comorbid primary sleep disorders, behavioral, and lifestyle factors and psychotropic medication-related sleep side effects that may negatively affect sleep in patients with depression.

Screen for Primary Sleep Disorders

Primary sleep disorders such as obstructive sleep apnea (OSA), restless legs syndrome (RLS), and circadian rhythm disorders coexist with major depression. These primary sleep disorders can also mimic depressive disorders due to shared symptoms including sleep disturbance, daytime fatigue, irritability, mood, and cognitive symptoms. Therefore, patients with depression should be routinely screened to adequately assess and treat primary sleep disorders. Patients with depression with a history and examination suggestive of primary sleep disorders should be considered for a referral to sleep clinic for further diagnostic evaluation and treatment.

Behavioral and Lifestyle Factors

It is important to assess behavioral and lifestyle factors that may cause or perpetuate sleep disturbances in patients with depression. Factors such as lack of structured activities, daytime naps, and irregular sleep patterns can worsen sleep difficulties by further disrupting circadian rhythms and homeostatic regulation of sleep. Therefore, it is important to understand the sleep-wake cycle across a full 24-hour day in patients with depression rather than focusing on their night time complaints only. Additionally, careful assessment of sleep hygiene is recommended to understand environmental and personal factors that may contribute to sleep disturbance in patients with depression. The assessment of effects of commonly used nonprescription substances is also essential for a comprehensive sleep assessment. Consumption of caffeine should be elicited due to adverse effects of caffeine intake on sleep. A detailed history of substance use patterns including smoking, alcohol, prescription, and illicit drug use must be sought as substance use disorders tend to worsen sleep disturbance and clinical outcomes in patients with depression.

Medication-Related Side Effects

The impact of medications, prescribed for both psychiatric and nonpsychiatric reasons, should be carefully assessed during evaluation of sleep dysfunction in depressive disorders. Psychotropic medications are often associated with sleep-related side effects due to their impact on sleep architecture and physiology. According to a meta-analysis, as compared to placebo, second-generation antidepressants are often associated with insomnia or hypersomnia depending upon their mode of action [51]. The authors noted highest incidence of insomnia was with bupropion and desvenlafaxine. Additionally, bupropion was the only antidepressant in the meta-analysis to be less likely to cause sedation than placebo. Agomelatine was the only antidepressant that was less likely to cause insomnia than placebo.

Mirtazapine and fluvoxamine were the most sedating, and were noted to have the highest incidence of hypersomnia [51].

Other sleep-related medication side effects of antidepressants include symptoms suggestive of RLS, REM sleep behavior disorder (RBD), sleepwalking and sleep-related eating disorder (SRED). RLS, in context of depression and antidepressant medications, has been covered in detail in the next section of this chapter. RBD is a parasomnia disorder characterized by REM sleep without atonia (RSWA) and dream enactment behaviors. A retrospective study at a tertiary-level sleep center compared RSWA in patients with traditional RBD (idiopathic and secondary to Parkinson's disease), antidepressant-induced RBD, psychiatric patients without RBD (including those untreated and treated with antidepressants), and controls [52]. RSWA was noted to be highest in traditional and antidepressant induced RBD, followed by psychiatric patients treated with antidepressants. RSWA was lowest in untreated psychiatric patients and controls. The authors noted that antidepressant treatment, and not depression, was associated with increased RSWA, even in psychiatric patients without dream enactment behaviors [52].

Sleepwalking is a NREM parasomnia behavior, which has been associated with antidepressant use including amitriptyline, paroxetine, fluoxetine, sertraline, mirtazapine, reboxetine, and bupropion. The exact mechanisms of sleepwalking associated with the use of antidepressants are not completely understood [53]. SRED is a variant of sleepwalking that is characterized by recurrent episodes of eating and drinking during sleep with problematic consequences. Patients with SRED have partial or full amnesia for their eating behavior. The pathophysiologic mechanisms of SRED are unclear, although dopaminergic dysfunction has been implicated [54]. Medications used in treatment of depression may also be associated with SRED. Mirtazapine was associated with SRED in a depressed female and discontinuation of mirtazapine led to a resolution of symptoms [54]. In contrast, melatonergic agents including agomelatine and melatonin have been reported to have beneficial effect in treating SRED in a female depressed patient with panic disorder and sleep apnea [55].

Given the complex interrelationships between sleep disorders and medications, it is critical to obtain a comprehensive history including a detailed chronology of both sleep disturbances and medication use. Polysomnography (PSG) study should be considered if there is a concern for a parasomnia disorder in a patient with depression, whether or not it may be caused or worsened by psychotropic medication use as it would be suggestive of underlying primary sleep disorders such as OSA and periodic limb movement disorder that can mimic or precipitate parasomnia symptoms in patients with depression.

ASSESSMENT

In this section, we summarize the literature on subjective and objective sleep findings associated with depressive disorders, primarily major depression.

Subjective Tests

Standardized screening tools routinely used to assess symptom severity and treatment response in depression include self-report scales such as the Patient Health Questionnaire (PHQ-9) [56] and Beck Depression Inventory (BDI) [57]. Montgomery-Asberg Depression Rating Scale (MADRS) [58], and Hamilton Rating Scale for Depression (HRSD) [59] are clinician-rated scales and may be used for patients experiencing difficulty with self-report instruments. Inventory of Depression Symptomatology (IDS) [60] and Quick Inventory of Depression Symptomatology (QIDS) [61] are alternative depression scales, with both clinician-administered and self-report versions, that include additional specific questions that are more helpful to quantify sleep disturbances such as insomnia, hypersomnolence, and fatigue.

However, these questionnaires may not be adequate for assessment of the severity or the response to treatment for specific sleep disturbances in patients with depression. Additionally, none of the previously mentioned depression scales assess for the presence of nightmares in patients with depression. The Pittsburgh Sleep Quality Index (PSQI), a self-reported measure of sleep behavior and symptoms, can be used in psychiatric settings to assess overall sleep quality and the frequency of nightmares as well [62]. Another self-report screening questionnaire, Insomnia Severity Index (ISI), is a validated tool to assess insomnia severity, patient satisfaction with sleep quality, daytime impairment, and overall distress caused by sleep dysfunction in patients with depression over the past 2 weeks [63]. This scale has seven items that measure insomnia symptom severity on a 5-point scale ranging from zero (not at all) to 4 (very much). A score of 10 on ISI scale

has been reported to be optimal for detection of insomnia with 86.1% sensitivity and 87.7% specificity in a community sample [64].

Epworth Sleepiness Scale (ESS) can be used for assessment of hypersomnolence associated with depression. ESS is a simple, self-administered questionnaire, which measures a person's general level of daytime sleepiness or their average sleep propensity in daily life. The questionnaire is based on retrospective reports of the likelihood of dozing off or falling asleep (0 = not at all; 3 = highly likely) in a variety of different situations with a maximum score of 24. Total ESS scores greater than 10 notably distinguish normal subjects from patients with various sleep disorders including narcolepsy, OSA, and idiopathic hypersomnia [65].

Objective Tests

Multiple sleep procedures have been used to objectively assess sleep disturbances in patients with depression in research settings. Objective electroencephalography (EEG) methods that have been used to measure sleep disturbance in patients with depression include polysomnography (PSG), power spectral (density) analysis, automated analysis of SWA and slow wave counts, measurement of the coherence of EEG rhythms, and topographic analysis using high density EEG (hd-EEG). The multiple sleep latency test (MSLT), another EEG-based sleep test typically used for diagnostic assessment of narcolepsy, has been used for assessment of hypersomnia associated with depression in research studies. Actigraphy is a noninvasive method of monitoring human rest and activity cycles. An actigraph, a device worn on wrist for a period of 1 to 2 weeks, counts the number of limb movements that occur for 1-minute epochs. Periods of relative absence of such movements are interpreted as sleep and periods of high activity as wakefulness. Actigraphy is a valid measure to assess sleep patterns in normal subjects and patients with sleep disorders such as circadian rhythm disorders. Actigraphy has been utilized in multiple studies for objective assessment of sleep quality and physical activity in patients with depression. Key sleep architectural changes in depressive disorders, based on PSG studies, are summarized in Table 17.1.

As compared to controls, patients with depression have altered sleep architecture with slow wave sleep (SWS) and REM sleep abnormalities. A recent meta-analytic study did not report changes in SWS between patients with depression and

TABLE 17.1. KEY POLYSOMNOGRAPHY FINDINGS OBSERVED IN DEPRESSIVE DISORDERS

Depressive Disorders	Polysomnography Findings
MDD	a. Decreased total amount of SWS and abnormal temporal distribution of SWS, reduced SWA, EEG power in the slow wave range (Delta frequency band, 1–4.5 Hz)
	b. Reduced REM latency, longer duration of the first REM sleep, increased percentage of REM sleep, and increased rapid eye movements during REM sleep periods (increased REM density)
MDD with seasonal pattern	a. Decreased sleep efficiency, decreased SWS percentage
	b. Increased REM density but normal REM latency
Persistent depressive disorder	a. Reduction in SWS
	b. No REM sleep abnormalities

Abbreviations: EEG, electroencephalography; MMD, major depressive disorder; SWA, slow-wave activity; SWS, slow-wave sleep; REM, rapid eye movement.

controls after controlling for first night effect for overnight PSG studies, although, the authors did confirm differences in REM sleep parameters in patients with depression [66]. Additionally, unaffected first degree relatives of patients with major depression are noted to have decreased REM latency which suggests a possible genetic link between REM sleep latency and major depression [67]. Further studies suggest increased REM density to be the most specific biological marker of depression [68, 69]. Sub-group analyses for gender reveal more severe sleep disturbances in male as compared to female patients with depression which deserves further research, as this finding may reflect gender differences in biological expression or the severity of depression at the time of presentation [66].

Sleep architectural changes vary across depressive disorders and may normalize with specific treatments. Patients with persistent depressive disorder (dysthymia) demonstrate reduction in SWS as compared to healthy controls [70]. Unlike major depression, REM sleep abnormalities have not been noted in persistent depressive disorder and the sleep architectural changes in these patients are similar to the changes noted in patients with generalized anxiety disorder [71]. Sleep architectural changes in major depression patients with seasonal pattern seem to normalize during summer time and after bright light therapy (BLT) [72].

The objective sleep findings in major depression may have both diagnostic and prognostic implications as well. Evidence suggests that decreased SWA in the first NREM sleep cycle is more commonly seen in atypical than melancholic depression. Studies employing power spectral analysis suggest that an increase in SWA after antidepressant treatment was associated with a greater likelihood of improvement in patients with MDD [73]. Additionally, reduced delta sleep ratio (measured by ratio of SWS counts per minute in the first NREM sleep period over counts in the second NREM period) has been correlated with decreased treatment response and increased likelihood of recurrent episodes of depression [74, 75].

Reduced coherence of EEG rhythms between different cortical regions (a marker of poor functional connectivity) has been noted in patients with depression as compared to healthy controls. Presence of reduced coherence may predict a risk of recurrence in depressed individuals particularly in adolescents and those at a high risk of depression [76, 77].

Despite the numerous studies over the years confirming these objective sleep alterations associated with depression, none of them are consistent enough to be used as a diagnostic test for the presence or absence of depression. Similarly, neither PSG nor actigraphy are clinically indicated to investigate sleep disturbances related to depression, although these diagnostic sleep tests are primarily used to rule out comorbid primary sleep disorders in patients with depression.

MANAGEMENT

In this section, we provide recommendations for management of key sleep disturbances either due to primary sleep disorders comorbid with depression or due to depressive disorders.

Obstructive Sleep Apnea and Major Depression

Patients with OSA present with symptoms of loud and disruptive snoring, poor sleep quality due to frequent arousals, dry mouth upon awakening, early morning headaches, and excessive daytime sleepiness/fatigue. OSA patients can present with mood changes, irritability, and cognitive dysfunction [78]. This constellation of OSA symptoms can be misdiagnosed as depression due to symptom overlap between OSA and depression. Additionally, both of these disorders coexist frequently as it has been noted that one in five patients with OSA are diagnosed with depression, and one in five patients with major depression are diagnosed with OSA [79].

A bidirectional link between the two disorders exists as supported by a large population based study where 6,427 OSA patients and 27,023 patients with depression were longitudinally followed for a period of 15 years, and each group of patients had significantly higher risk of developing the other disorder as compared to the controls [80]. According to a recent study ($n = 700$), the presence of insomnia in men with OSA further increases the prevalence and severity of depression as compared to men with either OSA or insomnia alone [81].

Ong and colleagues [82] reported a higher prevalence of OSA (39%) in patents with comorbid MDD and insomnia. According to this study, the risk factors for OSA included male gender, higher body mass index (BMI) and older age. Another retrospective study reported depression and insomnia severity, in addition to higher BMI, as the risk factors for OSA in 115 patients with unipolar and bipolar depression [83]. Based on MRI findings, OSA patients with elevated depressive symptoms have extensive neural injury especially in specific brain regions including bilateral hippocampi and caudate nuclei, anterior corpus callosum, right anterior thalamus, and medial pons as compared to patients with OSA alone [84].

Management

In a meta-analysis study by Stubbs and colleagues [85], the authors noted that 36.3% of the patients with major depression ($n = 525$) had OSA, as determined by PSG study that confirmed Apnea–Hypopnea Index (AHI) >5/hour. Increasing age and BMI were most significantly correlated with presence of OSA [85]. Understandably, presence of untreated OSA can lead to more severe and prolonged episodes of depression thus

leading to higher rates of treatment resistance [86]. Therefore, screening and treatment of OSA is very important to achieve optimal outcomes in patients with depression. Screening tools for OSA such as STOP-Bang questionnaire have been be used in psychiatric settings [87]. This questionnaire is named for and evaluates eight important risk factors for OSA including: loud snoring, tiredness, observed apneas, high blood pressure, BMI >35, age >50 years, neck circumference >16 inches, and gender (being male). Patients with depression with a high pretest probability for OSA (STOP-Bang questionnaire score equal or >3) should be considered for a referral to a sleep center for further diagnostic evaluation and treatment of possible comorbid OSA.

Hobzova and colleagues [88] investigated the effect of continuous positive airway pressure (CPAP) on depression and cognitive symptoms in patients with severe OSA ($n = 59$), recruited from a sleep center. As compared to the control group, CPAP use was associated with significant improvements in attention, working memory, and depressive symptoms [88]. However, in a meta-analysis by Gupta and colleagues [89], CPAP was shown to have a moderate clinical effect on symptoms of depression in OSA, but was not found to be superior to dental appliances or placebo (sham CPAP). The authors postulated that improvement in subjective symptoms of depression in patients OSA with CPAP use may be mediated by patient expectations and contact with healthcare providers [89]. On the contrary, in another meta-analysis by Povitz and colleagues [90], the authors suggested that treatments for OSA, such as CPAP and mandibular advancement device, may be useful components of treatment of depressive symptoms in individuals with OSA. The authors cited significant heterogeneity between trials and use of depressive symptom scales that have not been validated in OSA patients as study limitations [90]. Additionally, it must be noted that improvements in depression symptoms in OSA patients with CPAP use may take up to 6 months [91].

Limited research has been done to assess the comorbidity of OSA in primary psychiatric populations, especially in the psychiatric inpatient settings. Results from nationwide inpatient sample data showed prevalence of OSA equivalent to 2.24% ($n = 35,625$) in psychiatric inpatients hospitalized with a primary diagnosis of major depression ($n = 1,589,752$) between 2010 and 2014 [92]. As compared to those with major depression alone, patients with comorbid

OSA were noted to have increased length of inpatient stay, increased cost of hospitalization, increased prevalence of medical comorbidities (obesity, hypertension, diabetes mellitus, congestive heart failure, chronic obstructive pulmonary disease), increased morbidity, higher risk of inpatient mortality, and increased disposition to skilled nursing and short-term hospital facilities. Additionally, patients with OSA had significantly higher utilization of ECT, which likely is reflective of nonresponse to standard treatments and greater severity of depression in this group, and significant underutilization of CPAP use during inpatient stay (<5%). More systematic research is warranted to investigate the comorbidity and the effects of treatments for comorbid OSA on mood, sleep, and quality of life in patients with major depression recruited from psychiatric inpatient and outpatient settings.

Restless Legs Syndrome and Major Depression

RLS is a common clinical condition characterized by irresistible urge to move legs while in a resting position (sitting or lying), usually in evening or night time, and it frequently leads to trouble initiating sleep, nonrestorative sleep, and daytime fatigue. Based on epidemiological data, RLS patients have increased odds (OR 2.4) of major depression as compared to healthy controls [93]. Based on findings of a study examining relationship between RLS and depressive symptoms, it is apparent that RLS patients are more likely to endorse somatic symptoms of depression, particularly those related to the sleep disturbance, and not the cognitive symptoms of depression [94]. Additionally, patients with depression tend to have higher prevalence of RLS symptoms.

Probable shared mechanisms that explain the comorbidity of RLS and major depression include dopamine dysfunction, sleep disturbances, and the adverse effects of psychotropic medications. In a study comparing PSG variables among patients with major depression, RLS with depressive symptoms, and RLS alone, it was noted that RLS patients had the most significant sleep disturbances, and the presence of depression symptoms did not deteriorate sleep quality further [95]. Koo and colleagues [96] investigated the association of RLS and depression in a cross-sectional study including male participants (n = 982) with no RLS, mild RLS, and moderate-severe RLS. The authors noted that depression was significantly

associated with moderate-severe RLS versus those with no RLS. Based on the study findings, the authors postulated that this association was mediated by sleep disturbance and severity of periodic limb movements during sleep [96].

Management

The management of comorbid RLS and major depression can often be challenging as serotonergic antidepressants, lithium, and antipsychotics can cause or worsen RLS symptoms. Of note, serotonergic second-generation antidepressants (fluoxetine, paroxetine, citalopram, sertraline, escitalopram, venlafaxine, duloxetine, reboxetine, and mirtazapine) were associated with RLS in 9% of patients in a prospective study. The authors reported that mirtazapine had highest incidence of provoking or deteriorating RLS (28% of patients) whereas reboxetine was the only second-generation antidepressant not associated with RLS. Typically, RLS associated with antidepressants occurred during the initial days of treatment [97]. Nonpharmacological approaches include mental alerting activities, avoiding substances or medication that aggravate RLS, and addressing the possibility of iron deficiency as serum ferritin levels are inversely related to severity of RLS symptoms [98]. Readers are advised to refer to Chapter 14 of this volume on sleep-related movement disorders for detailed pharmacological management of RLS.

Circadian Rhythm Sleep Disorders and Major Depression

CRSDs arise from dysfunction of the circadian clock or misalignment between the timing of the endogenous circadian rhythm and externally imposed social and work cycles [99]. CRSDs manifest as chronic or recurrent sleep wake disturbance and lead to significant functional and mental health impairments. Screening for circadian rhythm disturbances is important during sleep evaluation in depressive disorders as CRSD patients not only present with insomnia, hypersomnia, or both as common sleep complaints, but these patients also have higher depressive comorbidity.

Based on sleep–wake cycles, behavioral patterns, and physiological rhythms, individuals can be described as early chronotypes (preference for morning or "morning larks") or delayed chronotypes (preference for evening or "night owls"). In a study by Chan and colleagues (n = 253) [100], patients with depression with evening type circadian preferences had higher insomnia severity, more depressive symptoms, and higher suicidality. Gaspar-Barba and colleagues [101] reported that, in a cross-sectional study of adults with major depression ($n = 100$), participants with an evening chronotype had more severe suicidal ideation and greater functional impairment relative to those with morning or intermediate chronotypes. Morning chronotypes are those people who consistently prefer diurnal activity, while evening types are those who prefer nocturnal activities and can be assessed using the Horne–Ostberg Morningness–Eveningness Questionnaire [102].

High psychiatric comorbidity has been reported in patients delayed sleep phase disorder (DSPD); a common CRSD characterized by stable delay in sleep onset relative to desired bedtime with resultant insomnia and daytime impairment. Reid and colleagues [103] systematically evaluated the prevalence of *Diagnostic and Statistical Manual of Mental Disorders* (fourth edition; DSM-IV) Axis I disorders in subjects with DSPD and those with an evening type circadian preference. The study findings were significant for a higher risk of anxiety, depressive, and substance use disorders in those with evening type circadian preference with or without formal diagnosis of DSPD. Murray and colleagues [104] compared subjects with circadian DSPD ($n = 103$) and noncircadian DSPD ($n = 79$), based on timing of salivary dim light melatonin onset (DLMO), in terms of mood and daytime functioning. A circadian DSPD phenotype was defined as having a DLMO time at or after desired bed time, while the noncircadian DSPD phenotype was defined as having a DLMO time greater than 30 minutes before desired bed time. The authors noted higher prevalence of moderate-severe depressive symptoms and higher odds of mild depressive symptoms in circadian DSPD group as compared to those with noncircadian DSPD [104]. Additionally, increased prevalence of major depression with seasonal pattern has been reported in patients with DSPD, and these disorders may share a common pathophysiological mechanism leading to delayed circadian phase [105].

Management

Patients with major depression exhibit major alterations in circadian rhythms as compared to nondepressed individuals [106]. For instance, findings such as decreased core body temperature (T-core), cortisol irregularities, sleep architecture abnormalities (REM and SWS), initial insomnia and early morning awakenings, diurnal variation in mood, and diurnal and seasonal variations in suicide rates are reflective of chrono-biological and circadian rhythm alterations in depression. Detailed history of sleep–wake pattern along with use of diagnostic tools such as sleep diary and actigraphy can help establish the diagnosis of coexisting CRSD's in patients with depression. Clinically valid tools such as Morningness–Eveningness Questionnaire (MEQ) [102] and Munich Chronotype Questionnaire (MCTQ) [107] can be useful to determine CRSDs. Readers are advised to refer to Chapter 13 of this volume for detailed management of CRSDs.

Insomnia and Major Depression

The DSM-5 definition of insomnia disorder is comprised of a predominant complaint of dissatisfaction with sleep quantity or quality, associated with one or more specific symptoms including difficulty initiating sleep, difficulty maintaining sleep, and early morning awakening with inability to return to sleep. The sleep difficulty should occur at least three times per week for a period of 3 months or more despite adequate opportunity for sleep for establishing a diagnosis of insomnia. The symptoms of insomnia are not better explained by other primary sleep disorders, physiological effects of substance, and coexisting psychiatric and medical conditions. From an objective perspective, absence of REM sleep abnormalities distinguishes primary insomnia from depression as insomnia patients present with increased SOL and SWS abnormalities similar to depression [18].

A meta-analysis by Baglioni and colleagues [14] suggests that nondepressed individuals with insomnia have a twofold risk of developing depression (OR 2.10, confidence interval [CI] 1.86–2.38) as compared with healthy controls. These results were substantiated by another meta-analysis study including 34 cohort studies ($n = 172,077$) indicating that insomnia is significantly associated with increased risk of depression (pooled relative risk = 2.27; 95 % CI 1.89–2.71) [108]. During acute depressive episodes, insomnia is the most common sleep complaint with trouble initiating sleep (initial insomnia), disrupted sleep (middle insomnia), early morning awakenings (terminal insomnia), and/or nonrestorative sleep. A bidirectional link between insomnia and depression is evident given substantial evidence that each condition predisposes towards the development of other [109].

In a study examining the effect of presleep rumination in patients with moderate-high depressive symptoms, actigraphy monitoring for a period of 1 week was suggestive of longer SOL, and these results were significant even after controlling for baseline sleep disturbance and depressive symptoms [110]. In a large sample (*n* = 711) of patients with depression, PSG-measured prolonged SOL (>30 minutes) has been associated with significantly increased risk of nonremission following pharmacological and/or psychological treatments for depression [111]. In contrast, subjective insomnia complaints alone were not associated with poor treatment outcomes in this study. Not only does insomnia increase the risk of depression and contribute to poor treatment outcomes, but the re-emergence of insomnia can predict the recurrence of a new depressive episode [112], and treatment of insomnia in depression is associated with improved depression outcomes [113].

Management

Insomnia associated with depressive disorders may be treated with psychotherapy, medications, or a combination of these treatment modalities.

Psychotherapy

Cognitive behavioral therapy for insomnia (CBT-I) is now considered the first-line psychotherapeutic intervention for management of primary insomnia [114] and may be preferable to pharmacotherapy for many patients. Treatment outcomes with CBT-I may differ based on the insomnia phenotype. CBT-I may serve as a more effective treatment for patients with insomnia with normal sleep duration and increased cognitive arousal as compared to those with short sleep duration (<6 hours) and physiological arousal. Stimulus control, sleep restriction, and cognitive restructuring are the key components of CBT-I [115].

Stimulus control techniques strengthen the association between sleep and bedroom environment. Patients are advised to go to bed only when sleepy and leave the bed if sleep is not attained within 15 to 20 minutes, in addition to maintaining a strict wake-time and avoiding daytime napping. Another technique, sleep restriction, aims to increase the SE in patients with depression and insomnia. Sleep efficiency is measured by total time slept divided by total time in bed, and a SE of less than 85% is considered abnormal. Patients are advised to limit the amount of time spent in bed and to reduce waking time in bed with goal of increasing the likelihood of sleeping while in bed. Total time in bed is then gradually increased until the desired TST is achieved. Cognitive restructuring techniques can be very helpful to address negative and counterproductive beliefs associated with sleep. Other components of CBT-I include relaxation and sleep hygiene techniques, but these techniques alone are generally not effective without the key CBT-I interventions.

Evidence suggests that CBT-I is efficacious in treatment of insomnia comorbid with depression [116] and also prevents relapse of depression. It is to be noted that individuals with both depression and insomnia may have difficulties adhering to CBT-I treatments, particularly those with severely reduced TST (<3.65 hours of sleep) who are at greatest risk for an early termination of CBT-I. Patients with more severe depression experience more difficulties adhering to a fixed wake-up time and restricting time in bed along with heightened sleep-related cognitive distortions as compared to those who are less depressed. CBT for depression (CBT-D) is an effective treatment that focusses on techniques such as behavioral activation and cognitive restructuring. CBT-D has also been associated with reduction of insomnia symptoms in patients with depression. To improve adherence to CBT-I and target depressive symptomatology, it is recommended to incorporate elements of both CBT-I and CBT-D to achieve optimal outcomes for insomnia treatment in patients who also have depression.

Pharmacological Management

Several medication strategies can be successfully used to resolve insomnia in patients with depression. These strategies include the use of antidepressants alone, the use of low-dose sedating antidepressant or hypnotic medications as adjuncts, and the use of atypical antipsychotic medications.

Antidepressant medications

Insomnia may improve in parallel with other depressive symptoms when patients are treated with standard antidepressant medications (selective serotonin reuptake inhibitors [SSRIs], serotonin-norepinephrine reuptake inhibitors [SNRIs]). However, for many patients, the insomnia is severe enough to be intolerable during the weeks required for an antidepressant effect, or the insomnia may persist despite improvement of other depressive symptoms. Pharmacological management of persistent insomnia in patients with depression can be challenging due to concerns of medication side effects and polypharmacy risks, as well as the refractory nature of insomnia for many. Additionally, some individuals may have a paradoxical response to medications, with worsened insomnia caused by medications that are typically considered sedating, and vice versa, with more stimulating medications. To minimize these concerns, thorough patient education about possible medication effects, and individually tailored medication trials are a critical part of the clinical approach.

Most classes of antidepressant drugs, including SSRIs, SNRIs, norepinephrine reuptake inhibitors (NRI), monoamine oxidase inhibitors (MAOI), and activating tricyclic antidepressants (TCA) may deteriorate sleep quality mainly due to activation of serotonergic 5-HT2 receptors and increased noradrenergic and dopaminergic neurotransmission [117]. On the other hand, antidepressants with antihistaminergic action such as sedating TCAs and mirtazapine or trazodone with antagonistic action at serotonergic 5-HT2 receptors could improve sleep [117]. Based on data from clinical trials, the average prevalence of treatment-emergent insomnia associated with SSRI was 17% as compared to 9% in the placebo arm. On the other hand, the rate of treatment-emergent hypersomnolence with SSRIs was noted to be 16% as compared to 8% in the placebo arm [118]. According to a meta-analysis examining sleep-related side effects of second-generation antidepressants, bupropion, and desvenlafaxine have the highest incidence of insomnia, whereas mirtazapine and fluvoxamine have highest incidence of somnolence [51]. In general, both the sleep-disrupting and sleep-promoting effects of the antidepressants are the strongest in the first few weeks of treatment; however, in some patients these sleep disturbances may persist, thus aggravating insomnia complaints or causing daytime somnolence [119].

In terms of effects on sleep architecture, antidepressants including SSRIs, SNRIs, and activating TCAs increase REM latency, cause suppression of REM sleep, and may impair sleep continuity, whereas sedating antidepressants decrease sleep latency, improve SE, increase SWS, and usually have little or no effect on REM sleep [118, 120, 121]. The effects of antidepressants on REM sleep are probably related to increased synaptic levels of monoamines, due to reuptake blockade, and are likely mediated by 5 HT-1 receptors in REM sleep initiating centers in the brain [121]. REM-suppressant activity was once considered

to be a vital mechanism of antidepressant effectiveness; however, the effectiveness of antidepressants such as bupropion and moclobemide, which increase REM sleep, questions this hypothesis [119, 122]. The effects of antidepressants on SWS are quite diverse as antidepressants having significant 5-HT2A/2C receptor antagonist properties increase SWS, whereas other drugs, such as SSRIs or MAOIs, either decrease SWS or cause no change [122].

The sedating antidepressants can be used either as monotherapy (if tolerated at full therapeutic doses) or as an adjunct to first line antidepressant treatments, such as SSRIs, especially early in the treatment [121]. In clinical practice, sedating antidepressants including mirtazapine, trazodone, and TCAs are often used to treat insomnia in addition to first-line antidepressant treatment; however, this practice has not yet been systematically substantiated and needs further investigation [121]. Clinicians prescribing adjunct sedating antidepressants, especially during the first 6 weeks of primary antidepressant trial, may consider discontinuing them to determine whether the patient's sleep disturbance has responded to the primary antidepressant [123] and to minimize the risk of oversedation in long-term [120]. Consideration of primary sleep disorders such as RLS and RBD must be taken in to account prior to choosing an antidepressant medication to treat insomnia as some of these medications can cause or worsen symptoms of RLS or RBD [118, 121]

Trazodone, an antidepressant with sedative action mainly due to 5-HT2 and alpha1 receptor blockade, is commonly used for management of insomnia in patients with depression [124]. Nirenberg and colleagues [125] investigated the hypnotic effects of trazodone for persistent, exacerbated, or new insomnia in patients with major depression ($n = 17$) who were taking either fluoxetine or bupropion [125]. In this double-blind, placebo-controlled crossover trial, sleep was assessed using PSQI scores and sleep items of Yale–New Haven Hospital Depressive Symptom Inventory. The authors noted that, as compared to placebo, improvements in subjective sleep duration and early morning awakenings were noted in patients taking trazodone. Only one patient dropped out in this study due to excessive daytime sedation associated with trazodone use. In an another placebo-controlled crossover trial ($n = 11$), the authors noted that, as compared to placebo, trazodone (100 mg) use was associated with increase in SE (primary target variable), TST, and SWS, as well as a decrease in early morning awakenings and stage N2. However, no significant changes in REM sleep were noted [126].

Low-dose mirtazapine (7.5–15 mg) at bedtime is another commonly used adjunct medication for management of insomnia in depression. Mirtazapine is a tetracyclic, atypical antidepressant with presynaptic norepinephrine and serotonin releasing properties and antagonistic actions at 5-HT2 and 5-HT3, alpha2-adrenergic, and histamine (H1) receptors [119]. Mirtazapine has a propensity to shorten SOL, improve SE, and increased TST [119]. In an open-label study, Winokur and colleagues [127] used PSG studies at baseline and follow-up to assess the effects of mirtazapine on sleep in patients with major depression (*n* = 6). As compared to baseline, mirtazapine (15–30 mg at bedtime) was associated with significantly decreased sleep latency and significantly increased TST and SE from baseline levels during week 1, with similar results observed after week 2. No significant changes in REM sleep parameters were noted in this study [127]. Mirtazapine is generally well tolerated, but does have possible side effects including daytime sedation, increased appetite, weight gain, and RLS. Worsening of sleep after initiation of mirtazapine should prompt an inquiry for RLS as mirtazapine is among the most likely antidepressants to cause or worsen RLS symptoms [128, 129].

Not all TCAs have favorable effects on sleep as secondary amine tricyclic medications, like desipramine and protriptyline, tend to increase wake after sleep onset (WASO) time and reduce SE [119]. On the other hand, other TCAs (clomipramine, amitriptyline, doxepin) preferentially act upon 5-HT inducing sleep and daytime somnolence [130, 131]. TCAs exert effects on neurotransmitter systems, including blockade of histamine H1, alpha1 adrenergic and muscarinic cholinergic receptors, and may lead to daytime sleepiness [130, 132]. Low-dose doxepin (3–6 mg), US Food and Drug Approval (FDA)-approved treatment for primary insomnia, selectively antagonizes H1 receptors thus promoting the initiation and maintenance of sleep [133]. No systematic evidence is available yet to support the use of low-dose doxepin in treatment of insomnia comorbid with depressive disorders. In general, TCAs can be associated with poor tolerability, due to anticholinergic and cardio-toxic side effects, and must be used with caution in patients with severe depression at a high risk of intentional overdose.

Other antidepressants with a potentially beneficial effect on sleep quality and architecture in patients with depression, but used rarely in clinical practice, deserve a mention here. Nefazodone, a 5-HT2 receptor antagonist, tends to improve sleep quality and maintenance in depression. Manber and colleagues [134] investigated the effects of nefazodone monotherapy (300–600 mg) as compared to psychotherapy (CBT-based) alone and combination therapy (nefazodone + psychotherapy) on mood and subjective sleep outcomes in adult patients with chronic major depression (*n* = 484). The authors noted significant improvements in sleep quality, WASO time, latency to sleep onset, and SE in each of the three treatment groups. However, these improvements occurred earlier in the course of treatment for participants receiving nefazodone, alone or in combination with psychotherapy. Moreover, only monotherapy with nefazodone improved early morning awakening and TST [134]. However, due to rare association with severe liver damage, this medication has largely been withdrawn from markets. Ritanserin, another specific 5-HT2 receptor antagonist, has been shown to increase SWS in healthy subjects and patients with major depression at a single dose of 5 mg daily [135]. Agomelatine, a novel antidepressant, which exerts antidepressant effect by agonism of melatonin receptors (MT1 and MT2) and antagonism of 5 HT2C receptors, has been shown to improve sleep quality and SE with increases in SWS and normalize REM sleep in patients with major depression at doses of 25 to 50 mg daily [136].

Hypnotics. Benzodiazepine receptor agonists (BzRAs) such as zolpidem, zaleplon, and eszopiclone are among the first-line agents for management of primary insomnia and are used increasingly in psychiatric patients. As compared to placebo, the addition of eszopiclone (3 mg) to antidepressant medication (fluoxetine) has been associated with statistically significant improvements in subjective sleep quality, WASO, TST, and SE in patients with depression. The authors noted a faster onset of antidepressant response and a greater magnitude of antidepressant effect with eszopiclone/fluoxetine co-therapy [137]. During 2-week follow-up, improvements in sleep and depression were maintained after stopping eszopiclone with no significant central nervous system or benzodiazepine withdrawal adverse effects [138].

Another multicenter, double-blind, randomized controlled study reported significant improvement in insomnia in MDD patients, taking escitalopram 10 mg/day, with concomitant use of zolpidem-extended release (12.5 mg) as compared to placebo [139]. The authors suggested that improvement in sleep measures was not associated with augmentation of antidepressant response of escitalopram. Asnis et al. [140] reported safe and efficacious use of zolpidem (10 mg) for management of persistent insomnia in patients with depression being treated with SSRIs (fluoxetine, sertraline, paroxetine). As compared to placebo, zolpidem use for a period of 4 weeks was associated with improved sleep quality, longer TST, and improved daytime functioning. Discontinuation of zolpidem led to pretreatment severity of insomnia but no withdrawal side effects.

BzRAs have less of an abuse potential as compared to benzodiazepines, although these medications should still be used with caution in patients with depression who also have a history of substance use disorders. Short-term use is generally recommended in patients with depression even without a history of substance use disorders due to habit forming potential of these drugs. Other side effects that may be concerning are amnesia and complex sleep-related behaviors such as sleep-relating eating disorder, sleepwalking, and sleep driving, particularly with the use of zolpidem [141]. In the United States, the FDA now recommends the use of zolpidem 5 mg (rather than 10 mg) in female patients for management of insomnia due a higher likelihood of adverse events (https://www.fda.gov/drugs/drugsafety/ucm334041.htm).

In a 10-year nationwide population based cohort study from Taiwan, the authors categorized patients with comorbid major depression and insomnia (n = 3,235) in to three groups based on mean dose of hypnotics at baseline. As compared to low and medium dosage patients, those with high dosage of hypnotics were noted to have highest rates of subsequent diagnosis of breathing-related sleep disorder (BRSD) and worse depression outcomes [142]. Therefore, it is important for clinicians to assess for coexisting BRSD in patients with major depression and insomnia both at baseline and at follow-up, especially with the use of high dosage of hypnotics.

Second-generation antipsychotics. Augmentation with second-generation atypical antipsychotics has been increasingly recognized as a treatment option for patients with refractory major depression [143]. Effects of second-generation antipsychotics on sleep architecture and sleep quality have been assessed in some studies of patients with major depression. Pooled data from two randomized placebo controlled studies suggest that adjunct administration of quetiapine extended release (XR; 150 mg/day and 300 mg/day) was associated with significant improvements in depressive symptoms and subjective sleep quality based on MADRS, Hamilton Depression Rating Scale sleep disturbance, and PSQI global scores [144]. Results from a single blind study using adjunctive quetiapine immediate release (100–200 mg/day) in patients with depression (unipolar and bipolar) were not suggestive of improvement in PSQI global scores in the treatment arm [145]. However, in the same study, objective monitoring of sleep with PSG studies at baseline and follow-up showed significant differences in sleep architecture including a decrease in REM sleep and an increase in stage N2 sleep, especially 2 to 4 days after quetiapine treatment [145].

Locklear and colleagues [146] investigated the effects of quetiapine XR monotherapy (flexible dosing 50–300 mg/day) on mood and sleep outcomes in elderly patients with major depression in a randomized double-blind placebo-controlled study. As compared to placebo (n = 173), those receiving quetiapine XR (n = 162) were noted to have significant improvements in mood, quality of life, and subjective sleep quality (measured by PSQI scores) [146]. In a study by Trivedi et al. [147], the authors investigated effects of quetiapine XR monotherapy on mood and sleep in patients with unipolar major depression. Pooled data, corresponding to 6 or 8 weeks of drug (n = 1,117) or placebo (n = 635) administration, were analyzed. The authors concluded that, as compared to placebo, quetiapine XR (50–300 mg/day) monotherapy significantly improved symptoms of subjective sleep disturbance in patients with MDD, including those with either high or low baseline sleep disturbance levels [147].

Another randomized placebo-controlled trial examined the effects of olanzapine augmentation on sleep quality and architecture in patients with major depression. The authors suggested that patients with depression taking olanzapine had significant improvements in terms of secondary outcome measures such as SE, TST, and sleep latency but not the primary outcome (increase in SWS) as measured by PSG studies at baseline and follow-up [148]. As compared to placebo, no significant changes in mood and cognition were noted in patients with depression taking olanzapine. However, in an open-label study of olanzapine augmentation (2.5–10 mg/day) in patients with MDD with unsatisfactory response to therapeutic doses of an SSRI ($n = 12$), the authors noted improvements in subjective sleep quality, improved SE and increased SWS as determined by PSG at baseline, 1 night, and 3 weeks after initiating olanzapine. The authors attributed the increase in SWS to 5-HT (2A/2C) receptor blockade, which has been identified as a relevant mechanism in the therapeutic effect of olanzapine in SSRI-resistant depressed patients [149].

In an open-label trial, the Krystal and colleagues [150] investigated the effects of adjunctive use of brexpiprazole (target dose: 3 mg/day) on sleep disturbances in patients with major depression with inadequate response to standard antidepressant treatment. Sleep parameters were assessed objectively by using PSG study at baseline and at 8 weeks. The ISI and the ESS were used for subjective assessment of insomnia and hypersomnolence respectively. The authors noted significant improvements in objective sleep measures including SOL, WASO, TST, and SE with adjunct brexpiprazole use. Similarly, significant improvements were noted in mood, insomnia, hypersomnolence ,and quality of life, based on subjective rating scales [150].

While prescribing atypical antipsychotics for management of insomnia in patients with major depression, it is important for clinicians to do a thorough risk–benefit analysis and monitor the patients for the emergence of adverse effects including daytime somnolence, akathisia, extrapyramidal symptoms, weight gain, dyslipidemia, and hyperglycemia [143]. Additionally, weight gain caused by antipsychotic medications can also increase the risk of OSA in this population. More recently, weight-independent mechanisms, such as potential effects on upper airway function, have been implicated in worsening of breathing events in patients taking atypical antipsychotics including olanzapine, risperidone and quetiapine [151].

Combination Treatments

CBT-I for management of insomnia has been shown to be effective in improving both insomnia and depressive symptoms. Patients with major depression receiving open-label antidepressant treatment (escitalopram) and CBT-I (seven sessions) had higher rates of remission of both depression and insomnia (61.5% and 50%, respectively) as compared to those receiving escitalopram alone and control therapy (33.3% and 7.7%, respectively) [152]. A randomized controlled trial comparing the effects of CBT-I delivered by a therapist versus self-help CBT-I (written materials only), after 6 weeks of antidepressant treatment in patients with comorbid insomnia and depression, suggests superiority of CBT-I compared to the self-help group. Patients who had received four sessions of CBT-I with a therapist had significantly higher remission rates (61%) for both depression and insomnia as compared to self-help group (5.6%), who received written CBT-I materials only for a period of eight weeks [153]. However, Lancee and colleagues [154] examined the effect of self-help CBT-I on insomnia outcomes in subjects with low ($n = 198$), mild ($n = 182$), and high depression symptoms ($n = 99$). Self-help CBT-I was similarly effective in all the three groups based on sleep outcomes that were assessed at 4 weeks and the improvements were noted to be sustained at 18 weeks posttreatment. The authors suggested that self-help CBT-I is an effective treatment strategy irrespective of depression severity [154].

Carney and colleagues [155] compared the efficacy of combined CBT-I and antidepressant therapy to interventions that targeted either insomnia or depression. Study participants ($n = 107$) were randomized to three categories: antidepressant (escitalopram) + CBT-I (four sessions), CBT-I + placebo, or antidepressant + four-session sleep hygiene control. Sleep diaries were used to monitor subjective sleep quality, and overnight PSG was done at baseline and posttreatment for objective sleep assessment. All the groups improved on subjective sleep measures, but only the CBT-I groups improved on objective sleep measures, and the AD + sleep hygiene group worsened in terms of objective sleep posttreatment. All the groups, including CBT-I + placebo, improved in terms of depression severity, which suggests antidepressant properties of CBT-I, an area that needs further investigation [155]. Overall, CBT-I has been noted to have small to medium effect in terms of improving depression symptomatology based on a systematic review of studies examining the impact of CBT-I on depression [156].

Hypersomnolence and Major Depression

The DSM-5 definition of hypersomnolence disorder includes self-reported excessive sleepiness despite a main sleep period lasting at least 7 hours, with at least one of the following symptoms:

1. Recurrent lapses of sleep or lapses into sleep during the same day.
2. A prolonged main sleep episode of more than 9 hours per day that is non restorative.
3. Difficulty being fully awake after abrupt awakening.

The hypersomnolence symptoms occur at least three times per week, for at least 3 months, and these symptoms are not attributable another primary sleep disorder (e.g., breathing related sleep disorder, narcolepsy, circadian rhythm sleep-wake disorder, or a parasomnia disorder), physiological effects of a substance (e.g., a drug of abuse, a medication), and coexisting mental and medical disorders. Hypersomnolence has been associated with an increased risk of incident depression in prospective studies such that individuals with hypersomnolence have higher odds (OR 2.46–2.91) of developing subsequent major depressive episode [12]. Hypersomnolence is considered as a highly treatment-resistant symptom that increases the risk of relapse [7] and the risk of suicide in patients with depression [157].

Patients with depression and hypersomnolence often present with long sleep time, sleep inertia, and excessive daytime sleepiness with long nonrefreshing naps. The objective findings of MSLT for evaluation of hypersomnolence in depressive disorders have been inconsistent [158, 159]. These findings suggest that MSLT is likely not particularly useful to assess hypersomnolence in mood disorders, as majority of these patients may not demonstrate a pathologic SOL on MSLT [160]. However, as compared to healthy controls, patients with depression and co-occurring hypersomnolence demonstrate significantly greater total sleep duration measured objectively using both *ad libitum* PSG and actigraphy [161]. These results have been corroborated by prior studies that suggest patients with co-occurring mood disorders and hypersomnolence may demonstrate increased sleep duration when measured by actigraphy measures [162, 163].

Prevalence estimates of hypersomnolence in major depression vary widely across ages and studies. Hypersomnolence has been reported amongst 10% to 20% of patients with major depression and up to 36.2% of the patients with atypical depressive features may complain of hypersomnolence

[164]. Additionally, females and younger patients with major depression seem to have higher prevalence of hypersomnolence [165]. Moreover, in a survey-based study of 201 opposite-sex twin pairs, female patients with depression reported significantly more hypersomnolence as compared to males, who endorsed more insomnia during depressive episodes [166]. In adults with depression with nonmelancholic features, hypersomnolence was reported to be more common than early morning awakening (terminal insomnia) [167]. Co-occurring insomnia and hypersomnolence symptoms, in patients with a major depressive episode within the past year, were more frequently observed in those with bipolar spectrum disorder or major depression with persistent depressive disorder ("double depression") [168].

As compared to insomnia, there has been little research to elucidate the role of biomarkers in hypersomnolence associated with major depression. Hypocretin-independent hypothalamic dysfunction has been implicated in hypersomnolence observed in patients with depression [163]. The results of Treatment with Exercise Augmentation for Depression (TREAD) trial indicate a relationship between changes in inflammatory and neurotrophic biomarkers and changes in hypersomnia, and not insomnia, in non-remitted MDD patients. Specifically, reductions in BDNF and IL-1β were correlated with reductions in hypersomnia in MDD patients in this study [169]. Evidence suggests that, in contrast to melancholic depression, patients with atypical depression may have reduced function of HPA axis [170]. Additionally, overactivity of the HPA axis in melancholic depression is associated with decreased BDNF levels [171]. Therefore, it is plausible that improvement in hypersomnia symptoms in atypical depression is associated with reduction in BDNF as evident by results of TREAD trial [169].

Management

Despite the reported treatment refractory nature of hypersomnolence and fatigue in patients with depression, much less research has been done on this topic. Similar to insomnia, treatment of hypersomnolence and fatigue may favorably impact depression outcomes [172]. To date, there are no pharmacological drugs that have been approved to manage hypersomnolence and fatigue in depressive disorders [160]. General principles of management include avoidance of sedating psychotropic medications and considering antidepressants with noradrenergic action due to favorable effects on the wake drive. "Alerting" antidepressants such as SSRIs, SNRIs, and bupropion may be considered for patients presenting with depression and complaints of hypersomnolence.

Bupropion has been noted to have greater efficacy in resolution of hypersomnolence and fatigue in patients with depression as compared to SSRIs and placebo based on pooled data from multiple double-blind randomized controlled trials [173]. Wake-promoting agents such as modafinil and armodafinil, which are FDA-approved for treatment of hypersomnolence associated with OSA, shift work disorder, and narcolepsy, have gained attention for management of hypersomnolence in mood disorders [160]. Modafinil is usually well tolerated with a low abuse potential as compared to conventional psychostimulants. Several open label studies have suggested efficacy of modafinil use in treatment of hypersomnolence and fatigue in depression. Two placebo-controlled trials failed to show improvement in hypersomnolence, fatigue, and depression severity with the use of modafinil as an adjunct to SSRI therapy for major depression. Pooled data from five studies included in a secondary endpoint analysis also suggested a lack of efficacy of modafinil and armodafinil to improve hypersomnolence in mood disorder patients [174].

Nightmares and Major Depression

The DSM-5 definition of nightmare disorder includes repeated occurrences of extended, extremely dysphoric, and well-remembered dreams that usually involve efforts to avoid threats to survival, security, or physical integrity and that generally occur during the second half of the major sleep episode. The individual rapidly becomes alert and oriented upon awakening from the dysphoric dreams. The resulting sleep disturbance causes clinically significant distress or impairment in social, occupational, or other areas of functioning. The nightmare symptoms are not attributable to the physiological effects of substances or coexisting mental and medical disorders.

Risk factors for nightmares in general adult population were examined in a cross-sectional population based survey [175]. The risk factors for nightmares include a depression-related negative attitude toward the self (OR 1.32 per 1-point increase), insomnia (OR 6.90), exhaustion, and fatigue (OR 6.86, $p < 0.001$ for all). Other risk factors including female sex, age, a self-reported

impaired ability to work, low life satisfaction, the use of antidepressants or hypnotics, and frequent heavy use of alcohol were also strongly associated with frequent nightmares ($p < 0.001$ for all) [175].

In another cross-sectional study ($n = 2,822$), nightmares occurred more frequently in individuals with insomnia as compared to those without insomnia. Nightmare frequency was assessed using an item for nightmares on the PSQI. Multiple regression analyses revealed that both nightmares and insomnia were associated with an increase in depression scores as measured by a 12-item version of the Center for Epidemiological Studies Depression scale (CES-D). Individuals with comorbid insomnia and nightmares had higher depression scores as compared to those with insomnia or nightmares alone. The authors concluded that insomnia and nightmares worsened the depression both independently and additively [176].

Nightmares have been reported more frequently in patients with melancholic depression, as compared to those without melancholic features, and depressed mood in the morning in these patients may be related to negative dream content [177]. Additionally, increased rates of nightmares and middle and terminal insomnia have been reported in melancholic patients who attempted suicide as compared to nonattempters with melancholia [178]. Despite the significant association of nightmares with a higher risk of suicide, the routinely used clinical scales for assessment of depression do not specifically query the presence of disturbing dreams or nightmares which may result in underestimation of the overall severity of sleep disturbance and possibly suicide risk in patients with depression.

Management

There seems to be lack of systematic research focusing on treatment of nightmares associated with depressive disorders. It is prudent to rule out iatrogenic causes of nightmares as the use of commonly prescribed medications including antidepressants, melatonin, nicotine supplements, and beta-blockers can be associated with nightmares [179]. Additionally, alcohol and illicit drug use or withdrawal can lead to nightmares as well [175]. Management strategies, derived mainly from the posttraumatic stress disorder (PTSD) literature, include medications (prazosin; dose: 1–16 mg), imagery rehearsal therapy, and exposure, relaxation, and rescripting therapy (ERRT) can be utilized for treatment of nightmares but their utilization in depressive disorders is not clear [180–182].

Sleep Therapies as Treatment of Major Depression

Disturbances in circadian rhythms play an important role in pathogenesis of mood disorders. Chronotherapy is based on a controlled exposure to environmental stimuli, which aims to normalize the disturbed biorhythms thus leading to therapeutic efficacy in treatment of depression [183]. The common chronotherapeutic modalities used in treatment of major depression include sleep deprivation, BLT, and sleep phase advance (SPA) therapy.

Sleep Deprivation

Several studies show positive effects of sleep deprivation in reducing symptoms of depression. Total sleep deprivation (TSD) may be particularly effective in patients with melancholic depression as compared to those with atypical and seasonal depression. Evidence suggests that neural changes identified in depression, including increased metabolism in the amygdala, orbital prefrontal gyrus, inferior temporal, and anterior cingulate cortices, normalize after a night of TSD in TSD responders [184]. One of the most rapid and effective treatments for depression, a single night of TSD, can be associated with improvement in depression in 50% of the patients with depression by the next day. However, the beneficial effects of TSD are not sustainable and tend to dissipate after recovery sleep, whether naps or nocturnal sleep.

Partial sleep deprivation (PSD), including deprivation of either REM sleep or SWS has not been shown to be as effective as TSD and is associated with mild-to-moderate improvements in depression. It is difficult to determine the component of TSD that is associated with therapeutic effects, since neither partial deprivation of NREM or REM sleep have equal efficacy, and since there are likely complex interrelationships between these sleep parameters [185]. Gradual rather than acute improvements tend to be associated with PSD and the effects may be sustainable for a longer period than TSD, although the improvement in depression diminishes after discontinuation of PSD therapy. Sleep deprivation therapies still remain experimental for regular clinical use, and more research is warranted to both understand the mechanism of action and how to implement these treatments into standard clinical practice.

Bright Light Therapy

BLT has been shown to be effective treatment of both seasonal and nonseasonal depression with effect sizes of 0.84 and 0.53, respectively [186]. The standard treatment requisites for BLT therapy include light intensities of 5,000 to 10,000 lux (measured at the level of the eyes) and a therapeutic distance of 60 to 80 cm from the light box. Morning treatments are recommended to enhance daytime wakefulness and to not exacerbate insomnia. Treatment is usually started with a dose of 30 minutes using a light intensity of 10,000 lux, and the duration of treatment can be extended in case of insufficient response [187].

The exact mechanism of action of BLT is unclear, although the chronobiological effects of BLT on the autonomic nervous system, with a potential to restore sympatho-vagal balance, seem to be the key to the antidepressant properties of BLT. Despite beneficial effects and remarkable safety profile of BLT, it seems to be underutilized for management of nonseasonal major depression [188]. Better response to chrono-therapeutic interventions has been reported in patients with depression who have a delayed chronotype and diurnal variation in mood [28]. Fritzsche and colleagues [189] demonstrated that a prior positive response to TSD could predict a beneficial outcome with BLT in patients with major depression [189]. In depressed youth, short-term improvements in sleep including longer sleep durations, advanced sleep onset, less time awake during night, and an improved SE have been reported in those receiving BLT and sleep deprivation (1 night), as compared to BLT alone [190].

In a double-blind, randomized placebo-controlled trial, Lieverse and colleagues [191] investigated the effects of BLT in elderly patients (>60 years) with major depression ($n = 89$). As compared to placebo (red light, 50 lux), early morning BLT (pale blue light, 7,500 lux) for 1 hour over a period of 3 weeks improved mood and enhanced SE. Additionally, BLT produced continuing improvement in mood and an attenuation of cortisol hyperexcretion even after discontinuation of treatment [191]. In another study, as compared to controls, beneficial effects of morning BLT (1 hour) were noted in terms of improved mood and decreased subjective sleepiness in major depression patients ($n = 13$) with seasonal pattern [192].

Sleep Phase Advance

Major depression is associated with phase delay due to chronobiological alterations in patients with depression [193]. SPA is a chronotherapy that has been primarily used to augment and sustain the effects of TSD and/or BLT in patients with depression [194]. As compared to sleep phase delay, it has been shown that the clinical effectiveness of TSD can be significantly improved in combination with SPA (time in bed scheduled from 5 PM–12 AM) [195, 196]. Additionally, combined chronotherapy (including TSD, BLT, and SPA) has been noted to be effective in improving clinical outcomes in patients with drug-refractory major depression (*n* = 13) in an open-label trial [194].

Chronotherapy and Medications

Both partial and TSD are known to potentiate the effects of SSRIs and tricyclic antidepressants [197]. In a 9-week randomized trial comparing chronotherapeutic interventions, (including sleep deprivation, BLT, and sleep time stabilization) to exercise in major depression patients treated with duloxetine (*n* = 75), the authors noted that both groups responded well to treatment. However, patients treated with chronotherapeutic interventions had an augmented and sustained antidepressant response and remission as compared to patients treated with exercise [198]. BLT is generally well tolerated; however, in a different study, BLT as an adjunct to trimipramine resulted in persistent restlessness, sleep disturbance, increased sedation, and decreased appetite in comparison to trimipramine therapy alone for major depression [199]. Triple chronotherapy including 1 night of TSD, followed by a 3-night SPA along with four sessions of 30-minute BLT has shown to cause rapid and sustained improvement in patients with depression and suicidal ideations in a small open-label pilot study. Six out of 10 patients (60%) achieved remission in 5 days of trial of triple chronotherapy as an adjunct to medication treatment [200]. More research is needed with larger numbers of subjects randomized to active or control treatments to confirm efficacy of this intervention.

SLEEP AND SOMATIC TREATMENTS FOR MAJOR DEPRESSION

Ketamine

Ketamine is gaining popularity as a fast-acting antidepressant, and it has been shown to induce sleep changes such as increased early night SWA as well as high-amplitude slow waves. These slow-wave changes are limited to the first night post ketamine infusion, although sleep changes such as decreased wake time and increased TST have been observed during the first and second night post infusion [201]. Additionally, concomitant increase in SWA (marker of central synaptic plasticity) and BDNF (peripheral marker of plasticity) has been associated with response to ketamine treatment in patients with treatment resistant major depression in another study [42].

Electroconvulsive Therapy (ECT)

Despite established efficacy of ECT in management of treatment refractory depression, there exists limited evidence of its effects on sleep disturbance in depression. One of the studies using PSG to compare REM latency before and after ECT suggested an increase in REM latency in patients with depression (*n* = 11). However, individuals showed significant variability in REM latency both during and after ECT, and the majority of the responders continued to have shortened REM latencies [202]. Findings from another study comparing ECT responders and nonresponders, using PSG studies pre- and post-ECT, were significant for association of sleep-onset REM periods with poor response to ECT [203]. ECT has not been associated with short-term changes in subjective and actigraphy-assessed sleep in patients with depression who were also noted to have profoundly underestimated their sleep duration [204]. Use of actigraphy to assess sleep and physical activity has been reported in patients with treatment-resistant depression undergoing electro-convulsive therapy (ECT) [205]. Improvements in physical activity rather than sleep were noted with the use of actigraphy despite significant improvements in depression after ECT treatments.

Repetitive Transcranial Magnetic Stimulation (rTMS)

Similar to pharmacological and ECT treatment for major depression, rTMS has been associated with improvements in REM sleep architectural changes, characteristic of major depression, with increase in REM sleep latency and prolongation of NREM–REM cycle length [206]. In healthy young adults receiving two sessions (sham and experimental treatment) of high-frequency rTMS applied to left dorsolateral prefrontal cortex (DLPFC), there was a decrease in stage N1 and a small enhancement in stage N3 during the first episode of NREM sleep [207]. In an open-label study, localized potentiation of slow-wave changes has been reported in patients with treatment resistant depression receiving high frequency rTMS over the DLPFC for 10 sessions. The authors hypothesized that localized increases in SWS may reflect locally enhanced neuroplasticity induced by rTMS [208]. An open-label study using actigraphy in patients with medication-resistant major depression (n = 14) showed that bilateral rTMS treatments involving DLPFC were associated with subjective improvements in sleep quality and mood but not in objective sleep measures [209]. The authors suggest future double blind sham-controlled studies to elucidate the effects of rTMS on sleep–wake cycle and sleep disturbance in major depression.

Vagal Nerve Stimulation (VNS)

In a study examining sleep architecture at baseline and 10 to 12 weeks follow-up in patients with treatment refractory depression (n = 7), VNS has been associated with improvements in depression symptoms and sleep architecture including decreased stage N1, increased stage N2, and decreased awake time. Additionally, the strength or amplitude of ultradian EEG rhythms was restored to normal range after VNS surgery [210]. However, VNS can cause increase in respiratory rate, decrease in respiratory amplitude, decrease in tidal volume, and decrease in oxygen saturation during periods of device activation. VNS stimulation has been associated with worsening of sleep apnea and can cause central and obstructive breathing events that may respond to adjustments in the VNS settings or using treatment modalities such as CPAP [211]. Patients with treatment refractory depression, undergoing VNS treatment, should be enquired about any such untoward sleep-related effects for timely and effective management.

Deep Brain Stimulation (DBS)

Deep brain stimulation (DBS) has been considered as an experimental treatment for management of treatment refractory depression. As compared to DBS responders, resting state EEG data in DBS nonresponders shows hemispheric EEG power asymmetry characterized by increased frontal theta waves in the right hemisphere and an increase in parietal synchronization in the left hemisphere [212]. The authors view these significant differences in DBS responders as a marker of treatment efficacy of DBS in major depression. Future studies investigating the efficacy of DBS should focus on the impact of DBS on comorbid sleep disturbances and sleep-related EEG parameters as additional indicators of clinical response in treatment-refractory depression.

SLEEP AND SUICIDE

Suicide is the tenth leading cause of death in the United States overall, and the suicide rates have been rising steadily in recent years. In 2016, suicide became the second most prevalent cause of death in those aged 10 to 34, and the fourth most prevalent for ages 35 to 54. In 2016 (the last year of data available from the Centers for Disease Control), there were 45,000 deaths by suicide in the United States, more than double the number of homicides in that year. Among multiple suicide risk factors, prior suicide attempts, age, ethnicity, and gender are nonmodifiable. On the other hand, many risk factors are potentially modifiable, including current depressive symptoms, drug and alcohol abuse, social isolation, psychological stress, and hopelessness. Additionally, recent and emerging evidence reliably identifies sleep disturbance as a modifiable risk factor for suicidal ideation, suicide attempts, and suicide [213].

Findings from a meta-analysis indicate that that sleep disturbance is associated with increased risk for suicidal ideation, suicide attempts and death by suicide (risk ratio = 2.79, 95% CI = 2.44–3.19). Depression did not seem to moderate the association between sleep and suicide variables, and this infers that there is an association of insomnia and suicide risk independent of depression [214]. These findings have been replicated in a systematic review by Bernert and colleagues [215] such that poor sleep quality, insomnia, and nightmares were noted to be independent and significant risk factors for increased risk of suicidal ideations, suicide attempts, and death by suicide. In another systematic review examining the association of sleep disturbances and suicidal behaviors in psychiatric patients, the authors noted that patients with psychiatric diagnoses and comorbid sleep disturbances were significantly more likely to report suicidal behaviors as compared to those without sleep disturbance (OR = 1.99, 95% CI 1.72, 2.30, p <0.001) [216]. This association was noted across several psychiatric conditions including depression (OR = 3.05, 95% CI 2.07, 4.48, p < 0.001), PTSD (OR = 2.56, 95% CI 1.91, 3.43, p <0.001), panic disorder (OR = 3.22, 95% CI 1.09, 9.45, p = 0.03), and schizophrenia (OR = 12.66, 95% CI 1.40, 114.44, p = 0.02) [216].

In the following section, we summarize the neurobiological mechanisms underlying the association of sleep and suicide, and discuss primary sleep disorders as potential and modifiable risk factors for suicidal thoughts, behaviors, and attempts.

Neurobiology

Serotonin (5-HT) is the key mediator in the regulation of sleep, and it has an intricate role in the regulation and maintenance of sleep [217]. Notably, the release of serotonin appears to be highest during waking states, reduced during SWS, and lowest during REM sleep [218]. Changes in sleep pattern could alter the dynamics of 5-HT as evident in a study conducted in rodents that showed chronic sleep deprivation causes gradual and persistent desensitization of the (5-HT) 1A receptor system [219], and this effect persisted despite unlimited time for sleep recovery. This serotonin desensitization was paralleled by blunted HPA axis stress reaction resulting in decreased pituitary cortisol response [220]. In humans, an in vivo study of cerebral serotonin receptors showed that sleep deprivation for as little as 24 hours duration induces global molecular alterations in the cortical serotonergic receptor system thereby leading to significant increase in the 5-HT 2A receptor binding potential [221].

Serotonergic dysregulation appears to play an important role in suicide risk. Low cerebrospinal fluid levels of serotonin's main metabolite, 5-Hydroxyindoleacetic acid (5-HIAA) have been consistently observed after death by suicide, and this finding predicts future attempts in suicide attempters [222]. Furthermore, PET studies have shown that patients with major depression who attempt suicide have lower midbrain serotonin transporter binding as compared to individuals with major depression lacking any past history of suicide attempts [223]. Therefore, low levels of 5-HT appears to be a marker of impulsivity and decreased decision-making skills, thus increasing the suicide risk. Serotonergic dysfunction in the prefrontal cortex is associated with poor decision-making and executive dysfunction, which in presence of comorbid insomnia and sleep reduction results in further increased risk of suicide [224].

Another important mechanism that shows the relationship between sleep and suicide is HPA axis dysfunction [225]. Cortisol release is a potential biomarker of suicide risk and particularly in the setting of a stress-related suicide. Stress activates the HPA axis system, which in turn releases a cascade of hormones including CRH, adrenocorticotropic hormone, and cortisol. Sleep deprivation also leads to changes in HPA axis that increases an individual's susceptibility to hyperarousal, alterations in REM sleep, and subsequent suicidal behavior [225].

The circadian drive for sleep may also be associated with suicide risk. A study investigating the timing of suicide deaths suggests that a 24-hour rhythm exists for the timing of suicide deaths, suggesting a connection to circadian rhythms. For all ages, there was a peak in deaths in the morning hours. This pattern varied by age, however, with a peak for older adults (>45 years old) in the morning, and for younger people (<25 years old), suicide deaths peak mostly in the evening [226]. Further research will be needed to confirm this pattern and to begin to unravel the neurobiological links between circadian regulation and suicide and depression. Dysregulation of several biomarkers like serotonin, melatonin, and cortisol have also been implicated in suicide circadian variations and a role of chronotherapeutics has been suggested in the reduction of suicidal behaviors [227]. Abnormalities of CLOCK gene expression may also be associated with an increased suicide risk. Scquiera and colleagues [228] reported a significant down-regulation in *per1*, one of the CLOCK genes, in the dorsolateral prefrontal cortex in deaths by suicide as compared to nonsuicide deaths in patients with depression [228].

Primary Sleep Disorders and Suicide
Insomnia

Although depression is a major risk factor for suicide, poor sleep quality independently increases the risk for suicide by 34% [229]. A longitudinal research study conducted among a large group of elderly subjects concluded that poor self-reported sleep quality at the study onset was associated with an increased risk of death by suicide during the 10-year follow-up period [230]. A similar study conducted in Japan in middle-aged adults concluded that the presence of any type of insomnia (initial, middle, or terminal) predicted a significantly increased risk of death by suicide 14 years later [231]. In both of these studies, the presence of depression was not a required criterion when examining the association between sleep and suicide deaths, strengthening the independent association of insomnia and suicide risk. CBT-I has been found to be an effective treatment option for significantly reducing suicidal ideation in a veteran population with insomnia, and the result was independent of changes in depressive symptom severity [232].

The individuals with chronic insomnia presumably become more hopeless about their sleep duration and the negative cognitions that follow it and hence are more likely to report suicidal ideations than individuals without insomnia [233]. Hopelessness is one of the strongest psychological risk factors for suicidal ideation and possibly attempts. A longitudinal study suggested that hopelessness contributed to suicidal ideation and was predictive of suicide attempts during a 10-year follow up period, even after controlling for a history of prior suicide attempts [234]. However, another study from the same group demonstrated a clear link between hopelessness and suicidal ideation but did not predict suicide attempts during the follow-up period [235].

Hopelessness is defined as pessimism or a "system of negative expectations" regarding oneself and one's future life [236]. It has also been shown to mediate the relationship between other suicide risk factors such as rumination, traumatic childhood, stress, depression, and suicidality [237]. It is an independent factor that distinguishes between depressive individuals with suicidal ideations and depressive individuals without suicidal ideations [238]. There are cognitive aspects of chronic insomnia with pessimistic connotation such as "When I don't get the proper amount of sleep on a given night, I need to catch up the next day by napping or the next night by sleeping longer" and "I need 8 hours of sleep to feel refreshed and function well during the day." These common misperceptions and pessimistic cognitions about sleep in patients with chronic insomnia can be rated using Dysfunctional Beliefs and Attitudes about Sleep (DBAS) scale [239, 240]. In a prospective study including 50 individuals with depressive disorders, the authors found that dysfunctional beliefs about sleep, evaluated with the DBAS, correlated to the intensity of suicidal ideation, as did the presence and severity of insomnia symptoms [241].

Nightmares

Research also suggests that patients with depression who self-report repetitive and frightening dreams are more likely to be suicidal when compared to those without frequent nightmares [242]. A prospective, population-based study was conducted in Finland to determine if there was an association between nightmare frequency at baseline and suicide deaths at follow-up, 14 years later [243]. The results indicated that subjects reporting occasional nightmares were 57% more likely to die by suicide when compared with subjects with no nightmares, and in those with frequent nightmares, the risk of suicide increased even more dramatically to 105% when compared to those without frightening dreams. Nadroff and colleagues [244] have reported that duration of nightmares and insomnia is associated with suicide risk independent of current insomnia symptoms or nightmares, anxiety symptoms, depressive symptoms, and PTSD symptoms.

Sleep Apnea

Several studies were done to assess the relationship between sleep apnea and suicide planning and attempts, in addition to suicidal ideation. One of the studies proposed that repeated arousals during sleep due to sleep-related breathing events may contribute to worsening of suicidality through the fragmentation of sleep and reduction of sleep quality [245]. Furthermore, chronic deprivation and disruption of sleep can significantly impact mental and physical energy and may potentially inhibit one's ability to efficiently cope with the stressors or existing mental health difficulties. Also, sleep apnea has been linked to the development of multiple general medical and psychiatric comorbidities (cardiovascular, pulmonary diseases, depression) that not only contribute to decreased quality of life but are independently associated with increased suicide risk [246].

CONCLUSIONS

Sleep disturbances are commonly present in depressive disorders and manifest as insomnia, poor sleep quality, nightmares, and hypersomnia/fatigue. Reduced SWS, decreased REM latency, and increased REM density are the most specific findings noted in major depression. Presence of untreated sleep disturbances not only pose a significant risk for new-onset major depression but also complicate the clinical course and prognosis thereby resulting in poor treatment response and increased risk of depressive relapse. Sleep disturbance, independent of depression severity, has been shown to be a potentially modifiable risk factor for suicide. Emerging evidence suggests that there are common neurobiological mechanisms underlying development of sleep and mood disturbances in major depression. Primary sleep disorders such as OSA, RLS, and circadian rhythm disorders not only increase the risk of depression but also complicate the treatment of depression.

It is imperative to comprehensively assess and treat sleep disturbances, either comorbid with depression or due to coexisting primary sleep disorders, to optimize remission, prevent relapse and reduce the risk of suicide in patients with depressive disorders. Medications, chronotherapies, and behavioral approaches, alone or in combination, may prove to be effective in treating sleep disturbances comorbid with depressive disorders. CBT-I is an effective treatment for insomnia in patients with depression and can be used in combination with antidepressant medications to achieve optimal outcomes in patients with depression. Despite their frequent prevalence and association with poorer prognosis for depression treatment, there is limited evidence guiding the treatment of nightmares and hypersomnia in depressive disorders.

FUTURE DIRECTIONS

The negative impact of sleep disturbances on depression outcomes is substantial but continues to present a timely opportunity to develop clinical strategies and research methodologies to adequately address this common and problematic comorbidity. At a clinical level, there needs to be a greater emphasis on training clinicians as behavioral sleep medicine specialists and providing easier access to sleep medicine services for optimal treatment of primary sleep disorders such as OSA. Optimal treatment of sleep disturbances should be viewed as an effective intervention in improving treatment outcomes in depressive disorders and a potential opportunity to prevent suicide. Greater utilization of standardized subjective tools and objective sleep measures, substantiated by research methodologies and unique to psychiatric patients, is needed for sleep assessment and measurement of treatment outcomes in depression. CBT-I, a promising treatment for management of insomnia comorbid with depression, needs wider implementation and more research to establish its efficacy in preventing suicide. Similarly, there needs to be a greater focus on the evaluation and management of nightmares, hypersomnia, and fatigue associated with depressive disorders to develop evidence-based strategies to improve clinical and safety outcomes.

KEY CLINICAL PEARLS

- Presence of sleep disturbances in depressive disorders is associated with increased depression severity, poor response to treatment, greater risk of relapse, and even suicide.
- A bidirectional link exists between sleep and depression due to shared neurobiological mechanisms.
- Sleep architectural changes in major depression include decreased SWS, decreased REM sleep latency, and increased REM density.
- Primary sleep disorders including OSA, RLS, and circadian rhythm disorders frequently co-exist with depression, and these disorders can mimic or worsen depressive symptoms.
- Untreated OSA can lead to treatment resistance in patients with depression, and optimal recognition and treatment of OSA can improve depression outcomes.
- Antidepressant medications can cause or worsen primary sleep disorders such as RLS, NREM and REM parasomnia behaviors.
- CBT-I is an effective treatment of insomnia comorbid with major depression.

CASE ILLUSTRATION

A 65-year-old male presented for the evaluation and management of chronic depression. He has multiple failed antidepressant medication trials for treatment of depression. He reported an unsuccessful trial of CBT for the management of depression. He denied any history suggestive of bipolar disorder or psychotic symptoms. He denied any history suggestive of anxiety disorders and PTSD. He denies any prior psychiatric hospitalization or suicide attempts. There was no history suggestive of alcohol and substance use disorders. His depression was partially treated with imipramine 75 mg at bedtime. He complained of poor sleep and feeling tired and unmotivated during the day. He reported a history suggestive of loud snoring. Medical history was suggestive of morbid obesity (BMI >35) and hypertension. Imipramine level was done and it was noted to be in therapeutic range. STOP-BANG screening questionnaire was suggestive of high pretest probability for OSA. A PSG study was ordered and findings were suggestive of moderately severe OSA. The patient noted significant improvements in mood, sleep quality, daytime functioning, and energy levels after initiation of CPAP therapy for OSA in conjunction with imipramine for treatment of depression.

Key Point

Consider diagnostic sleep testing in medication-refractory patients with depression who are at a high pretest probability of OSA.

SELF-ASSESSMENT QUESTIONS

1. Major depression is associated with all of the following sleep architectural changes *except*
   a. decreased REM latency.
   b. increased slow wave sleep.
   c. increased REM density.
   d. increased sleep onset latency.

Answer: b

2. A 52-year-old obese male presents for evaluation of depression with excessive daytime sleepiness and fatigue as his main complaints. He reports unrefreshing sleep with dry mouth and early morning headaches. He has been prescribed Sertraline 100 mg daily by his primary care physician for treatment of depression. He also takes Lisinopril for management of hypertension. He denies substance abuse issues. What is the next best step in management?
   a. Increase the dose of Sertraline.
   b. Add Bupropion.
   c. Refer for psychotherapy.
   d. Consider testing for sleep apnea.

Answer: d

3. A 40-year-old female with a history of RLS presents for evaluation and treatment of comorbid major depression. Which of the following antidepressants prescribed for depression management is least likely to worsen symptoms of RLS in this patient?
   a. Mirtazapine
   b. Fluoxetine
   c. Bupropion
   d. Venlafaxine

Answer: c

4. A 68-year-old male presents for evaluation of sleep complaints characterized by recurrent episodes of acting violently in his dreams leading to self-injury and accidentally hitting his wife. He remembers being attacked in his dreams. His antidepressant dose was recently increased for optimal management of major depression. He has served in the military in the past but denies any combat situations. His partner denies that he snores or loses consciousness during these episodes. Which of the following is the most likely diagnosis?
   a. Posttraumatic stress disorder
   b. REM sleep behavior disorder
   c. Seizures
   d. Nocturnal panic attacks

Answer: b

5. Which of the following techniques is least effective for management of insomnia?
   a. Sleep hygiene
   b. Sleep restriction
   c. Stimulus control
   d. Cognitive restructuring

Answer: a

REFERENCES

1. Topuzoglu, A., et al., *The epidemiology of major depressive disorder and subthreshold depression in Izmir, Turkey: prevalence, socioeconomic differences, impairment and help-seeking.* J Affect Disord, 2015. **181**: p. 78–86.
2. Silva, M.T., et al., *Prevalence of depression morbidity among Brazilian adults: a systematic review and meta-analysis.* Rev Bras Psiquiatr, 2014. **36**(3): p. 262–270.
3. Blazer, D.G., et al., *The prevalence and distribution of major depression in a national community sample: the National Comorbidity Survey.* Am J Psychiatry, 1994. **151**(7): p. 979–86.
4. Rush, A.J., et al., *Acute and longer-term outcomes in depressed outpatients requiring one or several treatment steps: a STAR*D report.* Am J Psychiatry, 2006. **163**(11): p. 1905–1917.
5. Hawton, K., et al., *Risk factors for suicide in individuals with depression: a systematic review.* J Affect Disord, 2013. **147**(1-3): p. 17–28.
6. Reynolds, C.F., 3rd and D.J. Kupfer, *Sleep research in affective illness: state of the art circa 1987.* Sleep, 1987. **10**(3): p. 199–215.
7. Kaplan, K.A. and A.G. Harvey, *Hypersomnia across mood disorders: a review and synthesis.* Sleep Med Rev, 2009. **13**(4): p. 275–285.
8. Peterson, M.J. and R.M. Benca, *Sleep in mood disorders.* Psychiatr Clin North Am, 2006. **29**(4): p. 1009–1032; abstract ix.
9. Franzen, P.L. and D.J. Buysse, *Sleep disturbances and depression: risk relationships for subsequent depression and therapeutic implications.* Dialogues Clin Neurosci, 2008. **10**(4): p. 473–481.
10. Reynolds, C.F., 3rd, et al., *Which elderly patients with remitted depression remain well with continued interpersonal psychotherapy after discontinuation of antidepressant medication?* Am J Psychiatry, 1997. **154**(7): p. 958–962.

11. Ford, D.E. and L. Cooper-Patrick, *Sleep disturbances and mood disorders: an epidemiologic perspective.* Depress Anxiety, 2001. **14**(1): p. 3–6.

12. Breslau, N., et al., *Sleep disturbance and psychiatric disorders: a longitudinal epidemiological study of young adults.* Biol Psychiatry, 1996. **39**(6): p. 411–418.

13. Chang, P.P., et al., *Insomnia in young men and subsequent depression. The Johns Hopkins Precursors Study.* Am J Epidemiol, 1997. **146**(2): p. 105–114.

14. Baglioni, C., et al., *Insomnia as a predictor of depression: a meta-analytic evaluation of longitudinal epidemiological studies.* J Affect Disord, 2011. **135**(1-3): p. 10–19.

15. Ford, D.E. and D.B. Kamerow, *Epidemiologic study of sleep disturbances and psychiatric disorders. An opportunity for prevention?* Jama, 1989. **262**(11): p. 1479–1484.

16. Li, S.X., et al., *Residual sleep disturbances in patients remitted from major depressive disorder: a 4-year naturalistic follow-up study.* Sleep, 2012. **35**(8): p. 1153–1161.

17. Pace-Schott, E.F. and J.A. Hobson, *The neurobiology of sleep: genetics, cellular physiology and subcortical networks.* Nat Rev Neurosci, 2002. **3**(8): p. 591–605.

18. Benca, R.M., et al., *Sleep and psychiatric disorders. A meta-analysis.* Arch Gen Psychiatry, 1992. **49**(8): p. 651–68; discussion 669–670.

19. Thase, M.E., *Depression, sleep, and antidepressants.* J Clin Psychiatry, 1998. **59 Suppl 4**: p. 55–65.

20. Argyropoulos, S.V. and S.J. Wilson, *Sleep disturbances in depression and the effects of antidepressants.* Int Rev Psychiatry, 2005. **17**(4): p. 237–245.

21. Pfleiderer, B., et al., *Effective electroconvulsive therapy reverses glutamate/glutamine deficit in the left anterior cingulum of unipolar depressed patients.* Psychiatry Res, 2003. **122**(3): p. 185–192.

22. Michael, N., et al., *Metabolic changes within the left dorsolateral prefrontal cortex occurring with electroconvulsive therapy in patients with treatment resistant unipolar depression.* Psychol Med, 2003. **33**(7): p. 1277–1284.

23. Zhang, J., et al., *Glutamate normalization with ECT treatment response in major depression.* Mol Psychiatry, 2013. **18**(3): p. 268–270.

24. Niciu, M.J., et al., *Glutamate and its receptors in the pathophysiology and treatment of major depressive disorder.* J Neural Transmission, 2014. **121**(8): p. 907–924.

25. Nechita, F., M.C. Pirlog, and A.L. ChiriTa, *Circadian malfunctions in depression - neurobiological and psychosocial approaches.* Rom J Morphol Embryol, 2015. **56**(3): p. 949–955.

26. Bunney, B.G., et al., *Circadian dysregulation of clock genes: clues to rapid treatments in major depressive disorder.* Mol Psychiatry, 2015. **20**(1): p. 48–55.

27. Hasler, B.P., et al., *Phase relationships between core body temperature, melatonin, and sleep are associated with depression severity: further evidence for circadian misalignment in non-seasonal depression.* Psychiatry Res, 2010. **178**(1): p. 205–7.

28. Bunney, B.G. and W.E. Bunney, *Rapid-acting antidepressant strategies: mechanisms of action.* Int J Neuropsychopharmacol, 2012. **15**(5): p. 695–713.

29. Mendlewicz, J., *Disruption of the circadian timing systems: molecular mechanisms in mood disorders.* CNS Drugs, 2009. **23 Suppl 2**: p. 15–26.

30. Du, L., et al., *MAO-A gene polymorphisms are associated with major depression and sleep disturbance in males.* Neuroreport, 2004. **15**(13): p. 2097–101.

31. Nestler, E.J., et al., *Neurobiology of depression.* Neuron, 2002. **34**(1): p. 13–25.

32. Gold, P.W. and G.P. Chrousos, *Organization of the stress system and its dysregulation in melancholic and atypical depression: high vs low CRH/NE states.* Mol Psychiatry, 2002. **7**(3): p. 254–275.

33. Wolkowitz, O.M. and V.I. Reus, *Neurotransmitters, neurosteroids and neurotrophins: new models of the pathophysiology and treatment of depression.* World J Biol Psychiatry, 2003. **4**(3): p. 98–102.

34. Sculthorpe, L.D. and A.B. Douglass, *Sleep pathologies in depression and the clinical utility of polysomnography.* Can J Psychiatry, 2010. **55**(7): p. 413–421.

35. Held, K., et al., *Treatment with the CRH1-receptor-antagonist R121919 improves sleep-EEG in patients with depression.* J Psychiatr Res, 2004. **38**(2): p. 129–136.

36. Karege, F., et al., *Decreased serum brain-derived neurotrophic factor levels in major depressed patients.* Psychiatry Res, 2002. **109**(2): p. 143–148.

37. Lampe, I.K., et al., *Association of depression duration with reduction of global cerebral gray matter volume in female patients with recurrent major depressive disorder.* Am J Psychiatry, 2003. **160**(11): p. 2052–2054.

38. Duman, R.S., J. Malberg, and J. Thome, *Neural plasticity to stress and antidepressant treatment.* Biol Psychiatry, 1999. **46**(9): p. 1181–1191.

39. Faraguna, U., et al., *A causal role for brain-derived neurotrophic factor in the homeostatic regulation of sleep.* J Neurosci, 2008. **28**(15): p. 4088–4095.

40. Giese, M., et al., *The interplay of stress and sleep impacts BDNF level.* PLoS One, 2013. **8**(10): p. e76050.

41. Tononi, G. and C. Cirelli, *Sleep and the price of plasticity: from synaptic and cellular homeostasis*

to memory consolidation and integration. Neuron, 2014. **81**(1): p. 12–34.

42. Duncan, W.C., et al., *Concomitant BDNF and sleep slow wave changes indicate ketamine-induced plasticity in major depressive disorder.* Int J Neuropsychopharmacol, 2013. **16**(2): p. 301–311.

43. Chang, C.H., et al., *Ventromedial prefrontal cortex regulates depressive-like behavior and rapid eye movement sleep in the rat.* Neuropharmacology, 2014. **86**: p. 125–132.

44. Ebdlahad, S., et al., *Comparing neural correlates of REM sleep in posttraumatic stress disorder and depression: a neuroimaging study.* Psychiatry Res, 2013. **214**(3): p. 422–428.

45. Aizawa, H., et al., *Hyperactivation of the habenula as a link between depression and sleep disturbance.* Front Human Neuroscience, 2013. **7**: p. 826.

46. Mulders, P.C., et al., *Resting-state functional connectivity in major depressive disorder: A review.* Neurosci Biobehav Rev, 2015. **56**: p. 330–344.

47. Kaiser, R.H., et al., *Large-scale network dysfunction in major depressive disorder: a meta-analysis of resting-state functional connectivity.* JAMA Psychiatry, 2015. **72**(6): p. 603–611.

48. Menon, V., *Large-scale brain networks and psychopathology: a unifying triple network model.* Trends Cogn Sci, 2011. **15**(10): p. 483–506.

49. Spiegelhalder, K., et al., *Neuroimaging insights into insomnia.* Curr Neurol Neurosci Rep, 2015. **15**(3): p. 9.

50. Liu, C.H., et al., *Increased salience network activity in patients with insomnia complaints in major depressive disorder.* Front Psychiatry, 2018. **9**: p. 93.

51. Alberti, S., et al., *Insomnia and somnolence associated with second-generation antidepressants during the treatment of major depression: a meta-analysis.* J Clin Psychopharmacol, 2015. **35**(3): p. 296–303.

52. McCarter, S.J., et al., *Antidepressants increase REM sleep muscle tone in patients with and without REM sleep behavior disorder.* Sleep, 2015. **38**(6): p. 907–917.

53. Stallman, H.M., M. Kohler, and J. White, *Medication induced sleepwalking: a systematic review.* Sleep Med Rev, 2018. **37**: p. 105–113.

54. Jeong, J.-H. and W.-M. Bahk, *Sleep-related eating disorder associated with mirtazapine.* J Clin Psychopharmacol, 2014. **34**(6): p. 752–753.

55. Zapp, A.A., E.C. Fischer, and M. Deuschle, *The effect of agomelatine and melatonin on sleep-related eating: a case report.* J Med Case Rep, 2017. **11**(1): p. 275.

56. Kroenke, K., R.L. Spitzer, and J.B. Williams, *The PHQ-9: validity of a brief depression severity measure.* J Gen Intern Med, 2001. **16**(9): p. 606–613.

57. Steer, R.A., et al., *Dimensions of the Beck Depression Inventory-II in clinically depressed outpatients.* J Clin Psychol, 1999. **55**(1): p. 117–128.

58. Muller, M.J., et al., *Differentiating moderate and severe depression using the Montgomery-Asberg depression rating scale (MADRS).* J Affect Disord, 2003. **77**(3): p. 255–260.

59. Hamilton, M., *A rating scale for depression.* J Neurol Neurosurg Psychiatry, 1960. **23**: p. 56–62.

60. Rush, A.J., et al., *The Inventory of Depressive Symptomatology (IDS): psychometric properties.* Psychol Med, 1996. **26**(3): p. 477–486.

61. Rush, A.J., et al., *The 16-Item Quick Inventory of Depressive Symptomatology (QIDS), clinician rating (QIDS-C), and self-report (QIDS-SR): a psychometric evaluation in patients with chronic major depression.* Biol Psychiatry, 2003. **54**(5): p. 573–83.

62. Buysse, D.J., et al., *The Pittsburgh Sleep Quality Index: a new instrument for psychiatric practice and research.* Psychiatry Res, 1989. **28**(2): p. 193–213.

63. Bastien, C.H., A. Vallieres, and C.M. Morin, *Validation of the Insomnia Severity Index as an outcome measure for insomnia research.* Sleep Med, 2001. **2**(4): p. 297–307.

64. Morin, C.M., et al., *The Insomnia Severity Index: psychometric indicators to detect insomnia cases and evaluate treatment response.* Sleep, 2011. **34**(5): p. 601–608.

65. Johns, M.W., *A new method for measuring daytime sleepiness: the Epworth sleepiness scale.* Sleep, 1991. **14**(6): p. 540–545.

66. Baglioni, C., et al., *Sleep and mental disorders: a meta-analysis of polysomnographic research.* Psychol Bull, 2016. **142**(9): p. 969–990.

67. Giles, D.E., et al., *Polysomnographic parameters in first-degree relatives of unipolar probands.* Psychiatry Res, 1989. **27**(2): p. 127–136.

68. Lauer, C.J., et al., *From early to late adulthood: changes in EEG sleep of depressed patients and healthy volunteers.* Biol Psychiatry, 1991. **29**(10): p. 979–993.

69. Berger, M. and D. Riemann, *Symposium: normal and abnormal REM sleep regulation: REM sleep in depression-an overview.* J Sleep Res, 1993. **2**(4): p. 211–223.

70. Arriaga, F., P. Rosado, and T. Paiva, *The sleep of dysthymic patients: a comparison with normal controls.* Biol Psychiatry, 1990. **27**(6): p. 649–656.

71. Arriaga, F. and T. Paiva, *Clinical and EEG sleep changes in primary dysthymia and generalized anxiety: a comparison with normal controls.* Neuropsychobiology, 1990. **24**(3): p. 109–114.

72. Anderson, J.L., et al., *Sleep in fall/winter seasonal affective disorder: effects of light and changing seasons.* J Psychosom Res, 1994. **38**(4): p. 323–337.

73. Luthringer, R., et al., *All-night EEG spectral analysis as a tool for the prediction of clinical response to antidepressant treatment.* Biol Psychiatry, 1995. **38**(2): p. 98–104.

74. Kupfer, D.J., et al., *Delta sleep ratio: a biological correlate of early recurrence in unipolar affective disorder.* Arch Gen Psychiatry, 1990. **47**(12): p. 1100–1105.

75. Jindal, R.D., et al., *Electroencephalographic sleep profiles in single-episode and recurrent unipolar forms of major depression: II. Comparison during remission.* Biol Psychiatry, 2002. **51**(3): p. 230–236.

76. Armitage, R., H.P. Roffwarg, and A.J. Rush, *Digital period analysis of EEG in depression: periodicity, coherence, and interhemispheric relationships during sleep.* Prog Neuropsychopharmacol Biol Psychiatry, 1993. **17**(3): p. 363–372.

77. Fulton, M.K., R. Armitage, and A.J. Rush, *Sleep electroencephalographic coherence abnormalities in individuals at high risk for depression: a pilot study.* Biol Psychiatry, 2000. **47**(7): p. 618–625.

78. Kerner, N.A. and S.P. Roose, *Obstructive sleep apnea is linked to depression and cognitive impairment: evidence and potential mechanisms.* Am J Geriatric Psychiatry, 2016. **24**(6): p. 496–508.

79. Ohayon, M.M., *The effects of breathing-related sleep disorders on mood disturbances in the general population.* J Clin Psychiatry, 2003. **64**(10): p. 1195–1200; quiz, 1274–1276.

80. Pan, M.L., et al., *Bidirectional association between obstructive sleep apnea and depression: a population-based longitudinal study.* Medicine (Baltimore), 2016. **95**(37): p. e4833.

81. Lang, C.J., et al., *Co-morbid OSA and insomnia increases depression prevalence and severity in men.* Respirology, 2017. **22**(7): p. 1407–1415.

82. Ong, J.C., et al., *Frequency and predictors of obstructive sleep apnea among individuals with major depressive disorder and insomnia.* J Psychosom Res, 2009. **67**(2): p. 135–141.

83. Cai, L., et al., *Evaluation of the risk factors of depressive disorders comorbid with obstructive sleep apnea.* Neuropsychiatr Dis Treat, 2017. **13**: p. 155–159.

84. Cross, R.L., et al., *Neural alterations and depressive symptoms in obstructive sleep apnea patients.* Sleep, 2008. **31**(8): p. 1103–1109.

85. Stubbs, B., et al., *The prevalence and predictors of obstructive sleep apnea in major depressive disorder, bipolar disorder and schizophrenia: A systematic review and meta-analysis.* J Affect Disord, 2016. **197**: p. 259–267.

86. Hobzova, M., et al., *Depression and obstructive sleep apnea.* Neuro Endocrinol Lett, 2017. **38**(5): p. 343–352.

87. Alam, A., K.N. Chengappa, and F. Ghinassi, *Screening for obstructive sleep apnea among individuals with severe mental illness at a primary care clinic.* Gen Hosp Psychiatry, 2012. **34**(6): p. 660–664.

88. Hobzova, M., et al., *Cognitive function and depressivity before and after CPAP treatment in obstructive sleep apnea patients.* Neuro Endocrinol Lett, 2017. **38**(3): p. 145–153.

89. Gupta, M.A., F.C. Simpson, and D.C. Lyons, *The effect of treating obstructive sleep apnea with positive airway pressure on depression and other subjective symptoms: A systematic review and meta-analysis.* Sleep Med Rev, 2016. **28**: p. 55–68.

90. Povitz, M., et al., *Effect of treatment of obstructive sleep apnea on depressive symptoms: systematic review and meta-analysis.* PLoS Med, 2014. **11**(11): p. e1001762.

91. Li, Y.Y., et al., *Anxiety and depression are improved by continuous positive airway pressure treatments in obstructive sleep apnea.* Int J Psychiatry Med, 2016. **51**(6): p. 554–562.

92. Patel, R., Kodya, S., and Chopra, A. (2010, November). Impact of Obstructive Sleep Apnea (OSA) on Hospital Outcomes of Patients with Major Depressive Disorder (MDD): a Nationwide Inaptient Sample Study. Poster session presented at Academy of Consultation-Liaison Psychiatry ACLP), Orlando, Florida.

93. Hornyak, M., *Depressive disorders in restless legs syndrome: epidemiology, pathophysiology and management.* CNS Drugs, 2010. **24**(2): p. 89–98.

94. Hornyak, M., et al., *Impact of sleep-related complaints on depressive symptoms in patients with restless legs syndrome.* J Clin Psychiatry, 2005. **66**(9): p. 1139–1145.

95. Brand, S., et al., *Comparison of sleep EEG profiles of patients suffering from restless legs syndrome, restless legs syndrome and depressive symptoms, and major depressive disorders.* Neuropsychobiology, 2010. **61**(1): p. 41–48.

96. Koo, B.B., et al., *Restless legs syndrome and depression: effect mediation by disturbed sleep and periodic limb movements.* Am J Geriatr Psychiatry, 2016. **24**(11): p. 1105–1116.

97. Rottach, K.G., et al., *Restless legs syndrome as side effect of second generation antidepressants.* J Psychiatr Res, 2008. **43**(1): p. 70–75.

98. Silber, M.H., et al., *An algorithm for the management of restless legs syndrome.* Mayo Clin Proc, 2004. **79**(7): p. 916–922.

99. Zhu, L. and P.C. Zee, *Circadian rhythm sleep disorders.* Neurol Clin, 2012. **30**(4): p. 1167–1191.

100. Chan, J.W., et al., *Eveningness and insomnia: independent risk factors of nonremission in*

major depressive disorder. Sleep, 2014. **37**(5): p. 911–917.

101. Gaspar-Barba, E., et al., *Depressive symptomatology is influenced by chronotypes.* J Affect Disord, 2009. **119**(1-3): p. 100–106.

102. Horne, J.A. and O. Ostberg, *A self-assessment questionnaire to determine morningness-eveningness in human circadian rhythms.* Int J Chronobiol, 1976. **4**(2): p. 97–110.

103. Reid, K.J., et al., *Systematic evaluation of Axis-I DSM diagnoses in delayed sleep phase disorder and evening-type circadian preference.* Sleep Med, 2012. **13**(9): p. 1171–1177.

104. Murray, J.M., et al., *Prevalence of circadian misalignment and its association with depressive symptoms in delayed sleep phase disorder.* Sleep, 2017. **40**(1).

105. Lee, H.J., et al., *Delayed sleep phase syndrome is related to seasonal affective disorder.* J Affect Disord, 2011. **133**(3): p. 573–579.

106. Germain, A. and D.J. Kupfer, *Circadian rhythm disturbances in depression.* Hum Psychopharmacol, 2008. **23**(7): p. 571–585.

107. Roenneberg, T., A. Wirz-Justice, and M. Merrow, *Life between clocks: daily temporal patterns of human chronotypes.* J Biol Rhythms, 2003. **18**(1): p. 80–90.

108. Li, L., et al., *Insomnia and the risk of depression: a meta-analysis of prospective cohort studies.* BMC Psychiatry, 2016. **16**(1): p. 375.

109. Buysse, D.J., *Insomnia, depression and aging. Assessing sleep and mood interactions in older adults.* Geriatrics, 2004. **59**(2): p. 47–51; quiz 52.

110. Pillai, V., et al., *A seven day actigraphy-based study of rumination and sleep disturbance among young adults with depressive symptoms.* J Psychosom Res, 2014. **77**(1): p. 70–75.

111. Troxel, W.M., et al., *Insomnia and objectively measured sleep disturbances predict treatment outcome in depressed patients treated with psychotherapy or psychotherapy-pharmacotherapy combinations.* J Clin Psychiatry, 2012. **73**(4): p. 478–485.

112. Manber, R. and A.S. Chambers, *Insomnia and depression: a multifaceted interplay.* Curr Psychiatry Rep, 2009. **11**(6): p. 437–442.

113. Howland, R.H., *Sleep interventions for the treatment of depression.* J Psychosoc Nurs Ment Health Serv, 2011. **49**(1): p. 17–20.

114. Wilson, S.J., et al., *British Association for Psychopharmacology consensus statement on evidence-based treatment of insomnia, parasomnias and circadian rhythm disorders.* J Psychopharmacol, 2010. **24**(11): p. 1577–1601.

115. Morin, C.M., et al., *Psychological and behavioral treatment of insomnia: update of the recent evidence (1998–2004).* Sleep, 2006. **29**(11): p. 1398–1414.

116. Manber, R., et al., *Cognitive behavioral therapy for insomnia enhances depression outcome in patients with comorbid major depressive disorder and insomnia.* Sleep, 2008. **31**(4): p. 489–495.

117. Wichniak, A., et al., *Effects of antidepressants on sleep.* Curr Psychiatry Rep, 2017. **19**(9): p. 63.

118. Doghramji, K. and W.C. Jangro, *Adverse effects of psychotropic medications on sleep.* Sleep Med Clin, 2016. **11**(4): p. 503–514.

119. Fava, M., *Daytime sleepiness and insomnia as correlates of depression.* J Clin Psychiatry, 2004. **65 Suppl 16**: p. 27–32.

120. Wichniak, A., A. Wierzbicka, and W. Jernajczyk, *Sleep and antidepressant treatment.* Curr Pharm Des, 2012. **18**(36): p. 5802–5817.

121. Wilson, S. and S. Argyropoulos, *Antidepressants and sleep: a qualitative review of the literature.* Drugs, 2005. **65**(7): p. 927–947.

122. Sharpley, A.L. and P.J. Cowen, *Effect of pharmacologic treatments on the sleep of depressed patients.* Biol Psychiatry, 1995. **37**(2): p. 85–98.

123. Clark, N.A. and B. Alexander, *Increased rate of trazodone prescribing with bupropion and selective serotonin-reuptake inhibitors versus tricyclic antidepressants.* Ann Pharmacother, 2000. **34**(9): p. 1007–1012.

124. Fagiolini, A., et al., *Rediscovering trazodone for the treatment of major depressive disorder.* CNS Drugs, 2012. **26**(12): p. 1033–1049.

125. Nierenberg, A.A., et al., *Trazodone for antidepressant-associated insomnia.* Am J Psychiatry, 1994. **151**(7): p. 1069–1072.

126. Saletu-Zyhlarz, G.M., et al., *Insomnia in depression: differences in objective and subjective sleep and awakening quality to normal controls and acute effects of trazodone.* Prog Neuropsychopharmacol Biol Psychiatry, 2002. **26**(2): p. 249–260.

127. Winokur, A., et al., *Acute effects of mirtazapine on sleep continuity and sleep architecture in depressed patients: a pilot study.* Biol Psychiatry, 2000. **48**(1): p. 75–78.

128. Chopra, A., D.S. Pendergrass, and J.M. Bostwick, *Mirtazapine-induced worsening of restless legs syndrome (RLS) and ropinirole-induced psychosis: challenges in management of depression in RLS.* Psychosomatics, 2011. **52**(1): p. 92–94.

129. Kolla, B.P., M.P. Mansukhani, and J.M. Bostwick, *The influence of antidepressants on restless legs syndrome and periodic limb movements: A systematic review.* Sleep Med Rev, 2018. **38**: p. 131–140.

130. DeMartinis, N.A. and A. Winokur, *Effects of psychiatric medications on sleep and sleep disorders.*

CNS Neurol Disord Drug Targets, 2007. **6**(1): p. 17–29.

131. Holshoe, J.M., *Antidepressants and sleep: a review.* Perspect Psychiatr Care, 2009. **45**(3): p. 191–197.

132. Wiegand, M.H., *Antidepressants for the treatment of insomnia: a suitable approach?* Drugs, 2008. **68**(17): p. 2411–2417.

133. Weber, J., et al., *Low-dose doxepin: in the treatment of insomnia.* CNS Drugs, 2010. **24**(8): p. 713–720.

134. Manber, R., et al., *The effects of psychotherapy, nefazodone, and their combination on subjective assessment of disturbed sleep in chronic depression.* Sleep, 2003. **26**(2): p. 130–136.

135. Staner, L., et al., *5-HT2 receptor antagonism and slow-wave sleep in major depression.* Acta Psychiatr Scand, 1992. **86**(2): p. 133–137.

136. De Berardis, D., et al., *The melatonergic system in mood and anxiety disorders and the role of agomelatine: implications for clinical practice.* Int J Mol Sci, 2013. **14**(6): p. 12458–12483.

137. Fava, M., et al., *Eszopiclone co-administered with fluoxetine in patients with insomnia coexisting with major depressive disorder.* Biol Psychiatry, 2006. **59**(11): p. 1052–1060.

138. Krystal, A., et al., *Evaluation of eszopiclone discontinuation after cotherapy with fluoxetine for insomnia with coexisting depression.* J Clin Sleep Med, 2007. **3**(1): p. 48–55.

139. Fava, M., et al., *Improved insomnia symptoms and sleep-related next-day functioning in patients with comorbid major depressive disorder and insomnia following concomitant zolpidem extended-release 12.5 mg and escitalopram treatment: a randomized controlled trial.* J Clin Psychiatry, 2011. **72**(7): p. 914–928.

140. Asnis, G.M., et al., *Zolpidem for persistent insomnia in SSRI-treated depressed patients.* J Clin Psychiatry, 1999. **60**(10): p. 668–676.

141. Perez-Diaz, H., A. Iranzo, and J. Santamaria, *[Zolpidem-induced sleep-related behavioural disorders].* Neurologia, 2010. **25**(8): p. 491–497.

142. Li, C.-T., et al., *High dosage of hypnotics predicts subsequent sleep-related breathing disorders and is associated with worse outcomes for depression.* Sleep, 2014. **37**(4): p. 803–809.

143. Wang, P. and T. Si, *Use of antipsychotics in the treatment of depressive disorders.* Shanghai Archives of Psychiatry, 2013. **25**(3): p. 134–140.

144. Bauer, M., et al., *Evaluation of adjunct extended-release quetiapine fumarate on sleep disturbance and quality in patients with major depressive disorder and an inadequate response to on-going antidepressant therapy.* Int J Neuropsychopharmacol, 2013. **16**(8): p. 1755–1765.

145. Gedge, L., et al., *Effects of quetiapine on sleep architecture in patients with unipolar or bipolar depression.* Neuropsychiatr Dis Treat, 2010. **6**: p. 501–508.

146. Locklear, J.C., et al., *Effects of once-daily extended release quetiapine fumarate (quetiapine XR) on quality of life and sleep in elderly patients with major depressive disorder.* J Affect Disord, 2013. **149**(1-3): p. 189–195.

147. Trivedi, M.H., et al., *Evaluation of the effects of extended release quetiapine fumarate monotherapy on sleep disturbance in patients with major depressive disorder: a pooled analysis of four randomized acute studies.* Int J Neuropsychopharmacol, 2013. **16**(8): p. 1733–1744.

148. Lazowski, L.K., et al., *Sleep architecture and cognitive changes in olanzapine-treated patients with depression: a double blind randomized placebo controlled trial.* BMC Psychiatry, 2014. **14**: p. 202.

149. Sharpley, A.L., et al., *Olanzapine increases slow wave sleep and sleep continuity in SSRI-resistant depressed patients.* J Clin Psychiatry, 2005. **66**(4): p. 450–454.

150. Krystal, A.D., et al., *Effects of adjunctive brexpiprazole on sleep disturbances in patients with major depressive disorder: an open-label, flexible-dose, exploratory study.* Prim Care Companion CNS Disord, 2016. **18**(5).

151. Khazaie, H., et al., *A weight-independent association between atypical antipsychotic medications and obstructive sleep apnea.* Sleep Breath, 2018. **22**(1): p. 109–114.

152. Manber, R., et al., *Cognitive behavioral therapy for insomnia enhances depression outcome in patients with comorbid major depressive disorder and insomnia.* Sleep, 2008. **31**(4): p. 489–495.

153. Ashworth, D.K., et al., *A randomized controlled trial of cognitive behavioral therapy for insomnia: an effective treatment for comorbid insomnia and depression.* J Couns Psychol, 2015. **62**(2): p. 115–123.

154. Lancee, J., et al., *Baseline depression levels do not affect efficacy of cognitive-behavioral self-help treatment for insomnia.* Depress Anxiety, 2013. **30**(2): p. 149–156.

155. Carney, C.E., et al., *Cognitive behavioral insomnia therapy for those with insomnia and depression: a randomized controlled clinical trial.* Sleep, 2017. **40**(4).

156. Taylor, D.J. and K.E. Pruiksma, *Cognitive and behavioural therapy for insomnia (CBT-I) in psychiatric populations: a systematic review.* Int Rev Psychiatry, 2014. **26**(2): p. 113–205.

157. Goldstein, T.R., J.A. Bridge, and D.A. Brent, *Sleep disturbance preceding completed suicide in adolescents.* J Consult Clin Psychol, 2008. **76**(1): p. 84–91.

158. Dolenc, L., A. Besset, and M. Billiard, *Hypersomnia in association with dysthymia in comparison with idiopathic hypersomnia and normal controls.* Pflugers Arch, 1996. **431**(6 Suppl 2): p. R303–R304.

159. Billiard, M., et al., *Hypersomnia associated with mood disorders: a new perspective.* J Psychosom Res, 1994. **38 Suppl 1**: p. 41–47.

160. Plante, D.T., *Hypersomnia in mood disorders: a rapidly changing landscape.* Curr Sleep Med Rep, 2015. **1**(2): p. 122–130.

161. Plante, D.T., J.D. Cook, and M.R. Goldstein, *Objective measures of sleep duration and continuity in major depressive disorder with comorbid hypersomnolence: a primary investigation with contiguous systematic review and meta-analysis.* J Sleep Res, 2017. **26**(3): p. 255–265.

162. Kofmel, N.C., et al., *Sleepiness and performance is disproportionate in patients with non-organic hypersomnia in comparison to patients with narcolepsy and mild to moderate obstructive sleep apnoea.* Neuropsychobiology, 2014. **70**(3): p. 189–194.

163. Bassetti, C., et al., *The narcoleptic borderland: a multimodal diagnostic approach including cerebrospinal fluid levels of hypocretin-1 (orexin A).* Sleep Med, 2003. **4**(1): p. 7–12.

164. Posternak, M.A. and M. Zimmerman, *Partial validation of the atypical features subtype of major depressive disorder.* Arch Gen Psychiatry, 2002. **59**(1): p. 70–76.

165. Posternak, M.A. and M. Zimmerman, *Symptoms of atypical depression.* Psychiatry Res, 2001. **104**(2): p. 175–181.

166. Khan, A.A., et al., *Gender differences in the symptoms of major depression in opposite-sex dizygotic twin pairs.* Am J Psychiatry, 2002. **159**(8): p. 1427–1429.

167. Parker, G., et al., *Sleeping in? The impact of age and depressive sub-type on hypersomnia.* J Affect Disord, 2006. **90**(1): p. 73–76.

168. Soehner, A.M., K.A. Kaplan, and A.G. Harvey, *Prevalence and clinical correlates of co-occurring insomnia and hypersomnia symptoms in depression.* J Affect Disord, 2014. **167**: p. 93–97.

169. Rethorst, C.D., et al., *IL-1beta and BDNF are associated with improvement in hypersomnia but not insomnia following exercise in major depressive disorder.* Transl Psychiatry, 2015. **5**: p. e611.

170. Juruena, M.F., et al., *Atypical depression and non-atypical depression: Is HPA axis function a biomarker? A systematic review.* J Affect Disord, 2018. **233**: p. 45–67.

171. Kunugi, H., et al., *Interface between hypothalamic-pituitary-adrenal axis and brain-derived neurotrophic factor in depression.* Psychiatry Clin Neurosci, 2010. **64**(5): p. 447–459.

172. Franzen, P.L. and D.J. Buysse, *Sleep disturbances and depression: risk relationships for subsequent depression and therapeutic implications.* Dial Clin Neuroscienc, 2008. **10**(4): p. 473–481.

173. Papakostas, G.I., et al., *Resolution of sleepiness and fatigue in major depressive disorder: A comparison of bupropion and the selective serotonin reuptake inhibitors.* Biol Psychiatry, 2006. **60**(12): p. 1350–1355.

174. Goss, A.J., et al., *Modafinil augmentation therapy in unipolar and bipolar depression: a systematic review and meta-analysis of randomized controlled trials.* J Clin Psychiatry, 2013. **74**(11): p. 1101–1107.

175. Sandman, N., et al., *Nightmares: risk factors among the Finnish general adult population.* Sleep, 2015. **38**(4): p. 507–514.

176. Nakajima, S., et al., *Impact of frequency of nightmares comorbid with insomnia on depression in Japanese rural community residents: a cross-sectional study.* Sleep Med, 2014. **15**(3): p. 371–374.

177. Besiroglu, L., M.Y. Agargun, and R. Inci, *Nightmares and terminal insomnia in depressed patients with and without melancholic features.* Psychiatry Res, 2005. **133**(2-3): p. 285–287.

178. Agargun, M.Y., et al., *Nightmares, suicide attempts, and melancholic features in patients with unipolar major depression.* J Affect Disord, 2007. **98**(3): p. 267–270.

179. Ahmed, A.I., et al., *[Hallucinations and vivid dreams by use of metoprolol].* Tijdschr Psychiatr, 2010. **52**(2): p. 117–121.

180. Kung, S., Z. Espinel, and M.I. Lapid, *Treatment of nightmares with prazosin: a systematic review.* Mayo Clinic Proceedings, 2012. **87**(9): p. 890–900.

181. Davis, J.L., et al., *Physiological predictors of response to exposure, relaxation, and rescripting therapy for chronic nightmares in a randomized clinical Trial.* J Clin Sleep Med, 2011. **7**(6): p. 622–631.

182. Casement, M.D. and L.M. Swanson, *A meta-analysis of imagery rehearsal for post-trauma nightmares: effects on nightmare frequency, sleep quality, and posttraumatic stress.* Clin Psychology Rev, 2012. **32**(6): p. 566–574.

183. Dopierala, E. and J. Rybakowski, *Sleep deprivation as a method of chronotherapy in the*

treatment of depression. Psychiatr Pol, 2015. **49**(3): p. 423–433.

184. Gillin, J.C., et al., *Sleep deprivation as a model experimental antidepressant treatment: findings from functional brain imaging*. Depress Anxiety, 2001. **14**(1): p. 37–49.

185. Giedke, H. and F. Schwarzler, *Therapeutic use of sleep deprivation in depression*. Sleep Med Rev, 2002. **6**(5): p. 361–377.

186. Golden, R.N., et al., *The efficacy of light therapy in the treatment of mood disorders: a review and meta-analysis of the evidence*. Am J Psychiatry, 2005. **162**(4): p. 656–662.

187. Pail, G., et al., *Bright-light therapy in the treatment of mood disorders*. Neuropsychobiology, 2011. **64**(3): p. 152–162.

188. Oldham, M.A. and D.A. Ciraulo, *Bright light therapy for depression: a review of its effects on chronobiology and the autonomic nervous system*. Chronobiol Int, 2014. **31**(3): p. 305–319.

189. Fritzsche, M., et al., *Sleep deprivation as a predictor of response to light therapy in major depression*. J Affect Disord, 2001. **62**(3): p. 207–215.

190. Kirschbaum, I., et al., *Short-term effects of wake- and bright light therapy on sleep in depressed youth*. Chronobiol Int, 2018. **35**(1): p. 101–110.

191. Lieverse, R., et al., *Bright light treatment in elderly patients with nonseasonal major depressive disorder: a randomized placebo-controlled trial*. Arch Gen Psychiatry, 2011. **68**(1): p. 61–70.

192. Partonen, T., *Effects of morning light treatment on subjective sleepiness and mood in winter depression*. J Affect Disord, 1994. **30**(1): p. 47–56.

193. Emens, J., et al., *Circadian misalignment in major depressive disorder*. Psychiatry Res, 2009. **168**(3): p. 259–261.

194. Echizenya, M., et al., *Total sleep deprivation followed by sleep phase advance and bright light therapy in drug-resistant mood disorders*. J Affect Disord, 2013. **144**(1-2): p. 28–33.

195. Riemann, D., et al., *How to preserve the antidepressive effect of sleep deprivation: A comparison of sleep phase advance and sleep phase delay*. Eur Arch Psychiatry Clin Neurosci, 1999. **249**(5): p. 231–237.

196. Albert, R., et al., *[Sleep deprivation and subsequent sleep phase advance stabilizes the positive effect of sleep deprivation in depressive episodes]*. Nervenarzt, 1998. **69**(1): p. 66–69.

197. Benedetti, F. and C. Colombo, *Sleep deprivation in mood disorders*. Neuropsychobiology, 2011. **64**(3): p. 141–151.

198. Martiny, K., et al., *A 9-week randomized trial comparing a chronotherapeutic intervention (wake and light therapy) to exercise in major depressive disorder patients treated with duloxetine*. J Clin Psychiatry, 2012. **73**(9): p. 1234–1242.

199. Muller, M.J., et al., *Side effects of adjunct light therapy in patients with major depression*. Eur Arch Psychiatry Clin Neurosci, 1997. **247**(5): p. 252–258.

200. Sahlem, G.L., et al., *Adjunctive triple chronotherapy (combined total sleep deprivation, sleep phase advance, and bright light therapy) rapidly improves mood and suicidality in suicidal depressed inpatients: an open label pilot study*. J Psychiatr Res, 2014. **59**: p. 101–107.

201. Duncan, W.C. and C.A. Zarate, *Ketamine, sleep, and depression: current status and new questions*. Curr Psychiatry Rep, 2013. **15**(9). doi:10.1007/s11920-013-0394-z.

202. Coffey, C.E., et al., *Effects of ECT on polysomnographic sleep: a prospective investigation*. Convuls Ther, 1988. **4**(4): p. 269–279.

203. Grunhaus, L., et al., *Sleep-onset rapid eye movement after electroconvulsive therapy is more frequent in patients who respond less well to electroconvulsive therapy*. Biol Psychiatry, 1997. **42**(3): p. 191–200.

204. Hoogerhoud, A., et al., *Short-term effects of electroconvulsive therapy on subjective and actigraphy-assessed sleep parameters in severely depressed inpatients*. Depress Res Treat, 2015. **2015**: p. 764649.

205. Winkler, D., et al., *Actigraphy in patients with treatment-resistant depression undergoing electroconvulsive therapy*. J Psychiatr Res, 2014. **57**: p. 96–100.

206. Cohrs, S., et al., *High-frequency repetitive transcranial magnetic stimulation delays rapid eye movement sleep*. Neuroreport, 1998. **9**(15): p. 3439–3443.

207. Graf, T., et al., *High frequency repetitive transcranial magnetic stimulation (rTMS) of the left dorsolateral cortex: EEG topography during waking and subsequent sleep*. Psychiatry Res, 2001. **107**(1): p. 1–9.

208. Saeki, T., et al., *Localized potentiation of sleep slow-wave activity induced by prefrontal repetitive transcranial magnetic stimulation in patients with a major depressive episode*. Brain Stimul, 2013. **6**(3): p. 390–396.

209. Nishida, M., et al., *Actigraphy in patients with major depressive disorder undergoing repetitive transcranial magnetic stimulation: an open label pilot study*. J ECT, 2017. **33**(1): p. 36–42.

210. Armitage, R., et al., *The effects of vagus nerve stimulation on sleep EEG in depression: a preliminary report*. J Psychosom Res, 2003. **54**(5): p. 475–482.

211. Parhizgar, F., K. Nugent, and R. Raj, *Obstructive sleep apnea and respiratory complications associated with vagus nerve stimulators.* J Clin Sleep Med, 2011. **7**(4): p. 401–407.

212. Quraan, M.A., et al., *EEG power asymmetry and functional connectivity as a marker of treatment effectiveness in DBS surgery for depression.* Neuropsychopharmacology, 2014. **39**(5): p. 1270–1281.

213. Perlis, M.L., et al., *Suicide and sleep: is it a bad thing to be awake when reason sleeps?* Sleep Med Rev, 2016. **29**: p. 101–107.

214. Pigeon, W.R., M. Pinquart, and K. Conner, *Meta-analysis of sleep disturbance and suicidal thoughts and behaviors.* J Clin Psychiatry, 2012. **73**(9): p. e1160–e1167.

215. Bernert, R.A., et al., *Sleep disturbances as an evidence-based suicide risk factor.* Curr Psychiatry Rep, 2015. **17**(3): p. 554.

216. Malik, S., et al., *The association between sleep disturbances and suicidal behaviors in patients with psychiatric diagnoses: a systematic review and meta-analysis.* Syst Rev, 2014. **3**: p. 18.

217. Monti, J.M., *Serotonin control of sleep-wake behavior.* Sleep Med Rev, 2011. **15**(4): p. 269–281.

218. Ursin, R., *Serotonin and sleep.* Sleep Med Rev, 2002. **6**(1): p. 55–67.

219. Novati, A., et al., *Chronically restricted sleep leads to depression-like changes in neurotransmitter receptor sensitivity and neuroendocrine stress reactivity in rats.* Sleep, 2008. **31**(11): p. 1579–1585.

220. Roman, V., et al., *Too little sleep gradually desensitizes the serotonin 1A receptor system.* Sleep, 2005. **28**(12): p. 1505–1510.

221. Elmenhorst, D., et al., *Sleep deprivation increases cerebral serotonin 2A receptor binding in humans.* Sleep, 2012. **35**(12): p. 1615–1623.

222. Chatzittofis, A., et al., *CSF 5-HIAA, cortisol and DHEAS levels in suicide attempters.* Eur Neuropsychopharmacology, 2013. **23**(10): p. 1280–1287.

223. Miller, J.M., et al., *Positron emission tomography quantification of serotonin transporter in suicide attempters with major depressive disorder.* Biol Psychiatry, 2013. **74**(4): p. 287–295.

224. Mann, J.J., *The serotonergic system in mood disorders and suicidal behaviour.* Phil Trans R Soc B, 2013. **368**(1615): p. 20120537.

225. Han, K.S., L. Kim, and I. Shim, *Stress and sleep disorder.* Exp Neurobiology, 2012. **21**(4): p. 141–150.

226. Preti, A. and P. Miotto, *Diurnal variations in suicide by age and gender in Italy.* J Affect Dis, 2001. **65**(3): p. 253–261.

227. Benard, V., P.A. Geoffroy, and F. Bellivier, *[Seasons, circadian rhythms, sleep and suicidal behaviors vulnerability].* Encephale, 2015. **41**(4 Suppl 1): p. S29–S37.

228. Sequeira, A., et al., *Gene expression changes in the prefrontal cortex, anterior cingulate cortex and nucleus accumbens of mood disorders subjects that committed suicide.* PLoS One, 2012. **7**(4): p. e35367.

229. Bernert, R.A. and T.E. Joiner, *Sleep disturbances and suicide risk: a review of the literature.* Neuropsychiatr Dis Treat, 2007. **3**(6): p. 735–43.

230. Turvey, C.L., et al., *Risk factors for late-life suicide: a prospective, community-based study.* Am J Geriatric Psychiatry, 2002. **10**(4): p. 398–406.

231. Fujino, Y., et al., *Prospective cohort study of stress, life satisfaction, self-rated health, insomnia, and suicide death in Japan.* Suicide Life-Threat Behav, 2005. **35**(2): p. 227–237.

232. Trockel, M., et al., *Effects of cognitive behavioral therapy for insomnia on suicidal ideation in veterans.* Sleep, 2015. **38**(2): p. 259–265.

233. Woznica, A.A., et al., *The insomnia and suicide link: toward an enhanced understanding of this relationship.* Sleep Med Rev, 2015. **22**: p. 37–46.

234. David Klonsky, E., et al., *Hopelessness as a predictor of attempted suicide among first admission patients with psychosis: a 10-year cohort study.* Suicide Life-Threat Behav, 2012. **42**(1): p. 1–10.

235. Qiu, T., E.D. Klonsky, and D.N. Klein, *Hopelessness predicts suicide ideation but not attempts: a 10-year longitudinal study.* Suicide Life Threat Behav, 2017. **47**(6): p. 718–722.

236. Beck, A.T., et al., *The measurement of pessimism: the hopelessness scale.* J Consult Clin Psychology, 1974. **42**(6): p. 861.

237. Smith, J.M., L.B. Alloy, and L.Y. Abramson, *Cognitive vulnerability to depression, rumination, hopelessness, and suicidal ideation: Multiple pathways to self-injurious thinking.* Suicide Life-Threat Behav, 2006. **36**(4): p. 443–454.

238. Nycr, M., et al., *Factors that distinguish college students with depressive symptoms with and without suicidal thoughts.* Ann Clin Psychiatry, 2013. **25**(1): p. 41–49.

239. Morin, C.M., et al., *Dysfunctional beliefs and attitudes about sleep among older adults with and without insomnia complaints.* Psychology Aging, 1993. **8**(3): p. 463.

240. Morin, C.M., A. Vallières, and H. Ivers, *Dysfunctional beliefs and attitudes about sleep (DBAS): validation of a brief version (DBAS-16).* Sleep, 2007. **30**(11): p. 1547–1554.

241. McCall, W.V., et al., *Nightmares and dysfunctional beliefs about sleep mediate the effect of*

insomnia symptoms on suicidal ideation. J Clin Sleep Med, 2013. **9**(2): p. 135.

242. Ağargün, M.Y., et al., *Repetitive and frightening dreams and suicidal behavior in patients with major depression.* Comp Psychiatry, 1998. **39**(4): p. 198–202.

243. Tanskanen, A., et al., *Nightmares as predictors of suicide.* Sleep, 2001. **24**(7): p. 845–848.

244. Nadorff, M.R., S. Nazem, and A. Fiske, *Insomnia symptoms, nightmares and suicide risk: duration of sleep disturbance matters.* Suicide Life-Threat Behav, 2013. **43**(2): p. 139–149.

245. Bishop, T.M., L. Ashrafioun, and W.R. Pigeon, *The association between sleep apnea and suicidal thought and behavior: an analysis of national survey data.* J Clin Psychiatry, 2017. **79**(1): 17m11480.

246. Krahn, L.E., B.W. Miller, and L.R. Bergstrom, *Rapid resolution of intense suicidal ideation after treatment of severe obstructive sleep apnea.* J Clin Sleep Med, 2008. **4**(1): p. 64–65.

18

Bipolar and Related Disorders

JACOB G. DINERMAN, BRETT J. DAVIS, JESSICA A. JANOS,
SAMANTHA L. WALSH, AND LOUISA G. SYLVIA

INTRODUCTION

Bipolar disorder is a debilitating, chronic mental health condition characterized by episodes of mania, hypomania, and depression. There are several categories of bipolar disorder ranging from the least severe, known as cyclothymia, to the most severe, bipolar I disorder with psychotic features (see Table 18.1). Individuals with bipolar disorder spend the majority of their time in a major depressive episode when ill; however, this depression differs from unipolar depression, as it is typically characterized with underlying restlessness and agitation as opposed to abnormally low energy and apathy.[1,2] A manic episode is on the opposite end of the bipolar spectrum and is characterized by overactivity, restlessness, acceleration of thought, and elevated or irritable mood.[1,3] Other symptoms include pressured speech, decreased need for sleep, impairment in verbal memory and executive functioning, and impulsivity. Psychotic features are sometimes present, but must occur predominantly within the context of a mood episode to maintain a diagnosis of bipolar disorder (see Table 18.1).[1] Hypomanic episodes are shorter, less severe, and less disruptive than manic episodes, but share similar symptoms to a manic episode. Bipolar disorder with mixed features is a specifier for when symptoms of manic and depressive episodes are present simultaneously.[1]

Bipolar disorder is recurrent and chronic, and typically emerges in young adults (18–25 years old) as depression.[4] Hypomanic symptoms can precede full manic episodes, such that a person diagnosed with bipolar II disorder may later develop bipolar I disorder.[5-7] If left untreated, symptoms and episodes of mania and depression can worsen over time, periods of "normality" between episodes often grow shorter, and episodes last longer, leading to greater impairment and poorer quality of life.[8,9] Individuals

with bipolar disorder also often experience a higher medical burden than the general population because they tend to have poorer lifestyles, take psychiatric medications that worsen their cardiovascular risk, and may have overlapping etiology with physiological processes responsible for medical conditions.[10]

The aim of this chapter is to understand the association between sleep disturbance and bipolar disorder as well as to review empirically validated treatments for sleep disturbance within this population. Sleep is an important treatment target for this psychiatric condition given that sleep disturbance increases the risk of developing bipolar disorder as well as worsens its course of illness.[11] Thus, the understanding of sleep disturbance in bipolar disorder is crucial to better treatment and outcomes.

SLEEP DISRUPTIONS IN BIPOLAR DISORDER

Sleep disturbance is a diagnostic criterion for both manic and depressive episodes observed in bipolar I and II disorders.[1] Sleep disturbance in bipolar disorder is either hypersomnia or insomnia. Patients with hypersomnia may sleep too much, experience persistent exhaustion even when sleeping an average of at least seven hours nightly, or have difficulty getting out of bed in the morning.[12] Patients with insomnia may struggle to fall asleep or to remain asleep.[13] For individuals with bipolar disorder, these types of sleep impairments are common throughout the course of illness, with the severity of the sleep disturbance often increasing leading up to and during mood episodes.[14-18] These disturbances are also clinically meaningful as bipolar patients with more severe sleep disturbances tend to report lower quality of life than bipolar patients with healthy sleep habits.[19-21]

TABLE 18.1. BIPOLAR DISORDERS

Disorder	Diagnostic Criteria
Bipolar I	Experiencing at least one manic episode over the course of one's lifetime. May or may not include episodes of major depression and/or psychosis.
Bipolar II	Experiencing at least one episode of major depression and at least one hypomanic episode over the course of one's lifetime.
Cyclothymia	Experiencing at least 2 years of both hypomanic and depressive periods without ever fulfilling the criteria for an episode of mania, hypomania, or major depression.
Unspecified bipolar and related disorder	Used when symptoms characteristic of a bipolar and related disorder predominate, but do not meet full criteria and clinician does not disclose the reason that presentation does not meet full criteria.

These are the primary diagnostic categories for bipolar and related disorders, but they are not all-inclusive. Other diagnoses include other specified bipolar and related disorder, substance/medication-induced bipolar and related disorder, bipolar and related disorder due to another medical condition.[1]

Characteristics of Sleep Disturbance and Bipolar Disorder

Sleep Disturbance between Mood Episodes

Evidence of chronic sleep disturbance in euthymic bipolar patients has been mixed, possibly due to differences between studies in how sleep disturbance is operationalized.[15-17,22,23] Despite conflicting findings, a recent meta-analysis concluded that adults with bipolar disorder do tend to experience insomnia, hypersomnia, and variability in sleep–wake cycles between mood episodes.[24]

Sleep Disturbance Preceding Mood Episodes

Sleep disturbances are the most common prodrome of mania, with 77% of participants reporting a disturbance in sleep habits 21 to 29 days (on average) before the onset of a manic episode.[25] Sleep disturbance is the sixth most common prodrome of bipolar depression, with 24% of bipolar adults reporting this symptom 11 to 19 days (on average) prior to a depressive episode.[25] Some evidence suggests that sleep impairment may also cause or contribute to the onset of a mood episode.[26,27] In summary, sleep disturbances reliably predict mood episodes for many bipolar patients and could serve as early treatment targets to prevent or lessen the severity of approaching mood episodes.[28]

Sleep Disturbance during Manic Episodes

According to the *Diagnostic and Statistical Manual of Mental Disorders* (fifth edition; DSM-V), a reduction in the need for sleep (i.e., "feels rested after only 3 hours of sleep") is one of the most common features of a manic episode.[1] Evidence suggests that between 69% and 99% of bipolar individuals experience sleep disturbance during a manic episode. This wide range may be attributable to methodological differences.[14] Individuals in manic episodes experience symptoms of insomnia, such that they have trouble falling asleep, sleep for short amounts of time, and/or wake up several hours earlier than they would prefer. Compared to controls, manic individuals exhibit shorter rapid eye movement (REM) latency, increased REM density, and decreased total sleep time.[14] Unlike patients with a primary insomnia diagnosis, manic individuals do not feel tired despite sleeping for only a few hours and/or have no desire to sleep.[3]

Sleep Disturbance during Depressive Episodes

Depressive episodes in bipolar disorder may be characterized by insomnia *or* hypersomnia nearly every night.[1,12,14,29-31] In a recent study, bipolar participants were asked to recall sleep disturbances over the past 5 years using a validated, retrospective life-charting assessment.[32] Participants reported that during depressive episodes, insomnia was present for 52% of months, and hypersomnia was present for 56% of months (participants were allowed to report experience of both within the same month). Several studies involving polysomnography have observed abnormal sleep architecture, such as reduced REM latency, in depressed bipolar patients compared to controls.[14]

Sleep Deprivation Can Cause Marked Changes in Mood

Sleep deprivation, even in healthy patients, is known to impair affect regulation and worsen mood.[33-35] The effects of experimentally-induced sleep deprivation are especially striking in bipolar populations. In one study, 40 hours of sleep deprivation caused seven of nine depressed, rapid-cycling bipolar adults to enter into a manic episode.[26] In a larger study, sleep deprivation induced mania or hypomania in 11% of 206 depressed bipolar subjects.[36] Another study found that 40% to 60% of depressed adults with bipolar disorder exhibited dramatic improvement in depressive symptoms during 40 hours of sleep deprivation, although symptoms returned shortly after sleep was resumed.[26] Other studies have corroborated the tendency of sleep deprivation to reduce depressive symptoms and/or induce manic symptoms.[25,37,38]

The Role of Circadian Rhythms in Bipolar Sleep Disruption

Circadian rhythms describe biological processes, such as the sleep–wake cycle, that repeat in near 24-hour cycles.[39] These rhythms operate even in the absence of environmental time cues such as changes in light and temperature, relying instead on endogenous timekeeping mechanisms.[40]

Disruptions in the sleep–wake cycle as well as other circadian processes including patterns of appetite, temperature regulation, metabolism, energy levels, activity, and hormone release are common in patients with bipolar disorder.[15,41–44] For example, bipolar patients are observed to have lower levels of melatonin—a key hormone in regulating the sleep–wake rhythms—and later melatonin peaks compared to healthy controls.[43,45] Further, bipolar adults are more likely than controls to have an "evening" chronotype, a preference for functioning at night rather than during the day (night-owls), which also reflects abnormal circadian rhythms.[46]

Many mood-regulating treatments for bipolar disorder, including use of mood stabilizers, bright light therapy (BLT), and sleep deprivation therapy, are known to alter circadian rhythms.[47–50] Lithium, for example, is shown to prolong the period of circadian rhythms (including sleep, temperature, and activity) in human and nonhuman trials.[51,52] These changes may contribute to the therapeutic effect of lithium and other common bipolar treatments.[53–55]

Unstable Social Zeitgebers May Cause Circadian Rhythm Disruptions

Zeitgebers are the "time-giving" external cues that help circadian rhythms align with changes in the environment. Social zeitgebers are the everyday activities that constitute daily routines, such as regular meals with family or the time at which one commutes to work or goes to bed. According to the social zeitgeber theory, when stressful life events, such as family illness or international travel, interrupt one's social routines, this leads to disruptions in one's biological rhythms, as well (e.g., sleep, temperature, cortisol).[56] Major life events are consistently observed to precede mood episodes,[57–59] and more specifically, life events have been found to be associated with disruption of social routines and sleep in adults with bipolar spectrum disorder more so compared to controls.[60]

Genetic Mechanisms for Circadian Disruptions

Circadian irregularities may also stem from genetic abnormalities.[61,62] For example, the CLOCK and BMAL1 genes are central to circadian regulation of biological functions, and certain polymorphisms in these genes are associated with bipolar disorder.[63–67] The behaviors of mice with a mutation in the CLOCK gene resemble human mania, including hyperactivity, an intensified pursuit of rewards from cocaine, and decreased need for sleep.[68] According to a recent review, findings of circadian rhythm disruptions' association with any one gene have been modest, suggesting that multiple genes are implicated in a genetic predisposition for weak or irregular circadian rhythms.[14]

TREATMENT OF SLEEP DISTURBANCE IN BIPOLAR DISORDER

Pharmacotherapy

There are many pharmacotherapy options for treating sleep disturbance in bipolar disorder, including psychiatric, nonpsychiatric, or over-the-counter medications, as well as supplements. Each pharmacotherapy option has pros (degree of treatment response) and cons (degree of side effects), but it is important to note that adding sleep aids for insomnia to the treatment regime of a bipolar patient may reduce his or her overall medication adherence, as many mood-stabilizing medications are already sedating.[69] Therefore, clinicians need to be very careful in considering the additive impact of side effects across medications, as bipolar patients tend to be on an average of at least three psychotropic medications.[70] The following is a brief review of some of the most commonly used medications to treat sleep disturbance in bipolar disorder.

Benzodiazepines

Benzodiazepines (e.g., alprazolam [Xanax], diazepam [Valium], clonazepam [Klonopin], lorazepam [Ativan]) are sedative-hypnotic medications classically used to treat adults with insomnia.[71,72] However, they can be highly addictive and are often associated with psychomotor and cognitive impairments. Rapid discontinuation of benzodiazepines can lead to "rebound insomnia," although this is less common in newer versions of the drug.[14] Benzodiazepines may be prescribed to alleviate insomnia more immediately in cases where mood stabilizers have been prescribed, but need time to take proper effect, and the interaction of these medications has not been extensively studied.[9] It is important to note that one study found no significant effects of benzodiazepine usage on clinical outcome of patients treated with lithium or quetiapine over 6 months, but longer-term effects are lesser known.[73]

Non-Benzodiazepine Sedatives

Non-benzodiazepine sedatives such as zolpidem (Ambien), zaleplon (Sonata), eszopiclone (Lunesta) raise levels of the amino acid gamma-aminobutyric acid (GABA) to slow down brain activity, allowing the body to relax and promoting sleep. They are preferred for short-term insomnia treatment using the lowest effective dose and have side effects including drowsiness, memory loss, and unusual sleep-related behaviors, like sleep driving or eating.[74] In bipolar patients, non-benzodiazepine sedatives have been demonstrated as effective and safe agents for outpatients with insomnia.[75]

Mood Stabilizers

Lithium is a widely used and effective mood-stabilizing treatment that also shows evidence of slowing down circadian periodicity and modifying circadian cycle length.[47] Thus, it may target dysregulated circadian rhythms to promote sleep in bipolar patients, in addition to regulating symptoms of mania and depression. Lithium toxicity is a concern, such that patients who are prescribed lithium must have their blood levels carefully monitored to avoid toxicity. Valproic acid (Depakote), lamotrigine (Lamictal), and carbamazepine (Tegretol) are also commonly prescribed to stabilize mood symptoms in bipolar disorder, but their relationship to sleep is not well studied, and to our knowledge, there are no clinical trials that have explored their effects on sleep in this population.

Antidepressants

While low doses of antidepressants are sometimes used in the general population to treat insomnia, it is important to note that use of antidepressant agents with hypnotic effects may be associated with a switch to mania or hypomania as well as long-term worsening of bipolar illness.[76] Thus, the use of antidepressants is generally recommended only to treat very severe depression in bipolar individuals (and prescribers are advised to discontinue their use after recovery from the severe depressive episode). These medications are not ideal for use as sleep aids in bipolar disorder.

Modafinil

Modafinil, a stimulant medication, is used to treat narcolepsy and has been used to treat hypersomnia in depressed patients with bipolar disorder.[77] As with other stimulants, side effects may be serious, ranging from cardiovascular to dermatologic effects.[78] Modafinil is associated with mania, psychosis, and suicidal ideation in patients with disorders other than bipolar disorder.[78] Therefore, caution is advised in the use of modafinil for bipolar patients who may be more susceptible to experiencing these psychiatric symptoms.

Melatonin

Melatonin is a neurohormonal byproduct of serotonin, a key neurotransmitter involved in mood disorders.[45] Melatonin is naturally present in the body and helps regulate the sleep–wake cycle. It is also sold as an over-the-counter supplement, as well as approved as a sleep aid. Bipolar patients have been shown to exhibit lower melatonin levels and a later peak time for melatonin during the night compared to healthy controls.[43] Thus, melatonin supplements may be particularly useful in this population, and serious side effects (e.g., headaches, sedation, and fatigue) are relatively uncommon.

Nonpharmacologic Treatments

Over the past three decades, nonpharmacological treatments have been developed to supplement medications for bipolar patients who experience sleep disturbances. These interventions include psychotherapies and chronotherapies, which generally include sleep hygiene techniques as core features of the intervention. Sleep hygiene is the culmination of positive habits that an individual can adopt to improve their sleep.[79] For example, having a comfortable sleeping environment is crucial to a good night's sleep, so optimizing temperature (68–72° F), eliminating noise (exception: white noise), improving bed comfortability, and comfortable clothes are all important components of practicing good sleep hygiene. For individuals with bipolar disorder, it is particularly important to establish a quiet, low-stimulation environment before sleep (e.g., limit screen time, conflicts with others, caffeine). This may need to be started several hours before bedtime given the challenges for bipolar patients to unwind (due to underlying agitation, restlessness, and irritability associated with bipolar episodes). Strategies to create a more structured routine may also help with sleep, such as getting in and out of bed at the same time every day. This is particularly important for individuals with bipolar disorder as they tend to have disrupted daily routines, or circadian rhythms, as well as phase shifted sleep cycles.[59] Thus, allowing for more flexible "target times" for activities (e.g., setting a goal to be in bed, but allowing 45 minutes before and after the target time to count toward hitting goals) as well as slightly shifted target times (e.g., set a target time of in bed by 12–1 AM and out of bed by 9–10 AM) may be especially helpful for patients with bipolar disorder.

Another way to help synchronize circadian rhythms is to eat at approximately the same time each day. Individuals with bipolar disorder may need to pay special attention to their diets to help their sleep and level of alertness as they tend to have reactive hyperglycemia. Reactive hyperglycemia occurs from eating simple carbohydrates in the morning, which then causes an excessive increase in blood sugar, quickly followed by a dramatic decrease.[4] This may cause an individual to feel tired, "fuzzy," or irritable. Consequently, bipolar patients will often continue consuming these simple carbohydrates in an effort to "chase" their blood sugar. This cycle can continue throughout the day, leaving individuals feeling drowsy when they should be alert and alert when they should be unwinding and getting ready to go to sleep. Exercise has also been shown to help synchronize the circadian clock, and thus, it is recommended that individuals exercise nearly every day.[4] Clinicians should encourage patients to keep a sleep log and/or purchase a mobile device that can estimate sleep quality for better tracking and monitoring of sleep. In sum, for individuals with bipolar disorder, it is important to assess, monitor, and counsel on the core aspects of sleep hygiene.

Psychotherapies
Interpersonal and Social Rhythms Therapy

Interpersonal and social rhythms therapy (IPSRT) builds upon the foundations of basic sleep hygiene in its assumption that bipolar individuals are particularly susceptible to disruptions in the social rhythms circadian, which cause sleep disturbance.[80] Thus, a central tenet of IPSRT is improving one's social rhythms, including interactions with others, physical activity, or meal times. With the assumption that synchronized social rhythms are "the hallmark of the euthymic state," IPSRT focuses on the perceived major pathways to social rhythm disruptions, such as managing stressful life events and regularizing social routines, particularly bed time and wake time (to improve one's sleep cycle and reduce sleep disturbance).[81] IPSRT uses four phases of treatment, which generally begin on a weekly basis and taper off as the patient progresses through the phases.[82]

The first phase consists of psychoeducation, assessment of interpersonal relationships and social routines, and, finally, a collaboration between therapist and patient to choose an interpersonal problem area to be the initial focus of therapy.[82] The second phase consists of efforts to regulate the patient's social rhythms with a particular focus on the selected interpersonal problem area. In the third phase, the aim is to build the patient's confidence regarding his/her ability to use techniques learned in the second phase of treatment, as well as to improve interpersonal relationships using techniques largely outlined in the interpersonal psychotherapy manual.[83] The final phase of IPSRT involves readying the patient for either reduction in visit frequency or the termination of therapy entirely, which generally begins on a weekly basis and tapers off as the patient progresses through the phases.[81]

IPSRT has been shown to improve social rhythms, with promising data on its ability to improve bipolar symptoms. Frank and colleagues[10] conducted the first large study of IPSRT in combination with pharmacotherapy for bipolar disorder. While no significant differences were observed between treatment strategies in terms of time to stabilization of acute episode, IPSRT was associated with longer time to recurrence of both manic and depressive episodes. Further, regulation of daily routines was inversely related to recurrence during the maintenance phase. Another study found that IPSRT improved recovery rates as well as yielded shorter times to recovery than the control group, but not more so than family-focused therapy or cognitive-behavioral therapy.[84] In sum, IPSRT is a suitable addition to treatment options for the management of sleep disruptions in bipolar disorder patients.

Cognitive Behavioral Therapy for Insomnia

Cognitive behavioral therapy for insomnia (CBT-I) has proven to be efficacious in adults with insomnia.[71,72,85,86] Given the previously discussed links between sleep and affective disorders, CBT-I is considered a good nonpharmacological treatment option for bipolar patients who are suffering from insomnia; however, several modifications have been suggested for bipolar disorder. For example, CBT-I recommends only going to bed when feeling tired and getting out of bed if not asleep in 20 minutes.[85] This improves insomnia in the nonbipolar population, but for individuals with bipolar disorder, waiting to go to bed until they are tired could inadvertently initiate sleep deprivation (as bipolar individuals often do not feel tired), which could trigger (hypo)manic symptoms.[87] Thus, researchers suggest that bipolar individuals should get into bed before they feel tired to begin the process of downregulating and unwinding (despite not feeling tired).[88] Furthermore, CBT-I recommends getting out of bed in the middle of the night after being awake for 20 to 30 minutes and returning to bed when sleepy, so that bed is used only for sleeping. The researchers caution that for individuals with bipolar disorder, getting out of bed in the middle of night when sleep is not being achieved could further encourage them to engage in arousing activities that contradict sleep (given the tendency for individuals with bipolar disorder to engage in goal-directed behaviors and to not feel tired).[88] Thus, teaching relaxation activities that bipolar individuals can do in bed is important (e.g., listening to mindfulness apps, recording positive mantras on their phone, performing breathing exercises).

Given these data on sleep and bipolar disorder, researchers have adapted the original CBT-I protocol for bipolar patients. Specifically, CBT-I for bipolar disorder includes three principles of CBT-I: (a) sleep hygiene; (b) daily tracking of mood, sleep, and routines; and (c) goal setting to regularize sleep and wake times, as well as two new principles: (a) activity scheduling to reduce disruptions of circadian rhythm and (b) the identification of and coping with prodromes of affective episodes (which may or may not include

sleep disturbances).[14] It is important to note that sleep restriction may not need to be omitted in all cases.[14]

Given the aforementioned concerns of using CBT-I for patients with bipolar disorder, one study examined the safety and efficacy of CBT-I modified for patients with bipolar disorder in a group of 15 euthymic subjects.[88] They observed that with this modified approach, which adjusted stimuli control to account for safety concerns, they were successful at improving sleep with only a small percentage of participants exhibiting mild elevation in mood.[88] To determine if CBT-I for bipolar disorder improved mood state, sleep, and functioning, another study randomized bipolar participants ($n = 58$) to either CBT-I for bipolar disorder or a psychoeducational control group.[89] This preliminary study suggests that CBT-I for bipolar disorder can improve both sleep dysregulation and mood symptoms associated with bipolar disorder.

Chronotherapies

Chronotherapeutic interventions aim to treat mood disorders and improve biological rhythms through exposure to environmental stimuli.[90] These interventions are nonpharmaceutical and include three types: sleep deprivation or wake therapy, sleep phase advance, and light and dark therapy.[90]

Sleep Deprivation

There are several theorized mechanisms of action for sleep deprivation. Mood disorders are often characterized by abnormal sleep patterns, appetite, and circadian rhythms.[39,91] Based on these characteristics, several theories about the mechanisms of action of sleep deprivation therapy have been proposed, including serotonergic factors,[92] the release of monoamines,[93] and increase in cerebral adenosine concentration.[94]

Sleep deprivation has been shown to improve depressive symptoms in about 60% of patients within 24 hours after the night of sleep deprivation.[95] However, symptom reduction may last for only a few hours or until the end of the following day.[95] It is unclear how many hours of sleep deprivation are necessary to yield positive outcomes; however, a typical sleep deprivation treatment involves staying awake for approximately 36 hours (or "total" sleep deprivation).[49,96] A noticeable change in mood is not generally seen until the end of the wake period during sleep deprivation treatment.[97] Partial sleep deprivation involves withholding sleep during the second half of the night and is effective but not as effective as total sleep deprivation.[98,99] Sleep deprivation as a therapy has been associated with a number of adverse effects, including the onset of (hypo)mania in some patients[26] as well as the development of poor eating habits and substance use.[100] While not practiced as frequently as a single therapy for mood disorders, adjunctive sleep deprivation has been shown to decrease depressive symptoms the day after the night of sleep deprivation.[101] Depressive symptoms did relapse after the night of recovery sleep, but the relapse rate was lower for those taking antidepressants or mood stabilizer like lithium in conjunction with the sleep deprivation therapy compared to those who were not also taking medications.[101] Due to the nature of sleep deprivation therapy, this intervention has not been studied recently, especially in bipolar patients (given that it can precipitate manic/hypomanic episodes).

Sleep Phase Advance

Sleep phase advance involves waking up about 6 hours earlier than usual and has been shown to improve mood in bipolar depressed patients.[102] This chronotherapeutic intervention has not been popular in routine care given the challenges of adapting one's schedule.[103] However, sleep phase advance has been shown to enhance the clinical impact of sleep deprivation over a short period of time when compared to other antidepressant treatment options, such as electroconvulsive therapy or pharmacotherapy.[104] The combination of sleep deprivation and sleep phase advance has also been shown to prevent the relapse on returning to a typical night's sleep often associated with chronotherapeutic treatment modalities.[104]

Bright Light Therapy

Sunlight can be very influential in changing one's circadian rhythm. Thus, artificial light, or BLT, may be a powerful method of resetting circadian rhythm disruptions, such as sleep disturbance, and may be a way to catalyze a robust and stable antidepressant response in depressed bipolar patients. Currently, there are no clear guidelines on the best light dosage (intensity and duration) and time of the day to maximize the efficacy of BLT for bipolar disorder.[105,106] However, researchers suggest that a 7,000 lux light may be optimum.[105,106] Further, this research suggests that beginning with 15 minutes of light therapy midday that is increased by 15 minutes each week either to response or a maximum of 45 to 60 minutes per day may yield the best results in bipolar disorder or reduce the likelihood of triggering manic symptoms.

Other studies suggest that BLT may be beneficial for bipolar disorder. BLT is an effective treatment for seasonal affective disorder[107-111] and nonseasonal depression.[112-114] Specific to bipolar depression, the results of BLT have been more mixed.[37,105,106,115-118] While more trials examining BLT's effect on bipolar depression are warranted, BLT does appear to be a promising treatment due to its preliminary efficacy, accessibility and affordability, lack of side effects, lack of drug–drug interactions, and a provider's ability to adjust dosage based on side effects and mood fluctuations.[105]

Dark Therapy

Dark therapy, or extended time in bed, may also have beneficial effects for those with bipolar disorder experiencing sleep disturbances, especially those experiencing rapid cycling (i.e., experiencing at least four mood episodes in 1 year). Two case reports have noted that mood swings in rapid cycling patients are improved when wake–sleep and light–dark rhythms are regimented.[119,120] In a later study, 16 consecutively admitted manic patients were given dark therapy in addition to treatment as usual.[121] These patients were then compared to inpatients matched for age, sex, age at onset, number of previous illness episodes, and duration of current episode and were treated with therapy as usual. It was noted that dark therapy was associated with a rapid reduction in mania; however, if the patient had already been experiencing mania for more than 2 weeks then dark therapy had no clinical effect. These data are very preliminary and require replication for bipolar disorder in randomized and controlled samples prior to being implemented clinically.

CONCLUSION AND FUTURE DIRECTIONS

Sleep disruptions (insomnia or hypersomnia) are present across the course of bipolar disorder and occur before, during, and in between mood episodes (i.e., mania, hypomania, depression). These disruptions may trigger mood episodes as well as worsen the course of illness. Moreover, maintaining good sleep habits and ameliorating sleep disturbances may prevent mood relapse in bipolar patients.

Evidence-based clinical recommendations for managing sleep disturbance in bipolar disorder are summarized in Table 18.2. In terms of psychopharmacological treatment, hypnotics

TABLE 18.2. SLEEP RECOMMENDATIONS FOR BIPOLAR DISORDER

Sleep Tip	Why Important for Bipolar Disorder
Establish a regular sleep routine	Bipolar disorder is particularly susceptible to circadian rhythm disruptions.
Optimize circadian rhythm disruptions	Creating a regular work, meal, exercise and interactions with others may help to improve the sleep/wake cycle
Consider medication interactions/side effects	Adding a sleep aid may compound the sedating effects of other medications for bipolar disorder (e.g., mood stabilizers, antipsychotics) and thus, should be used carefully as this may reduce overall medication adherence.
Allow more time to relax before bed	Individuals with bipolar disorder are more likely to feel underlying restlessness, agitation, and irritability.
Shift sleep phase slowly	Individuals with bipolar disorder may be more likely to have phase shifted sleep (bed times between 12–3 AM) and although it is ideal to align sleep cycle with the light/dark cycle; shifts in sleep routine should occur slowly (as they will be difficult for the individual) and will likely remain slightly shifted.
Go to bed even when not feeling sleepy	Individuals with bipolar disorder often do not feel tired, even when getting very little sleep, therefore it is important for them to get into bed despite not feeling tired.
Use stimulants sparingly	For hypersomnia, be cautious in using stimulants given their risk for triggering an elevated mood state in bipolar disorder.
Do not encourage getting out of bed in the middle of the night	This could increase the likelihood that bipolar individuals will engage in arousing activities given their tendency to do goal-directed behaviors and not to feel tired.
Teach relaxation strategies to do while in bed	These strategies can help bipolar patients relax while in bed, (e.g., mindfulness activities and meditations).
Do not use sleep restriction to shift sleep routine	Sleep restriction could cause hypomanic or manic symptoms.
Gradual dosing of bright light (7,000 lux) to 45–60 minutes per day	Light therapy shows preliminary evidence to improve mood in bipolar patients as well as to help phase shift sleep.

and sedating antidepressants are widely used in the nonbipolar population to treat insomnia, but adverse effects and lack of studies that investigate their interactions with other psychiatric drugs warrant caution when prescribing them for bipolar disorder. Hypersomnia may be alleviated by stimulants such as modafinil, but stimulants must be used carefully in individuals with bipolar disorder given that they can trigger a manic episode. In summary, clinicians should be cautious when prescribing medications for insomnia or hypersomnia in a bipolar patient and be vigilant in monitoring the dosage, use, and overall risk–benefit ratio.

Psychological interventions and chronotherapies have been developed to improve sleep in bipolar disorder. IPSRT and CBT-I for bipolar disorder can reduce sleep disruptions in bipolar disorder (several specific aspects of these treatments are summarized in Table 18.2). The field of chronotherapeutics has further advanced these nonpharmacological treatment interventions by introducing sleep deprivation or wake therapy, sleep phase advance, light therapy, and dark therapy, but results from these treatments tend to be mixed. Of these, sleep deprivation has shown some efficacy but may trigger manic or hypomanic episodes; sleep phase advance as an adjunctive therapy has been able to reduce relapse and increase clinical effects of sleep deprivation; and BLT is approved to treat unipolar depression, with recent evidence suggesting that it can alleviate bipolar depressive symptoms.

In summary, sleep is an important treatment target for bipolar disorder, as good sleep may prevent future episodes as well as improve the current course of the illness. Given the unique characteristics of bipolar disorder, clinicians need to be thoughtful in how they apply empirically validated treatments for insomnia and hypersomnia to this clinical population and use modified treatments for bipolar disorder when possible. Future studies are needed to further develop and refine treatments to address sleep disturbances, which are a common and clinically significant feature of bipolar disorder.

KEY CLINICAL PEARLS

- Sleep disturbance is a diagnostic criterion for both manic and depressive episodes observed in bipolar I and II disorders.
- Bipolar patients with more severe sleep disturbances tend to report lower quality of life than bipolar patients with healthy sleep habits.
- Sleep disturbances reliably predict mood episodes for many bipolar patients and could serve as early treatment targets to prevent or lessen the severity of approaching mood episodes.
- Unlike patients with a primary insomnia diagnosis, manic individuals do not feel tired despite sleeping for only a few hours and/or have no desire to sleep.
- Adults with bipolar disorder are more likely than controls to have an "evening" chronotype, a preference for functioning at night rather than during the day (night-owls), which also reflects abnormal circadian rhythms.
- Bipolar patients have been shown to exhibit lower melatonin levels and a later peak time for melatonin during the night compared to healthy controls.
- Lithium may target dysregulated circadian rhythms to promote sleep in bipolar patients.
- IPSRT and CBT-I can reduce sleep disruptions in bipolar disorder.

SELF-ASSESSMENT QUESTIONS

1. Bipolar depressive episodes are characterized by what type of sleep disturbance?
   a. Hypersomnia
   b. Insomnia
   c. Both a and b
   d. Neither a or b

Answer: c

2. Which medication class has shown to be both safe and effective for treating sleep in bipolar disorder?
   a. Benzodiazepines
   b. Anti-depressants
   c. Mood stabilizers
   d. Non-benzodiazepine sedatives and mood stabilizers

Answer: d

3. All the following are examples of good sleep hygiene for bipolar disorder except
   a. creating a regular work, meal, exercise and social routines.
   b. allowing for ample time to relax before bed.
   c. getting out of bed in the middle of the night if you can't sleep.
   d. establishing a regular work routine.

Answer: c

4. An important modification for CBT-I for bipolar disorder is
   a. going to bed when you feel tired.
   b. monitoring your sleep and mood symptoms.
   c. not getting out of bed in the middle of the night, even if you are having trouble sleeping.
   d. not allowing for any flexibility in the target bed and wake times.

Answer: c

5. While there are currently no clear guidelines for bright light therapy for treating bipolar disorder, recent research suggests that the most efficacious guidelines are
   a. starting with 10,000 lux in the morning for 15 minutes.
   b. gradual dosing to 7,000 lux for 45 to 60 minutes.
   c. less than 5,000 lux of light exposure per day.
   d. exposure to 7,000 lux multiple times throughout the day.

Answer: b

REFERENCES

1. American Psychiatric Association. *Diagnostic and Statistical Manual of Mental Disorders.* 5th ed. Arlington, VA: American Psychiatric Association; 2013.
2. Judd LL, Akiskal HS, Schettler PJ, et al. The long-term natural history of the weekly symptomatic

status of bipolar I disorder. *Archives of General Psychiatry.* 2002;59(6):530–537.

3. Snook E, Mosely-Dendy K, Hirschfeld RMA. Presentation, clinical course, and diagnostic assessment of bipolar disorder. In: Yildiz A, Ruiz P, Nemeroff CB, eds. *The Bipolar Book: History, Neurobiology, and Treatment.* New York, NY: Oxford University Press; 2015:35–48.

4. Goodwin FK, Jamison KR. *Manic-Depressive Illness: Bipolar Disorders and Recurrent Depression.* 2nd ed. New York, NY: Oxford University Press; 2007.

5. Eaton WW, Anthony JC, Gallo J, et al. Natural history of Diagnostic Interview Schedule/DSM-IV major depression. The Baltimore Epidemiologic Catchment Area follow-up. *Archives of General Psychiatry.* 1997;54(11):993–999.

6. Angst J, Preisig M. Outcome of a clinical cohort of unipolar, bipolar and schizoaffective patients. Results of a prospective study from 1959 to 1985. *Schweizer Archiv fur Neurologie und Psychiatrie.* 1995;146(1):17–23.

7. Coryell W, Endicott J, Keller M. Outcome of patients with chronic affective disorder: a five-year follow-up. *American Journal of Psychiatry.* 1990;147(12):1627–1633.

8. Cutler NR, Post RM. Life course of illness in untreated manic-depressive patients. *Comprehensive Psychiatry.* 1982;23(2):101–115.

9. Newman CF, Leahy RL, Beck AT, Reilly-Harrington NA, Gyulai L. *Bipolar Disorder: A Cognitive Therapy Approach.* Washington, DC: American Psychological Association; 2002.

10. Frank E, Kupfer DJ, Thase ME, et al. Two-year outcomes for interpersonal and social rhythm therapy in individuals with bipolar I disorder. *Archives of General Psychiatry.* 2005;62(9):996–1004.

11. Ritter PS, Hofler M, Wittchen HU, et al. Disturbed sleep as risk factor for the subsequent onset of bipolar disorder: data from a 10-year prospective-longitudinal study among adolescents and young adults. *Journal of Psychiatric Research.* 2015;68:76–82.

12. Akiskal HS, Van Valkenburg C. Mood disorders. In: Segal DL, ed. *Diagnostic Interviewing.* New York, NY: Springer; 1994:79–107.

13. Soehner AM, Kaplan KA, Harvey AG. Prevalence and clinical correlates of co-occurring insomnia and hypersomnia symptoms in depression. *J Affect Disord.* 2014;167:93–97.

14. Harvey AG. Sleep and circadian rhythms in bipolar disorder: seeking synchrony, harmony, and regulation. *American Journal of Psychiatry.* 2008;165(7):820–829.

15. Jones SH, Hare DJ, Evershed K. Actigraphic assessment of circadian activity and sleep patterns in bipolar disorder. *Bipolar Disorders.* 2005;7(2):176–186.

16. Millar A, Espie CA, Scott J. The sleep of remitted bipolar outpatients: a controlled naturalistic study using actigraphy. *Journal of Affective Disorders.* 2004;80(2-3):145–153.

17. Ritter PS, Marx C, Lewtschenko N, et al. The characteristics of sleep in patients with manifest bipolar disorder, subjects at high risk of developing the disease and healthy controls. *Journal of Neural Transmission.* 2012;119(10):1173–1184.

18. Tal JZ, Primeau M. Circadian rhythms, sleep, and their treatment impact. In: Yildiz A, Ruiz P, Nemeroff CB, eds. *The Bipolar Book: History, Neurobiology, and Treatment.* New York, NY: Oxford University Press; 2015:35–48.

19. Bradley AJ, Webb-Mitchell R, Hazu A, et al. Sleep and circadian rhythm disturbance in bipolar disorder. *Psychological Medicine.* 2017;47(9):1678–1689.

20. Gruber J, Miklowitz DJ, Harvey AG, et al. Sleep matters: sleep functioning and course of illness in bipolar disorder. *Journal of Affective Disorders.* 2011;134(1–3):416–420.

21. Sylvia LG, Dupuy JM, Ostacher MJ, et al. Sleep disturbance in euthymic bipolar patients. *Journal of Psychopharmacology.* 2012;26(8):1108–1112.

22. Gershon A, Thompson WK, Eidelman P, McGlinchey EL, Kaplan KA, Harvey AG. Restless pillow, ruffled mind: sleep and affect coupling in interepisode bipolar disorder. *Journal of Abnormal Psychology.* 2012;121(4):863–873.

23. St-Amand J, Provencher MD, Belanger L, Morin CM. Sleep disturbances in bipolar disorder during remission. *Journal of Affective Disorders.* 2013;146(1):112–119.

24. Ng TH, Chung KF, Ho FY, Yeung WF, Yung KP, Lam TH. Sleep–wake disturbance in interepisode bipolar disorder and high-risk individuals: a systematic review and meta-analysis. *Sleep Medicine Reviews.* 2015;20:46–58.

25. Jackson A, Cavanagh J, Scott J. A systematic review of manic and depressive prodromes. *Journal of Affective Disorders.* 2003;74(3):209–217.

26. Wehr TA, Goodwin FK, Wirz-Justice A, Breitmaier J, Craig C. 48-hour sleep–wake cycles in manic-depressive illness: naturalistic observations and sleep deprivation experiments. *Archives of General Psychiatry.* 1982;39(5):559–565.

27. Barbini B, Colombo C, Benedetti F, Campori E, Bellodi L, Smeraldi E. The unipolar-bipolar dichotomy and the response to sleep deprivation. *Psychiatry Research.* 1998;79(1):43–50.

28. Plante DT, Winkelman JW. Sleep disturbance in bipolar disorder: therapeutic

implications. *American Journal of Psychiatry.* 2008;165(7):830–843.

29. Benazzi F. Clinical differences between bipolar II depression and unipolar major depressive disorder: lack of an effect of age. *Journal of Affective Disorders.* 2003;75(2):191–195.

30. Benazzi F, Rihmer Z. Sensitivity and specificity of DSM-IV atypical features for bipolar II disorder diagnosis. *Psychiatry Research.* 2000;93(3):257–262.

31. Forty L, Smith D, Jones L, et al. Clinical differences between bipolar and unipolar depression. *British Journal of Psychiatry.* 2008;192(5):388–389.

32. Kanady JC, Soehnera AM, Harvey AG. A retrospective examination of sleep disturbance across the course of bipolar disorder. *Journal of Sleep Disorders and Therapy.* 2015;4(2):1000193.

33. Dinges DF, Pack F, Williams K, et al. Cumulative sleepiness, mood disturbance, and psychomotor vigilance performance decrements during a week of sleep restricted to 4–5 hours per night. *Sleep.* 1997;20(4):267–277.

34. Drake CL, Roehrs TA, Burduvali E, Bonahoom A, Rosekind M, Roth T. Effects of rapid versus slow accumulation of eight hours of sleep loss. *Psychophysiology.* 2001;38(6):979–987.

35. Zohar D, Tzischinsky O, Epstein R, Lavie P. The effects of sleep loss on medical residents' emotional reactions to work events: a cognitive-energy model. *Sleep.* 2005;28(1):47–54.

36. Colombo C, Benedetti F, Barbini B, Campori E, Smeraldi E. Rate of switch from depression into mania after therapeutic sleep deprivation in bipolar depression. *Psychiatry Research* 1999;86(3):267–270.

37. Leibenluft E, Turner EH, Feldman-Naim S, Schwartz PJ, Wehr TA, Rosenthal NE. Light therapy in patients with rapid cycling bipolar disorder: preliminary results. *Psychopharmacology Bulletin.* 1995;31(4):705–710.

38. Wehr TA, Sack DA, Rosenthal NE. Sleep reduction as a final common pathway in the genesis of mania. *American Journal of Psychiatry.* 1987;144(2):201–204.

39. Grandin LD, Alloy LB, Abramson LY. The social zeitgeber theory, circadian rhythms, and mood disorders: review and evaluation. *Clinical Psychology Review.* 2006;26(6):679–694.

40. Minors DS, Waterhouse JM. Introduction to circadian rhythms. In: Folkard S, TMonk TH, eds. *Hours of Work: Temporal Factors in Work-Scheduling.* New York, NY: Wiley; 1985:1–14.

41. Geoffroy PA, Boudebesse C, Henrion A, et al. An ASMT variant associated with bipolar disorder influences sleep and circadian rhythms:

a pilot study. *Genes, Brain, and Behavior.* 2014;13(3):299–304.

42. Kennedy SH, Kutcher SP, Ralevski E, Brown GM. Nocturnal melatonin and 24-hour 6-sulphatoxymelatonin levels in various phases of bipolar affective disorder. *Psychiatry Research.* 1996;63(2):219–222.

43. Nurnberger JI, Jr., Adkins S, Lahiri DK, et al. Melatonin suppression by light in euthymic bipolar and unipolar patients. *Archives of General Psychiatry.* 2000;57(6):572–579.

44. Souetre E, Salvati E, Wehr TA, Sack DA, Krebs B, Darcourt G. Twenty-four-hour profiles of body temperature and plasma TSH in bipolar patients during depression and during remission and in normal control subjects. *American Journal of Psychiatry.* 1988;145(9):1133–1137.

45. Lanfumey L, Mongeau R, Hamon M. Biological rhythms and melatonin in mood disorders and their treatments. *Pharmacol Therapy.* 2013;138(2):176–184.

46. Melo MC, Abreu RL, Neto VBL, de Bruin PF, de Bruin VM. Chronotype and circadian rhythm in bipolar disorder: a systematic review. *Sleep Medicine Reviews.* 2017;34:46–58.

47. Abe M, Herzog ED, Block GD. Lithium lengthens the circadian period of individual suprachiasmatic nucleus neurons. *Neuroreport.* 2000;11(14):3261–3264.

48. Basturk M, Karaaslan F, Esel E, Sofuoglu S, Tutus A, Yabanoglu I. Effects of short and long-term lithium treatment on serum prolactin levels in patients with bipolar affective disorder. *Progress in Neuro-Psychopharmacology and Biological Psychiatry.* 2001;25(2):315–322.

49. McClung CA. Circadian genes, rhythms and the biology of mood disorders. *Pharmacology and Therapeutics.* 2007;114(2):222–232.

50. Ogden CA, Rich ME, Schork NJ, et al. Candidate genes, pathways and mechanisms for bipolar (manic-depressive) and related disorders: an expanded convergent functional genomics approach. *Molecular Psychiatry.* 2004;9(11):1007–1029.

51. Johnsson A, Engelmann W, Pflug B, Klemke W. Period lengthening of human circadian rhythms by lithium carbonate, a prophylactic for depressive disorders. *International Journal of Chronobiology.* 1983;8(3):129–147.

52. Welsh DK, Moore-Ede MC. Lithium lengthens circadian period in a diurnal primate, Saimiri sciureus. *Biological Psychiatry.* 1990;28(2):117–126.

53. McCarthy MJ, Le Roux MJ, Wei H, Beesley S, Kelsoe JR, Welsh DK. Calcium channel genes associated with bipolar disorder modulate

lithium's amplification of circadian rhythms. *Neuropharmacology*. 2016;101:439–448.

54. Moreira J, Geoffroy PA. Lithium and bipolar disorder: impacts from molecular to behavioural circadian rhythms. *Chronobiology International*. 2016;33(4):351–373.

55. Noguchi T, Lo K, Diemer T, Welsh DK. Lithium effects on circadian rhythms in fibroblasts and suprachiasmatic nucleus slices from Cry knockout mice. *Neuroscience Letters*. 2016;619:49–53.

56. Ehlers CL, Frank E, Kupfer DJ. Social zeitgebers and biological rhythms. A unified approach to understanding the etiology of depression. *Archives of General Psychiatry*. 1988;45(10):948–952.

57. Johnson SL. Life events in bipolar disorder: towards more specific models. *Clinical Psychology Review*. 2005;25(8):1008–1027.

58. Johnson SL, Miller I. Negative life events and time to recovery from episodes of bipolar disorder. *Journal of Abnormal Psychology*. 1997;106(3):449–457.

59. Sylvia LG, Alloy LB, Hafner JA, Gauger MC, Verdon K, Abramson LY. Life events and social rhythms in bipolar spectrum disorders: a prospective study. *Behavior Therapy*. 2009;40(2):131–141.

60. Boland EM, Bender RE, Alloy LB, Conner BT, LaBelle DR, Abramson LY. Life events and social rhythms in bipolar spectrum disorders: an examination of social rhythm sensitivity. *Journal of Affective Disorders*. 2012;139(3):264–272.

61. Harvey AG, Schmidt DA, Scarna A, Semler CN, Goodwin GM. Sleep-related functioning in euthymic patients with bipolar disorder, patients with insomnia, and subjects without sleep problems. *American Journal of Psychiatry*. 2005;162(1):50–57.

62. Murray G, Harvey A. Circadian rhythms and sleep in bipolar disorder. *Bipolar Disorders*. 2010;12(5):459–472.

63. Benedetti F, Serretti A, Colombo C, et al. Influence of CLOCK gene polymorphism on circadian mood fluctuation and illness recurrence in bipolar depression. *American Journal of Medical Genetics Part B, Neuropsychiatric Genetics*. 2003;123b(1):23–26.

64. Lee KY, Song JY, Kim SH, et al. Association between CLOCK 3111T/C and preferred circadian phase in Korean patients with bipolar disorder. *Progress in Neuro-Psychopharmacology and Biological Psychiatry*. 2010;34(7):1196–1201.

65. Mansour HA, Monk TH, Nimgaonkar VL. Circadian genes and bipolar disorder. *Annals of Medicine*. 2005;37(3):196–205.

66. Nievergelt CM, Kripke DF, Barrett TB, et al. Suggestive evidence for association of the circadian genes PERIOD3 and ARNTL with bipolar disorder. *American Journal of Medical Genetics Part B, Neuropsychiatric Genetics*. 2006;141b(3):234–241.

67. Serretti A, Benedetti F, Mandelli L, et al. Genetic dissection of psychopathological symptoms: insomnia in mood disorders and CLOCK gene polymorphism. *American Journal of Medical Genetics Part B, Neuropsychiatric Genetics*. 2003;121b(1):35–38.

68. Roybal K, Theobold D, Graham A, et al. Mania-like behavior induced by disruption of CLOCK. *Proceedings of the National Academy of Sciences of the United States of America*. 2007;104(15):6406–6411.

69. Yildiz A, Ruiz P, Nemeroff C. *The Bipolar Book: History, Neurobiology, and Treatment*. New York, NY: Oxford University Press; 2015.

70. Weinstock LM, Gaudiano BA, Epstein-Lubow G, Tezanos K, Celis-Dehoyos CE, Miller IW. Medication burden in bipolar disorder: a chart review of patients at psychiatric hospital admission. *Psychiatry Research*. 2014;216(1):24–30.

71. Buscemi N, Vandermeer B, Friesen C, et al. Manifestations and management of chronic insomnia in adults: summary. 2005;125:1–10.

72. National Institutes of Health. National Institutes of Health state of the science conference statement: manifestations and managements of chronic insomnia in adults, June 13-15, 2005. *Sleep*. 2005;28(9):1049–1057.

73. Bobo WV, Reilly-Harrington NA, Ketter TA, et al. Effect of adjunctive benzodiazepines on clinical outcomes in lithium- or quetiapine-treated outpatients with bipolar I or II disorder: results from the Bipolar CHOICE trial. *Journal of affective disorders*. 2014;161:30–35.

74. Zolpidem and related agents. Thomson Micromedex; 2017. Accessed October 11, 2017.

75. Schaffer CB, Schaffer LC, Miller AR, Hang E, Nordahl TE. Efficacy and safety of nonbenzodiazepine hypnotics for chronic insomnia in patients with bipolar disorder. *Journal of Affective Disorders*. 2011;128(3):305–308.

76. Ghaemi SN, Hsu DJ, Soldani F, Goodwin FK. Antidepressants in bipolar disorder: the case for caution. *Bipolar Disorders*. 2003;5(6):421–433.

77. Frye MA, Grunze H, Suppes T, et al. A placebo-controlled evaluation of adjunctive modafinil in the treatment of bipolar depression. *American Journal of Psychiatry*. 2007;164(8):1242–1249.

78. Modafinil. Thomson Micromedex; 2017. www.micromedexsolutions.com. Accessed October 11, 2017.

79. Miklowitz DJ, Goldstein MJ. *Bipolar Disorder: A Family-Focused Treatment Approach*. New York, NY: Guilford Press; 1997.

80. Ehlers CL, Kupfer DJ, Frank E, Monk TH. Biological rhythms and depression: the role of zeitgebers and zeitstorers. *Depression.* 1993;1(6):285–293.

81. Frank E. *Treating bipolar disorder: a clinician's guide to interpersonal and social rhythm therapy.* New York, NY: Guilford Press; 2005.

82. Frank E. Interpersonal and social rhythm therapy: a means of improving depression and preventing relapse in bipolar disorder. *Journal of Clinical Psychology.* 2007;63(5):463–473.

83. Klerman GL, Weissman MM, Rounsaville BJ, Chevron E. *Interpersonal Psychotherapy of Depression.* New York, NY: Basic Books; 1984.

84. Miklowitz DJ, Otto MW, Frank E, et al. Psychosocial treatments for bipolar depression: a 1-year randomized trial from the Systematic Treatment Enhancement Program. *Archives of General Psychiatry.* 2007;64(4):419–426.

85. Edinger JD, Means MK. Cognitive-behavioral therapy for primary insomnia. *Clinical psychology Review.* 2005;25(5):539–558.

86. Morin CM, Bootzin RR, Buysse DJ, Edinger JD, Espie CA, Lichstein KL. Psychological and behavioral treatment of insomnia: update of the recent evidence (1998–2004). *Sleep.* 2006;29(11):1398–1414.

87. Wehr TA. Improvement of depression and triggering of mania by sleep deprivation. *JAMA.* 1992;267(4):548–551.

88. Kaplan KA, Harvey AG. Behavioral treatment of insomnia in bipolar disorder. *American Journal of Psychiatry.* 2013;170(7):716–720.

89. Harvey AG, Soehner AM, Kaplan KA, et al. Treating insomnia improves mood state, sleep, and functioning in bipolar disorder: A pilot randomized controlled trial. *Journal of Consulting and Clinical Psychology.* 2015;83(3):564–577.

90. Benedetti F, Barbini B, Colombo C, Smeraldi E. Chronotherapeutics in a psychiatric ward. *Sleep Medicine Reviews.* 2007;11(6):509–522.

91. Boivin DB. Influence of sleep–wake and circadian rhythm disturbances in psychiatric disorders. *Journal of Psychiatry and Neuroscience.* 2000;25(5):446–458.

92. Smeraldi E, Benedetti F, Barbini B, Campori E, Colombo C. Sustained antidepressant effect of sleep deprivation combined with pindolol in bipolar depression. A placebo-controlled trial. *Neuropsychopharmacology.* 1999;20(4):380–385.

93. Ebert D, Berger M. Neurobiological similarities in antidepressant sleep deprivation and psychostimulant use: a psychostimulant theory of antidepressant sleep deprivation. *Psychopharmacology.* 1998;140(1):1–10.

94. Demet EM, Chicz-Demet A, Fallon JH, Sokolski KN. Sleep deprivation therapy in depressive illness and Parkinson's disease. *Progress in Neuro-Psychopharmacology and Biological Psychiatry.* 1999;23(5):753–784.

95. Giedke H, Schwärzler F. Therapeutic use of sleep deprivation in depression. *Sleep Medicine Reviews.* 2002;6(5):361–377.

96. Benedetti F, Colombo C. Sleep deprivation in mood disorders. *Neuropsychobiology.* 2011;64(3):141–151.

97. Haug HJ, Fahndrich E. A turning point for mood during sleep deprivation therapy—does it exist? *Pharmacopsychiatry.* 1988;21(6):418–419.

98. Schilgen B, Tolle R. Partial sleep deprivation as therapy for depression. *Archives of General Psychiatry.* 1980;37(3):267–271.

99. Wirz-Justice A, Benedetti F, Berger M, et al. Chronotherapeutics (light and wake therapy) in affective disorders. *Psychological Medicine.* 2005;35(7):939–944.

100. Harvey AG, Talbot LS, Gershon A. Sleep disturbance in bipolar disorder across the lifespan. *Clinical Psychology: Science and Practice.* 2009;16(2):256–277.

101. Wu JC, Bunney WE. The biological basis of an antidepressant response to sleep deprivation and relapse: review and hypothesis. *American Journal of Psychiatry.* 1990;147(1):14–21.

102. Wehr TA, Wirz-Justice A, Goodwin FK, Duncan W, Gillin JC. Phase advance of the circadian sleep–wake cycle as an antidepressant. *Science.* 1979;206(4419):710–713.

103. Benedetti F. Antidepressant chronotherapeutics for bipolar depression. *Dialogues in clinical neuroscience.* 2012;14(4):401–411.

104. Berger M, Vollmann J, Hohagen F, Konig A. Sleep deprivation combined with consecutive sleep phase advance as a fast-acting therapy in depression: an open pilot trial in medicated and unmedicated patients. *American Journal of Psychiatry.* 1997;154(6):870.

105. Sit D, Wisner KL, Hanusa BH, Stull S, Terman M. Light therapy for bipolar disorder: a case series in women. *Bipolar Disorders.* 2007;9(8):918–927.

106. Sit DK, McGowan J, Wiltrout C, et al. Adjunctive bright light therapy for bipolar depression: a randomized double-blind placebo-controlled trial. *American Journal of Psychiatry.* 2018;175(2):131–139.

107. Lewy AJ, Bauer VK, Cutler NL, et al. Morning vs evening light treatment of patients with winter depression. *Archives of General Psychiatry.* 1998;55(10):890–896.

108. Terman M, Terman JS, Ross DC. A controlled trial of timed bright light and negative air ionization

for treatment of winter depression. *Archives of General Psychiatry*. 1998;55(10):875–882.

109. Melrose S. Seasonal Affective Disorder: An Overview of Assessment and Treatment Approaches. *Depression Research and Treatment*. 2015;2015:178564.

110. Nussbaumer B, Kaminski-Hartenthaler A, Forneris CA, et al. Light therapy for preventing seasonal affective disorder. *Cochrane Database of Systematic Reviews*. 2015(11):Cd011269.

111. Rohan KJ, Mahon JN, Evans M, et al. Randomized trial of cognitive-behavioral therapy versus light therapy for seasonal affective disorder: acute outcomes. *American Journal of Psychiatry*. 2015;172(9):862–869.

112. Chojnacka M, Antosik-Wójcińska AZ, Dominiak M, et al. A sham-controlled randomized trial of adjunctive light therapy for non-seasonal depression. *Journal of Affective Disorders*. 2016;203:1–8.

113. Goel N, Terman M, Terman JS, Macchi MM, Stewart JW. Controlled trial of bright light and negative air ions for chronic depression. *Psychological Medicine*. 2005;35(7):945–955.

114. Golden RN, Gaynes BN, Ekstrom RD, et al. The efficacy of light therapy in the treatment of mood disorders: a review and meta-analysis of the evidence. *American Journal of Psychiatry*. 2005;162(4):656–662.

115. Papatheodorou G, Kutcher S. The effect of adjunctive light therapy on ameliorating breakthrough depressive symptoms in adolescent-onset bipolar disorder. *Journal of Psychiatry and Neuroscience*. 1995;20(3):226–232.

116. Benedetti F, Barbini B, Fulgosi MC, et al. Combined total sleep deprivation and light therapy in the treatment of drug-resistant bipolar depression: acute response and long-term remission rates. *Journal of Clinical Psychiatry*. 2005;66(12):1535–1540.

117. Dauphinais DR, Rosenthal JZ, Terman M, DiFebo HM, Tuggle C, Rosenthal NE. Controlled trial of safety and efficacy of bright light therapy vs. negative air ions in patients with bipolar depression. *Psychiatry Research*. 2012;196(1):57–61.

118. Zhou T, Dang W, Ma Y, et al. Clinical efficacy, onset time and safety of bright light therapy in acute bipolar depression as an adjunctive therapy: A randomized controlled trial. *Journal of Affective Disorders*. 2018;227:90–96.

119. Wehr TA, Turner EH, Shimada JM, Lowe CH, Barker C, Leibenluft E. Treatment of a rapidly cycling bipolar patient by using extended bed rest and darkness to stabilize the timing and duration of sleep. *Biological Psychiatry*. 1998;43(11):822–828.

120. Wirz-Justice A, Van den Hoofdakker RH. Sleep deprivation in depression: what do we know, where do we go? *Biological Psychiatry*. 1999;46(4):445–453.

121. Barbini B, Benedetti F, Colombo C, et al. Dark therapy for mania: a pilot study. *Bipolar Disorders*. 2005;7(1):98–101.

19

Anxiety, Obsessive-Compulsive, and Related Disorders

BRUCE ROHRS, BENJAMEN GANGEWERE, ALICIA KAPLAN, AND AMIT CHOPRA

INTRODUCTION

Anxiety disorders are the most common group of psychiatric disorders in the United States, with a life time prevalence of 28.8% [1]. Insomnia is a widespread public health issue, affecting almost one-third of the population, with substantial comorbidity with other psychiatric disorders [2, 3]. It is estimated that 70% to 90% of the anxiety disorder patients exhibit insomnia [4]. As compared to primary insomnia, patients with anxiety disorders and comorbid insomnia demonstrate significantly reduced sleep efficiency (SE) and slow-wave sleep [5]. Despite significant comorbidity of sleep disturbances and anxiety disorders, much of the available research has focused on sleep disturbances in affective disorders. Additionally, only generalized anxiety disorder (GAD) and separation anxiety disorder include sleep disturbances as a part of the *Diagnostic and Statistical Manual of Mental Disorders* (fifth edition; DSM-5) diagnostic criteria.

However, the expanding investigation into the convergence of sleep and anxiety disorders has yielded a number of clinically significant findings. Prospective research examining the relative temporal onset of sleep disturbance in anxiety disorders reveals that in a majority of individuals (43%) the anxiety disorder precedes the onset of insomnia or occurs at about the same time (39%). In a substantial minority of cases (18%), the insomnia actually precedes the development of the anxiety disorder [6]. Additionally, prospective studies suggest that self-reported sleep disturbance is linked to the later development of anxiety disorders, suggesting that sleep issues, specifically insomnia, may be either a risk factor or a prodromal symptom for anxiety disorders [7]. Poor sleep can mediate the level of overall functional impairment in individuals with anxiety disorders

thus leading to significantly worse mental health-related quality of life and increased disability relative to those with anxiety disorders alone [8, 9].

Furthermore, sleep dysfunction at baseline can predict poor treatment outcomes in anxiety disorder patients. In a study examining cognitive-behavioral therapy (CBT) and D-cycloserine treatment outcomes in social anxiety disorder (SAD), individuals with poor sleep at baseline had worse treatment outcomes as compared to those without sleep disturbances [10]. Evidence based clinical guidelines suggest that CBT for insomnia (CBT-I) is both effective and superior as compared to medications [11–13]. However, there is a dearth of research examining the efficacy of CBT-I in the treatment of insomnia associated with anxiety disorders. Therefore, comprehensive understanding of both the comorbidity and impact of sleep disturbances in anxiety disorders is needed to guide development of effective treatment strategies.

Due to recent nosological and organizational changes in the DSM-5, the conditions that have historically been considered as anxiety disorders have been redistributed into three distinct categories: obsessive-compulsive (OCD) and related disorders, anxiety disorders, and trauma and stressor-related disorder. Furthermore, many disorders that were formerly included in the category of "Disorders First Occurring in Infancy, Childhood, and Adolescence" have now been redistributed among the previously listed categories such that separation anxiety disorder and selective mutism are now included under the section of "Anxiety Disorders" while reactive attachment disorder is classified as a "Trauma- and Stressor-Related Disorder." Virtually all of the anxiety disorders have a high degree of comorbidity with other anxiety disorders and with mood disorders, particularly major depressive disorder. While it is beyond the scope of this chapter to explore this comorbidity in depth, it is clear that the diagnostic overlap makes it more difficult to sort out "pure types" of anxiety disorders for research purposes. For the purposes of this chapter, we will review sleep disturbances in GAD, panic disorder (PD), and OCD, with lesser attention on the diagnoses including social phobia, trichotillomania/excoriation disorder, and hoarding due to limited research on these topics.

PATHOPHYSIOLOGY

Emotional Dysregulation

While authors have suggested shared underlying neurological substrates that can lead to sleep disturbances and anxiety disorders, this link is still speculative. In healthy individuals, fronto-limbic circuits are involved in processing emotional stimuli. These fronto-limbic circuits encompass four key regions of the brain including hippocampus, amygdala, insula, and prefrontal complex (PFC) [14–19]. Within the PFC, the structures implicated in emotional regulation include medial PFC, ventromedial PFC (vmPFC), dorsomedial PFC (dmPFC) [20–22] and dorsal anterior cingulate cortex (dACC) [14, 17]. Evidence suggests that the activity of hippocampus, amygdala, and insula is increased in anxious adults [23–25]. Hyperresponsiveness of mPFC, dACC, and dmPFC along with hypo-activity of vmPFC during conscious appraisal of fear [20–22, 26] potentially explains the diminished modulation of fear response in anxious individuals.

Sleep deprivation has a negative impact on emotional regulation in response to negative stimuli. An functional magnetic resonance (fMRI) investigation study compared healthy and anxious adolescents on a measure of sleep amount and neural response to faces with negatively valence. Group differences were noted in terms of neural response to negative faces especially in dACC and hippocampus. In both these regions, the correlation between sleep amounts with BOLD activation was positive in anxious adolescents but negative in healthy adolescents. Additionally, the functional connectivity between brain regions including dACC and dorsomedial PFC, and between hippocampus and insula was correlated negatively with sleep amount in anxious adolescents, whereas it correlated positively in healthy adolescents [27]. These findings may suggest that sleep plays a role

in emotional dysregulation in individuals predisposed to emotional difficulties.

Impaired Executive Functioning

Ample evidence suggests that sleep deprivation leads to impaired executive functioning [28, 29] and deficits in inhibition [30], attention [31] and memory [32]. Following 1 night of sleep deprivation, increased amygdala activity in response to negative stimulus and decreased connectivity between the amygdala and mPFC has been reported [33]. It is plausible that impaired executive functioning associated with sleep deprivation may lead to a diminished ability to regulate or inhibit anxiety related processes such maladaptive repetitive thoughts including worries, ruminations, and obsessions [34]. The association of impaired executive functioning with repetitive thoughts and attentional and inhibitory deficits in GAD and OCD patients further attests the hypothesis that sleep loss may impair executive functioning leading to diminished ability to regulate or inhibit anxiety symptoms [34].

Cortisol Dysregulation

Another important mechanism that links sleep disturbance with anxiety and related disorders is dysregulated cortisol [34]. It is evident that healthy individuals have steep increase in cortisol secretion in the morning followed by gradual decline during the day and a nadir during sleep [35, 36]. Additionally, in response to an acute stressor, cortisol levels increase in healthy individuals [37]. However, poor sleep has been implicated in dysregulated diurnal cortisol with consequences such as blunted morning cortisol secretion, elevated evening cortisol [35], and blunted cortisol reactivity to stressors [38].

Dysregulated diurnal cortisol has been associated with impaired executive dysfunction, inhibition, and memory [39–41]. It has been suggested that over time the downstream effects of dysregulated cortisol, due to sleep disturbance, may contribute to the development of an anxiety-related disorder [34]. Not surprisingly, individuals with GAD exhibit blunted wakening cortisol response [42] and higher total cortisol output [43], whereas individuals with OCD have been noted to have elevated overnight cortisol secretion [44] and blunted cortisol reactivity to stressors [45].

Anxiety Sensitivity

AS is a transdiagnostic factor that contributes to both anxiety disorders [46, 47] and sleep disturbance [48]. AS is defined as a trait-like fear of anxiety-related feelings and sensations and comprises of three separate dimensions: physical concerns (i.e., heart racing is a sign of an impending heart attack), cognitive concerns (i.e., mind going blank is a sign of mental incapacitation or insanity), and social concerns (i.e., observable symptoms, such as blushing, will result in social rejection) [49]. Specifically, high AS and its dimensions have been associated with sleep disturbance, short sleep duration, poor sleep quality, sleep dysfunction, prolonged sleep onset latency (SOL), and sleep-related impairment, even after accounting for relevant psychological factors [50–54].

In a study examining the association between AS and sleep disturbance in anxious patients, the authors noted that AS was associated with increased sleep disturbance across anxiety disorders including GAD, PD, and SAD. The primary anxiety disorder diagnosis was significantly associated with sleep disturbance; however, this association was no longer significant after controlling for AS [55]. The authors suggested AS being a transdiagnostic factor that appears to be an important predictor of sleep disturbance in anxiety disorders. Moreover, reductions in AS have been found to contribute to positive treatment outcomes for patients with anxiety disorders [56] and insomnia [57]. Finally, evidence suggests that targeting AS, using CBT strategies, may be an effective way to reduce co-occurring insomnia symptoms in anxiety disorder patients [52, 58].

CLINICAL APPROACH

Patients with anxiety, OCD, and related disorders can present with a range of sleep disturbances including sleep initiation and maintenance insomnia, nocturnal panic attacks, nightmares, poor sleep quality, and daytime fatigue. The majority of evidence suggests that anxiety disorders are associated with insomnia, but one study utilizing subjective reports of total sleep time (TST) found that slightly over 8% of individuals with PD reported hypersomnia (sleeping more than 9 hours per night). The presence of co-occurring depression in the sample influenced this finding, but individuals without depression also reported excessive sleepiness [59]. This finding has not been replicated and warrants further investigation.

It is important to comprehensively assess the sleep disturbance in anxious patients at the time of initial presentation and to determine the temporal relationship between sleep disturbance and anxiety symptoms. Assessment of comorbid psychiatric disorders, especially mood disorders, is crucial for a thorough understanding and treatment of sleep disturbance in this population. Presence of co-occurring psychiatric disorders in general has been correlated with a higher risk of sleep disturbance. For example, as compared to individuals with no psychiatric disorder, the risk of sleep disturbance increases by 2.2 to 3.2 times for individuals with two psychiatric disorders and 4.6 to 6.3 times for individuals with three or more psychiatric disorders [60]. As compared to young depressed patients without sleep disturbance, those with sleep disturbances may experience a greater burden of comorbid anxiety symptoms, hyperarousal, and poor cognitive and physical functioning [61].

Assessment of substance use in anxious patients is an important part of evaluation process and includes the consumption of caffeine, nicotine, alcohol, and recreational drugs. Epidemiological studies suggest high comorbidity of anxiety disorders among individuals with substance use disorders (SUD) ranging from 17.7% to 29.9% [62, 63]. Evidence suggests that anxiety disorders, SUDs, and sleep disturbance co-occur commonly and contribute to worse clinical outcomes. However, remarkably few studies have investigated factors leading to sleep disturbance among adults with co-occurring anxiety disorders and SUD. In a study, the authors noted that AS, particularly the cognitive concerns, may represent an important transdiagnostic mechanism underlying sleep disturbance in patients with co-occurring anxiety disorders and SUD [48]. Lifestyle and environmental factors leading to poor sleep hygiene and resulting sleep disturbance also need to be fully explored.

Primary sleep disorders, such as obstructive sleep apnea (OSA), can coexist with anxiety disorders. Findings suggest that, as compared to men, women are more likely to have comorbid OSA and anxiety. Presence of OSA may precipitate and perpetuate anxiety, whereas anxiety negatively impacts quality of life in patients with OSA. Treatment of OSA may improve anxiety symptoms, whereas anxiety symptoms can be a deterrent to appropriate treatment of OSA [64]. For example, claustrophobic tendencies have been noted in 63% of the participants in a study examining continuous positive airway pressure (CPAP) compliance in OSA. Claustrophobia negatively affects short-term and longer-term compliance CPAP thus leading to treatment nonadherence [65].

New-onset sleep problems after initiation of pharmacological treatment may likely be suggestive of iatrogenic side effects including insomnia, vivid dreams, nightmares, daytime sedation, restless legs syndrome (RLS), parasomnia behaviors, and worsening of breathing-related sleep disorders. For example, antidepressant medications can worsen or cause RLS and benzodiazepine medications can potentially worsen OSA. Clinical use of standard sleep procedures such as polysomnography (PSG) and actigraphy is indicated when there is a suspicion for coexisting primary sleep disorders in anxious patients such as OSA, parasomnias, and circadian rhythm disorders. Treatment of sleep disturbances associated with anxiety disorders (GAD and PD) and OCD has been summarized in Table 19.1 and also has been discussed in detail in the context of specific anxiety, OCD, and related disorders.

ASSESSMENT

None of the commonly used subjective questionnaires for assessment of anxiety, OCD, and related disorders, including Generalized Anxiety Disorder 7-item scale (GAD-7) scale for GAD assessment, Panic Disorder Severity Scale (PDSS) for PD assessment, and Yale–Brown Obsessive Compulsive Severity (Y-BOCS) scale for OCD assessment include subjective sleep measures. Hamilton Anxiety Rating scale (HAM-A), a clinician-rated scale for assessment of GAD [66], can be used for assessment of insomnia in GAD patients. The Pittsburgh Sleep Quality Index (PSQI) [67] and Insomnia Severity Index (ISI) [68] are commonly used in research studies to assess sleep quality and insomnia severity in patients with anxiety disorders. Sleep diaries can be used to subjectively monitor sleep duration and patterns in anxious patients.

The objective measures used for assessment of sleep in anxiety disorders include PSG and actigraphy. Sleep parameters including SOL, wake after sleep onset time (WASO), SE, and TST can be estimated by using both PSG and actigraphy studies. Since actigraphy does not include electroencephalography (EEG) monitoring, only PSG studies can evaluate sleep architectural changes including nonrapid eye movement (NREM) and rapid eye movement (REM) sleep alterations in patients with anxiety disorders. It must be noted that, in patients with anxiety disorders, the current use of PSG and actigraphy is limited to research studies only.

TABLES 19.1. EVIDENCE-BASED TREATMENTS FOR SLEEP DISTURBANCE ASSOCIATED WITH GENERALIZED ANXIETY DISORDER, PANIC DISORDER, AND OBSESSIVE-COMPULSIVE DISORDER

GAD	CBT (for GAD)
	Modified CBT-I for nonresponders
	• Avoid sleep restriction
	Eszopiclone + Escitalopram
	Pregabalin
	Melatonergic agents (including Ramelteon and Agomelatine)
PD	Modified CBT (psychoeducation, breathing retraining)
	Conventional CBT for PD
	CBT-I
	• Avoid sleep restriction, meditative relaxation and hypnotic imagery in nocturnal panic attacks
	Escitalopram (improvement in subjective sleep only)
	CPAP (if patient has comorbid OSA)
	Benzodiazepines
	• Prefer short-term use
OCD	Concentrated exposure response prevention
	• Intervention not targeting sleep
	• Patients with higher baseline sleep disturbance had better overall outcomes

Abbreviations: CBT: cognitive-behavioral therapy; CBT-I: Cognitive behavioral therapy for insomnia; CPAP, continuous positive airway pressure; GAD, generalized anxiety disorder; OCD, obsessive-compulsive disorder; OSA: obstructive sleep apnea; PD, panic disorder.

Current evidence points to a degree of incongruity between the objective and subjective measures in at least some of the anxiety and related disorders [5]. This could suggest that the afflicted individuals are unreliable or erroneous in their self-reporting of sleep disturbance. This issue was examined in more depth, by authors who drew on many years of clinical observation as well as extant research [4]. The authors suggest that some patients with co-occurring anxiety and sleep disorders have more difficulty distinguishing between sleep and wakefulness and show sleep state misperception, such that relatively brief periods of nocturnal wakefulness are perceived as lasting for a much longer period of time. The authors concluded that PSG may be unreliable as a measure of insomnia because it fails to fully account for gradations of consciousness between wakefulness and sleep in this population [4].

Additionally, the authors suggest a need to develop new physiological and neuroimaging markers to distinguish these gradations to increase diagnostic precision as well as improving our understanding of the underlying mechanisms to explain the sleep disturbance in patients with anxiety disorders. Several in-depth reviews examine the sleep architectural changes in patients with anxiety disorders, pointing to a number of contradictory findings between studies [34, 69]. However, the three consistent findings across anxiety disorders are increased SOL, decreased TST, and potentially reduced SE. Table 19.2 summarizes the subjective and objective sleep findings in GAD, PD, and OCD.

PANIC DISORDER (PD) AND NOCTURNAL PANIC ATTACKS

Individuals with PD frequently report sleep disturbance, including insomnia, restlessness, non-restorative sleep with frequent awakenings, and nocturnal panic attacks. The latter are instances where the individual awakens abruptly from a sound sleep with panic symptoms, including heart palpitations, shortness of breath, chest discomfort, and feelings of impending disaster and/or terror. The majority of patients with PD (65%–70%) report at least one nocturnal episode, a substantial minority (30%–45%) have recurrent nocturnal panic attacks, and a few individuals (2%) with PD present only nocturnal attacks [70].

The nocturnal panic attacks usually occur within the first 3 hours of sleep onset, are short lived (lasting approximately 2–8 minutes), and devoid of dreams, cognitions and imagery. PD patients with nocturnal panic attacks report higher rates of insomnia as well as depression as compared to those without nocturnal panic

TABLE 19.2. SUMMARY OF SUBJECTIVE AND OBJECTIVE SLEEP DISTURBANCES IN GENERALIZED ANXIETY DISORDER, PANIC DISORDER, AND OBSESSIVE COMPULSIVE DISORDER

	Subjective Sleep Complaints	Sleep Architecture Changes based on Polysomnography)
GAD	• Worse subjective sleep quality • Subjective sleep disturbance associated with development of GAD over time	• ↑ SOL • ↓ TST • NREM sleep alterations • Evidence on SE is mixed. • Evidence suggesting REM sleep changes is inconclusive
PD	• Insomnia, restlessness, non-restorative sleep with frequent awakenings • Nocturnal panic attacks • PD patients with nocturnal panic and lifetime history of depression report worst subjective sleep disturbance	• ↑ SOL • ↓ SE • ↓ TST • NREM abnormalities, though less robust, include ↑ N1 and ↓ stage N2 and N3. • Evidence supporting REM abnormalities is limited
OCD	• 45%–50% of OCD patients may complain of sleep disturbance • More symptomatic individuals complain of higher sleep disturbance • Associated with circadian rhythm disorders	• ↓ TST • ↑ WASO • ↓ SE • Evidence for NREM and REM alterations mixed

Abbreviations: GAD, generalized anxiety disorder; NREM: Non rapid-eye movement; OCD, obsessive-compulsive disorder; PD, panic disorder; REM: Rapid eye movement; SE: Sleep Efficiency; SOL: Sleep onset latency; TST: Total sleep time; WASO: Wake after sleep onset.

attacks [5]. An association between sleep paralysis and nocturnal panic attacks has been noted with 35% of subjects with isolated sleep paralysis reporting wake panic attacks (unrelated to sleep paralysis) and 16% of these subjects met full criteria of PD [71]. While the patients with sleep paralysis have an increased risk of PD, the reverse association does not appear to be true [71].

Etiology

A review of recent advances in the field of anxiety and sleep considers nocturnal panic attacks to be the major cause of sleep difficulties in PD [69]. This finding is mediated through a variety of potential mechanisms including sleep difficulties caused by the nocturnal panic attacks and a behavioral conditioning paradigm whereby the afflicted individuals pair sleep and high anxiety awakenings, thus rendering comfortable sleep increasingly difficult. The authors also suggest that cognitive distortions associated with sleep have a potential influence on the development and maintenance of nocturnal panic attacks. These cognitive distortions negatively affect SOL as well as the ability to return to sleep following an event, thus leading to decreased overall sleep time. Rather than being restorative, sleep becomes an occasion of increasing dread for such patients, and almost 30% of patients with nocturnal panic attacks develop severe sleep restriction with TST of less than 5 hours per night [59]. Additionally, AS may play a role as an intervening variable. AS leads to higher selective attention to abnormal and potentially problematic (or interpreted as such) physical sensations noted in individuals with anxiety disorders. This sensitivity can amplify cognitive distortions that may impair sleep. AS is significantly higher in individuals with PD and has been correlated with increased sleep-onset latency [52].

Differential Diagnosis

Nocturnal panic attacks are distinguishable from other problematic sleep events such as parasomnias (night terrors), sleep apnea, awakening related to posttraumatic stress disorder (PTSD), and nocturnal epilepsy. Unlike sleep terrors, which occur mostly in N3 sleep, nocturnal panic attacks usually occur in late N2 or early N3 sleep [72]. Additionally, individuals with sleep terrors usually have no recollection of the event and will often resume peaceful sleep without fully awakening, whereas in nocturnal panic the individual will have a vivid recollection of awakening and will often have difficulty resuming sleep [73]. While

some authors have suggested a link between nocturnal panic and sleep apnea [74], there are important distinctions. Sleep apnea is a much more repetitive phenomenon with multiple episodes that occur NREM and REM sleep whereas PSG studies have not found this to be the case in nocturnal panic. However, it should be noted that presence of sleep apnea confers a higher risk of future development of PD [75]. Unlike nocturnal epilepsy, no EEG abnormalities have been reported during nocturnal panic episodes [76]. Finally, PTSD-related awakening typically occurs in the context of nightmares, which occur during REM sleep, whereas nocturnal panic attacks are not associated with nightmares and typically occur during NREM sleep [5].

Subjective Sleep Changes in PD

Individuals with PD report increased sleep disturbance as compared to healthy controls [77]. Additionally, PD patients with nocturnal panic and lifetime history of depression report significantly greater subjective sleep disturbance as compared to those with PD alone, PD with nocturnal panic attacks, and PD with history of lifetime depression [59].

Sleep Architectural Changes in PD

As compared to healthy controls, PD patients exhibit sleep architectural changes including increased SOL [78, 79], decreased SE [78–80], and decreased TST [81]. These sleep findings overall were not affected by presence of nocturnal panic according to one study [81]. Evidence supporting REM abnormalities in PD is limited and NREM abnormalities, although less robust, include increased stage N1 and decreased stage N2 and N3 [34].

Treatments
Psychotherapy

There is a paucity of studies looking at the effects of treatment of sleep disturbance in PD, although limited evidence suggests that psychological treatment of panic and nocturnal panic utilizing a modified CBT intervention is effective in both reducing both daytime and nocturnal panic [82]. These interventions posit that individuals with nocturnal panic are more sensitive to physiological changes during sleep and are more likely to misinterpret these changes as indicative of a potentially dangerous physiological state (similar to AS, as previously mentioned). Common misinterpretations include physiological changes being indicative of potential cardiac arrest or of nocturnal suffocation. In addition to psychoeducation and breathing retraining, patients are encouraged to voluntarily induce panic-like symptoms through hyperventilation. Patients are also awoken at different times of the night to simulate being awoken by internal cues so that the classically conditioned associations are weakened. Finally, poor sleep habits such as inconsistent sleep/wake times are targeted.

Results are promising with over 70% of participants being free of nocturnal panic and a significant number having remission of both daytime and nighttime panic at the end of a 10-week treatment intervention, a treatment effect that was maintained at the end of a 9-month follow-up [83]. Another study that examined the efficacy of conventional CBT versus nocturnally adapted CBT, admittedly using a small subject group, found that both interventions were about equally effective in producing symptom remission, an effect that lasted through a 1-year follow-up [82]. However, a third study reported that sleep parameters did not improve after conventional treatment of panic [84].

Taken together, these findings suggests that specifically targeted interventions may not be necessary to treat both panic and co-occurring sleep disturbance; however, it should not be assumed that sleep disturbance resolves with successful treatment of panic. Patients should be evaluated for resolution of sleep disturbance as well as resolution of panic; this evaluation should then guide the need for further specialized intervention. When necessary, specific sleep-targeted interventions do appear to be helpful for achieving a positive treatment outcome. There are certain behavioral interventions that may not be helpful in PD patients due to potential worsening of anxiety symptoms. Of note, individuals with nocturnal panic attacks are significantly more distressed by conditions that resemble sleep, such as meditative relaxation and hypnotic imagery [85, 86]. Additionally, sleep deprivation in PD has been associated with worsening of panic attacks [87].

Medications
Evidence suggests effectiveness of paroxetine, venlafaxine, sertraline, citalopram, fluoxetine, and escitalopram in treatment of PD [88]. Unfortunately, limited evidence exists to ascertain the efficacy of first-line pharmacological treatments for PD in improving associated sleep disturbance. Treatment with escitalopram has been associated with improvement in subjective sleep quality in female patients with PD whereas the objective sleep measures remained unchanged during treatment [89].

Benzodiazepines (BZD) have documented efficacy in treatment of PD, and BZDs are equally efficacious and may be better tolerated than tricyclic/selective serotonin reuptake inhibitor antidepressants [90]. As compared to controls, PD patients taking alprazolam were noted to have increase in SE, TST, and stage N2. Additionally, decrease in wakefulness during the total sleep period, stage N3, and the oxygen desaturation and periodic limb movement indices and improved subjective sleep quality, somatic complaints, drive, affectivity, and drowsiness in the morning were reported in patients taking alprazolam [91]. However, the duration of use of BZD medications should be limited due to concerns including addiction potential, increased fall risk in the elderly, increased risk for cognitive impairment, and rebound anxiety [92]. No evidence exists to support efficacy of benzodiazepine receptor agonists (BzRAs) in treatment of sleep disturbance associated with PD.

Other Modalities
In patients with comorbid PD and OSA, as compared to sham treatment, the use of therapeutic CPAP for OSA management has been shown to reduce the frequency of both nocturnal and daytime panic attacks, the PDSS score, and use of alprazolam to alleviate panic attacks. Therefore, it is recommended to optimally treat coexisting OSA in PD patients to achieve best clinical outcomes [93].

GENERALIZED ANXIETY DISORDER (GAD)
GAD is one of the few anxiety disorder diagnoses that specifically include sleep disturbance (difficulty falling asleep, staying asleep, or having restless and unsatisfying sleep) as one of its potential diagnostic criteria (DSM-5). As many as 70% of patients with GAD have significant complaints of insomnia, and it appears that the relationship between sleep disturbance and anxiety disorders is higher in GAD than in most other anxiety disorders [8]. The temporal relationship between the development of insomnia and the onset of GAD is unclear, with some studies suggesting that in some individuals, insomnia may be a prodromal feature for GAD [2, 94]. Not surprisingly, daytime dysfunction is strongly associated with insomnia and

GAD, even when the presence of a mood disorder is factored out.

In a cross-sectional, prospective, observational, and multicenter study, the severity of the GAD was most strongly associated with the presence of insomnia (odds ratio [OR] 9.253 for severe GAD; 95% confidence interval [CI] 1.914–44.730; $p = 0.006$). Other factors included pain interference and symptoms of depression [95]. In a cross-sectional study in a university setting ($n = 462$), the authors assessed sleep and anxiety using the ISI, PSQI, Epworth Sleepiness Scale, and GAD-7 [96]. The prevalence of clinically significant insomnia was noted to be 10.6% (95% CI 7.8%–13.4%), more frequent in first-year students. GAD was more frequent in students suffering from insomnia ($p = 0.006$) and in poor sleepers ($p = 0.003$). The authors noted that 50.8% of the participants with GAD reported hypersomnolence as compared to 30.9% of those with no clinically significant anxiety ($p < 0.0001$) [96].

Etiology

In a study of individuals without a GAD diagnosis, those characterized as "worriers" reported increased sleep disturbance as compared to "nonworriers" [97]. Another study examining a nonclinical sample indicated that ruminations at baseline were associated with poor sleep quality among individuals with high levels of worry and reduction in sleep quality at follow-up [98]. Further research examining the association between sleep disturbance and GAD symptoms such as rumination and worry in GAD may help in the development of targeted interventions to improve sleep outcomes in GAD patients [69]. Emotional dysregulation, characterized by mood lability or difficulty modulating emotional responses, may also play a role in sleep disturbance associated with GAD [69]. As compared to healthy controls, individuals with GAD and emotional dysregulation were noted to have greater sleep disturbance, increased nightmare frequency, difficulty waking in the morning, daytime sleepiness, and notably poor daytime functioning [99].

Subjective Sleep Changes in GAD

As compared to healthy controls, GAD patients report worse subjective sleep and are more likely to have a sleep disorder [100–102]. On the other hand, subjective sleep disturbance has been associated with development of GAD over time, which is suggestive of the role of sleep disturbance in the etiology of GAD [103]. Additionally, adult patients with GAD have higher odds of sleep disturbance despite controlling for comorbid major depression [104].

Sleep Architectural Changes in GAD

PSG findings in GAD suggest significantly longer SOL, decreased TST, and NREM sleep alterations as compared to healthy controls [69]. The evidence on decreased SE seems to be somewhat mixed in GAD patients as most studies, except one, do not report decreased SE in GAD patients as compared to healthy controls. Similarly, evidence suggesting REM sleep changes in GAD patients seems to be inconclusive [34].

Treatments
Psychotherapy

Research on the effectiveness of psychotherapeutic interventions on insomnia in individuals with GAD has been somewhat mixed. An earlier study found that subjects with GAD who were treated with CBT showed significant improvement in both anxiety and sleep following intervention, even though sleep was not specifically targeted in the intervention, suggesting that a broader-based treatment strategy may be effective [105]. However, later research determined that while some sleep issues (global sleep quality and SOL) improved, other aspects of sleep (subjective sleep quality, sleep duration, SE, and daytime dysfunction) did not improve. The authors concluded that significant sleep disturbance remains at the end of treatment in GAD patients [106]. The authors further suggested that targeted interventions specifically aimed at improving sleep prior to or during CBT may be beneficial for poor sleepers [106]. An ancillary finding of significance is that individuals with baseline sleep disturbance showed a worse overall anxiety treatment response to CBT intervention. The reasons for this observation are unclear; it could indicate that pronounced insomnia represents a more symptomatic form of GAD, or it could suggest that secondary characteristics of insomnia (e.g., poorer concentration) impaired the ability of participants to focus on aspects of the CBT treatment.

In a study examining sequential treatments of comorbid insomnia and GAD, 10 women with chronic insomnia and GAD were randomly assigned to CBT for GAD followed by CBT for insomnia, or to CBT for insomnia followed by CBT for GAD. The authors found that initiating treatment for GAD first resulted in superior clinical benefits in anxiety and sleep and subsequent insomnia-specific treatment then led to additional improvements in worry and sleep quality [107]. For the clinician, the implications are fairly straight forward. An alert clinician will assess the patient's sleep quality at both the onset of treatment and as treatment progresses. Positive changes in sleep quality may result from a more general, anxiety-targeted intervention, and specific sleep-targeted intervention may not be required. However, if necessary, a more sleep-specific targeted intervention should be instituted as residual sleep disturbances increase the risk of relapse of anxiety disorders [6].

However, it has been suggested that highly anxious patients may poorly tolerate sleep restriction, a core component of CBT-I, due to increased anxiety about not getting enough sleep thus compromising TST [108]. On the other hand, CBT-I techniques such as stimulus control may be beneficial for GAD patients such as scheduled worry time and getting out of bed when unable to control anxious thoughts [108]. Further research is warranted to identify positive predictors of response to CBT-I and develop treatment protocols that incorporate CBT-I for successful outcomes in GAD patients with significant sleep disturbance [69].

Medications

In a randomized controlled study, citalopram (20 mg) and doxepin (12.5 mg) significantly improved sleep quality in anxiety patients. As compared to those taking citalopram, significantly greater improvements in sleep latency, measured subjectively, were noted in patients taking doxepin. The authors suggested that citalopram and doxepin could have a beneficial effect in treatment of patients with comorbid insomnia and anxiety disorders [109]. The combination of eszopiclone (benzodiazepine receptor agonist) and escitalopram (SSRI) has been shown to significantly improve anxiety, sleep disturbance, and daytime functioning in GAD patients in a placebo-controlled study [110]. Another study reported efficacy and tolerability of pregabalin in significantly reducing daytime anxiety and insomnia in GAD patients [111]. However, dose-related sedation has been reported in approximately 10% to 30% of patients typically in the first 2 weeks of pregabalin treatment likely associated with the dose and the speed of titration. Citalopram 20 to 40 mg daily has been associated with additional improvements in subjective sleep disturbance (as measured by PSQI rating scale) in patients with late-life anxiety disorders (age >60 years), primarily GAD, in a 32-week study trial [112].

Ramelteon, a melatonin receptor agonist, has been associated with increased TST and reduced SOL in a 12-week open-label study in 27 adult patients with GAD [113]. Similarly, agomelatine, a melatonin agonist and serotonergic antagonist, has been noted to be effective in improving insomnia and daytime symptoms in GAD patients in a randomized, double-blind placebo-controlled study for a period of 12 weeks [114]. These findings, taken together, may suggest the role of circadian rhythm disruption in pathogenesis and treatment of sleep–wake disturbances in GAD.

Newer Treatments

Repetitive transcranial magnetic stimulation (rTMS), an emerging and promising technique for treatment of neuropsychiatric disorders, has been noted for efficacy in treatment of comorbid GAD and insomnia in a randomized, double-blind, sham controlled pilot study [115]. The rTMS treatment was administered over the right posterior parietal cortex at a frequency of 1 Hz and an intensity of 90% of the rTMS motor threshold for a period of 10 days. Significant improvements in GAD and insomnia symptoms were noted in the treatment group ($n = 18$) with low frequency stimulation as compared to the sham group. Currently, rTMS is US Food and Drug Administration–approved for management of major depressive disorder and future studies are needed to establish the efficacy of rTMS in management of GAD.

SOCIAL ANXIETY DISORDER (SAD)

The comorbidity of SAD and sleep disturbance has not been extensively studied. Limited evidence suggests between 30% and 60% of individuals with SAD have moderate to marked sleep impairment [116]. Buckner and colleagues [117] compared insomnia in SAD patients ($n = 23$) to healthy controls ($n = 23$) using the Social Interaction Anxiety Scale and the ISI. Individuals with SAD reported increased insomnia symptoms, and social anxiety correlated with sleep dissatisfaction, sleep-related functional impairment, perception of a sleep problem to others, and distress about sleep problems. Additionally, depressive symptoms, measured using Beck Depression Inventory, mediated the relationship between social anxiety and insomnia [117]. Sleep quality has been noted to predict the outcomes of CBT for generalized SAD [10] as patients with poor baseline sleep quality had slower improvement and higher posttreatment social anxiety symptom severity. The SAD patients with self-report of "rested" sleep during the night following CBT had reported lower social anxiety symptoms and global severity. Therefore, it is important to address sleep quality prior to initiation and during acute CBT treatment for SAD to achieve optimal treatment outcomes.

Subjective Sleep Findings in SAD
As compared to healthy controls, patients with generalized type of SAD reported impairment in sleep quality, longer sleep latency, increased sleep disturbance, and greater daytime dysfunction [116]. The authors suggested that these findings are similar to those in patients with anxiety disorders such as PD and deserve further clinical and research attention.

Sleep Architectural Changes in SAD
According to one study, there appears to be no significant polysomnographic findings that define the sleep disturbances in SAD patients. No alterations of sleep parameters including TST, SOL, SE, and REM measures were noted in SAD patients as compared to healthy controls [118].

Treatments
Psychotherapy
Reports of sleep difficulties show a significant positive correlation with severity of SAD, even after controlling for the effect of coexisting mood symptoms [119]. Individuals with both SAD and subjective insomnia show greater clinical severity at the start of cognitive-behaviorally oriented treatment and continue to show greater impairment at the end of the treatment. Finally, while there was an overall general treatment effect (reduction in anxiety), this effect did not extend to improved sleep, which remained problematic [119]. Brief CBT-I (five sessions) for insomnia was noted to be efficacious in improving sleep quality in a patient with comorbid insomnia and SAD [120]. Future research focusing on incorporating CBT-I in to existing behavioral and medication treatments may prove to be beneficial to optimize clinical outcomes in SAD.

Medications
There is a lack of evidence-based pharmacological treatment strategies for management of sleep disturbances associated with SAD. To our knowledge, no studies have been done to examine the comparative effectiveness of behavioral and psychopharmacological treatment either singly or in combination on sleep disturbance in individuals with SAD.

OBSESSIVE-COMPULSIVE DISORDER (OCD)
OCD is characterized by obsessions (intrusive and repetitive thoughts, urges or images) and compulsions (repetitive behaviors or mental acts) that can be debilitating. It is estimated that approximately 2% to 3% of the general population suffers from this complex and debilitating disorder [1]. There is a well-established correlation between OCD and sleep; however, the exact nature of this link is unclear. Some studies have reported that up to 75% of their subjects with OCD have clinically significant coexisting sleep disturbance, although figures in the 40% to 50% range are more common [121, 122]. Additionally, the relationship between sleep disturbance and OCD appears to be linear, with more symptomatic individuals having a higher level of sleep disturbance [53], and this relationship holds for individuals with subclinical OCD symptoms [123].

Etiology
Some authors have hypothesized common underlying biological factors responsible for sleep disturbance and OCD that include abnormalities in the brain serotonergic system [124] and aberrant activation of the locus coerulus, which disrupts alertness and exacerbates OCD [125]. Others have examined the impact of specific OCD symptoms on sleep disturbance. For instance, a study reported that the severity of compulsions was negatively correlated to TST in children with primary OCD as compared to healthy controls. Sleep disturbance was measured using home-based actigraphy monitoring for a period of 7 days in this study [126]. In another study, the authors reported that obsessions, rather than compulsions, were independently linked to insomnia (despite controlling for depression) in adult OCD patients [127]. These results were replicated by Raines and colleagues [53] who reported that the unacceptable thoughts domain of OCD was significantly associated with insomnia symptoms, whereas the contamination concerns, responsibility for harm, and symmetry/completeness domains were not. The authors further hypothesized that AS, particularly cognitive concerns, is a shared risk factor that could potentially explain the association between OCD and sleep disturbances [53]. The hypothesis that sleep difficulties exacerbate

OCD symptoms has not yet been explored in a prospective study. However, Cox and Olatunji [123] examined the link between the severity of sleep issues and the severity of subclinical OCD symptoms in a nationally representative sample (n = 2,073). The authors concluded that individual with sleep disturbance reported increased obsessive-compulsive symptom severity as compared to those without sleep disturbance.

There is a growing evidence to suggest circadian rhythm sleep-wake alterations in patients with OCD. Delayed sleep phase disorder (DSPD) is a pattern of delayed sleep onset and offset sleep relative to desired bed and wake times, which results in significant distress or dysfunction. Based on retrospective data, patients with severe OCD show a prevalence of DSPD at a rate at least twice that of the general population (17.6% vs. 0.17%–8.9%) [128]. OCD patients with DSPD in this study were younger and had earlier age of onset of OCD, and all of them were unemployed. A meta-analytic study confirmed the higher rate of DSPD in individuals with OCD, although after the effects of comorbid depression were ruled out this association remained a trend but lost statistical significance [129]. Further exploration of the association with DSPD and OCD, using objective measures and biological markers, may not only help consolidate our understanding of sleep disturbance in OCD but also offer insights in to potentially new treatment targets [128].

Subjective Sleep Changes in OCD

Subjective sleep changes in OCD is an area of further study as there is only one study to date that compares subjective sleep in adult OCD patients to healthy controls [130]. The authors compared OCD patients with and without comorbid depression to healthy controls and concluded that OCD patients without depressive symptoms had sleep patterns similar to healthy controls (who also met criteria for poor sleep). Another study noted that OCD patients had increased likelihood of sleep disturbance, but this association was not significant after controlling for comorbid mood and SUDs [8].

Sleep Architectural Changes in OCD

As compared to healthy controls, OCD patients exhibit alterations in sleep parameters including reduced TST [124, 131], increased WASO [124],[132], and reduced SE [124, 132]. The evidence for NREM and REM alterations in OCD patients is mixed as the results are not consistent across the studies [34]. Some earlier findings suggestive of changes in REM efficiency and latency in individuals with OCD, were later attributed to comorbid depression [69].

Treatments
Psychotherapy
Limited literature is available to examine the impact of psychotherapeutic treatments of OCD on co-occurring sleep disturbance. One study, utilizing a concentrated exposure and response prevention protocol for OCD, reported that approximately 70% of the sample showed evidence of significant sleep disturbance at the start of treatment. The authors concluded that majority of patients showed significant symptom reduction, including improvement in sleep difficulties, even though the intervention did not specifically target sleep [121]. Interestingly, sleep disturbance at baseline did not impair treatment outcome; on the contrary, patients with higher degree of baseline sleep disturbance had better OCD treatment outcomes. Furthermore, the sleep changes were independent of changes in comorbid depressive symptoms.

Medications
First-line pharmacological treatment for OCD includes SSRIs and the tricyclic antidepressant, clomipramine. Higher doses and longer treatment trials for at least 3 months are often needed. Atypical antipsychotics, such as risperidone and aripiprazole, can be used for management of refractory OCD [133]. To our knowledge, sleep outcomes have not been systematically well studied with the use of pharmacological treatments for management of OCD.

Neurostimulation Treatments
Despite emerging evidence to support the efficacy of deep brain stimulation in the management of refractory OCD [134], the impact of co-occurring sleep disturbances on OCD outcomes has not been systematically studied. However, presence of circadian rhythm sleep disturbances, and not insomnia, has been associated with poor clinical response in OCD patients who received rTMS as an experimental therapy in a research study [135].

OCD-RELATED DISORDERS

Hoarding Disorder
Hoarding disorder is relatively new psychiatric classification that has been characterized as a

complex clinical phenomenon characterized by an accumulation of and failure to discard a large number of possessions resulting in debilitating clutter. It was once thought to be rare but is now estimated to affect between 2% and 6% of the population. One study explores the connection between hoarding and sleep difficulties [136]. The authors determined that 50% of the sampled clinical population had insomnia. As individuals with pathological hoarding often live in a decreasing amount of space in their residence, many activities increasingly occur in the same limited area that can potentially interfere with sleep hygiene practices thus leading to stimulus dyscontrol. The authors originally hypothesized that insomnia in patients with hoarding disorder would be correlated with the degree of clutter, using a stimulus dyscontrol model of insomnia, whereby activities not associated with sleep in the sleeping area interfere with the sleep-promoting process.

However, the study findings did not support this hypothesis. The authors noted that insomnia predicted hoarding severity, which was true after the effects of co-occurring mood disorders were factored out. However, the authors determined that insomnia was correlated with acquiring and difficulty discarding possessions rather than with clutter per se. The authors hypothesized that this finding was related to sleep-deprivation activation of reward sensitive areas in the brain (leading to increased acquisition) as well as decreasing decisional capacity, which is also affected by sleep deprivation (leading to increased difficulty discarding possessions).

Trichotillomania/Excoriation Disorder

The body-focused repetitive behavior disorders of trichotillomania (hair pulling disorder) and excoriation (skin picking) disorder were recently reclassified from impulse-control disorders to obsessive-compulsive related disorders in the DSM- 5. The prevalence of trichotillomania is estimated to fall between 1% and 4%; the prevalence of excoriation disorder is between 0.2% and 12%, depending on criteria used [137]. The disorders are thought to share underlying illness features, and both can take a significant toll on afflicted individuals in terms of damaging physical effects, emotional effects, and social isolation.

There are only a few studies that examine sleep disturbance in trichotillomania and excoriation disorder. Survey data indicates that individuals with these disorders differed significantly from a control group (but not from each other) on a measure of sleep problems [137]. An additional study found significant sleep disturbance among dermatological patients with and without pathological excoriation when compared to normal controls [138]. Only in dermatological patients with pathological excoriation, the sleep disturbance was correlated with anxiety symptoms. Taken together, these studies suggest some level of sleep disturbance in individuals with trichotillomania and excoriation disorder, although the extent and nature of this association needs further exploration.

Psychological treatment of these disorders is challenging and includes an increased awareness of the problematic behavior as well as response prevention. The clinical challenges increase when the manifestation of the disorder occurs during sleep. Slightly over 12% of individuals with trichotillomania report some hair-pulling while asleep, and approximately 27% of individuals with excoriation disorder report some skin picking while asleep [137]. Body-focused repetitive behavioral disorders that occur only during sleep are considered quite rare, although a survey of dermatologists indicated that approximately 11% had treated at least one patient with trichotillomania that occurred only during sleep over the course of a career [139].

Two published case studies provide some additional information on association of trichotillomania and sleep. In the first case study, a young woman with an essentially noncontributory psychiatric history presented with symptoms of hair picking only while asleep. Polysomnography showed that she only engaged in this behavior during N3 sleep; the authors hypothesized that she had a rare form of NREM parasomnia that improved with imipramine treatment [140]. Angulo-Franco and colleagues [141] reported a middle-aged woman with symptoms of nocturnal epileptic seizures and trichotillomania who had a long history of psychiatric management, including treatment for severe childhood abuse. The authors determined, using PSG with video monitoring, that the nocturnal epileptic seizures and trichotillomania in this case were associated with sleep-related dissociative disorder. The patient showed gradual improvement on a regimen of sertraline, clonazepam, and supportive psychotherapy. This latter case, while technically meeting diagnostic criteria for trichotillomania, would probably be more appropriately classified as an example of a dissociative disorder with self-injurious behavior, thus reflecting the potential clinical complexity in some of these patients.

Additionally, trichotillomania has been reported as compulsive behaviors associated with dopamine agonists use in two patients with RLS [142]. The authors suggested increased stress, depression, and sleep disturbance to be the clinical correlates associated with compulsive behaviors in RLS patients.

Treatments
Evidence related to treatment of sleep disturbance in hoarding disorder, trichotillomania, and excoriation disorder is almost nonexistent except for the case studies discussed earlier.

CONCLUSIONS
While sleep disturbance frequently coexist with anxiety, obsessive-compulsive, and related disorders, the nature of this relationship remains unclear. However, there is some emerging evidence pointing to the role of serotonergic system, circadian rhythm disruption, cortisol abnormalities, emotional dysregulation, impaired executive functioning, and AS as underlying factors for sleep disturbance in anxiety disorders; this evidence is far from being conclusive and warrants further exploration. There is substantial evidence suggesting that individuals with co-occurring anxiety disorders and sleep disturbance represent a clinically challenging and treatment refractory subset of this patient population. There is an imminent need to systematically assess the impact of sleep disturbance on symptom severity and treatment outcomes in this population. Limited evidence is available for medications and targeted psychotherapeutic interventions for management of sleep disturbance, thus warranting the development of robust sleep interventions to achieve optimal clinical outcomes.

FUTURE DIRECTIONS
There are a number of areas for future research. The outcome literature for treatment of anxiety disorders has largely overlooked sleep outcomes as a treatment variable of interest. To illustrate, a recent literature review of cognitive-behavioral treatments of anxiety disorders suggests that only 25 (2%) of the 1,205 studies reported sleep data, and even in these studies the sleep outcomes were often inadequately measured. First, the priority is to routinely incorporate the baseline and final assessments of sleep disturbance in research studies examining the efficacy of pharmacological or psychological treatments of anxiety disorders. Second, more research is warranted to understand the neurobiology and identify the clinical risk factors associated with sleep disturbances in patients with anxiety disorders. Third, very limited research exists to discern the optimal treatment of sleep disturbance co-occurring with anxiety disorders. Research focus on developing optimal treatment modalities for sleep disturbance is urgently needed to develop clinical strategies that fully address the management of anxiety, OCD, and related disorders.

CLINICAL PEARLS
- Sleep disturbance is frequently comorbid with anxiety and related disorders and leads to poor clinical outcomes and worse quality of life in patients with anxiety disorders.
- Three consistent objective findings across anxiety disorders are increased SOL, decreased TST, and potentially reduced SE.
- Anxiety sensitivity is considered to be a trans-diagnostic factor that leads to sleep disturbance in patients with anxiety disorders.
- Differential diagnosis of nocturnal panic attacks includes OSA, nocturnal seizures, parasomnias (night terrors), and PTSD.
- Nocturnal panic attacks usually occur in late stage N2 or early stage N3 sleep.
- Sleep quality has been noted to predict the outcomes of CBT for SAD.
- OCD has been associated with higher prevalence of delayed sleep phase circadian rhythm disorder
- CBT for specific anxiety disorders (not targeting sleep) may result in improvement with sleep disturbance; targeted sleep interventions are needed in anxious patients with continued sleep disturbance
- Among CBT-I, sleep restriction may be poorly tolerated in patients with anxiety disorders and sleep disturbance.

SELF-ASSESSMENT QUESTIONS
1. Which of the following should be considered in the differential diagnosis of nocturnal panic attacks?
   a. Night terrors
   b. Obstructive sleep apnea
   c. Nocturnal seizures
   d. All of the above

Answer: d

2. Which of the following sleep architectural changes distinguishes depressive disorders from anxiety disorders?
   a. Increased wake after sleep onset time (WASO)
   b. Increased sleep onset latency (SOL)
   c. Decreased REM latency (REML)
   d. Decreased sleep efficiency (SE)

Answer: c

3. Nocturnal panic attacks typically occur during which of the following sleep stage transitions?
   a. Stage N1 to N2
   b. Stage N2 to N3
   c. Stage N2 to REM
   d. REM to stage N2

Answer: b

4. Treatment of comorbid obstructive sleep apnea has been shown to improve outcomes of which of the following anxiety disorders?
   a. Generalized Anxiety Disorder
   b. Social anxiety Disorder
   c. Panic Disorder
   d. None of the above

Answer: c

5. Which of the following techniques in cognitive behavioral treatment for insomnia (CBT-I) is the least well tolerated in patients with anxiety disorders?
   a. Sleep restriction
   b. Stimulus control
   c. Cognitive restructuring
   d. Relaxation techniques

Answer: a

REFERENCES

1. Kessler, R.C., et al., *Lifetime prevalence and age-of-onset distributions of DSM-IV disorders in the National Comorbidity Survey Replication.* Arch Gen Psychiatry, 2005. **62**(6): p. 593–602.
2. Breslau, N., et al., *Sleep disturbance and psychiatric disorders: a longitudinal epidemiological study of young adults.* Biol Psychiatry, 1996. **39**(6): p. 411–8.
3. Ancoli-Israel, S. and T. Roth, *Characteristics of insomnia in the United States: results of the 1991 National Sleep Foundation Survey. I.* Sleep, 1999. **22 Suppl 2**: p. S347–S353.
4. Uhde, T.W., B.M. Cortese, and A. Vedeniapin, *Anxiety and sleep problems: emerging concepts and theoretical treatment implications.* Curr Psychiatry Rep, 2009. **11**(4): p. 269–76.
5. Papadimitriou, G.N. and P. Linkowski, *Sleep disturbance in anxiety disorders.* Int Rev Psychiatry, 2005. **17**(4): p. 229–36.
6. Ohayon, M.M. and T. Roth, *Place of chronic insomnia in the course of depressive and anxiety disorders.* J Psychiatr Res, 2003. **37**(1): p. 9–15.
7. Neckelmann, D., A. Mykletun, and A.A. Dahl, *Chronic insomnia as a risk factor for developing anxiety and depression.* Sleep, 2007. **30**(7): p. 873–80.
8. Ramsawh, H.J., et al., *Relationship of anxiety disorders, sleep quality, and functional impairment in a community sample.* J Psychiatr Res, 2009. **43**(10): p. 926–33.
9. Soehner, A.M. and A.G. Harvey, *Prevalence and functional consequences of severe insomnia symptoms in mood and anxiety disorders: results from a nationally representative sample.* Sleep, 2012. **35**(10): p. 1367–75.
10. Zalta, A.K., et al., *Sleep quality predicts treatment outcome in CBT for social anxiety disorder.* Depress Anxiety, 2013. **30**(11): p. 1114–20.
11. Smith, M.T., et al., *Comparative meta-analysis of pharmacotherapy and behavior therapy for persistent insomnia.* Am J Psychiatry, 2002. **159**(1): p. 5–11.
12. Sivertsen, B., et al., *Cognitive behavioral therapy vs zopiclone for treatment of chronic primary insomnia in older adults: a randomized controlled trial.* Jama, 2006. **295**(24): p. 2851–8.
13. Schutte-Rodin, S., et al., *Clinical guideline for the evaluation and management of chronic insomnia in adults.* J Clin Sleep Med, 2008. **4**(5): p. 487–504.
14. Etkin, A., T. Egner, and R. Kalisch, *Emotional processing in anterior cingulate and medial prefrontal cortex.* Trends Cogn Sci, 2011. **15**(2): p. 85–93.
15. Hartley, C.A. and E.A. Phelps, *Changing fear: the neurocircuitry of emotion regulation.* Neuropsychopharmacology, 2010. **35**(1): p. 136–46.
16. Milad, M.R., et al., *A role for the human dorsal anterior cingulate cortex in fear expression.* Biol Psychiatry, 2007. **62**(10): p. 1191–4.
17. Ochsner, K.N., et al., *For better or for worse: neural systems supporting the cognitive down- and up-regulation of negative emotion.* Neuroimage, 2004. **23**(2): p. 483–99.
18. Phelps, E.A., *Human emotion and memory: interactions of the amygdala and hippocampal complex.* Curr Opin Neurobiol, 2004. **14**(2): p. 198–202.
19. Shin, L.M. and I. Liberzon, *The neurocircuitry of fear, stress, and anxiety disorders.* Neuropsychopharmacology, 2010. **35**(1): p. 169–91.
20. Morgan, M.A., L.M. Romanski, and J.E. LeDoux, *Extinction of emotional learning: contribution of medial prefrontal cortex.* Neurosci Lett, 1993. **163**(1): p. 109–13.

21. Quirk, G.J. and J.S. Beer, *Prefrontal involvement in the regulation of emotion: convergence of rat and human studies.* Curr Opin Neurobiol, 2006. **16**(6): p. 723–7.

22. Quirk, G.J., et al., *Stimulation of medial prefrontal cortex decreases the responsiveness of central amygdala output neurons.* J Neurosci, 2003. **23**(25): p. 8800–7.

23. Etkin, A. and T.D. Wager, *Functional neuroimaging of anxiety: a meta-analysis of emotional processing in PTSD, social anxiety disorder, and specific phobia.* Am J Psychiatry, 2007. **164**(10): p. 1476–88.

24. Hattingh, C.J., et al., *Functional magnetic resonance imaging during emotion recognition in social anxiety disorder: an activation likelihood meta-analysis.* Front Hum Neurosci, 2012. **6**: p. 347.

25. Kalisch, R. and A.M. Gerlicher, *Making a mountain out of a molehill: on the role of the rostral dorsal anterior cingulate and dorsomedial prefrontal cortex in conscious threat appraisal, catastrophizing, and worrying.* Neurosci Biobehav Rev, 2014. **42**: p. 1–8.

26. Vogt, B.A., *Pain and emotion interactions in subregions of the cingulate gyrus.* Nat Rev Neurosci, 2005. **6**(7): p. 533–44.

27. Carlisi, C.O., et al., *Sleep-amount differentially affects fear-processing neural circuitry in pediatric anxiety: A preliminary fMRI investigation.* Cogn Affect Behav Neuroscience, 2017. **17**(6): p. 1098–1113.

28. Harrison, Y. and J.A. Horne, *The impact of sleep deprivation on decision making: a review.* J Exp Psychol Appl, 2000. **6**(3): p. 236–49.

29. Nilsson, J.P., et al., *Less effective executive functioning after one night's sleep deprivation.* J Sleep Res, 2005. **14**(1): p. 1–6.

30. Drummond, S.P., J.C. Gillin, and G.G. Brown, *Increased cerebral response during a divided attention task following sleep deprivation.* J Sleep Res, 2001. **10**(2): p. 85–92.

31. Drummond, S.P., M.P. Paulus, and S.F. Tapert, *Effects of two nights sleep deprivation and two nights recovery sleep on response inhibition.* J Sleep Res, 2006. **15**(3): p. 261–5.

32. Goel, N., et al., *Neurocognitive consequences of sleep deprivation.* Semin Neurol, 2009. **29**(4): p. 320–39.

33. Yoo, S.S., et al., *The human emotional brain without sleep--a prefrontal amygdala disconnect.* Curr Biol, 2007. **17**(20): p. R877–R878.

34. Cox, R.C. and B.O. Olatunji, *A systematic review of sleep disturbance in anxiety and related disorders.* J Anxiety Disord, 2016. **37**: p. 104–129.

35. Omisade, A., O.M. Buxton, and B. Rusak, *Impact of acute sleep restriction on cortisol and leptin levels in young women.* Physiol Behav, 2010. **99**(5): p. 651–656.

36. Spiegel, K., R. Leproult, and E. Van Cauter, *Impact of sleep debt on metabolic and endocrine function.* Lancet, 1999. **354**(9188): p. 1435–1439.

37. Dickerson, S.S. and M.E. Kemeny, *Acute stressors and cortisol responses: a theoretical integration and synthesis of laboratory research.* Psychol Bull, 2004. **130**(3): p. 355–391.

38. Wright, C.E., et al., *Poor sleep the night before an experimental stress task is associated with reduced cortisol reactivity in healthy women.* Biol Psychol, 2007. **74**(3): p. 319–327.

39. Stawski, R.S., et al., *Associations between cognitive function and naturally occurring daily cortisol during middle adulthood: timing is everything.* J Gerontol B Psychol Sci Soc Sci, 2011. **66 Suppl 1**: p. i71–i81.

40. Gomez, R.G., et al., *Effects of major depression diagnosis and cortisol levels on indices of neurocognitive function.* Psychoneuroendocrinology, 2009. **34**(7): p. 1012–1018.

41. Buss, C., et al., *Autobiographic memory impairment following acute cortisol administration.* Psychoneuroendocrinology, 2004. **29**(8): p. 1093–1096.

42. Hek, K., et al., *Anxiety disorders and salivary cortisol levels in older adults: a population-based study.* Psychoneuroendocrinology, 2013. **38**(2): p. 300–305.

43. Mantella, R.C., et al., *Salivary cortisol is associated with diagnosis and severity of late-life generalized anxiety disorder.* Psychoneuroendocrinology, 2008. **33**(6): p. 773–781.

44. Kluge, M., et al., *Increased nocturnal secretion of ACTH and cortisol in obsessive compulsive disorder.* J Psychiatr Res, 2007. **41**(11): p. 928–933.

45. Gustafsson, P.E., et al., *Diurnal cortisol levels and cortisol response in youths with obsessive-compulsive disorder.* Neuropsychobiology, 2008. **57**(1-2): p. 14–21.

46. Boswell, J.F., et al., *Anxiety sensitivity and interoceptive exposure: a transdiagnostic construct and change strategy.* Behav Ther, 2013. **44**(3): p. 417–431.

47. Naragon-Gainey, K., *Meta-analysis of the relations of anxiety sensitivity to the depressive and anxiety disorders.* Psychol Bull, 2010. **136**(1): p. 128–150.

48. Dixon, L.J., et al., *Anxiety sensitivity and sleep disturbance: Investigating associations among patients with co-occurring anxiety and substance use disorders.* J Anxiety Disord, 2018. **53**: p. 9–15.

49. Taylor, S., et al., *Robust dimensions of anxiety sensitivity: development and initial validation of the Anxiety Sensitivity Index-3.* Psychol Assess, 2007. **19**(2): p. 176–188.

50. Alcantara, C., et al., *Anxiety sensitivity and racial differences in sleep duration: Results from a national survey of adults with cardiovascular disease.* J Anxiety Disord, 2017. **48**: p. 102–108.

51. Calkins, A.W., et al., *Psychosocial predictors of sleep dysfunction: the role of anxiety sensitivity, dysfunctional beliefs, and neuroticism.* Behav Sleep Med, 2013. **11**(2): p. 133–143.

52. Hoge, E.A., et al., *The role of anxiety sensitivity in sleep disturbance in panic disorder.* J Anxiety Disord, 2011. **25**(4): p. 536–538.

53. Raines, A.M., et al., *Obsessive-compulsive symptom dimensions and insomnia: The mediating role of anxiety sensitivity cognitive concerns.* Psychiatry Res, 2015. **228**(3): p. 368–372.

54. Weiner, C.L., et al., *Anxiety sensitivity and sleep-related problems in anxious youth.* J Anxiety Disord, 2015. **32**: p. 66–72.

55. Baker, A.W., et al., *Examining the Role of Anxiety Sensitivity in Sleep Dysfunction Across Anxiety Disorders.* Behav Sleep Med, 2017. **15**(3): p. 216–227.

56. Smits, J.A.J., et al., *The efficacy of cognitive-behavioral interventions for reducing anxiety sensitivity: A meta-analytic review.* Behav Res Ther, 2008. **46**(9): p. 1047–1054.

57. Short, N.A., et al., *The effects of an anxiety sensitivity intervention on insomnia symptoms.* Sleep Med, 2015. **16**(1): p. 152–159.

58. Short, N.A., et al., *A randomized clinical trial examining the effects of an anxiety sensitivity intervention on insomnia symptoms: Replication and extension.* Behav Res Ther, 2017. **99**: p. 108–116.

59. Singareddy, R. and T.W. Uhde, *Nocturnal sleep panic and depression: relationship to subjective sleep in panic disorder.* J Affect Disord, 2009. **112**(1–3): p. 262–266.

60. Roth, T., et al., *Sleep problems, comorbid mental disorders, and role functioning in the national comorbidity survey replication.* Biol Psychiatry, 2006. **60**(12): p. 1364–1371.

61. Nyer, M., et al., *Relationship between sleep disturbance and depression, anxiety, and functioning in college students.* Depress Anxiety, 2013. **30**(9): p. 873–880.

62. Conway, K.P., et al., *Lifetime comorbidity of DSM-IV mood and anxiety disorders and specific drug use disorders: results from the National Epidemiologic Survey on Alcohol and Related Conditions.* J Clin Psychiatry, 2006. **67**(2): p. 247–257.

63. Grant, B.F., et al., *Prevalence and co-occurrence of substance use disorders and independent mood and anxiety disorders: results from the National Epidemiologic Survey on Alcohol and Related Conditions.* Arch Gen Psychiatry, 2004. **61**(8): p. 807–816.

64. Diaz, S.V. and L.K. Brown, *Relationships between obstructive sleep apnea and anxiety.* Curr Opin Pulm Med, 2016. **22**(6): p. 563–569.

65. Edmonds, J.C., et al., *Claustrophobic tendencies and continuous positive airway pressure therapy non-adherence in adults with obstructive sleep apnea.* Heart Lung, 2015. **44**(2): p. 100–106.

66. Thompson, E., *Hamilton Rating Scale for Anxiety (HAM-A).* Occup Med (Lond), 2015. **65**(7): p. 601.

67. Buysse, D.J., et al., *The Pittsburgh Sleep Quality Index: a new instrument for psychiatric practice and research.* Psychiatry Res, 1989. **28**(2): p. 193–213.

68. Morin, C.M., et al., *The Insomnia Severity Index: psychometric indicators to detect insomnia cases and evaluate treatment response.* Sleep, 2011. **34**(5): p. 601–8.

69. Boland, E.M. and R.J. Ross, *Recent advances in the study of sleep in the anxiety disorders, obsessive-compulsive disorder, and posttraumatic stress disorder.* Psychiatr Clin North Am, 2015. **38**(4): p. 761–776.

70. Mellman, T.A. and T.W. Uhde, *Sleep panic attacks: new clinical findings and theoretical implications.* Am J Psychiatry, 1989. **146**(9): p. 1204–7.

71. Bell, C.C., D.D. Dixie-Bell, and B. Thompson, *Panic attacks: relationship to isolated sleep paralysis.* Am J Psychiatry, 1986. **143**(11): p. 1484.

72. Landry, P., et al., *Electroencephalography during sleep of patients with nocturnal panic disorder.* J Nerv Ment Dis, 2002. **190**(8): p. 559–62.

73. Craske, M.G. and J.C. Tsao, *Assessment and treatment of nocturnal panic attacks.* Sleep Med Rev, 2005. **9**(3): p. 173–84.

74. Edlund, M.J., M.E. McNamara, and R.P. Millman, *Sleep apnea and panic attacks.* Compr Psychiatry, 1991. **32**(2): p. 130–2.

75. Su, V.Y., et al., *Sleep apnea and risk of panic disorder.* Ann Fam Med, 2015. **13**(4): p. 325–30.

76. Craske, M.G., et al., *Presleep attributions about arousal during sleep: nocturnal panic.* J Abnorm Psychol, 2002. **111**(1): p. 53–62.

77. Overbeek, T., et al., *Sleep complaints in panic disorder patients.* J Nerv Ment Dis, 2005. **193**(7): p. 488–93.

78. Lauer, C.J., et al., *Panic disorder and major depression: a comparative electroencephalographic sleep study.* Psychiatry Res, 1992. **44**(1): p. 41–54.

79. Lydiard, R.B., et al., *Electroencephalography during sleep of patients with panic disorder.* J Neuropsychiatry Clin Neurosci, 1989. **1**(4): p. 372–6.

80. Sloan, E.P., et al., *Nocturnal and daytime panic attacks--comparison of sleep architecture, heart rate variability, and response to sodium lactate challenge.* Biol Psychiatry, 1999. **45**(10): p. 1313–20.

81. Mellman, T.A. and T.W. Uhde, *Electroencephalographic sleep in panic disorder. A focus on sleep-related panic attacks.* Arch Gen Psychiatry, 1989. **46**(2): p. 178–84.

82. Marchand, L., et al., *Efficacy of two cognitive-behavioral treatment modalities for panic disorder with nocturnal panic attacks.* Behav Modif, 2013. **37**(5): p. 680–704.

83. Craske, M.G., et al., *Cognitive behavioral therapy for nocturnal panic.* Behav Ther, 2005. **36**(1): p. 43–54.

84. Cervena, K., et al., *Sleep disturbances in patients treated for panic disorder.* Sleep Med, 2005. **6**(2): p. 149–53.

85. Craske, M.G., et al., *Reactivity to interoceptive cues in nocturnal panic.* J Behav Ther Exp Psychiatry, 2001. **32**(3): p. 173–90.

86. Tsao, J.C. and M.G. Craske, *Reactivity to imagery and nocturnal panic attacks.* Depress Anxiety, 2003. **18**(4): p. 205–13.

87. Roy-Byrne, P.P., T.W. Uhde, and R.M. Post, *Effects of one night's sleep deprivation on mood and behavior in panic disorder. Patients with panic disorder compared with depressed patients and normal controls.* Arch Gen Psychiatry, 1986. **43**(9): p. 895–899.

88. Freire, R.C., et al., *Current pharmacological interventions in panic disorder.* CNS Neurol Disord Drug Targets, 2014. **13**(6): p. 1057–1065.

89. Todder, D. and B.T. Baune, *Quality of sleep in escitalopram-treated female patients with panic disorder.* Hum Psychopharmacol, 2010. **25**(2): p. 167–173.

90. Offidani, E., et al., *Efficacy and tolerability of benzodiazepines versus antidepressants in anxiety disorders: a systematic review and meta-analysis.* Psychother Psychosom, 2013. **82**(6): p. 355–362.

91. Saletu-Zyhlarz, G.M., et al., *Nonorganic insomnia in panic Disorder: comparative sleep laboratory studies with normal controls and placebo-controlled trials with alprazolam.* Hum Psychopharmacol, 2000. **15**(4): p. 241–254.

92. Chouinard, G., *Issues in the clinical use of benzodiazepines: potency, withdrawal, and rebound.* J Clin Psychiatry, 2004. **65 Suppl 5**: p. 7–12.

93. Takaesu, Y., et al., *Effects of nasal continuous positive airway pressure on panic disorder comorbid with obstructive sleep apnea syndrome.* Sleep Med, 2012. **13**(2): p. 156–160.

94. Ford, D.E. and D.B. Kamerow, *Epidemiologic study of sleep disturbances and psychiatric disorders. An opportunity for prevention?* JAMA, 1989. **262**(11): p. 1479–1484.

95. Ferre Navarrete, F., et al., *Prevalence of Insomnia and Associated Factors in Outpatients With Generalized Anxiety Disorder Treated in Psychiatric Clinics.* Behav Sleep Med, 2017. **15**(6): p. 491–501.

96. Choueiry, N., et al., *Insomnia and relationship with anxiety in university students: a cross-sectional designed study.* PLoS One, 2016. **11**(2): p. e0149643.

97. Kertz, S.J. and J. Woodruff-Borden, *Human and economic burden of GAD, subthreshold GAD, and worry in a primary care sample.* J Clin Psychol Med Settings, 2011. **18**(3): p. 281–90.

98. Takano, K., Y. Iijima, and Y. Tanno, *Repetitive thought and self-reported sleep disturbance.* Behav Ther, 2012. **43**(4): p. 779–89.

99. Tsypes, A., A. Aldao, and D.S. Mennin, *Emotion dysregulation and sleep difficulties in generalized anxiety disorder.* J Anxiety Disord, 2013. **27**(2): p. 197–203.

100. Brenes, G.A., et al., *Insomnia in older adults with generalized anxiety disorder.* Am J Geriatr Psychiatry, 2009. **17**(6): p. 465–72.

101. Tempesta, D., et al., *Neuropsychological functioning in young subjects with generalized anxiety disorder with and without pharmacotherapy.* Prog Neuropsychopharmacol Biol Psychiatry, 2013. **45**: p. 236–41.

102. Wetherell, J.L., H. Le Roux, and M. Gatz, *DSM-IV criteria for generalized anxiety disorder in older adults: distinguishing the worried from the well.* Psychol Aging, 2003. **18**(3): p. 622–7.

103. Batterham, P.J., N. Glozier, and H. Christensen, *Sleep disturbance, personality and the onset of depression and anxiety: prospective cohort study.* Aust N Z J Psychiatry, 2012. **46**(11): p. 1089–98.

104. Ramsawh, H.J., et al., *Relationship of anxiety disorders, sleep quality, and functional impairment in a community sample.* J Psychiatric Res, 2009. **43**(10): p. 926–933.

105. Belanger, L., et al., *Insomnia and generalized anxiety disorder: effects of cognitive behavior therapy for gad on insomnia symptoms.* J Anxiety Disord, 2004. **18**(4): p. 561–71.

106. Ramsawh, H.J., et al., *Sleep quality improvement during cognitive behavioral therapy for anxiety disorders.* Behav Sleep Med, 2016. **14**(3): p. 267–78.

107. Belleville, G., et al., *Sequential treatment of comorbid insomnia and generalized anxiety disorder.* J Clin Psychol, 2016. **72**(9): p. 880–96.

108. Smith, M.T., M.I. Huang, and R. Manber, *Cognitive behavior therapy for chronic insomnia occurring within the context of medical and psychiatric disorders.* Clin Psychol Rev, 2005. **25**(5): p. 559–92.

109. Wu, J., F. Chang, and H. Zu, *Efficacy and safety evaluation of citalopram and doxepin on sleep quality in comorbid insomnia and anxiety disorders.* Exp Ther Med, 2015. **10**(4): p. 1303–1308.

110. Pollack, M., et al., *Eszopiclone coadministered with escitalopram in patients with insomnia and comorbid generalized anxiety disorder.* Arch Gen Psychiatry, 2008. **65**(5): p. 551–62.

111. Holsboer-Trachsler, E. and R. Prieto, *Effects of pregabalin on sleep in generalized anxiety disorder.* Int J Neuropsychopharmacol, 2013. **16**(4): p. 925–36.

112. Blank, S., et al., *Outcomes of late-life anxiety disorders during 32 weeks of citalopram treatment.* J Clin Psychiatry, 2006. **67**(3): p. 468–72.

113. Gross, P.K., R. Nourse, and T.E. Wasser, *Ramelteon for insomnia symptoms in a community sample of adults with generalized anxiety disorder: an open label study.* J Clin Sleep Med, 2009. **5**(1): p. 28–33.

114. Stein, D.J., A.A. Ahokas, and C. de Bodinat, *Efficacy of agomelatine in generalized anxiety disorder: a randomized, double-blind, placebo-controlled study.* J Clin Psychopharmacol, 2008. **28**(5): p. 561–6.

115. Huang, Z., et al., *Repetitive transcranial magnetic stimulation of the right parietal cortex for comorbid generalized anxiety disorder and insomnia: A randomized, double-blind, sham-controlled pilot study.* Brain Stimul, 2018;11(5):1103–1109.

116. Stein, M.B., C.D. Kroft, and J.R. Walker, *Sleep impairment in patients with social phobia.* Psychiatry Res, 1993. **49**(3): p. 251–6.

117. Buckner, J.D., et al., *Social anxiety and insomnia: the mediating role of depressive symptoms.* Depress Anxiety, 2008. **25**(2): p. 124–30.

118. Brown, T.M., B. Black, and T.W. Uhde, *The sleep architecture of social phobia.* Biol Psychiatry, 1994. **35**(6): p. 420–1.

119. Kushnir, J., et al., *The link between social anxiety disorder, treatment outcome, and sleep difficulties among patients receiving cognitive behavioral group therapy.* Sleep Med, 2014. **15**(5): p. 515–21.

120. Tang, N.K., *Brief CBT-I for insomnia comorbid with social phobia: A case study.* Behav Cogn Psychother, 2010. **38**(1): p. 113–22.

121. Nordahl, H., et al., *Sleep disturbances in treatment-seeking OCD-patients: Changes after concentrated exposure treatment.* Scand J Psychol, 2018. **59**(2): p. 186–191.

122. Paterson, J.L., et al., *Sleep and obsessive-compulsive disorder (OCD).* Sleep Med Rev, 2013. **17**(6): p. 465–74.

123. Cox, R.C. and B.O. Olatunji, *Sleep disturbance and obsessive-compulsive symptoms: Results from the national comorbidity survey replication.* J Psychiatr Res, 2016. **75**: p. 41–5.

124. Voderholzer, U., et al., *Sleep in obsessive compulsive disorder: polysomnographic studies under baseline conditions and after experimentally induced serotonin deficiency.* Eur Arch Psychiatry Clin Neurosci, 2007. **257**(3): p. 173–82.

125. Kalanthroff, E., et al., *What underlies the effect of sleep disruption? The role of alertness in obsessive-compulsive disorder (OCD).* J Behav Ther Exp Psychiatry, 2017. **57**: p. 212–213.

126. Alfano, C.A. and K.L. Kim, *Objective sleep patterns and severity of symptoms in pediatric obsessive compulsive disorder: a pilot investigation.* J Anxiety Disord, 2011. **25**(6): p. 835–9.

127. Timpano, K.R., et al., *Obsessive compulsive symptoms and sleep difficulties: exploring the unique relationship between insomnia and obsessions.* J Psychiatr Res, 2014. **57**: p. 101–7.

128. Mukhopadhyay, S., et al., *Delayed sleep phase in severe obsessive-compulsive disorder: a systematic case-report survey.* CNS Spectr, 2008. **13**(5): p. 406–13.

129. Nota, J.A., K.M. Sharkey, and M.E. Coles, *Sleep, arousal, and circadian rhythms in adults with obsessive-compulsive disorder: a meta-analysis.* Neurosci Biobehav Rev, 2015. **51**: p. 100–7.

130. Bobdey, M., et al., *Reported sleep patterns in obsessive compulsive disorder (OCD).* Int J Psychiatry Clin Pract, 2002. **6**(1): p. 15–21.

131. Insel, T.R., et al., *The sleep of patients with obsessive-compulsive disorder.* Arch Gen Psychiatry, 1982. **39**(12): p. 1372–7.

132. Hohagen, F., et al., *Sleep EEG of patients with obsessive-compulsive disorder.* Eur Arch Psychiatry Clin Neurosci, 1994. **243**(5): p. 273–8.

133. Veale, D., et al., *Atypical antipsychotic augmentation in SSRI treatment refractory obsessive-compulsive disorder: a systematic review and meta-analysis.* BMC Psychiatry, 2014. **14**: p. 317.

134. Alonso, P., et al., *Deep brain stimulation for obsessive-compulsive disorder: a meta-analysis of treatment outcome and predictors of response.* PLoS One, 2015. **10**(7): p. e0133591.

135. Donse, L., et al., *Sleep disturbances in obsessive-compulsive disorder: Association with non-response to repetitive transcranial magnetic stimulation (rTMS).* J Anxiety Disord, 2017. **49**: p. 31–39.

136. Raines, A.M., et al., *An Initial Investigation of the Relationship Between Insomnia and Hoarding.* J Clin Psychol, 2015. 71(7): p. 707–14.

137. Ricketts, E.J., et al., *Sleep functioning in adults with trichotillomania (hair-pulling disorder), excoriation (skin-picking) disorder, and a non-affected comparison sample.* J Obsessive-Compulsive Related Dis, 2017. **13**: p. 49–57.

138. Singareddy, R., et al., *Skin picking and sleep disturbances: relationship to anxiety and need for research.* Depress Anxiety, 2003. **18**(4): p. 228–32.

139. Murphy, C., et al., *Sleep-isolated trichotillomania: a survey of dermatologists.* J Clin Sleep Med, 2007. **3**(7): p. 719–721.

140. Murphy, C., T. Valerio, and S.N. Zallek, *Trichotillomania: an NREM sleep parasomnia?* Neurology, 2006. **66**(8): p. 1276.

141. Angulo-Franco, M., et al., *Trichotillomania and non-epileptic seizures as sleep-related dissociative phenomena.* J Clin Sleep Med, 2015. **11**(3): p. 271–273.

142. Pourcher, E., S. Remillard, and H. Cohen, *Compulsive habits in restless legs syndrome patients under dopaminergic treatment.* J Neurol Sci, 2010. **290**(1-2): p. 52–56.

20

Trauma- and Stressor-Related Disorders

JANEESE A. BROWNLOW, KATHERINE E. MILLER,
PHILIP R. GEHRMAN, AND RICHARD J. ROSS

INTRODUCTION

Trauma- and stressor-related disorders (TSRD) are debilitating psychiatric disorders in which exposure to a traumatic or stressful event is an essential diagnostic criterion.[1] Five psychiatric disorders are included in TSRD: reactive attachment disorder (RAD), a disorder of infancy or early childhood characterized by an array of severely disturbed and developmentally inappropriate attachment behaviors; disinhibited social engagement disorder (DSES), a childhood disorder marked by a pattern of behavior that comprises culturally inappropriate, overly familiar behavior with relative strangers; posttraumatic stress disorder (PTSD), a disorder characterized by the development of distinct symptoms following exposure to one or more traumatic events; acute stress disorder (ASD), a disorder defined by the development of characteristic symptomatology lasting 3 days to 1 month following exposure to one or more traumatic events; and adjustment disorder (AD), a disorder marked by the presence of emotional and/or behavioral symptoms in response to a recognizable stressor. Children with RAD and DSES may be susceptible to sleep-related difficulties (e.g., sleep onset delay or a desire to have a guardian present at sleep onset)[2]; however, there are limited data on this topic. This chapter will focus on the management of sleep disturbances in PTSD, ASD, and AD.

Data accumulated over the last 20 years provide evidence that trauma-exposed populations report disturbed sleep at greater rates than individuals in the general population.[3] Specifically, trauma-exposed populations endorse difficulty initiating sleep,[4,5] difficulty maintaining sleep,[4,6] atypical sleep-disruptive behaviors,[7] and recurrent nightmares.[4,8]

This chapter presents an overview of sleep disturbances in TSRD, and summarizes the evidence for empirically supported psychotherapeutic and pharmacological interventions for these disturbances. First, we provide a succinct description of each disorder in TSRD and elaborate on its characteristic sleep disturbance(s). We then review the different forms of psychotherapy and pharmacotherapy that have shown utility in treating these sleep disturbances.

CLINICAL APPROACHES TO SLEEP DYSFUNCTION IN TSRD

The most frequent sleep disturbances identified in TSRD are distressing dreams (nightmares) related to a traumatic event and insomnia, one manifestation of hyperarousal.[1] Although nightmares that replay a traumatic experience are quite specific to ASD and PTSD, insomnia can occur in a range of mental disorders, including mood, anxiety, and substance use disorders. These are often comorbid with TSRD. Therefore, a comprehensive mental health assessment is required for individuals presenting with TSRD and sleep complaint(s). A medical evaluation, including polysomnography (PSG), may need to be carried out when there is any suspicion that sleep-disordered breathing is the cause of insomnia or when there is a report that distressing dreams are being enacted and a diagnosis of rapid eye movement (REM) sleep behavior disorder (RBD) is being considered.

POSTTRAUMATIC STRESS DISORDER

PTSD occurs in the aftermath of exposure to actual or threatened death, serious injury, or sexual violence in one or more of the following ways: directly experiencing the traumatic event, witnessing the event, learning that such an event happened to a close family member or friend, or experiencing repeated or extreme exposure to adverse details of the event.[1] Diagnostic criteria comprise four symptom clusters: intrusive re-experiencing in the form of memories, nightmares, or flashbacks (Criterion B), persistent avoidance of certain stimuli (Criterion C), negative alterations in cognitions and mood (Criterion D), and marked alterations in arousal and reactivity (Criterion E).[1] The duration of these symptoms is greater than 1 month; they cause clinically significant distress or impairment in social, occupational or other important areas of functioning; and they cannot be attributed to the physiological effects of a substance or medical condition[1].

Estimates of the lifetime, past 12-month, and past 6-month prevalence of PTSD in the US population, using the *Diagnostic and Statistical Manual* (fifth edition) criteria, were 8.3%, 4.7%, and 3.8%, respectively.[9] The most endorsed Criterion A traumatic exposures were disaster (50.5%), physical or sexual assault (53.1%), and death of a family member or close friend due to violence/accident/disaster (51.8%).[9]

SLEEP DISTURBANCES IN PTSD

Sleep disturbances, in the form of insomnia and recurrent nightmares, are core features of PTSD, and nightmares are a hallmark symptom.[10] Obstructive sleep apnea (OSA),[11] periodic limb movement disorder (PLMD),[12,13] and RBD[14] have also been linked to PTSD. These associations are discussed further in the following text.

Subjective sleep disturbances have been well documented in PTSD and are consistently endorsed by more individuals with PTSD as compared to healthy controls.[15] This relation has been reported across diverse samples, including military veterans, sexual assault survivors, and mixed trauma groups. In daily sleep diaries, individuals with PTSD compared to healthy controls reported decreased total sleep time (TST), decreased sleep efficiency (SE), increased wake after sleep onset (WASO), and increased sleep onset latency (SOL).[16–18]

Objective PSG findings in PTSD have been mixed. However, a meta-analysis provided evidence for increased stage N1 sleep, reduced stage N3 sleep (i.e., slow-wave sleep), and greater REM density (number of REMs/REM sleep time) in PTSD subjects compared to controls.[19] Another meta-analysis found that PTSD was linked to poorer sleep continuity, reduced sleep depth, and increased REM sleep pressure (as defined by shorter REM latency [the time from the sleep onset to the first epoch of REM sleep]), increased REM density, and increased REM sleep.[20] One theory of the discrepancy between objective and subjective sleep measures in PTSD invokes sleep misperception, that is, a tendency to underestimate TST and

overestimate SOL compared to objective data.[21] Another hypothesis invokes the heterogeneity of hyperarousal symptoms across diverse participant samples. Using a median split of the Clinically Administered PTSD Scale (CAPS) Criterion E scores (PTSD + hyperarousal defined as scores ≥ 25; PTSD – hyperarousal defined as scores <25), Van Wyk and colleagues[22] found that patients with PTSD + hyperarousal experienced reduced SE, had greater WASO, and reported poorer sleep quality compared to patients with PTSD – hyperarousal.

PTSD AND INSOMNIA

Approximately 70% of individuals diagnosed with PTSD endorse difficulty initiating and/or maintaining sleep.[4] Recent data indicate that insomnia may be an important predictor of, or independent risk factor for, the development and maintenance of PTSD.[23–25] Gehrman and colleagues[24] found that predeployment insomnia symptoms in military personnel significantly increased the risk of developing PTSD, depression, and anxiety disorders following deployment. Wright and colleagues[25] showed that insomnia symptoms at 4 months postdeployment were significant predictors of PTSD symptoms as well as symptoms of depression at 12 months postdeployment. Further, insomnia in subjects with PTSD has been linked to increased psychiatric comorbidity, including alcohol use, major depressive disorder (MDD), and generalized anxiety disorder (GAD).[26] Collectively, these findings highlight the importance of the assessment and treatment of insomnia in both subjects at high risk for the development of PTSD and those with established PTSD.

PTSD AND NIGHTMARES

Recurrent nightmares are another highly prevalent and distressing feature of PTSD. Two distinct types of posttraumatic nightmares, replicative and symbolic, have been reported in the literature.[27,28] Replicative nightmares, often viewed as highly specific to PTSD, appear to replicate part or all of the traumatic event(s); in this way, their content is more logical than, and lacking in the distortions of, normal dreaming.[28,29] Symbolic nightmares contain distortions, eidetic images, and irrational structures, with some symbolic representations of the trauma. The reported prevalence of recurrent nightmares in PTSD varies in relation to differences in methodology, in particular, the criteria and tools used to define and assess nightmares across studies.[30] Another source of heterogeneity is the population studied (e.g., civilian vs. military).[31] By self-report, 19% to 96% of individuals with PTSD endorsed experiencing nightmares.[5,32] Nightmares are difficult to capture during objective monitoring, as they are reported to occur infrequently in the sleep laboratory setting.[33,34]

Like insomnia, recurrent nightmares in the wake of a traumatic event may predict the subsequent development of PTSD and other psychiatric disorders.[5,7,35] For instance, nightmares within 1 month of experiencing a traumatic event predicted PTSD symptoms 6 weeks and 1 year following the event.[36,37] Persistent nightmares have been associated with poor sleep quality,[38,39] depression, and heightened risk for suicide.[40-42] For example, Sjostrom and colleagues[42] showed that nightmare sufferers had a five-fold increase in suicidality even after controlling for psychiatric diagnosis. Recurrent nightmares, particularly those seen in PTSD, frequently require targeted treatment interventions.[43]

PTSD AND OBSTRUCTIVE SLEEP APNEA (OSA)

OSA is characterized by partial or complete reductions in airflow during sleep, hypopneas and apneas, respectively. These are due to blockage of the upper airway, and they lead to arousals and sleep fragmentation.[44,45] OSA prevalence estimates in the general population range from 3% to 7% in men and 2% to 5% in women.[46] OSA reportedly is prevalent in PTSD and other trauma-exposed populations, with high estimates ranging from 40% to 90%.[47-50] Further, a recent study found that 69% of a group of veterans with PTSD had an Apnea–Hypopnea Index (AHI) greater than 10, indicating at least mild OSA.[51] Sharafkhaneh and colleagues[11] found that individuals with OSA had a higher prevalence of PTSD, depression, and anxiety compared to controls. The etiology, consequences, and possible mechanisms of the reported link between OSA and PTSD, as well as the implications for treating this comorbidity, requires further examination.[11,52]

PTSD AND SLEEP-RELATED MOVEMENT DISORDERS

PLMD is characterized by periodic, highly stereotyped limb movements during sleep, primarily non-REM sleep; these are often associated with partial arousal or awakening.[44] The prevalence estimates for PLMD in the general adult population range from 4% to 11%,[53] but there is evidence that the rate in individuals with PTSD is much higher. Mellman and colleagues[13] reported

that 33% of individuals with PTSD had periodic limb movements (PLM), with frequencies ranging from 2 to 33 per hour. In another study, 76% of Vietnam veterans with PTSD had clinically significant PLMs.[12] Other studies have found an elevated PLM index in PTSD patients compared to controls.[54,55] It is important to note that these findings are limited to combat-related PTSD and to understand that antidepressant medications commonly used to treat the PTSD symptom complex can increase PLMs during sleep and possibly exacerbate insomnia[56].

PTSD AND RAPID EYE MOVEMENT SLEEP BEHAVIOR DISORDER

RBD is characterized by REM sleep without atonia on PSG and dream enactment behavior.[44] Approximately 60% of cases of RBD are idiopathic. RBD often is a harbinger of the neurodegenerative disorders Parkinson's disease and Lewy body dementia. Individuals with PTSD often endorse prominent, sometimes injurious, movement during sleep,[4] and there is much evidence to support a fundamental REM sleep abnormality in PTSD[10,19,57]; however, there are limited data on the relationship between RBD and PTSD. One study reported that 56% of RBD patients had comorbid PTSD.[14] Further investigations are needed to better understand the relation of RBD and PTSD.

Recently, Mysliwiec and colleagues[7] proposed a novel diagnosis, trauma-associated sleep disorder (TSD), which incorporates trauma-related nightmare enactment associated with specific clinical characteristics, extreme nocturnal manifestations of traumatic experiences, including disruptive nocturnal behaviors (e.g., striking at or choking bed partner). Unlike RBD, TSD is characterized by an onset in close proximity to a trauma, and "sympathetic overdrive" in REM sleep. Further, nightmares in TSD may be observed in REM sleep or non-REM sleep, and the dreams may not be recalled upon awakening.

TREATMENT OF SLEEP DISTURBANCES IN PTSD

Treatments for PTSD are generally less effective in ameliorating the sleep disturbances than the waking symptoms. Few studies have examined the efficacy and mechanisms of psychotherapeutic and pharmacological interventions for disturbed sleep in PTSD. Here, we provide a succinct summary of modalities used for treating disturbed sleep in PTSD (see Table 20.1).

TABLE 20.1. RANDOMIZED CONTROLLED TRIALS OF PSYCHOTHERAPEUTIC AND PHARMACOLOGICAL INTERVENTIONS FOR DISTURBED SLEEP IN POSTTRAUMATIC STRESS DISORDER, PUBLISHED SINCE 2010

First Author, Year	Study Characteristics	Study Design	Treatment Duration	Control Group	Primary Outcome Measures	Reported Findings
Cook et al[126]	0% Female; PTSD-diagnosed Veterans	IR (*n* = 61)	6 sessions × 90 mins.	Active condition (Sleep and nightmare management) (*n* = 63)	NFQ, PSQI-A	Both IR and active control groups showed improvements in sleep quality; however, neither group reported significant change in nightmare frequency.
Davis et al[127]	82% Female; PTSD-diagnosed civilians	ERRT (*n* = 17)	3 sessions × 180 mins.	Waitlist (*n* = 18)	TAA, CAPS, TSI, PSQI, TRNS, PILL, PTCSS	Compared to waitlist controls, ERRT group showed greater improvements in nightmare frequency and severity, and related psychopathology
Germain et al[128]	14% Female; PTSD-diagnosed Veterans	Prazosin (*n* = 18) BSI (*n* = 17)	8.9mg (5.7) 8 sessions × 45 mins.	Placebo (*n* = 15)	CGI-I, ISI, PSQI, PSQI-A, PghSD	Both active treatment groups exhibited greater reductions in insomnia severity and waking PTSD symptoms than the control group.
Margolies et al[70]	10% Female; PTSD-diagnosed Veterans	CBT-I + IR (*n* = 20)	4 sessions × 60 mins.	Waitlist (*n* = 20)	SD, ACT, PSQI, PSQI-A, DBAS, PTSD-SR, PHQ-9, POMS	Compared to waitlist controls, CBT-I + IR group endorsed greater improvements on self-report and objective sleep measures, PTSD severity, depression, and overall distress.

Study	Sample characteristics	Intervention	Dose/Sessions	Control	Measures	Results
Raskind et al.[89]	19% Female; PTSD-diagnosed active-duty soldiers	Prazosin (n = 32)	Morning 4mg (1.4) Evening 15.6 mg (6) 15 weeks	Placebo (n = 35)	CAPS nightmare item, PSQI, CGI change item	Prazosin group reported greater improvements on posttraumatic nightmares, sleep quality, and global status compared to the control group.
Talbot et al.[60]	68.9% Female; Adults w/PTSD and insomnia	CBT-I (n = 29)	8 sessions	Waitlist (n = 16)	SD, PSG, ISI, PSQI, ESS, PSQI-A, CAPS nightmare item	Compared to waitlist controls, CBT-I group reported improvements on subjective sleep, disruptive nocturnal behaviors, and work and interpersonal functioning. Also, both groups endorsed reductions in daytime PTSD symptoms and posttraumatic nightmares.
Thunker et al.[129]	27% Female; PTSD-diagnosed civilians	IR (3 subgroups) Primary nightmare sufferers (n = 22), Depressive patients (n = 21), PTSD patients (n = 26)	8 sessions × 50 mins.	Waitlist (n = 12)	NF ADN	Primary nightmare sufferers, Depressive patients, and PTSD patients reported reductions in nightmare frequency compared to the waitlist control group.

Abbreviations: ACT, actigraphy; ADN, anxiety during nightmares; BSI, behavioral sleep intervention; CAPS, clinician administered PTSD scale; CBT-I, cognitive behavioral therapy; CGI-I, clinical global impression improvement; DBAS, Dysfunctional Beliefs and Attitudes about Sleep Scale; ESS, Epworth Sleepiness Scale; IR, imagery rehearsal; ISI, insomnia severity index; NF, nightmare frequency; PghSD, Pittsburgh Sleep Diary; PHQ-9, Patient Health Questionnaire-9; PILL, Physical Health and Quality of Life Pennebaker Inventory of Limbic Languidness; POMS, Profile of Mood States; PSG, polysomnography; PSQI, Pittsburgh Sleep Quality Index; PSQI-A, Pittsburgh Sleep Quality Index–Addendum; PTCSS, Post Treatment Clinical Significance Survey; PTSD, posttraumatic stress disorder; PTSD-SR, PTSD Symptom Scale–Self Report; SD, sleep diary; TAA, Trauma Assessment for Adults: Self-Report Version; TSI, Trauma Symptom Inventory; TRNS, Trauma-Related Nightmare Survey

Psychotherapeutic Interventions for Disturbed Sleep in PTSD

Cognitive behavioral therapy for insomnia (CBT-I) is an intervention aimed at enhancing overall sleep quality.[58,59] CBT-I includes instruction in stimulus control and sleep restriction, cognitive restructuring, sleep hygiene education, and relaxation training.[59]

There is some evidence that CBT-I is effective for insomnia related to PTSD. In a pilot study of CBT-I in patients with PTSD, Gellis and Gehrman[60] found significant improvements in self-reported sleep quality and insomnia severity (assessed with the Insomnia Severity Index (ISI)]. Recently, Talbot and colleagues[61] conducted the first randomized clinical trial (RCT) of an 8-week course of CBT-I in a community sample seeking treatment for PTSD. Compared to waitlist controls, the CBT-I group had superior responses on all sleep diary measures, sleep quality assessed with the Pittsburgh Sleep Quality Index (PSQI), and PSG-derived TST; these effects remained significant at 6-month follow-up. Insomnia assessed with the ISI remitted in 41% of the CBT-I group. However, both groups reported reductions in PTSD severity and posttraumatic nightmares. Trials with an active treatment control group are warranted to establish the relation of these responses to the therapeutic elements of CBT-I specifically.

There has been some progress in the development and implementation of targeted treatments for TSRD, particularly trauma-related recurrent nightmares. Recently, the clinical practice guidelines for PTSD developed by the American Psychological Association[62] and the Department of Veterans Affairs/Department of Defense (VA/DOD)[63] reported that no clear recommendation can be provided in regard to psychotherapeutic approaches to nightmare treatment due to the inconsistent evidence and the quality of study designs. Given this caveat, we highlight the present state of the literature.

Imagery rehearsal therapy (IRT)[64–66] is the best studied psychotherapeutic intervention for posttraumatic nightmares. There is evidence that it leads to increased mastery of nightmare content and experiences.[67] A variety of treatment protocols that share the following basic components of IRT have been investigated: choosing a repetitive nightmare, rescripting it during waking, and imaginally rehearsing the new dream script at bedtime. Two recent meta-analyses with data from predominantly uncontrolled trials summarized the results of studies of IRT for posttraumatic nightmares.[66,68] They reported large effect sizes for nightmare frequency, sleep quality, and overall PTSD severity. It is important to acknowledge that these meta-analyses combined findings from a variety of treatment protocols with diverse populations (not necessarily diagnosed with PTSD). Recently, Harb and colleagues[69] emphasized the limitations of the extant IRT literature and identified strategies for advancing the field, in particular using Consolidated Standards of Reporting Trials (CONSORT) guidelines for conducting and reporting on trials and considering differences among treatment protocols and study populations.

Some RCTs have reported positive findings using a combination of CBT-I and IRT to treat insomnia and recurrent nightmares in patients with PTSD.[70] Margolies and colleagues[71] conducted the first RCT of a 6-week course of CBT-I + adjunctive IRT in Operation Enduring Freedom (OEF) and Operation Iraqi Freedom (OIF) veterans with PTSD. Compared to waitlist controls, the CBT-I + IRT group reported improvements in subjectively and objectively measured sleep, a reduction in PTSD symptom severity, and a reduction in posttraumatic nightmares. Also, there were reductions in depression and distressed mood.

Exposure, relaxation, and rescripting therapy (ERRT) is a variant of IRT that has shown promise in reducing posttraumatic nightmares and insomnia predominantly in civilians with PTSD symptoms.[72-74] In an uncontrolled study that used imagery rescripting and exposure therapy (IRET), a variant of ERRT, Long and colleagues[75] showed reductions in nightmare frequency and PTSD severity and an increase in sleep time.

Pharmacological Interventions for Disturbed Sleep in PTSD

There are few studies on the benefits of pharmacotherapy for insomnia in PTSD patients.[76] One small, single-blinded, placebo-controlled trial found no significant advantage of the benzodiazepine clonazepam.[77] However, clonazepam is the mainstay of pharmacotherapy for RBD[77] and may have a place in the treatment of dream enactment in PTSD. In a series of case reports, the non-benzodiazepine benzodiazepine receptor agonist (NBRA) zolpidem was reported to be beneficial for insomnia related to PTSD.[78] In a randomized placebo controlled trial, Pollack and colleagues[79] found that a 3-week treatment with the NBRA eszopiclone led to increased improvements in PTSD symptomatology, including disturbed sleep.

Trazodone, a selective serotonin reuptake inhibitor (SSRI) that also acts as a 5-HT$_2$ receptor antagonist, is often used in low doses for treating insomnia.[80] Warner and colleagues[81] found that 72% of PTSD patients treated with trazodone found the drug to be beneficial in decreasing nightmares and reducing SOL. Trazodone also improved the sleep disturbance and other PTSD symptoms in a group of veterans with PTSD.[82] Nefazodone, another SSRI/5-HT2 antagonist, led to changes in dream content in PTSD subjects.[83] Neither trazodone nor nefazodone has been tested in an RCT in a PTSD population.

Other pharmacotherapies have been classified as having low level evidence for efficacy in managing recurrent nightmares; these include topiramate, low-dose cortisol, and gabapentin.[65] Perhaps the most important advance in the pharmacotherapy of posttraumatic nightmares is prazosin, an alpha-1 adrenoceptor antagonist approved by the US Food and Drug Administration for the treatment of hypertension. Several studies in military[84-88] and civilian[89] populations have reported on the efficacy of prazosin in the treatment of nightmares, finding decreases in posttraumatic nightmares, non-nightmare distressed awakenings, and other sleep disturbances, and improvements in sleep quality and overall PTSD symptoms. In a recent meta-analysis of placebo-controlled trials of prazosin for PTSD-related sleep disturbances, George and colleagues[90] reported significant improvements in nightmare frequency and sleep quality as well as PTSD severity. Despite the promising results of studies of prazosin for the treatment of posttraumatic nightmares, Khacatryan and colleagues[91] highlighted the potential limitations of these studies, including the enrollment of predominantly male veterans or service members. Further, most of the studies were conducted by a single group of researchers. Prazosin must be administered prior to each sleep period to avoid the recurrence of nightmares; it is not known whether there could be a lasting beneficial effect after drug discontinuation. Recently, a large multisite study[92] examining the effectiveness of prazosin for combat-related PTSD found that it did not differ from placebo in reducing nightmare frequency or PTSD severity. As a result, the new VA/DOD clinical practice guidelines make no recommendation for or against prazosin for the treatment of recurrent nightmares.[63]

Other Therapeutic Interventions for Disturbed Sleep in PTSD

Continuous positive airway pressure (CPAP) is the recommended therapy for OSA.[93] CPAP acts as a pneumatic splint to prevent the upper airway soft tissue from collapsing[94]; it uses air under pressure to maintain airway patency during sleep. In a recent study of CPAP, El-Solh and colleagues[94] found that veterans with severe to very severe PTSD had a larger reduction in PTSD symptom distress compared to those with mild-to-moderate PTSD, and these improvements were greater with prolonged use of CPAP. In addition to alleviating breathing and snoring problems in PTSD patients, CPAP has also been found to be beneficial in improving the nightmare disturbance. Two recent studies[95,96] found that a reduction in nightmare frequency was associated with CPAP adherence.

ACUTE STRESS DISORDER (ASD)

Similar to PTSD, ASD follows exposure to actual or threatened death, serious injury, or sexual violation.[1] In contrast to PTSD, ASD refers to an initial, potentially transient, reaction. Symptoms must persist for at least 3 days, but no longer than a month, following trauma exposure. Individuals must meet criteria for at least nine of fourteen symptoms across the following categories: intrusion, negative mood, dissociation, avoidance, and hyperarousal.[1]

Prevalence estimates of ASD are difficult to ascertain due to the fluctuating nature of the symptoms and the challenge posed by distinguishing between normal and pathological responses during a brief time frame.[97,98] Fewer than 20% of individuals experiencing a non-interpersonal trauma (e.g., motor vehicle accident, severe burns, industrial accident) are estimated to meet diagnostic criteria for ASD. In contrast, survivors of interpersonal violence (e.g., rape, assault) have a high prevalence of ASD (20%–50%).[1] Approximately 50% of individuals with ASD will subsequently develop PTSD; however, a majority of PTSD-diagnosed individuals will not have met criteria for ASD.[98] Therefore, ASD is currently considered a moderate predictor for the development of PTSD.[99]

Sleep Disturbances in ASD

Similar to the difficulty with ascertaining prevalence rates for ASD, there are challenges with identifying the prevalence of sleep disturbances in the immediate aftermath of trauma exposure. Difficulty falling and staying asleep are among the most frequently reported symptoms of ASD in survivors of traumatic injuries,[100,101] and greater sleep severity in this acute phase has been associated with the development of PTSD.[102] PSG studies conducted in recent traumatic injury survivors have identified significantly more fragmented REM sleep in individuals who go on to develop PTSD.[102,103] It has been theorized that this early disruption in REM sleep compromises the adaptive role of sleep in emotional processing, thereby increasing the vulnerability to symptom chronicity.[103]

ASD and Insomnia

Stress is widely recognized as a component of the pathophysiology of insomnia.[104] ASD has a limited time frame (<1 month), and it is difficult to determine whether sleep disturbance shortly after trauma exposure will resolve or develop into a full diagnosis of insomnia, which requires the persistence of symptoms for at least 3 months.[1] The sleep onset and maintenance difficulties commonly reported soon after a trauma may be associated with elevated nocturnal arousal, as previously discussed in the PTSD section.

ASD and Nightmares

Dreams, nightmares in particular, may be a component of the early trauma response.[105] It has been argued that dreams following trauma may serve an adaptive function in the emotional processing and assimilation of the experience.[105,106] On the other hand, a high level of distress associated with the dream report or the similarity of the dream content to the trauma may identify individuals at risk for further symptom progression. For example, a study of dream diary reports from recently hospitalized accident survivors found that 30% of the participants reported remembering a dream, and 46% of their dream reports were considered trauma-related.[107] At a 6-week follow-up, those who had initially endorsed trauma-related dreams reported significantly more severe PTSD symptoms.

Treatment of Sleep Disturbance in ASD

Although there is evidence that trauma-focused CBT soon after trauma exposure may be helpful in reducing chronic PTSD symptoms, the effect on sleep, specifically, is not known.[108] The efficacy of sleep-specific interventions for reducing insomnia or nightmares in the early aftermath of trauma is also not known. Psychoeducation about avoiding maladaptive strategies for coping with

insomnia and reassessment of treatment readiness if symptoms persist may be an appropriate alternative.[109]

A recent meta-analysis limited to RCTs found no evidence for the usefulness of any drug in inhibiting the development of ASD or preventing the associated sleep disturbance.[110] The use of benzodiazepines, which are often prescribed to improve sleep in the aftermath of trauma, has been discouraged because of the absence of evidence of the effectiveness of these drugs and their known adverse effects.[111] A small, uncontrolled case series[109] provided evidence that prazosin could reduce nightmare frequency and improve sleep in soldiers deployed to an active war zone, but more research is required.

ADJUSTMENT DISORDER (AD)

AD is characterized by amplified responses occurring within 3 months, but not lasting longer than 6 months, following a stressful event or events.[1] AD may be diagnosed following a traumatic event if the response does not meet the criteria for PTSD or ASD. Symptoms must be out of proportion to the severity or intensity of the stressor and cannot represent a normal bereavement response. There are several diagnostic specifiers (e.g., with depressed mood, with anxiety, with disturbance of conduct) that characterize the symptom profile.

As with ASD, the prevalence estimates for AD are difficult to determine because of study population heterogeneity, potential symptom overlap with other disorders, and the lack of specific diagnostic criteria.[112] Rates of a primary AD diagnosis are estimated to lie between 5% and 20% in outpatient mental health settings and frequently estimated to reach 50% in a hospital psychiatric consultation setting.[1] A recent longitudinal study found the prevalence of AD following trauma exposure to be 19% at 3 months, with the mixed depression and anxiety profile the most common.[113] Individuals with new medical diagnoses have the highest rates of AD.[114] AD is also frequently diagnosed among military personnel.[115]

Sleep Disturbances in AD

Although sleep-related symptoms are not necessary for a diagnosis of AD, they are prevalent in a large proportion of individuals with this disorder. For example, 86% of cancer patients meeting criteria for AD in the preceding month reported sleep disturbances,[114] and sleep disturbance was the most commonly reported AD symptom among accident and assault injury survivors at a 3-month postinjury assessment[113] Acute insomnia, conceptualized as the sleep disturbance that occurs from 3 days to 3 months following a stressor, may parallel an AD response.[115] Individuals with a prior vulnerability to insomnia or other sleep disturbance are the most susceptible to acute insomnia.[116]

Little is known about the dream and nightmare disturbance in AD. Some studies indicate that individuals may recall more dreams or report an increase in distressing dreams during periods of heightened stress or life transition,[105,117–119] but this change may arise without an AD diagnosis. The course of this dream change is unclear, as is the degree of associated functional impairment.

Treatment of Sleep Disturbance in AD

There is limited research on the treatment of sleep disturbance in AD. The efficacy of CBT-I for acute insomnia is unclear,[115] and whether early CBT-I might prevent the development of chronic insomnia is not known. Addressing maladaptive coping, such as substance use, may be appropriate as an initial intervention. The use of psychotropic medications in AD is not well understood.[120] Psychotherapeutic approaches may be considered first. Additionally, the efficacy of nightmare treatment protocols for an acute dream disturbance in AD is not known.

CONCLUSIONS

TSRD are disabling psychiatric disorders with prominent sleep disturbances that may meet criteria for comorbid sleep disorders. Several recent reviews[64,121–123] and meta-analyses[66,68,124,125] have reported on the treatment of disturbed sleep in PTSD and conclude that psychotherapeutic and pharmacological interventions show promise. Currently, there are limited data on the efficacy of psychotherapeutic and pharmacological interventions for disturbed sleep in ASD and AD.

FUTURE DIRECTIONS

Over the last several decades, there has been an increasing interest in understanding the role of sleep in the pathophysiology of TSRD. Challenges remain in identifying the nature and course of sleep changes following trauma and other stressors. Such information will be essential to the implementation of personalized sleep-focused interventions in the aftermath of psychological stress. There is promise for both innovative psychotherapeutic and pharmacologic strategies.

KEY CLINICAL PEARLS

- Sleep disturbances may be early symptoms following trauma or other stress exposure. These symptoms are considered "hallmark" symptoms of PTSD and may contribute to the development and maintenance of the disorder.
- It is essential to focus on sleep-related symptoms of TSRD in addition to the broadly defined psychiatric disorder.
- A comprehensive assessment approach is recommended to develop an appropriate treatment plan.

SELF-ASSESSMENT QUESTIONS

1. Which of the following interventions has the strongest empirical support for improving sleep quality in PTSD-diagnosed populations?
   a. Prazosin
   b. Cognitive-behavioral therapy for insomnia
   c. Imagery rehearsal therapy
   d. Trazodone

Answer: b

2. Which one of these medications is most effective in the treatment of nightmares in patients with PTSD?
   a. Nefazodone
   b. Clonazepam
   c. Prazosin
   d. Venlafaxine

Answer: c

3. Identify the sleep disorder, aside from insomnia or recurrent nightmares, that has the greatest comorbidity in trauma-exposed populations.
   a. Obstructive sleep apnea
   b. Periodic limb movement disorder
   c. Night terrors
   d. Sleep paralysis

Answer: a

4. Which of these statements is true regarding acute stress disorder and PTSD?
   a. Both disorders can occur at any time following a traumatic event.
   b. Acute stress disorder occurs only in children, while PTSD occurs at any age.
   c. PTSD is not diagnosed until one month following the traumatic event.
   d. Acute stress disorder describes symptoms in individuals who were not present

for the traumatic incident, while PTSD occurs in those who were present.

Answer: c

5. What is the best psychotherapeutic intervention for treating posttraumatic nightmares?
a. Prolonged exposure therapy
b. Sleep dynamic therapy
c. Dialectical behavior therapy
d. Imagery rehearsal therapy

Answer: d

REFERENCES

1. American Psychiatric Association. Diagnostic and Statistical Manual of Mental Disorders. 5th ed. Washington, DC: American Psychiatric Association; 2013.
2. Gregory AM, Sadeh A. Annual research review: sleep problems in childhood psychiatric disorders-A review of the latest science. J Child Psychol Psychiatry. 2016;57(3):296–317.
3. Sinha SS. Trauma-induced insomnia: a novel model for trauma and sleep research. Sleep Med Rev. 2016;25:74–83.
4. Ohayon MM, Shapiro CM. Sleep disturbance and psychiatric disorder associated with posttraumatic stress disorder in the general population. Compr Psychiatry. 2000; 41(6): 469–478.
5. Neylan TC, Marmar, CR, Metzler TJ, et al. Sleep disturbances in the Vietnam generation: findings from a nationally representative sample of male Vietnam veterans. Am J Psychiatr. 1998;155(7):929–933.
6. Mellman TA, David, D, Kulick-Bell R, Hebding J, Nolan B. Sleep disturbance and its relationship to psychiatric morbidity after Hurricane Andrew. Am J Psychiatri. 1995;152(11):1659–1663.
7. Mysliwiec V, Brock MS, Creamer JL, O'Reilly B, Germain A, Roth B. Trauma associated sleep disorder: a parasomnia induced by trauma. Sleep Med Rev. 2017; 1–11.
8. Davis JL, Byrd P, Rhudy JL, Wright DC. Characteristics of chronic nightmares in a trauma-exposed treatment-seeking sample. Dreaming. 2007;17(4):187–198.
9. Kilpatrick DG, Resnick HS, Milanak ME, Miller MW, Keyes KM, Friedman MJ. National estimates of exposure to traumatic events and PTSD prevalence using DSM-IV and DSM-5 criteria. J Traumatic Stress. 2013; 26:537–547.
10. Ross RJ et al. Sleep disturbance as the hallmark of posttraumatic stress disorder. Am J Psychiatriy. 1989;146:697–707.
11. Sharafkhaneh A Giray N, Richardson P, et al. Association of psychiatric disorders and sleep apnea in a large cohort. Sleep. 2005;28(11):1405–1411.
12. Brown TM, Boudewyns PA. Periodic limb movements of sleep in combat veterans with posttraumatic stress disorder. J Trauma Stress. 1996;9(1):129–136.
13. Mellman TA, Kulick-Bell R, Ashlock LE, et al. Sleep events among veterans with combat-related posttraumatic stress disorder. Am J Psychiatry. 1995; 152:110–115.
14. Husain AM, Miller PP, Carwile ST. REM sleep behavior disorder: potential relationship to posttraumatic stress disorder. J Clin Neurophysiol. 2001; 18(2):148–157.
15. Cox, R. C., Tuck, B. M., Olatunji, B. O. Sleep disturbance in posttraumatic stress disorder: epiphenomenon or causal factor? Curr Psychiatry Rep. 2017;19(4):22.
16. Straus LD, Drummond SPA, Nappi CM, Jenkins MM, Norman SB. Sleep variability in military-related PTSD: a comparison to primary insomnia and healthy controls. J Trauma Stress. 2015;28:8–16.
17. Wallace DM, Shafazand S, Ramos AR, Carvalho DZ, Gardener H, Lorenzo D, et al. Insomnia characteristics and clinical correlates in Operation Enduring Freedom/Operation Iraqi Freedom veterans with post-traumatic stress disorder and mild traumatic brain injury: an exploratory study. Sleep Med. 2011;12:850–859.
18. van Liempt S, van Zuiden M, Westenberg H, Super A, Vermetten E. Impact of impaired sleep on the development of PTSD symptoms in combat veterans: a prospective longitudinal cohort study. Depress Anxiety. 2013;30:469–474.
19. Kobayashi, I., Boarts, J. M., & Delahanty, D. L. Polysomnographically measured sleep abnormalities in PTSD: A meta-analytic review. Psychophysiology, 2007;44:660–669.
20. Baglioni C, Nanovska S, Regen W, et al. Sleep and mental disorders: a meta-analysis of polysomnographic research. Psychol Bull. 2016; 142(9):969–990.
21. Werner KB, Griffin MG, Galovski TE. Objective and subjective measurement of sleep disturbance in female trauma survivors with posttraumatic stress disorder. Psychiatry Res. 2016;240:234–240.
22. Van Wyk M, Thomas KGF, Solms M, Lipinska G. Prominence of hyperarousal symptoms explains variability of sleep disruption in posttraumatic stress disorder. Psychological Trauma. 2016; 8(6):688–696.

23. Bryant RA et al. Sleep disturbance immediately prior to trauma predicts subsequent psychiatric disorders. Sleep. 2010; 33(1):69–74.

24. Gehrman, P et al. Predeployment sleep duration and insomnia symptoms as risk factors for new-onset mental health disorder following military deployment. Sleep. 2013; 36(7):1009–1018.

25. Wright, KM, Britt TW, Bliese PD, Adler AB, Picchioni D, Moore D. Insomnia as predictor versus outcome of PTSD and depression among Iraq combat veterans. J Clin Psychol. 2011; 67:1240–1258.

26. Belleville G, Guay S, Marchand A. Impact of sleep disturbances on PTSD symptoms and perceived health. J. Nerv Ment Dis. 2009;192(2):126–132.

27. Phelps AJ, Forbes D, Creamer M. Understanding posttraumatic nightmares: an empirical and conceptual review. Clin Psycholo Rev. 2008;28(2):338–355.

28. Schreuder BJ, Igreja V, van Dijk J, et al. Intrusive re-experiencing of chronic strife or war. Adv Psychiatr Treat. 2001;7:102–108.

29. Mellman TA, Hipolito MS. Sleep disturbance in the aftermath of trauma and posttraumatic stress disorder. CNS Spectr. 2006; 11(18):611–615.

30. Hasler B, Germain A. Correlates and treatments of nightmares in adults. Sleep Med Clin. 2009;4(4):507–517.

31. Robert G, Zandra A. Measuring nightmare and bad dream frequency: impact of retrospective and prospective instruments. J Sleep Res. 2008;17(2):132–139.

32. Leskin GA, Woodward SH, Young HE, Sheikh JI. Effects of comorbid diagnoses on sleep disturbance in PTSD. J Psychiatr Res. 2002;36(6):449–452.

33. Blagrove M, Haywood S. Evaluating the awakening criterion in the definition of nightmares: how certain are people in judging whether a nightmare woke them up? J Sleep Res. 2006;15(2):117–124.

34. Woodward SH, Arsenault NJ, Murray C, Bliwise, DL. Laboratory sleep correlates of nightmare complaint in PTSD inpatients. Biol Psychiatry, 2000;48(11):1081–1087.

35. van Liempt S., Vermetten E, Geuze E. et al. Pharmacotherpy for disordered sleep in post-traumatic stress disorder: a systematic review. Int Clin Psychopharmacol. 2006;21:193–202.

36. Mellman TA, David D, Bustamante V, et al. Dreams in the acute aftermath of trauma and their relationship to PTSD. J Trauma Stress. 2001;14(1)241–247.

37. Kobayashi I, Sledjesk EM, Spoonster, E, et al. Effects of early nightmares on the development of sleep disturbances in motor vehicle accident victims. J Trauma Stress. 2008;21(6):548–555.

38. Paul F, Schredl M, Alpers GW. Nightmares affect the experience of sleep quality but not sleep architecture: an ambulatory polysomnographic study. Borderline Personality Disord Emot Dysregul. 2015; 2:3.

39. Levin R, Fireman G. Nightmare prevalence, nightmare distress, and self-reported psychological disturbance. Sleep. 2002;25(2):205–212.

40. Nadorff MR, Nazem S, Fiske A. Insomnia symptoms, nightmares, and suicidal ideation in a college student sample. Sleep. 2011;34(1):93–98.

41. Bernert RA Joiner TE, Cukrowicz KC. et al. Suicidality and sleep disturbances. Sleep 2005; 28(9):1135–1141.

42. Sjostrom N, Waern M, Hetta J. Nightmares and sleep disturbances in relation to suicidality in suicide attempters. Sleep. 2007;30(1):91–95.

43. Morin CM, Espie CA. The Oxford Handbook of Sleep and sleep Disorders. New York: Oxford University Press, 2012.

44. American Academy of Sleep Medicine. International Classification of Sleep: Diagnostic and Coding Manual. Rev ed. Westchester, IL: American Academy of Sleep Medicine; 2001.

45. American Academy of Sleep Medicine. International Classification of Sleep Disorders: Diagnostic and Coding Manual. 2nd ed. Westchester, IL: American Academy of Sleep Medicine; 2005.

46. Punjabi NM. The epidemiology of adult obstructive sleep apnea. Proc Am Thorac Soc. 2008;5(2):136–143.

47. Lydiard RB Hamner MH. Clinical importance of sleep disturbance as a treatment target in PTSD. Focus. 2009;8(2):176–183.

48. Krakow B. et al. Nightmares, insomnia, and sleep-disordered breathing in fire evacuees seeking treatment for posttraumatic sleep disturbance. J Trauma Stress. 2004;17(3):257–268.

49. Krakow B et al. Complex insomnia: insomnia and sleep-disordered breathing in a consecutive series of crime victims with nightmares and PTSD. Biol Psychiatry. 2013;49:948–953.

50. Krakow B et al. Signs and symptoms of sleep-disordered breathing in trauma survivors: a matched comparison with classic sleep apnea patients. J Nerv Ment Dis. 2006;194(6):433–439.

51. Yesavage JA et al. Sleep-disordered breathing in Vietnam veterans with posttraumatic stress disorder. Am J Geriatr Pschiatr. 2012;20:199–204.

52. Ehrmann DE, Pitt B, Deldin PJ. Sleep-disordered breathing and psychopathology: a complex web of questions and answers. J Sleep Disord Ther. 2013;2(6):1–3.

53. Hornyak M, Feige B, Riemann D, et al. Periodic leg movements in sleep and periodic limb movement

disorder: prevalence, clinical significance and treatment. Sleep Med Rev. 2006;10:169–177.

54. Ross RJ et al. Motor dysfunction during sleep in posttraumatic stress disorder. Sleep. 1994;17(8):723–732.

55. Germain A, Nielsen TA. Sleep pathophysiology in posttraumatic stress disorder and idiopathic nightmare sufferers. Biol Psychiatry. 2003;54:1092–98.

56. Desautels A, Michaud M, Lanfranchi P, et al. Periodic limb movements in sleep. In Chokroverty S, Allen R, Waters A, Montagna P, eds. Sleep and Movement Disorders. Oxford: Oxford University Press, pp. 650–663.

57. Mellman TA, Kobayashi I, Lavela J, et al. A relationship between REM sleep measures and the duration of posttraumatic stress disorder in a young adult urban minority population. Sleep. 2014; 37(8):1321–1326.

58. Morin CM, Benca R. Chronic insomnia. Lancet. 2012;379:1129–1141.

59. Morin, CM, Epsie CA. Insomnia: A Clinical Guide to Assessment and Treatment. New York: Kluwer Academic/Plenum; 2003.

60. Gellis LA, Gehrman PR. Cognitive behavioral treatment for insomnia in veterans with long-standing posttraumatic stress disorder: a pilot study. J Aggress Maltreat Trauma. 2011;20:904–916.

61. Talbot LS, Maguen S, Metzler TJ et al. Cognitive behavioral therapy for insomnia in posttraumatic stress disorder: A randomized controlled trial. Sleep. 2014;37(2):327–341.

62. American Psychological Association. Clinical Practice Guidelines for the Treatment of Posttraumatic Stress Disorder (PTSD) in Adults. Washington, DC: American Psychological Association; 2017.

63. Department of Veterans Affairs. VA/DOD Clinical practice guidelines for the management of posttraumatic stress disorder and acute stress disorder. Washington, DC: Department of Veteran Affairs; 2017.

64. Nappi CM. Drummond SP, Hall JM. Treating nightmares and insomnia in posttraumatic stress disorder: A review of current evidence. Neuropharmacology. 2012;62:576–585.

65. Aurora et al. Best practice guide for the treatment of nightmare disorder in adults. J Clin Sleep Med. 2010;6(4):389–401.

66. Hansen K, Hoflin V, Kroner-Borowik T et al. Efficacy of psychological interventions aiming to reduce chronic nightmares: a meta-analysis. Clin Psychol Rev. 2013;33:146–155.

67. Germain A, Krakow B, Faucher B, et al. Increased mastery elements associated with imagery rehearsal treatment for nightmares in

sexual assault survivors with PTSD. Dreaming. 2004;14:195–206.

68. Casement MD, Swanson LM. A meta-analysis of imagery rehearsal for post-traumatic nightmares: effects on nightmare frequency, sleep quality, and posttraumatic stress. Clin Psychol Rev. 2012;32:566–574.

69. Harb GC, Phelp AJ, Forbes D, et al. A critical review of the evidence base of imagery rehearsal for posttraumatic nightmares: pointing the way for the future research. J Trauma Stress. 2013; 26: 570–579.

70. Ulmer CS, Edinger JD, Calhoun PS. A multicomponent cognitive-behavioral intervention for sleep disturbance in veterans with PTSD: A pilot study. J Clin Sleep Med. 2011; 7(1):57–68.

71. Margolies SO, Rybarczyk B, Vrana SR, Leszczysz DJ, Lynch J. Efficacy of a cognitive-behavioral treatment for insomnia and nightmares in Afghanistan and Iraq veterans with PTSD. J Clin Psychology. 2013;69(10):1026–1042.

72. Davis, JL, Wright DC. Exposure, relaxation, and rescripting treatment for trauma-related nightmares. J Trauma Dissociation. 2006;7(1):5–18.

73. Davis JL, Wright DC. Randomized clinical trial for treatment of chronic nightmares in trauma-exposed adults. J Trauma Stress. 2007;20(2):123–133.

74. Rhudy JL et al. Cognitive-behavioral treatment for chronic nightmares in trauma-exposed persons: assessing physiological reactions to nightmare-related fear. J Clin Psyholo. 2010;66:365–382.

75. Long ME, Hammons ME, Davis JL, et al. Imagery rescripting and exposure group treatment of post-traumatic nightmares in Veterans with PTSD. J Anxiety Disord. 2011;25:531–535.

76. Schutte-Rodin S, Broch L, Buyssee D, et al. Clinical guideline for the evaluation and management of chronic insomnia in adults. J Clin Sleep Med. 2008;4(5):487–504.

77. Cates ME, Bishop MH, Davis LL, et al. Clonazepam for treatment of sleep disturbances associated with combat-related posttraumatic stress disorder. Ann Pharmacother. 2004;38:1395–1399.

78. Dieperink ME, Drogemuller, L. Zolpidem for insomnia related to PTSD. Psychiatr Serv. 1999;50(3):421.

79. Pollack MH et al. Eszopiclone for the treatment of posttraumatic stress disorder and associated insomnia: a randomized, double-blind, placebo controlled trial. J Clin Psychiatry. 2011;72(7):892–897.

80. Saletu-Zyhlarz GM, Abu-Bakker MH, Anderer P, et al. Insomnia in depression: differences in objective and subjective sleep and awakening quality to normal controls and acute effects of trazodone.

Prog Neuropsychopharmacol Biol Psychiatry. 2002;26(2):249–260.

81. Warner MD, Dom MR, Peabody CA. Survey on the usefulness of trazodone in patients with PTSD with insomnia or nightmares. Pharmacopsychiatry. 2001;34(4):128–131.

82. Hertzberg MA, Feldman ME, Beckham JC, et al. Trial of trazodone for posttraumatic stress disorder suing a multiple baseline group design. J Clin Psychopharmacol 1996;16(4):294–298.

83. Mellman TA, David D, Barza I. Nefazodone treatment and dream reports in chronic PTSD. Depress Anxiety. 1999;9(3):146–148.

84. Raskind MA, Dobie DJ, Kanter ED, et al. The alpha-adrenergic antagonist prazosin ameliorates combat trauma nightmares in veterans with post-traumatic stress disorder: a report of 4 cases. J Clin Psychiatry. 2000;61(2):129–133.

85. Raskind MA, Peskind ER, Kanter ED, et al. Reduction of nightmares and other PTSD symptoms in combat veterans by prazosin: a placebo-controlled study. PsychiatryOnline. 2003;160(2):371–373.

86. Raskind MA, Peskind ER, Hoff DJ et al. A parallel group placebo controlled study of prazosin for trauma nightmares and sleep disturbance in combat veterans with post-traumatic stress disorder. Biol Psychiatry. 2007;61:928–934.

87. Raskind MA, Peterson K, Williams T, et al. A trial of prazosin for combat trauma PTSD with nightmares in active-duty soldiers returned from Iraq and Afghanistan. Am J Psychiatry.2013; 170:1003–1010.

88. Thompson CE, Talyor FB, McFall ME, et al. Non nightmare distressed awakenings in veterans with posttraumatic stress disorder: response to prazosin. J Trauma Stress. 2008;21(4):417–420.

89. Taylor et al. Prazosin effects on objective sleep measures and clinical symptoms in civilian trauma posttraumatic stress disorder: a placebo-controlled study. Biol Psychiatry. 2008;63:629–632.

90. George KC, Kebejian L, Ruth LJ, Miller CW, Himelhoch S. Meta-analysis of the efficacy and safety of prazosin versus placebo for the treatment of nightmares and sleep disturbances in adults with posttraumatic stress disorder. J Trauma Dissociation. 2016;17(4):494–510.

91. Khachatryan D, Groll D, Booij L, Sepehry AA, Schutz CG. Prazosin for treating sleep disturbances in adults with posttraumatic stress disorder: a systematic review and meta-analysis of randomized controlled trials. Gen Hosp Psychiatry.2016;39:46–52.

92. Raskind MA, Chow, PB, Harris C et al. Trial of Prazosin for posttraumatic stress disorder in military veterans. N Engl J Med. 2018;378:507–517.

93. Cao MT, Sternbach JM, Guilleminault C. Continuous positive airway pressure therapy in obstructive sleep apnea: benefits and alternatives. Expert Rev. Respir. Med. 2017;11:259–272.

94. El-Solh AA, Vermont L, Homish GG, Kufel T. The effects of continuous positive airway pressure on post-traumatic stress disorder symptoms in veterans with post-traumatic stress disorder and obstructive sleep apnea: a prospective study. Sleep Med. 2017;33:145–150.

95. Collen JF, Lettieri CJ, Hoffman M. The impact of posttraumatic stress disorder on CPAP adherence in patients with obstructive sleep apnea. J Clin Sleep Med. 2012;8:667–672.

96. Gharaibeh K, Tamanna S, UJllah M, Geraci SA. Effects of continuous positive airway pressure therapy on nightmares in patients with post-traumatic stress disorder and obstructive sleep apnea. J Invest Med. 2013;61:480–481.

97. Bryant RA. Acute stress disorder. Curr Opin Psychology. 2017;14:127–131.

98. Bryant RA, Freidman MJ, Spigel D, Ursano R, Strain J. A review of acute stress disorder in DSM-5. Depression Anxiety. 2011;28(9):802–817.

99. Bryant RA, Creamer M, O'Donnell et al. A comparison of the capacity of DSM-IV and DSM-5 acute stress disorder definitions to predict posttraumatic stress disorder and related disorders. J Clin Psychiatry. 2015;76(4):391–397.

100. Difede J, Ptacek J, Roberts J et al. Acute stress disorder after burn injury: a predictor of posttraumatic stress disorder? Psychosomatic Med. 2002;64(5):826–834.

101. Koren D, Arnon I, Lavie P, Klein E. Sleep complaints as early predictors of posttraumatic stress disorder: a 1-year prospective study of injured survivors of motor vehicle accidents. Am J Psychiatr. 2002; 159(5):855–857.

102. Mellman TA, Bustamante V, Fins AI et al. REM sleep and the early development of posttraumatic stress disorder. Am J Pschiatr. 2002;159(10):241–247.

103. Mellman TA, Pigeon WR, Nowell PD et al. Relationships between REM sleep findings and PTSD symptoms during the early aftermath of trauma. J Trauma Stress. 2007;20(5):893–901.

104. Levenson JC, Kay DB, Buysse DJ. The pathophysiology of insomnia. Chest. 2015;147(4):1179–1192.

105. Hartmann E. Nightmare after trauma as paradigm for all dreams: A new approach to the nature and functions of dreaming. Psychiatry. 1998;61(3):223–238.

106. Newell PT, Cartwright RD. Affect and cognition in dreams: A critique of the cognitive role

in adaptive dream functioning and support for associative models. Psychiatry.2000;63(1):34–44.

107. Mellman TA, David D, Bustamante V et al. Dreams in the acute aftermath of trauma and their relationship to PTSD. J Trauma Stress.2001;14(1):241–247.

108. Bryant RA, Mastrodomenico J, Felmingham KL et al. Treatment of acute stress disorder: a randomized controlled trial. Arch Gen Psychiatr.2008;65(6):659–667.

109. Smith MT, Perilis ML. Who is a candidate for cognitive-behavioral therapy for insomnia? Health Psychology. 2006;25(1):15.

110. Sijbrandij M, Kleiboer A, Bisson JI et al. Pharmacological prevention of post-traumatic stress and acute stress disorder: A systematic review and meta-analysis. The Lancet Psychiatr. 2015;2(5):413–421.

111. Guina J, Rossetter SR, DeRhodes BJ et al. Benzodiazepines for PTSD: a systematic review and meta-analysis. J Psychiatric Practice. 2015;21(4):281–303.

112. Casey P. Adjustment disorder: new developments. Curr Psychiatr Rep. 2014;16(6):451.

113. O'Donnell ML, Alkemade N, Creamer M et al. A longitudinal study of adjustment disorder after trauma exposure. Am J Psychiatr. 2016;173(12):1231–1238.

114. Hund B, Reuter K, Harter M et al. Stressors, symptoms profile, and predictors of adjustment disorder in cancer patients. Results from an epidemiological study with the composite international diagnostic interview, adaptation for oncology (CIDI-O). Depress Anxiety.2016;33(2):153–161.

115. Ellis JG, Gehrman P, Epsie CA et al. Acute insomnia: current conceptualization and future direction. Sleep Med Rev. 2012;16(1):5–14.

116. Drake CL, Pillai V, Roth T. Stress and sleep reactivity: a prospective investigation of the stress-diathesis model of insomnia. Sleep. 2014;37(8):1295–1304.

117. Cartwright R, Agargun MY, Kirby J et al. Relation of dreams to waking concerns. Psychiatry Res. 2006;141(3):261–270.

118. Schredl M. Factors affecting the continuity between waking and dreaming: emotional intensity and emotional tone of the waking-life event. Sleep Hypnosis. 2006;8(1):1–5.

119. Van Rijn E, Eichenlaub JB, Lewis PA et al. The dream-lag effect: selective processing of personally significant events during rapid eye movements sleep, but not during slow wave sleep. Neurobiol Learn Mem. 2015;122:98–109.

120. Carta MG, Balestrieri M, Murru A, et al. Adjustment disorder: epidemiology, diagnosis, and treatment. Clin Pract Epidemiol Ment Health. 2009;5(1):15.

121. Brownlow JA, Harb GC, Ross, RJ. Treatment of sleep disturbances in posttraumatic stress disorder: a review of the literature. Curr Psychiatry Rep. 2015;17:41.

122. Miller KE, Brownlow JA, Woodward S et al. Sleep and dreaming in posttraumatic stress disorder. Curr Psychiatry Rep. 2017;19:71.

123. Koffel E, Khawaja IS, Germain A. Sleep disturbances in posttraumatic stress disorder: updated review and implications for treatment. Psychiatr Ann. 2016;46(3):173–176.

124. Seda G, Sanchez-Ortuno MM, Welsh CH et al. Comparative meta-analysis of prazosin and imagery rehearsal therapy for nightmare frequency, sleep quality, and posttraumatic stress. J Clin Sleep Med. 2015;11(1):11–22.

125. Ho FY, Chan CS, Tang KN. Cognitive-behavioral therapy for sleep disturbances in treating posttraumatic stress disorder symptoms: A meta-analysis of randomized controlled trials. Clin Psychology Rev. 2016;43:90–102.

126. Cook JM, Cary MS, Gamble GM, et al. Imagery rehearsal for posttraumatic nightmares: A randomized controlled trial. J Trauma Stress. 2010; 23(5):553–563.

127. Davis JL, Rhudy JL, Pruiksma KE, et al. Physiological predictors of response to exposure, relaxation, and rescripting therapy for chronic nightmares in a randomized clinical trial. J Clin Sleep Med. 2011;7(6):622–631.

128. Germain A, Richardson R, Moul DE, et al. Placebo-controlled comparison of prazosin and cognitive-behavioral treatments for sleep disturbances in US military veterans. J Psychosom Res. 2012; 72(2): 89–96.

129. Thunker J, Pietrowsky R. Effectiveness of a manualized imagery rehearsal therapy for patients suffering from nightmare disorders with and without a comorbidity of depression or PTSD. Behav Res Ther. 2012; 50: 558–564.

21

Schizophrenia Spectrum and Other Psychotic Disorders

CHI-HUNG AU, MAN-SUM CHAN, AND KA-FAI CHUNG

INTRODUCTION

Based on the *Diagnostic and Statistical Manual of Mental Disorders* (fifth edition; DSM-5) classification, schizophrenia spectrum and other psychotic disorders include schizophrenia, delusional disorder, brief psychotic disorder, schizophreniform disorder, schizoaffective disorder, substance and medication-induced psychotic disorder, psychotic disorder due to another medical condition, and schizotypal personality disorder. Characteristic features of psychotic disorders include delusions, hallucinations, disorganized thinking and speech, grossly disorganized or abnormal motor behavior, and negative symptoms.

Historically, sleep disturbances have been reported in schizophrenia since their first clinical descriptions [1]. Emil Kraepelin noted that individuals with dementia praecox, the earlier definition of schizophrenia, had disrupted sleep and also recognized that rest in bed and care for food and sleep are the most valuable treatment interventions in such patients. Eugen Bleuler, who first coined the term *schizophrenia* in 1908, suggested that sleep is altered in psychotic patients as these patients were afraid that something or someone will attack them while asleep. In 1960s, Finberg and colleagues studied sleep patterns in patients with schizophrenia and noted that, as compared to controls, those with schizophrenia required a significantly longer time to fall asleep and showed greater variability in the amount of sleep occurring prior to the onset of first dream. Additionally, schizophrenia patients with hallucinations were noted to have higher density of rapid eye movement (REM) activity as compared to those without hallucinations [2].

Over the last 50 years, progress has been made to understand the comorbidity, neurobiology, and impact of sleep disturbances on acute and chronic outcomes in schizophrenia. Current empirical evidence suggests that sleep disturbance occurs in 30% to 80% of patients with schizophrenia and is associated with positive and negative symptoms, cognitive deficits, poorer outcome, and impaired quality of life [3]. Difficulty falling or maintaining asleep has been associated with symptoms severity and considered as a prodromal symptom of psychotic relapse. Sleep disturbances in schizophrenia may arise during the acute phase of illness and in many cases persists in the chronic phase [4]. Sleep architectural abnormalities in schizophrenia have been implicated in symptomatology, neurocognitive function, and clinical outcome [3, 5].

Noncompliance with medications is not uncommon in clinical course of schizophrenia. For those patients who experience insomnia prior to discontinuation of antipsychotic medications, the severity of insomnia has been strongly associated with severity of psychotic symptoms after discontinuation of antipsychotic medications [6].

Additionally, major primary sleep disorders including insomnia, breathing-related sleep disorders, hypersomnolence disorders, parasomnia disorders, sleep-related movement, and circadian rhythm sleep disorders are commonly prevalent in patients with schizophrenia [7].

Despite the frequent comorbidity and the negative outcomes associated with sleep disturbance in patients with schizophrenia, sleep is rarely the direct focus of treatment. This chapter provides an overview of the current understanding of the neurobiology, diagnosis, and management of key comorbid primary sleep disorders in patients with schizophrenia.

NEUROBIOLOGY

A number of neural mechanisms, neurotransmitter pathways, brain regions, and body systems are implicated in sleep initiation and maintenance;

hence, a multifactorial model is needed to explain the sleep disturbance in schizophrenia.

Neurotransmitters

Dysfunction in specific neural circuits including dopaminergic and serotoninergic pathways has been implicated in both schizophrenia and sleep disorders [7]. While overactivity of the D_2 receptors in the striatum is linked to positive symptoms of schizophrenia, dopamine is also implicated in increased wakefulness eventually leading to insomnia [7, 8]. Thus, it can be inferred that the co-occurrence of insomnia and schizophrenia likely share a common pathophysiology. Difficulties initiating and maintaining sleep as well as circadian rhythm disorders are commonly reported in schizophrenia [9]. These sleep disturbances are thought to be related to a presumed hyperactivity of the dopaminergic system and dysfunction of the GABAergic system, both associated with signaling in sleep-wake promoting brain regions and with core features of schizophrenia [10].

Neural Substrates

Sleep spindles are waxing/waning, 12 to 16 Hz oscillations that are characteristic of N2 sleep. Sleep spindles are generated by the thalamic reticular nucleus (TRN) in combination with the dorsal thalamus and are then transferred to the cortex, via thalamic relay neurons, where spindle oscillations are synchronized and sustained over time [1]. TRN is an inhibitory shell made of GABAergic neurons that envelops a large portion of the thalamus [11]. Deficits in thalamic function have been implicated in the neurobiology of schizophrenia [11, 12]. For example, as compared to healthy controls and psychiatric control groups, marked reductions of spindle activity have been demonstrated in medicated patients with chronic schizophrenia, medicated adolescents with early-onset schizophrenia, and antipsychotic drug-naïve patients with early-course schizophrenia and their first-degree relatives [1]. Taken together, these findings suggest the possibility of thalamo-cortical dysfunction in pathophysiology of schizophrenia, particularly related to GABAergic and N-methyl-D-aspartate receptor (NMDA) mediated glutamatergic neurotransmission [1]. Manoach and colleagues [13] have proposed that reduced spindle activity may be considered as an endophenotype of schizophrenia as the sleep spindle deficit may impair sleep-dependent memory consolidation and contribute to psychotic symptoms such that

it may represent a novel treatment biomarker for schizophrenia.

Inflammatory Biomarkers

Extensive data showing that schizophrenia is associated with chronic low-grade systemic inflammation. Sleep disorders are considered to be a risk factor for several systemic inflammation-related diseases [14]. Additionally, the sleep-inflammation link has been noted to be stronger in women within the general population [15]. In a cross-sectional case control study, Lee and colleagues [15] compared community dwelling outpatients with schizophrenia ($n = 144$, 46% women) and controls ($n = 134$, 52% women) in terms of reported sleep disturbances, mental and physical health, cognitive status, and inflammatory biomarkers including proinflammatory cytokines (high sensitivity C-reactive protein [hs-CRP], interleukin [IL]-6, tumor necrosis factor-α [TNF-α]) and an anti-inflammatory cytokine (IL-10). As compared to controls, patients with schizophrenia had had longer sleep duration, worse sleep quality, and increased levels of hs-CRP, IL-6, and TNF-α. The authors noted that worse sleep quality and global cognitive functioning were associated with higher hs-CRP and IL-6 levels in the schizophrenia group. Moreover, females with schizophrenia were less likely to have good sleep quality and had elevated levels of hs-CRP and IL-6 compared to males with schizophrenia [15].

In another study, Fang and colleagues [14] examined the associations between sleep quality and inflammatory markers in patients with schizophrenia. Sleep quality was measured objectively using actigraphy in schizophrenia inpatients ($n = 199$). The blood concentration of white blood cells (WBC) and neutrophils, together with neutrophil-lymphocyte ratio (NLR), and platelet–lymphocyte ratio (PLR) were used to measure the state of inflammation. The authors noted that total sleep time (TST) was negatively associated with NLR and PLR, and sleep efficiency (SE) was negatively associated with neutrophil counts and NLR. Sleep onset latency (SOL), total activity counts, wake after sleep onset (WASO), and number of awakenings were positively associated with WBC and neutrophil counts. The average length of awakening was positively associated with NLR and PLR. The authors suggested that improving sleep quality may modulate the state of inflammation in patients with schizophrenia [14].

Circadian Rhythm Abnormalities

Circadian rhythm sleep–wake disorders (CRSWDs) in patients with schizophrenia appear to be independent of the amount of daytime sleep and daytime activities [16], suggesting that there might be an intrinsic circadian system abnormality in schizophrenia. Patients with schizophrenia exhibit an irregular pattern of melatonin secretion, which is indicative of a disruption in the circadian rhythmicity of melatonin [17]. Moreover, recent evidence suggests a loss of circadian expression of certain clock genes in patients with schizophrenia as compared to healthy controls [18, 19]. Johansson and colleagues [18] reported a loss of rhythmic expression of CRY1 and PER2 in fibroblasts obtained from patients with chronic schizophrenia, as compared to cells from healthy controls. The sleep quality in patients with chronic schizophrenia was noted to be poor in comparison with the healthy controls. Additionally, the authors found, in another patient sample, that mononuclear blood cells from patients with schizophrenia experiencing their first episode of psychosis had decreased expression of CLOCK, PER2 and CRY1 as compared to blood cells from healthy controls. Sun and colleagues [19] reported that disruptions in diurnal rhythms of the expression of PER1 and PER3, despite 8 weeks of clozapine treatment, may contribute to the vulnerability to recurrence of psychosis and efficacy of long-term maintenance treatment in schizophrenia.

Genetic Variations

Both schizophrenia and sleep disorders are characterized by a strong genetic component with shared genetic loci [20, 21], Significant genetic associations have been reported to establish the comorbidity of schizophrenia and sleep disorders [22]. For example, antipsychotic-induced restless legs syndrome (RLS) has been linked to polymorphisms located on CLOCK, BTB domain containing 9 (*BTBD9*), G protein subunit beta 3 (*GNB3*), and tyrosine hydroxylase (*TH*) genes. Clozapine-induced hypersomnolence was correlated with polymorphisms of histamine-*N*-methyltransferase (*HNMT*) gene, whereas insomnia was associated with variants of the melatonin receptor 1 (*MTNR1*) gene [22]. TH is a key component of dopamine metabolism and has been implicated in schizophrenia, antipsychotic-induced extrapyramidal side effects and RLS [23–25]. HNMT is another enzyme implicated in neurotransmission by inactivating histamine in the central nervous system [26]. Research suggests that histamine is involved in sleep–wake regulation and levels of HNMT demonstrate a circadian rhythmicity [27]. Similarly, GNB3 enhances signal transduction and ion transport [28]. GNB3 is likely implicated in dopaminergic and serotoninergic transmission as polymorphisms of GNB3 gene have been linked to depression, efficacy of antipsychotic medications, and neuroleptic-associated weight gain [29–31]. Finally, BTBD9 encodes a protein, whose exact function has not yet been identified, and it may be involved in interneuronal and intraneuronal signal transduction [22]. In summary, these genetic variations implicate the circadian system, dopamine, and histamine metabolism and signal transduction pathways in schizophrenia and comorbid sleep disorders [22].

SLEEP ASSESSMENT TOOLS

Subjective Questionnaires

Subjective questionnaires can be used for screening and assessment of sleep disorders. Table 21.1 presents the commonly used questionnaires for assessment of a range of primary sleep disorders.

TABLE 21.1. QUESTIONNAIRES FOR SCREENING AND ASSESSMENT OF SLEEP DISORDERS

Sleep Problem/ Sleep Disorders	Name of Questionnaires
General sleep disturbance	Pittsburgh Sleep Quality Index [32]
Insomnia disorder	Insomnia Severity Index [33] Athens Insomnia Scale [34]
Hypersomnia	Epworth Sleepiness Scale [35]
Obstructive sleep apnea	STOP-Bang Questionnaire [36] Berlin Questionnaire [37]
Circadian rhythm sleep wake disorder	Morningness–Eveningness Questionnaire [38]
Parasomnia	Mayo Sleep Questionnaire [39] Munich Parasomnia Screening [40]
Restless leg syndrome	Cambridge–Hopkins Questionnaire [41]

Sleep Diary

Sleep diaries are used to establish the pattern of sleep on a nightly basis. Sleep diary records the pattern and quality of sleep, meal times, any caffeine or alcohol use, daily activities including naps and exercise, and the use of medications. Sleep diaries should be used for at least 7 consecutive days to examine differences in sleep pattern on weekdays and weekend. Sleep diaries are used to assess the severity of sleep dysfunction and treatment response in patients receiving cognitive-behavioral therapy for insomnia (CBT-I) and those with circadian rhythm sleep disorders.

Polysomnography (PSG)

PSG is clinically indicated in schizophrenia patients to investigate comorbid sleep disorders such as obstructive sleep apnea (OSA), periodic limb movement disorder (PLMD), narcolepsy, parasomnias, and refractory insomnia. Research driven PSG results indicate that reduced SE and TST, as well as increased sleep latency, are found in most patients with schizophrenia. Additionally, some studies report alterations of N2 sleep, N3, and REM sleep (reduced REM latency and REM density). Clinical variables such as severity of illness, positive symptoms, negative symptoms, outcome, neurocognitive impairment, and brain structure are likely implicated in sleep architectural changes in schizophrenia [42].

Actigraphy

Although PSG remains the gold standard, actigraphy has been recognized to be a useful method to study sleep–wake pattern in patients with psychotic disorders [43]. Actigraphy can record long-term ambulatory pattern of sleep over several nights [44]. Actigraphy does not measure actual sleep stages but allows an estimation of the overall sleep quality and quantity [45]. Therefore, actigraphy data can serve as an outcome measure for changes in sleep-wake pattern in patients receiving antipsychotic treatment. Actigraphy is also indicated to assess CRSWDs that may be present in schizophrenia patients. Patients with schizophrenia typically demonstrate a reduced level of motor activity, prolonged time in bed, increased sleep latency, more disrupted nocturnal sleep, more daytime sleep, and a less distinct circadian rhythm [46].

CLINICAL APPROACH

Sleep symptoms must be actively enquired as schizophrenia patients do not often volunteer to report sleep disturbances. A comprehensive sleep history not only helps to identify specific sleep complaints but also guides further sleep-specific investigations. It is important to assess the negative consequences of sleep disturbances such as daytime sleepiness, fatigue, poor concentration and memory, low mood, irritability, reduced motivation, and impaired social function. Primary sleep disorders such as OSA, RLS, and sleep-related eating disorders (SRED) are common in schizophrenia. Patients with schizophrenia are at a higher risk of obesity, a recognized risk factor for OSA, due to genetic factors and unhealthy lifestyle [47]. Effects of antipsychotic medications on sleep should always be considered for any negative sleep-related consequences. Intriguingly, antipsychotic medications appear to be a risk factor of OSA independent of obesity [48]. Both RLS and SRED are exacerbated by antipsychotics [49, 50], possibly due to dopaminergic and serotoninergic antagonism, respectively.

Patients with schizophrenia are at higher risks of substance abuse (nicotine, cannabis, alcohol, and cocaine) compared to the general population [51]. The underlying mechanism is not completely clear. Patients with schizophrenia might self-medicate with substances to relieve disabling symptoms such as anhedonia and insomnia [52]. Substance use could also be due to an imbalance of hippocampal-prefrontal regulation of dopamine release in nucleus accumbens, which is implicated in both the rewarding mechanism and the pathophysiology of psychotic symptoms [53]. There have been limited studies on the impact of substance use on sleep in schizophrenia. Generally, the use of substances worsens sleep quality [54]. Although cannabis acutely reduces sleep latency and increases slow-wave sleep (SWS) [55, 56], these effects vanish on chronic use. Sleep disturbance occurs upon withdrawal of cannabis and can last up to 7 weeks [57]. While both nicotine and alcohol use are associated with OSA [58, 59], opioids increase the risk of central sleep apnea [60].

This section focuses on assessment and management of comorbid primary sleep disorders in patients with schizophrenia.

Obstructive Sleep Apnea (OSA)

OSA is a condition characterized by recurrent episodes of airflow reduction or cessation caused by varying degrees of upper airway occlusion. Risk factors for OSA include obesity, short and thick neck, small and receding jaw, oropharyngeal crowding, male gender, advanced age, hypertension, and postmenopausal status. The prevalence of OSA in schizophrenia ranges from 1.6% to 52% [61]. Obesity, worsened by lack of exercise and atypical antipsychotic use, are the likely culprit for the high rates of OSA in schizophrenia patients [62]. Apart from causing weight gain, atypical antipsychotics appear to increase the risk of OSA risk with other mechanisms such as decreasing upper airway tone and an alternation of respiratory control secondary to dopamine receptor antagonism [63]. Therefore, identification and treatment of OSA in schizophrenia patients is important for improving clinical outcomes.

There are several questionnaires that have been developed for screening of OSA such as STOP-Bang questionnaire and Berlin questionnaire. However, there is uncertainty about the accuracy and clinical utility of all potential screening tools due to variations in sample characteristics and OSA diagnostic procedure in the validation studies [64]. Use of screening questionnaires alone for clinical evaluation of OSA can yield false-positive results, which can lead to unnecessary investigations. On the other hand, the diagnosis of OSA can be missed in case the results are false-negative. Therefore, it is not recommended to use these screening tools alone for diagnosis of OSA.

Overnight polysomnography (PSG) is the gold standard for diagnosis of OSA. Home sleep apnea testing (HSAT) is recommended for individuals whose symptoms and signs are significant enough to suggest presence of underlying moderate to severe risk of OSA [65]. A minimum of 4 hours of good quality data are necessary for diagnosis. HSAT is more convenient and comfortable and has a much lower cost than PSG [65]. A negative or inconclusive HSAT warrants in-lab PSG to definitely rule out OSA.

Antipsychotics are associated with weight gain, which causes or worsens OSA in patients with schizophrenia. A RCT demonstrated that a switch from olanzapine, quetiapine, or risperidone to aripiprazole resulted in an improvement in triglycerides and weight reduction [66]. Therefore, it is worthwhile to review the antipsychotic regimen and consider weight-neutral antipsychotic medication options once diagnosis of OSA is established [67], although there is a lack of studies on the impact of antipsychotic-switch on OSA. However, the clinician should be cautious when switching antipsychotic medications due to the risk of relapse of psychosis.

Specific treatments like continuous positive airway pressure (CPAP) therapy are usually necessary for optimal treatment of OSA. CPAP is the gold standard for the treatment of OSA that works by maintaining the upper airway opened mechanically with a column of air [68]. CPAP use of at least 6 hours per night is associated with reduction in sleepiness and improvement in mood, cognitive function, and quality of life [69]. Data on CPAP use in schizophrenia patients with OSA are very limited. A majority of the case reports [70, 71] found that psychotic symptoms improved with CPAP, but there was a case report on a 52-year old male with schizophrenia who developed a psychotic episode 5 days after commencing CPAP and the psychotic symptoms resolved after ceasing CPAP and commencing antipsychotics [72]. CPAP may offer novel benefits to address cognitive impairment and sleep disturbance in patients with schizophrenia [73]. In a pilot study from Australia, the authors investigated the impact of CPAP use in management of severe OSA (AHI >30/hour) in patients with treatment refractory schizophrenia ($n = 8$) [73]. As compared to baseline, marked improvements were noted in terms of sleep architecture (improved SWS and REM sleep), metabolic parameters (improved blood pressure control and weight loss), and cognition were associated with CPAP use in patients with schizophrenia [73].

CPAP is associated with side effects including dry mouth, sneezing, nasal drips, facial allergy, and air leak. The adherence with CPAP treatment can be as low as 50% in the general population. CPAP adherence may be lower in patients with psychotic disorders as reflected by their poor adherence to physical health medications [74]; however, empirical data are lacking. Evidence suggests that educational, supportive, and behavioral interventions might be effective in improving CPAP compliance [75].

Patients' view on CPAP machine, including any associated delusion, should be sought. Psychiatrists should explain the needs and benefits of CPAP, possible obstacles, and ways to deal with them. The most appealing benefit might be a reduction in psychotic symptoms and an improvement in sleep, daytime tiredness, and cognitive function, which allows patients to function better. Other treatment options for OSA include weight loss, positional therapy, oral appliances, nasal expiratory positive airway pressure, surgery, and hypoglossal nerve stimulation; however, their use in schizophrenia patients with OSA has not been well examined. Readers are advised to refer to the chapter on breathing-related sleep disorders for details about these treatment options for general management of OSA.

Narcolepsy

Narcolepsy is a rare sleep disorder affecting 0.025% to 0.05% of the population. It is characterized by a sudden intrusion of sleep (with reduced REM latency) into wakefulness resulting in sleep attacks, excessive sleepiness, and REM sleep-related phenomena like sleep paralysis, cataplexy, and hypnagogic hallucinations [3]. Sleep paralysis appears a few months after the onset of excessive sleepiness, but some cases may take years to develop, and it usually occurs when patients are drifting off to sleep or waking up. Cataplexy is a sudden loss of muscle tone bilaterally, which is usually induced by strong emotional response such as laughter and anger. It typically develops over seconds and lasts up to 1 to 2 minutes. Hypnagogic hallucinations, defined as vivid dreamlike experiences occurring at the transition from wake to sleep, are present in 33% to 80% of narcolepsy patients.

Typically, hypnagogic hallucinations have a multimodal characteristic, combining visual, auditory, and tactile phenomena [3]. Hypnagogic hallucinations usually last up to a minute, but are so vivid that patients cannot distinguish them from reality. Patients with narcolepsy can mix up their lucid dreams with reality, resulting in delusional memories, or "dream delusions" [76]. Dream delusions can persist after the treatment with stimulants and in patients with good insight about narcolepsy [77]. While the exact mechanism is unclear, it may be related to their dreams being more frequent and vivid than in healthy individuals [78] or due to an inability to differentiate the source of memory [76].

Narcolepsy has high prevalence of comorbid conditions including depression, anxiety, obesity, diabetes mellitus, hypertension, chronic obstructive pulmonary disease, OSA, PLMD, RLS, and non-REM (NREM) parasomnias [79]. Although the risk of narcolepsy is not increased in schizophrenia, it is sometimes misdiagnosed as schizophrenia due to presence of hypnagogic hallucinations [80]. A case-control study of 148 patients with narcolepsy, 21 patients with acute exacerbation of schizophrenia, and 128 healthy controls found some differences in the hallucinatory experience between patients with narcolepsy and schizophrenia (Table 21.1) [81].

Management

As described by Kishi and colleagues [82], there are three diagnostic possibilities that exist when symptoms of psychosis and narcolepsy occur in the same individual. The first scenario is that the patient has a psychotic features associated with narcolepsy as evident by several case reports and clinical studies report that hypnagogic and hypnopompic hallucinations can be misinterpreted as the active psychotic state of schizophrenia thus leading to misdiagnoses and inappropriate treatment [83–85]. In such cases, narcolepsy tends to have no response to antipsychotics, which can lead to a diagnosis of refractory schizophrenia. The psychopathology characterizing such patients has been described as multimodal hallucinations, lack of formal thought disorder, appropriate affect, retention of ability to relate to others, and a striking degree of insight into their illness [84, 86]. The psychotic features usually abate with appropriate treatment of narcolepsy using psycho-stimulants and not antipsychotics [82].

Stimulant-induced psychosis is the second diagnostic possibility in patients with narcolepsy and concurrent psychosis. Evidence suggests that pharmacological management of narcolepsy patients with stimulant-induced psychosis can be complicated [82]. It has been demonstrated that long-term use of psychostimulants such as methamphetamine, as needed for the treatment of narcolepsy, can cause reduction of dopamine transporter density in the brain, even after stopping the use of psycho-stimulants [87]. This phenomenon can be associated with the development of persistent psychotic symptoms [87]. However, most patients with narcolepsy do not develop stimulant-induced psychosis even on a high dose of methylphenidate over a prolonged period [88]. Data obtained from long-term follow-up (mean follow up: 15.4 years) in narcolepsy patients ($n = 329$) suggest that only 3.2% of narcolepsy patients developed signs of stimulant induced psychosis.

The third diagnostic possibility is that both schizophrenia and narcolepsy can present concurrently in an individual. Based on independent prevalence, it has been estimated that 1 to 18 individuals in a population of 2 million may have combination of schizophrenia and narcolepsy [82]. In such cases, treatment of both schizophrenia and narcolepsy are advised while keeping an eye on signs of stimulant-induced psychosis [82]. It may be a consideration to use wake-promoting agents such as modafinil and armodafinil to treat narcolepsy in patients with schizophrenia to prevent worsening of psychotic symptoms. However, based on a review study, adjunctive use of modafinil has been associated with small risk of exacerbation of psychosis in patients with schizophrenia (6%). It must be noted that worsening of narcolepsy symptoms can occur with antipsychotic use, potentially due to D2 antagonism as dopamine is implicated in the maintenance of wakefulness [89]. Based on current literature, which relies on use of stimulants and first-generation antipsychotics, the prognosis of individuals with comorbid schizophrenia and narcolepsy seems to be poor [82]. In such cases, the combination including atypical antipsychotics and wake-promoting agents such as modafinil and armodafinil may be considered; however, empirical data are lacking for such combination treatments.

Hypersomnolence

Hypersomnolence disorders comprise of a diverse group of conditions with excessive daytime sleepiness (EDS). Based on a naturalistic study, up to 32% of the patients with schizophrenia ($n = 100$) reported EDS [90]. The symptoms of EDS have been understudied and can be attributed to multiple causes including a symptom of schizophrenia, primary sleep disorders, or a medication side effect [90]. Sleep can be used a coping strategy by patients with schizophrenia to provide important respite from distressing psychotic experiences [91]. Common primary sleep disorders such as OSA, already covered in detail, can cause excessive daytime somnolence in schizophrenia [61].

Kluge and colleagues [92] reported that, as compared to baseline, patients with schizophrenia had increased sleep propensity with use of clozapine and olanzapine, based on multiple sleep latency testing (MSLT). Both antipsychotics induced caused shortened sleep latency and more sleep onsets during the MSLT daytime nap tests as compared to baseline. These antipsychotic-induced effects on sleep propensity were noted to be strongest in the morning. Interestingly, objective short sleep latency on MSLT was not necessarily associated with subjective sleepiness [92]. In a 6-week double-blind study, treatment with lurasidone 80 mg or 160 mg, administered once daily in the evening, was associated with a reduction in subjective daytime sleepiness similar in magnitude to placebo, while quetiapine extended release 600 mg/day was associated with a significant increase in daytime sleepiness, compared to both lurasidone dose groups and placebo [93].

Management

In an 8-week randomized double-blind placebo-controlled study, the authors investigated the efficacy of and safety of modafinil on parkinsonism and EDS, as well as on negative symptoms and cognitive abilities in patients with schizophrenia or schizoaffective disorder [94]. The authors noted that modafinil (50–200 mg) improved antipsychotic-induced parkinsonism but not EDS (subjectively reported), psychiatric symptoms or cognition in patients with schizophrenia and schizoaffective disorder. In a review study, examining the efficacy of modafinil as an adjunctive treatment of sedation, negative symptoms, and cognition in schizophrenia, the authors suggested that modafinil is generally well tolerated and may have some efficacy in the treatment of antipsychotic-induced sedation and cognitive domains; however, well-powered, prospective, randomized placebo-controlled trials are necessary to elucidate the efficacy and effectiveness modafinil as an adjunctive treatment for sedation, negative symptoms, and cognitive deficits in schizophrenia [95].

Parasomnias

Parasomnias are abnormal events that occur during sleep and classified as NREM-related, REM-related, and other parasomnias. Studies on parasomnias in schizophrenia are scarce. A recent study indicated that the prevalence of parasomnia symptoms, including sleepwalking, night terrors, dream enactment, and nightmares, was 9.1% among 120 schizophrenia patients, compared to 13.8% in patients with mood disorders and 19.0% in those with anxiety disorders [96].

Common NREM-related parasomnias include sleepwalking and SRED. The former has a lifetime prevalence of 18.3% and point prevalence of 4.3% in adults, while SRED occurs in 4.6% of an unselected university student sample. Both sleepwalking and SRED are recurrent episodes of incomplete awakening from sleep that occur during the first third of the night. Sleepwalking is associated with ambulation and other complex behaviors out of bed, while SRED is associated with involuntary eating. Both disorders are associated with injuries and accidents. For sleepwalkers, they are prone to bumping into objects or falling down, while agitated sleepwalking, panicky running, self-injury, and other dangerous behaviors can occur. Eating of inedible or toxic substances, sleep disturbance due to night eating, sleep-related injury from obtaining or cooking food,

TABLE 21.2. DIFFERENCES IN THE CHARACTERISTICS OF SLEEP-RELATED HALLUCINATION BETWEEN NARCOLEPSY AND SCHIZOPHRENIA

	Narcolepsy	Schizophrenia
Sleep-related hallucinations	Common (81%)	Common (80%)
Occurring ≥3/week	Uncommon (17%)	Common (81%)
Visual hallucination	Common (83%)	Less common (29%)
Auditory hallucination	Less common (45%)	Common (81%)
Kinetic hallucination	Common (71%)	Rare (5%)

TABLE 21.3. MAJOR DIFFERENCES BETWEEN SLEEPWALKING AND SLEEP-RELATED EATING DISORDER

	Sleepwalking	SRED
Age at episode onset	Childhood	Middle age
Identified triggering factor (e.g., trauma, stress)	Uncommon (19%)	Common (62%)
Nocturnal episodes nightly or almost nightly	Uncommon (10%)	Common (73%)
Total loss of awareness during episode	Common (39%)	Rare (7%)
Presence of dream-like mentation	Common (67%)	Rare (0%)
Injuries	Common (52%)	Rare (7%)
History of eating disorder	Uncommon (14%)	Common (60%)
Current insomnia	Rare (5%)	Common (73%)
Psychiatric disorders	Uncommon (21%)	Common (62%)

Abbreviation: SRED, sleep-related eating disorder.

and increased weight are possible complications of SRED [97]. Table 21.3 highlights major differences between sleep walking and sleep-related eating disorder.

A recent study comparing 15 patients with SRED and 21 patients with sleepwalking detected several differences in their nocturnal episodes and psychiatric history (Table 21.2) [98]. Nocturnal confusion in patients with dementia or due to medical conditions, such as epilepsy and hypoglycemia, should be ruled out. SRED should be differentiated from other conditions that are associated with increased eating such as Kleine–Levin syndrome, dissociative disorder, bulimia nervosa, night eating disorder, and binge eating disorder. Several psychiatric drugs are associated with NREM-related parasomnias, such as olanzapine, quetiapine, risperidone, ziprasidone, mirtazapine, benzodiazepines (BDZ; triazolam), and zolpidem [99, 100].

Common REM-related parasomnias include sleep paralysis, nightmares, and REM sleep behavior disorder (RBD). Sleep paralysis is characterized by transient and generalized inability to move (atonia) and speak during the transition from sleep to wakefulness. While eye movements are intact, patients may have breathing difficulties when they try to breathe deeply. Choking and suffocation feelings are common. It can be associated with hypnic hallucinations. Attacks are short lasting (from seconds to 20 minutes) with a mean duration of 6 minutes. The lifetime prevalence of sleep paralysis is 15% to 40% in the general population [3], 22% in psychiatric patients [101],

and 9% in schizophrenia [102]. Current evidence suggests that the prevalence of sleep paralysis does not appear to be increased in patients with schizophrenia [101, 102]. Patients might interpret the experience of hypnagogic hallucinations and sleep paralysis with spiritual explanations, which are prevalent in some cultures [103, 104].

The prevalence of nightmares in patients with schizophrenia is unclear. One study reported the prevalence of nightmares in patients with schizophrenia spectrum disorders ($n = 388$) to be 9%. The authors reported that comorbidity of nightmares and insomnia, and not nightmares alone, was associated with the risk of suicide attempt over follow-up in these patients (adjusted hazard ratio [HR] 11.10, 95% confidence interval [CI] 1.68–73.43, $p < 0.05$) [105]. Nightmares can be associated with medications such as beta-blockers (e.g., atenolol, propranolol), antidepressants (e.g., escitalopram, paroxetine, sertraline, venlafaxine), antipsychotics (risperidone), agents acting through GABA pathway (gabapentin, triazolam, and zopiclone), anticholinesterase inhibitor (donepezil and rivastigmine), dopamine agonists (e.g., levodopa, bupropion), and others [106]. RBD can occur in the context of psychotropic medication use (selective serotonin reuptake inhibitors [SSRIs]), OSA, and narcolepsy. There have been case reports on the association between TCAs, SSRIs, and serotonin and noradrenaline reuptake inhibitors (SNRIs) and RBD, but the association between antipsychotics and REM parasomnias is unclear [107].

The diagnosis of NREM- and REM-related parasomnias is based on clinical history, but PSG should be considered if disorders such as OSA, PLMD, and seizures are suspected and if the parasomnia episodes are associated with injuries.

Management

No clinical trials exist that assess the efficacy of specific treatments for sleepwalking. A prospective study of 50 adults with chronic sleepwalking showed that the acceptance and effectiveness of BZDs and psychiatric medications were poor, while the treatment of breathing-related sleep disorder by CPAP or surgery resulted in resolution of sleepwalking [108]. Due to the limited data, no recommendations can be made for schizophrenia with sleepwalking, except that the inciting psychotropic agent, that led to sleepwalking, may be replaced by an alternative agent. For idiopathic SRED, the first-line treatment includes SSRIs (fluoxetine 20–60 mg/day; paroxetine 20–30 mg/day), and topiramate (100–300 mg/day) and clonazepam (0.5–2 mg/day) can be used as second-line agents [100]. Drug-induced SRED can usually resolve by withdrawing the offending agent [109–112]. Behavioral treatments such as maintaining a safe sleep environment, sleep hygiene education, and stress management can be helpful for both sleepwalking and SRED.

In most cases of sleep paralysis, psycho-education, reassurance, and advice on sleep hygiene with particular emphasis on adequate duration of sleep are sufficient. Nightmares as a drug side effect can usually resolve by withdrawing the offending agent. The American Academy of Sleep Medicine recommends imagery rehearsal therapy for nightmare disorder (Level A evidence) [113].

Circadian Rhythm Sleep Disorder (CRSD)

CRSD is characterized by a chronic misalignment of the endogenous circadian rhythm to the external environment that results in sleep–wake disturbances, distress, and functional impairment [3]. Disrupted circadian rhythm in schizophrenia is characterized by delayed or non-24-hour sleep-wake phase, sleep onset difficulty, prolonged sleep, and reduced daytime activity [16]. Environmental cues such as social activities and light–dark cycle play a role in the alignment of the endogenous circadian rhythm with sleep–wake cycle. Dysfunction of neurotransmitters systems, including dopamine and glutamate, may be one of the causes for CRSD [102]. The circadian rhythm of melatonin in schizophrenia patients with CRSD appears to be blunted and disturbed [16].

Delayed sleep–wake disorder (DSPD) accounts for 80% of the CRSD cases attending sleep clinics [114, 115]. DSPD is reportedly more common in adolescents and young adults, but the prevalence in patients with schizophrenia is unclear. A study of 22 schizophrenia patients with DSPD, 22 patients with delayed sleep phase (but not meeting the criteria of disorder) and 22 patients with normal sleep–wake phase showed that DSPD was significant for a greater severity of negative symptoms, longer sleep latency, poorer sleep quality, higher hypnotic use, more irregular social rhythm, poorer functioning, and higher unemployment rate than patients with delayed sleep phase and normal sleep–wake phase [116].

A comprehensive sleep history, sleep diary, and actigraphy are necessary to make a definite diagnosis of CRSD. Standardized chronotype questionnaires, such as the Composite Scale of Morningness, can be used to assess an individual's circadian preference. Salivary dim light melatonin onset (DLMO) can be useful for confirming the diagnosis and for determining the optimal timing of treatment with light and melatonin [117].

Management

It is common for patients with CRSD to have problems with the regulation of circadian rhythm and sleep homeostasis. Therefore, treatment that targets at both circadian and homeostatic process of sleep regulation is recommended [118]. No previous studies have been conducted on the treatment of CRSD in patients with schizophrenia. In general, low-dose exogenous melatonin at 0.5 mg given 5 hours before habitual sleep onset or 2 to 4 hours before DLMO can be used for the treatment of DSPD. Evening light restriction and 2 hours of bright (5,000 lux) light on awakening is effective in advancing sleep phase by 2 to 3 hours. A combination of melatonin and bright light therapy generally attains the best outcomes. Since bright light therapy has been associated with an induction of manic/hypomanic and mixed state in patients with bipolar disorder, caution should as well taken in patients with schizoaffective disorder [119]. In an open label study, Omori and colleagues [120] noted that low dose of aripiprazole (0.5–3 mg), a second-generation antipsychotic, which is effective in treatment of depression and schizophrenia, advanced the sleep rhythm and reduced nocturnal sleep time in the subjects with DSPD [120]. Efficacy of aripiprazole in treating circadian rhythm disorders, particularly DSPD, in schizophrenia remains to be determined.

Sleep-Related Movement Disorders

Sleep-related movement disorders are characterized by relatively simple, usually stereotyped movements that disturb sleep onset and maintenance. Sleep-related movement disorders are common, particularly RLS, in schizophrenia due to the use of antipsychotics [49]. The prevalence of RLS and RLS symptoms in patients with schizophrenia has been shown to be 21.4% and 47.8%, respectively, which is significantly higher than the prevalence of 9.3% and 19.5%, respectively, in healthy controls [121]. Apart from being associated with iron deficiency, RLS has a close relationship with the dopaminergic system [122]. While RLS symptoms are relieved with iron supplements, these symptoms are worsened by the use of dopamine antagonists, especially antipsychotics. Given that RLS is a common condition in patients with schizophrenia and has negative consequences, it is important to identify and treat RLS. Despite disabling

symptoms of RLS, patients usually find it difficult to describe the uncomfortable feeling and the diagnosis is often delayed [123], especially in patients with schizophrenia with cognitive deficits and apathy [124]. Restlessness and fidgetiness are the most frequent complaints in patients with schizophrenia and RLS [121]. The symptomatology of RLS overlaps with that of akathisia, a known side effect of antipsychotics. As compared to akathisia, RLS symptoms tend to be worse at night and get better with movement. In addition to antipsychotics, antiemetics, antihistamines, TCAs, SSRIs, SNRIs, mirtazapine, and lithium can cause RLS [125]. PSG is not necessary to make a diagnosis of RLS. Objective sleep findings in RLS patients include increased SOL, high arousal index, and significant periodic limb movements [126].

PLMD is characterized by periodic episodes of repetitive, highly stereotyped limb movements during sleep that causes sleep disturbances. To confirm the diagnosis PLMD, PLM index should be ≥5 per hour in children and ≥15 per hour in adults. PLMD is a diagnosis of exclusion and overnight PSG is indicated for confirming the diagnosis. Dopaminergic impairment and/or diminished inhibition of the central pattern generator for PLMs have been proposed as etiological factors [127]. The prevalence and association of PLMD with age and antipsychotic treatment are controversial [128–130]. Table 21.4 presents a comparison between RLS, PLMD, and akathisia due to antipsychotics.

TABLE 21.4. CLINICAL FEATURES OF RESTLESS LEG SYNDROME, PERIODIC LIMB MOVEMENT DISORDER, AND AKATHISIA

	Timing	Motor	Sensory
RLS	Occurs both awake and during sleep (as PLMs) Worse at night and at rest	Voluntary movements Frequency depends on severity Stretching, kicking, or walking	Urge to move and uncomfortable sensation of lower limbs Relieved with movement
PLMD	Only occurs during sleep Usually during first half of sleep	Involuntary, brief muscle twitches, jerky movements, or upward flexion (every 20-40 seconds)	No urge to move No uncomfortable sensation
Akathisia	Not related to the time of day Can last for a whole day Disappears during sleep	Usually voluntary Pacing, walking, inability to stand still, rocking, crossing/uncrossing legs	Inner urge to move all or part of the body No focal sensory complaints

Abbreviation: RLS, restless leg syndrome; PLM, periodic limb movement; PLMD, periodic limb movement disorder.

Management

Since antidepressant and antipsychotic use can potentially worsen RLS, careful inquiry in to RLS symptoms is recommended while deciding treatment modalities for management of schizophrenia and comorbid mood/anxiety disorders. Caution is advised when dopamine agonists are used for management of RLS symptoms in schizophrenia patients due to the risk of exacerbation of psychotic symptoms [127]. Alpha-2-delta calcium channel ligands, such as pregabalin and gabapentin, might be better treatment options for initial RLS treatment in patients with schizophrenia as these medications do not aggravate psychotic symptoms and are preferred when insomnia, anxiety, or pain symptoms are present [131]. The American Academy of Sleep Medicine practice guideline 2012 update on RLS and PLMD pointed out that randomized controlled trials evaluating treatment options for patients with PLMD are lacking; however, treatments for RLS have been shown to decrease PLM indices in subjects with RLS and are likely to be effective in treating the sleep dysfunction of PLMD [132].

Insomnia

The prevalence of insomnia in patients with schizophrenia is estimated to range between 30% and 80% [42]. In acute stage of schizophrenia, patients can suffer from severe insomnia and even total sleeplessness. Despite antipsychotic treatment, approximately 30% patients reported residual insomnia [133]. Lunsford-Avery [134] showed that adolescents with ultra-high risk for psychosis and poor sleep were at higher risk of worsening positive symptoms in the next 12 months than those without sleep disturbance. Poor sleep quality adversely affects quality of life, cognitive function, and mood and increases suicidal behaviors in schizophrenia. A longitudinal study demonstrated that baseline insomnia symptoms might be associated with increased suicidal behaviors in patients with schizophrenia spectrum disorders [105].

Insomnia is seldom the presenting complaint in patients with schizophrenia. The duration, frequency, and severity of insomnia symptoms and the associated daytime consequences are essential to the diagnosis of insomnia disorder. Dysfunctional sleep-related cognitions and behaviors are important areas of assessment. Distorted appraisal of a transient sleep problem may lead to cognitive and emotional hyperarousal and counterproductive coping, such as poor sleep hygiene, which forms vicious cycles that perpetuate insomnia. Comorbid psychiatric conditions like mood disorders, anxiety disorders and posttraumatic stress disorder (PTSD) should be assessed for comprehensive evaluation of sleep dysfunction in schizophrenia patients. Substance use disorders are prevalent in schizophrenia, which makes it essential to assess the consumption of caffeine, tobacco, illicit drugs, and alcohol. Sleep–wake patterns should be assessed to determine whether the sleep phase is delayed, advanced, or irregular. Lastly, prior history of insomnia and pertinent medical history and concomitant medication use should be assessed. Collateral information from a bed partner is often necessary to exclude primary sleep disorders such as OSA and PLMD. Table 21.5 summarizes the differential diagnoses of insomnia in patients with schizophrenia.

A recent systematic review and meta-analysis of the PSG findings in schizophrenia showed an increase of SOL, WASO, and the number of nocturnal awakenings and a reduced TST and SE, compared to healthy controls [5]. The latency and duration of REM and SWS were reduced in schizophrenia patients. Only the percentage of N2 sleep and length of the first REM period did not differ between patients with schizophrenia and healthy controls. Furthermore, absence of sleep architectural abnormalities in medication-naïve patients was reported, while patients with antipsychotic withdrawal for longer than 8 weeks had less sleep architectural abnormalities compared to shorter duration of withdrawal, although abnormalities in sleep continuity were similar in the two groups.

The differences between medication-naïve, medication-withdrawn, and medicated patients in sleep continuity and architecture suggest that sleep architectural abnormalities in schizophrenia are largely related to antipsychotic medications, while sleep onset difficulty is a characteristic feature of schizophrenia patients irrespective of medication status. The systematic review also found SWS deficit especially in schizophrenia patients with illness duration greater than 3 years as compared to those with shorter duration of illness [5].

Although PSG studies are not routinely performed in patients with schizophrenia, these findings suggest that PSG measures (among other neurophysiological parameters) are potential candidates for a better understanding of the neurobiology of schizophrenia. Currently, PSG studies are indicated in schizophrenia patients with high suspicion of comorbid primary sleep disorders such

TABLE 21.5. DIFFERENTIAL DIAGNOSES OF INSOMNIA
IN PATIENTS WITH SCHIZOPHRENIA

Insomnia disorder

Comorbid psychiatric disorders

    Depressive disorder

    Bipolar disorder

    Anxiety disorders

    Posttraumatic stress disorder

    Acute stress and adjustment disorders

    Drugs and alcohol related disorder

        Antidepressants (e.g., selective serotonin reuptake inhibitors, serotonin and noradrenaline reuptake inhibitors, bupropion)

        Stimulants (e.g., amphetamine, dexamphetamine, methylphenidate, cocaine, caffeine, nicotine)

        Withdrawal of alcohol, cannabis, opiates and hypnotics

    Neurocognitive disorders

Comorbid medical disorders

    Pain conditions

    Endocrine dysfunction (e.g., hyperthyroidism, pheochromocytoma)

    Menopausal transition

Comorbid specific sleep disorders

    Delayed/advanced/irregular sleep-wake phase disorders

    Obstructive sleep apnea

    Periodic limb movement disorder

    Parasomnias

as OSA, PLMD, narcolepsy, and parasomnias and in cases of refractory insomnia.

Management

The recommended treatments for chronic insomnia include pharmacological and psycho-behavioral therapies [135]. In this section, we focus on evidence based pharmacological and psychological treatments of insomnia in patients with insomnia.

Pharmacotherapy

Short and immediate-acting BZDs and non-BDZ hypnotics (Z-drugs) are generally recommended for short-term use only for insomnia due to the risk of adverse effects, tolerance, abuse, and dependence [136]. These medications should also be used with caution in schizophrenia patients especially those with OSA due to risk of decrease in minimum overnight saturation [137]. Of concern,

the use of BZDs and Z-drugs has been associated with an increased risk of mortality in patients with schizophrenia based on two large studies [138, 139]. The results from a Finnish study ($n = 2,588$) suggest that, as compared to antipsychotic poly-pharmacy and antidepressant use, BDZ use was associated with a substantial increase in mortality in patients with schizophrenia (HR 1.91, 95% CI 1.13–3.22), and this was attributable to suicidal deaths (HR 3.83, 95% CI 1.45–10.12) and to non-suicidal deaths (HR 1.60, 95% CI 0.86–2.97). In a retrospective study ($n = 18,953$), Fontanella et al. [139] reported that the hazard of mortality was 208% higher for patients using BZDs without an antipsychotic (HR 3.08, 95% CI 2.63–3.61; $p < 0.001$) and 48% higher for patients using BZDs with antipsychotics (HR 1.48, 95% CI 1.15–1.91, $p = 0.002$). The authors noted that the patients using BDZ were at a greater risk of death by suicide and accidental poisoning as well as from natural causes.

Ramelteon is a short-acting melatonin receptor agonist that reduces sleep latency and improves sleep quality, whereas TST is not increased. It is considered relatively safe due to minimal side effects [140]. Studies with small sample size have been conducted in schizophrenia patients and showed that ramelteon is safe and might be associated with improvement in cognitive function and lipid profile [141, 142]. Suvorexant suppresses wakefulness by blocking the hypothalamic neuropeptides, orexin A, and orexin B from binding to orexin OX1R and OXR2 receptors. It is approved by the US Food and Drug Administration (FDA) for the treatment of sleep onset and/or sleep maintenance insomnia [143]. Suvorexant dosages range from 5 mg to 20 mg (recommended starting dose is 10 mg) and should be taken within 30 minutes before bedtime with at least 7 hours remaining before planned awakening [143]. It is associated with low dependency potential and rebound insomnia. To date, only one case report on the use of suvorexant for treating insomnia in schizophrenia is available [144]. Sedating low-dose antidepressant can be used alone for the treatment of insomnia. Low-dose doxepin (3 mg and 6 mg) has FDA approval for the treatment of insomnia characterized by difficulties with sleep maintenance [145]. To our knowledge, there has been no study on the use of doxepin in patients with schizophrenia.

Off-Label Drugs for the Treatment of Insomnia

Mirtazapine, a noradrenergic and specific serotonergic antidepressant (NaSSA), has a sleep-promoting effect [146]. The side effects of mirtazapine may be dose-dependent; for example, a study showed that the use of mirtazapine 15 mg caused greater impairment in road-tracking tasks compared to mirtazapine 7.5 mg, but both doses did not differ in subjective somnolence [147]; therefore, low-dose mirtazapine should be used if it is chosen as an off-label agent for insomnia. Mirtazapine has been shown to improve negative symptoms and cognitive functioning in schizophrenia [148, 149]. Weight gain, daytime sedation, dizziness, and constipation are potential side effects; however, the risk of manic switch by using low-dose sleep-promoting antidepressants in schizoaffective disorder and bipolar disorder is low [150], especially in combination with antipsychotics [151].

Both typical and atypical antipsychotic drugs are recognized to have sleep-promoting effect in healthy subjects and patients with schizophrenia [3]. Typical antipsychotic drugs including haloperidol, thiothixene, and flupentixol reduced SOL and increased TST, SE, and REM latency, while SWS remained unchanged [3]. Administration of atypical antipsychotics including clozapine, olanzapine, and paliperidone decreased SOL, increased TST and SE, and may ameliorate insomnia in patients with schizophrenia. In contrast, the effects of quetiapine and risperidone are inconsistent, and no PSG studies have been published on the effects of aripiprazole, asenapine, iloperidone, and lurasidone. Furthermore, olanzapine and ziprasidone increased SWS, although changes in REM sleep were inconsistent [152].

A study of 92 inpatients with schizophrenia reported an improvement in subjective sleep quality after switching from first-generation antipsychotics (haloperiodol, chlorpromazine, and levomepromazine) to second-generation antipsychotics (risperidone, quetiapine, and olanzapine) [153]. The authors also found that sleep improvement was predicted by baseline sleep quality and the improvement of sleep quality was significantly correlated with improvement in negative symptoms. However, a recent systematic review found only one double-blind randomized controlled trial on the effectiveness of atypical antipsychotic for insomnia; furthermore, the study was rated as very low quality and showed no significant difference between quetiapine and placebo on sleep measures after 2 weeks of treatment [154]. Although antipsychotics may improve sleep, the medications can cause sedation, weight gain, and extrapyramidal side effects. Limited data are currently available on the benefits and risks of switching antipsychotic therapies for the treatment of insomnia in schizophrenia; hence, no recommendations can be made at this time.

Melatonin is a hormonal product of pineal gland. A meta-analysis demonstrated that melatonin reduced SOL, increased TST, and improved sleep quality [155]. Due to its minimal side effects, even if it is a weak hypnotic agent, schizophrenia patients with poor sleep quality may benefit from melatonin, based on two double-blind randomized controlled trials [156, 157]. In one study, authors reported that melatonin 2 mg (controlled release) was superior to placebo in terms of improving SE in patients with schizophrenia whose sleep quality is low [156]. In another study, relative to placebo, melatonin (3–12 mg) significantly improved the quality and depth of nighttime sleep, reduced the number of nighttime awakenings, and increased the duration of sleep without producing a morning hangover ($p < 0.05$) [157].

Cognitive-Behavioral Therapy for Insomnia

CBT-I is an effective treatment for comorbid insomnia in a number of psychiatric conditions including depressive disorder, anxiety disorders, PTSD, and substance use disorders [158]. Recent evidence showed that CBT-I was effective in patients with schizophrenia in alleviating insomnia. Eight sessions of CBT-I over 12 weeks plus standard care (medication and contact with the local clinical team) compared to standard care were offered to 50 schizophrenia patients with insomnia and persistent distressing delusions and hallucinations. More than 40% of patients receiving CBT-I no longer had insomnia by week 12, whereas only 4% of patients receiving standard care were insomnia-free [159]. The treatment effect for CBT covered a range from reducing but also increasing delusions and hallucinations [159]. The CBT-I program in this study included sleep hygiene education, stimulus control therapy, relaxation training, and cognitive therapy, but sleep restriction therapy was avoided due to the worsening effects of sleep loss on psychotic symptoms [160, 161]. More studies are needed to examine the role of gradual sleep restriction; that is, a minimal of 6.5 hours is used to reduce the risk of sleep deprivation instead of a drastic cut of sleep duration based on patient's TST. There has been limited data on the role of different CBT-I components in patients with schizophrenia (e.g., whether cognitive therapy is less effective due to patient's neurocognitive impairment), while the main therapeutic techniques should be sleep hygiene education, stimulus control therapy, and relaxation training.

CONCLUSIONS

Comprehensive sleep assessment is essential for healthcare professionals to understand primary sleep disorders and sleep dysfunction inherent in schizophrenia. Common primary sleep disorders, such as OSA, RLS, and SRED, should be vigilantly assessed. Particular attention should be paid to sleep dysfunction caused by antipsychotic medications. Accurate identification and treatment of sleep dysfunction in schizophrenia can significantly enhance clinical outcomes. More research is warranted to elucidate the prevalence and treatment of comorbid sleep disorders in schizophrenia. In view of the close relationship between schizophrenia and sleep disorders, sleep research is likely to advance our understanding of the neurobiology of schizophrenia.

FUTURE DIRECTIONS

Genetic and longitudinal studies are necessary to examine the link between schizophrenia and

comorbid sleep disorders. Interventions such as cognitive behavioral therapy for insomnia have recently been used in patients with schizophrenia, and the results are promising; however, further clinical trials are needed to examine the treatment of other comorbid sleep disorders (e.g., chronotherapy for DSPD and CPAP for OSA). Finally, electrophysiological abnormalities such as sleep spindle deficit might become a valuable target for novel therapies for patients with schizophrenia.

KEY CLINICAL PEARLS

1. Sleep disorders including insomnia, OSA, RLS, and SRED are common in schizophrenia, but they are often underrecognized and undertreated.
2. Sleep disorders in schizophrenia are often associated with worse clinical course of illness and physical morbidities.
3. Antipsychotic medications can worsen or cause symptoms of primary sleep disorders such as OSA, RLS, and SRED.
4. Use of benzodiazepine medications for treatment of insomnia has been associated with increased mortality in patients with schizophrenia.
5. Accurate identification and treatment of sleep dysfunction in schizophrenia can significantly enhance clinical outcomes.
6. CBT-I can be effective in alleviating insomnia.in patients with schizophrenia; however, sleep-restriction technique should be preferably avoided.

SELF-ASSESSMENT QUESTIONS

1. Which of the following medications for treatment of insomnia have been associated with increased mortality in patients with schizophrenia?
   a. Benzodiazepines.
   b. Ramelteon
   c. Suvorexant
   d. Sedating antidepressants

Answer: a

2. Which of the following techniques should be avoided when using cognitive behavioral treatment for insomnia (CBT-I) in schizophrenia?
   a. Stimulus control
   b. Relaxation techniques
   c. Sleep restriction
   d. Cognitive restructuring

Answer: c

3. 45 year old Caucasian non-obese male with schizophrenia complains of episodes of food consumption at night with lack of awareness of these episodes with resultant weight gain soon after a recent switch to atypical antipsychotic treatment. He and his partner do not endorse symptoms of breathing-related sleep disorder, restless legs syndrome and periodic limb movement disorder. He denies any eating issues during daytime. He denies any pertinent medical history. Which of the following is the most likely diagnosis?

  a. Night eating syndrome
  b. Sleep related eating disorder
  c. Binge eating disorder
  d. Nocturnal hypoglycemia

Answer: b

4. All primary sleep disorders reportedly have higher prevalence in schizophrenia except following?

  a. Obstructive sleep apnea
  b. Restless legs syndrome
  c. Sleep-related eating disorder
  d. REM sleep behavior disorder

Answer: d

5. Which of the following can help distinguish restless legs syndrome from akathisia associated with antipsychotic use?

  a. Relief in RLS symptoms with movement
  b. Circadian rhythmicity of RLS symptoms
  c. Both of the above
  d. None of the above

Answer: c

REFERENCES

1. Ferrarelli, F. and G. Tononi, *What are sleep spindle deficits telling us about schizophrenia?* Biol Psychiatry, 2016. **80**(8): p. 577–578.
2. Feinberg, I., R.L. Koresko, and F. Gottlieb, *Further observations on electrophysiological sleep patterns in schizophrenia.* Compr Psychiatry, 1965. **6**: p. 21–24.
3. Monti, J.M. and D. Monti, *Sleep in schizophrenia patients and the effects of antipsychotic drugs.* Sleep Med Rev, 2004. **8**(2): p. 133–148.
4. Afonso, P., V. Viveiros, and T. Vinhas de Sousa, *[Sleep disturbances in schizophrenia].* Acta Med Port, 2011. **24 Suppl 4**: p. 799–806.
5. Chan, M.S., et al., *Sleep in schizophrenia: a systematic review and meta-analysis of polysomnographic findings in case-control studies.* Sleep Med Rev, 2017. **32**: p. 69–84.
6. Chemerinski, E., et al., *Insomnia as a predictor for symptom worsening following antipsychotic withdrawal in schizophrenia.* Compr Psychiatry, 2002. **43**(5): p. 393–396.
7. Kaskie, R.E., B. Graziano, and F. Ferrarelli, *Schizophrenia and sleep disorders: links, risks, and management challenges.* Nat Sci Sleep, 2017. **9**: p. 227–239.
8. Oishi, Y. and M. Lazarus, *The control of sleep and wakefulness by mesolimbic dopamine systems.* Neurosci Res, 2017. **118**: p. 66–73.
9. Staedt, J., et al., *[Sleep disorders in schizophrenia].* Fortschr Neurol Psychiatr, 2010. **78**(2): p. 70–80.
10. Monti, J.M., et al., *Sleep and circadian rhythm dysregulation in schizophrenia.* Prog Neuropsychopharmacol Biol Psychiatry, 2013. **43**: p. 209–216.
11. Ferrarelli, F. and G. Tononi, *The thalamic reticular nucleus and schizophrenia.* Schizophr Bull, 2011. **37**(2): p. 306–315.
12. Pratt, J.A. and B.J. Morris, *The thalamic reticular nucleus: a functional hub for thalamocortical network dysfunction in schizophrenia and a target for drug discovery.* J Psychopharmacol, 2015. **29**(2): p. 127–137.
13. Manoach, D.S., et al., *Reduced sleep spindles in schizophrenia: a treatable endophenotype that links risk genes to impaired cognition?* Biol Psychiatry, 2016. **80**(8): p. 599–608.
14. Fang, S.H., et al., *Associations between sleep quality and inflammatory markers in patients with schizophrenia.* Psychiatry Res, 2016. **246**: p. 154–160.
15. Lee, E.E., et al., *Sleep disturbances and inflammatory biomarkers in schizophrenia: focus on sex differences.* Am J Geriatr Psychiatry, 2018.
16. Wulff, K., et al., *Sleep and circadian rhythm disruption in schizophrenia.* Br J Psychiatry, 2012. **200**(4): p. 308–316.
17. Almoguera, B., et al., *Association of common genetic variants with risperidone adverse events in a Spanish schizophrenic population.* Pharmacogenomics J, 2013. **13**(2): p. 197–204.
18. Johansson, A.S., et al., *Altered circadian clock gene expression in patients with schizophrenia.* Schizophr Res, 2016. **174**(1-3): p. 17–23.
19. Sun, H.Q., et al., *Diurnal neurobiological alterations after exposure to clozapine in first-episode schizophrenia patients.* Psychoneuroendocrinology, 2016. **64**: p. 108–116.
20. Lane, J.M., et al., *Genome-wide association analysis identifies novel loci for chronotype in 100,420 individuals from the UK Biobank.* Nat Commun, 2016. **7**: p. 10889.
21. Lane, J.M., et al., *Genome-wide association analyses of sleep disturbance traits identify new loci and highlight shared genetics with neuropsychiatric*

   and metabolic traits. Nat Genet, 2017. **49**(2): p. 274–281.

22. Assimakopoulos, K., et al., *Genetic variations associated with sleep disorders in patients with schizophrenia: a systematic review.* Medicines (Basel), 2018. **5**(2).

23. Rice, M.W., et al., *Mapping dopaminergic deficiencies in the substantia nigra/ventral tegmental area in schizophrenia.* Brain Struct Funct, 2016. **221**(1): p. 185–201.

24. Dauvilliers, Y. and J. Winkelmann, *Restless legs syndrome: update on pathogenesis.* Curr Opin Pulm Med, 2013. **19**(6): p. 594–600.

25. Kunugi, H., et al., *Association study of structural mutations of the tyrosine hydroxylase gene with schizophrenia and Parkinson's disease.* Am J Med Genet, 1998. **81**(2): p. 131–133.

26. Ogasawara, M., et al., *Recent advances in molecular pharmacology of the histamine systems: organic cation transporters as a histamine transporter and histamine metabolism.* J Pharmacol Sci, 2006. **101**(1): p. 24–30.

27. Solismaa, A., et al., *Histaminergic gene polymorphisms associated with sedation in clozapine-treated patients.* Eur Neuropsychopharmacol, 2017. **27**(5): p. 442–449.

28. Hamm, H.E., *The many faces of G protein signaling.* J Biol Chem, 1998. **273**(2): p. 669–672.

29. Kang, S.G., et al., *Possible association between G-protein beta3 subunit C825T polymorphism and antipsychotic-induced restless legs syndrome in schizophrenia.* Acta Neuropsychiatr, 2007. **19**(6): p. 351–356.

30. Lee, H.J., et al., *Association between a G-protein beta 3 subunit gene polymorphism and the symptomatology and treatment responses of major depressive disorders.* Pharmacogenomics J, 2004. **4**(1): p. 29–33.

31. Muller, D.J., et al., *Suggestive association between the C825T polymorphism of the G-protein beta3 subunit gene (GNB3) and clinical improvement with antipsychotics in schizophrenia.* Eur Neuropsychopharmacol, 2005. **15**(5): p. 525–531.

32. Buysse, D.J., et al., *The Pittsburgh Sleep Quality Index: A new instrument for psychiatric practice and research.* Psychiatry Research, 1989. **28**(2): p. 193–213.

33. Bastien, C.H., A. Vallières, and C.M. Morin, *Validation of the Insomnia Severity Index as an outcome measure for insomnia research.* Sleep medicine, 2001. **2**(4): p. 297–307.

34. Soldatos, C.R., D.G. Dikeos, and T.J. Paparrigopoulos, *Athens Insomnia Scale: validation of an instrument based on ICD-10 criteria.* Journal of psychosomatic research, 2000. **48**(6): p. 555–560.

35. Johns, M.W., *A new method for measuring daytime sleepiness: the Epworth Sleepiness Scale.* sleep, 1991. **14**(6): p. 540–545.

36. Chung, F., H.R. Abdullah, and P. Liao, *STOP-BANG questionnaire: a practical approach to screen for obstructive sleep apnea.* Chest, 2016. **149**(3): p. 631–638.

37. Netzer, N.C., et al., *Using the Berlin Questionnaire to identify patients at risk for the sleep apnea syndrome.* Ann Intern Med, 1999. **131**(7): p. 485–491.

38. Horne, J.A. and O. Östberg, *A self-assessment questionnaire to determine morningness-eveningness in human circadian rhythms.* Int J Chronobiol, 1976;4(2):97–110.

39. Boeve, B.F., et al., *Validation of the Mayo Sleep Questionnaire to screen for REM sleep behavior disorder in a community-based sample.* J Clin Sleep Med, 2013. **9**(05): p. 475–480.

40. Bosch, P., et al., *The Munich Parasomnia Screening in psychiatry.* Somnologie: Schlafforschung und Schlafmedizin, 2012. **16**(4): p. 257–262.

41. Allen, R.P., et al., *Validation of the self-completed Cambridge–Hopkins questionnaire (CH-RLSq) for ascertainment of restless legs syndrome (RLS) in a population survey.* Sleep Med, 2009. **10**(10): p. 1097–100.

42. Cohrs, S., *Sleep disturbances in patients with schizophrenia: impact and effect of antipsychotics.* CNS Drugs, 2008. **22**(11): p. 939–962.

43. Baandrup, L. and P.J. Jennum, *A validation of wrist actigraphy against polysomnography in patients with schizophrenia or bipolar disorder.* Neuropsychiatr Dis Treat, 2015. **11**: p. 2271–2277.

44. Sadeh, A., *The role and validity of actigraphy in sleep medicine: an update.* Sleep Med Rev, 2011. **15**(4): p. 259–267.

45. Wulff, K., et al., *The suitability of actigraphy, diary data, and urinary melatonin profiles for quantitative assessment of sleep disturbances in schizophrenia: a case report.* Chronobiol Int, 2006. **23**(1-2): p. 485–495.

46. Tahmasian, M., et al., *Clinical application of actigraphy in psychotic disorders: a systematic review.* Curr Psychiatry Rep, 2013. **15**(6): p. 359.

47. Mitchell, A.J., et al., *Prevalence of metabolic syndrome and metabolic abnormalities in schizophrenia and related disorders: a systematic review and meta-analysis.* Schizophr Bull, 2013. **39**(2): p. 306–318.

48. Khazaie, H., et al., *A weight-independent association between atypical antipsychotic medications and obstructive sleep apnea.* Sleep Breath, 2018. **22**(1): p. 109–114.

49. Aggarwal, S., S. Dodd, and M. Berk, *Restless leg syndrome associated with atypical antipsychotics: current status, pathophysiology, and*

clinical implications. Curr Drug Saf, 2015. **10**(2): p. 98–105.

50. Inoue, Y., *Sleep-related eating disorder and its associated conditions.* Psychiatry Clin Neurosci, 2015. **69**(6): p. 309–320.

51. Volkow, N.D., *Substance use disorders in schizophrenia: clinical implications of comorbidity.* Schizophrenia bulletin, 2009. **35**(3): p. 469–472.

52. Khantzian, E.J., *The self-medication hypothesis of addictive disorders: focus on heroin and cocaine dependence.* Am J Psychiatry, 1985. **142**(11): p. 1259–1264.

53. Chambers, R.A., J.H. Krystal, and D.W. Self, *A neurobiological basis for substance abuse comorbidity in schizophrenia.* Biol Psychiatry, 2001. **50**(2): p. 71–83.

54. Horn, W.T., S.C. Akerman, and M.J. Sateia, *Sleep in schizophrenia and substance use disorders: a review of the literature.* J Dual Diag, 2013. **9**(3): p. 228–238.

55. Barratt, E.S., W. Beaver, and R. White, *The effects of marijuana on human sleep patterns.* Biol Psychiatry, 1974. **8**(1): p. 47–54.

56. Cousens, K. and A. DiMascio, *(-)δ9 THC as an hypnotic: an experimental study of three dose levels.* Psychopharmacologia. 1973;33(4):355–364.

57. Budney, A.J., et al., *The time course and significance of cannabis withdrawal.* J Abnorm Psychol, 2003. **112**(3): p. 393–402.

58. Lin, Y.N., Q.Y. Li, and X.J. Zhang, *Interaction between smoking and obstructive sleep apnea: not just participants.* Chin Med J (Engl), 2012. **125**(17): p. 3150–3156.

59. Simou, E., J. Britton, and J. Leonardi-Bee, *Alcohol and the risk of sleep apnoea: a systematic review and meta-analysis.* Sleep Med, 2018. **42**: p. 38–46.

60. Correa, D., et al., *Chronic opioid use and central sleep apnea: a review of the prevalence, mechanisms, and perioperative considerations.* Anesth Analg, 2015. **120**(6): p. 1273–1285.

61. Myles, H., et al., *Obstructive sleep apnea and schizophrenia: a systematic review to inform clinical practice.* Schizophr Res, 2016. **170**(1): p. 222–225.

62. Winkelman, J.W., *Schizophrenia, obesity, and obstructive sleep apnea.* J Clin Psychiatry, 2001. **62**(1): p. 8–11.

63. Rishi, M.A., et al., *Atypical antipsychotic medications are independently associated with severe obstructive sleep apnea.* Clin Neuropharmacol, 2010. **33**(3): p. 109–113.

64. Jonas, D.E., et al., *Screening for obstructive sleep apnea in adults: evidence report and systematic review for the US Preventive Services Task Force.* JAMA, 2017. **317**(4): p. 415–433.

65. Kapur, V.K., et al., *Clinical practice guideline for diagnostic testing for adult obstructive sleep apnea: an American Academy of Sleep Medicine clinical practice guideline.* J Clin Sleep Med, 2017. **13**(3): p. 479–504.

66. Stroup, T.S., et al., *A randomized trial examining the effffectiveness of switching from olanzapine, quetiapine, or risperidone to aripiprazole to reduce metabolic risk: comparison of antipsychotics for metabolic problems (CAMP).* Am J Psychiatry, 2011. **168**(9): p. 947–956.

67. Krystal, A.D., H.W. Goforth, and T. Roth, *Effects of antipsychotic medications on sleep in schizophrenia.* Int Clin Psychopharmacol, 2008. **23**(3): p. 150–160.

68. Epstein, L.J., et al., *Clinical guideline for the evaluation, management and long-term care of obstructive sleep apnea in adults.* J Clin Sleep Med, 2009. **5**(3): p. 263–276.

69. Giles, T.L., et al., *Continuous positive airways pressure for obstructive sleep apnoea in adults.* Cochrane Database Syst Rev, 2006(3): p. Cd001106.

70. Karanti, A. and M. Landen, *Treatment refractory psychosis remitted upon treatment with continuous positive airway pressure: a case report.* Psychopharmacol Bull, 2007. **40**(1): p. 113–117.

71. Hiraoka, T. and N. Yamada, *Treatment of psychiatric symptoms in schizophrenia spectrum disorders with comorbid sleep apnea syndrome: a case report.* Seishin Shinkeigaku Zasshi, 2013. **115**(2): p. 139–146.

72. Kalucy, M.J., et al., *Obstructive sleep apnoea and schizophrenia--a research agenda.* Sleep Med Rev, 2013. **17**(5): p. 357–365.

73. Myles, H., et al., *Cognition in schizophrenia improves with treatment of severe obstructive sleep apnoea: A pilot study.* Schizophr Res Cogn, 2019. **15**: p. 14–20.

74. Velligan, D.I., et al., *Assessment of adherence problems in patients with serious and persistent mental illness: recommendations from the Expert Consensus Guidelines.* J Psychiatr Pract, 2010. **16**(1): p. 34–45.

75. Wozniak, D.R., T.J. Lasserson, and I. Smith, *Educational, supportive and behavioural interventions to improve usage of continuous positive airway pressure machines in adults with obstructive sleep apnoea.* Cochrane Database Syst Rev, 2014(1): p. Cd007736.

76. Wamsley, E., et al., *Delusional confusion of dreaming and reality in narcolepsy.* Sleep, 2014. **37**(2): p. 419–422.

77. Hays, P., *False but sincere accusations of sexual assault made by narcoleptic [correction of narcotic] patients.* Med Leg J, 1992. **60 (Pt 4)**: p. 265–271.

78. Dodet, P., et al., *Lucid dreaming in narcolepsy.* Sleep, 2015. **38**(3): p. 487–497.

79. Jennum, P., et al., *Comorbidity and mortality of narcolepsy: a controlled retro- and prospective national study.* Sleep, 2013. **36**(6): p. 835–840.

80. Bhat, S.K. and R. Galang, *Narcolepsy presenting as schizophrenia.* Am J Psychiatry, 2002. **159**(7): p. 1245.

81. Dahmen, N., et al., *Narcoleptic and schizophrenic hallucinations: implications for differential diagnosis and pathophysiology.* Eur J Health Econ, 2002. **3 Suppl 2**: p. S94–S98.

82. Kishi, Y., et al., *Schizophrenia and narcolepsy: a review with a case report.* Psychiatry Clin Neurosci, 2004. **58**(2): p. 117–124.

83. Shapiro, B. and H. Spitz, *Problems in the differential diagnosis of narcolepsy versus schizophrenia.* Am J Psychiatry, 1976. **133**(11): p. 1321–1323.

84. Douglass, A.B., et al., *Florid refractory schizophrenias that turn out to be treatable variants of HLA-associated narcolepsy.* J Nerv Ment Dis, 1991. **179**(1): p. 12–17; discussion 18.

85. Douglass, A.B., et al., *Schizophrenia, narcolepsy, and HLA-DR15, DQ6.* Biol Psychiatry, 1993. **34**(11): p. 773–780.

86. Coren, H.Z. and J.J. Strain, *A case of narcolepsy with psychosis (paranoid state of narcolepsy).* Compr Psychiatry, 1965. **6**: p. 191–199.

87. Sekine, Y., et al., *Methamphetamine-related psychiatric symptoms and reduced brain dopamine transporters studied with PET.* Am J Psychiatry, 2001. **158**(8): p. 1206–1214.

88. Pawluk, L.K., et al., *Psychiatric morbidity in narcoleptics on chronic high dose methylphenidate therapy.* J Nerv Ment Dis, 1995. **183**(1): p. 45–48.

89. Narendran, R., et al., *Is psychosis exacerbated by modafinil?* Arch Gen Psychiatry, 2002. **59**(3): p. 292–293.

90. Sharma, P., et al., *Excessive daytime sleepiness in schizophrenia: a naturalistic clinical study.* J Clin Diagn Res, 2016. **10**(10): p. Vc06–vc08.

91. Waite, F., et al., *Treating sleep problems in patients with schizophrenia.* Behav Cogn Psychother, 2016. **44**(3): p. 273–287.

92. Kluge, M., et al., *Sleep propensity at daytime as assessed by multiple sleep latency tests (MSLT) in patients with schizophrenia increases with clozapine and olanzapine.* Schizophr Res, 2012. **135**(1-3): p. 123–127.

93. Loebel, A.D., et al., *Daytime sleepiness associated with lurasidone and quetiapine XR: results from a randomized double-blind, placebo-controlled trial in patients with schizophrenia.* CNS Spectr, 2014. **19**(2): p. 197–205.

94. Lohr, J.B., et al., *Modafinil improves antipsychotic-induced parkinsonism but not excessive daytime sleepiness, psychiatric symptoms or cognition in schizophrenia and schizoaffective disorder: a randomized, double-blind, placebo-controlled study.* Schizophr Res, 2013. **150**(1): p. 289–296.

95. Saavedra-Velez, C., et al., *Modafinil as an adjunctive treatment of sedation, negative symptoms, and cognition in schizophrenia: a critical review.* J Clin Psychiatry, 2009. **70**(1): p. 104–112.

96. Hombali, A., et al., *Prevalence and correlates of sleep disorder symptoms in psychiatric disorders.* Psychiatry Res, 2019;279:116–122.

97. American Academy of Sleep Medicine, *International classification of sleep disorders.* 3rd ed. Darien, IL: American Academy of Sleep Medicine; 2014.

98. Brion, A., et al., *Sleep-related eating disorder versus sleepwalking: a controlled study.* Sleep Med, 2012. **13**(8): p. 1094–1101.

99. Stallman, H.M., M. Kohler, and J. White, *Medication induced sleepwalking: a systematic review.* Sleep Med Rev, 2018. **37**: p. 105–113.

100. Chiaro, G., M.T. Caletti, and F. Provini, *Treatment of sleep-related eating disorder.* Curr Treat Options Neurol, 2015. **17**(8): p. 361.

101. Waters, F., U. Moretto, and T.T. Dang-Vu, *Psychiatric illness and parasomnias: a systematic review.* Curr Psychiatry Rep, 2017. **19**(7): p. 37.

102. Sansa, G., et al., *Exploring the presence of narcolepsy in patients with schizophrenia.* BMC Psychiatry, 2016. **16**: p. 177.

103. Gangdev, P., *Relevance of sleep paralysis and hypnic hallucinations to psychiatry.* Australas Psychiatry, 2004. **12**(1): p. 77–80.

104. Hufford, D.J., *Sleep paralysis as spiritual experience.* Transcult Psychiatry, 2005. **42**(1): p. 11–45.

105. Li, S.X., et al., *Sleep disturbances and suicide risk in an 8-year longitudinal study of schizophrenia-spectrum disorders.* Sleep, 2016. **39**(6): p. 1275–1282.

106. Pagel, J.F. and P. Helfter, *Drug induced nightmares: an etiology based review.* Hum Psychopharmacol, 2003. **18**(1): p. 59–67.

107. Manni, R., P.L. Ratti, and M. Terzaghi, *Secondary "incidental" REM sleep behavior disorder: do we ever think of it?* Sleep Med, 2011. **12 Suppl 2**: p. S50–S53.

108. Guilleminault, C., et al., *Adult chronic sleepwalking and its treatment based on polysomnography.* Brain, 2005. **128**(Pt 5): p. 1062–1069.

109. Park, Y.M. and H.W. Shin, *Zolpidem induced sleep-related eating and complex behaviors in a*

patient with obstructive sleep apnea and restless legs syndrome. Clin Psychopharmacol Neurosci, 2016. **14**(3): p. 299–301.

110. Jeong, J.H. and W.M. Bahk, *Sleep-related eating disorder associated with mirtazapine.* J Clin Psychopharmacol, 2014. **34**(6): p. 752–753.

111. Lu, M.L. and W.W. Shen, *Sleep-related eating disorder induced by risperidone.* J Clin Psychiatry, 2004. **65**(2): p. 273–274.

112. Paquet, V., et al., *Sleep-related eating disorder induced by olanzapine.* J Clin Psychiatry, 2002. **63**(7): p. 597.

113. Aurora, R.N., et al., *Best practice guide for the treatment of nightmare disorder in adults.* J Clin Sleep Med, 2010. **6**(4): p. 389–401.

114. Dagan, Y. and M. Eisenstein, *Circadian rhythm sleep disorders: toward a more precise definition and diagnosis.* Chronobiol Int, 1999. **16**(2): p. 213–222.

115. Yamadera, W., et al., *Clinical features of circadian rhythm sleep disorders in outpatients.* Psychiatry Clin Neurosci, 1998. **52**(3): p. 311–316.

116. Patricia Yuan-Ping Poon, Y., et al., *Delayed sleep-wake phase disorder and delayed sleep-wake phase in schizophrenia: clinical and functional correlates.* Schizophr Res. 2018;202:412–413.

117. Abbott, S.M., K.J. Reid, and P.C. Zee, *Circadian rhythm sleep–wake disorders.* Psychiatr Clin North Am, 2015. **38**(4): p. 805–823.

118. Harvey, A.G., et al., *A transdiagnostic sleep and circadian treatment to improve severe mental illness outcomes in a community setting: study protocol for a randomized controlled trial.* Trials, 2016. **17**(1): p. 606.

119. Pail, G., et al., *Bright-light therapy in the treatment of mood disorders.* Neuropsychobiology, 2011. **64**(3): p. 152–162.

120. Omori, Y., et al., *Low dose of aripiprazole advanced sleep rhythm and reduced nocturnal sleep time in the patients with delayed sleep phase syndrome: an open-labeled clinical observation.* Neuropsychiatr Dis Treat, 2018. **14**: p. 1281–1286.

121. Kang, S.G., et al., *Characteristics and clinical correlates of restless legs syndrome in schizophrenia.* Prog Neuropsychopharmacol Biol Psychiatry, 2007. **31**(5): p. 1078–1083.

122. Guo, S., et al., *Restless legs syndrome: from pathophysiology to clinical diagnosis and management.* Front Aging Neurosci, 2017. **9**: p. 171.

123. Allen, R.P., P. Stillman, and A.J. Myers, *Physician-diagnosed restless legs syndrome in a large sample of primary medical care patients in western Europe: Prevalence and characteristics.* Sleep Med, 2010. **11**(1): p. 31–37.

124. Harvey, P.D., et al., *Negative symptoms and cognitive deficits: what is the nature of their relationship?* Schizophrenia Bulletin, 2006. **32**(2): p. 250–258.

125. Picchietti, D.L., et al., *Achievements, challenges, and future perspectives of epidemiologic research in restless legs syndrome (RLS).* Sleep Med, 2017. **31**: p. 3–9.

126. Hornyak, M., et al., *Polysomnography findings in patients with restless legs syndrome and in healthy controls: a comparative observational study.* Sleep, 2007. **30**(7): p. 861–865.

127. Rizzo, G., et al., *Brain imaging and networks in restless legs syndrome.* Sleep Med, 2017. **31**: p. 39–48.

128. Ohayon, M.M. and T. Roth, *Prevalence of restless legs syndrome and periodic limb movement disorder in the general population.* J Psychosomatic Res, 2002. **53**(1): p. 547–554.

129. Hoque, R. and A.L. Chesson, Jr., *Pharmacologically induced/exacerbated restless legs syndrome, periodic limb movements of sleep, and REM behavior disorder/REM sleep without atonia: literature review, qualitative scoring, and comparative analysis.* J Clin Sleep Med, 2010. **6**(1): p. 79–83.

130. Hornyak, M., et al., *Periodic leg movements in sleep and periodic limb movement disorder: prevalence, clinical significance and treatment.* Sleep Medicine Reviews, 2006. **10**(3): p. 169–177.

131. Garcia-Borreguero, D., et al., *The long-term treatment of restless legs syndrome/Willis-Ekbom disease: evidence-based guidelines and clinical consensus best practice guidance: a report from the International Restless Legs Syndrome Study Group.* Sleep Med, 2013. **14**(7): p. 675–684.

132. Aurora, R.N., et al., *Update to the AASM clinical practice guideline: The treatment of restless legs syndrome and periodic limb movement disorder in adults—an update for 2012: practice parameters with an evidence-based systematic review and meta-analyses.* Sleep, 2012. **35**(8): p. 1037.

133. Lieberman, J.A., et al., *Effectiveness of antipsychotic drugs in patients with chronic schizophrenia.* N Engl J Med, 2005. **353**(12): p. 1209–1223.

134. Lunsford-Avery, J.R., et al., *Actigraphic-measured sleep disturbance predicts increased positive symptoms in adolescents at ultra high-risk for psychosis: a longitudinal study.* Schizophr Res, 2015. **164**(1-3): p. 15–20.

135. Schutte-Rodin, S., et al., *Clinical guideline for the evaluation and management of chronic*

insomnia in adults. J Clin Sleep Med, 2008. **4**(5): p. 487–504.

136. Wilson, S.J., et al., *British Association for Psychopharmacology consensus statement on evidence-based treatment of insomnia, parasomnias and circadian rhythm disorders.* J Psychopharmacol, 2010. **24**(11): p. 1577–1601.

137. Mason, M., C.J. Cates, and I. Smith, *Effects of opioid, hypnotic and sedating medications on sleep-disordered breathing in adults with obstructive sleep apnoea.* Cochrane Database Syst Rev, 2015(7): p. Cd011090.

138. Tiihonen, J., et al., *Polypharmacy with antipsychotics, antidepressants, or benzodiazepines and mortality in schizophrenia.* Arch Gen Psychiatry, 2012. **69**(5): p. 476–483.

139. Fontanella, C.A., et al., *Benzodiazepine use and risk of mortality among patients with schizophrenia: a retrospective longitudinal study.* J Clin Psychiatry, 2016. **77**(5): p. 661–667.

140. Kuriyama, A., M. Honda, and Y. Hayashino, *Ramelteon for the treatment of insomnia in adults: a systematic review and meta-analysis.* Sleep Med, 2014. **15**(4): p. 385–392.

141. Borba, C.P.C., et al., *Placebo-controlled pilot study of ramelteon for adiposity and lipids in patients with schizophrenia.* Journal of clinical psychopharmacology, 2011. **31**(5): p. 653–658.

142. Shirayama, Y., et al., *Effects of add-on ramelteon on cognitive impairment in patients with schizophrenia: an open-label pilot trial.* Clinical Psychopharmacology and Neuroscience, 2014. **12**(3): p. 215–217.

143. Lee-Iannotti, J.K. and J.M. Parish, *Suvorexant: a promising, novel treatment for insomnia.* Neuropsychiatr Dis Treat, 2016. **12**: p. 491–495.

144. Suzuki, H., et al., *Reduced insomnia following short-term administration of suvorexant during aripiprazole once-monthly treatment in a patient with schizophrenia.* Asian J Psychiatr, 2017. **28**: p. 165–166.

145. Yeung, W.F., et al., *Doxepin for insomnia: a systematic review of randomized placebo-controlled trials.* Sleep Med Rev, 2015. **19**: p. 75–83.

146. Karsten, J., et al., *Low doses of mirtazapine or quetiapine for transient insomnia: A randomised, double-blind, cross-over, placebo-controlled trial.* J Psychopharmacol, 2017. **31**(3): p. 327–337.

147. Iwamoto, K., et al., *Effects of low-dose mirtazapine on driving performance in healthy volunteers.* Hum Psychopharmacol, 2013. **28**(5): p. 523–528.

148. Delle Chiaie, R., et al., *Add-on mirtazapine enhances effects on cognition in schizophrenic patients under stabilized treatment with clozapine.* Exp Clin Psychopharmacol, 2007. **15**(6): p. 563–568.

149. Zoccali, R., et al., *The effect of mirtazapine augmentation of clozapine in the treatment of negative symptoms of schizophrenia: a double-blind, placebo-controlled study.* Int Clin Psychopharmacol, 2004. **19**(2): p. 71–76.

150. Wichniak, A., et al., *Low risk for switch to mania during treatment with sleep promoting antidepressants.* Pharmacopsychiatry, 2015. **48**(3): p. 83–88.

151. Yatham, L.N., et al., *Canadian Network for Mood and Anxiety Treatments (CANMAT) and International Society for Bipolar Disorders (ISBD) collaborative update of CANMAT guidelines for the management of patients with bipolar disorder: update 2013.* Bipolar Disord, 2013. **15**(1): p. 1–44.

152. Monti, J.M., P. Torterolo, and S.R. Pandi Perumal, *The effects of second generation antipsychotic drugs on sleep variables in healthy subjects and patients with schizophrenia.* Sleep Med Rev, 2017. **33**: p. 51–57.

153. Yamashita, H., et al., *Effects of changing from typical to atypical antipsychotic drugs on subjective sleep quality in patients with schizophrenia in a Japanese population.* J Clin Psychiatry, 2004. **65**(11): p. 1525–1530.

154. Thompson, W., et al., *Atypical antipsychotics for insomnia: a systematic review.* Sleep Med, 2016. **22**: p. 13–17.

155. Ferracioli-Oda, E., A. Qawasmi, and M.H. Bloch, *Meta-analysis: melatonin for the treatment of primary sleep disorders.* PLoS One, 2013. **8**(5): p. e63773.

156. Shamir, E., et al., *Melatonin improves sleep quality of patients with chronic schizophrenia.* J Clin Psychiatry, 2000. **61**(5): p. 373–377.

157. Suresh Kumar, P.N., et al., *Melatonin in schizophrenic outpatients with insomnia: a double-blind, placebo-controlled study.* J Clin Psychiatry, 2007. **68**(2): p. 237–241.

158. Brasure, M., et al., *Psychological and behavioral interventions for managing insomnia disorder: an evidence report for a clinical practice guideline by the American College of Physicians.* Ann Intern Med, 2016. **165**(2): p. 113–124.

159. Freeman, D., et al., *Efficacy of cognitive behavioural therapy for sleep improvement in patients*

with persistent delusions and hallucinations (BEST): *a prospective, assessor-blind, randomised controlled pilot trial.* Lancet Psychiatry, 2015. **2**(11): p. 975–983.

160. Reeve, S., et al., *Disrupting sleep: the effects of sleep loss on psychotic experiences tested in an experimental study with mediation analysis.* Schizophr Bull, 2018. **44**(3): p. 662–671.

161. Reeve, S., B. Sheaves, and D. Freeman, *The role of sleep dysfunction in the occurrence of delusions and hallucinations: A systematic review.* Clin Psychol Rev, 2015. **42**: p. 96–115.

22

Substance Use Disorders

SHIRSHENDU SINHA, BHANU PRAKASH KOLLA,
AND MEGHNA P. MANSUKHANI

SLEEP TERMINOLOGY

Homeostatic sleep drive: The drive to sleep that progressively builds with continued wakefulness.

Insomnia: A sleep disorder in which the quantity or quality of sleep is less than desired, usually characterized by difficulty falling and/or staying asleep, and/or waking too early, with ensuing daytime sequelae like fatigue.

Polysomnography (PSG): A procedure that involves recording multiple physiological channels in order to determine sleep-related parameters and diagnose sleep disorders.

Rapid eye movement (REM) sleep: Stage of sleep characterized by conjugate eye movements, paralysis of muscles, and brain activity that is most similar to wakefulness.

REM density: The frequency of rapid eye movements occurring during REM sleep. REM density increases over the course of the sleep period and is greatest when homeostatic sleep drive (sleep pressure) is lowest.

REM latency: Time from sleep onset to the onset of REM sleep.

REM rebound: The characteristic increase in percentage of REM sleep after prior REM sleep deprivation.

Sleep architecture: The structure of sleep, including non-REM (stages N1, N2, and N3) and REM (stage R) sleep percentages.

Sleep efficiency (SE): Total sleep time divided by the time in bed.

Sleep fragmentation: Disruption in sleep characterized by awakenings and arousals (transitions to lighter stages of sleep from deeper sleep).

Sleep latency (SL): The amount of time from lights out to sleep onset.

Slow-wave sleep (SWS): Sleep stage characterized by low frequency and high amplitude waves, also called stage N3.

Total sleep time (TST): The amount of sleep obtained, usually reported in minutes.

Wake after sleep onset (WASO): The amount of time awake after the onset of sleep and before the final awakening.

INTRODUCTION

Addictive substances such as alcohol and other drugs can have immediate and persistent effects on sleep architecture. About 70% of patients admitted for detoxification report sleep disturbances at the time of admission and 80% of those who report sleep disturbances relate them to their substance use.[1] Sleep disturbances can occur in the form of sleep onset and maintenance insomnia or hypersomnia. There appears to be a significant bidirectional relationship between substance use and sleep disturbances.[2] Sleep disturbances with or without a primary psychiatric disorder can increase the risk of emergence or relapse of substance use disorder.[3,4] Conversely, both short- and long-term use of substances could lead to acute and chronic disturbances in sleep.[5] There is evidence to suggest that long-term sobriety from substance use may lead to restoration of a normal sleep architecture.[6]

This narrative review describes the characteristics and trajectory of sleep disturbances seen in the context of substance use. We explore the relationship between sleep disturbances and clinical and patient-reported outcomes. We describe subjective and objective sleep disturbances seen during the period of substance use and abstinence. We also discuss evidenced-based therapeutic options aimed at modulating sleep disturbances in individuals struggling with comorbid substance use and sleep disturbances or disorders. This review primarily focuses on the effects of the use of alcohol, cannabis, cocaine and opioids on sleep.

CO-OCCURRENCE OF SLEEP DISTURBANCES AND SUBSTANCE USE DISORDER

Both sleep disturbances and substance use disorders are extremely common in the general population. Sleep disruptions, specifically insomnia or hypersomnolence, can predispose subjects to overuse substances with a view to mitigate these symptoms. Some sleep disorders such as sleep apnea can be significantly exacerbated by the use of certain substances such as alcohol and opioids. Conversely, most addictive substances significantly alter the neuro chemistry of the brain and, in turn, impact centers responsible for the regulation of sleep initiation, maintenance, and the regulation of breathing. The sleep disruptions occur in the context of substance use, intoxication, and withdrawal. They can persist for weeks to months following abstinence and potentially increase the risk of relapse thus perpetuating a cycle that results in maintaining both the addiction and sleep disturbance.

In this chapter, we discuss the common sleep disorders that are associated with the use of addictive substances. The evidence with regards the prevalence of these disorders in the context of substance intoxication, withdrawal, and early recovery is presented when available. We review the studies that examine the impact of the sleep disturbances on relapse risk in addictive disorders. The nascent literature examining the utility of treating the sleep disturbances to reduce relapse risk and improve outcomes is also presented. However, the studies are limited by the use of small samples, short durations of follow-up and significant heterogeneity.

CLINICAL APPROACH

Substance use disorders are highly prevalent in the general population and frequently encountered in patients presenting to mental health professionals.

Evidenced-based screening for potential substance use disorders is an integral part of all initial assessments. Clinicians should also consider retaking a substance use history in patients with refractory sleep disorders.

A thorough clinical history is the cornerstone for the detection of substance use disorders. Open-ended, nonjudgmental questions about the use of alcohol, its frequency and quantity, and potential consequences should be part of an initial sleep medicine evaluation. Patients should also be queried about the use of other illicit drugs and the misuse/overuse of prescription medication(s). Screening tools such as the Alcohol Use Disorders Identification Test (AUDIT) or the Alcohol Use Disorders Identification Test–Concise (AUDIT-C) can help identify patients at increased risk of alcohol use disorders. When appropriate, urine drug screens should be part of a sleep evaluation. This is especially important when evaluating patients presenting with hypersomnia. Clinicians should be aware of the type of drug screens available and reporting times. Most common addictive substances can be detected in the urine for about 2 to 3 days. Cannabis is detectable for about 7 days in intermittent uses and for up to 28 days in regular users. Alcohol, because of its short half-life, can be detected for 12 to 24 hours. However, clinicians should be aware of nuances associated with drug testing that are specific to their local toxicology laboratories.

Patients with substance use disorders can present with excessive sleepiness or insomnia in the context of both intoxication and withdrawal depending on the substance. The majority of these sleep disturbances may resolve upon the resolution of intoxication/withdrawal symptoms.

SLEEP AND ALCOHOL USE DISORDER

There has been a significant increase in the use of alcohol in the general population. The prevalence of alcohol use disorders has also increased substantially in the recent years. About 13% of the general population in the united states meets criteria for an alcohol use disorder making it an extremely common condition.[7]

Subjective Findings

Alcohol use affects sleep quality and duration and has become a targeted area of interest for researchers and clinicians. Sleep disturbances are common among alcohol users with prevalence rates ranging between 35% and 70%.[8] These rates are substantially higher than those observed in the general population (~15%–30%).[6] Alcohol is commonly considered to be a sleep-promoting agent. Around 20% to 30% of individuals with chronic insomnia use alcohol to promote sleep onset/induction. However, with chronic use, tolerance may develop to the sleep-inducing effects of alcohol.[9] Sleep disturbances could range from sleep onset and maintenance insomnia, **early morning awakening**, and nonrestorative sleep, to reduced daytime alertness and hypersomnia. These symptoms are often treatment-refractory in individuals with an alcohol use disorder (AUD).[8] Sleep disturbance is frequently the primary symptom once individuals with AUD reduce or stop drinking alcohol.[10]

Objective Findings
Sleep Latency
In healthy nonalcoholics, acute consumption of alcohol before bedtime shortens SL, while subjects who use of alcohol chronically exhibit a prolonged SL. SL is further prolonged during early (e.g., weeks 1 and 2 of abstinence) and late withdrawal (e.g., weeks 2 through 8 of abstinence), even when other variables such as age and sex are adjusted for.[9] SL may not normalize until after several months (e.g., months 5 through 9) of abstinence.[11]

Total Sleep Time (TST)
Consistent with increased SL, TST is reduced in individuals with AUD during chronic use, as well as during early and postacute withdrawal, compared to healthy controls.[5] Studies have shown that TST in individuals with AUD may improve after a period of sustained abstinence of weeks or months. Length of sobriety from alcohol appears to correlate with improvement in TST.[11]

Slow-Wave Sleep (SWS)
Studies have shown a reduction in SWS in alcoholics,[6] particularly in the phase of early abstinence.[5] There is uncertainty as to when SWS completely recovers following sustained abstinence and may be in the range of 3 to 14 months or longer. SWS deficits in chronic alcoholics during periods of prolonged abstinence are reversed by the acute use of alcohol.[6]

Rapid Eye Movement (REM) Sleep
Acute consumption of alcohol suppresses REM sleep, both in healthy controls as well in individuals with AUD.[5] In alcoholics, REM rebound usually occurs after a period of abstinence.[6] Additionally, shortened REM latency, higher REM density, an increase in the number of REM periods, and shorter intervals between REM cycles may be noted. REM rebound has been observed after early (2–3 weeks) and prolonged abstinence (27 months).[12]

REM Latency
Reports regarding REM latency are inconsistent in the medical literature. Individuals with AUD and comorbid depression tend to have shorter REM latencies compared to individuals with AUD without depressive symptoms.[13]

Breathing Parameters during Sleep
Alcohol is a muscle relaxant and can potentially worsen sleep apnea by relaxing upper airway muscles. Recent meta-analytic data have suggested that alcohol results in an increase in the Apnea–Hypopnea Index (AHI), particularly in snorers and those with a prior diagnosis of obstructive sleep apnea. Alcohol consumption also results in a reduction in the mean oxygen saturation.[14]

Correlation between Subjective and Objective Sleep Findings in AUD
The data on the relationship between subjective sleep complaints and objective sleep parameters in patients with AUD are limited. In a study of 172 individuals with AUDs, of whom 104 had insomnia as assessed by the Sleep Disorders Questionnaire, the results indicated individuals with baseline sleep disturbances who were abstinent from alcohol had prolonged SL and reduced SE at 1 month of abstinence compared to those without sleep disturbances, indicating consistency between self-report and objective findings.[15]

Clinical Implications
Increased SL in individuals with AUD has been shown to be associated with lower melatonin levels as well as delayed onset and peak melatonin levels.[16] Presence of sleep disordered breathing can lead to increased WASO and reduced SE in individuals with AUD.[17] Lastly, in patients with AUD, insomnia correlates with severity of AUD, self-report of alcohol use as a sleep aid, as well as severity of self-reported depression symptoms.[15]

Self-reported sleep onset insomnia, and sleep disturbances in general, have been found to be a major risk factor for relapse.[12] Sleep disturbances in the early period of abstinence were shown to predict relapse to alcohol at 5 months in one study.[15] In addition, patients who report using alcohol to help them fall asleep appear to be at increased risk of relapse.[18]

Objective sleep measurements can serve as predictors of clinical outcomes in AUD. One study noted that prolonged SL during the initial period of abstinence could predict relapse to alcohol use within the following 5 months.[19] One other study failed to show any such relationship; that is, relapse to alcohol was independent of SL.[13] There appears to be a correlation between SWS and clinical outcomes in AUD. Reduced SWS predicts severity of withdrawal symptoms during subacute withdrawal (8–32 days of abstinence).[20] Additionally, reduced SWS during abstinence has been noted to be a factor influencing relapse.[19]

There are conflicting studies on REM sleep measurements and AUD prognosis. One large study noted that increased REM latency was associated with sobriety from alcohol.[19] Another smaller study failed to show an association, especially when REM latency was measured later in the course of sobriety (i.e., at 19 weeks).[11] It may be reasonable to surmise that physiological measurements of sleep later in the course of abstinence, in general, would be better predictors of clinical outcomes than those observed during early sobriety.

Treatments

There is no US Food and Drug Administration (FDA)-approved pharmacotherapy to treat sleep disturbances in individuals with AUD. A number of studies have explored the use of sleep-promoting medications to target sleep disturbances in individuals with AUD.[21] One such agent is gabapentin, which has been shown to have therapeutic utility in treating sleep disturbances as well as facilitating abstinence in individuals with AUD.[22]

Melatonin levels have been found to be decreased in some alcoholics.[16] Studies have evaluated the therapeutic benefits of melatonin receptor agonists (i.e., ramelteon and agomelatine) in this target population. During the early course of abstinence, ramelteon use was found to be beneficial in reducing scores on the Insomnia Severity Index (ISI), decreasing SL, and improving TST as measured by actigraphy in one study.[23]

Trazodone, a commonly prescribed sleep aid, has also been studied in this context. The results of studies on the effects of trazodone are mixed. Trazodone has been shown to result in improvements in subjective measurements of sleep.[24] However, the improvements in objective measurements of sleep did not appear to correlate with clinical improvement. This study suggested that treating insomnia with trazodone in patients with AUD might impede improvements in alcohol consumption and lead to increased drinking when trazodone is stopped. However, a subsequent study indicated that use of trazodone was not associated with increased risk of relapse.[25]

Antipsychotic medications with sedative properties such quetiapine have been studied for use in patients with AUD and sleep disturbances. Quetiapine has been noted to be beneficial for sleep maintenance insomnia.[26] Improvement was noted in the insomnia subscale of the Hamilton Depression Rating Scale (HAM-D) in one study. However, the evidence regarding benefit of quetiapine for sleep-related outcomes in patients with AUD is inconsistent. One study noted improved abstinence rates with the use of quetiapine, while another study showed an increased risk of rehospitalization.[27,28] Benzodiazepine and benzodiazepine-like agents are not preferred pharmacotherapies in individuals with AUD because of their addictive potential and elevated risk of accidental overdose when combined with alcohol.

There are three medications approved by FDA for the treatment of alcohol use disorders: disulfiram, naltrexone (oral and long-acting injectable), and acamprosate. PSG and clinical data noted potential beneficial role of acamprosate in reversal alcohol-related changes in sleep architecture.[29]

The nonpharmacological treatment intervention such as cognitive-behavioral therapy for insomnia (CBT-I) in underutilized in alcohol related disorders; thus, the evidence for efficacy remains inconclusive.[30]

SLEEP AND CANNABIS USE DISORDER

There has been a substantial increase in cannabis use in the general population. Close to 9.5% of US adults reported using cannabis in the previous month, and 2.9% met criteria for a cannabis use disorder.[31]

Subjective Findings

With short-term use, cannabis can have a sleep inducing effect. Studies have shown cannabis to be helpful in initiating sleep as self-reported by participants in one study.[32] However, sleep disturbances have been noted in chronic users of cannabis, experienced mostly during withdrawal phase.[33,34] Commonly reported sleep disturbances include strange dreams, insomnia, and poor quality of sleep, with a varying degree of occurrence of these symptoms, from 32% to 76%.[34] These sleep disturbances have been noted in both inpatient (residential)[34] and outpatient settings.[35,36] Placebo-controlled studies have examined resultant sleep disturbances after discontinuation of oral tetrahydrocannabinol (THC) use and smoked marijuana. These studies have consistently shown self-reported sleep disturbances during abstinence in comparison to baseline.[34,37]

One of the common self-reported sleep disturbances experienced during early withdrawal is strange dreams, which could be experienced as early as 1 to 3 days after cannabis discontinuation, reaching a peak after 2 to 6 days and lasting for up to 2 weeks. These symptoms generally occur in conjunction with other subjective sleep disturbances.[38] Longer periods (6–7 weeks) of sleep disturbances have been noted in large studies with strange dreams in particular lasting for as long as 45 days.[38] Chronic users tend to develop tolerance to the sleep-promoting effects of cannabis.[39]

Objective Findings

Findings of objective sleep disturbances in cannabis users vary across studies. One PSG study noted reduced SL and decreased WASO. Several other PSG studies report increased SWS, REM sleep, and REM density, but these findings are not consistent.[40] Chronic users develop tolerance to most of the effects observed in naïve users, including sleep-promoting effects, SWS enhancement, and increased sleep efficiency. There is considerable variability in the impact of cannabis on REM sleep time, with studies reporting decreased, no change, or increase in REM sleep time.[5]

PSG studies of cannabis withdrawal have noted increase in SL and WASO, while TST, SE, and SWS time are reduced. REM rebound and shorter REM latency have also been noted.[5] At the outset of withdrawal, a decrease in SWS time has been observed. These sleep changes during withdrawal are better appreciated among heavy cannabis users (cannabis use ≥5 times per week over the past 3 months).[41] A decrease in TST, SE, and REM sleep and an increase in WASO start appearing over the first 2 weeks of abstinence and can persist for more than 45 days during continued abstinence from cannabis.[38]

REM sleep tends to rebound early in abstinence but decreases over time during abstinence.[42] Recent studies have shown a statistically significant but clinically insignificant reduction in the AHI following the administration of a synthetic THC analog.[43] However, there is significant heterogeneity in the response and the use of cannabis as a therapeutic option for obstructive sleep apnea is a premature consideration at this time. The American Academy of Sleep Medicine specifically recommends against the use of cannabis and/or its synthetic extracts for the treatment of obstructive sleep apnea.[44]

Correlation between Subjective and Objective Sleep Findings in Cannabis Use Disorder

Chronic users develop tolerance to the sleep promoting effects of cannabis.[42] Sleep disturbances and strange dreams are associated with abstinence.[42] These subjective complaints have been noted to be consistent across studies, with prolonged SL, reduced SWS, and REM rebound observed on PSG during abstinence.[45]

Clinical Implications

Sleep disturbances appear to be a trigger for cannabis use; baseline sleep disturbances double the risk of future use.[46] Patients may self-medicate with cannabis to treat their sleep disturbances.[47] Sleep disturbances along with other withdrawal symptoms have been correlated with a higher probability of relapse.[48] A study conducted in military personnel noted that perceived poor quality of sleep before a quit attempt was associated with increased use of cannabis later.[47] Sleep disturbances experienced during abstinence also play a critical role in relapse.[49,50] The presence of periodic limb movements during abstinence may correlate with increased severity of cannabis use.[41]

Treatments

There is no FDA-approved medication to treat sleep disturbances in cannabis users. Oral THC can improve sleep disturbances during withdrawal and may result in relapse with resumption of cannabis use.[51] THC targets withdrawal symptoms in a dose-dependent manner.[51] However, it should be noted that tolerance to the sleep-promoting effect of THC may be noted in chronic users. In general, sleep disturbances continue to worsen with long-term use of THC.

One study indicated that combination pharmacotherapy of lofexidine (an alpha-2 agonist recently FDA-approved to treat opioid withdrawal in the adult population) and oral THC can target sleep disturbances and mitigate relapse compared to oral THC alone.[52] Nabilone, a FDA-approved synthetic analog of THC, appears to have promising effects in the treatment of irritability and sleep disturbances experienced during withdrawal and can thus facilitate abstinence.[53] Nabiximol, a synthetic combination of THC and cannabidiol, has been shown to have limited benefit in this context.[54] The studies need replication and larger clinical samples before these medications can be recommended.

Mood stabilizers such as valproic acid have shown no benefit and, in fact, have been noted to result in worsening of sleep disturbances in chronic cannabis users. Medications such as zolpidem, mirtazapine, gabapentin, and quetiapine have been shown to improve subjective sleep disturbances and/or objective sleep parameters in cannabis users. However, these medications have not been shown to reduce the rates of relapse.[5,49]

While behavior treatments such as CBT-I might be beneficial in this population currently, there is no evidence suggesting its efficacy in this specific indication.

SLEEP AND OPIOID USE DISORDER

There has been a steady increase in the prevalence of opioid use disorders in the general population in the United States. Roughly 0.1% of the population endorses using heroin in the last 1 month and close to 2 million adults meet criteria for an opioid use disorder.[55]

Subjective Findings

Sedation and daytime drowsiness are commonly experienced during short-term use of opioids.[56] Other common side effects of opioid pharmacotherapy include dizziness.[57] Tolerance to the sedative effects of opioids can develop as early as 2 to 3 days while on a stable dose.[58] Sleep onset and maintenance insomnia along with daytime sedation have been reported in the early stages of methadone detoxification.[59] A variety of sleep disturbances such as insomnia, hypersomnia, increased SL, and reduced sleep duration have been noted in the early phase of opioid withdrawal.[60]

Objective Findings

Opioids, even in a single dose, can alter the sleep architecture of individuals without preexisting sleep disturbances. Electroencephalography (EEG) and electromyography (EMG) studies have demonstrated an increase in arousals during acute intoxication with heroin, morphine, or methadone. Heroin use has been shown to reduce theta waves and percentage of REM sleep.[61] Morphine and methadone may reduce SWS and increase stage N2 sleep.[62]

Short-term use of opioids generally results in increased REM latency, decreased REM sleep time, an increase in stages N1 and N2, and reduced SWS. Increase in SL and WASO with a concomitant decrease in TST and SE have also been noted with the acute use of opioids.[5] Chronic use of opioids results in tolerance to the sleep disturbances described above.[63] Abnormal PSG findings such as increased SL, increased awakenings, decreased TST, and decreased SE are usually observed in chronic opioid users despite the development of tolerance. SWS time and REM sleep are reduced compared to baseline. Duration of stage N2 sleep is increased similar that seen with acute use.[5] Actigraphy data from individuals with prescription opioid use disorder are consistent with a variety of sleep disturbances noted in the total sleep time, SE, SL, total time awake, and time spent moving.[64]

Sleep parameters change during the period of abstinence from opioids. Within a week of abstinence from chronic opioid use, there is a decrease in TST, SWS, REM, and stage N2 with an increase in SL, WASO, and REM latency compared to healthy controls.[65] During the first 3 weeks of abstinence, prolonged SL, decreased SE, decreased TST, increased arousal index, increased stages N1 and 2, and decreased SWS have been observed in subjects using opioids compared to healthy sleepers.[60]

Correlation between Subjective and Objective Sleep Findings in Opioid Use Disorder

There appears to be an inverse relationship between the Epworth Sleepiness Scale scores and SWS time in individuals with heroin use disorder during early phase of treatment in methadone maintenance treatment (MMT).[59] Pittsburgh Sleep Quality Index (PSQI) scores have also been found to significantly correlate with average diary-reported sleep time, subjective ratings of feeling rested, and PSG sleep efficiency in MMT patients.[66]

Clinical Implications

One study indicated that a higher methadone dose (defined as greater than 120 mg/day) was associated with poor sleep quality, higher rates of sleep disturbances, more frequent use of sleeping medications, and higher rates of daytime dysfunction.[67] Another study failed to show any correlation between the dose of methadone and sleep-related outcomes. Severity of opioid use disorder at baseline was associated with sleep disturbances seen in individuals with MMT.

Poor sleep quality is predictive of relapse to opioid use. Comorbid psychiatric conditions, nicotine and benzodiazepine use, chronic pain, and unemployment are associated with sleep disturbances in patients with MMT.[67]

Unintentional opioid overdose is a significant concern, especially in the context of use of high dose or extended release opioids for the management of noncancer chronic pain. The causes of overdose are typically multifactorial.[68] Studies have indicated that chronic opioid use is associated with several abnormalities including nocturnal oxygen desaturation and abnormal breathing patterns, including cluster breathing and ataxic or Biot's respiratory patterns as well as hypercapnia.[63] Chronic opioid treatment (COT), particularly with extended release preparations is associated with increased risk of central and obstructive sleep apnea compared to body mass index (BMI) and age-matched controls.[69] Between 30% and 90% of patients on COT develop central apnea in a dose-dependent fashion. The risk factors for central sleep apnea in patients on COT include a daily morphine equivalent dose (MED) of >200 mg, low or normal BMI, and combining of opioids and benzodiazepines or hypnotics. While opioids can reduce respiratory rate, benzodiazepines can reduce that tidal volume, thus compounding the risk of respiratory arrest. This risk appears to be particularly acute in the first 6 months of combined use of both medications.[70] Several studies have indicated that chronic opioid use is an independent risk factor for irregular breathing patterns, central apneas, and hypopneas.[69]

Walker et al.[71] performed a retrospective cohort study examining 60 patients receiving COT matched for age, sex, and BMI with 60 patients not on opioids to examine the effect of MED on breathing patterns during sleep. Results indicated that the AHI was greater in the opioid group (43.5 per hour vs. 30.2 per hour, $p < 0.05$) as a result of increased central sleep apnea. After controlling for BMI, age, and sex, there was a significant dose–response relationship between MED and AHI ($p < 0.001$), obstructive apnea ($p < 0.001$), hypopnea ($p < 0.001$), and central apnea ($p < 0.001$) indices. Ataxic breathing was seen in 92% of patients receiving an MED dose of ≥ 200 mg. These findings suggest a dose-dependent relationship between COT and the development of CSA and ataxic breathing.

Treatments

There is no FDA-approved medication to treat sleep disturbances in opioid users. Optimization of management of pain with evidenced-based use of opioid medications may improve sleep disturbances associated with pain.[72] Opioids such as oxycodone and methadone can be used as last resort pharmacotherapy for treatment-refractory restless legs syndrome.[73]

On the other hand, there is compelling evidence that sleep disordered breathing is a common occurrence in individuals on COT, and there appears to be a strong association between sleep disordered breathing and risk for unintentional opioid-related overdose.[74] The previously noted risk factors should be identified and appropriately addressed throughout the course of opioid treatment. Preemptive PSG can be considered for patients identified at risk for sleep disordered breathing and on COT or being considered for opioid therapy. There are a number of evidence-based safe practice guidelines to help clinicians reduce the chances of accidental opioid-related mortality and morbidity. Some of these recommendations include using the lowest possible clinically effective dose of opioids for an optimal duration, use of alternative pharmacotherapies (nonopioid analgesics, antiepileptic medications, antidepressants), and other modalities of therapy such as physical therapy and cognitive behavioral therapy especially for conditions associated with noncancer chronic pain; avoidance of co-prescription of other central nervous system depressants such as sedatives, hypnotics, or anxiolytic benzodiazepines; and advice against the use of alcohol. Adaptive servo-ventilation (ASV) is an evidenced-based treatment for opioid-induced central sleep apnea.[75] However, assessment for discontinuation of opioid use and substitution of other forms of pain relief should be considered over ASV especially since strength of evidence for use of ASV for opioid induced central sleep apnea is poor.

SLEEP AND COCAINE USE DISORDER
About 4.8 million adults reported using cocaine in the last year in 2015. Close to 18.6% of them met criteria for a cocaine use disorder.[76]

Subjective Findings
The early phase of cocaine withdrawal is characterized by sleep disturbances such as hypersomnia and bad dreams.[77] Persistent abstinence from cocaine leads to normalization of sleep patterns over the course of several weeks.[78] A number of self-rated sleep-related parameters such as sleep quality and depth of sleep, daytime alertness, and cognitive functions such as attention and concentration improve over the first few weeks of abstinence from cocaine.[79,80] Chronic users of cocaine tend to have persistent sleep disturbances as measured by the PSQI. Sleep onset and maintenance insomnia are commonly seen in active users as cocaine is a psychoactive stimulant.

Objective Findings
Interestingly, PSG findings in the abstinence phase indicate insomnia like states, inconsistent with self-reported improvement in sleep disturbances during this time period.[81,82] It is postulated that perception of sleep quality is altered in chronic users of cocaine relative to healthy controls evidenced by association of abnormal PSG findings with impaired sleep dependent learning and cognitive function.[81]

Sleep Latency (SL)
SL is increased with acute use of cocaine.[83] SL is decreased in early abstinence but could be prolonged later in the course of abstinence.

Total Sleep Time (TST)
TST appears to be the longest in the first week of abstinence.[84] TST decreases over time during abstinence.[84] Studies have reported insomnia in the third week of abstinence with eventual restoration of normal sleep patterns with long-term abstinence from cocaine.[79]

Slow-Wave Sleep (SWS)
SWS is significantly reduced in chronic users of cocaine relative to age-matched healthy controls.[79]

SWS increases during abstinence but remains suboptimal, at about 50% lower than age-matched healthy controls at the week three of abstinence.[79,82]

REM Sleep
Administration of cocaine results in acute suppression of REM sleep followed by REM rebound.[83] REM sleep eventually decreases in chronic use of cocaine.[82] REM sleep could be increased in the first week of abstinence but is reduced during second and third week of abstinence from cocaine.[82]

Correlation between Subjective and Objective Sleep Findings in Cocaine Use Disorder
As previously noted, PSG findings in abstinence phase actually indicate insomnia like states inconsistent with self-reported improvement of sleep disturbances during this time period.[81,85] However, an increase in REM sleep in early phase of withdrawal correlates with subjective symptoms of dreaming.[77]

Clinical Implications
There appears to be a correlation between sleep disturbances during abstinence from chronic use with poor performance in cognitive tasks such as attention, focus, concentration, and vigilance. Studies have indicated a significant correlation between objectively measured sleep disturbances (SWS, REM time, and stage N2 sleep) and sleep-dependent procedural learning.[81] Acute intake of cocaine restores these cognitive deficits in the short-term.[81] Consequently, from the perspective of addictive disorders, these deficits are risk factors for relapse on cocaine. Persistent sleep disturbances during abstinence impair sleep-dependent performance in cognitive tasks and could lead to relapse to cocaine use.[79] One study noted that abstinence from cocaine was associated with restoration of normal sleep architecture, especially SWS, REM sleep time, and TST.[79]

Treatments
There is no FDA-approved medication to treat sleep disturbances in cocaine users. Studies have looked into the use of lisuride, a high-affinity D2 and D3 receptor agonist, to treat REM rebound that occurs with initial withdrawal of cocaine.[86] Lisuride was found to be effective in decreasing REM sleep and increasing REM latency, but had no therapeutic benefits in addressing other symptoms present during early abstinence.

Tiagabine, a GABA-reuptake inhibitor, is an agent that enhances SWS; disturbances of SWS have been associated with impairment in cognitive tasks. Tiagabine was noted to alter sleep architecture in that it enhanced SWS throughout the sleep period, with no benefits observed with regard to TST or cognitive tasks.[87]

Modafinil, an alertness-promoting agent, has been studied in the treatment of sleep disturbances secondary to cocaine use disorder.[88] Modafinil acts partially through the dopamine transporter system, has much less abuse potential, and, with its procognitive effects, theoretically makes for an ideal pharmacotherapeutic agent in treating sleep disturbances seen in chronic users of cocaine. Modafinil not only seems to restore SWS but also addresses other sleep disturbances in chronic cocaine users.[84] However, the effects of modafinil on clinical outcomes have been mixed,[88] and this medication has not yet been approved by the FDA to treat sleep disturbances seen in cocaine use disorder.

CONCLUSIONS

Sleep disturbances are common in the context of substance use. They occur during intoxication and withdrawal. Depending on the substance, these sleep disturbances can persist for weeks to months. In addition, certain substances like alcohol, cannabis, and opioids can also influence breathing parameters during sleep. These changes, especially in the context of opioids, can result in significant morbidity. Sleep disturbances also significantly impact the patient's quality of life during abstinence and can potentially increase the risk of relapse. Thus far, the research into treating these sleep disruptions with a view to reducing relapse risk is limited. There are currently no FDA-approved medications to treat sleep disturbances in the context of substance use disorders. Given the significant comorbidity between substance use and sleep disruption, this is an unmet need. Future research into identifying specific patient subgroups that are at risk for sleep disruption following cessation of substance use and treatment options that improve sleep related outcomes and mitigate relapse risk is required.

FUTURE DIRECTIONS

Given the considerable overlap between sleep disturbances and addictions future studies must identify specific sleep disturbances occurring

in the context of substance use and withdrawal that might increase risk for relapse. Specifically, the types of sleep disturbances in early alcohol recovery that might increase the risk of relapse should be identified. Studies examining whether treating these sleep disturbances can reduce the risk of relapse are required. Similarly, studies examining whether interventions directed at improving sleep quality in early cannabis recovery can result in increased abstinence are urgently needed. Given the high rates of sleep disordered breathing in opioid users, studies examining whether there are specific patient populations that are at risk are necessary. Sleep disruptions provide an easy, accessible group of symptoms that can be readily assessed and treated. However, whether such interventions result in improved substance use related outcomes is unclear. Future studies should address this gap in evidence.

KEY CLINICAL PEARLS
- Sleep disturbances are commonly prevalent in subjects with substance use disorders.
- Alcohol use results in worsening of sleep apnea and change in sleep architecture. Cessation of alcohol use results in a REM rebound that can last for many months.
- Sleep disturbances are among the most common symptoms of cannabis withdrawal and can result in relapse.
- Opioids can result in a worsening of both obstructive and central sleep apnea.
- While patients experience subjective improvement in sleep during early cocaine abstinence, objective measures indicate significant sleep disruption.

CLINICAL CASE ILLUSTRATION

A 32-year-old single female with a history of prescription opioid use disorder currently on 20 mg 3 times daily of OxyContin for chronic pain disorder presented to the sleep center for an evaluation of excessive sleepiness during the daytime. She completed an Epworth Sleepiness Scale where she scored 20/24. Her bed partner described moderate snoring and some pauses in her respiration. Her screening overnight oximetry was significantly abnormal and suggestive of central sleep apnea (Figure 22.1). She underwent a sleep study, which revealed severe central sleep apnea with an AHI of 30 per hour and a central apnea index of

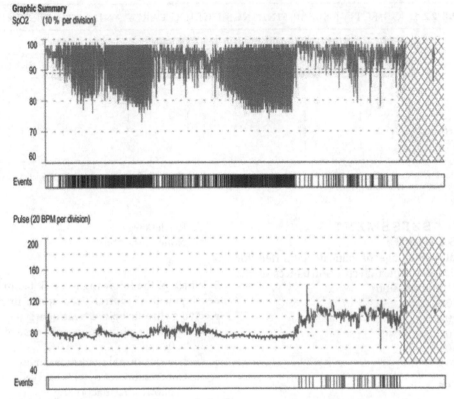

FIGURE 22.1. Abnormal overnight pulse oximetry findings associated with opioid medication use.

28 per hour. CPAP was ineffective in controlling the disordered breathing events. Following the evaluation, the patient was referred to a pain rehabilitation center with an explicit goal to taper and discontinue her opioid medication and explore behavior treatment options and physical therapy to help reduce symptoms of chronic pain.

The patient has successfully completed her treatment program and discontinued all opioid use. Her daytime sleepiness resolved. A screening oximetry that was performed following the discontinuation of her opioid medication indicated complete resolution of disordered breathing events (Figure 22.2).

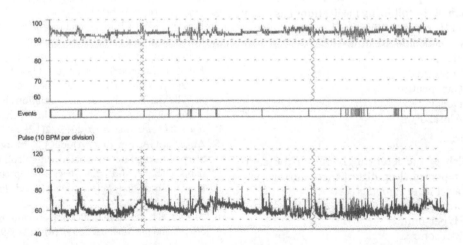

FIGURE 22.2. Normalization of overnight pulse oximetry findings after discontinuation of opioid medication.

TABLE 22.1. OBJECTIVE SLEEP FINDINGS DURING EARLY AND LATE ABSTINENCE

	Alcohol		Cannabis		Opioids		Cocaine	
	Early Abs	Late Abs	Early Abs	Late Abs	Early Abs	Late Abs	Early Abs	Late Abs
SL	↑	↑	↑	↑	↑	↑	↓	↑
TST	↓	↓	↓	↓	↓	↓	↑	↓
SWS	↓	↓	↓	?	↓	↓	↓	↓
REM sleep	↑	↑	↑	↓	↓	?	↑	↓
REM latency	?	?	↓	?	↑	?	↑	?

Abbreviations: ↑, increased; ↓, decreased, ?, data inconclusive; Abs, abstinence; REM, rapid eye movement; SL, sleep latency; SWS, slow-wave sleep; TST, total sleep time.

SELF-ASSESSMENT QUESTIONS

1. What percentage of patients admitted for detoxification report sleep disturbances at the time of the admission?
   a. 10%
   b. 20%
   c. 30%
   d. 50%
   e. 70%

Answer: e

2. Which of the following statements correctly describes the relationship between alcohol use and sleep latency (SL; the amount of time from lights out to sleep onset)?
   a. Chronic alcohol use shortens SL
   b. Chronic alcohol use does not affect SL
   c. The effect of alcohol use on SL is unpredictable
   d. Chronic alcohol use prolongs SL
   e. Acute alcohol use prolongs SL

Answer: d

3. Which of the following medications has a dual therapeutic role in addressing both sleep disturbances and alcohol use disorder?
   a. Naltrexone
   b. Topiramate
   c. Gabapentin
   d. Depakote
   e. Alprazolam

Answer: c

4. Which of the following is one of the commonly reported sleep disturbances during early withdrawal from cannabis use?
   a. Strange dreams
   b. Hypersomnia
   c. Parasomnia
   d. Restless legs
   e. None of the above

Answer: a

5. Which of the following is a risk factor for the development of central sleep apnea in patients receiving chronic opioid treatment?
   a. Daily morphine equivalent dose of >200 mg
   b. Low or normal body mass index
   c. Combination of opioids and sedative-hypnotic pharmacotherapy
   d. All of the above
   e. None of the above

Answer: d

REFERENCES

1. Roncero C, Grau-Lopez L, Diaz-Moran S, Miquel L, Martinez-Luna N, Casas M. [Evaluation of sleep disorders in drug dependent inpatients]. *Medicina clinica.* 2012;138(8):332–335.
2. Johnson EO, Breslau N. Sleep problems and substance use in adolescence. *Drug and Alcohol Dependence.* 2001;64(1):1–7.
3. Breslau N, Roth T, Rosenthal L, Andreski P. Sleep disturbance and psychiatric disorders: a longitudinal epidemiological study of young adults. *Biological Psychiatry.* 1996;39(6):411–418.
4. Haario P, Rahkonen O, Laaksonen M, Lahelma E, Lallukka T. Bidirectional associations between insomnia symptoms and unhealthy behaviours. *Journal of Sleep Research.* 2013;22(1):89–95.
5. Angarita GA, Emadi N, Hodges S, Morgan PT. Sleep abnormalities associated with alcohol, cannabis, cocaine, and opiate use: a comprehensive review. *Addiction Science & Clinical Practice.* 2016;11(1):9.
6. Brower KJ. Insomnia, alcoholism and relapse. *Sleep Medicine Reviews.* 2003;7(6):523–539.

7. Grant BF, Chou S, Saha TD, et al. Prevalence of 12-month alcohol use, high-risk drinking, and DSM-IV alcohol use disorder in the united states, 2001–2002 to 2012–2013: Results from the national epidemiologic survey on alcohol and related conditions. *JAMA Psychiatry.* 2017;74(9):911–923.

8. Chakravorty S, Chaudhary NS, Brower KJ. Alcohol dependence and Its relationship with insomnia and other sleep disorders. *Alcoholism, Clinical and Experimental Research.* 2016;40(11):2271–2282.

9. Roehrs T, Roth T. Insomnia as a path to alcoholism: tolerance development and dose escalation. *Sleep.* 2018;41(8).

10. Logan RW, Williams WP 3rd, McClung CA. Circadian rhythms and addiction: mechanistic insights and future directions. *Behavioral neuro,science.* 2014;128(3):387–412.

11. Drummond SP, Gillin JC, Smith TL, DeModena A. The sleep of abstinent pure primary alcoholic patients: natural course and relationship to relapse. *Alcoholism, Clinical and Experimental Research.* 1998;22(8):1796–1802.

12. Foster JH, Peters TJ. Impaired sleep in alcohol misusers and dependent alcoholics and the impact upon outcome. *Alcoholism, Clinical And experimental Research.* 1999;23(6):1044–1051.

13. Gillin JC, Smith TL, Irwin M, Butters N, Demodena A, Schuckit M. Increased pressure for rapid eye movement sleep at time of hospital admission predicts relapse in nondepressed patients with primary alcoholism at 3-month follow-up. *Archives of General Psychiatry.* 1994;51(3):189–197.

14. Kolla BP, Foroughi M, Saeidifard F, Chakravorty S, Wang Z, Mansukhani MP. The impact of alcohol on breathing parameters during sleep: A systematic review and meta-analysis. *Sleep Medicine Reviews.* 2018.

15. Brower KJ, Aldrich MS, Robinson EA, Zucker RA, Greden JF. Insomnia, self-medication, and relapse to alcoholism. *The American Journal of Psychiatry.* 2001;158(3):399–404.

16. Kuhlwein E, Hauger RL, Irwin MR. Abnormal nocturnal melatonin secretion and disordered sleep in abstinent alcoholics. *Biological Psychiatry.* 2003;54(12):1437–1443.

17. Aldrich MS, Shipley JE, Tandon R, Kroll PD, Brower KJ. Sleep-disordered breathing in alcoholics: association with age. *Alcoholism, Clinical and Experimental Research.* 1993;17(6):1179–1183.

18. Kolla BP, Schneekloth T, Mansukhani MP, et al. The association between sleep disturbances and alcohol relapse: a 12-month observational cohort study. *The American Journal on Addictions.* 2015;24(4):362–367.

19. Brower KJ, Aldrich MS, Hall JM. Polysomnographic and subjective sleep predictors of alcoholic relapse. *Alcoholism, Clinical and Experimental Research.* 1998;22(8):1864–1871.

20. Gillin JC, Smith TL, Irwin M, Kripke DF, Brown S, Schuckit M. Short REM latency in primary alcoholic patients with secondary depression. *The American Journal of Psychiatry.* 1990;147(1):106–109.

21. Kolla BP, Mansukhani MP, Schneekloth T. Pharmacological treatment of insomnia in alcohol recovery: a systematic review. *Alcohol and Alcoholism.* 2011;46(5):578–585.

22. Mason BJ, Quello S, Goodell V, Shadan F, Kyle M, Begovic A. Gabapentin treatment for alcohol dependence: a randomized clinical trial. *JAMA Internal Medicine.* 2014;174(1):70–77.

23. Brower KJ, Conroy DA, Kurth ME, Anderson BJ, Stein MD. Ramelteon and Improved Insomnia in Alcohol-Dependent Patients: A Case Series. *Journal of Clinical Sleep Medicine.* 2011;7(3):274–275.

24. Friedmann PD, Rose JS, Swift R, Stout RL, Millman RP, Stein MD. Trazodone for sleep disturbance after alcohol detoxification: a double-blind, placebo-controlled trial. *Alcoholism, Clinical and Experimental Research.* 2008;32(9):1652–1660.

25. Kolla BP, Schneekloth TD, Biernacka JM, et al. Trazodone and alcohol relapse: a retrospective study following residential treatment. *The American Journal on Addictions.* 2011;20(6):525–529.

26. Chakravorty S, Hanlon AL, Kuna ST, et al. The effects of quetiapine on sleep in recovering alcohol-dependent subjects: a pilot study. *Journal of Clinical Psychopharmacology.* 2014;34(3):350–354.

27. Monnelly EP, Ciraulo DA, Knapp C, LoCastro J, Sepulveda I. Quetiapine for treatment of alcohol dependence. *Journal of Clinical Psychopharmacology.* 2004;24(5):532–535.

28. Monnelly EP, Locastro JS, Gagnon D, Young M, Fiore LD. Quetiapine versus trazodone in reducing rehospitalization for alcohol dependence: a large data-base study. *Journal of Addiction Medicine.* 2008;2(3):128–134.

29. Mason BJ. Acamprosate, alcoholism, and abstinence. *The Journal of Clinical Psychiatry.* 2015;76(2):e224–e225.

30. Brooks AT, Wallen GR. Sleep disturbances in individuals with alcohol-related disorders: a review of cognitive-behavioral therapy for insomnia (CBT-I) and associated non-pharmacological therapies. *Substance Abuse: Research and Treatment.* 2014;8:55–62.

31. Hasin DS, Saha TD, Kerridge BT, et al. Prevalence of marijuana use disorders in the united states between 2001–2002 and 2012–2013. *JAMA Psychiatry.* 2015;72(12):1235–1242.

32. Chait LD. Subjective and behavioral effects of marijuana the morning after smoking. *Psychopharmacology.* 1990;100(3):328–333.

33. Crowley TJ, Macdonald MJ, Whitmore EA, Mikulich SK. Cannabis dependence, withdrawal, and reinforcing effects among adolescents with conduct symptoms and substance use disorders. *Drug and Alcohol Dependence.* 1998;50(1):27–37.

34. Haney M, Ward AS, Comer SD, Foltin RW, Fischman MW. Abstinence symptoms following oral THC administration to humans. *Psychopharmacology.* 1999;141(4):385–394.

35. Budney AJ, Hughes JR, Moore BA, Novy PL. Marijuana abstinence effects in marijuana smokers maintained in their home environment. *Archives of General Psychiatry.* 2001;58(10):917–924.

36. Budney AJ, Vandrey RG, Hughes JR, Thostenson JD, Bursac Z. Comparison of cannabis and tobacco withdrawal: severity and contribution to relapse. *Journal of Substance Abuse Treatment.* 2008;35(4):362–368.

37. Haney M, Ward AS, Comer SD, Foltin RW, Fischman MW. Abstinence symptoms following smoked marijuana in humans. *Psychopharmacology.* 1999;141(4):395–404.

38. Budney AJ, Moore BA, Vandrey RG, Hughes JR. The time course and significance of cannabis withdrawal. *Journal of Abnormal Psychology.* 2003;112(3):393–402.

39. Chait LD, Zacny JP. Reinforcing and subjective effects of oral delta 9-THC and smoked marijuana in humans. *Psychopharmacology.* 1992;107(2-3):255–262.

40. Nicholson AN, Turner C, Stone BM, Robson PJ. Effect of Delta-9-tetrahydrocannabinol and cannabidiol on nocturnal sleep and early-morning behavior in young adults. *Journal of Clinical Psychopharmacology.* 2004;24(3):305–313.

41. Bolla KI, Lesage SR, Gamaldo CE, et al. Polysomnogram changes in marijuana users who report sleep disturbances during prior abstinence. *Sleep Medicine.* 2010;11(9):882–889.

42. Bolla KI, Lesage SR, Gamaldo CE, et al. Sleep disturbance in heavy marijuana Users. *Sleep.* 2008;31(6):901–908.

43. Carley DW, Prasad B, Reid KJ, et al. Pharmacotherapy of Apnea by Cannabimimetic Enhancement, the PACE clinical trial: effects of dronabinol in obstructive sleep apnea. *Sleep.* 2018;41(1).

44. Ramar K, Rosen IM, Kirsch DB, et al. Medical cannabis and the treatment of obstructive sleep apnea: an American Academy of Sleep Medicine position statement. *J Clin Sleep Med.* 2018;14(4):679–681.

45. Vorspan F, Guillem E, Bloch V, et al. Self-reported sleep disturbances during cannabis withdrawal in cannabis-dependent outpatients with and without opioid dependence. *Sleep Medicine.* 2010;11(5):499–500.

46. Mednick SC, Christakis NA, Fowler JH. The spread of sleep loss influences drug use in adolescent social networks. *PloS One.* 2010;5(3):e9775.

47. Babson KA, Boden MT, Harris AH, Stickle TR, Bonn-Miller MO. Poor sleep quality as a risk factor for lapse following a cannabis quit attempt. *Journal of Substance Abuse Treatment.* 2013;44(4):438–443.

48. Allsop DJ, Norberg MM, Copeland J, Fu S, Budney AJ. The Cannabis Withdrawal Scale development: patterns and predictors of cannabis withdrawal and distress. *Drug and Alcohol Dependence.* 2011;119(1-2):123–129.

49. Vandrey R, Smith MT, McCann UD, Budney AJ, Curran EM. Sleep disturbance and the effects of extended-release zolpidem during cannabis withdrawal. *Drug and Alcohol Dependence.* 2011;117(1):38–44.

50. Budney AJ, Vandrey RG, Hughes JR, Moore BA, Bahrenburg B. Oral delta-9-tetrahydrocannabinol suppresses cannabis withdrawal symptoms. *Drug and Alcohol Dependence.* 2007;86(1):22–29.

51. Haney M, Hart CL, Vosburg SK, et al. Marijuana withdrawal in humans: effects of oral THC or divalproex. *Neuropsychopharmacology.* 2003; 29:158.

52. Haney M, Hart CL, Vosburg SK, Comer SD, Reed SC, Foltin RW. Effects of THC and lofexidine in a human laboratory model of marijuana withdrawal and relapse. *Psychopharmacology.* 2008;197(1):157–168.

53. Haney M, Cooper ZD, Bedi G, Vosburg SK, Comer SD, Foltin RW. Nabilone decreases marijuana withdrawal and a laboratory measure of marijuana relapse. *Neuropsychopharmacology.* 2013;38(8):1557–1565.

54. Allsop DJ, Copeland J, Lintzeris N, et al. Nabiximols as an agonist replacement therapy during cannabis withdrawal: a randomized clinical trial. *JAMA Psychiatry.* 2014;71(3):281–291.

55. Rudd RA, Seth P, David F, Scholl L. Increases in drug and opioid-involved overdose deaths: United States, 2010–2015. *MMWR Morbidity and mortality weekly report.* 2016;65(50-51):1445–1452.

56. Young-McCaughan S, Miaskowski C. Definition of and mechanism for opioid-induced sedation. *Pain Management Nursing.* 2001;2(3):84–97.

57. Kantor TG, Hopper M, Laska E. Adverse effects of commonly ordered oral narcotics. *Journal of Clinical Pharmacology.* 1981;21(1):1–8.

58. Jacox A, Carr DB, Payne R. New clinical-practice guidelines for the management of pain in patients with cancer. *The New England Journal of Medicine.* 1994;330(9):651–655.

59. Xiao L, Tang YL, Smith AK, et al. Nocturnal sleep architecture disturbances in early methadone treatment patients. *Psychiatry Research.* 2010;179(1):91–95.

60. Asaad TA, Ghanem MH, Abdel Samee AM, El-Habiby MM. Sleep profile in patients with chronic opioid abuse: a polysomnographic evaluation in an Egyptian sample. *Addictive Disorders & Their Treatment.* 2011;10(1):21–28.

61. Kay DC, Pickworth WB, Neidert GL, Falcone D, Fishman PM, Othmer E. Opioid effects on computer-derived sleep and EEG parameters in nondependent human addicts. *Sleep.* 1979;2(2):175–191.

62. Dimsdale JE, Norman D, DeJardin D, Wallace MS. The effect of opioids on sleep architecture. *J Clin Sleep Med.* 2007;3(1):33–36.

63. Wang D, Teichtahl H. Opioids, sleep architecture and sleep-disordered breathing. *Sleep Medicine Reviews.* 2007;11(1):35–46.

64. Hartwell EE, Pfeifer JG, McCauley JL, Maria MM-S, Back SE. Sleep disturbances and pain among individuals with prescription opioid dependence. *Addictive Behaviors.* 2014;39(10):1537–1542.

65. Howe RC, Hegge FW, Phillips JL. Acute heroin abstinence in man: I. Changes in behavior and sleep. *Drug and Alcohol Dependence.* 1980;5(5):341–356.

66. Hsu W-Y, Chiu N-Y, Liu J-T, et al. Sleep quality in heroin addicts under methadone maintenance treatment. *Acta Neuropsychiatrica.* 2012;24(6):356–360.

67. Peles E, Schreiber S, Adelson M. Variables associated with perceived sleep disorders in methadone maintenance treatment (MMT) patients. *Drug and Alcohol Dependence.* 2006;82(2):103–110.

68. Webster LR, Cochella S, Dasgupta N, et al. An analysis of the root causes for opioid-related overdose deaths in the United States. *Pain Medicine.* 2011;12 Suppl 2:S26–S35.

69. Correa D, Farney RJ, Chung F, Prasad A, Lam D, Wong J. Chronic opioid use and central sleep apnea: a review of the prevalence, mechanisms, and perioperative considerations. *Anesthesia and Analgesia.* 2015;120(6):1273–1285.

70. Sun EC, Dixit A, Humphreys K, Darnall BD, Baker LC, Mackey S. Association between concurrent use of prescription opioids and benzodiazepines and overdose: retrospective analysis. *BMJ.* 2017;356:j760.

71. Walker JM, Farney RJ, Rhondeau SM, et al. Chronic opioid use is a risk factor for the development of central sleep apnea and ataxic breathing. *Journal of Clinical Sleep Medicine.* 2007;3(5):455–461.

72. Argoff CE, Silvershein DI. A comparison of long- and short-acting opioids for the treatment of chronic noncancer pain: tailoring therapy to meet patient needs. *Mayo Clinic Proceedings.* 2009;84(7):602–612.

73. Silber MH, Becker PM, Buchfuhrer MJ, et al. The appropriate use of opioids in the treatment of refractory restless legs syndrome. *Mayo Clinic Proceedings.* 2018;93(1):59–67.

74. Cheatle MD, Webster LR. Opioid therapy and sleep disorders: risks and mitigation strategies. *Pain Medicine.* 2015;16 Suppl 1:S22–S26.

75. Shapiro CM, Chung SA, Wylie PE, et al. Home-use servo-ventilation therapy in chronic pain patients with central sleep apnea: initial and 3-month follow-up. *Sleep & breathing/Schlaf & Atmung.* 2015;19(4):1285–1292.

76. Grant BF, Saha TD, Ruan WJ, et al. Epidemiology of DSM-5 drug use disorder: results from the National Epidemiologic Survey on Alcohol and Related Conditions–III. *JAMA Psychiatry.* 2016;73(1):39–47.

77. Cottler LB, Shillington AM, Compton WM, III, Mager D, Spitznagel EL. Subjective reports of withdrawal among cocaine users: recommendations for DSM-IV. *Drug & Alcohol Dependence.* 1993;33(2):97–104.

78. Gawin FH, Kleber HD. Abstinence symptomatology and psychiatric diagnosis in cocaine abusers: clinical observations. *Archives of General Psychiatry.* 1986;43(2):107–113.

79. Angarita GA, Canavan SV, Forselius E, Bessette A, Pittman B, Morgan PT. Abstinence-related changes in sleep during treatment for cocaine dependence. *Drug and Alcohol Dependence.* 2014;134:343–347.

80. Coffey SF, Dansky BS, Carrigan MH, Brady KT. Acute and protracted cocaine abstinence in an outpatient population: a prospective study of mood, sleep and withdrawal symptoms. *Drug and Alcohol Dependence.* 2000;59(3):277–286.

81. Morgan PT, Pace-Schott EF, Sahul ZH, Coric V, Stickgold R, Malison RT. Sleep, sleep-dependent procedural learning and vigilance in chronic cocaine users: Evidence for occult insomnia. *Drug and Alcohol Dependence.* 2006;82(3):238–249.

82. Matuskey D, Pittman B, Forselius E, Malison RT, Morgan PT. A multistudy analysis of the effects of early cocaine abstinence on sleep. *Drug and Alcohol Dependence.* 2011;115(1-2):62–66.

83. Johanson CE, Roehrs T, Schuh K, Warbasse L. The effects of cocaine on mood and sleep in

cocaine-dependent males. *Experimental and Clinical Psychopharmacology.* 1999;7(4):338–346.

84. Morgan PT, Pace-Schott E, Pittman B, Stickgold R, Malison RT. Normalizing effects of modafinil on sleep in chronic cocaine users. *The American Journal of Psychiatry.* 2010;167(3):331–340.

85. Morgan PT, Pace-Schott EF, Sahul ZH, Coric V, Stickgold R, Malison RT. Sleep architecture, cocaine and visual learning. *Addiction (Abingdon, England).* 2008;103(8):1344–1352.

86. Gillin JC, Pulvirenti L, Withers N, Golshan S, Koob G. The effects of lisuride on mood and sleep during acute withdrawal in stimulant abusers: a preliminary report. *Biological Psychiatry.* 1994;35(11):843–849.

87. Morgan PT, Malison RT. Pilot study of lorazepam and tiagabine effects on sleep, motor learning, and impulsivity in cocaine abstinence. *American Journal of Drug and Alcohol Abuse.* 2008;34(6):692–702.

88. Sangroula D, Motiwala F, Wagle B, Shah VC, Hagi K, Lippmann S. Modafinil Treatment of Cocaine Dependence: A Systematic Review and Meta-Analysis. *Substance Use and Misuse.* 2017;52(10):1292–1306.

23

Neurodevelopmental Disorders

ALTHEA ROBINSON SHELTON, JESSICA DUIS, AND BETH MALOW

INTRODUCTION

Sleep plays an important role in synaptic maturation and brain development.[1,2] Chronic sleep deprivation may contribute to disrupted memory consolidation and disrupted synaptic plasticity.[3] Sleep deprivation has been observed to affect the neural circuitry underlying emotional regulation, including abnormal connectivity of the amygdala and prefrontal cortex.[4] Thus, in the developing child, sleep likely serves many purposes, including memory consolidation, emotional regulation, and cognition.

In typically developing (TD) children, chronic sleep deprivation has been shown to cause, hyperactivity, a decrease in attention span, and problems with behavior.[5-7] Sleep disturbance is a common concern that parents express to their children's pediatrician. Approximately 10% to 25% of TD children have sleep problems pertaining to sleep onset delay and nocturnal awakenings.[8,9] However, sleep disturbances are even more prevalent in children with neurodevelopmental disorders (NDD). In NDD, the prevalence of sleep disorders has been reported to be as high as 86%.[10,11] In fact, sleep disturbances are included in the diagnostic criteria for many NDDs. In addition, sleep disturbances are significantly higher than in age-matched TD children,[12] and unlike TD individuals, sleep disorders in children with NDD commonly last into adolescence and adulthood.[13]

Common sleep complaints in NDD are insomnia (sleep onset and sleep maintenance difficulty) and hypersomnia (excessive daytime sleepiness). Sleep disturbances in children with NDD likely represent a complex interaction of biological and environmental factors.[14] There are several disorders of neurodevelopment with prominent sleep disturbances (Table 23.1). This chapter will focus on assessment and treatment of common sleep disturbances associated with NDD including autism spectrum disorders (ASD), Down syndrome (DS), Prader–Willi syndrome (PWS), Angelman syndrome (AS), Rett syndrome, fragile X syndrome (FXS), Williams syndrome (WS), and Smith–Magenis syndrome (SMS).

AUTISM SPECTRUM DISORDER (ASD)

ASD is not a disease but a syndrome with multiple nongenetic and genetic causes.[15] Within this are a group of clinically heterogeneous NDDs sharing common features related to impaired social and communication abilities in addition to stereotyped behaviors.[16] In 2013, the fifth edition of the *Diagnostic and Statistical Manual* (DSM-V) combined autism, Asperger's syndrome, and persuasive development disorder into a single diagnosis of ASD.[17] ASD is characterized by impairments in social communication and the presence of restricted and repetitive behavioral (RRB) patterns. In the United States, it affects 1 in 68 children.[17]

Sleep disturbance is a common comorbidity in ASD. Estimates of the prevalence of sleep disturbances in ASD range from 40% to 80%.[18] Sleep disturbances are prevalent across spectrum diagnoses and cognitive levels (including children with normal/high IQs).[19,20] Sleep disturbances in ASD may occur as a result of a complex interaction between biological, psychological, social/environmental, and family factors. A combination of these problems or just one may contribute to sleep disturbances.[20] Autism symptom severity, gastrointestinal (GI) problems, and anxiety has been shown to be the main risk factors for sleep problems.[21]

Much headway has been made in understanding the underlying genetics of autism that may play a role in insomnia. Focus has been drawn to genes that control the circadian rhythm and abnormal melatonin production as underlying causes for insomnia in ASD.[22,23]

In mammals, the suprachiasmatic nucleus (SCN) in the anterior hypothalamus is the pacemaker of the circadian rhythm. The SCN entrains

TABLE 23.1. SLEEP DISORDERS ASSOCIATED WITH NEURODEVELOPMENTAL DISORDERS

Sleep Symptoms	Autism	Down Syndrome	Prader-Willi Syndrome	Angelman Syndrome	Fragile X Syndrome	Williams Syndrome	Rett Syndrome	Smith-Magenis Syndrome
Sleep onset insomnia	+++			+	++	++	++	
Sleep maintenance insomnia	+	+		++	++	++	+++	+++
Obstructive sleep apnea		+++	+++		+			
Central sleep apnea			+				+++	
Daytime sleepiness		+	+++			+		+++
Nocturnal seizures	+			+++				

+ mild; ++ moderate; +++ severe.

circadian clocks via neural and neuro-endocrine pathways.[24] The circadian clock gene abnormalities have been hypothesized as a causative factor for ASD. Mutations affecting gene function in circadian-relevant genes are more frequent in patients with ASD than in controls.[25] Clock gene abnormalities have been theorized to be the causative factor in deficits seen in social engagement and communication in ASD.[23]

The pineal gland produces melatonin, which is an important regulator of the circadian rhythm.[24] Melatonin is involved in many functional processes including regulation of the sleep–wake cycle in humans.[26] There are several studies that show a decrease in the amount of melatonin or the major metabolite of melatonin (urinary 6-sulphatoxymelatonin) in children and adolescents with ASD compared to controls in the serum, saliva and/or urine.[27–29] It has been postulated that the sleep problems found in ASD may be due to genetic abnormalities associated with melatonin synthesis and melatonin's role in modulating synaptic changes.[22] A combination of abnormal receptor sites, decreased melatonin production, and increased breakdown may explain insomnia in ASD.[30,31]

Sleep Disturbances in ASD

Parent reported sleep problems in ASD range from 40% to 80% depending on the study.[18–20,32–34]

A study of 167 children with ASD revealed that 86% of subjects had at least one sleep problem. These included parasomnias, insomnia, bedtime resistance, sleep disordered breathing, morning rising difficulties, and daytime sleepiness. Out of all these sleep problems, the most common was insomnia (56%).[35]

In ASD, insomnia presents as sleep onset delay, or frequent nocturnal awakenings and/or reduced sleep duration.[36] In children with ASD, insomnia is 10 times more frequent than in TD children and often persists into adolescence.[37] Difficulty settling down and prolonged sleep onset are common parent complaints. Studies focusing on parent report show that children with ASD can take several hours to fall asleep.[12,32,33] In addition, multiple prolonged nocturnal awakenings are commonly reported. Parents report awakenings that can last up to 3 hours where the child will often play or lay in bed laughing or talking.[33,38] Sleep problems have been shown to persist into adulthood and effect daytime functioning.[39] Subjective reports of sleep disturbances in ASD have been supported by polysomnography (PSG) data that showed low sleep efficiencies, prolonged sleep latency, increased N1 sleep, decreased N2 and N3 sleep, and frequent nocturnal awakenings.[40] Several studies using PSG have shown that there are abnormalities in rapid eye movement

(REM) sleep in children with ASD. Studies show a decrease in total REM sleep and the frequency of REMs in children with ASD.[20,41] Even when compared to children with developmental delay without ASD, children with ASD have lower REM sleep percentage.[42]

In patients with ASD, daily functioning can be impaired due to poor sleep, which can affect patients' behavior, communication, socialization, development, and cognitive functioning. More and more research indicates that sleep disturbances in ASD worsen core ASD symptoms, such as repetitive behaviors, poor social interactions ,and communication difficulties.[43,44] In addition, short sleep duration has been correlated with decreased IQ scores in children with ASD.[45] There are multiple causes for insomnia, but communication and emotional difficulties may prevent children with ASD from following a parent's instructions on falling asleep.[46] Veatch et al.[45] reported that severity scores for social/communication impairment and RRB were increased for children with ASD who were reported to sleep ≤420 minutes per night (lower 5th percentile) compared to children sleeping ≥660 minutes (upper 95th percentile). In addition, patients with short sleep duration were less likely to develop peer relationships,[45] whereas reduction in sleep disturbance over time has been associated with improved social skills and ability.[47]

Sleep disturbances can affect daytime behavior in ASD. Children with ASD described by their parents as poor sleepers, as opposed to good sleepers, had higher scores related to affective problems on the Child Behavior Checklist.[43] In addition, short sleep duration in children with ASD has been shown to be associated with stereotypic behaviors and social skill deficits.[20] Sikora et al.[48] evaluated a large cohort of 3,452 children with ASD using multiple measures of behavior. The results showed that children with ASD and sleep problems had more internalizing and externalizing behavioral problems and poor adaptive functioning compared to children with ASD and no sleep problems.[48]

Treatment

It has been recommended that all children with ASD be screened for insomnia. Medical and neurological comorbidities (epilepsy, obstructive sleep apnea [OSA], GI issues) need to be assessed and treated since these often contribute to insomnia. Once excluded, the first-line treatment is behavioral through parent education,[49] with studies documenting improvement in sleep, daytime behavior, or both.[50,51] Behavioral intervention starts with assessing the patient's sleep hygiene. Sleep hygiene is a person's daytime and evening habits that contribute to successful sleep. Once those habits are addressed, the sleep clinician can help the family and patient develop a consistent sleep routine. Ensuring that the amount of sleep and timing of sleep is age appropriate. There are also different behavioral interventions based on whether the patient has a sleep onset versus a sleep maintenance insomnia. Although there are no approved medications by the US Food and Drug Administration (FDA) for pediatric insomnia, if behavioral interventions are unsuccessful, pharmacological intervention may be warranted.[49] Melatonin has been shown to increase sleep time in children with ASD.[52] Although, there is limited data on efficacy, antiepileptics and antidepressants may be used, especially if there is comorbid epilepsy and/or mood disorder.[52] There is evidence for the use of gabapentin for sleep maintenance in ASD.[53] Antidepressants (mirtazapine, amitriptyline, doxepin, trazodone) may promote sleep by decreasing sleep onset latency and increasing total sleep time.[54]

GENETIC SYNDROMES

Down Syndrome (DS)

DS is the most common genetic disorder occurring in 1 out of 691 births.[55] The majority of cases occur due to an extra chromosome 21.[56] In 5% of individuals, one copy of chromosome 21 is translocated to another acrocentric chromosome, and, in 2% to 4% of cases, there is a mosaicism of trisomy.[56]

Sleep Disturbances in DS

There are several physical attributes that predispose patients with DS to having sleep disturbances. Patients with DS have a smaller bony dimension of the upper airway due to midface and maxillary hypoplasia, as well as relative macroglossia.[57] In addition, children with DS are hypotonic, and this hypotonia causes an increase in laryngomalacia.[58]

Sleep disorders are often underrecognized in children with DS.[59] Compared to TD children, those with DS are reported to have more excessive daytime sleepiness, fragmented sleep, early awakening, and sleep maintenance insomnia.[60] Patients with DS and OSA have been shown to prefer to sleep sitting cross-legged flopped-forward with head resting on the bed.[61] Likely due to their fragmented sleep, patients with DS have a decreased REM sleep and decreased sleep efficiency.[62,63]

DS is a NDD that presents primarily with excessive daytime sleepiness due to untreated/undertreated OSA. Patients with DS are also at risk for central sleep apnea (CSA) and hypoventilation.[64] There appears to be greater risk for CSA during infancy and an increased risk for OSA as patients get older.[64] Approximately, 50% to 80% of children with DS are affected by OSA.[64–66] The prevalence of OSA in adults with DS is estimated to be 35% to 42%.[67] Craniofacial and upper airway abnormalities are primarily responsible for this higher prevalence of OSA. Comorbidities, such as hypothyroidism and cardiac abnormalities, are associated with more severe OSA.[68]

Untreated OSA has multiple health-related consequences, including increased risks for cardiovascular disease and impaired cognitive function. The cardiovascular consequences of untreated OSA in DS include congestive heart failure, left ventricular hypertrophy, cor pulmonale, and pulmonary hypertension.[69]

Untreated OSA can lead to cognitive dysfunction. Children with OSA may present with hyperactivity, behavioral disruptions, and poor school performance.[70] One study showed that children with DS and OSA performed worse on cognitive flexibility tasks than those without OSA.[60] In addition, DS patients with higher apnea indices on PSG have been shown to have reduced visuoperceptual skills.[71] Untreated OSA can also affect mood in these patients. In adolescents with DS, comorbid depression and OSA have been associated with functional decline.[70]

Treatment

The American Academy of Pediatrics has recommended that at least once in the first 5 years of life, symptoms of OSA, including daytime sleepiness, heavy breathing, snoring, uncommon sleep positions, frequent night awakenings, apneic pauses, and behavior problems, be discussed with parents of children with DS.[72] Given the poor correlation between PSG results and parental report, all children with DS were recommended to have an overnight PSG by 4 years of age regardless of symptoms.[73] In addition, every cardiologic follow-up should include screening for OSA, even after age 4. Patients should be screened not only for nocturnal symptoms (snoring, gasping, restless sleep) but also for daytime symptoms, such as worsening of daytime behavior, mood changes, learning regression, and excessive daytime sleepiness.

Adenotonsillectomy is the gold standard first-line treatment for OSA in all children. Although adenotonsillectomy will often reduce the obstructive Apnea–Hypopnea Index in children with DS, it usually does not normalize it.[74] Also, there is often residual/persistent OSA status post adenotonsillectomy.[74,75] Thus, repeat PSG 3 months after adenotonsillectomy is often necessary. If OSA persists, re-evaluation by ENT for possible higher level upper airway surgery is warranted. Continuous positive airway pressure (CPAP) is another treatment option; however, CPAP adherence has been reported to be low in children in several studies.[76,77] In the authors' experience, having time to acclimate to CPAP in association with reward based behavioral interventions helps improve adherence. CPAP should be considered as first-line treatment for adults with DS and OSA.

Prader–Willi Syndrome (PWS)

Prader–Willi syndrome (PWS) is a neuroendocrine disorder present in approximately 1/15,000 individuals.[78] Hypothalamic dysfunction in these individuals is thought to be the cause of appetite dysregulation, hypogonadism, short stature, abnormal control of body temperature, and sleep disordered breathing including central and OSA with daytime hypersomnolence.[79] Other features in some individuals include narcolepsy and cataplexy-like phenotype that is not well defined. Infants are hypotonic at birth, and this improves over time. Individuals with PWS progress through defined nutritional stages. There are two nutritional stages: poor feeding, frequently with failure to thrive (FTT) in infancy (Stage 1), followed by hyperphagia leading to obesity in later childhood (Stage 2). The onset of hyperphagia begins at approximately age 8.[80]

PWS is caused by lack of paternal expression of the genes in the region of 15q11.2-q13.[81] A deletion from the paternal copy of chromosome 15q11.2-q13 is the most common cause and occurs in about 70% of cases. Maternal uniparental disomy can be detected in approximately 25% of cases. An imprinting defect is present in <5% of cases.[81]

Sleep Disturbances in PWS

Abnormalities in ventilatory control are common in PWS. In a large proportion of individuals with PWS, there is blunted or no hypoxic ventilator response. Apnea is one cause of hypoxia and more common in PWS when compared to the general population.[82] In addition, the hypercapneic ventilatory response is blunted in obese individuals with PWS.[83] These findings contribute to sleep-disordered breathing in PWS. Sleep-disordered breathing is common in PWS. CSA is more common in infancy, and it improves with age.[84] Data suggest that starting from age 2, OSA is more common.[85] From 3 to 6 years of age, OSA is reported in approximately 80% of children with PWS.[86]

Hypersomnia can be a debilitating feature of PWS. In a study of 60 adults with PWS, 67% reported daytime sleepiness. Narcolepsy was diagnosed in 35%, hypersomnia in 12%, and a suggestive, but unclear diagnosis was present in 53%.[87] One important caveat that makes the diagnosis of narcolepsy difficult is that daytime sleepiness can be related to poorly managed OSA likely due to poor CPAP adherence. In NT patients with narcolepsy type 1 (formerly narcolepsy with cataplexy) concentrations of hypocretin (HCRT-1) in cerebrospinal fluid (CSF) are often undetectable. A loss of 73% of hypocretin type-1 neurons causes a 50% decline in CSF hypocretin. Thus, in a narcoleptic patient with undetectable CSF Hcrt-1, virtually all of the hypocretin neurons have been lost.[88] Hypocretin levels in the CSF of PWS patients were noted to be in the intermediate range when compared to individuals diagnosed with narcolepsy. These levels also had a negative correlation with Epworth Sleepiness Scale scores in the PWS group suggesting that low CSF hypocretin levels may play a role in hypersomnia in PWS.[89] Case reports also suggest an increased incidence of cataplexy in PWS. Of the cases reported in the literature, only one-third of cases possessed the HLADQB1*0602 haplotype.[90] On the other hand, 98% of narcoleptics with low hypocretin are positive for DQB1*06:02 compared to 25% of the normal white population, 12% of the Japanese population, and 38% of the black population.[91]

In 70% to 90% of patients with PWS, a characteristic behavioral profile develops. This behavior often involves tantrums, stubbornness, insistence on sameness, and compulsivity.[92] Excessive daytime sleepiness has associated with an increase in these behavioral disturbances in children and adolescents with PWS.[93] In addition, attention deficit-hyperactivity disorder (ADHD) symptoms and insistence on sameness are common in PWS.[94] Untreated OSA worsens ADHD symptoms.[6] To summarize, sleep-disordered breathing and hypersomnia contribute to irritability and impulsivity of actions with worsening behavioral outbursts and reduced threshold to tantrums in patients with PWS.

Treatment

Growth hormone (GH) therapy is a standard FDA-approved treatment for children with PWS. Guidelines require PSG prior to the initiation of GH and then 8 to 10 weeks postinitiation. This suggested approach is related to increased concerns regarding sudden death in PWS individuals with untreated OSA while taking GH. Increased risk is noted in individuals during the first 9 months of treatment, especially in morbidly obese individuals.[95] Any new onset of behavioral concerns is an indication for PSG in individuals with PWS.

Modafinil is a successful treatment in many individuals with hypersomnia in this population. It is best to start at lower doses (50–100 mg in the morning) and increase based on if excessive daytime sleepiness persists. Care should be exercised due to possible increased risk of anxiety and the rare but life-threatening Stevens–Johnson syndrome. In some individuals with PWS, modafinil has helped both behavioral and sleep concerns.[96,97]

Angelman Syndrome (AS)

AS occurs in approximately 1/12,000 to 1/24,000 people. It is characterized by intellectual disability, gait ataxia, tremor of the limbs, and seizures with characteristic findings on electroencephalography (EEG). Individuals feature a happy demeanor that is characterized by inappropriate laughter, excitability, and smiling. Progressive microcephaly is often noted by the age of 2. Hypotonia may be noted at birth and developmental delays are often noted around 6 months of age.[98]

AS is caused by lack of maternal expression of *UBE3A*. Methylation studies of chromosome 15q11.2-q13 detect 80% of cases. The most common cause is a deletion on chromosome 15q11.2-q13 (70%). Paternal uniparental disomy is present in 3% of cases. An imprinting center defect causes 6% of cases. Approximately 11% of cases are due to a mutation in the maternally inherited allele of UBE3A, and these cases have normal methylation studies.[99]

Sleep Disturbances in AS

Overall sleep is not well characterized with large studies conducted with PSGs due to the difficulty in obtaining studies in this population. There is a high prevalence of sleep disorders in AS, which is reported to be between 20% to 80%.

The diagnostic criteria for AS include sleep disturbance as an associated characteristic.[100] Studies have primarily focused on parent-reported questionnaires to characterize sleep and the prevalence of sleep disturbance in these studies ranges from 25% to 100%.[101–103] Sleep problems appear to be more severe in early childhood. In adolescents and adults with AS, total sleep time often reaches above normal in some individuals. Overall, sleep problems are maximal between the ages of 2 and 6 years.[102]

Frequent nocturnal awakenings are perhaps the biggest concern reported by parents.[103] Studies also suggest that abnormalities in circadian rhythm play a role.[104] The most commonly reported problems are difficulty with sleep initiation, frequent nocturnal awakenings, and a decreased need for sleep.[102,105–107] Total sleep time is, on average, 5 to 6 hours per day. However, daytime sleepiness is not reported.[102] PSG studies are few but show that the percentage of REM sleep is reduced and that slow-wave sleep may be increased.[108,109] Periodic leg movements was a feature of interest in one PSG study and showed periodic leg movements to be present in 7/10 participants.[109] Seizure activity is not noted to correlate with total sleep time in AS,[106] but the possibility of sleep fragmentation due to overt or subclinical seizures should be considered in the differential diagnosis.[110]

Approximately 90% of patients with AS present with epileptic seizures; seizures disrupt sleep architecture and alter REM sleep.[111] Sleep, particularly non-REM stages, can activate clinical seizures.[112] Given that the majority of children with AS have epilepsy, sleep fragmentation from seizures is to be expected.[105] Conant et al.[113] found that 69% of AS patients with epilepsy reported sleep problems. In addition, the severity of seizures correlated with sleep disturbances.

As stated earlier, 70% of AS cases are caused by the deletion of the 15q11-q13 region of the maternally inherited chromosome 15.[99] This deletion disrupts the gene that encodes for the B3 subunit of the GABA$_A$ receptor. This receptor plays an important role in seizure disorders, motor control, and cognitive processing.[114,115] Alterations in the GABA$_A$ receptor may cause thalamocortical disruptions that lead to the abnormal sleep patterns in AS.[108,114]

Treatment

There is a relationship between disruptive behaviors and sleep onset. Targeted treatment to improve sleep environment, sleep hygiene, and parent–child interactions during sleep times improves disruptive behaviors in a sustainable way.[116] Treatment may include a trial of melatonin for help in initially falling asleep.[117] Melatonin should be given 35 to 45 minutes before desired bedtime. The starting dose can range from 1 to 3 mg. It is not successful in preventing nighttime awakenings. GABA$_A$ receptor agonists, such as benzodiazepines, may be helpful for nocturnal awakenings and to treat seizures. Clonazepam is a commonly used benzodiazepine for this indication. A standard starting dose is 0.01 mg/kg/day given 30 to 35 minutes before bed.

Rett Syndrome (RS)

RS is present in 1/8,500 individuals. In its classical form, it is characterized by normal development initially followed by regression in language and motor skills. Repetitive stereotypic hand movements replace purposeful hand use. Additional features include seizures, progressive microcephaly, dysautonomia, bruxism, autistic features, ataxia, tremors, breath-holding spells, and apnea. Girls may have episodes of screaming and crying and panic-like attacks.[118]

Rett syndrome is caused by loss-of-function mutation in Methyl-CpG-binding protein 2 (MeCP2) located on the X chromosome. MECP2-related disorders include an expanded spectrum including atypical Rett syndrome and a phenotype that includes severe neonatal encephalopathy. Diagnosis is by sequencing and deletion/duplication studies of MECP2.[119]

Sleep Disturbances in Rett Syndrome

Impaired sleep pattern is included in the supportive criteria for Rett syndrome.[118] In a large study that included 320 families, 80% of individuals experienced sleep problems with frequent nocturnal awakenings, bruxism, and difficulty falling asleep. Night laughing was present in 77% of individuals, and this occurred more often in persons with a deletion in MECP2. Age was associated with a decreased prevalence of sleep concerns. Sleep problems did not improve with treatment, but improvement over time was noted.[120]

Individuals with Rett syndrome have apnea and hypoventilation with bradycardia followed by exaggerated tachycardia. During episodes of cyanosis, these patients appear well despite the occurrence. A study of the PSG characteristics of Rett syndrome showed wakeful hypoventilation, central apnea, and hypoxia in 67% of girls with none of these during sleep.[121] This resulted in speculation of normal brain stem influence but faulty cortical influence on ventilation in patients with Rett's syndrome. Individuals with Rett syndrome may be at increased risk of CSA-hypopnea syndrome associated with hypoventilation. A study of 13 girls with Rett syndrome compared to 40 healthy controls showed ventilatory impairment during sleep.[122]

Treatment

Melatonin may be helpful for difficulties falling asleep in patients with Rett syndrome.[123] When used for its hypnotic effect, melatonin should be given 35 to 45 minutes before desired bedtime. A double-blind, placebo-controlled crossover study showed that melatonin (2.5 to 7.5 mg) used nightly reduced mean sleep latency in girls with Rett syndrome.[123] In several case reports, CPAP use for 1 to 2 hours during waking was shown to help treat daytime respiratory symptoms.[124] Positive airway pressure (mainly bilevel positive airway pressure) also is essential for management of CSA.

Fragile X Syndrome (FXS)

FXS is one of the most common genetic causes of intellectual disability.[125] Typically, the boys are affected more than girls.[126] It is estimated that 1 in 4,000 males and 1 in 6,000 to 8,000 females are born with the condition.[127] In addition to intellectual disability (mild to severe), there can be language abnormalities, communication difficulties, hyperactivity, and stereotypic behaviors. Patients with FXS have a characteristic physical appearance which includes hypotonia, a prominent forehead, an elongated face, high-arched palate, protruding ears, and macro-orchidism.[128] FXS is the most common single gene mutation known to cause ASD.[129]

Fragile X is an X-linked NDD involving an unstable trinucleotide repeat expansion of cytosine guanine (CGG) in the first exon of the FMR1 gene. This causes a reduction in the fragile X mental retardation protein. Individuals with the full mutation of fragile X have >200 CGG repeats with premutation carriers having 55 to 200 GG repeats.[128,130]

Sleep Disturbances in FXS

The literature on sleep disturbances in FXS is burgeoning. Kronk and colleagues[131] have performed two different studies examining sleep disturbances in FXS. A smaller study to evaluate sleep problems in 90 children with FXS using the Child Sleep Habits Questionnaire (CSHQ)

showed the prevalence of sleep problems to be 47%. Approximately, a fifth of the patients (19%) were on a sleep aid, although this did not decrease the amount of sleep disturbance.[131] In another study, a large cohort of 1,295 children with FXS was evaluated using a parental survey. Thirty-two percent of caregivers reported that their children had sleep difficulties. Common complaints were difficulty falling asleep (sleep onset insomnia) and frequent nocturnal awakenings (sleep maintenance insomnia).[14]

Hypotonia along with their facial morphology (high-arched palate) increase the risk of patients with FXS developing OSA. The Fragile X Clinical and Research Consortium Database showed a 7% prevalence of OSA in patients with FXS.[126] FMR 1 premutation carriers that have fragile X ataxia tremor syndrome have been shown to have an increased prevalence of OSA and are 3.4 times more likely to develop OSA.[132]

Treatment

In a thorough review of FXS, Kidd et al.[126] recommended that the primary care physician ask about sleep problems in children with FXS at every well child visit. Behavioral interventions with or without medical treatment may be warranted. A referral to a sleep specialist may be needed.[126] Behavioral intervention for sleep problems (mainly difficulty falling and staying asleep) may be effective in these patients.[133]

Williams Syndrome (WS)

WS is present in 1/7,500 individuals.[134] It is often recognized due to a diagnosis of congenital heart disease (supravalvular aortic stenosis, peripheral pulmonic stenosis). Additional features include intellectual disabilities, overfriendliness, anxiety, ADHD, endocrinopathies (hypercalcemia, hypothyroidism, and precocious puberty), FTT, hypotonia, hyperflexibility, and typical facies (e.g., stellate iris pattern).[135]

WS is caused by a contiguous gene deletion on chromosome 7q11.23. Diagnosis is by chromosomal microarray or fluorescent in situ hybrization. The critical gene appears to be the *elastin* (*ELN*)gene.[134]

Sleep Disturbances in WS

Sleep disturbances are reported in 65% of patients with WS.[136] Parent reported questionnaires completed for 64 participants with WS showed that 97% had sleep concerns. This included resistance to bedtime, sleep anxiety, frequent awakenings, and excessive daytime somnolence. Sleeps disorders have been correlated to daytime behavioral disturbances and learning difficulties in WS.[137] Studies based on parent-report demonstrated a correlation between language development scores in children with WS and nighttime sleep duration. Although age was correlated with language development, nighttime sleep duration accounted for 10% of the variance in a measure of language development.[138]

Patients with WS have increased sleep latency and decreased sleep efficiency.[136] Difficulty falling asleep and increased restlessness in WS patients compared to controls has been reported.[139] A study of nine adolescents with WS and nine controls confirmed these findings and found increased non-REM percentage, increased slow-wave sleep, decreased REM sleep percentage, increased number of periodic leg movements, and irregular sleep cycles.[140] Another study reported increased respiratory-related arousals and decreased sleep efficiency on PSG.[139]

Treatment

Abnormal or absent nocturnal melatonin peak is reported.[141,142] In particular, individuals with WS had increased bedtime cortisol and less pronounced rise in melatonin levels before sleep. This may suggest benefit with melatonin treatment

Smith–Magenis Syndrome (SMS)

SMS is present in 1/15,000 individuals. Typical features include developmental delays, significant sleep disturbance, maladaptive and self-injurious behaviors (often recognized after 18 months of age), feeding difficulties, FTT, hypotonia, sleepiness, and listlessness.[143]

SMS is caused by a deletion of chromosome 17p11.2 or by a mutation in retinoic acid induced 1 (RAI1 gene). Diagnostic work-up most often includes a chromosomal microarray, although fluorescence in situ hybridization (FISH) analysis can be completed. If the diagnosis is suspected and these studies are negative, molecular genetic testing of RAI1 should be performed.

Sleep Disturbances in SMS

Sleep disturbances in SMS are characterized by shortened sleep cycles with frequent nocturnal awakenings. Often, this is first noted after 18 months of age along with additional behavioral disturbances.[144] The more severe sleep disturbances are associated with increased severity of behavioral concerns. Delays in speech

development correlate in severity to sleep disorders as well.[145]

Treatment

It has been known for some time that children with SMS have shift in their circadian rhythm of melatonin. Peak time was 12 PM (compared to 3:30 AM in a control group).[146] Excessive daytime sleepiness is typical. Individuals with SMS have reversed circadian rhythms. While melatonin may be helpful, abnormalities in the metabolism of melatonin are not the sole cause of abnormal sleep in SMS.[147] Nonetheless, treatment is aimed at inversion of circadian rhythm, for example, with a beta-blocker, such as acebutolol 10mg/kg, in the morning to halt daily melatonin secretion. In addition, extended release melatonin (titrate 1 to 3 mg every 1 to 2 weeks to a maximum of 10 mg) should be given in the evening.[148]

CONCLUSIONS

Understanding of the unique features of sleep problems in patients with NDD is essential to formulate an appropriate treatment plan. Sleep problems and sleep disturbances in children with NDD are pervasive and a public health concern. Different interventions can be recommended depending on the type of developmental disorder, although behavioral intervention should be provided to all patients.

KEY CLINICAL PEARLS

- Prevalence of sleep disorders in children with NDD has been reported to be as high as 86%.
- Sleep disturbances in children with NDD likely represent a complex interaction of biological and environmental factors.
- Insomnia is the most common sleep problem in children with ASD.
- Evidence suggests a decrease in the amount of melatonin or the major metabolite of melatonin (urinary 6-sulphatoxymelatonin) in children and adolescents with ASD compared to controls.
- PSG data in ASD shows prolonged sleep latency, increased N1 sleep, decreased N2 and N3 sleep, lower REM sleep percentage, low sleep efficiency. and frequent nocturnal awakenings.
- Short sleep duration in children with ASD has been shown to be associated with stereotypic behaviors and social skill deficits.

- Children with DS presenting primarily with excessive daytime sleepiness should be evaluated for OSA, CSA, and hypoventilation.
- Craniofacial and upper airway abnormalities are primarily responsible for this higher prevalence of OSA in children with DS.
- All children with DS were recommended to have an overnight PSG by 4 years of age regardless of symptoms. In addition, every cardiologic follow-up should include screening for OSA, even after age 4.
- Hypersomnia can be a debilitating feature, which can exacerbate behavioral disturbances in children with PWS.
- GH therapy, a standard treatment for individuals with PWS, has been associated with increased risk of sudden death in patients with PWS and untreated OSA.
- Severity of seizures correlates with sleep disturbances in patients with Angelman syndrome.

SELF-ASSESSMENT QUESTIONS

A research study is being conducted evaluating sleep in children with NDD. It is a case control study using multiple validated pediatric questionnaires along with objective data from blood work and overnight PSG.

1. An 8-year old boy with ASD presents for a screening visit as part of the study protocol. His parents want him to be part of the study because he takes hours to fall asleep. He often will not fall asleep for 2 to 3 hours. His parents state that "he can't shut his brain down." He drinks caffeinated soda with dinner and plays video games after dinner. He can't settle down to go to sleep and leaves his room repeatedly to find his parents. Once asleep, he stays asleep. He does not have sleep-disordered breathing symptoms. He does not have symptoms concerning for seizures or reflux disorder. What should be used first line to treat this patient?
   a. Melatonin 1 to 3 mg by mouth 30 to 45 minutes before bed
   b. A sedating antidepressant 30 to 45 minutes before bed
   c. A sedating antiepileptic 30 to 45 minutes before bed
   d. Behavioral interventions

Answer: d

2. A 4-year old-boy with a history of Down syndrome meets the study entry criteria and is sent for an overnight polysomnogram. On the overnight polysomnogram, he is found to have moderate obstructive sleep apnea. What should be the next step in treating him?
   a. Referral to ENT for evaluation for adenotonsillectomy
   b. Referral back to the sleep lab for a CPAP titration
   c. Referral to a sleep dentist for evaluation for a dental appliance
   d. Watchful waiting

Answer: a

3. An 11-year-old girl with a history of Rett syndrome meets the study entry criteria and is sent for an overnight polysomnogram. Her parents deny snoring. However, she does have periods of respiratory pauses and gasping in sleep. She is not a sweaty sleeper. She does not have morning nasal congestion or headache. What is a common finding on polysomnogram in patients with Rett syndrome?
   a. A high percentage of REM sleep
   b. Central sleep apnea with associated hypoventilation
   c. Obstructive sleep apnea
   d. A normal sleep study

Answer: b

4. A 9-year-old girl with Smith–Magenis syndrome presents for a screening visit. Her parents want her in the study because she is having excessive daytime sleepiness along with difficulty falling and staying asleep at night. When she is asleep, they deny hearing snoring or respiratory pauses in sleep. She is not a sweaty sleeper. She does not have morning nasal congestion or headache. What is the most likely cause of her sleep symptoms?
   a. Central sleep apnea associated with hypoventilation
   b. Obstructive sleep apnea
   c. An inverted circadian rhythm
   d. Narcolepsy type 2 (formerly narcolepsy without cataplexy)

Answer: c

5. A 16-year-old boy with a history of Prader–Willi syndrome presents for a screening visit as part of the study protocol. His parents want him in the study because of his excessive daytime sleepiness. He has a history of OSA. He is status

post an adenotonsillectomy, and now he is using CPAP to treat his residual OSA. His adherence to CPAP is checked, and he is wearing CPAP nightly for 8 hours. His residual apnea hypopnea index in 0.9 (excellent adherence and effective treatment). What is a known effective treatment for his excessive daytime sleepiness?

a. Increase his CPAP pressure
b. Initiate modafinil to be taken in the morning
c. Initiate a traditional stimulant in the morning
d. No treatment

Answer: b

REFERENCES

1. Peirano PD, Algarin CR. Sleep in brain development. *Biol Res.* 2007;40(4):471–478.
2. Maquet P. The role of sleep in learning and memory. *Science.* 2001;294(5544):1048–1052.
3. Picchioni D, Reith RM, Nadel JL, Smith CB. Sleep, plasticity and the pathophysiology of neurodevelopmental disorders: the potential roles of protein synthesis and other cellular processes. *Brain Sci.* 2014;4(1):150–201.
4. Maski KP, Kothare SV. Sleep deprivation and neurobehavioral functioning in children. *Int J Psychophysiol.* 2013;89(2):259–264.
5. Cassoff J, Bhatti JA, Gruber R. The effect of sleep restriction on neurobehavioural functioning in normally developing children and adolescents: insights from the Attention, Behaviour and Sleep Laboratory. *Pathologie-biologie.* 2014;62(5):319–331.
6. Gozal D. Sleep-disordered breathing and school performance in children. *Pediatrics.* 1998;102(3 Pt 1):616–620.
7. Gregory AM, Sadeh A. Sleep, emotional and behavioral difficulties in children and adolescents. *Sleep Med Rev.* 2012;16(2):129–136.
8. Owens JA, Witmans M. Sleep problems. *Curr Probl Pediatr Adolesc Health Care.* 2004;34(4):154–179.
9. Mindell JA, Meltzer LJ, Carskadon MA, Chervin RD. Developmental aspects of sleep hygiene: findings from the 2004 National Sleep Foundation Sleep in America poll. *Sleep Med.* 2009;10(7):771–779.
10. Didden R, Sigafoos J. A review of the nature and treatment of sleep disorders in individuals with developmental disabilities. *Res Dev Disabil.* 2001;22(4):255–272.
11. Harvey MT, Kennedy CH. Polysomnographic phenotypes in developmental disabilities. *Int J Dev Neurosci.* 2002;20(3–5):443–448.
12. Cotton S, Richdale A. Brief report: parental descriptions of sleep problems in children with autism, Down syndrome, and Prader–Willi syndrome. *Res Dev Disabil.* 2006;27(2):151–161.
13. Angriman M, Caravale B, Novelli L, Ferri R, Bruni O. Sleep in children with neurodevelopmental disabilities. *Neuropediatrics.* 2015;46(3):199–210.
14. Kronk R, Bishop EE, Raspa M, Bickel JO, Mandel DA, Bailey DB Jr. Prevalence, nature, and correlates of sleep problems among children with fragile X syndrome based on a large scale parent survey. *Sleep.* 2010;33(5):679–687.
15. Spence SJ. The genetics of autism. *Sem Ped Neurol.* 2004;11(3):196–204.
16. Grigg-Damberger M, Ralls F. Treatment strategies for complex behavioral insomnia in children with neurodevelopmental disorders. *Curr Op Pulmonary Med.* 2013;19(6):616–625.
17. American Psychiatric Association. *Diagnostic and Statistical Manual of Mental Disorders.* 5th ed. Washington, DC: American Psychiatric Association; 2013.
18. Souders MC, Mason TB, Valladares O, et al. Sleep behaviors and sleep quality in children with autism spectrum disorders. *Sleep.* 2009;32(12):1566–1578.
19. Allik H, Larsson JO, Smedje H. Sleep patterns of school-age children with Asperger syndrome or high-functioning autism. *J Autism Dev Disord.* 2006;36(5):585–595.
20. Richdale AL, Schreck KA. Sleep problems in autism spectrum disorders: prevalence, nature, & possible biopsychosocial aetiologies. *Sleep Med Rev.* 2009;13(6):403–411.
21. Hollway JA, Aman MG, Butter E. Correlates and risk markers for sleep disturbance in participants of the Autism Treatment Network. *J Autism Dev Disord.* 2013;43(12):2830–2843.
22. Bourgeron T. The possible interplay of synaptic and clock genes in autism spectrum disorders. *Cold Spring Harbor Sym Quant Biol.* 2007;72:645–654.
23. Wimpory D, Nicholas B, Nash S. Social timing, clock genes and autism: a new hypothesis. *J Intellect Disabil Res.* 2002;46(Pt 4):352–358.
24. Rosenwasser AM, Turek FW. Neurobiology of circadian rhythm regulation. *Sleep Med Clin.* 2015;10(4):403–412.
25. Yang Z, Matsumoto A, Nakayama K, et al. Circadian-relevant genes are highly polymorphic in autism spectrum disorder patients. *Brain Dev.* 2016;38(1):91–99.
26. Ackermann K, Stehle JH. Melatonin synthesis in the human pineal gland: advantages, implications, and difficulties. *Chronobiol Int.* 2006;23(1–2):369–379.
27. Tordjman S, Anderson GM, Pichard N, Charbuy H, Touitou Y. Nocturnal excretion of

6-sulphatoxymelatonin in children and adolescents with autistic disorder. *Biol Psychiatry.* 2005;57(2):134–138.

28. Melke J, Goubran Botros H, Chaste P, et al. Abnormal melatonin synthesis in autism spectrum disorders. *Mole Psychiatry.* 2008;13(1):90–98.

29. Mulder EJ, Anderson GM, Kemperman RF, Oosterloo-Duinkerken A, Minderaa RB, Kema IP. Urinary excretion of 5-hydroxyindoleacetic acid, serotonin and 6-sulphatoxymelatonin in normoserotonemic and hyperserotonemic autistic individuals. *Neuropsychobiology.* 2010;61(1):27–32.

30. Veatch OJ, Goldman SE, Adkins KW, Malow BA. Melatonin in children with autism spectrum disorders: how does the evidence fit together? *J Nature Science.* 2015;1(7):e125.

31. Souders MC, Zavodny S, Eriksen W, et al. Sleep in children with autism spectrum disorder. *Curr Psychiatry Rep.* 2017;19(6):34.

32. Krakowiak P, Goodlin-Jones B, Hertz-Picciotto I, Croen LA, Hansen RL. Sleep problems in children with autism spectrum disorders, developmental delays, and typical development: a population-based study. *J Sleep Res.* 2008;17(2):197–206.

33. Schreck KA, Mulick JA. Parental report of sleep problems in children with autism. *J Autism Dev Disord.* 2000;30(2):127–135.

34. Richdale AL, Prior MR. The sleep/wake rhythm in children with autism. *Eur Child Adolesc Psychiatry.* 1995;4(3):175–186.

35. Liu X, Hubbard JA, Fabes RA, Adam JB. Sleep disturbances and correlates of children with autism spectrum disorders. *Child Psychiatry Hum Dev.* 2006;37(2):179–191.

36. Kotagal S, Broomall E. Sleep in children with autism spectrum disorder. *Pediatric Neurol.* 2012;47(4):242–251.

37. Sivertsen B, Posserud MB, Gillberg C, Lundervold AJ, Hysing M. Sleep problems in children with autism spectrum problems: a longitudinal population-based study. *Autism.* 2012;16(2):139–150.

38. Reynolds AM, Malow BA. Sleep and autism spectrum disorders. *Ped Clin N Am.* 2011;58(3):685–698.

39. Baker EK, Richdale AL. Sleep patterns in adults with a diagnosis of high-functioning autism spectrum disorder. *Sleep.* 2015;38(11):1765–1774.

40. Limoges E, Mottron L, Bolduc C, Berthiaume C, Godbout R. Atypical sleep architecture and the autism phenotype. *Brain.* 2005;128(Pt 5):1049–1061.

41. Miano S, Bruni O, Elia M, et al. Sleep in children with autistic spectrum disorder: a questionnaire and polysomnographic study. *Sleep Med.* 2007;9(1):64–70.

42. Buckley AW, Rodriguez AJ, Jennison K, et al. Rapid eye movement sleep percentage in children with autism compared with children with developmental delay and typical development. *Arch Ped Adolesc Med.* 2010;164(11):1032–1037.

43. Malow BA, Marzec ML, McGrew SG, Wang L, Henderson LM, Stone WL. Characterizing sleep in children with autism spectrum disorders: a multidimensional approach. *Sleep.* 2006;29(12):1563–1571.

44. Cohen S, Conduit R, Lockley SW, Rajaratnam SM, Cornish KM. The relationship between sleep and behavior in autism spectrum disorder (ASD): a review. *J Neurodev Disord.* 2014;6(1):44.

45. Veatch OJ, Sutcliffe JS, Warren ZE, Keenan BT, Potter MH, Malow BA. Shorter sleep duration is associated with social impairment and comorbidities in ASD. *Autism Res.* 2017;10(7):1221–1238.

46. Johnson KP, Malow BA. Assessment and pharmacologic treatment of sleep disturbance in autism. *Child Adolesc Psychiatric Clin N Am.* 2008;17(4):773–785, viii.

47. May T, Cornish K, Conduit R, Rajaratnam SM, Rinehart NJ. Sleep in high-functioning children with autism: longitudinal developmental change and associations with behavior problems. *Behav Sleep Med.* 2015;13(1):2–18.

48. Sikora DM, Johnson K, Clemons T, Katz T. The relationship between sleep problems and daytime behavior in children of different ages with autism spectrum disorders. *Pediatrics.* 2012;130(Suppl 2):S83–S90.

49. Malow BA, Byars K, Johnson K, et al. A practice pathway for the identification, evaluation, and management of insomnia in children and adolescents with autism spectrum disorders. *Pediatrics.* 2012;130(Suppl 2):S106–S124.

50. Malow BA, Adkins KW, Reynolds A, et al. Parent-based sleep education for children with autism spectrum disorders. *J Autism Dev Disord.* 2014;44(1):216–228.

51. Johnson CR, Turner KS, Foldes E, Brooks MM, Kronk R, Wiggs L. Behavioral parent training to address sleep disturbances in young children with autism spectrum disorder: a pilot trial. *Sleep Med.* 2013;14(10):995–1004.

52. Guenole F, Godbout R, Nicolas A, Franco P, Claustrat B, Baleyte JM. Melatonin for disordered sleep in individuals with autism spectrum disorders: systematic review and discussion. *Sleep Med Rev.* 2011;15(6):379–387.

53. Robinson AA, Malow BA. Gabapentin shows promise in treating refractory insomnia in children. *J Child Neurol.* 2013;28(12):1618–1621.

54. McCall C, McCall WV. What is the role of sedating antidepressants, antipsychotics, and

anticonvulsants in the management of insomnia? *Curr Psychiatry Rep.* 2012;14(5):494–502.

55. Parker SE, Mai CT, Canfield MA, et al. Updated National Birth Prevalence estimates for selected birth defects in the United States, 2004-2006. *Birth Def Res Part A, Clin Mol Teratol.* 2010;88(12):1008–1016.

56. Hassold T, Sherman S. Down syndrome: genetic recombination and the origin of the extra chromosome 21. *Clin Genet.* 2000;57(2):95–100.

57. de Miguel-Diez J, Alvarez-Sala JL, Villa-Asensi JR. Magnetic resonance imaging of the upper airway in children with Down syndrome. *Am J Resp Crit Care Med.* 2002;165(8):1187; author reply 1187.

58. Bertrand P, Navarro H, Caussade S, Holmgren N, Sanchez I. Airway anomalies in children with Down syndrome: endoscopic findings. *Ped Pulmonol.* 2003;36(2):137–141.

59. Hoffmire CA, Magyar CI, Connolly HV, Fernandez ID, van Wijngaarden E. High prevalence of sleep disorders and associated comorbidities in a community sample of children with Down syndrome. *J Clin Sleep Med.* 2014;10(4):411–419.

60. Breslin J, Spano G, Bootzin R, Anand P, Nadel L, Edgin J. Obstructive sleep apnea syndrome and cognition in Down syndrome. *Dev Med Child Neurol.* 2014;56(7):657–664.

61. Senthilvel E, Krishna J. Body position and obstructive sleep apnea in children with Down syndrome. *J Clin Sleep Med.* 2011;7(2):158–162.

62. Mims M, Thottam PJ, Kitsko D, Shaffer A, Choi S. Characterization of sleep architecture in Down syndrome patients pre and post airway surgery. *Cureus.* 2017;9(1):e983.

63. Nisbet LC, Phillips NN, Hoban TF, O'Brien LM. Characterization of a sleep architectural phenotype in children with Down syndrome. *Sleep Breath/Schlaf & Atmung.* 2015;19(3):1065–1071.

64. Fan Z, Ahn M, Roth HL, Li L, Vaughn BV. Sleep apnea and hypoventilation in patients with Down syndrome: analysis of 144 polysomnogram studies. *Children (Basel, Switzerland).* 2017;4(7).

65. de Miguel-Diez J, Villa-Asensi JR, Alvarez-Sala JL. Prevalence of sleep-disordered breathing in children with Down syndrome: polygraphic findings in 108 children. *Sleep.* 2003;26(8):1006–1009.

66. Dyken ME, Lin-Dyken DC, Poulton S, Zimmerman MB, Sedars E. Prospective polysomnographic analysis of obstructive sleep apnea in down syndrome. *Arch Ped Adolesc Medic.* 2003;157(7):655–660.

67. Hill EA. Obstructive sleep apnoea/hypopnoea syndrome in adults with Down syndrome. *Breathe (Sheffield, England).* 2016;12(4):e91–e96.

68. Maris M, Verhulst S, Wojciechowski M, Van de Heyning P, Boudewyns A. Outcome of adenotonsillectomy in children with Down syndrome and obstructive sleep apnoea. *Arch Dis Child.* 2017;102(4):331–336.

69. Cua CL, Blankenship A, North AL, Hayes J, Nelin LD. Increased incidence of idiopathic persistent pulmonary hypertension in Down syndrome neonates. *Ped Cardiol.* 2007;28(4):250–254.

70. Carskadon MA, Pueschel SM, Millman RP. Sleep-disordered breathing and behavior in three risk groups: preliminary findings from parental reports. *Child Nerv Syst.* 1993;9(8):452–457.

71. Andreou G, Galanopoulou C, Gourgoulianis K, Karapetsas A, Molyvdas P. Cognitive status in Down syndrome individuals with sleep disordered breathing deficits (SDB). *Brain Cogn.* 2002;50(1):145–149.

72. Bull MJ. Health supervision for children with Down syndrome. *Pediatrics.* 2011;128(2):393–406.

73. Goffinski A, Stanley MA, Shepherd N, et al. Obstructive sleep apnea in young infants with Down syndrome evaluated in a Down syndrome specialty clinic. *Am J Med Genet A.* 2015;167A(2):324–330.

74. Shete MM, Stocks RM, Sebelik ME, Schoumacher RA. Effects of adeno-tonsillectomy on polysomnography patterns in Down syndrome children with obstructive sleep apnea: a comparative study with children without Down syndrome. *Int J Pediatr Otorhinolaryngol.* 2010;74(3):241–244.

75. Goldstein NA, Armfield DR, Kingsley LA, Borland LM, Allen GC, Post JC. Postoperative complications after tonsillectomy and adenoidectomy in children with Down syndrome. *Arch Otolaryngol Head Neck Surg.* 1998;124(2):171–176.

76. Marcus CL, Rosen G, Ward SL, et al. Adherence to and effectiveness of positive airway pressure therapy in children with obstructive sleep apnea. *Pediatrics.* 2006;117(3):e442–e451.

77. Hawkins SM, Jensen EL, Simon SL, Friedman NR. Correlates of Pediatric CPAP Adherence. *J Clin Sleep Med.* 2016;12(6):879–884.

78. Driscoll DJ, Miller JL, Schwartz S, Cassidy SB. Prader–Willi syndrome. In: Pagon RA, Adam MP, Ardinger HH, et al., eds. *GeneReviews*. https://www.ncbi.nlm.nih.gov/books/NBK1330/. October 6, 1998; last revision: December 14, 2017.

79. Swaab DF. Prader–Willi syndrome and the hypothalamus. *Acta Paed.* 1997;423(Suppl):50–54.

80. Miller JL, Lynn CH, Driscoll DC, et al. Nutritional phases in Prader–Willi syndrome. *Am J Med Genet A.* 2011;155A(5):1040–1049.

81. State MW, Dykens EM. Genetics of childhood disorders: XV. Prader–Willi syndrome: genes,

brain, and behavior. *J Am Acad Child Adolesc Psychiatry.* 2000;39(6):797–800.

82. Arens R, Gozal D, Omlin KJ, et al. Hypoxic and hypercapnic ventilatory responses in Prader–Willi syndrome. *J Appl Physiol (1985–).* 1994;77(5):2224–2230.

83. Gillett ES, Perez IA. Disorders of sleep and ventilatory control in Prader–Willi syndrome. *Diseases (Basel, Switzerland).* 2016;4(3).

84. Khayat A, Narang I, Bin-Hasan S, Amin R, Al-Saleh S. Longitudinal evaluation of sleep disordered breathing in infants with Prader–Willi syndrome. *Arch Dis Child.* 2017;102(7):638–642.

85. Cohen M, Hamilton J, Narang I. Clinically important age-related differences in sleep related disordered breathing in infants and children with Prader–Willi Syndrome. *PLoS One.* 2014;9(6):e101012.

86. Sedky K, Bennett DS, Pumariega A. Prader–Willi syndrome and obstructive sleep apnea: co-occurrence in the pediatric population. *J Clin Sleep Med.* 2014;10(4):403–409.

87. Ghergan A, Coupaye M, Leu-Semenescu S, et al. Prevalence and phenotype of sleep disorders in 60 adults with Prader-Willi syndrome. *Sleep.* 2017:zsx162-zsx162.

88. Mignot E, Lammers GJ, Ripley B, et al. The role of cerebrospinal fluid hypocretin measurement in the diagnosis of narcolepsy and other hypersomnias. *Arch Neurol.* 2002;59(10):1553–1562.

89. Omokawa M, Ayabe T, Nagai T, et al. Decline of CSF orexin (hypocretin) levels in Prader–Willi syndrome. *Am J Med Genet A.* 2016;170A(5):1181–1186.

90. Tobias ES, Tolmie JL, Stephenson JB. Cataplexy in the Prader–Willi syndrome. *Arch Dis Child.* 2002;87(2):170.

91. Mignot E, Thorsby E. Narcolepsy and the HLA system. *N Engl J Med.* 2001;344(9):692.

92. Dykens EM, Cassidy SB, King BH. Maladaptive behavior differences in Prader–Willi syndrome due to paternal deletion versus maternal uniparental disomy. *Am J Mental Retard.* 1999;104(1):67–77.

93. Richdale AL, Cotton S, Hibbit K. Sleep and behaviour disturbance in Prader–Willi syndrome: a questionnaire study. *J Intellect Disabil Res.* 1999;43 (Pt 5):380–392.

94. Wigren M, Hansen S. ADHD symptoms and insistence on sameness in Prader–Willi syndrome. *J Intellect Disabil Res.* 2005;49(Pt 6):449–456.

95. Craig ME, Cowell CT, Larsson P, et al. Growth hormone treatment and adverse events in Prader–Willi syndrome: data from KIGS (the Pfizer International Growth Database). *Clin Endocrinol.* 2006;65(2):178–185.

96. De Cock VC, Diene G, Molinas C, et al. Efficacy of modafinil on excessive daytime sleepiness in Prader–Willi syndrome. *Am J Med Genet A.* 2011;155A(7):1552–1557.

97. Weselake SV, Foulds JL, Couch R, Witmans MB, Rubin D, Haqq AM. Prader–Willi syndrome, excessive daytime sleepiness, and narcoleptic symptoms: a case report. *J Med Case Rep.* 2014;8:127.

98. Dagli AI, Mueller J, Williams CA. Angelman syndrome. In: Adam MP, Ardinger HH, Pagon RA, et al., eds. *GeneReviews®.* https://www.ncbi.nlm.nih.gov/books/NBK1144/. September 15, 1998; last revision: December 21, 2017

99. Mabb AM, Judson MC, Zylka MJ, Philpot BD. Angelman syndrome: insights into genomic imprinting and neurodevelopmental phenotypes. *Trends Neurosci.* 2011;34(6):293–303.

100. Williams CA, Beaudet AL, Clayton-Smith J, et al. Angelman syndrome 2005: updated consensus for diagnostic criteria. *Am J Med Genet A.* 2006;140(5):413–418.

101. Zori RT, Hendrickson J, Woolven S, Whidden EM, Gray B, Williams CA. Angelman syndrome: clinical profile. *J Child Neurol.* 1992;7(3):270–280.

102. Clayton-Smith J. Clinical research on Angelman syndrome in the United Kingdom: observations on 82 affected individuals. *Am J Med Genet.* 1993;46(1):12–15.

103. Summers JA, Allison DB, Lynch PS, Sandler L. Behaviour problems in Angelman syndrome. *J Intellect Disabil Res.* 1995;39 (Pt 2):97–106.

104. Shi SQ, Bichell TJ, Ihrie RA, Johnson CH. Ube3a imprinting impairs circadian robustness in Angelman syndrome models. *Curr Biol.* 2015;25(5):537–545.

105. Pelc K, Cheron G, Boyd SG, Dan B. Are there distinctive sleep problems in Angelman syndrome? *Sleep Med.* 2008;9(4):434–441.

106. Walz NC, Beebe D, Byars K. Sleep in individuals with Angelman syndrome: parent perceptions of patterns and problems. *American J Ment Retard.* 2005;110(4):243–252.

107. Bruni O, Ferri R, D'Agostino G, Miano S, Roccella M, Elia M. Sleep disturbances in Angelman syndrome: a questionnaire study. *Brain Dev.* 2004;26(4):233–240.

108. Dan B, Boyd SG. Angelman syndrome reviewed from a neurophysiological perspective: the UBE3A-GABRB3 hypothesis. *Neuropediatrics.* 2003;34(4):169–176.

109. Miano S, Bruni O, Elia M, Musumeci SA, Verrillo E, Ferri R. Sleep breathing and periodic leg movement pattern in Angelman Syndrome:

a polysomnographic study. *Clin Neurophysiol.* 2005;116(11):2685–2692.

110. Robinson-Shelton A, Malow BA. Sleep Disturbances in Neurodevelopmental Disorders. *Curr Psychiatry Rep.* 2016;18(1):6.

111. Nunes ML, Ferri R, Arzimanoglou A, Curzi L, Appel CC, Costa da Costa J. Sleep organization in children with partial refractory epilepsy. *J Child Neurol.* 2003;18(11):763–766.

112. Herman ST, Walczak TS, Bazil CW. Distribution of partial seizures during the sleep--wake cycle: differences by seizure onset site. *Neurology.* 2001;56(11):1453–1459.

113. Conant KD, Thibert RL, Thiele EA. Epilepsy and the sleep-wake patterns found in Angelman syndrome. *Epilepsia.* 2009;50(11): 2497–2500.

114. Huntsman MM, Porcello DM, Homanics GE, DeLorey TM, Huguenard JR. Reciprocal inhibitory connections and network synchrony in the mammalian thalamus. *Science.* 1999;283(5401):541–543.

115. DeLorey TM, Handforth A, Anagnostaras SG, et al. Mice lacking the beta3 subunit of the GABAA receptor have the epilepsy phenotype and many of the behavioral characteristics of Angelman syndrome. *J Neurosci.* 1998;18(20): 8505–8514.

116. Allen KD, Kuhn BR, DeHaai KA, Wallace DP. Evaluation of a behavioral treatment package to reduce sleep problems in children with Angelman Syndrome. *Res Dev Disabil.* 2013;34(1):676–686.

117. Zhdanova IV, Wurtman RJ, Wagstaff J. Effects of a low dose of melatonin on sleep in children with Angelman syndrome. *J Pediatr Endocrinol Metab.* 1999;12(1):57–67.

118. Christodoulou J, Ho G. MECP2-related disorders. In: Adam MP, Ardinger HH, Pagon RA, et al., eds. *GeneReviews®*. https://www.ncbi.nlm. nih.gov/books/NBK1497/. October 3, 2001; last revision: September 19, 2019

119. Amir RE, Van den Veyver IB, Wan M, Tran CQ, Francke U, Zoghbi HY. Rett syndrome is caused by mutations in X-linked MECP2, encoding methyl-CpG-binding protein 2. *Nature Genet.* 1999;23(2):185–188.

120. Wong K, Leonard H, Jacoby P, Ellaway C, Downs J. The trajectories of sleep disturbances in Rett syndrome. *J Sleep Res.* 2015;24(2):223–233.

121. Marcus CL, Carroll JL, McColley SA, et al. Polysomnographic characteristics of patients with Rett syndrome. *J Pediatr.* 1994;125(2): 218–224.

122. Carotenuto M, Esposito M, D'Aniello A, et al. Polysomnographic findings in Rett syndrome:

a case-control study. *Sleep Breath.* 2013;17(1): 93–98.

123. McArthur AJ, Budden SS. Sleep dysfunction in Rett syndrome: a trial of exogenous melatonin treatment. *Dev Med Child Neurol.* 1998;40(3):186–192.

124. Julu PO, Witt Engerstrom I, Hansen S, Apartopoulos F, Engerstrom B. Treating hypoxia in a feeble breather with Rett syndrome. *Brain Dev.* 2013;35(3):270–273.

125. Hersh JH, Saul RA. Health supervision for children with fragile X syndrome. *Pediatrics.* 2011;127(5):994–1006.

126. Kidd SA, Lachiewicz A, Barbouth D, et al. Fragile X syndrome: a review of associated medical problems. *Pediatrics.* 2014;134(5):995–1005.

127. Keysor CS, Mazzocco MM. A developmental approach to understanding Fragile X syndrome in females. *Microsc Res Tech.* 2002;57(3):179–186.

128. McLennan Y, Polussa J, Tassone F, Hagerman R. Fragile x syndrome. *Curr Genom.* 2011;12(3):216–224.

129. Won J, Jin Y, Choi J, et al. Melatonin as a Novel interventional candidate for fragile X syndrome with autism spectrum disorder in humans. *Int J Mole Sci.* 2017;18(6).

130. Willemsen R, Oostra BA, Bassell GJ, Dictenberg J. The fragile X syndrome: from molecular genetics to neurobiology. *Ment Retard Dev Disabil Res Rev.* 2004;10(1):60–67.

131. Kronk R, Dahl R, Noll R. Caregiver reports of sleep problems on a convenience sample of children with fragile X syndrome. *Am J Intellect Dev Disabil.* 2009;114(6):383–392.

132. Hamlin A, Liu Y, Nguyen DV, Tassone F, Zhang L, Hagerman RJ. Sleep apnea in fragile X premutation carriers with and without FXTAS. *Am J Med Genet Part B, Neuropsychiatric Genet.* 2011;156b(8):923–928.

133. Weiskop S, Richdale A, Matthews J. Behavioural treatment to reduce sleep problems in children with autism or fragile X syndrome. *Dev Med Child Neurol.* 2005;47(2):94–104.

134. Morris CA. Williams syndrome. In: Adam MP, Ardinger HH, Pagon RA, et al., eds. *GeneReviews®*. https://www.ncbi.nlm.nih.gov/ books/NBK1249/. April 9, 1999; last revision: March 23, 2017.

135. Martens MA, Wilson SJ, Reutens DC. Research review: Williams syndrome: a critical review of the cognitive, behavioral, and neuroanatomical phenotype. *J Child Psychology Psychiatry All Disc.* 2008;49(6):576–608.

136. Goldman SE, Malow BA, Newman KD, Roof E, Dykens EM. Sleep patterns and daytime sleepiness in adolescents and young adults

with Williams syndrome. *J Intellect Disabil Res.* 2009;53(2):182–188.

137. Annaz D, Hill CM, Ashworth A, Holley S, Karmiloff-Smith A. Characterisation of sleep problems in children with Williams syndrome. *Res Dev Disabil.* 2011;32(1):164–169.

138. Axelsson EL, Hill CM, Sadeh A, Dimitriou D. Sleep problems and language development in toddlers with Williams syndrome. *Res Dev Disabil.* 2013;34(11):3988–3996.

139. Mason TB, Arens R, Sharman J, et al. Sleep in children with Williams syndrome. *Sleep Med.* 2011;12(9):892–897.

140. Gombos F, Bodizs R, Kovacs I. Atypical sleep architecture and altered EEG spectra in Williams syndrome. *J Intellect Disabil Res.* 2011;55(3):255–262.

141. Sniecinska-Cooper AM, Iles RK, Butler SA, Jones H, Bayford R, Dimitriou D. Abnormal secretion of melatonin and cortisol in relation to sleep disturbances in children with Williams syndrome. *Sleep Med.* 2015;16(1): 94–100.

142. Santoro SD, Giacheti CM, Rossi NF, Campos LM, Pinato L. Correlations between behavior, memory, sleep-wake and melatonin in Williams-Beuren syndrome. *Physiol Behav.* 2016;159:14–19.

143. Smith ACM, Boyd KE, Elsea SH, et al. Smith–Magenis syndrome. In: Adam MP, Ardinger HH, Pagon RA, et al., eds. *GeneReviews®.* https://www.ncbi.nlm.nih.gov/books/NBK1310/. October 22, 2001; last revision: September 5, 2019.

144. Gropman AL, Duncan WC, Smith AC. Neurologic and developmental features of the Smith–Magenis syndrome (del 17p11.2). *Pediatr Neurol.* 2006;34(5):337–350.

145. Poisson A, Nicolas A, Sanlaville D, et al. [Smith–Magenis syndrome is an association of behavioral and sleep/wake circadian rhythm disorders]. *Arch Pediatr.* 2015;22(6):638–645.

146. De Leersnyder H, De Blois MC, Claustrat B, et al. Inversion of the circadian rhythm of melatonin in the Smith–Magenis syndrome. *J Pediatr.* 2001;139(1):111–116.

147. Novakova M, Nevsimalova S, Prihodova I, Sladek M, Sumova A. Alteration of the circadian clock in children with Smith–Magenis syndrome. *J Clin Endocrinol Metab.* 2012;97(2):E312–E318.

148. Carpizo R, Martinez A, Mediavilla D, Gonzalez M, Abad A, Sanchez-Barcelo EJ. Smith–Magenis syndrome: a case report of improved sleep after treatment with beta1-adrenergic antagonists and melatonin. *J Pediatr.* 2006;149(3):409–411.

24

Delirium

KOTARO HATTA

INTRODUCTION

The fundamental aspect of delirium is altered consciousness and its fluctuation.[1] Delirium represents a disturbance in attention, awareness, and cognition, which develops over a short period of time and tends to fluctuate.[2] The diagnostic criteria of delirium, based on the *Diagnostic and Statistical Manual of Mental Disorders* (fifth edition; DSM-5,[2] include the following:

A. A disturbance in attention (i.e., reduced ability to direct, focus, sustain, and shift attention) and awareness (reduced orientation to the environment).

B. The disturbance develops over a short period of time (usually hours to a few days), represents a change from baseline attention and awareness and tends to fluctuate in severity during the course of a day.

C. An additional disturbance in cognition (e.g., memory deficit, disorientation, language, visuospatial ability, or perception).

D. The disturbances in Criteria A and C are not better explained by another pre-existing, established, or evolving neurocognitive disorder and do not occur in the context of a severely reduced level of arousal, such as coma.

E. There is evidence from the history, physical examination, or laboratory findings that the disturbance is a direct physiological consequence of another medical condition, substance intoxication or withdrawal (i.e., due to a drug of abuse or to a medication), or exposure to a toxin, or is due to multiple etiologies.

In addition, sleep–wake cycle disturbance is one of clinical core features of delirium.[3] Excessive release of dopamine, noradrenaline, and glutamate and reduced availability of acetylcholine are considered physiological factors leading to sleep–wake cycle fragmentation in delirium.[4] Simultaneously, anxiety due to change in environment, such as hospitalization, can lead to sleep–wake cycle fragmentation in elderly patients with mild cognitive impairment or dementia.[5]

The prevalence of delirium is 18% to 50% on admission, and the incidence during hospitalization is 10% to 82% in general medical and geriatric wards, the intensive care unit (ICU), postoperative, and palliative care settings.[6] Furthermore, increase in the incidence of delirium seems likely with the increase in the aging population. Delirium used to be considered as a transient phenomenon; however, growing literature shows that necessarily may not be true. Delirium has been shown to be independently associated with an increased risk of death (odds ratio [OR] 2.0; 95% confidence interval [CI] 1.5–2.5).[7] Delirium reportedly increased the risk of incident dementia (OR 8.7, 95% CI 2.1–35), and was associated with worsening dementia severity (OR 3.1, 95% CI 1.5–6.3), deterioration in global function score (OR 2.8, 95% CI 1.4–5.5), and loss of 1 or more Mini-Mental State Examination points per year (95% CI 0.11–1.89) than those with no history of delirium.[8]

The initial management of people with delirium includes identification and management of the possible underlying causes, effective communication and reorientation techniques, provision of suitable care environment, and provision of reassurance to patients and family.[9] For management of agitation associated with delirium, it is recommended to use verbal and nonverbal de-escalation techniques and to consider an antipsychotic medication, at the lowest effective dose, on a short-term basis. The need for effective sleep-focused treatment strategies for prevention and treatment of delirium is clearly evident. As nonpharmacologic prevention, a multicomponent intervention strategy with proven effectiveness includes early mobilization and promoting sleep.[6] Some evidence exists that psychotropic medications with hypnotic properties including antipsychotics[9,10] and antidepressants, such as trazodone[11] and mianserin,[12] reportedly having beneficial treatment effects on delirium.[13-16] However, there is an apparent lack of synthesized literature that guides the psychiatrists to learn sleep-focused prevention and treatment strategies for delirium, including new developments in this field. This chapters aims to further our understanding of the role of sleep in the pathophysiology and management of delirium.

SLEEP AND DELIRIUM: PATHOPHYSIOLOGY

Delirium is a neurobehavioral syndrome caused by dysregulation of neuronal activity secondary to systemic disturbances. So far, several hypotheses such as neuroinflammatory, neuronal aging, oxidative stress, neurotransmitter deficiency, neuroendocrine, diurnal dysregulation, and network disconnectivity have been proposed.[4] Sleep–wake cycle disturbances are plausible contributing factors toward pathophysiology of delirium given that hospitalized patients experience multiple sleep alterations including sleep loss, sleep fragmentation, and sleep–wake cycle disorganization. Also, there is some emerging literature suggesting that *PER* clock gene function may be disturbed in delirium.[17,18] Additionally, diurnal sleep/melatonin dysregulation and orexin neurotransmission deserve further mention here due to their key role in sleep–wake cycle regulation.[4]

Melatonin

Melatonin is synthesized primarily in the pineal gland from L-tryptophan by way of serotonin. Melatonin has a variety of physiological functions such as regulation of circadian rhythms, vasomotor responses, sleep, retinal neuromodulation, inflammatory and immune processes, and scavenging oxidative stress.[19] Melatonin shows these functions via binding with various proteins, such as MT_1 and MT_2 receptors. The MT_1 receptor plays a role in acute inhibition of firing from the suprachiasmatic nucleus, and the MT_2 receptor plays a role in phase-shifting effects on circadian rhythms. Plasma melatonin begins to increase in the evening and reaches its peak around 2 AM. Such nocturnal secretion is a major characteristic of melatonin that promotes sleep with nocturnal hypotensive, vasodilating, and hypothermic action. However, the nocturnal secretion of melatonin decreases with age. Nair et al.[20] reported plasma melatonin secretion with low peak among elderly men (mean age = 68 years) as compared to the high peak among young men (mean age =

24 year). These findings may have clinical implications such that the hospitalized elderly patients are vulnerable to circadian related sleep–wake disturbances, and hence to delirium, due much lower peak of melatonin secretion.

The anti-inflammatory properties of melatonin deserve a mention here due to the relationship between neuroinflammation and development of delirium. Melatonin is derived from L-tryptophan through the methoxyindole pathway. Neuroinflammation can activate the kynurenine pathway and decrease the biosynthesis of melatonin,[21] Interestingly, reduced levels of endogenous melatonin have also been established in various delirium-risk conditions, such as ischemic heart disease, advanced diabetes, and certain types of cancers.[22-24] In addition, not only neuroprotective but neurotoxic metabolites are also produced through the kynurenine pathway. Adams-Wilson et al.[25] examined the relationship between kynurenine/tryptophan ratio and delirium/coma free days and found a significant negative correlation.

Fink et al.[26] reported effects of melatonin and ramelteon on survival rate after sepsis in rats. In this placebo-controlled study, the administration of melatonin or ramelteon significantly improved median survival time. In addition, this effect was completely antagonized by co-administration of luzindole, a potent melatonin receptor antagonist. Furthermore, the authors reported that melatonin, ramelteon, or luzindole had no significant effect on survival time in MT_1 and MT_2 receptor knockout mice. Interestingly, prolongation of survival time by melatonin was dose-dependent.

Finally, potent antioxidant ability of melatonin should be mentioned. Reduced levels of endogenous melatonin have been established in various conditions such as ischemic brain disease[27] and ischemic heart disease.[28] In a study by our group, described later, the admission diagnoses in patients receiving ramelteon were consistent with such medical conditions. It is plausible that melatonin agonist ramelteon may have worked as a potent antioxidant and contributed to delirium prevention in our study.

Orexin

Orexin is an alerting neuropeptide produced by neurons located predominantly in lateral hypothalamic area, perifornical area, and posterior hypothalamus.[29] The orexin-A levels in cerebrospinal fluid (CSF) during active wake state are highest during the dark phase in nocturnal rodents and highest during the light phase in diurnal species.[30] As a primary arousal signal in wake control, orexin signaling is necessary for normal circadian regulation of consolidated wakefulness. Accordingly, as compared to melatonin, orexin is predominantly secreted during daytime in humans.[29] In contrast to melatonin, orexin secretion decreases by 10% only in older adults, as compared to younger adults.[31]

Interestingly, as compared to controls, patients with moderate to severe Alzheimer disease were shown to have higher mean orexin levels in CSF. Additionally, these patients had significantly impaired nocturnal sleep compared to controls and patients with mild Alzheimer's disease.[32] Furthermore, significantly higher levels of orexin in the brain of rats with acute pancreatitis were reportedly found when compared to healthy controls.[33] As dementia and inflammation are risk factors for delirium, it is possible that patients with delirium have increased orexin levels thus accounting for the resultant sleep–wake disturbance.[34]

CLINICAL APPROACH

Sleep disturbances in delirium can present as insomnia, sleep fragmentation, daytime somnolence, and reversal of sleep–wake phases.[35] However, a recent review suggests that it may be difficult to ascertain whether poor sleep is casually related to delirium or to determine unequivocally whether treatment interventions actually improve objective sleep quality; it is well known that patients experience poor quality sleep in the ICU and that sleep promotion represents a low-risk intervention with potential to improve delirium outcomes.[36] A more recent cohort study, including 145 consecutive newly admitted elderly acute general hospital patients, has shown that delirium-only group had significantly higher sleep disturbance, as measured by the Delirium Rating Scale-Revised-98 (DRS-R-98) sleep item scores ≥2, as compared with the other subgroups: dementia only, comorbid delirium–dementia, and no-delirium/no-dementia subgroups. Additionally, the severity of sleep–wake cycle disturbance over time was significantly associated with the diagnosis of delirium but not with age, sex, or dementia. These findings suggest that observer-rated more severe sleep–wake cycle disturbances are highly associated with delirium irrespective of dementia status, consistent with being a core feature of delirium.[35]

Therefore, addressing the underlying clinical and environmental factors plays an important role in improvement of sleep and delirium. However, medical conditions can not necessarily resolve immediately, and some may be irreversible. Also, medication side effects can not necessarily be removed. For example, glucocorticoids or opioids are essential for systemic lupus erythematosus or cancer pain. Accordingly, we need prevention and treatment methods for management of sleep disturbance and delirium.[7]

MANAGEMENT

Nonpharmacological Interventions

Hshieh et al.[37] identified 14 studies assessing effectiveness of multicomponent (e.g., reorientation, early mobilization, therapeutic activities, hydration, nutrition, sleep strategies, and hearing and vision adaptations) nonpharmacologic delirium interventions and reported reductions in delirium incidence (OR 0.47) in 11 studies, reductions in delirium incidence by 44% in 4 randomized or matched studies, reductions in rate of falls in 4 studies (OR 0.38), reductions in rate of falls by 64% in 2 studies, and a trend toward decreases in lengths of stay (mean difference –0.16 days) and institutionalization rates (5% decreased odds of institutionalization).[37] Martinez et al.[38] identified seven randomized trials of diverse quality assessing effectiveness of multicomponent nonpharmacologic delirium interventions and reported reductions in delirium incidence (relative risk [RR] 0.73) and reductions in accidental falls during the hospitalization (RR 0.39) without evidence of differential effectiveness according to ward type or dementia rates, but nonsignificant reductions in delirium duration, hospital stay, and mortality.[38] Thus, multicomponent nonpharmacologic delirium prevention interventions are effective in reducing delirium incidence and preventing falls, with trend toward decreasing length of stay; however, these interventions are associated with nonsignificant reductions in mortality.

Interestingly, Litton et al.[39] identified nine studies assessing the efficacy of earplugs as an ICU strategy for reducing delirium and reported reductions in delirium incidence (RR 0.59) and reductions in hospital mortality (RR 0.77). Thus, one of methods for sleep hygiene improvement is effective in reducing delirium incidence. Hunter et al.[40] reported with a total of 26 articles referenced that early mobilization suggested a decrease in delirium by 2 days, reduced risk of readmission or death, and reduced ventilator-assisted pneumonia, central line, and catheter infections. In contrast, Galanakis et al.[41] reported that although hydration is a believed to be a key component of delirium reversibility, yet there are conflicting results on its efficacy as an intervention for delirium management. Sanford and Flaherty[42] reported that knowledge on how overall nutritional status and individual nutrients predispose or directly lead to the development of delirium is currently very limited as most studies in the area of nutrition and cognition still describe mental status changes using the term dementia and do not specifically address nutrition and delirium.

Pharmacological Interventions
Melatonin Receptor Agonists

As mentioned before, hospitalized elderly patients may be vulnerable to circadian-related sleep–wake disturbances, and hence to delirium, due much lower peak of melatonin secretion. Therefore, effects of supplying melatonin to hospitalized elderly patients on delirium prevention have been investigated. The incidence of delirium in the melatonin group was significantly lower than that in the placebo group in the trials by Sultan[43] (5 mg of melatonin 90 minutes before operative time and at night of operation) and Al-Aama et al.[44] (0.5 mg of melatonin every night). In the trial by de Jonghe et al.,[45] as compared to placebo, use of melatonin (3 mg in the evening) did not reduce the incidence of delirium; however, lesser proportion of patients taking melatonin had experienced a long-lasting episode of delirium, compared to the placebo group.

Ramelteon is an US Food and Drug Administration (FDA)-approved drug for management of insomnia, and has six- and three-fold higher affinity for MT_1 and MT_2 receptors, respectively, than melatonin.[46] Similar to melatonin, ramelteon reduces core temperature and modulates skin temperature.[47] To assess the efficacy of ramelteon in the prevention of delirium, our group conducted a multicenter, rater-blinded, placebo-controlled RCT in ICUs and acute-phase wards. Eligible patients were aged 65 to 89 years, who were newly admitted due to medical and surgical emergency, able to take medicine orally, and expected to stay less than 48 hours. Study participants were randomly assigned to ramelteon (8 mg/day; $n = 33$) or placebo ($n = 34$) nightly for 7 days. Main outcome measure was incidence of delirium according to the *Diagnostic and Statistical Manual of Mental Disorders* (fourth edition; DSM-IV-TR).[48] Our results showed that patients taking ramelteon developed delirium less frequently than those taking placebo.[49] Patients in this study had at least two risk factors for delirium, like age 65 years or older and a severe illness that is deteriorating or at risk of deterioration.[10] Dementia is a major risk factor for delirium, and, as compared to placebo, the incidence of delirium in patients with dementia (Clinical Dementia Rating score ≥0.5) receiving ramelteon turned out to be lower

in the subanalysis of our study.[50] Additionally, there were no adverse events potentially attributable to ramelteon as a delirium prevention drug.

The improved delirium prevention outcomes with the use of ramelteon, as compared to melatonin, could potentially be explained by higher affinity of ramelteon for MT_1 and MT_2 receptors. Another reason for improved outcomes may be the standardization of dosage used for ramelteon. Furthermore, we used 8 mg of ramelteon, whereas the dose of melatonin in the previous melatonin studies ranged from 0.5 to 5 mg. With respect to anti-inflammatory effects of melatonin, survival time after sepsis in rats was significantly improved dose-dependently up to 1.0 mg/kg melatonin.[27] It is possible that melatonin doses (0.5 to 5 mg) may be considerably low for humans in terms of delirium prevention. Such dose-dependency could be applicable to effects of delirium prevention due to our better results with use of ramelteon (8 mg) which is a high dose for melatonin neurotransmission. Considering these points, melatonin neurotransmission in our ramelteon study may have been much more potent than that in the previous melatonin studies. Thus, it may be speculated that melatonin neurotransmission is correlated with degree of delirium prevention.

More recently, Nishikimi et al.[51] reported results of a single-center, triple-blinded, randomized placebo-controlled trial to examine whether the use of ramelteon could prevent delirium and shorten the duration of ICU stay in critically ill patients. In this study, the patients, who could take medicines orally or through a nasogastric tube during the first 48 hours of admission in the ICU setting, were randomly assigned to ramelteon (8 mg/day; $n = 45$) or placebo ($n = 43$) at 8:00 PM every day until discharge from the ICU. The authors found that, as compared to the placebo group, there was a trend toward decrease in the duration of ICU stay (4.56 days vs. 5.86 days), the primary endpoint of study, in the ramelteon group ($p = 0.082$ and $p = 0.028$ before and after adjustments, respectively). In terms of secondary endpoints, decrease in the incidence (24.4% vs 46.5%; $p = 0.044$) and duration (0.78 vs 1.40 days; $p = 0.048$) of delirium were observed in the ramelteon group in this study. The authors also noted that nonintubated patients receiving ramelteon showed statistically significant fewer awakenings per night and a higher proportion of nights without awakenings. In contrast, our group did not report significant differences in any sleep parameters with use of ramelteon and lack of statistical power could be a possible explanation for such an observation in our study.[49]

To summarize, melatonin and ramelteon, have effects on delirium prevention in varying degrees. The possible mechanisms for therapeutic effects include regulation of sleep–wake cycle, inflammatory processes, and scavenging oxidative stress associated with delirium.

Orexin Receptor Antagonist

Suvorexant, a potent and highly selective for orexin-1 receptor and orexin-2 receptor antagonist, is an FDA-approved treatment for primary insomnia in the United States. Suvorexant has been associated with improvements in subjective measures of total sleep time, time to sleep onset, and wake after sleep onset,[52] without altering non-rapid eye movement and rapid eye movement sleep architecture as assessed by electroencephalographic monitoring.[53] The scientific rationale for using suvorexant for delirium prevention is its ability to promote natural sleep that could improve sleep–wake cycle disturbance in delirium. High selectivity for orexin-1 and orexin-2 receptor antagonism[54] and little affinity for acetylcholine receptors (Ki >10μM)[55] may be advantage for delirium prevention. Reportedly, another dual orexin receptor antagonist did not lower hippocampal acetylcholine.[56] Thus, we hypothesized that suvorexant would have preventive effects on delirium.

To assess the efficacy of suvorexant in prevention of delirium, our group conducted a multi-center, rater-blinded, placebo-controlled RCT in ICUs and acute-phase wards. Eligible patients were aged 65 to 89 years, who were newly admitted due to medical and surgical emergency, able to take medicine orally, and expected to stay less than 48 hours. Study participants were randomly assigned to suvorexant (15 mg/day) ($n = 36$) or placebo ($n = 36$) nightly for 3 days. The main outcome measure was incidence of delirium according to the DSM-5. Patients taking suvorexant developed delirium less frequently than those taking placebo (suvorexant, 0% ($n/N = 0/36$) vs. placebo, 17% (6/36), $p = 0.025$).[57] With respect to changes in sleep–wake cycle disturbance score (item 1) of DRS-R-98, analysis of variance revealed a tendency for main effect of treatment, suggesting the potential of suvorexant to improve sleep–wake cycle disturbance that is a core feature of delirium.

Another RCT examining the effects suvorexant on delirium prevention in ICU setting showed that, as compared to placebo, suvorexant led to significant reduction in incidence of both clinical delirium (14.7% vs. 33.3%, $p = 0.069$) and subsyndromal delirium symptoms (17.6% vs. 47.2%, $p = 0.011$).[58] Furthermore, Kaplan–Meier estimates revealed that time to delirium onset

was significantly longer in the suvorexant group as compared to the placebo group. These findings suggest that suvorexant has beneficial effects on delirium prevention and highlight the importance of correcting sleep–wake cycle disturbance in prevention of delirium. The efficacy of suvorexant may seem to be comparable to melatonergic agents; however, future head-to-head comparison studies are recommended.

Antipsychotics

Teslyar et al.[59] identified five studies examining older postsurgical patients and reported that, as compared to placebo, those receiving antipsychotic medication had a 50% reduction in the relative risk of delirium (RR 0.51). Serafim et al.[60] identified 15 studies (12 RCTs and 3 cohort studies) and reported 81% reduction in delirium prevalence in surgical patients receiving antipsychotics.[60] In contrast, Neufeld et al.[61] identified seven studies comparing antipsychotics to placebo or no treatment for delirium prevention in postoperative patients and reported no significant effect on delirium incidence (OR 0.56).

Schrijver et al.[62] identified four RCT using haloperidol for the prevention of delirium in adult hospitalized patients. The authors reported protective effect of haloperidol for delirium in older patients scheduled for surgery. Among them, two studies reported a significant reduction in ICU delirium incidence (noncardiac surgery patients; haloperidol 15.3% vs. saline 23.2%, $p = 0.031$[63]; elective gastrointestinal surgery patients, haloperidol 10.5% vs. saline 32.5%, $p = 0.019$[64]), and one study found a significant reduction in delirium severity and duration (acute and elective [73.5%] hip-surgery patients; incidence: haloperidol 15.1% vs. placebo 16.5%, $p = 0.687$; duration: haloperidol < placebo, mean difference 6.4 days, $p = 0.001$; severity: haloperidol < placebo, mean difference DRS-Max 4.0, $p = 0.001$[65]). Santos et al.[66] identified three RCTs and one cohort study evaluating the effectiveness of haloperidol prophylaxis in critically ill patients with a high risk for delirium. The authors reported a reduction in the incidence of delirium in elderly patients admitted to ICUs after noncardiac surgery and in general ICU patients; however, the results in mechanically ventilated critically ill adults were contradictory.[66]

Santos et al.[66] concluded that, balancing the benefits and low side effects associated with haloperidol prophylaxis, the preventive intervention may be useful to reduce the incidence of delirium in critically ill adults in ICUs. However, our prospective observational study in 2,453 patients receiving antipsychotics for delirium has shown the rate of extrapyramidal symptoms at 5.6%.[67]

In a systematic review, Kishi et al.[68] identified 15 studies (mean duration of study: 9.8 days) with 949 total participants (amisulpride = 20, aripiprazole = 8, chlorpromazine = 13, haloperidol = 316, intramuscular olanzapine or haloperidol injection = 62, olanzapine = 144, placebo = 75, quetiapine = 125, risperidone = 124, usual care = 30, ziprasidone = 32) and reported the superiority of antipsychotics to placebo/usual care in terms of response rate (RR 0.22; the number-needed-to-treat = 2), delirium severity scales scores (standardized mean difference [SMD] = −1.27), Clinical Global Impression Severity Scale scores (SMD = −1.57), and time to response (SMD = −1.22).[68] The authors also reported a higher incidence of dry mouth (RR 13.0; the number needed to harm [NNH] = 5) and sedation (RR 4.59; NNH = 5) in the antipsychotic group compared with placebo/usual care. Additionally, the pooled second-generation antipsychotics were associated with shorter time to response (SMD = −0.27) and a lower incidence of extrapyramidal symptoms (RR 0.31; NNH = 7) compared with haloperidol. However, Agar et al.[69] recently reported the inferiority of antipsychotics to placebo in improvement of delirium symptom scores for 72 hours and overall survival in a randomized trial in palliative care. It must be noted that, in this study, antipsychotics with long half-lives (haloperidol and risperidone) were administered every 12 hours and daytime administration of such antipsychotics could potentially worsen sleep–wake disturbances in delirious patients thus leading to suboptimal clinical outcomes. Similarly Girard et al.[70] reported that the use of haloperidol or ziprasidone in the ICU setting, as compared with placebo, did not significantly alter the duration of delirium, and the study drugs were administered at 12-hour intervals. Additionally, the majority of patients in this study had hypoactive delirium, for which the antipsychotic drugs may not have a beneficial effect.[71]

Our group conducted a real-world prospective observational study over a 1-year period at 33 general hospitals that included delirium patients in medical and surgical settings, who received antipsychotics for management of delirium and were evaluated by psychiatrists.[67] Among 2,834 patients who developed delirium, 2,453 patients received antipsychotics, such as risperidone (34%), quetiapine (32%), and parenteral haloperidol (20%), for delirium. As a result, the mean Clinical Global Impressions–Improvement Scale score was 2.02 (SD 1.09), and that the rate of serious adverse events such as aspiration pneumonia was only 0.9%. Thus, by virtue of dosage adjustment and early detection of side effects, the risk of side effects associated with the use of antipsychotics for older patients with delirium might be low in general hospital settings.

Gabapentin

In an RCT, gabapentin has shown to improve sleep by increasing slow-wave sleep (gabapentin: 19.4 ± 4.2%; control: 11.3 ± 4.4%; $p = 0.0009$) and has resulted in greater polysomnography and participant-reported sleep duration, following a 5-hour phase advance on day 1 and day 28 of use. without evidence of next-day impairment and greater sleep duration during at-home use.[72] Leung et al.[73] conducted a RCT to examine effects of gabapentin as an add-on agent to intravenous anesthetics such as fentanyl and propofol in the treatment of postoperative pain on delirium and reported a reduction in delirium incidence with the use of gabapentin as compared to placebo. In contrast, other RCTs did not find a difference between gabapentin and placebo in reducing the incidence or duration of postoperative delirium among elective total knee arthroplasty patients[74] and patients 65 years of age or older who were undergoing surgery involving the spine or arthroplasty of hips or knees.[75] Further studies that examine the efficacy of gabapentin in delirious patients, other than postoperative delirium, are needed.

CONCLUSIONS

Delirium is a neurobehavioral syndrome caused by dysregulation of neuronal activity secondary to systemic disturbances. As sleep–wake cycle disturbance is one of core features for delirium, it is essential to evaluate clinical factors such as medical illnesses, psychiatric disorders, substance use disorders, medication side effects, and environmental factors leading to sleep disturbance in delirious patients. In addition, multicomponent nonpharmacologic delirium prevention interventions are effective in reducing delirium incidence and preventing falls, with trend toward decreasing length of stay, but lead to nonsignificant reductions in mortality. Pharmacological interventions targeting melatonin or orexin to improve sleep–wake disturbance have shown beneficial effects on delirium prevention. Antipsychotics are essential for the treatment of delirium in real practice, but outcomes from RCTs are controversial.

FUTURE DIRECTIONS

Delirium is associated with significant morbidity and mortality and prevention of delirium is a key clinical priority. Fortunately, multicomponent nonpharmacologic delirium prevention interventions have been established, and preventive effects of a melatonin receptor agonist and an orexin receptor antagonist on delirium have been shown. Therefore, the significance of predictive methods is increasing for delirium. Multicomponent non-pharmacologic delirium prevention interventions include prediction process from evaluating delirium risk factors. Additionally, research focused on understanding the etiology of delirium is gaining momentum. For example, an increase in blood natural killer cell activity may be associated with developing delirium.[76] Moreover, Shinozaki et al.[77] has shown that the bispectral electroencephalography index was determined to be a significant indicator of delirium, with sensitivity 80% and specificity 87.7%, suggesting the possibility of bispectral electroencephalography to distinguish delirious patients from nondelirious patients and the feasibility of the technology for mass screening of delirium in hospitals. Further studies with larger sample size are needed to justify the use of preventive methods for patients to reduce incidence of delirium in hospital settings. Thus, development of comprehensive models that focus on prediction, prevention, and treatment of delirium are desired.

KEY CLINICAL PEARLS

- Multicomponent nonpharmacologic delirium prevention interventions are effective in reducing delirium incidence and preventing falls.
- Age-related change in melatonin rhythm causes decrease in nocturnal secretion of melatonin.
- This causes disturbed sleep–wake cycle, which is a core feature of delirium.
- Melatonin has effects on delirium prevention to some extent.
- Ramelteon, a potent melatonin agonist, has more pronounced effects on delirium prevention probably due to higher affinity for MT_1 and MT_2 receptors than melatonin and more standardized dosing that melatonin.
- Suvorexant, a potent and selective orexin antagonist, also has effects on delirium prevention. The potential is similar to that of ramelteon.
- Antipsychotics are essential for the treatment of delirium in real practice in contrast to controversial outcomes from RCTs.

ACKNOWLEDGMENT

This work was supported by Japan Society for the Promotion of Science (JSPS KAKENHI Grant-in-Aid for Scientific Research (C): 17K10342).

SELF-ASSESSMENT QUESTIONS

1. Which of the following is a feature of delirium?
   a. Delirium represents a disturbance in attention, awareness, and cognition, which does not fluctuate.
   b. Sleep–wake cycle fragmentation
   c. A multicomponent intervention strategy includes sleep deprivation
   d. None of the above

Answer: b

2. Which of the following is true about biosynthesis of melatonin?
   a. It is synthesized from L-tryptophan through the kynurenine pathway.
   b. It increases due to neuroinflammation.
   c. It decreases at night-time.
   d. None of the above

Answer: d

3. Which of the following is true about Ramelteon?
   a. Is not FDA approved for management of primary insomina
   b. Does not have effects on delirium prevention unlike melatonin
   c. Has higher affinity for MT_1 and MT_2 receptors as compared to melatonin
   d. None of the above

Answer: c

4. Which of the following is a characteristic of orexin?
   a. Orexin is an alerting neuropeptide produced in pons.
   b. Orexin-A levels in cerebrospinal fluid are highest during the light phase in diurnal species.
   c. Orexin expression with normal human increases according to age.
   d. None of the above

Answer: b

5. Which of the following is true about suvorexant, a drug for insomnia treatment?
   a. Is a potent and selective orexin-1 and orexin-2 receptor antagonist as assessed by EEG
   b. Is a potent and selective $5-HT_{2A}$ receptor antagonist
   c. Does not have effects on delirium prevention
   d. None of the above

Answer: a

REFERENCES

1. European Delirium Association and American Delirium Society. The DSM-5 criteria, level of arousal and delirium diagnosis: inclusiveness is safer. BMC Med. 2014;12:141.

2. American Psychiatric Association. Diagnostic and Statistical Manual of Mental Disorder, 5th ed. Washington, DC: American Psychiatric Association; 2013.

3. Trzepacz PT, Meagher DJ. Neuropsychiatric aspects of delirium, in Textbook of Neuropsychiatry 5th ed. Edited by Yudofsky SC, Hales RE. Washington, DC: American Psychiatric Press, 2008, pp 445–518.

4. Maldonado JR. Neuropathogenesis of delirium: review of current etiologic theories and common pathways. Am J Geriatr Psychiatry. 2013;21(12):1190–1222.

5. Kabeshita Y, Adachi H, Matsushita M, et al. Sleep disturbances are key symptoms of very early stage Alzheimer disease with behavioral and psychological symptoms: a Japan multi-center cross-sectional study (J-BIRD). Int J Geriatr Psychiatry. 2017;32(2):222–230.

6. Inouye SK, Westendorp RG, Saczynski JS. Delirium in elderly people. Lancet. 2014;383 (9920):911–922.

7. Witlox J, Eurelings LS, de Jonghe JF, Kalisvaart KJ, Eikelenboom P, van Gool WA. Delirium in elderly patients and the risk of postdischarge mortality, institutionalization, and dementia: a meta-analysis. JAMA. 2010;304(4):443–451.

8. Davis DH, Muniz Terrera G, Keage H, et al. Delirium is a strong risk factor for dementia in the oldest-old: a population-based cohort study. Brain. 2012;135(Pt 9):2809–2816.

9. Young J, Murthy L, Westby M, Akunne A, O'Mahony R; Guideline Development Group. Diagnosis, prevention, and management of delirium: summary of NICE guidance. BMJ. 2010;341:c3704.

10. American Geriatrics Society Expert Panel on Postoperative Delirium in Older Adults. American Geriatrics Society abstracted clinical practice guideline for postoperative delirium in older adults. J Am Geriatr Soc. 2015;63(1):142–150.

11. Okamoto Y, Matsuoka Y, Sasaki T, Jitsuiki H, Horiguchi J, Yamawaki S. Trazodone in the treatment of delirium. J Clin Psychopharmacol. 1999;19(3):280–282.

12. Uchiyama M, Tanaka K, Isse K, Toru M. Efficacy of mianserin on symptoms of delirium in the aged: an open trial study. Prog Neuropsychopharmacol Biol Psychiatry. 1996;20(4):651–656.

13. Stahl SM. Stahl's Essential Psychopharmacology., 4th ed. Cambridge, UK: Cambridge University Press; 2013.

14. Yamadera H, Nakamura S, Suzuki H, Endo S. Effects of trazodone hydrochloride and imipramine on polysomnography in healthy subjects. Psychiatry Clin Neurosci. 1998;52(4):439–443.

15. Everitt H, Baldwin DS, Stuart B, et al. Antidepressants for insomnia in adults. Cochrane Database Syst Rev. 2018;5:CD010753.

16. Palomäki H, Berg A, Meririnne E, et al. Complaints of poststroke insomnia and its treatment with mianserin. Cerebrovasc Dis. 2003;15(1-2): 56–62.

17. Azama T, Yano M, Oishi K, et al. Altered expression profiles of clock genes hPer1 and hPer2 in peripheral blood mononuclear cells of cancer patients undergoing surgery. Life Sci. 2007;80(12):1100–1108.

18. Tamiya H, Ogawa S, Ouchi Y, Akishita M. Rigid cooperation of Per1 and Per2 proteins. Sci Rep. 2016;6:32769.

19. Pandi-Perumal SR, BaHammam AS, Brown GM, et al. Melatonin antioxidative defense: therapeutical implications for aging and neurodegenerative processes. Neurotox Res. 2013;23(3):267–300.

20. Nair NP, Hariharasubramanian N, Pilapil C, Isaac I, Thavundayil JX. Plasma melatonin--an index of brain aging in humans? Biol Psychiatry. 1986;21(2):141–150.

21. Lovelace MD, Varney B, Sundaram G, et al. Recent evidence for an expanded role of the kynurenine pathway of tryptophan metabolism in neurological diseases. Neuropharmacology. 2017;112(Pt B):373–388.

22. Yaprak M, Altun A, Vardar A, Aktoz M, Ciftci S, Ozbay G. Decreased nocturnal synthesis of melatonin in patients with coronary artery disease. Int J Cardiol. 2003;89(1):103–107.

23. Hikichi T, Tateda N, Miura T. Alteration of melatonin secretion in patients with type 2 diabetes and proliferative diabetic retinopathy. Clin Ophthalmol. 2011;5:655–660.

24. Schernhammer ES, Hankinson SE. Urinary melatonin levels and postmenopausal breast cancer risk in the Nurses' Health Study cohort. Cancer Epidemiol Biomarkers Prev. 2009;18(1):74–79.

25. Adams Wilson JR, Morandi A, Girard TD, et al. The association of the kynurenine pathway of tryptophan metabolism with acute brain dysfunction during critical illness. Crit Care Med. 2012;40(3):835–841.

26. Fink T, Glas M, Wolf A, et al. Melatonin receptors mediate improvements of survival in a model of polymicrobial sepsis. Crit Care Med. 2014;42(1):e22–e31.

27. Chen HY, Chen TY, Lee MY, et al. Melatonin decreases neurovascular oxidative/nitrosative damage and protects against early increases in the blood-brain barrier permeability after transient

focal cerebral ischemia in mice. J Pineal Res. 2006 Sep;41(2):175–182.

28. Petrosillo G, Colantuono G, Moro N, et al. Melatonin protects against heart ischemia-reperfusion injury by inhibiting mitochondrial permeability transition pore opening. Am J Physiol Heart Circ Physiol. 2009;297(4):H1487–H1493.

29. Ohno K, Sakurai T. Orexin neuronal circuitry: role in the regulation of sleep and wakefulness. Front Neuroendocrinol. 2008;29(1):70–87.

30. Gotter AL, Winrow CJ, Brunner J, et al. The duration of sleep promoting efficacy by dual orexin receptor antagonists is dependent upon receptor occupancy threshold. BMC Neurosci. 2013;14:90.

31. Hunt NJ, Rodriguez ML, Waters KA, Machaalani R. Changes in orexin (hypocretin) neuronal expression with normal aging in the human hypothalamus. Neurobiol Aging. 2015;36(1):292–300.

32. Liguori C, Romigi A, Nuccetelli M, et al. Orexinergic system dysregulation, sleep impairment, and cognitive decline in Alzheimer disease. JAMA Neurol. 2014;71(12):1498–1505.

33. Hamasaki MY, Barbeiro HV, Barbeiro DF, et al. Neuropeptides in the brain defense against distant organ damage. J Neuroimmunol. 2016;290:33–35.

34. Krystal AD, Benca RM, Kilduff TS. Understanding the sleep–wake cycle: sleep, insomnia, and the orexin system. J Clin Psychiatry. 2013;74 Suppl 1:3–20.

35. FitzGerald JM, O'Regan N, Adamis D, et al. Sleep–wake cycle disturbances in elderly acute general medical inpatients: Longitudinal relationship to delirium and dementia. Alzheimers Dement (Amst). 2017;7:61–68.

36. Kamdar BB, Martin JL, Needham DM, Ong MK. Promoting Sleep to Improve Delirium in the ICU. Crit Care Med. 2016;44(12):2290–2291.

37. Hshieh TT, Yue J, Oh E, et al. Effectiveness of multicomponent nonpharmacological delirium interventions: a meta-analysis. JAMA Intern Med. 2015;175(4):512–20.

38. Martinez F, Tobar C, Hill N. Preventing delirium: should non-pharmacological, multicomponent interventions be used? A systematic review and meta-analysis of the literature. Age Ageing. 2015;44(2):196–204.

39. Litton E, Carnegie V, Elliott R, Webb SA. The Efficacy of Earplugs as a Sleep Hygiene Strategy for Reducing Delirium in the ICU: A Systematic Review and Meta-Analysis. Crit Care Med. 2016;44(5):992–999.

40. Hunter A, Johnson L, Coustasse A. Reduction of intensive care unit length of stay: the case of early mobilization. Health Care Manag. 2014;33(2):128–135.

41. Galanakis C, Mayo NE, Gagnon B. Assessing the role of hydration in delirium at the end of life. Curr Opin Support Palliat Care. 2011;5(2):169–173.

42. Sanford AM, Flaherty JH. Do nutrients play a role in delirium? Curr Opin Clin Nutr Metab Care. 2014;17(1):45–50.

43. Sultan SS. Assessment of role of perioperative melatonin in prevention and treatment of postoperative delirium after hip arthroplasty under spinal anesthesia in the elderly. Saudi J Anaesth. 2010;3:169–173.

44. Al-Aama T, Brymer C, Gutmanis I, Woolmore-Goodwin SM, Esbaugh J, Dasgupta M. Melatonin decreases delirium in elderly patients: A randomized, placebo-controlled trial. Int J Geriatr Psychiatry. 2011;26(7):687–694.

45. de Jonghe A, van Munster BC, Goslings JC, et al.; Amsterdam Delirium Study Group. Effect of melatonin on incidence of delirium among patients with hip fracture: a multicentre, double-blind randomized controlled trial. CMAJ. 2014;186(14):E547–E556.

46. Miyamoto M. Pharmacology of ramelteon, a selective MT1/MT2 receptor agonist: a novel therapeutic drug for sleep disorders. CNS Neurosci Ther. 2009;15(1):32–51.

47. Markwald RR, Lee-Chiong TL, Burke TM, Snider JA, Wright KP Jr. Effects of the melatonin MT-1/MT-2 agonist ramelteon on daytime body temperature and sleep. Sleep. 2010;33(6):825–831.

48. American Psychiatric Association. Diagnostic and Statistical Manual of Mental Disorders. 4th ed. Washington, DC: American Psychiatric Association; 1994.

49. Hatta K, Kishi Y, Wada K, Takeuchi T, Odawara T, Usui C, Nakamura H; DELIRIA-J Group. Preventive effects of ramelteon on delirium: a randomized placebo-controlled trial. JAMA Psychiatry. 2014;71(4):397–403.

50. Hatta K, Kishi Y, Wada K. Ramelteon for Delirium in Hospitalized Patients. JAMA. 2015;314(10):1071–1072.

51. Nishikimi M, Numaguchi A, Takahashi K, et al. Effect of administration of ramelteon, a aelatonin receptor agonist, on the duration of stay in the ICU: a single-center randomized placebo-controlled trial. Crit Care Med. 2018;46(7):1099–1105.

52. Michelson D, Snyder E, Paradis E, et al. Safety and efficacy of suvorexant during 1-year treatment of insomnia with subsequent abrupt treatment discontinuation: a phase 3 randomised, double-blind, placebo-controlled trial. Lancet Neurol. 2014;13(5):461–471.

53. Ma J, Svetnik V, Snyder E, Lines C, Roth T, Herring WJ. Electroencephalographic power spectral density profile of the orexin receptor antagonist suvorexant in patients with primary insomnia and healthy subjects. Sleep. 2014;37(10):1609–1619.

54. Winrow CJ, Gotter AL, Cox CD, et al. Promotion of sleep by suvorexant-a novel dual orexin receptor antagonist. J Neurogenet. 2011;25(1-2):52–61.

55. BELSOMRA® package insert. Pharaceuticals and Medical Devices Agency. http://www.info.pmda.go.jp/downfiles/ph/PDF/170050_1190023F1024_1_06.pdf.

56. Yao L, Ramirez AD, Roecker AJ, et al. The dual orexin receptor antagonist, DORA-22, lowers histamine levels in the lateral hypothalamus and prefrontal cortex without lowering hippocampal acetylcholine. J Neurochem. 2017;142(2):204–214.

57. Hatta K, Kishi Y, Wada K, et al.; DELIRIA-J Group. Preventive effects of suvorexant on delirium: A randomized placebo-controlled trial. J Clin Psychiatry. 2017;78(8):e970–e979.

58. Azuma K, Takaesu Y, Soeda H, et al. Ability of suvorexant to prevent delirium in patients in the intensive care unit: a randomized controlled trial. Acute Med Surg. 2018;5(4):362–368.

59. Teslyar P, Stock VM, Wilk CM, Camsari U, Ehrenreich MJ, Himelhoch S. Prophylaxis with antipsychotic medication reduces the risk of postoperative delirium in elderly patients: a meta-analysis. Psychosomatics. 2013;54(2):124–131.

60. Serafim RB, Bozza FA, Soares M, et al. Pharmacologic prevention and treatment of delirium in intensive care patients: A systematic review. J Crit Care. 2015;30(4):799–807.

61. Neufeld KJ, Yue J, Robinson TN, Inouye SK, Needham DM. Antipsychotic Medication for Prevention and Treatment of Delirium in Hospitalized Adults: A Systematic Review and Meta-Analysis. J Am Geriatr Soc. 2016;64(4):705–14.

62. Schrijver EJ, de Graaf K, de Vries OJ, Maier AB, Nanayakkara PW. Efficacy and safety of haloperidol for in-hospital delirium prevention and treatment: A systematic review of current evidence. Eur J Intern Med. 2016 Jan;27:14–23. doi:10.1016/j.ejim.2015.10.012. Epub 2015 Nov 6.

63. Wang W, Li HL, Wang DX, et al. Haloperidol prophylaxis decreases delirium incidence in elderly patients after noncardiac surgery: a randomized controlled trial. Crit Care Med. 2012;40(3):731–739.

64. Kaneko T, Cai J, Ishikura T, Kobayashi M, Naka T, Kaibara N. Prophylactic consecutive administration of haloperidol can reduce the occurrence of postoperative delirium in gastrointestinal surgery. Yonago Acta Med 1999;42:179–184.

65. Kalisvaart KJ, de Jonghe JF, Bogaards MJ, et al. Haloperidol prophylaxis for elderly hip-surgery patients at risk for delirium: a randomized placebo-controlled study. J Am Geriatr Soc. 2005;53(10):1658–1666.

66. Santos E, Cardoso D, Neves H, Cunha M, Rodrigues M, Apóstolo J. Effectiveness of haloperidol prophylaxis in critically ill patients with a high risk of delirium: a systematic review. JBI Database System Rev Implement Rep. 2017;15(5):1440–1472.

67. Hatta K, Kishi Y, Wada K, et al. Antipsychotics for delirium in the general hospital setting in consecutive 2453 inpatients: a prospective observational study. Int J Geriatr Psychiatry. 2014;29(3):253–262.

68. Kishi T, Hirota T, Matsunaga S, Iwata N. Antipsychotic medications for the treatment of delirium: a systematic review and meta-analysis of randomised controlled trials. J Neurol Neurosurg Psychiatry. 2016;87(7):767–774.

69. Agar MR, Lawlor PG, Quinn S, et al. Efficacy of Oral Risperidone, Haloperidol, or Placebo for Symptoms of Delirium Among Patients in Palliative Care: A Randomized Clinical Trial. JAMA Intern Med. 2017;177(1):34–42.

70. Girard TD, Exline MC, Carson SS, et al.; MIND-USA Investigators. Haloperidol and ziprasidone for treatment of delirium in critical illness. N Engl J Med. 2018 Oct 22. doi:10.1056/NEJMoa1808217. [Epub ahead of print]

71. Bleck TP. Dopamine Antagonists in ICU Delirium. N Engl J Med. 2018 Oct 22. doi:10.1056/NEJMe1813382. [Epub ahead of print]

72. Furey SA, Hull SG, Leibowitz MT, Jayawardena S, Roth T. A randomized, double-blind, placebo-controlled, multicenter, 28-day, polysomnographic study of gabapentin in transient insomnia induced by sleep phase advance. J Clin Sleep Med. 2014;10(10):1101–1109.

73. Leung JM, Sands LP, Rico M, et al. Pilot clinical trial of gabapentin to decrease postoperative delirium in older patients. Neurology. 2006;67(7):1251–1253.

74. Dighe K, Clarke H, McCartney CJ, Wong CL. Perioperative gabapentin and delirium following total knee arthroplasty: a post-hoc analysis of a double-blind randomized placebo-controlled trial. Can J Anaesth. 2014;61(12):1136–1137.

75. Leung JM, Sands LP, Chen N, et al.; Perioperative Medicine Research Group. Perioperative Gabapentin Does Not Reduce Postoperative Delirium in Older Surgical Patients: A Randomized Clinical Trial. Anesthesiology. 2017;127(4):633–644.

76. Hatta K, Kishi Y, Takeuchi T, Wada K, Odawara T, Usui C, Machida Y, Nakamura H; DELIRIA-J Group. The predictive value of a change in natural killer cell activity for delirium. Prog Neuropsychopharmacol Biol Psychiatry. 2014;48:26–31.

77. Shinozaki G, Chan AC, Sparr NA, et al. Delirium detection by a novel bispectral electroencephalography device in general hospital. Psychiatry Clin Neurosci. 2018;72(12):856–863.

25

Neurocognitive Disorders

THOMAS GOSSARD AND ERIK K. ST. LOUIS

INTRODUCTION

Over the past two decades, evidence for a strong bidirectional relationship between sleep and neurocognitive disorders (NCD) has emerged. One of the key functions of sleep for brain health appears to be drainage of metabolites and toxins such as beta-amyloid that accumulate with continued wakefulness, making insufficient sleep and sleep disorders of significant concern to the development of neurodegeneration. Sleep disturbances are frequent in patients with dementia and NCDs, including poor sleep efficiency and architecture, more frequent comorbidities such as sleep disordered breathing, excessive sleep-related limb movements, and the parasomnias. This chapter highlights current Diagnostic and Statistical Manual of Mental Disorders (fifth edition; DSM-5) constructs and classifications for the major and mild NCDs, including Alzheimer's disease (AD), dementia with Lewy bodies (DLB), and Parkinson's disease dementia (PDD), and the related prodromal states of amnestic and nonamnestic mild cognitive impairment (MCI). Next, several less common neurodegenerative dementias are discussed, including frontotemporal dementia (FTD), Huntington's disease (HD), and nondegenerative alternative pathologies including Creutzfeld–Jacob disease (CJD), vascular dementia, human immunodeficiency virus (HIV) encephalopathy, and traumatic brain injury (TBI). Each topical section reviews major sleep disturbances and comorbidities and relevant diagnostic and therapeutic approaches toward these disorders, with respect to the frequency of key sleep disturbances such as insomnia, hypersomnia, sleep-disordered breathing, nocturnal movements, and parasomnias. The chapter concludes with a case vignette of a patient with the major NCD of DLB, in which sleep disturbances and comorbidities are especially prominent and relevant to the clinical approach to the evaluation, diagnosis, and treatment of the patient.

DEFINITIONS AND CLASSIFICATION

DSM-5 Neurocognitive Disorders Classification

The framework for NCDs provided in the DSM-5 includes three major syndromes: delirium and major and mild NCDs. The cluster of cognitive disorders in the DSM-5 are defined by a disorder of cognition as the most prominent and defining characteristic for these clinical disorders. Major NCDs are dementia syndromes, with modification in the current DSM-5 so that learning and memory deficits are not required, and other cognitive domains can be chiefly involved and impacted. Subtypes are divided etiologically, with diagnostic confidence in the etiology being classified as probable or possible. Delirium is discussed in detail in Chapter 24 of this volume.

Major and Mild Neurocognitive Disorders

Major and mild NCDs are broad categories of neurodegenerative disorders in which attentional disturbances are not the central feature. Patients with either mild or major NCD experience a decline in one or more cognitive domains, but the primary difference between the two classifications is derived from whether or not the patient is able to independently perform everyday tasks. Under the DSM-5 guidelines, a continuum exists between the two definitions, rather than two distinct categories.[1] Official DSM-5 diagnostic criteria for mild NCD are "evidence of modest cognitive decline from a previous level in one or more cognitive domains,"[2] but these impairments do not significantly impact independent daily activities. This decline is not solely a result of delirium, nor should it be explained primarily by another psychiatric disorder (e.g., major depressive disorder or schizophrenia). A diagnosis of mild NCD does not require that there be further decline over time, although mild NCD usually indicates heightened risk for subsequent evolution to a major NCD. The DSM-5 definition of mild NCD is similar to previously defined diagnostic criteria of MCI.[3-6]

Once a patient experiences cognitive decline to the point where they can no longer perform independent tasks, a diagnosis of major NCD is warranted. Major NCD includes most of the disorders previously categorized as dementias, such as AD, DLB, and PDD. In the DSM-5 guidelines, major NCD represents an alternative definition for dementia. This definition change was enacted for several reasons: to encompass more variations of cognitive decline, to include cognitive decline in younger populations (as associated with HIV and TBI), and in an attempt to eliminate the negative stigma often associated with the term of dementia.[1] Compared to the previous definition of dementia in the *Diagnostic and Statistical Manual of Mental Disorders* (fourth edition; DSM-IV), major NCD has more inclusive diagnostic criteria.[7] In addition to requiring cognitive decline in only one cognitive domain, a symptom of memory loss is not necessary for diagnosis of a NCD. In both mild and major NCD, "significant cognitive decline" is based on the observations of the clinician or concern expressed by an individual or informant.

In clinical practice, once a judgment is made between major and mild NCD, the subtypes of NCD can be explored. Cognitive decline is often one of the first symptoms to arise in the course of a severe disease and most often results from etiologies such as AD, DLB, or other NCDs. DSM-5 criteria allow physicians to make this distinction between etiologies, alongside the determination of levels of severity, and also with regard to level of diagnostic certainty such as "possible" or "probable" cases. We will now discuss the most common subtypes of major and mild NCD.

ALZHEIMER'S DISEASE (AD)

Since its discovery in 1911, AD has been the principal cause of irreversible NCDs in advanced age. For a DSM-5 diagnosis of major NCD as a result of AD, deterioration of memory and learning ability and an additional cognitive feature are necessary.[2] For mild NCD as a result of AD, a decline in memory and learning alone is sufficient for diagnosis.[2] A defining feature of AD in both mild and major NCD is the gradual and insidious progression of cognitive decline, which is often the most difficult for family members or loved ones to observe.

A 1989 study of AD in the community reported a high prevalence of probable AD in the elderly population, impacting an estimated 10.3% of adults over the age of 65 years.[8] This prevalence increased with advancing age, with 47.2% of the population over the age of 85 diagnosed with probable AD.[8] Since then, several groups have attempted to estimate and forecast AD prevalence. More recently, a multistate model and systematic review was utilized to estimate the current prevalence of AD in the population (3.65%), and forecast the future prevalence of AD in 2060 (9.30%).[9] The authors propose that this projected increase is due to the large number of people currently living with preclinical AD. This indicates the importance of developing secondary interventions to slow or stop the progression of AD.

The cognitive decline observed in AD patients is associated with the accumulation of beta-amyloid peptides and tau protein in the brain. Both of these proteins are normal constituents in the brain; however, in AD they form abnormal proteinaceous aggregate deposits. The buildup of these proteins is a result of an inability of the brain to maintain homeostasis between the production and clearance of these proteins. The reason for loss of normal homeostatic function varies between patients, but includes risk factors such as genetic (APOE allele, family history), lifestyle (weight, sleep quality, lack of exercise), and more.

Common biomarkers in AD patients include tau, beta-amyloid, and signs of neuronal loss and synaptic injury, such as neurofilament light chains, alpha-2-macroglobulin, neurogranulin, synaptosomal protein-25 (SNAP-25), and visinin-like protein 1 (VILIP-1). Pathologically, findings include neurofibrillary tangles, neuritic plaques, and neuronal loss. A simple biomarker classification system recently was proposed to classify the presence of biomarkers in AD,[10] known as the "A/T/N" system, in which the *A* refers to beta-amyloid, *T* for tau, and *N* for neurodegeneration or neuronal injury.[10] Highly affected structures early in the course of AD include the entorhinal cortex, hippocampus, amygdala, and the nucleus basalis of Meynert, with eventual more diffuse involvement of the suprachiasmatic nucleus (SCN), intralaminar nuclei of the thalamus, locus coeruleus, raphe nuclei, central autonomic regulators, and the neocortex.

In addition to biomarker evaluation, the quality and architecture of sleep in AD patients has been a developing field of interest over the past several years. The frequency of sleep disturbances in mild to moderate AD is believed to be about 25%, but may be up to 50% in patients with severe AD.[11] Polysomnographic features of AD patients include low-amplitude slow-wave activity in sleep and wake, decreased rapid eye movement (REM) sleep latency duration, concomitant increased percentage of N1, reduced percentages of slow-wave sleep (SWS; N3) and REM sleep, and poorly formed sleep spindles and K complexes.[12-14] Interestingly, reduction in fast spindles has been linked to impaired immediate recall in AD patients.[15]

Several sleep disturbances are associated with AD, such as sleep architecture alterations, disrupted nocturnal sleep, sleep–wake cycle alteration, restless leg syndrome (RLS), sleep-related breathing disorders, and frequent presence of daytime sleepiness and insomnia.[16] Perhaps the most common sleep disturbance in AD patients is a result of a disturbance in the circadian timing of the sleep–wake cycle regulated by the biological clock in the SCN.[17] This phenomenon, known as sun-downing, is a frequent consequence of AD and other major NCDs, and is characterized by confusion, agitation, anxiety, and frequent aggressiveness occurring in the late afternoon and extending into the night.[11] The risk for obstructive sleep apnea (OSA) and RLS appears to be higher for patients with AD in comparison to normal controls.[18-20] REM sleep behavior disorder (RBD) has been rarely documented in association with AD, but appears to most often and typically reflect an accompanying symptom of synucleinopathies in Parkinson's disease (PD) or DLB instead of tauopathies and other proteinopathies.[21]

Sleep disturbances often cause daytime sleepiness in AD patients and have been shown to have a negative effect on independent cognitive ability, regardless of the level of AD severity.[22] In addition, recent research has found that sleep loss may lead to higher levels of amyloid[23] with accumulation of beta-amyloid in the brain,[24] suggesting that the diagnosis and treatment of sleep disturbances in patients with mild and major NCDs including AD should be a priority in the management of these patients. Sleep disturbances associated with neurodegeneration such as sun-downing are difficult to therapeutically treat, but there are treatments available for several sleep comorbidities. A safe, tolerable, and effective pharmaceutical treatment remains elusive, as many sedative/hypnotic agents have no effect or undesirable side effects for patients with AD. Functional impairments of AD patients with OSA can improve significantly with (CPAP) continuous positive airway pressure therapy.[25] Treatment for RLS includes medications such as dopamine agonists, but the efficacy and safety of these medications is yet to be demonstrated in major NCD patients.[11]

A better understanding of the neurodegenerative biomarkers, risk factors, and sleep characteristics of AD has enabled exploration into possible treatments and even potential future cures of mild and major NCDs. Biomarkers have allowed for an earlier detection of prodromal AD. The future of AD treatment will likely rely on individualized medicine, allowing the physician to treat heterogeneous pathologies within AD and other mild and major NCDs.[26]

LEWY BODY DISEASE (LBD)

NCD due to LBD is another etiological subtype in the DSM-5 classification. The large scope of these diagnostic criteria allows this subtype to encompass PDD and DLB. Symptoms are similar to those with AD, but the DSM-5 classification and other diagnostic consortiums[27] have determined that LBD is its own subtype of NCDs. The onset is insidious with a gradual progression. However, the primary cognitive functions that are affected in LBD are nonamnestic, typically impacting complex attention and executive function rather than memory and learning early in the disease course. Diagnosis of LBD requires three core features: fluctuating cognition with pronounced variations of attention and alertness; detailed, well-formed, and recurrent hallucinations; and features of parkinsonism (here with a small *p*, meaning a clinical motor syndrome of parkinsonian signs that may include bradykinesia, rigidity, postural instability, and rest tremor, which may be associated not only with underlying synucleinopathies such as PD, DLB, and multiple system atrophy, but also in tauopathies such as progressive supranuclear palsy (PSP) or cortiocobasal degeneration (CBD), as well as other etiologic pathologies).[1] In addition, the DSM-5 lists RBD as only a suggestive feature,[2] while RBD is considered to be a core clinical feature of Lewy body diseases by most neurologists and by the most recent consensus diagnostic criteria for DLB.[27]

The prevalence of LBD is not well defined, but there have been many studies examining the rate of DLB and PDD in the population. The second most common neurodegenerative cause of dementia in old age, DLB, had been a relatively underdiagnosed form of dementia in the past. The uncertainty of prevalence is evident in various epidemiologic studies. A study in 2005 estimated the incidence of DLB to be 0.1% per year, accounting for 3.2% of the incidence of all new dementia cases within a year.[28] A more recent study in 2014 found similar results and determined the incidence rate to be 3.8% of all new dementia cases, with a prevalence of 4.2% of all dementia cases in the community.[29] A systematic review of the prevalence of DLB diagnosed by the updated diagnostic standards is yet to be performed, but many believe that the true DLB prevalence is higher than the literature has reported.[29] PD is perhaps the most well-known movement disorder. A recent systematic review of 47 epidemiologic studies demonstrated a continuous rise in PD diagnosis with age: 0.17% for 55 to 64 years, 0.43% in 65 to 69 years, 1.09% for 70 to 79 years, and 1.9% in those who are older than age 80.[30] In addition to physical symptoms of PD, 80% of PD patients develop dementia over the course of 8 years.[31]

Distinguishing PDD and DLB can be difficult for clinicians. There are clinical, pathological, and genetic criteria that guide distinction between the two diagnoses, although differentiating these entities remains difficult given their overlapping and highly similar clinical features. The most common distinguishing feature is the temporal course of the disease.[32] In general, DLB is diagnosed in patients who have a "cognitive first" presentation in which features of a major NCD occur early, either in advance of motor symptom appearance (generally by a 1 year or greater time interval) or even may occur simultaneously or within the same one year period following the evolution of motor impairments of parkinsonism. On the other hand, PDD is diagnosed when patients have a "motor first" presentation, with motor impairments occurring prior to major neurocognitive features by at least 1 year.[32] Along with the earlier onset of dementia, fluctuations in attention and hallucinations are more pronounced in DLB patients compared to PD. In contrast, defining symptoms of PD include rigidity, rest tremor, bradykinesia, and an impairment of postural reflexes and gait that is caused in part by degeneration of dopaminergic cells in the midbrain substantia nigra. Advanced PDD is clinically similar to DLB, with fluctuations in consciousness and vivid hallucinations. Some consider these two highly similar diseases to lie within a unitary LDB spectrum (i.e., "lumping" rather than "splitting") given highly similar, overlapping genetics, neuropathology, neurochemistry, and neuropsychological deficits.[33,34]

The pathology of both diseases is also similar. LBD is categorized by presence of Lewy bodies in limbic structures, accompanied by neocortical structures. Lewy bodies contain aggregates of misfolded α-synuclein protein. The aggregation of Lewy bodies leads to reduced dopamine transporter uptake in the basal ganglia, which may be demonstrated by a dopamine transport uptake scan (DaTscan), which demonstrates dopamine in presynaptic nerve terminals of the striatum; an abnormal DaTscan therefore shows reduced uptake of dopaminergic neurons in the brain's striatum. DaTscan can be useful in distinguishing LBD from AD (77.7% sensitivity and 90.4% specificity),[35] since computer tomography (CT) and magnetic resonance imaging (MRI) studies alone most often cannot differentiate between LBD and AD without sophisticated off-line volumetric analyses.[32] Postganglionic sympathetic cardiac innervation is reduced in LBD, which can be quantified with iodine-meta-iodobenzylguanidine (MIBG) myocardial scintigraphy. PSG confirmation of RBD is also beneficial to quantify REM sleep without atonia in those with suspected RBD.[36]

RBD is the most common sleep disturbance in patients with synucleinopathies such as PDD or DLB.[37] RBD is characterized by loss or dysregulation of normal REM sleep atonia, leading to increased muscle activity during REM sleep (known as REM sleep without atonia [RSWA]), and clinical dream enactment behavior. The association between RBD and LBD has continued to develop over recent years, with estimates that 67% to 91.9% of patients at risk for phenoconversion from RBD to DLB or PDD may develop a defined neurodegenerative disease over an 8 to 15 year period.[38-40] Patients with RBD and PD may also have a higher chance of developing major NCD, as indicated by several studies.[41,42] RBD is symptomatically treated by use of melatonin or clonazepam, which appear to reduce the frequency and severity of dream enactment episodes and reduce the potential for injury.[43,44] Unfortunately, there are currently no known treatments capable of reducing the risk or delaying the progression of RBD to NCD. Given that RBD is thought to represent a prodromal stage of covert synucleinopathy with a high risk toward progressing in the future into PD or DLB, RBD presents a unique opportunity for future disease-modifying trials[45] of neuroprotective therapies. Regular follow-up with a sleep neurologist is recommended to enable injury prevention and monitoring patients for symptoms and signs of progression so that early symptomatic therapy for cognitive and motor impairments may be offered.

In patients with LBD, the incidence of sleep disturbances, daytime sleepiness, and movement disorders is higher than patients with AD.[46] In addition to RBD, RLS, hypersomnia, and insomnia, nocturnal arousals and awakenings are also common in LBD. Polysomnographic findings indicate reduced sleep spindle density and greater theta frequency power in patients with PDD, while in DLB, PSG indicates increased theta activity, loss of alpha waves, and a variability of electroencephalography (EEG) power, especially indicative of fluctuating cognition of DLB patients.[47-50] OSA, periodic leg movements of sleep, and nonspecific frequent cortical arousals are frequent findings at polysomnography in DLB patients.[50]

Symptomatic therapies such as cholinesterase inhibitors that may improve cognitive impairment and reduce hallucinations may be helpful in DLB and PDD, even more so than in AD. However, DLB and PDD remain irreversible and relentlessly progressive neurodegenerative diseases for which specific treatment options to alter the disease course are lacking. A better understanding of biomarkers, disease molecular progression, and risk factors is necessary to make significant steps to treat or slow the advancement of LBDs.

OTHER NEURODEGENERATIVE DISEASES

NCD due to frontotemporal degeneration is a DSM-5 classification including frontotemporal dementia (FTD), corticobasal degeneration (CBD), and progressive supranuclear palsy (PSP). These diseases are relatively uncommon and generally somewhat neglected in the scope of more common and better known neurodegenerative major NCD such as AD, PDD, and DLB, but FTD, PSP, or CBD have an incidence of 10.8 cases out of every 100,000 people.[51] Similar to other NCDs, prevalence peaks in the age range of 65 to 69 at 42.6 cases per 100,000 people. A majority of behavior variant FTD (bvFTD) diagnoses appear earlier than AD or DLB, between 60 and 64 years of age, followed by PSP (70–74 years) and CBD and nonfluent/agrammatic variant primary progressive aphasia (nfvPPA; 75–79 years).[51] Like AD, DLB, and PDD, the onset of these neurodegenerative diseases is insidious with gradual progression, primarily affecting neurobehavioral aspects of cognition such as language, social awareness, and disinhibition. Most FTD, PSP, and CBD cases are pathologically tauopathies.

NCD Due to Frontotemporal Degeneration (FTD)

FTD is a neurobehavioral syndrome associated with underlying tauopoathy or TAR DNA-binding protein molecular weight 43 (TDP-43)-opathies. FTD is likely underdiagnosed due to its similarities with AD, mental illness, and other common NCDs. Despite hypothesized underdiagnoses, FTD is the second most common neurodegenerative dementia in patients under the age of 65, after AD, which remains the most common dementia in both younger and older patients, and vascular dementia.[52] The average age of onset is anywhere from 45 and 65, but there have also been documented cases in the elderly and those under the age of 30.[52]

The three core clinical subtypes of FTD are bvFTD, nfvPPA, and semantic variant primary progressive aphasia (svPPA). FTD is often classified into one of these subtypes based on which symptoms first manifest. In bvFTD, patients demonstrate changes in behavior, personality, emotion, and executive control. The bvFTD can be easily misdiagnosed as a psychiatric illness, due to analogous manifestation of these early symptoms.[53] Diagnostic criteria for bvFTD include the necessity of at least three different symptoms from five categories: disinhibition, lack of empathy, compulsions, hyperorality, or executive dysfunction. Evidenced by its most common symptoms, bvFTD affects areas in the brain that are responsible for behavior and decision-making such as the medial frontal, orbital frontal, anterior cingulate, and frontoinsular cortices.[54] The two other subtypes of FTD are types of primary progressive aphasia (PPA), which have the hallmark of language impairment. svPPA has a relatively slow progression, often affecting one temporal lobe of the brain before spreading to the other side. The anterior and inferior temporal lobes are often first affected, followed by pathologic spread to other areas of the temporal lobe and the ventromedial frontal cortex and insula.[53] Patients with svPPA first experience anomia (difficulty finding words to name the objects) and comprehension deficits with single words. Over time, patients lose semantic knowledge of particular words. For example, a patient with advanced svPPA may not recognize the word "dog" even when given the clue "man's best friend." Grammar, executive function, and visuospatial skills remain relatively intact, demonstrating the specific nature of this disease to first impact the anatomically distinct dominant cortical language areas. The third recognized subtype of FTD is nfvPPA. This subtype is similar to svPPA, but language impairments in nfvPPA are characterized by severely nonfluent, effortful speech and word-finding problems, rather than loss of semantic knowledge. Comprehension remains intact, and anomia is rare in patients with the nfvPPA variant of the disease. The progression is slow and begins with minor speech problems such as substitutions, deletions, or additions of speech sounds. Eventually, patients become non-verbal, when the lesion in the brain spreads from the left inferior frontal gyrus and the anterior insula to other surrounding areas of the brain.[55]

Sleep disturbances in patients with FTD are similar to those seen in AD patients.[56] For example, FTD may have disturbances in the sleep–wake cycle, alpha rhythms in the EEG, and sleep-related breathing disorders.[56-58] However, REM sleep parameters in FTD are less altered than in AD.[59] There are some defined discrepancies between variants of FTD, such as higher nighttime activity in patients with bvFTD (85%) compared to svPPA (3%).[58]

NCD due to Corticobasal Degeneration (CBD)

CBD is pathologically and clinically distinct from other NCDs. CBD was first defined by a set of symptoms that included motor impairments such as limb rigidity, bradykinesia, falls, abnormal gait, tremor, and limb dystonia. However, many of these symptoms were later found to be due to other underlying tauopathies. There are now four defined phenotypes that CBD may encompass: corticobasal syndrome (CBS), frontal behavioral-spatial syndrome, nfvPPA, and PSP syndrome. However, to be definitively diagnosed as CBD, symptoms must be caused by widespread deposition of hyperphosphorylated 4-repeat tau in neurons and glia.[60] Postmortem tissue examination is the gold standard of diagnosis in CBD. Clinically, homogeneity of the symptoms makes this a difficult disease to diagnose, with an estimate of only 56% of cases being diagnosed correctly.[61] For a clinical diagnosis of CBS, the chief phenotypical manifestation of CBD, two of the following indicators are required: asymmetric presentation of limb rigidity/akinesia, limb dystonia, limb myoclonus in addition to either oro-buccal or limb apraxia, cortical sensory deficit, or alien limb phenomena.[60] CBS is rarely diagnosed due to prevailing diagnostic uncertainty; epidemiologic studies found that only 1 case out of 534 cases of parkinsonism (i.e., signs of bradykinesia,

rigidity, postural instability, and rest tremor) was due to CBD,[62] with no cases identified in a population study of over 100,000 people.[63] Since CBS is so rare, much of the information is based on case reports rather than large cohort studies. Periodic leg movements of sleep and insomnia may be prevalent in those with CBS.[64]

NCD Due to Progressive Supranuclear Palsy (PSP)

Another phenotype of CBD is PSP syndrome. This condition was originally considered as its own NCD before the discovery of the 4R-tau protein as the pathologic cause. PSP is more accurately diagnosed than CBS, with an 80% accuracy of clinical diagnosis.[53] PSP is also more common than CBS, with estimates of prevalence ranging from 0.15 to 6.4 patients out of every 100,000.[63,65] Typically, patients with early PSP will present with vertical supranuclear gaze palsy and postural instability with falls. Falls are often severe because of the impairment of postural reflexes and bradykinesia. In addition to these motor symptoms, patients can also present with other frontotemporal symptoms, such as behavioral changes, reduced executive function, and attention deficits. There are currently no identified biomarkers that help distinguish PSP from the other frontotemporal disorders. PSP has a dynamic relationship with other FTD diseases; bvFTD or nfvPPA can progress to PSP, or vice versa.[66] For patients with PSP, sleep disturbances are common (60%),[67] circadian rhythm and REM sleep architecture are severely disrupted, often leading to daytime sleepiness and sleep deprivation.[68,69] Sleep disturbances and impaired electroretinogram in patients with CBD are an atypical manifestation,[70] and continued research of sleep disorders in FTD and CBD is necessary to characterize common sleep problems in these disorders.

NCD DUE TO VASCULAR DISEASE

Updates to DSM-5 diagnostic criteria include disorders in which cerebrovascular disease is the dominant or exclusive etiology for neurocognitive impairments. Predominantly known as multi-infarct dementia in the past, the definition of NCD due to vascular disease is more inclusive than it once was.[1,7] Hemorrhagic and ischemic lesions, as well as small vessel disease, are each now included. The diagnosis can also be made in the absence of physical signs of stroke.[2] Common symptoms include impairment in processing speed, executive function, hemiparesis, pseudobulbar palsy, and visual field deficits. Neuroimaging using MRI or CT, or various risk factors such as atrial fibrillation, hypertension, diabetes mellitus, and hypercholesteremia[71] are used as supporting evidence for vascular disease.

Vascular disease causes about 15% of NCD cases every year, second only to AD.[72] Epidemiologic studies demonstrated that vascular dementia was the sole cause in 9% to 33% of patients with dementia.[72] There remains no specifically effective therapy for brain damage caused by vascular disease other than rehabilitation. Vascular NCD most often occur spontaneously and have stepwise deterioration with sudden and precipitous decline followed by periods of stability, in contrast to the slow, insidious progression of other NCDs due to neurodegeneration.

Sleep disorders in the scope of vascular disease are similar to those seen in AD but are often more severe in NCD due to vascular disease. A greater disruption of sleep–wake cycles, poorer sleep quality, and a stronger association with OSA was demonstrated in vascular NCDs in comparison to AD.[73,74] Sleep disorders have a dynamic relationship with vascular disease, as numerous studies have demonstrated that OSA is a risk factor for stroke and NCD due to vascular disease.[75] Polysomnographic evidence of vascular neurodegeneration includes lower occipital EEG frequencies with higher theta and delta power, and lower alpha and beta power, as compared to healthy controls.[76–78]

In terms of pathobiology of the disease, vascular neurodegeneration is primarily caused by atherosclerotic cerebral blood vessels that impair blood flow to the brain, leading to cerebral infarction. Because of high energy needs, the brain requires a continuous and regulated supply of blood to deliver the oxygen and nutrients necessary for proper ionic and neuronal function. If blood flow regulation is impeded, neuronal dysfunction or death may then occur, leading to neurocognitive impairments. Minimizing risk factors for cardiovascular problems are the mainstays of preventing further cognitive decline in the setting of vascular disease, with usual recommendations including smoking cessation; optimizing control of hypertension, diabetes, and hyperlipidemia; managing obesity through weight loss; and treatment of OSA with nasal CPAP. However, there have yet to be any specific treatments for improving cognitive impairments due to vascular disease.[71]

HUNTINGTON'S DISEASE (HD)

HD is an autosomal-dominant progressive neurodegenerative disorder. The genetic mutation underlying HD is hereditary and can be unknowingly passed along to offspring, as symptoms often do not appear until after the patient has had children. HD affects an estimated 5 to 7 individuals per 100,000 people.[79] Every child of a parent with HD has a 50/50 chance of carrying the faulty gene. Only about 3% to 4% of patients at high risk for HD (at least one parent who carries the mutant allele) choose to be genetically screened for HD.[80] About 8% of patients do not have a known affected family member due to germline HD mutations.[79] Common clinical symptoms of HD include chorea, dystonia, incoordination, cognitive decline, and behavioral difficulties.[81] Although symptoms typically first begin to appear in middle age, they can manifest anytime from 1 to 80 years of age. Genetic testing for the *HTT* gene that encodes the protein huntingtin can confirm a diagnosis of HD. An expanded cytosine–adenine–guanine (CAG) trinucleotide repeat copy number (normal 10–35, with HD patients typically over 40–50) is diagnostic of HD, and the disease may become more severe in phenotype in successive generations as copy number variants increase, a phenomena known as anticipation.

As with most NCD classified by the DSM-5, the difference between mild and major severity for cognitive impairment exists as a continuum between the two classifications. Mild cognitive decline due to HD first appears through subtle changes in personality, cognition, and motor control. Patients often present complaining of difficulties in doing simple tasks at home or at work. Over time, these features worsen, leading to severe impairment of planning, organizing, and delayed acquisition of new skills. Behavioral symptoms including psychosis can become severe as well.

HD is caused by a mutation in the *mhTT* gene on chromosome number 4 that leads to a larger than normal huntingtin protein. The large protein is produced in the brain and aggregates, causing nerve damage and death, particularly in the basal ganglia. Other regions that are affected are wide-ranging including the substania nigra; cortical regions 3, 5, and 6; the CA1 region of the hippocampus; the angular gyrus in the parietal lobe; Purkinje cells of the cerebellum; lateral tuberal nuclei; and the centromedial-parafascicular complex of the thalamus.[81] However, in the early symptomatic stages of the disease, huntingtin aggregation is not yet prolific, and there is a lack of neurodegeneration despite significant neurological dysfunction. In major NCD due to HD, affected regions are full of the mutant huntingtin protein, and cell atrophy and neurodegeneration are abundant. Ultimately, the protein does not directly prove to be fatal, but rather the drastic neuronal loss leads to fatal falls, aspiration, inanition, or dysphagia.

Most sleep disturbances in HD stem from an altered sleep–wake cycle. Patients often have a significantly disrupted night–day activity pattern, most likely a result of an imbalance of melatonin.[82] However, it is yet to be defined whether sleep disorders are specifically caused by the genetic pathology of HD, or if they result from having a NCD.[83] If the sleep–wake cycle can be maintained, it may alleviate daytime sleepiness and allow for more functional independence in HD patients. There are also some sleep architecture disturbances to note in HD patients including longer sleep latency, lower sleep efficiency, frequent nocturnal awakenings, and less SWS than controls.[84,85] However, severity of sleep disturbances does not seem to correlate with the severity of NCD due to HD.[84,86] Much like other NCD, treatment of sleep disorders often includes behavioral therapy and possibly prescription of melatonin or clonazepam. Bright light treatment and restricted periods of voluntary exercise have been shown to be effective in maintaining a healthy sleep–wake rhythm in mice with the HD gene.[87] In addition, there have been promising studies on mouse models that have shown hypnotic drugs may have a corrective effect on the sleep–wake cycle and EEG abnormalities of HD mice.[88]

PRION DISEASE

The three main phenotypes of human transmissible spongiform encephaopathies—CJD disease, Gerstman Strausser Scheinker (GSS), and fatal familial insomnia (FFI)—are progressive neurodegenerative diseases of adults caused by PRNP, the human prion protein.[89] These are extremely rare diseases, typically with an approximate 1 per million worldwide incidence rate. Mutations in the prion protein PRNP gene on chromosome 20 are causative for these disorders, leading to accumulation of abnormally folded proteins, which cause neuronal apoptosis and death. These diseases are relentlessly progressive and uniformly fatal, without any known effective treatment other than supportive care and symptomatic treatment of myoclonus and seizures. Prion diseases may be inherited, with an autosomal dominant pattern, or

sporadic due to de novo mutation. Age of onset is usually between 30 and 50 years, but later onset in elderly is also frequent, and earlier onset in the teens or 20s is possible. Neuropathology shows amyloid plaques that stain positive for PRNP, which are diffuse in CJD and GSS and focal in the thalamus in FFI, with eventual diffuse spongiform encephalopathy in advanced and diffuse disease, especially in CJD. Several genetic mutations of the PRNP for the three main prion disease phenotypes have been described.

CJD most often presents subacutely over a time course of weeks to months, with predominant subacute dementia, myoclonus (often with startle), and ataxia. Features of parkinsonism, or even alien-limb syndrome with hemiapraxia, may also be seen. EEG often shows generalized periodic sharp wave complexes within 2 months of disease development, and brain MRI may show fluid-attenuated inversion recovery (FLAIR) signal hyperintensities in the basal ganglia and nonenhancing gyriform diffusion weighted imaging (DWI) signal abnormalities of the cerebral cortex (aka cortical ribbon sign, or "ribboning"). Cerebrospinal fluid characteristically shows 14-3-3 protein, a marker of acute neuronal cell death that is not specific for CJD, but helpful and supportive for the diagnosis in the appropriate clinical context.

GSS disease is characterized by progressive degeneration of the cerebellum and neocortex, with clinical signs of progressive ataxia, dysarthria, nystagmus, dysphagia, spasticity, visual disturbances including blindness, hearing loss and deafness, variable features of parkinsonism, and dementia. The disease course may range from a few months, to between 2 and 12 years.

FFI has subacute or insidious onset of insomnia as its predominant initial feature, with later evolution to cognitive impairment, autonomic and thermoregulatory instability, and ataxia with variable brain stem involvement. Each of the prion disease phenotypes may also have prominent sleep disturbances, especially initial and sleep maintenance insomnia, but also excessive sleep-related movements including periodic leg movements of sleep and REM sleep atonia loss with excessive elementary leg jerking and even RBD with complex motor, dream enactment behaviors. FFI and prion diseases ultimately progress to a state that some experts have described as agrypnia excitata, with status dissociatus (severely deranged sleep architecture with severe REM sleep atonia loss, and altered NREM sleep architecture with loss of K complexes, sleep spindles, and delta waves, but persistence of N1 stage features, leading to extreme difficulty discriminating sleep–wake states).[90] The possibility of an autoimmune disorder that can mimic FFI, such as autoimmune encephalopathies resulting from antivoltage gated potassium channel antibodies (i.e., Morvan syndrome), should also be considered since these disorders may be treatable.

HIV-ASSOCIATED NEUROCOGNITIVE DISORDER (HAND)

HIV-associated NCD (HAND), also known as HIV encephalopathy, is due to neurocognitive dysfunction associated with direct HIV infection of the central nervous system (CNS), which occurs early in the course of HIV infection.[91] HIV can enter the CNS during early stages of infection, and persistent CNS HIV infection and inflammation probably contribute to the development of HAND. Combination antiretroviral therapy (CART) has fortunately led to a substantial increase in prolonged survival in patients with HIV infection, changing the spectrum of clinical presentations of HAND. The CNS appears to be a relative sanctuary for HIV replication and a reservoir for persisting HIV infection despite CART therapy efficacy, so that HAND manifestations may evolve in patients otherwise effectively treated by CART. HAND risk appears to increase with advancing age and presence of cardiovascular risk factors such as atherosclerosis, hyperlipidemia, diabetes, and positive smoking history.[91] An estimated 15% to 55% of HIV-infected patients have HAND, with increasingly milder phenotypes of manifestations in the CART era since the 1990s. Asymptomatic neurocognitive impairments are seen in approximately 30% of HIV-infected patients, mild NCD due to HIV in 20% to 30% of individuals, and HIV associated major NCD in 2% to 8% or less today.[91]

The pathophysiology of HAND is thought to involve a combination of influences resulting from direct HIV infection of the CNS, associated immune and inflammatory phenomena, and even CART therapies, mediating additional alterations and impairments in neuronal metabolism and function, altered neurotransmission, and neuronal injury and loss. Clinical manifestations of HAND include neurovegetative problems with reduced mood, motivation, and appetite. Neuropsychological deficits include psychomotor slowing with impairments in memory, attention, and executive dysfunction.

There has been limited literature specifically focused on sleep disturbances associated with HAND, with most studies focused on symptoms of insomnia, hypersomnia, and sleep-disordered breathing.[92–94] In one large cross-sectional study of HIV-infected military beneficiaries, there was no evidence that symptoms of sleep disturbance were specifically associated with HIV infection. Forty-six percent of HIV-infected patients endorsed insomnia symptoms on the Pittsburgh Sleep Quality Index (PSQI), and 30% reported daytime hypersomnolence using the Epworth Sleepiness Scale, but these were similar in frequency to the reported sleep disturbance symptoms in an age- and sex-matched control group without HIV infection.[93] Factors associated with insomnia in the HIV-infected patients in that study included depression, higher waist size, and lower education status, but neurocognitive impairment was not associated with symptoms of sleep disturbance. However, there was evidence that sleep disturbance impacted the daily functioning of HIV infected patients with insomnia, who were threefold more likely to have a decline in activities of daily living than those without insomnia. Eighteen percent of HIV-infected patients used a sleep medication weekly.

A nearly identical frequency of insomnia and poor sleep quality, 47%, was reported in a large French survey based study of HIV patients.[95] Poor sleep quality was associated with HIV infection duration, and nevirapine and efavirenz treatment as specific disease-related factors.[95] Other nonspecific factors associated with insomnia in HIV-positive patients included depression, male sex, active employment, living single, and tobacco smoking. Another large survey based study of HIV-infected patients in China found that 43.1% of patients reported insomnia symptoms on the PSQI, which was again most prominently associated with anxiety and depression history.[96]

Insomnia in HAND has been associated primarily with psychological and psychiatric factors, and evidence of whether insomnia is more frequent compared to the general population has been conflicting. However, there may be even greater severity insomnia in those with HIV infection. One small case-control study utilizing objective sleep assessment with polysomnography comparatively analyzed HIV-infected insomnia patients with HIV seronegative insomniacs, which suggested that the HIV-infected insomnia patients had poorer sleep, manifested by longer sleep latencies, lower sleep efficiency, and a reduced REM sleep time, after adjusting for age, sex, and psychiatric co-morbidity.[92,94] Early in the course of HIV infection, adenotonsillar hypertrophy associated with infection may be a principal cause for OSA and resultant hypersomnia symptoms.[97]

There is evidence in HIV populations that sleep disturbance may have direct impact on cognitive functioning. In one large survey based study of 218 HIV-positive patients that also utilized objective home sleep patterns and duration with wrist actigraphy monitoring, poorer reported sleep quality and shorter (<7 hours) or longer (>8 hours vs. 7–8 hours) sleep times were associated with lower self-reported cognitive functioning.[98] Another small scale but comprehensive study analyzing subjective and objective sleep and cognitive measures involved 36 HIV-infected patients, 75% of whom were cognitively impaired. This study found that 37% of patients had chronic partial sleep deprivation; better cognitive performance on attention, psychomotor speed, and executive function neuropsychological tasks was associated with better objective sleep measures indexed by reduced wake after sleep onset time and greater sleep efficiency and total sleep time.[99]

In summary, evidence for specific sleep disturbances in patients with HAND has been mixed, but available data suggest that insomnia is the main sleep comorbidity and is principally driven by mental health comorbidities in mood and anxiety spectrum, highly similar to the general population. There may be smaller contributions resulting from direct HIV CNS infection and CART therapies for HIV. Sleep comorbidities in HIV infection may impact cognitive functioning, so when there is a suspicion for insomnia or sleep disordered breathing, prompt evaluation and treatment is indicated to optimize functioning and quality of life, similar to other patient populations with sleep comorbidity. Additional studies of HIV-positive patients focused on the full range of sleep disturbances using objective sleep measures are needed to determine whether there are specific problems in sleep due to HIV infection, and how sleep disorders in patients with HAND should be treated.

NCD DUE TO TRAUMATIC BRAIN INJURY (TBI)
In TBI, the onset of symptoms most often occurs immediately following the traumatic event. Additionally, symptoms often do not worsen, but rather a partial or complete recovery may occur. For an injury to be considered a TBI according to DSM-5, at least one of the following criteria

must be met: loss of consciousness, posttraumatic amnesia, or confusion or disorientation after the event.[2] To be considered a major TBI, evidence for one or more neurological deficits must be present, and the patient must have impaired functional independence. Symptoms can vary greatly, but impaired cognitive functions such as communication, motor, and social skills are most common. In major NCD due to TBI, these impairments cause the patient to be unable to function in everyday life without assistance. This can lead to mental health symptoms such as anxiety and depression for an estimated 42% of patients who experience TBI.[100] Interestingly, mental health issues and functional independence appear to have a reciprocal relationship.[100]

TBIs in the United States are relatively common. In 2008, the overall prevalence for individuals between zero to 25 years of age was about 30%, with an incidence of 1.10 to 2.36 per 100 people per year.[101] In those who experience a TBI, an estimated 43.3% have residual disability 1 year after injury.[102] In comparison to that, an estimated 1.1% of the population have a long-term disability as a result of TBI.[103]

Unfortunately, TBI can have drastic and various effects on sleep quality and architecture. Several sleep disorders have been classified strictly as posttraumatic, including posttraumatic insomnia, posttraumatic excessive daytime sleepiness, posttraumatic pleiosomnia, and posttraumatic sleep–wake disorders.[104] Posttraumatic insomnia occurs in between 5% to 70% of TBI patients[105] and may be mediated by multiple factors including pain, adverse reactions to pharmaceuticals, depression, or trauma-induced brain damage.[104] The working definition of pleiosomnia is an additional sleep need of 2 hours per 24 hours,[106] likely caused by traumatic damage to neuronal systems that control wakefulness. As discussed in other NCD, daytime sleepiness due to OSA can cause severe cognitive problems. Mood disorders, medications, and other comorbidities that accompany TBI can also result in daytime sleepiness. Modafinil 200 to 400 mg daily can improve subjective daytime sleepiness.[107,108]

DIAGNOSIS AND TREATMENT OF COMMON SLEEP COMORBIDITIES IN PATIENTS WITH NEUROCOGNITIVE DISORDERS
The most common sleep disturbances in patients with mild and major NCDs are chronic insomnia,

hypersomnia, OSA, and RBD. Cognitive behavioral therapy (CBT) is considered to be the current treatment for chronic insomnia, but may be challenging to employ in patients with NCDs. Patients with sufficient cognitive capacity and attention to still participate in CBT for insomnia (CBT-I) measures can still be offered this as a first-line intervention as in other populations, although evidence basis for the use of CBT-I in cognitively impaired populations per se remains limited. Use of sedative-hypnotic medications chronically should be utilized only with great caution in patients with cognitive disorders, as in other populations. There has been recent emerging evidence that bright light therapy (2,500–10,000 Lux given in various regimens including for 1 hour in the morning, twice daily in morning and afternoon, evening, or even all day) may be beneficial for treatment of both hypersomnia and insomnia, as well as improving sleep, depression, and agitation, in patients with neurodegenerative disorders such as PD and AD, yet evidence remains mixed and further high-quality large clinical trials are needed to clarify its true efficacy and optimal schedules and doses for delivery. Sleep apnea may benefit from treatment with nasal CPAP or, when compliance/adherence to CPAP therapy is not feasible, by sleep repositioning with avoidance of sleep in the supine position or mandibular dental appliance therapies. Last, RBD may benefit from treatment with melatonin, 3 to 6 mg nightly, with higher doses up to 12 mg occasionally being necessary, and clonazepam 0.25 to 1.0 mg can be used for cases that do not respond to melatonin, yet has more adverse effects of sedation, dizziness, and imbalance.

CASE VIGNETTE

A 77-year-old man with a 20-year history of depression presents for psychiatric follow-up. His depression has been treatment resistant, with past failed trials of amitriptyline, doxepin, trazodone, fluoxetine, sertraline, and, most recently, bupropion currently administered at a 300-mg daily dose in the morning. He returns now with a 1-year history of worsened "depressive" symptoms, manifested chiefly by worsened apathy with increased social withdrawal, disinterest in usual hobbies, and lack of self-care. His wife provides collateral history and notes that he has fallen off from regular morning coffee with his friends and no longer accepts invitations to get together with them to play cards in the evenings. Previously an

avid and productive wood worker, he no longer seems to have the initiative to go to the garage to work on projects. He has become more disheveled and will sit in his pajamas until the afternoon unless his wife insists and supervises his dressing for the day. Six months ago, addition of paroxetine 40 mg daily brought no further improvement in symptoms.

His sleep has been especially poor for the last 6 months. He has difficulty initiating sleep at his usual habitual 11:00 PM bedtime, sometimes for as long as hours, and in contrast to prior years, he has difficult maintaining sleep with multiple nighttime awakenings for uncertain reasons. He would previously awaken at 6:00 AM without an alarm, but he now tends to remain in bed until 8:30 AM or 9:00 AM and often then his wife will need to rouse him for the day.

She reports that he has been snoring heavily for years, with occasional witnessed breathing pauses. He endorses occasional snort or gasp arousals and awakens with a dry mouth regularly. He seems to make frequent leg-kicking movements at night, but they don't awaken him, and he denies any uncomfortable urge to move the legs at night or other times.

For the last 6 years, there has been occasional dream enactment behavior occurring a few times per year, characterized by screaming or shouting, arm flailing, or punching movements. If awakened during these episodes, he will report nightmares in which he is defending himself against attackers or being chased by human or animal characters. During one of these episodes he inadvertently struck his wife and fell out of bed, bruising his shoulder and arm.

Additionally, for the last 2 years, he has been sleepier during the daytime, frequently dozing off if watching television or reading. He will nap for about an hour each day, which seems to help him remain awake for the rest of the day and evening until bedtime. His wife completed the Epworth Sleepiness Scale for him, with a score of 14 (scores >10 considered abnormal), indicating excessive daytime sleepiness and the possibility of an underlying primary sleep disorder rather than nonspecific contextual fatigue symptoms.

On a few occasions over the last 3 months, he has had episodes of awakening from sleep at night with vivid complex formed hallucinations. He reported seeing a person standing by the right foot of his bed, which lasted a minute or two in duration. The person did not speak, and each time he awakened his wife who verified that there was nobody there. He put on his glasses and went off to use the bathroom, and when he turned on the bathroom light, he looked back to the foot of the bed and the person he had seen was no longer there. On two occasions, he awakened hearing someone calling his name and awakened his wife to see if she had called him (she had not). This also happened once in the daytime after one of his naps. Aside from these concerns, his wife notes that he seems to walk much slower than before, and he has fallen twice in the last year.

In addition to bupropion 300 mg daily, his only other medications are losartan and simvastatin. He drinks a tumbler of bourbon once or twice per week and quit smoking (1/2 pack daily × 20 years) 20 years ago. There is a family history of an older brother with PD, but no other neurological or psychiatric disorders.

On examination, he was mildly disheveled and appeared somewhat drowsy but alerted readily to voice. He was withdrawn, made poor eye contact, and had soft, poorly articulated speech with hypokinetic dysarthria. On mental status examination, he had poor attention on digit span, calculation, and visuospatial construction abilities on the 10-point clock test and stated that it was October while it was currently July, but was otherwise oriented to self, year, and place. Cranial nerves were intact, including normal vertical gaze, with mildly reduced visual acuity, 20/40 bilaterally with correction (although only 20/200 without correction). There were mild and early bilateral cataracts. Motor survey showed symmetrically increased tone with mild cogwheel rigidity in both arms and legs and symmetrical bradykinesia with slowing of rapid alternating movements for finger and foot tapping. There was no tremor, and strength was normal throughout. Muscle stretch reflexes were intact and symmetric, with flexor plantar responses. Gait was slow with reduced stride length, and there was no postural instability on "pull" test or Romberg. A palmomental sign in the left submental region was elicited by stroking the right palm with the reflex hammer, and Meyerson's glabellar tap sign was present.

Neuropsychological testing demonstrated multimodal cognitive impairment, with evidence for moderate dysexecutive, attentional, and visuoperceptual abnormalities and psychomotor slowing consistent with mild and early dementia. Brain MRI showed only mild generalized cerebral atrophy. Fluorodeoxyglucose positron emission tomography (PET) showed diffuse hypometabolism in the frontotemporal regions, most prominent in the bitemporal regions, with sparing of the occipital region and posterior cingulate cortex. A dopamine transporter uptake scan showed reduced uptake in bilateral putamen.

PSG study demonstrated decreased sleep efficiency of 68%, and total sleep time 6.2 hours. Apnea–Hypopnea Index was 31 per hour, with especially frequent supine position dependent obstructive apneas and hypopneas. There was clear cut loss of REM sleep atonia (aka REM sleep without atonia; Figure 25.1), although there were no recorded abnormal behaviors during the sleep study. Periodic limb movement index was 110/hour, but movement arousals were limited at only 8/hour. A CPAP treatment trial was effective and well tolerated at 12 cm H$_2$0 pressure using a nasal pillow interface.

A diagnosis of DLB was made, and he was offered trials of Sinemet 25/100 mg three times daily and donepezil 5 mg each morning. Sleep diagnoses included severe OSA, chronic insomnia, multifactorial hypersomnia, and RBD. He was prescribed nasal CPAP, and a therapeutic trial of melatonin 3 mg at bedtime was recommended.

On follow-up visit 3 months later, he was largely stable with regard to daytime functioning, but his wife reported mild improvement in his social activities and reduced frequency of nocturnal and daytime hallucinations and nighttime behaviors during sleep. He was using nasal CPAP well and reported some improvement in daytime alertness.

This case demonstrates the myriad of sleep disturbances present in DLB, including prominent insomnia, hypersomnia, periodic leg movements of sleep, and RBD and demonstrates that teasing apart these issues and offering specific, targeted therapies for each can help the patient and their caregiver toward an improved quality of life and functioning.

CONCLUSIONS
Sleep and NCDs appear to have a strong bidirectional relationship. Patients with AD, DLB, and PDD and related prodromal states of amnestic and nonamnestic MCI may each have prominent sleep disturbances, and there is concern that chronic sleep deprivation and sleep disorders may contribute to neurodegenerative disease risk. Comorbid sleep disturbances are frequent in patients with dementia and NCDs, including poor sleep efficiency and architecture, sleep disordered breathing, excessive sleep-related limb movements, and the parasomnias. Less common neurodegenerative dementias such as FTD, HD, and

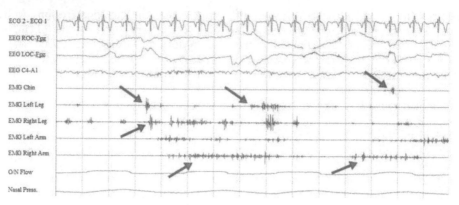

FIGURE 25.1. REM sleep without atonia. This figure displays a 15-second polysomnography epoch of rapid eye movement (REM) sleep. Electromyogram channels include the submentalis (chin, channel 5), left and right anterior tibialis (left leg, channel 6; right leg channel 7), and left and right flexor digitorum superficialis (right arm, channel 8, and left arm, channel 9). Phasic bursts of REM sleep without atonia are shown in the limbs, with a minimal burst also in the chin, as labeled by blue arrows. By contrast, normal background levels of physiologic REM sleep atonia are shown in the majority of the chin channel and in between bursts of phasic muscle activity in the limbs. Polysomnographic findings of RSWA together with a history of dream enactment behavior are required for the diagnosis of REM sleep behavior disorder.

CJD, vascular dementia, HIV encephalopathy, and TBI may also each have prominent sleep disturbances. Polysomnography should be considered early in the course of evaluation in patients with mild or major NCDs and sleep disturbance since recognition and treatment of sleep disturbances can improve functioning and quality of life for both patients and their caregivers alike.

FUTURE DIRECTIONS

Recent preclinical evidence has shown compelling evidence for the role of sleep in normal brain health, contributing to drainage of potentially neurotoxic proteins by the brain's glymphatic system during sleep, and suggests that sleep and neurodegeneration have bidirectional relationships; that is, poor sleep quantity and quality may contribute to neurodegenerative risk, while neurodegenerative disease also in turn causes poor sleep quality and sleep disturbance. However, direct evidence for the existence of a glymphatic system in human brain (similar to that shown in rodents) is thus far lacking, as the role for sleep clearance of neurotoxic proteins has, to date, relied on indirect cerebrospinal fluid markers and brain amyloid PET studies. Development of methods for demonstrating existence of a glymphatic system and its function in humans would be a pivotal advance. Most large-scale studies suggesting the association between sleep disturbance and neurodegeneration have also

been cross-sectional, so additional future large-scale prospective longitudinal cohort studies and critically intervention studies targeting improvement in sleep quantity and quality are needed to determine whether sleep is crucial to the prevention of neurodegenerative disorders. There is also evidence for the use of armodafinil 150–250 mg daily as a psychostimulant for the treatment of hypersomnia associated with dementia with Lewy bodies, with associated improvements in hypersomnia, visual hallucinations, agitation, and quality of life.[109]

KEY CLINICAL PEARLS
- Sleep and NCDs appear to be reciprocally related; poor sleep quantity and quality may influence development of neurodegeneration in the brain, while neurodegenerative and both mild and major NCDs lead to sleep disturbances.
- Key and treatable sleep disturbances in NCDs in include insomnia, hypersomnia, sleep-disordered breathing, and parasomnias.
- OSA is an especially important comorbidity in those with NCDs, since there is evidence it may lead to incident mild and major NCDs. Early treatment with CPAP may help prevent worsening cognitive decline and improve alertness and daytime functioning.

- RBD is strongly associated with the synucleinopathies, which include DLB and PD dementia.
- Treatment of RBD with melatonin can help prevent its injurious consequences and is generally well tolerated by those with NCDs.
- Polysomnography should be considered early in the evaluation of patients with NCDs and sleep disturbance, since diagnosis and treatment of sleep disorders may lead to improved functioning and quality of life in both patients with NCDs and their caregivers.

SELF-ASSESSMENT QUESTIONS

1. Which of the following clinical characteristics is a usual feature of REM sleep behavior disorder?
   a. Onset after age 50 years
   b. Highly stereotypic clinical behaviors
   c. Occurrence in first third of night
   d. A strong association with frontotemporal dementia

Answer: a

2. Which of the following is most commonly seen during polysomnography in patients with Alzheimer's disease?
   a. Increased N3 (slow wave) sleep
   b. Decreased REM sleep
   c. Increased sleep efficiency
   d. Decreased total sleep time

Answer: b

3. Which of the following is considered as a first-line treatment for REM sleep behavior disorder associated with dementia with Lewy bodies?
   a. Antidepressants
   b. Antipsychotics
   c. Melatonin
   d. Memantine

Answer: c

4. Which of the following is the most frequent sleep disorder encountered in patients with HIV-associated neurocognitive disorder?
   a. Restless legs syndrome
   b. Obstructive sleep apnea
   c. Insomnia
   d. REM sleep behavior disorder

Answer: c

5. Which of the following may be considered as an evidence based therapy for the treatment of hypersomnia associated with traumatic brain injury?
   a. Memantine
   b. Modafinil
   c. Melatonin
   d. Mycophenylate

Answer: b

REFERENCES

1. Sachdev PS, Blacker D, Blazer DG, et al. Classifying neurocognitive disorders: the DSM-5 approach. *Nature reviews Neurology.* 2014;10(11):634–642.
2. American Psychiatric Association. *Diagnostic and Statistical Manual of Mental Disorders.* 5th ed. Arlington, VA: American Psychiatric Association; 2013.
3. Blazer D. Neurocognitive disorders in DSM-5. *American Journal of Psychiatry.* 2013;170(6):585–587.
4. Petersen RC, Smith GE, Waring SC, Ivnik RJ, Tangalos EG, Kokmen E. Mild cognitive impairment: clinical characterization and outcome. *Archives of Neurology.* 1999;56(3):303–308.
5. Winblad B, Palmer K, Kivipelto M, et al. Mild cognitive impairment—beyond controversies, towards a consensus: report of the International Working Group on Mild Cognitive Impairment. *Journal of Internal Medicine.* 2004;256(3):240–246.
6. Petersen RC. Mild cognitive impairment as a diagnostic entity. *Journal of Internal Medicine.* 2004;256(3):183–194.
7. Bell CC. DSM-IV: Diagnostic and statistical manual of mental disorders. *JAMA.* 1994;272(10):828–829.
8. Evans DA, Funkenstein H, Albert MS, et al. Prevalence of Alzheimer's disease in a community population of older persons: higher than previously reported. *JAMA.* 1989;262(18):2551–2556.
9. Brookmeyer R, Abdalla N, Kawas CH, Corrada MM. Forecasting the prevalence of preclinical and clinical Alzheimer's disease in the United States. *Alzheimer's & Dementia.* 2018;14(2):121–129.
10. Jack CR, Jr., Bennett DA, Blennow K, et al. A/T/N: An unbiased descriptive classification scheme for Alzheimer disease biomarkers. *Neurology.* 2016;87(5):539–547.
11. Petit D, Montplaisir J, Boeve BF. Alzheimer's disease and other dementias. In: *Principles and Practice of Sleep Medicine.* 5th ed. 2010:1038–1047.
12. Prinz PN, Vitaliano PP, Vitiello MV, et al. Sleep, EEG and mental function changes in senile dementia of the Alzheimer's type. *Neurobiology of Aging.* 1982;3(4):361–370.

13. Montplaisir J, Petit D, Lorrain D, Gauthier S, Nielsen T. Sleep in Alzheimer's disease: further considerations on the role of brainstem and forebrain cholinergic populations in sleep-wake mechanisms. *Sleep.* 1995;18(3):145–148.

14. Ktonas PY, Golemati S, Xanthopoulos P, et al. Potential dementia biomarkers based on the time-varying microstructure of sleep EEG spindles. *Conference Proceedings.* 2007;2007:2464–2467.

15. Rauchs G, Schabus M, Parapatics S, et al. Is there a link between sleep changes and memory in Alzheimer's disease? *Neuroreport.* 2008;19(11):1159–1162.

16. Peter-Derex L, Yammine P, Bastuji H, Croisile B. Sleep and Alzheimer's disease. *Sleep Medicine Reviews.* 2015;19:29–38.

17. Zhou JN, Hofman MA, Swaab DF. No changes in the number of vasoactive intestinal polypeptide (VIP)-expressing neurons in the suprachiasmatic nucleus of homosexual men; comparison with vasopressin-expressing neurons. *Brain Research.* 1995;672(1–2):285–288.

18. Hoch CC, Reynolds Iii CF, Kupfer DJ, Houck PR, Berman SR, Stack JA. Sleep-disordered breathing in normal and pathologic aging. *Journal of Clinical Psychiatry.* 1986;47(10):499–503.

19. Ancoli-Israel S, Butters N, Parker L, Kripke DF. Dementia in Institutionalized Elderly: Relation to Sleep Apnea. *Journal of the American Geriatrics Society.* 1991;39(3):258–263.

20. Rose KM, Beck C, Tsai PF, et al. Sleep disturbances and nocturnal agitation behaviors in older adults with dementia. *Sleep.* 2011;34(6):779–786.

21. Boeve BF, Silber MH, Ferman TJ, et al. Clinicopathologic correlations in 172 cases of rapid eye movement sleep behavior disorder with or without a coexisting neurologic disorder. *Sleep Medicine.* 2013;14(8):754–762.

22. Lee JH, Bliwise DL, Ansari FP, et al. Daytime sleepiness and functional impairment in Alzheimer disease. *American Journal of Geriatric Psychiatry.* 2007;15(7):620–626.

23. Xie L, Kang H, Xu Q, et al. Sleep drives metabolite clearance from the adult brain. *Science.* 2013;342(6156):373–377.

24. Shokri-Kojori E, Wang G-J, Wiers CE, et al. β-Amyloid accumulation in the human brain after one night of sleep deprivation. *Proceedings of the National Academy of Sciences.* 2018;115(17):4483–4488.

25. Ancoli-Israel S, Palmer BW, Cooke JR, et al. Cognitive effects of treating obstructive sleep apnea in Alzheimer's disease: a randomized controlled study. *Journal of the American Geriatric Society.* 2008;56(11):2076–2081.

26. Bondi MW, Edmonds EC, Salmon DP. Alzheimer's Disease: Past, Present, and Future. *Journal of the International Neuropsychological Society.* 2017;23(9-10):818–831.

27. McKeith IG, Boeve BF, Dickson DW, et al. Diagnosis and management of dementia with Lewy bodies: Fourth consensus report of the DLB Consortium. *Neurology.* 2017;89(1):88–100.

28. Zaccai J, McCracken C, Brayne C. A systematic review of prevalence and incidence studies of dementia with Lewy bodies. *Age and Ageing.* 2005;34(6):561–566.

29. Vann Jones SA, O'Brien JT. The prevalence and incidence of dementia with Lewy bodies: a systematic review of population and clinical studies. *Psychological Medicine.* 2014;44(4):673–683.

30. Pringsheim T, Jette N, Frolkis A, Steeves TDL. The prevalence of Parkinson's disease: A systematic review and meta-analysis. *Movement Disorders.* 2014;29(13):1583–1590.

31. Aarsland D, Andersen K, Larsen JP, Lolk A, Kragh-Sorensen P. Prevalence and characteristics of dementia in Parkinson disease: an 8-year prospective study. *Archives of Neurology.* 2003;60(3):387–392.

32. McKeith IG, Dickson DW, Lowe J, et al. Diagnosis and management of dementia with Lewy bodies. *Third Report of the DLB Consortium.* 2005;65(12):1863–1872.

33. Aldridge GM, Birnschein A, Denburg NL, Narayanan NS. Parkinson's disease dementia and dementia with Lewy bodies have similar neuropsychological profiles. *Frontiers in Neurology.* 2018;9:123.

34. Jellinger KA, Korczyn AD. Are dementia with Lewy bodies and Parkinson's disease dementia the same disease? *BMC Medicine.* 2018;16(1):34.

35. McKeith I, O'Brien J, Walker Z, et al. Sensitivity and specificity of dopamine transporter imaging with 123I-FP-CIT SPECT in dementia with Lewy bodies: a phase III, multicentre study. *The Lancet Neurology.* 2007;6(4):305–313.

36. McCarter SJ, St Louis EK, Duwell EJ, et al. Diagnostic thresholds for quantitative REM sleep phasic burst duration, phasic and tonic muscle activity, and REM atonia index in REM sleep behavior disorder with and without comorbid obstructive sleep apnea. *Sleep.* 2014;37(10):1649–1662.

37. Boeve BF, Silber MH, Ferman TJ, et al. REM sleep behavior disorder and degenerative dementia: an association likely reflecting Lewy body disease. *Neurology.* 1998;51(2):363–370.

38. Postuma RB, Gagnon JF, Bertrand JA, Genier Marchand D, Montplaisir JY. Parkinson risk in idiopathic REM sleep behavior disorder:

preparing for neuroprotective trials. *Neurology.* 2015;84(11):1104–1113.

39. Iranzo A, Fernandez-Arcos A, Tolosa E, et al. Neurodegenerative disorder risk in idiopathic REM sleep behavior disorder: study in 174 patients. *PloS One.* 2014;9(2):e89741.

40. Postuma R, Iranzo A, Hu M, et al. Predictors of neurodegeneration in idiopathic REM sleep behavior disorder: a multicenter cohort study (CCI.003). *Neurology.* 2018;90(15 Suppl).

41. Massicotte-Marquez J, Decary A, Gagnon JF, et al. Executive dysfunction and memory impairment in idiopathic REM sleep behavior disorder. *Neurology.* 2008;70(15):1250–1257.

42. Marion MH, Qurashi M, Marshall G, Foster O. Is REM sleep behaviour disorder (RBD) a risk factor of dementia in idiopathic Parkinson's disease? *Journal of Neurology.* 2008;255(2):192–196.

43. Jung Y, St Louis EK. Treatment of REM Sleep Behavior Disorder. *Current Treatment Options in Neurology.* 2016;18(11):50.

44. McCarter SJ, St Louis EK, Boswell CL, et al. Factors associated with injury in REM sleep behavior disorder. *Sleep Medicine.* 2014;15(11):1332–1338.

45. Howell MJ, Schenck CH. Rapid eye movement sleep behavior disorder and neurodegenerative disease. *JAMA Neurology.* 2015;72(6):707–712.

46. Grace JB, Walker MP, McKeith IG. A comparison of sleep profiles in patients with dementia with lewy bodies and Alzheimer's disease. *International Journal of Geriatric Psychiatry.* 2000;15(11):1028–1033.

47. Bonanni L, Thomas A, Tiraboschi P, Perfetti B, Varanese S, Onofrj M. EEG comparisons in early Alzheimer's disease, dementia with Lewy bodies and Parkinson's disease with dementia patients with a 2-year follow-up. *Brain.* 2008;131(Pt 3):690–705.

48. Calzetti S, Bortone E, Negrotti A, Zinno L, Mancia D. Frontal intermittent rhythmic delta activity (FIRDA) in patients with dementia with Lewy bodies: a diagnostic tool? *Neurological Sciences.* 2002;23(Suppl 2):S65–S66.

49. Walker MP, Ayre GA, Cummings JL, et al. Quantifying fluctuation in dementia with Lewy bodies, Alzheimer's disease, and vascular dementia. *Neurology.* 2000;54(8):1616–1625.

50. Pao WC, Boeve BF, Ferman TJ, et al. Polysomnographic findings in dementia with Lewy bodies. *The Neurologist.* 2013;19(1):1–6.

51. Coyle-Gilchrist ITS, Dick KM, Patterson K, et al. Prevalence, characteristics, and survival of frontotemporal lobar degeneration syndromes. *Neurology.* 2016;86(18):1736–1743.

52. Snowden JS, Neary D, Mann DM. Frontotemporal dementia. *British Journal of Psychiatry.* 2002;180:140–143.

53. Olney NT, Spina S, Miller BL. Frontotemporal dementia. *Neurologic Clinics.* 2017;35(2):339–374.

54. Seeley WW, Crawford R, Rascovsky K, et al. Frontal paralimbic network atrophy in very mild behavioral variant frontotemporal dementia. *Archives of Neurology.* 2008;65(2):249–255.

55. Gorno-Tempini ML, Ogar JM, Brambati SM, et al. Anatomical correlates of early mutism in progressive nonfluent aphasia. *Neurology.* 2006;67(10):1849–1851.

56. McCarter SJ, St Louis EK, Boeve BF. Sleep Disturbances in Frontotemporal Dementia. *Current Neurology and Neuroscience Reports.* 2016;16(9):85.

57. Merrilees J, Hubbard E, Mastick J, Miller BL, Dowling GA. Rest-activity and behavioral disruption in a patient with frontotemporal dementia. *Neurocase.* 2009;15(6):515–526.

58. Merrilees J, Hubbard E, Mastick J, Miller BL, Dowling GA. Sleep in persons with frontotemporal dementia and their family caregivers. *Nursing Research.* 2014;63(2):129–136.

59. Kundermann B, Thum A, Rocamora R, Haag A, Krieg JC, Hemmeter U. Comparison of polysomnographic variables and their relationship to cognitive impairment in patients with Alzheimer's disease and frontotemporal dementia. *Journal of Psychiatric Research.* 2011;45(12):1585–1592.

60. Armstrong MJ, Litvan I, Lang AE, et al. Criteria for the diagnosis of corticobasal degeneration. *Neurology.* 2013;80(5):496–503.

61. Litvan I, Agid Y, Goetz C, et al. Accuracy of the clinical diagnosis of corticobasal degeneration: a clinicopathologic study. *Neurology.* 1997;48(1):119–125.

62. Winter Y, Bezdolnyy Y, Katunina E, et al. Incidence of Parkinson's disease and atypical parkinsonism: Russian population-based study. *Movement Disorders.* 2010;25(3):349–356.

63. Schrag A, Ben-Shlomo Y, Quinn NP. Prevalence of progressive supranuclear palsy and multiple system atrophy: a cross-sectional study. *Lancet.* 1999;354(9192):1771–1775.

64. Roche S, Jacquesson JM, Destee A, Defebvre L, Derambure P, Monaca C. Sleep and vigilance in corticobasal degeneration: a descriptive study. *Neurophysiologie clinique/Clinical Neurophysiology.* 2007;37(4):261–264.

65. Golbe LI, Davis PH, Schoenberg BS, Duvoisin RC. Prevalence and natural history of progressive supranuclear palsy. *Neurology.* 1988;38(7):1031–1034.

66. Donker Kaat L, Boon AJ, Kamphorst W, Ravid R, Duivenvoorden HJ, van Swieten JC. Frontal presentation in progressive supranuclear palsy. *Neurology.* 2007;69(8):723–729.

67. Arena JE, Weigand SD, Whitwell JL, et al. Progressive supranuclear palsy: progression and survival. *Journal of neurology.* 2016;263(2):380–389.

68. Walsh CM, Ruoff L, Varbel J, et al. Rest-activity rhythm disruption in progressive supranuclear palsy. *Sleep Medicine.* 2016;22:50–56.

69. Walsh CM, Ruoff L, Walker K, et al. Sleepless Night and Day, the Plight of Progressive Supranuclear Palsy. *Sleep.* 2017;40(11).

70. Armstrong RA. Visual signs and symptoms of corticobasal degeneration. *Clinical & Experimental Optometry.* 2016;99(6):498–506.

71. Gorelick PB, Scuteri A, Black SE, et al. Vascular contributions to cognitive impairment and dementia: a statement for healthcare professionals from the American Heart Association/American Stroke Association. *Stroke.* 2011;42(9):2672–2713.

72. Amar K, Wilcock G. Vascular dementia. *BMJ (Clinical Research Ed).* 1996;312(7025):227–231.

73. Aharon-Peretz J, Masiah A, Pillar T, Epstein R, Tzischinsky O, Lavie P. Sleep-wake cycles in multiinfarct dementia and dementia of the Alzheimer type. *Neurology.* 1991;41(10):1616–1619.

74. Erkinjuntti T, Partinen M, Sulkava R, Telakivi T, Salmi T, Tilvis R. Sleep apnea in multiinfarct dementia and Alzheimer's disease. *Sleep.* 1987;10(5):419–425.

75. Culebras A, Anwar S. Sleep Apnea Is a Risk Factor for Stroke and Vascular Dementia. *Current Neurology and Neuroscience Reports.* 2018;18(8):53.

76. Sato K, Kamiya S, Okawa M, Hozumi S, Hori H, Hishikawa Y. On the EEG component waves of multi-infarct dementia seniles. *International Journal of Neuroscience.* 1996;86(1-2):95–109.

77. Signorino M, Pucci E, Belardinelli N, Nolfe G, Angeleri F. EEG spectral analysis in vascular and Alzheimer dementia. *Electroencephalography and Clinical Neurophysiology.* 1995;94(5):313–325.

78. van Straaten EC, de Haan W, de Waal H, et al. Disturbed oscillatory brain dynamics in subcortical ischemic vascular dementia. *BMC Neuroscience.* 2012;13:85.

79. Almqvist EW, Elterman DS, MacLeod PM, Hayden MR. High incidence rate and absent family histories in one quarter of patients newly diagnosed with Huntington disease in British Columbia. *Clinical Genetics.* 2001;60(3):198–205.

80. Laccone F, Engel U, Holinski-Feder E, et al. DNA analysis of Huntington's disease: five years of experience in Germany, Austria, and Switzerland. *Neurology.* 1999;53(4):801–806.

81. Walker FO. Huntington's disease. *The Lancet.* 2007;369(9557):218–228.

82. Aziz NA, Pijl H, Frolich M, et al. Delayed onset of the diurnal melatonin rise in patients with Huntington's disease. *Journal of Neurology.* 2009;256(12):1961–1965.

83. Morton AJ. Circadian and sleep disorder in Huntington's disease. *Experimental Neurology.* 2013;243:34–44.

84. Hansotia P, Wall R, Berendes J. Sleep disturbances and severity of Huntington's disease. *Neurology.* 1985;35(11):1672–1674.

85. Wiegand M, Moller AA, Lauer CJ, et al. Nocturnal sleep in Huntington's disease. *Journal of Neurology.* 1991;238(4):203–208.

86. Baker CR, Dominguez DJ, Stout JC, et al. Subjective sleep problems in Huntington's disease: A pilot investigation of the relationship to brain structure, neurocognitive, and neuropsychiatric function. *Journal of the Neurological Sciences.* 2016;364:148–153.

87. Cuesta M, Aungier J, Morton AJ. Behavioral therapy reverses circadian deficits in a transgenic mouse model of Huntington's disease. *Neurobiology of Disease.* 2014;63:85–91.

88. Kantor S, Varga J, Morton AJ. A single dose of hypnotic corrects sleep and EEG abnormalities in symptomatic Huntington's disease mice. *Neuropharmacology.* 2016;105:298–307.

89. Mastrianni JA. Genetic prion diseases. In: Adam MP, Ardinger HH, Pagon RA, et al., eds. *GeneReviews®.* https://www.ncbi.nlm.nih.gov/books/NBK1229/. March 27, 2003; last revision: January 2, 2014.

90. Provini F. Agrypnia excitata. *Current Neurology and Neuroscience Reports.* 2013;13(4):341.

91. Saylor D, Dickens AM, Sacktor N, et al. HIV-associated neurocognitive disorder: pathogenesis and prospects for treatment. *Nature Reviews Neurology.* 2016;12(5):309.

92. Reid S, Dwyer J. Insomnia in HIV infection: a systematic review of prevalence, correlates, and management. *Psychosomatic Medicine.* 2005;67(2):260–269.

93. Crum-Cianflone NF, Roediger MP, Moore DJ, et al. Prevalence and factors associated with sleep disturbances among early-treated HIV-infected persons. *Clinical Infectious Diseases.* 2012;54(10):1485–1494.

94. Low Y, Goforth HW, Omonuwa T, Preud'homme X, Edinger J, Krystal A. Comparison of polysomnographic data in age-, sex- and Axis I psychiatric diagnosis matched HIV-seropositive and HIV-seronegative insomnia patients. *Clinical Neurophysiology.* 2012;123(12):2402–2405.

95. Allavena C, Guimard T, Billaud E, et al. Prevalence and risk factors of sleep disturbance in a large HIV-infected adult population. *AIDS and Behavior.* 2016;20(2):339–344.

96. Huang X, Li H, Meyers K, et al. Burden of sleep disturbances and associated risk factors: A cross-sectional survey among HIV-infected persons on antiretroviral therapy across China. *Scientific Reports.* 2017;7(1):3657.

97. Epstein LJ, Strollo PJ, Jr., Donegan RB, Delmar J, Hendrix C, Westbrook PR. Obstructive sleep apnea in patients with human immunodeficiency virus (HIV) disease. *Sleep.* 1995;18(5):368–376.

98. Byun E, Gay CL, Lee KA. Sleep, fatigue, and problems with cognitive function in adults living with HIV. *Journal of the Association of Nurses in AIDS Care.* 2016;27(1):5–16.

99. Gamaldo CE, Gamaldo A, Creighton J, et al. Evaluating sleep and cognition in HIV. *Journal of Acquired Immune Deficiency Syndromes (1999).* 2013;63(5):609–616.

100. Kreutzer JS, Seel RT, Gourley E. The prevalence and symptom rates of depression after traumatic brain injury: a comprehensive examination. *Brain Injury.* 2001;15(7):563–576.

101. McKinlay A, Grace RC, Horwood LJ, Fergusson DM, Ridder EM, MacFarlane MR. Prevalence of traumatic brain injury among children, adolescents and young adults: Prospective evidence from a birth cohort. *Brain Injury.* 2008;22(2):175–181.

102. Corrigan JD, Selassie AW, Orman JA. The epidemiology of traumatic brain injury. *Journal of Head Trauma Rehabilitation.* 2010;25(2):72–80.

103. Zaloshnja E, Miller T, Langlois JA, Selassie AW. Prevalence of long-term disability from traumatic brain injury in the civilian population of the United States, 2005. *Journal of Head Trauma Rehabilitation.* 2008;23(6):394–400.

104. Baumann CR. Sleep and traumatic brain injury. *Sleep Medicine Clinics.* 2016;11(1):19–23.

105. Zeitzer JM, Friedman L, O'Hara R. Insomnia in the context of traumatic brain injury. *Journal of Rehabilitation Research and Development.* 2009;46(6):827–836.

106. Sommerauer M, Valko PO, Werth E, Baumann CR. Excessive sleep need following traumatic brain injury: a case-control study of 36 patients. *Journal of Sleep Research.* 2013; 22(6):634–639.

107. Kaiser PR, Valko PO, Werth E, et al. Modafinil ameliorates excessive daytime sleepiness after traumatic brain injury. *Neurology.* 2010;75(20):1780–1785.

108. Jha A, Weintraub A, Allshouse A, et al. A randomized trial of modafinil for the treatment of fatigue and excessive daytime sleepiness in individuals with chronic traumatic brain injury. *Journal of Head Trauma Rehabilitation.* 2008;23(1):52–63.

109. Lapid MI, Kuntz KM, Mason SS, et al. Efficacy, Safety, and Tolerability of Armodafinil Therapy for Hypersomnia Associated with Dementia with Lewy Bodies: A Pilot Study. *Dementia and geriatric cognitive disorders.* 2017;43(5–6):269–280.

26

Neurological Disorders

RIKINKUMAR S. PATEL, MURUGA LOGANATHAN, ERIK K. ST. LOUIS,
AND AMIT CHOPRA

SLEEP DISORDERS AND STROKE

Stroke is the second leading cause of death worldwide and has significant personal, societal and economic consequences [1]. Most strokes are ischemic (approximately 85%), rather than hemorrhagic and result from a transient or permanent reduction in cerebral blood flow to a specific territory of the brain. The traditional risk factors for stroke include male sex, ethnicity, age, hypertension and atrial fibrillation [1]. Sleep deprivation and sleep disorders are known risk factor for cardiovascular events including stroke [2, 3]. Both short and long sleep durations have been associated with an increased risk of stroke [4]. Sleep disorders including sleep apnea (obstructive and central), insomnia, and sleep-related movement disorders have been implicated as risk factors for or consequences of stroke [5–7].

Conversely, cerebrovascular events can lead to impairments in sleep drive and sleep disorders such as breathing-related sleep disorders (BRSDs), insomnia, hypersomnia, restless legs syndrome (RLS), and parasomnias. Sleep architecture is disturbed in stroke patients, regardless of BRSD. Terzoudi and colleagues [8] reported that stroke patients without BRSD have reductions in total sleep time (TST) and sleep efficiency, reduced stage II and slow-wave sleep (SWS), increased wake after sleep onset (WASO) time, and increased sleep latency. Untreated sleep disturbances have been associated with greater symptom severity and poor clinical outcomes in stroke patients. Treatment of sleep disorders may also improve recovery from stroke and may help prevent future stroke events [9].

In this section, we will focus on evaluation and management of common sleep disorders in stroke patients including BRSD, circadian rhythm sleep–wake disorders, RLS, and insomnia.

Breathing-Related Sleep Disorders (BRSDs)

As compared to the general population, patients with history of stroke or transient ischemic attack (TIA) have significantly higher frequency of sleep apnea syndromes [10]. In a meta-analysis study ($n = 2,343$), including patients with hemorrhagic stroke and TIA, the authors noted that the frequency of BRSDs with an apnea–hypopnea index (AHI) >5 was 72% and those with an AHI >20 was 38% in stroke patients. Only 7% of the BRSDs were due to primary central sleep apnea (CSA) and most patients had obstructive sleep apnea (OSA). Patients with recurrent strokes had higher incidence of BRSD as compared to those with initial strokes. Several prospective studies have reported that snoring and other symptoms seen in OSA are independent risk factors for stroke, especially ischemic stroke [11]. After adjusting for potential confounders, patients with OSA are twice as likely to suffer a stroke compared to patients without OSA over a 3½-year follow-up [5]. Results from the Wisconsin Sleep Cohort study indicate that patients with AHI of 20 per hour had a fourfold increased risk of stroke over 4-year follow-up [12].

Pathophysiologic factors that likely mediate the association between OSA and stroke include metabolic derangements, coagulopathics, endothelial dysregulation, inflammation, worsened hypertension, and cardiac arrhythmias [13]. Some of the putative causes of vascular disease in patients with OSA include nocturnal hypertension, hypoxemia, and sympathetic surges. During obstruction of the upper airway large variations in blood pressure (BP) and persistent increase in BP during sleep result in increased turbulence and stress within the vessel walls [14]. Additionally, apneic episodes of OSA can cause oxidative stress during hypoxemia, damaging endothelial cells [15]. Moreover, in patients with acute ischemic stroke, as compared to those without sleep-disordered breathing (SDB), those with SDB had significant peripheral endothelial dysfunction at baseline. Interestingly, as compared with patients with persisting SDB, peripheral endothelial function improved in stroke patients with normalized SDB ($p < 0.05$). The authors suggested a mechanistic link between peripheral endothelial dysfunction and SDB in stroke patients [16].

Altered cerebral hemodynamic flow and impaired cerebral autoregulation may occur during obstructive apneas in OSA, thereby reducing cerebral blood flow [17]. Obstructive events cause variations in intra-thoracic pressure, thereby decreasing cerebral blood flow and increasing stroke risk [17]. Transcranial doppler has demonstrated decreased cerebral blood flow velocity in the middle cerebral artery during periods of apnea [17]. Therefore, obstructive apnea episodes in patients with OSA can cause subclinical cerebrovascular damage, which over time can result in cerebral small vessel and white matter disease [18].

Management

OSA is a potentially important modifiable risk factor for stroke. Sleep apnea has a high frequency in patients with TIA and stroke, particularly in older patients with high body mass index (BMI), diabetes, and severe stroke. According to Bassetti and Aldrich [19], multiple regression analysis identified age, BMI, diabetes, and stroke severity as independent predictors of AHI. After the acute phase of stroke, there may be a decrease in the severity of OSA. This could possibly be due to less sleep time in the supine position and recovery from stroke associated complications [13]. Continuous positive airway pressure (CPAP) is the primary treatment modality for OSA as it decreases the risk of cardiovascular events and metabolic effects of OSA. CPAP use can lead to mild decrements in systolic and diastolic BP in OSA thus potentially decreasing the stroke risk in these patients [20]. During the follow-up period, severity of cardiovascular disease and associated mortality are higher in patients with untreated OSA. Better cognitive function and quality of life is seen in OSA patients treated with CPAP when compared to controls [12, 19, 21].

Insomnia

Insomnia is common in stroke patients. In a study assessing insomnia in patients with ischemic stroke, 277 patients underwent a comprehensive psychiatric evaluation 3 to 4 months after ischemic stroke. The authors reported that 56.7% reported any insomnia complaint, and 37.5% of the patients fulfilled the *Diagnostic and Statistical Manual of Mental Disorders* (fourth edition; DSM-IV) criteria of insomnia. In 38.6% of the patients, insomnia complaint or insomnia had already been present prior to the stroke, and it was a consequence of the stroke in 18.1% of the patients. Anxiety and the use of psychotropic drug were independent predictors for any insomnia complaint or insomnia, and anxiety, use of psychotropic drugs, disability after stroke, and dementia were noted to be independent correlates of insomnia complaint or insomnia poststroke [22].

Based on prospective data, insomnia has been identified as an independent risk factor for subsequent stroke. As compared to those without insomnia, individuals with insomnia ($n = 21,438$) had 54% higher risk of developing stroke (adjusted hazard ratio [HR] 1.54; 95% confidence interval [CI] 1.38–1.72). Furthermore, those with persistent insomnia had a higher 3-year cumulative incidence rate of stroke than those in the remission group ($p = 0.024$) [23]. In another study, 508 patients underwent psychiatric and sleep assessment at 3 months after acute stroke. Insomnia was reported in 168 (36.6%) patients and 64 [12.6%] patients had insomnia with daytime consequences. Depression scores and frontal lobe infarctions were significant predictors of insomnia, whereas depression and diabetes were predictors of insomnia with daytime consequences [24].

Additionally, in a similar cross-sectional study, 787 patients underwent mental status and insomnia assessment at 3 months after acute ischemic stroke. Eighty-seven (11.1%) patients reported suicidality (SI), and frequent awakenings from sleep were significantly higher in those with SI than the non-SI group, despite adjusting for potential confounders [25]. Other factors such as fatigue and pain have also been associated with SI in patients following acute ischemic stroke [26, 27]. Furthermore, stroke patients with SI were found to be more likely to have cerebral microbleeds (CMBs) in any brain region (36.6% vs. 20.2%, $p = 0.017$), specifically more lobar (29.3% vs. 13.5%, $p = 0.008$) and thalamic CMBs (19.5% vs. 7.5%, $p = 0.018$) [28], than non-SI patients.

Management

A practical approach towards insomnia management generally in stroke patients includes a thorough assessment of co-occurring psychiatric, cognitive, and medical symptomatology for optimal treatment outcomes. Other primary sleep disorders such as BRSD, RLS, and parasomnia behaviors should be thoroughly assessed. Additionally, iatrogenic causes, behavioral, and lifestyle factors that may cause or worsen insomnia should be explored. There exists very limited literature documenting efficacy of medications in treatment of insomnia in stroke patients. A randomized double-blind study comparing lorazepam (0.5–1 mg) and zolpidem (3.75–7.5 mg) showed no differences in efficacy in treating insomnia in patients with stroke and brain injury [29]. However, sedative-hypnotic agents should be used cautiously in stroke patients given increased risk of memory impairment, disorientation, and falls [9], as well as concern for worsening BRSD, especially if benzodiazepines are used. Cognitive-behavioral therapy for insomnia (CBT-I) may be effective in treating insomnia associated with several central neurological disorders, including stroke [30]. In a small study, CBT-I has shown efficacy in community dwelling individuals ($n = 5$) with poststroke insomnia. The authors collected daily sleep diaries over 11 weeks, including a 2-week baseline, 7-week intervention, and 2-week follow-up. At posttreatment follow-up, three participants no longer met diagnostic criteria for insomnia, and all participants showed improvements on two or more sleep parameters, including sleep duration and sleep onset latency (SOL). Additionally, three participants showed a reduction in daytime sleepiness, increased quality of life, and reduction in unhelpful beliefs about sleep [31].

Circadian Rhythm Sleep Disorders (CRSDs)

Shift work sleep disorder is the most common circadian rhythm abnormality that increases morbidity in the adult population. Workers having night shifts or evening shifts who make an effort to sleep during the day have a disturbed and interrupted sleep cycle due to noise, sunlight, unrecognized sleep disorders (due to low likelihood of having a sleeping partner during daytime), and circadian misalignment [32]. Diabetes mellitus, hypertension, obesity, cardiovascular disease, and an increase in mortality are some of the health hazards seen in workers with persistent and consecutive shifts, but its association with increased stroke risk is debatable [61–65]. A cohort study of more than 80,000 registered female nurses (Nurses' Health Study) indicated that after controlling vascular risk factors, rotating night shifts had a 4% increased risk of ischemic stroke for every 5 years of shift work [33], but there was no association between shift work and stroke in another case-control study conducted by Hermansson and colleagues [34].

Normally, the BP peaks twice during the day (i.e. around 9 AM and 7 PM and reaches a nadir during sleep [35]. During the nonrapid eye movement (NREM) sleep cycle, there is a 10% to 20% decrease in BP compared to the daytime values [35], a phenomenon often referred to as a normal physiologic nocturnal "dipping" of BP during sleep. Sometimes, the nocturnal BP may have abnormal fluctuations, and its value may vary from <0% (reversed dippers, sometimes exceeding the daytime BP), <10% (non-dippers), TO >20% (extreme dippers) as compared to daytime BP [36].

Myocardial infarction, left ventricular hypertrophy, congestive heart failure, stroke, and vascular dementia were some of the risks observed in patients without a typical dipping BP pattern during sleep [35–39]. Ischemic strokes, stroke deaths, silent brain infarcts, and intracranial hemorrhages were seen in patients with nondipper, extreme dipper, and reverse dipper BP patterns [36–38, 40, 41]. The risk of stroke in the elderly increased by two to seven folds in patients with extreme BP surges in the morning [42]. A population based study of the prognostic value of ambulatory BP monitoring of more than 1,500 Japanese men and women demonstrated a 20% increased risk of cardiovascular mortality in patients with a 5% decrease in the nocturnal systolic BP in hypertensive patients after a 9-year follow up period [39]. Therefore, variations in the diurnal BP pattern without nocturnal BP dipping is an important risk factor for cardiovascular incidents and strokes [18].

Restless Legs Syndrome (RLS)

RLS is a sleep-related movement disorder defined as an urge to move the legs, usually accompanied with abnormal sensations in the legs, and are typically worst in the evening at or following bedtime and relieved at least partially by movement and especially by getting up to walk [43]. Population-based surveys reported RLS as a common sleep disorder in 5% to 10% of the North American and European population [43–47]. The prevalence rises with age up to 60 to 70 years, after which it declines. RLS is twice as prevalent in women as compared to men [46, 47]. The deficiency in the central dopaminergic transmission, which is responsible for spinal excitability, is thought to underlie development of RLS [48], although the pathophysiology of RLS remains ill-defined.

According to three single case reports, RLS and periodic limb movement in sleep (PLMS) can manifest as immediate effects of stroke [49–51]. These cases demonstrated weakness, which was contralateral to the lesion, based on which many authors reported that these events supported that RLS and especially PLMS emerge due to suprasegmental disinhibition of the lower spinal circuitry. RLS is associated with PLMS and autonomic arousal, and some evidence has suggested that RLS and PLMS may be another risk factor for stroke [49–51] and cardiovascular disease [44, 52]. RLS severity and frequency has been associated with stroke and cardiovascular diseases [45, 53]. The Sleep Heart Health Study indicated that patients with coronary artery disease who developed RLS symptoms approximately every other day in a month had a strong association between their medical condition and RLS [53]. Repeated sympathetic arousals, associated with periodic leg movements, lead to a rise in heart rate and BP, which could also possibly explain this association [53]. Association between RLS and an increased risk for hypertension, cardiovascular disease, and strokes may be due to cyclical nocturnal autonomic arousals analogous to that identified patients with OSA [54].

In a study of 306 stroke patients, 35 (10.11%) met diagnostic criteria for RLS and the RLS symptoms had existed for an average of 60 ± 40 months before stroke. The mean age of onset was 52.94 (±10.32) years. Twenty-four patients (68%) had RLS symptoms contralateral to the hemisphere involved in the stroke, and 82.86% of the patients had imaging evidence of subcortical stroke. Patients with prestroke RLS differed from those without it only by subcortical location of the stroke (82.9% vs. 31.5% respectively, $p < 0.001$). As compared to those with cortical stroke, patients with subcortical stroke had prestroke RLS (22.83% vs 2.74%, $p < 0.001$), history of hypertension, and hemorrhagic stroke type [55].

Woo and colleagues [56] examined clinical characteristics of patients with poststroke RLS and PLMS in six patients. The authors found that poststoke RLS was more often bilateral, and lesions in both the pontine base and tegmentum together were associated with unilateral poststroke PLMS. Lesions in the corona radiata and adjacent basal ganglia were associated with bilateral RLS, whereas lesions confined to the corona radiata resulted in either unilateral or bilateral RLS [56].

In another single-center prospective study ($n = 94$), the authors reported that 24.4% of the minor stroke/TIA patients met diagnostic criteria for RLS using a questionnaire based on International RLS Study Group criteria. Of these patients, 12 had RLS preceding the index stroke/TIA and 11 were newly diagnosed with RLS. The authors reported that RLS patients had more depressive symptoms at follow-up ($p = 0.007$). Additionally, RLS was negatively associated with quality of life at baseline (odds ration [OR] 0.28, $p = 0.010$) and at follow-up (OR 0.14, $p = 0.029$), independent of functional outcome and depressive symptoms [57].

Management

No specific guidelines exist for RLS in stroke patients. Dopamine agonist therapy is considered to be the gold standard treatment for RLS and PLM disorders [44]. Pramipexole (0.25–1 mg) and ropinirole (0.25–2.0 mg) are the two nonergotamine dopamine agonists currently approved by the US Food and Drug Administration (FDA) for the treatment of RLS [58]. Gabapentin enacarbil (600–1,200 mg), a gabapentin prodrug in the alpha-2 delta ligand class, has proven to be efficacious in treating RLS. Rotigotine is a transdermal dopamine agonist patch for RLS therapy that confers the advantage of a longer duration of effect and a theorized lower risk for augmentation syndrome, a worsening of RLS symptom intensity, and topographic distribution with symptoms that occur ever earlier into the daytime and frequently spread from the legs to the arms [58]. Some of the other treatment modalities for RLS include clonazepam(0.25–1 mg), gabapentin (300–1,200 mg), and pregabalin (100–500 mg) [58]. Levodopa/carbidopa (25–100 mg) may be used on as needed basis for infrequent RLS symptoms, but it is ill-advised for regular daily usage given its high risk for augmentation (earlier onset, greater intensity of RLS symptoms, often with spread to the arms or upper body). In case of such side effects, dopamine agonist drugs should be switched to a nondopaminergic drugs such as an alpha-2-delta ligand medication or an opioid [59, 60].

Parasomnias

Rapid eye movement (REM) sleep behavior disorder (RBD) is a parasomnia disorder, characterized by dream enactment behaviors and associated with loss of normal skeletal muscle atonia during REM sleep, which is detected during polysomnography (PSG) to clinch the diagnosis. The behaviors associated with RBD are typically violent, with a significant potential for injury to the patient or the bed partner. RBD typically manifests in older adults with a prevalence 0.4 to 0.5% in this population [61]. RBD may be idiopathic or associated with neurodegenerative conditions particularly Parkinson's disease (PD), dementia with Lewy bodies, and multiple system atrophy with a prevalence ranging from 13% to 100% in these conditions [61, 62].

The prevalence and pathophysiology of RBD in stroke has been unclear [63]. According to some case reports and small case series, RBD in stroke has been related to brainstem lesions [64–68]. Tang and colleagues [63] examined the frequency of RBD in a prospective cohort of patients with acute ischemic stroke using the 13-item REM Sleep Behavior Disorder Questionnaire–Hong Kong (RBDQ-HK). The authors noted that among 119 stroke patients, 10.9% exhibited RBD as evident by RBDQ-HK score of 19 or above. As compared to those without RBD, the stroke patients with RBD had higher incidence of acute brain stem infarcts and smaller infarct volumes. Based on a multivariate analysis, the authors noted that brainstem infarcts were an independent predictor of RBD in stroke patients [63].

Management

Bedroom safety is crucial to the prevention of potential injuries to the patients and their partners. Patients with RBD can be treated to prevent sleep-related injury with either melatonin 3 to 12 mg or clonazepam 0.5 to 2.0 mg to limit injury potential.

SLEEP DISORDERS AND PARKINSON'S DISEASE (PD)

PD is the second most common neurodegenerative disorder, characterized by resting tremor, rigidity, bradykinesia, and postural instability. Sleep disorders are common nonmotor symptoms in PD and were first noted in an original monograph by James Parkinson. According to some studies, the prevalence of sleep disturbance in patients with PD is nearly 100% [69, 70]. Sleep disturbances in PD include sleep apnea, excessive daytime sleepiness (EDS) and sleep attacks, insomnia, RLS, and RBD.

Sleep disturbances negatively impact on health related quality of life in PD patients. In a recent Brazilian study, sleep quality was associated with depressive and anxious symptoms, poorer cognitive performance, and greater severity of PD

symptoms. In multivariate analysis, older age, disease severity, and anxiety symptoms were noted to be significant predictors of poorer sleep quality in PD patients [71].

A population-based cohort study from Taiwan ($n = 91,273$) found that the presence of nonapnea sleep disorders was an independent risk factor for the development of PD (crude HR 1.63, 95% CI 1.54–1.73, $p < 0.001$; adjusted HR 1.18, 95% CI 1.11–1.26, $p < 0.001$). In a subgroup analysis, individuals with chronic insomnia (lasting more than 3 months) had the greatest risk (crude HR 2.91, 95% CI 2.59–3.26, $p < 0.001$; adjusted HR 1.37, 95% CI 1.21–1.55, $p < 0.001$) [72]. Another population based cohort study indicated that patients with OSA, comorbid with insomnia, were at a significantly higher risk of PD onset. The authors compared 5,864 patients with newly diagnosed OSA and 23,269 subjects without OSA and followed the two cohorts for a period of up to 11 years [73]. The sex- and age-specific analysis revealed that female OSA patients aged 50 to 69 years were at the highest risk of developing PD (adjusted HR 2.82). These findings, taken together, are suggestive of a bidirectional link between sleep disorders and PD.

PSG studies indicate significant changes in sleep architecture in PD patients including decreased TST, and decreased SWS (N3) relative to lighter N1 and N2 sleep [74, 75]. Sleep architectural changes may serve as biomarkers for cognitive decline in PD patients. Latreille and colleagues [76] recently examined the relationship between sleep spindles and slow waves at baseline and increased likelihood of developing dementia in PD patients. The authors followed 68 nondemented PD patients and 47 healthy controls for a mean period of 4.5 years. All the participants underwent PSG recording and a comprehensive neuropsychological assessment at baseline. In the PD group, 18 patients developed dementia and 50 patients remained dementia-free. As compared to healthy controls and dementia-free PD patients, those patients with PD who developed dementia were noted to have lower sleep spindle density and amplitude, mostly in posterior cortical regions ($p < 0.05$) [76].

In this section, we focus on frequency, risk factors, clinical features, and management of common sleep disorders associated with PD.

Breathing-Related Sleep Disorders (BRSDs)

Prior studies have reported a frequency of BRSDs ranging between 43% and 66% [77–79], although some authors reported similar or lesser frequency of obstructive apneas and hypopneas during sleep in PD patients as compared to controls [80, 81].

Others have investigated the effects of antiparkinsonian medications on BRSDs in PD patients. A retrospective case-control study comparing PD patients ($n = 119$) and controls with OSA, showed that 57 (48%) of the PD patients had BRSDs [82]. The authors noted that PD patients with predominant central apnea episodes had higher AHI as compared to PD patients with predominant obstructive apnea episodes. All PD patients with predominant central episodes were treated with a combination of levodopa and dopamine agonists, whereas only 56% of PD patients with predominant obstructive apnea episodes were on that combined treatment. In a retrospective analysis, Gros and colleagues [83] compared the severity of OSA in PD inpatients with and without levodopa-carbidopa controlled-released (CR) formulation at bedtime. The authors reported that levodopa-carbidopa CR appeared to be associated with reduced OSA severity, predominantly in the second half of the night in PD patients [83].

Management

CPAP, bilevel positive airway pressure (BiPAP), and weight loss are some of the treatment modalities for management of OSA. Results of a randomized placebo-controlled trial with a crossover design showed that CPAP was effective in reducing apnea events, improving oxygen saturation, and increasing SWS in patients with PD and OSA. Additionally, CPAP treatment resulted in reduced daytime sleepiness in PD patients as measured by a multiple sleep latency test (MSLT) [84]. PD patients with daytime sleepiness, despite CPAP treatment for OSA, have showed significant improvement in hypersomnolence with combination of modafinil and CPAP therapy [85]. CPAP use has been associated with improvements in attention and vigilance [86], although the effect on executive function and memory is still debated in OSA patients [86, 87]. CPAP therapy was not associated with an improvement in cognition in PD patients after 3 and 6 weeks of CPAP use [88]. However, Kaminska and colleagues reported improvements in cognition in PD patients after 12 months of CPAP use for OSA management. The authors noted that Montreal Cognitive assessment (MoCA) scores improved by 1.6 ± 1.9 points ($p = 0.043$) and improvement in other non-motor symptoms including sleep quality and anxiety were also associated with CPAP use at 12 months follow-up in PD patients [89].

Hypersomnolence and Sleep Attacks

Hypersomnolence and EDS are commonly reported symptoms in PD patients, with frequency ranging from 20% to 60% [90–92]. The variability in sleepiness in PD is attributable to multiple definitions of hypersomnolence and cut-off scores for EDS, differences in measures used to assess EDS, variability of medication regimens, and comorbidities in PD patients [90]. Additionally, subjective complaints may not correlate well to objective measures of hypersomnolence in PD patients. In one study, 46.3% of the 134 PD patients reported subjective sleepiness, and only 13.4% of the patients had a weak negative correlation between subjective sleepiness and objective sleepiness as indexed by SOL on MSLT [93].

According to a large study, as compared to controls, EDS was noted more commonly in PD patients with higher age, higher dopamine agonist dose, more severe disease, autonomic dysfunction, and comorbid psychiatric symptoms [92]. Disturbed hypocretin signaling has been implicated in causing hypersomnolence in PD. Weinecke and colleagues prospectively compared PD patients with early and advanced PD to patients with narcolepsy and cataplexy, and matched controls. Sleep laboratory tests and cerebrospinal fluid (CSF) hypocretin levels were obtained. As compared to other groups, nocturnal sleep efficiency was most decreased in patients with advanced PD, whereas narcolepsy patients had the most severe hypersomnolence. Objective sleepiness in PD patients was correlated with decreased CSF hypocretin levels in this study [94].

Chung and colleagues [95] reported that subjective daytime sleepiness was associated with dosage of dopaminergic medications in a study of PD patients ($n = 128$). Additionally, presence of OSA predicted shorter sleep onset latencies during daytime MSLT in PD patients [95]. The antiparkinsonian drugs, especially dopamine agonists (ropinirole, pramipexole), may also cause dose-dependent somnolence. According to many studies, PD patients taking dopamine agonists have a higher frequency of hypersomnolence as compared to those taking levodopa [96–99].

Some of the other contributing factors toward somnolence in PD include alterations in the sleep-wake cycle, disturbed sleep due to motor and non-motor factors, and the disease itself [100]. Suzuki and colleagues demonstrated that PD patients with Hoehn & Yahr stage 4 had significantly more daytime sleepiness than stages 1, 2, or 3, using the Parkinson's Disease Sleep Scale (PDSS) [101]. Evidence from multiple studies suggests that EDS is related to disease duration and severity in PD [90].

Sleep attacks can occur during anytime of the day without a warning. Sleep attacks are defined as an event of overwhelming sleepiness that occurs without warning or with a prodrome that is sufficiently short or overpowering to prevent the patient from taking appropriate protective measures [100]. Sleep attacks occur with antiparkinsonian drugs like dopamine agonists, levodopa, and entacapone [102]. According to a retrospective review study, about 6.6% of patients on dopamine agonists manifested sleep attacks. Around 23% of patients were noted to fall asleep while driving according to a study conducted by Ondo [97]. Use of levodopa (OR 2.96, 95% CI 1.21–7.24), use of any dopamine agonist (OR 3.08, 95% CI 1.47–6.42), and older age (OR 0.96, 95% CI 0.93–0.99) were some of the significant factors associated with falling asleep while driving [97].

Management

Hypersomnolence and EDS have multifactorial origins in PD patients, and a treatment plan should be devised after a comprehensive review of underlying factors in individual PD patients. Sleepiness is routinely associated with PD but may also be seen due to medications and sleep disorders. Therefore, patients with PD should be counseled about safety during driving, especially those who present with hypersomnolence and EDS [100]. PD patients should be started on the lowest possible dose of dopaminergic medications with careful titration of these drugs and forewarning of the possibility of unpredictable sleep attacks as a possible adverse effect, and EDS and hypersomnolence symptoms should be carefully reviewed during clinical visits [100]. Dosage of antiparkinsonian medications should either be reduced, or the offending medication should be discontinued if an iatrogenic cause is suspected [100]. If EDS persists despite making medication changes, patients should have an overnight PSG to rule out treatable causes for sleepiness like sleep apnea or periodic limb movement disorder (PLMD) [100].

There is reasonable evidence basis for utilizing modafinil for treatment of EDS in patients with PD, since its therapeutic efficacy has been demonstrated in several studies [103–105]. Two out of three studies have shown significant improvement in subjective EDS symptoms, using the Epworth Sleepiness Scale (ESS), in PD patients taking modafinil [103–105]. Sodium oxybate, a drug used in treatment of narcolepsy, showed subjective improvement of fatigue and daytime sleepiness in PD patients in an open label study [106]. There has been an emerging focus on effective nonpharmacological interventions for treatment of EDS, such as light therapy [107]. The results of a randomized placebo-controlled trial demonstrated significant improvement in ESS score, sleep fragmentation, and sleep quality after 14 days in PD patients who received the active intervention, consisting of bright light therapy at 10,000 Lux for 1-hour duration given twice daily, between 9 AM and 11 AM and between 5 PM and 7 PM ($n = 31$). The authors also reported that light therapy was associated with increased daily physical activity as assessed by actigraphy [108].

Insomnia

Insomnia is a commonly reported complaint in PD patients with multifactorial origins [109]. Sleep fragmentation is the most common sleep disturbance in PD patients, affecting up to 74% to 88% of patients [110, 111]. Changes in sleep parameters such as decrease in TST and an increase in the number of awakenings and WASO are associated with sleep fragmentation in PD. Based on cross-sectional studies, subjective poor sleep is reported in 20% to 80% of PD patients [109, 112, 113]. Risk factors for insomnia in PD include disease duration, comorbid depression, and female sex [109]. In a case-control study, PD patients were noted to have significantly shorter TST ($p = 0.01$), lower sleep efficiency ($p = 0.001$), and increased REM latency ($p = 0.007$). The authors concluded that reduced TST was significantly associated with increased age ($p=0.001$) and increased levodopa dose ($p = 0.032$) in PD patients [79].

Several disease related factors (including motor and nonmotor symptoms) and comorbid primary sleep disorders can lead to insomnia in PD patients. In a study comparing drug-naïve and advanced PD patients to controls, using both subjective and objective measures, the authors noted that nocturia, nighttime cramps, dystonia, tremor, and daytime somnolence may lead to sleep initiation difficulties in drug-naïve PD patients [114]. In a PSG-based study comparing PD patients and controls, impaired bed mobility associated with rigidity and bradykinesia has been implicated in sleep maintenance insomnia and poor sleep efficiency in PD patients [115]. Additionally, wearing-off effects of dopaminergic medications can be associated with sleep maintenance insomnia in PD patients [116].

Nonmotor psychiatric symptoms and comorbid sleep disorders have been associated with sleep disturbances in PD patients. In a multicenter cross-sectional study including PD patients ($n = 188$) and controls ($n = 144$), correlation between depressive symptoms and nocturnal disturbances was examined in PD patients. Assessments were done using the PDSS for nocturnal sleep disturbances and Zung Self-Rating Depression Scale (SDS) for depressive symptoms. As compared to controls, significantly higher depressive symptoms (SDS score ≥40) were reported by 122 (64.9%) of PD patients. The authors indicated that depressive symptoms in PD correlated significantly with nocturnal disturbances including dystonia, tremor, and sleep fragmentation [117]. Visual hallucinations occur more frequently in elderly PD patients with longer duration of illness, cognitive impairment, and sleep disturbances [118]. Nomura and colleagues [119] used objective sleep measures to compare PD patients with and without visual hallucinations and found that nocturnal visual hallucinations in PD were likely to be related to RBD.

Multiple studies demonstrate that insomnia has a significant negative impact on quality of life in PD patients [120–123]. At least 10% of advanced PD patients consider sleep problems as their most bothersome symptom [124]. In a study examining the impact of insomnia and depression on quality of life in moderate-severe PD patients, the authors noted that 80% of the PD patients ($n = 102$) reported insomnia. Moderate to severe depressive symptoms were reported by approximately 50% of the patients, and PD patients with either insomnia or depression had a significantly lower quality of life as measured by Short Form Health Survey (SF-36) scale [125]. The authors concluded that pain and depressive symptoms were significantly related to insomnia in PD patients.

Management

Insomnia in PD patients is often multifactorial and exploration of all possible contributing factors is the first step to develop an effective treatment plan. Conservative management strategies include discontinuation of the medications causing insomnia, prescribing levodopa/carbidopa or a dopamine agonist just before bedtime if patients experience painful dystonia during their sleep [99], and addressing symptoms such as nocturia and nocturnal PD motor symptoms.

The current evidence base to support the treatment of insomnia in PD is considered insufficient per Movement Disorders Society Task Force guidelines [126]. In a 6-week, randomized placebo-controlled trial of eszopiclone in PD patients and insomnia ($n = 30$), the authors noted that use of eszopiclone was not associated with improvement in TST, the primary outcome measure. However, significant differences favoring eszopiclone were noted in number of awakenings ($p = 0.035$), quality of sleep ($p = 0.018$), and in physician-rated Clinical Global Impression improvement ($p = 0.035$) [127]. Similarly, as compared to placebo, melatonin improved subjective quality of sleep but not the objective sleep parameters in PD patients with insomnia [128]. However, as compared to placebo, use of rotigotine (2–16 mg/24 hour transdermal patch) in PD patients ($n = 190$) with unsatisfactory early-morning motor control resulted in significant improvements in control of both motor control and subjective nocturnal sleep disturbances [129].

Deep brain stimulation (DBS), an FDA-approved treatment for medication refractory PD, has been associated with significant improvements in subjective and objective sleep quality in PD patients [130–132]. In a study comparing sleep quality before and 3 months after subthalamic nucleus (STN) DBS, the authors reported that active DBS stimulation was associated with significant improvements in TST, sleep efficiency, and the duration of SWS, whereas sleep disturbances were similar to those observed before surgery in the absence of DBS stimulation [130]. In another study, as compared to baseline, STN DBS was associated with improved subjective sleep quality, sleep continuity, and nocturnal mobility but no change in RBD in PD patients [131]. Similarly, Arnulf and colleagues [132] reported improvements in sleep quality and nocturnal motor symptoms with STN DBS, but DBS had no effects on PLMS or RBD [132].

Treatment of comorbid depression can result in improved sleep outcomes in PD patients. Placebo-controlled studies of nortriptyline, paroxetine, and venlafaxine suggest that treatment of depression improves symptoms of insomnia in PD patients [133–135, 204–206]. Specific evidence-based treatments targeting other psychiatric symptoms such as anxiety, nocturnal panic attacks, and nocturnal hallucinations would be helpful for optimal treatment outcomes of insomnia in PD patients.

Restless Legs Syndrome (RLS)

Most current evidence suggests that PD is a risk factor for onset of RLS, but not vice versa [90], although evidence remains mixed; one recent large (n = 3.5 million) prospective study of US veterans that analyzed those with prevalent RLS for incident PD risk found a twofold increased risk for PD in those with RLS. The incidence rate for PD in those with prevalent RLS was 4.72 (95% CI 4.09–5.45)/10,000 patient-years, as compared to a propensity matched PD negative control group who had a PD incidence rate of 1.87 (95% CI 1.48–2.37)]/10,000 patient years [136]. The prevalence of RLS in PD patients is estimated to be between 3% to 20% [137]. Lee and colleagues [138] examined the factors contributing to RLS in PD patients (n = 447). The authors noted that, as compared to PD patients without RLS, those with RLS had severe PD disability, prolonged PD symptoms and anti-parkinsonian therapy, and greater cognitive impairment. The authors concluded that the long term duration of anti-parkinsonian therapy was the most important factor associated with the development of RLS in PD [138]. Additionally, PD patients with RLS tend to have delayed sleep onset, daytime sleepiness and overall poor sleep quality [115, 126, 127].

RLS patients have been noted to have a diminished dopaminergic activity in the striatum as demonstrated by a PET functional imaging study [139, 140]. A recent imaging study, using single-photon emission computed tomography (SPECT), demonstrated the evidence for different pathophysiological pathways between RLS and PD at the level of nigro-striatal presynaptic function. The authors found that striatal dopamine transporter binding measured by SPECT is reduced in PD but not in primary RLS [141] In a genotyping study of RLS patients (n = 258) as compared to controls, those with RLS were noted to have significantly decreased frequency of the alpha-synuclein promoter Rep1 allele 2, an allele variant known to confer higher PD risk [142].

Diagnosis of RLS in PD patients can be challenging; thus, a thorough clinical interview is essential to differentiate between RLS and PD-specific symptoms that mimic RLS. These PD-specific symptoms include akathisia, motor restlessness, nocturnal leg restlessness, and sensory complaints [143]. As an example, in a cohort of unmedicated PD patients (n = 200), 40% of PD patients had RLS as compared to the controls,

whereas only 15% of PD patients met criteria for the diagnosis of RLS in this study [144]. On the other hand, dopaminergic medications can mask coexistent RLS, which makes it difficult to interpret the studies that focus on assessment of RLS in medicated PD patients [90].

Management

The general approach toward treatment of RLS includes assessment and correction of coexisting iron deficiency and reduction of medication that can potentially worsen RLS such as antidepressants [90]. FDA has approved dopamine agonists (ropinirole, pramipexole) for moderate to severe RLS, although, there are no controlled trials that support this in PD patients with RLS [100]. Rotigotine, a dopamine agonist, has been approved as a 24-hour transdermal patch treatment with favorable clinical efficacy and tolerability in management of both PD and RLS [145].

REM Sleep Behavior Disorder (RBD)

The frequency of RBD, defined by PSG, occurs in between 39% to 46% in PD patients [146, 147]. The risk factors for RBD in PD patients include older age, greater PD severity, higher levodopa dosage, more falls, increased motor fluctuations, and greater psychiatric comorbidity [147]. The diagnosis of RBD requires PSG evidence of REM sleep without atonia (RSWA) in combination with either demonstration of dream enactment behavior during PSG study or history of dream enactment behaviors or both.

Clinically, RBD must be differentiated from apnea-related arousals during REM sleep and PLMS. Additionally, emergence of RBD has been reported in association with antidepressant use. In a prospective cohort study, the authors compared patients with idiopathic RBD (n = 100) with healthy controls (n = 45). RBD patients taking antidepressants (n = 27) were noted to have markers of prodromal neurodegeneration similar to those without antidepressants. However, RBD patients taking antidepressants had a lower risk of developing neurodegenerative disease than those without antidepressant use (5-year risk = 22% vs. 59%; RR = 0.22, 95% CI = 0.06–0.74) [148]. D

Dream enactment behaviors in RBD are associated with significant risk of accidental injury both to the patient and the bed partner. RBD symptoms can precede or follow the onset of PD and RBD is considered as one of the strongest risk factors of future development of PD [90]. Within

2 decades, approximately 50% to 70% or more of patients with idiopathic RBD will convert to a parkinsonian disorder [149]. According to a 16-year follow-up study of idiopathic RBD patients (n = 29), 81% of 26 patients (three patients were lost to follow-up) developed parkinsonism or a defined neurodegenerative disease [150]. RBD predicts a nontremor-predominant subtype, gait freezing, and an aggressive clinical course in PD patients. Presence of RBD has been associated with more severe nonmotor symptoms, including hallucinations and cognitive impairment and poor quality of life in PD patients [151, 152].

Management

Bedroom safety with environmental modifications aimed to reduce potential injury to the patient and bed partner is an integral part of management of RBD. These measures include removal of sharp objects, placing the mattress on the floor, and securing windows in the bedroom [153]. Treatments for idiopathic RBD, including clonazepam and melatonin, lack robust data to support their efficacy in management of RBD comorbid with a neurodegenerative disorder [90]. In a randomized placebo-controlled trial, memantine (20 mg/day) decreased symptoms of probable RBD in patients with PD and dementia of Lewy bodies over a 24-week follow-up period [154].

SLEEP DISORDERS AND MULTIPLE SCLEROSIS

Multiple sclerosis (MS) is an autoimmune disorder of the central nervous system characterized by inflammation and destruction of the brain and spinal cord [155]. MS is a chronic and debilitating neurological disorder that affects nearly half a million Americans and is a leading cause of nontraumatic disability in young adults [155]. There seems to be a disproportionately high frequency of primary sleep disorders in MS patients that play a key role in development of debilitating fatigue and poor functional outcomes [155]. The most common sleep disorders in MS include insomnia, RLS, PLMD, and BRSDs.

Presence of sleep disorders has been associated with fatigue, a common and disabling symptom of MS. In a cross-sectional study, 96% of MS patients with fatigue had a relevant sleep disorder, and having a sleep disorder was associated with an increased risk of fatigue (OR 18.5; 95% CI 1.6–208, p = 0.018) [156]. In a community-based longitudinal study of MS patients (n = 489), fatigue and sleep disturbance predicted onset of probable major depression on the Patient Health Questionnaire (PHQ-9) instrument 3½ years later among nondepressed patients at baseline [157]. Sleep disturbances, fatigue, and depression have been correlated with poor quality of life in MS patients [158, 159].

Despite their high prevalence and negative impact in MS, sleep disorders remain underrecognized and undertreated. In a cross-sectional survey based study of MS patients (n = 2,375), 898 (37.8%) screened positive for OSA, 746 (31.6%) for moderate to severe insomnia, and 866 (36.8%) for RLS. In contrast, only 4%, 11%, and 12% of the cohort reported being diagnosed by a healthcare provider with OSA, insomnia, and RLS, respectively. EDS was noted in 30% of respondents and more than 60% of the respondents reported abnormal fatigue. Therefore, greater attention to recognition and treatment of sleep disorders is warranted in MS patients [160]. In this section, we summarize the frequency, clinical characteristics and approach to management of common primary sleep disorders in MS patients.

Breathing-Related Sleep Disorders (BRSDs)

MS patients experience BRSDs which may manifest as OSA, CSA, and sleep-related hypoventilation syndrome [161]. The reported frequency of BRSDs varies between 0% and 87%, with variability explained by differences in study design, study population, and methodology [162]. Major risk factors for OSA in general population including age, male sex, and obesity also seem to be applicable in MS patients despite higher prevalence of MS in women.

BRSDs can increase oxidative stress and may worsen neuronal loss in people with MS due to intermittent hypoxia caused by apneas during the night [162]. On the other hand, inflammation in MS may also play a role in the occurrence of BRSDs. MS is an autoimmune disorder characterized with elevation of cytokine levels of tumor necrosis factor alpha (TNF-α), interleukin (IL)-6, and IL-1b, among others [163]. Additionally, systemic cytokine levels of TNF-α, IL-6, C-reactive protein, IL-1b, reactive oxygen species, and adhesion molecules are increased in OSA patients [164, 165].

In a study comparing MS patients (n = 48) with controls, the authors reported that mean AHI and mean central apnea index (CAI) were higher in the MS group. The authors concluded that MS patients, particularly those with brainstem involvement, have higher predilection for obstructive and central apnea events [166]. These findings have been replicated such that brainstem plaques in MS patients have been associated with CSA and central alveolar hypoventilation syndrome [166–168]. Therefore, presence of signs suggestive of brainstem dysfunction, such as dysarthria or dysphagia, may signal high risk of BRSD [155].

MS patients with comorbid OSA and those at elevated risk for OSA report increased fatigue as compared to MS patients with undiagnosed or low-risk of OSA [156, 160, 169, 170]. Presence of OSA predicts diminished quality life in MS patients [171]. Additionally, preliminary data suggest that apnea severity may correlate with impaired cognition in MS [172]. MS patients should be routinely screened for symptoms of BRSD including snoring, witnessed apneas, poor sleep quality, daytime hypersomnolence, and cognitive impairment [155]. Physical signs and symptoms associated with OSA including obesity, increased neck circumference, crowded oropharyngeal inlet, retrognathia, or micronathia, in conjunction with the previous symptoms, should prompt clinicians to consider diagnostic testing for BRSD [155].Use of screening tools such as the STOP-Bang questionnaire can aid in recognition of MS patients at high risk of OSA [173] and diagnosis of BRSD is confirmed with an overnight PSG study.

Management

Optimal management of BRSDs includes consideration of variables including apnea subtype (obstructive versus central), apnea severity, MS-specific symptoms, and limitations in individual MS patients [155]. Use of positive airway pressure (PAP) therapy has been associated with improvement in fatigue in MS patients with OSA, according to a noncontrolled prospective follow-up study [174]. A simplistic mask interface should be used in MS patients with hemiparesis and dexterity issues to improve PAP therapy compliance [155].

Oral appliances may be used to treat OSA in MS patients, especially when PAP compliance is an issue. However, MS patients with trigeminal neuralgia may not tolerate oral appliances due to worsening of pain [155]. Anti-inflammatory therapy with etanercept (a TNF-α antagonist) can improve OSA severity and hypersomnolence in the general population, based on a placebo-controlled double blind study [175]. These results may have implications that disease-modifying therapy using anti-inflammatory agents in MS

may also have beneficial effects on OSA. However, this remains to be proven in future systematic research studies [175]. Use of medications including opiates and antispasmodics in MS patients can worsen CSA; therefore, the use of such medications should be minimized if possible [155].

Narcolepsy

Narcolepsy patients mainly complain of hypersomnolence and EDS with accompanying symptoms like cataplexy, sleep paralysis, hallucinations (hypnagogic/hypnopompic), and disrupted nocturnal sleep [176]. Narcolepsy is further categorized as narcolepsy type I and narcolepsy type II. The prevalence rates of narcolepsy in MS patients are unknown. Hypocretin deficiency in narcolepsy type 1 can be established by presence of cataplexy or CSF hypocretin levels ≤110 pg/dL. Whereas, narcolepsy type II is associated with normal hypocretin levels. PSG and MSLT studies are required to establish the diagnosis of narcolepsy [177], which must confirm a mean sleep latency of up to 8 minutes and at least two sleep-onset REM periods (SOREMPs) during MSLT.

Although the exact cause of narcolepsy is still not determined, narcolepsy is considered to be an immune-mediated disorder with selective loss of hypothalamic hypocretin neurons [178]. Evidence for an immune basis of narcolepsy include factors such as strong association with HLA-DQB1*0602, a strong protective effect of DRB1*13:01-DQB1*06:03 haplotype [179], a recent discovery of circulating TRIB2-specific antibodies reactive to hypocretin neurons [180], and a genome-wide association with a T-cell receptor α chain [181]. MS is considered to be the fourth most common cause of secondary narcolepsy after inherited disorders, tumors, and head trauma [182]. Focal hypothalamic brain lesions have been correlated with development of narcolepsy in MS patients by multiple authors [183–186].

Management

As there is no permanent cure for narcolepsy, treatment should be directed toward symptom reduction. Counseling and lifestyle changes like following a systematic sleep–wake cycle regularly with scheduled naps during the day are some of the nonpharmacological treatment modalities for narcolepsy [187]. Medication treatments are used to alleviate symptoms of hypersomnolence and cataplexy in narcolepsy patients [188]. Wake-promoting agents such as modafinil and armodafinil are FDA-approved medications for treatment of hypersomnolence associated with narcolepsy. Due to their REM suppressant effects, antidepressant medications including selective serotonin reuptake inhibitors (SSRIs) and serotonin-norepinephrine reuptake inhibitors (SNRIs) can be used for treatment of cataplexy and sleep paralysis associated with narcolepsy [187, 189]. Sodium oxybate is now FDA-approved for treatment of both hypersomnolence and cataplexy in narcolepsy patients [190]. Due to risk of respiratory depression, it is recommended to avoid the concurrent use of central nervous system suppressants medications and alcohol in narcolepsy patients using sodium oxybate. In MS patients with hypothalamic lesions, trial of high doses of steroids can be effective to alleviate the symptoms of narcolepsy [191].

Circadian Rhythm Sleep Disorders (CRSDs)
Disruption in the internal (biological) circadian rhythm and the external 24-hour environment can lead to circadian rhythm sleep disorders (CRSDs) [192]. Patients complain of an exaggerated level of sleepiness or sleepiness adversely impacting important daily functions such as social and occupational activities [192]. The most common examples of CRSDs are shift work disorder and jetlag disorder. Delayed sleep–wake phase disorder is the most common CRSD seen in adolescents and younger adults, while advanced sleep–wake phase disorder is seen instead in the elderly population [193]. MS patients may have a disorganized sleep–wake cycle associated with demyelination of the afferent and efferent nerve pathways from the suprachiasmatic nucleus, the biological pacemaker in the human brain [194]. Although magnetic resonance imaging (MRI) is used to detect MS lesions in the hypothalamus, histologically [195, 196], there are no published studies which demonstrate a possible association between the specific localizations of radiological lesions and/or histopathological characteristics to CRSDs in MS. An accurate patient history and data based on sleep diaries is very useful in diagnosing CRSDs, as these are clinical diagnoses. Some of the details that should be taken into consideration during a clinical interview include details of hours of alertness during mornings and evenings, sleep–wake pattern during vacations, any functional difficulties, family history of CRSDs, head injuries, and side effects of drugs, especially psychotropic drugs [192].

Management
Proper evaluation of the circadian phase is crucial before initiating treatment to accomplish the appropriate circadian phase shift (i.e., resetting the clock) [192]. The treatment of CRSDs in MS patients consists of melatonin, timed bright light exposure, and scheduled daytime sleep which is similar to patients without MS [197].

Insomnia
Insomnia is a commonly reported sleep complaint in MS patients. Based on cross-sectional data from a Portuguese study, 22.3% of MS patients (n = 206) met criteria for chronic insomnia [198]. Others have reported that up to 40% of the MS patients may be at risk of insomnia disorder [160]. Risk factors associated with insomnia in MS patients include female sex, nocturnal symptoms, medical comorbidities, and higher levels of anxiety, depression and fatigue [198]. Insomnia has been correlated with a significantly lower quality of life in MS patients [198, 199]. A careful and precise sleep, psychiatric, and MS symptom history is essential for a comprehensive assessment of insomnia in MS patients. Specific consideration should be given to symptoms including frequency and severity of nocturnal pain, spasticity, urinary frequency, depression, and anxiety during sleep assessment. Common comorbid primary sleep disorders such as OSA and RLS should be explored in MS patients due to their negative impact on sleep. Additionally, medications used for treatment of MS symptoms can potentially interfere with sleep. Screening tools such as the Insomnia Severity Index (ISI) can be useful to assess the nature, severity, and impact of insomnia on daily functioning and to monitor treatment response. Sleep habits, lifestyle factors, and environmental factors should be assessed to ensure that poor sleep hygiene is not contributing to the sleep disturbance. Such data regarding the sleep routine and hygiene of patients can be obtained by maintaining a sleep diary for a period of 1 to 2 weeks [200].

Management
Currently, there are no definitive treatments for management of insomnia in MS patients. Practical strategies include adequate treatment of nocturnal MS symptoms such as pain and urinary urgency to improve insomnia. Iatrogenic causes of insomnia must be addressed and the dose of medications that can impact sleep onset and maintenance, especially wake-promoting agents, should

be reduced or discontinued if possible [155]. Use of immunotherapy such as beta-interferon has been associated with flu-like symptoms, fatigue, insomnia, and reduced sleep efficiency [201, 202] and these side effects may be reduced by switching from an evening to a morning administration schedule [203].

In a study incorporating telephone-administered cognitive-behavioral therapy (T-CBT) versus telephone-administered supportive emotion-focused therapy for treatment of depression in MS patients (n = 127), improvements in sleep-onset insomnia were associated with improvement in depression and anxiety. The type of psychotherapy did not predict improvement in sleep outcomes in this study. However, nearly a half of participants continued to report insomnia, and the authors recommend that additional treatment of insomnia is needed beyond the treatment of comorbid psychiatric disorders [204]. Evidence suggests that CBT-I is an effective treatment for insomnia in MS patients [205, 206]. In a case series (n = 11), CBT-I was effective for management of insomnia symptoms and improved depression and fatigue in MS patients [207].

Sleep-Related Movement Disorders

Restless legs syndrome (RLS) and Periodic limb movement disorder (PLMD) are the most common sleep-related movement disorders in MS patients [208, 209]. RLS is further classified as idiopathic or primary if no other cause can be identified or secondary if caused by another comorbid medical condition known to increase vulnerability, such as MS [155]. Disruptions in the dopaminergic pathway transmission and iron deficiency anemia have been associated with RLS [210, 211]. PLMD is diagnosed when there are frequent and sleep-disturbing PLMS recorded during PSG, that are associated with clinical symptoms of insomnia or daytime hypersomnolence in the absence of subjective RLS symptoms. PLMD is considered an endophenotype of RLS [212], and it has been associated with reduced serum ferritin levels and iron stores similar to RLS [213, 214].

As compared to controls, the prevalence of RLS in MS patients is two to six times higher based on large-scale epidemiological studies [215–217]. Another study reported the frequency of PLMD in MS patients to be 36%, as compared to 8% in healthy controls [209]. This study also demonstrated that MS patients with PLMD had greater MRI lesion loads in the infratentorial regions, particularly in the cerebellum and brainstem [209].

Primary progressive MS, higher degree of disability, cervical lesions, and older age are some of the risk factors associated with RLS in MS patients [215, 218, 219]. According to a recent large cross-sectional study, as compared to controls, women with MS had a greater incidence of RLS and daytime sleepiness [220]. MS patients presenting with severe RLS symptoms may present with disrupted sleep, daytime fatigue, and EDS [218].

Diagnosis of RLS in MS patients can be complicated due to the presence of MS-related sensory and motor symptoms, such as paresthesias and leg spasms that can mimic RLS [221]. Spinal cord MRI should be considered in evaluating RLS in MS patients due to association of RLS with cervical myelopathies and borrelia-induced myelitis [221]. Current evidence does not support iron deficiency as a risk factor for RLS in MS. In a case–control study, Manconi and colleagues [222] demonstrated no significant difference in serum ferritin levels between patients with MS and controls and no difference in ferritin levels between patients with MS with and without RLS. RLS is a clinical diagnosis, although PSG is necessary for diagnosing PLMD [197].

Management

No specific guidelines exist for management for RLS or PLMD in MS patients. General strategies include reduction or discontinuation of medications and substances that can cause or worsen RLS or PLMD. These include dopamine antagonists, lithium, SSRIs, SNRIs, antihistamines, tricyclic antidepressants, alcohol, tobacco, and caffeine [223–225]. Despite lack of association of iron deficiency in RLS comorbid with MS, iron studies are still recommended and iron supplementation should be considered for serum ferritin levels less than 75 ng/mL [155]. Current FDA-approved medications for management of moderate-severe RLS include dopamine agonists (pramipexole, ropinirole, and rotigotine) and α-2-δ ligand gabapentin enacarbil. Other α-2-δ ligand drugs gabapentin and pregabalin have also been shown to be efficacious treatments for RLS [226] and may be ideally suited for MS patients with concomitant conditions such as neuropathic pain or seizures [155].

REM Sleep Behavior Disorder (RBD)

RBD has been rarely associated with nonsynuclein structural lesions affecting the pons, medulla, or limbic system [227, 228]. A few case reports confirm the presence of RBD in MS patients.

Tippman-Peikert and colleagues [229] reported a case of 51-year-old female who developed RBD in the context of dorsal pontine demyelination secondary to MS. Plazzi and colleagues [230] reported onset of RBD as a heralding sign for MS in a 25-year-old female with periventricular and pontine demyelinating lesions. Interestingly, RBD disappeared with adrenocorticotropic hormone (ACTH) treatment and authors suggested use of brain imaging and longer-term follow-up in young patients presenting with RBD [230]. Additionally, new-onset RBD in known MS patients should also be evaluated for signs of radiographic progression. Video PSG not only confirms the diagnosis of RBD but also can be helpful to rule out conditions that mimic RBD, such as sleep apnea and seizures [155]. Management options for RBD include bedroom safety to prevent injurious behaviors, which is also aided by use of clonazepam or melatonin.

Sleep Disorders and Epilepsy

Epilepsy is a neurological disorder characterized by hyperexcitability and hypersynchrony of neuronal networks leading to recurrent seizures [231]. On the basis of cortical location, the epileptic seizures can be differentiated as generalized or focal (formerly known as partial). Epileptic seizures exhibit temporal patterns and have been further divided as diurnal, nocturnal, and diffuse types (those with temporal unpredictability) [232]. One-third of epilepsy patients have seizures during sleep [233].

As compared to the general population, sleep disorders are two to three times more common in adult epilepsy patients [234, 235]. Moreover, sleep disturbances including poor sleep quality, EDS, and insomnia are more common in epilepsy patients, and factors such as depressive mood, anxiety, and perceived sleep insufficiency are likely contributing factors [236]. Several sleep disorders may exacerbate the epileptic state, causing spikes and nocturnal seizures resulting in EDS and decreased quality of life and daytime activities [237]. In a large study, the presence of sleep disturbance in focal epilepsy patients has been associated with the greatest impairment in quality of life [233].

There exists a well-established reciprocal relationship between sleep and epilepsy; seizures may influence sleep, and sleep may influence seizure activity as well [238]. In the last two decades, considerable progress has been made in the understanding of the pathophysiology of sleep-related interictal and ictal phenomena and comorbidity between various sleep conditions and epilepsies

[239]. Nearly half of focal seizures may occur during sleep, with a majority of sleep-related seizures occurring during NREM, especially N1 or N2 sleep [240]. Herman and colleagues [240] suggested that frontal lobe seizures are most likely to occur during sleep, while patients with temporal lobe seizures have intermediate sleep seizure rates. Additionally, NREM sleep, particularly N2 sleep, promotes secondary generalization of focal seizures. Alterations in neurotransmitters (GABA, acetylcholine, and serotonin) and hyperpolarization of excitatory thalamo-cortical connections may provide a rationale for activation of focal seizures during NREM sleep [241]. Sleep spindles, short bursts of electrical activity from reticulo-thalamo-cortical circuitry, may also trigger epileptiform discharges (IEDs) during N2 sleep [241].

In this section, we summarize the common sleep disorders with a focus on their frequency, risk factors, clinical implications, and management in the setting of epilepsy. Sleep disturbances associated with psychogenic non-epileptic seizures (PNES) have also been included in this section.

Breathing-Related Sleep Disorders (BRSDs)

According to a recent meta-analysis, epilepsy patients are more susceptible to have OSA as compared to healthy controls (OR 2.36; 95 % CI 1.33–4.18). Approximately a third of epilepsy patients (33.4%) have mild-severe OSA, and men are more susceptible to OSA than women (OR 3.00; 95 % CI 2.25–3.99). The authors indicated that the frequency of OSA in patients with refractory epilepsy is not higher than that seen in epilepsy patients overall (17.5 vs 33.4 %). Additionally, OSA was not correlated to factors such as seizure type and number of antiepileptic drugs (AEDs) [242].

As compared to OSA, CSA has received much less attention in epilepsy patients [238]. In a large cohort study ($n = 416$), the majority of epilepsy patients had OSA (75%) whereas a minority had CSA (4%) and complex sleep apnea (8%), which is similar to the general population [243]. Epilepsy patients with CSA may present with less severe symptoms, as compared to those with OSA [243]. However, multiple authors have suggested a relationship between CSA and seizure activity, such that central apnea events can precede or occur during or following an episode of nocturnal or diurnal seizure events [244–248]. Additionally, Devinsky et al. [249] observed that BRSDs might lead to sudden unexpected death in epilepsy (SUDEP) individuals, during night time or in association with sleep.

Similar to the general population, evidence suggests that EDS is a consequence of OSA in epilepsy patients [250, 251]. Manni and colleagues [250] reported that approximately 23% of epilepsy patients with OSA endorsed EDS as compared to 9% of those without OSA. In another study by Gammino et al. [251], epilepsy patients with hypersomnolence were deemed to be at a higher risk of OSA as compared to those without hypersomnolence. The results of a pivotal study examining hypersomnolence in epilepsy patients suggested that primary sleep disorders (e.g., sleep apnea and RLS) and not epilepsy related factors (such as nocturnal seizures, AEDs, type of epilepsy) were significantly associated with hypersomnolence [252]. Piperidou and colleagues [253] reported that epilepsy patients with OSA symptoms endorsed more cognitive problems (using a self-report measure) than epilepsy patients without OSA symptoms.

The Sleep Apnea Scale of the Sleep Disorders Questionnaire (SA-SDQ) has a good sensitivity and specificity as a screening tool for patients with epilepsy at high risk of OSA [254, 255]. Other screening tools for OSA include the Berlin Questionnaire and the STOP-Bang questionnaire. Male sex, age >50 years, increased neck circumference and high BMI are some of the risk factors considered by these screening tools. Use of simple and easily administered screening questionnaires can identify patients at increased risk of OSA who can benefit from OSA treatment. According to a recent study, as compared to sleep history and physical assessment, the number of referrals to sleep medicine increased from 1.7% to 41.6% while using the STOP-Bang questionnaire for screening OSA in epilepsy patients in an outpatient setting [256].

Management

Among sleep disorders, sleep apnea is most likely to exacerbate seizures [257]. CPAP therapy has beneficial effects in patients with OSA as it decreases daytime sleepiness and enhances quality of life by improving mood, cognitive functions (attention, executive functions and memory) [87, 258–260], glucose control and BP [261]. In a recent meta-analysis, Lin and colleagues [262] demonstrated that epilepsy patients with comorbid and treated OSA had a measurable decrease in the seizure episodes and daytime sleepiness

by >fivefold as compared to untreated patients. Patients who received CPAP treatment were four times more likely to be seizure-free than the untreated patients [242]. Use of CPAP has also been associated with improved seizure control even in patients with medically refractory epilepsy [262].

The effects of CPAP therapy on interictal IEDs in patients with focal epilepsy and coexisting OSA during sleep were demonstrated by two studies [263, 264]. Decreased spiking during SWS has been noted after 2 to 3 days [263], and during all stages of NREM sleep after 1 month of CPAP use [264]. Oxygen-saturation levels during sleep improved significantly with CPAP therapy [263, 264]. CPAP decreases electroencephalography (EEG) arousals and hypoxemia associated with sleep apnea, decreases seizure susceptibility, stabilizes sleep, and can reduce OSA consequences such as cognitive impairment and neuronal, cardiovascular and metabolic dysfunction [238].

Vagal nerve stimulation (VNS) is a FDA-approved treatment of medication-refractory epilepsy. VNS causes an increase in respiratory rate and a decrease in respiratory amplitude, tidal volume, and oxygen saturation during periods of VNS activation [265]. Both central and obstructive respiratory events can occur in epilepsy patients and most patients have increase in AHI with VNS treatment. Respiratory events can be reduced with changes in VNS parameters or with the use of CPAP. Epilepsy patients seeking VNS are recommended to have sleep apnea screening both before and after VNS implantation [265].

Insomnia

About 10% of individuals experience the full clinical syndrome of chronic insomnia disorder, whereas 30% to 35% have transient insomnia amidst the general population [266]. Macedo et al. [267], in a recent literature review, noted that almost half of the patients with epilepsy had insomnia, but with variable frequency based on the inclusion criteria. However, frequency of insomnia in patients with epilepsy is 36% to 74%, and moderate-to-severe insomnia (ISI ≥15) is seen in about 15% to 51% of epilepsy patients [268]. Insomnia was associated with greater impairment in quality of life and higher degree of depressive symptoms in several studies, and was inconsistently related to female gender, poor seizure control, and AED poly-therapy [268]. In a cross-sectional study (n = 90), Yang and colleagues [269] demonstrated that insomnia severity in epilepsy patients is correlated with comorbid medical and depressive symptoms and not directly to the epilepsy [269]. Similarly, Vendrame et al. [270] noted that insomnia severity and poor sleep quality were significantly associated with depressive symptoms, number of antiepileptic medications, and poor quality of life in epilepsy patients.

During assessment of insomnia in epilepsy patients, iatrogenic causes of insomnia deserve consideration, as many antiepileptic medications including phenobarbital, phenytoin, and valproic acid can also disrupt sleep [271]. DBS is currently being explored as a potential treatment for medically refractory epilepsy. According to one study, epilepsy patients undergoing DBS, directed to the anterior nuclear thalami, experienced significantly more electro-clinical arousals during DBS stimulation periods. Additionally, the number of arousals was correlated positively with DBS voltage parameters in epilepsy patients [272].

In epilepsy patients, circadian rhythms can affect the frequency of seizures as the evolution of seizures into different phases cluster at specific times of day and at specific phases of the sleep–wake cycle [273]. As compared to healthy controls, patients with idiopathic generalized epilepsy have been noted to have delayed circadian phase [274]. Circadian rhythm disorders should therefore be assessed in epilepsy patients as these disorders can also mimic insomnia in clinical settings. Delayed sleep–wake phase disorder, particularly common in adolescents and young adults, may account for 10% of patients with chronic insomnia.

Standardized screening instruments such as the ISI and the Pittsburgh Sleep Quality Index (PSQI) can be implemented to assess insomnia symptoms and overall sleep quality in epilepsy patients. Scores >8 indicate mild insomnia symptoms, whereas scores >15 suggest moderate insomnia symptoms on the ISI scale. Scores >5 on PSQI scale indicate poor sleep quality [210].

Management

Treatment of insomnia in epilepsy patients is challenging due to disease severity, comorbid sleep and psychiatric disorders, and possible drug-related effects that can potentially lower the seizure threshold. Therefore, treatment of insomnia need to be individualized, comprehensive, and multimodal in patients with epilepsy [238]. Clinicians may choose antiepileptic medications with favorable effects on sleep while treating epilepsy patients with insomnia. Strategic choices of antiepileptic medications that may improve

sleep in addition to seizures include gabapentin, tiagabine, pregabalin, clobazam, and carbamazepine, which can reduce sleep latency and/or improve sleep efficiency [271]. In a randomized double-blind crossover study ($n = 9$), pregabalin was associated with decreased N1 sleep, increased SWS, and improved daytime attention in patients with epilepsy and insomnia [275]. VNS has been associated with a significant increase in SWS and a decrease in sleep latency and N1 sleep in pediatric patients with medically refractory epilepsy [276]. Additionally, VNS at low stimulus intensities has been noted to reduce daytime sleepiness in epilepsy patients, even in those without reductions in seizure frequency [277].

No specific guidelines exist for pharmacological treatment of insomnia in epilepsy patients. Benzodiazepines may be considered, but the benefits of treatment should be weighed against the risks such as tolerance, risk of falls, cognitive impairment, rebound insomnia, withdrawal seizures, and possibly worsening of comorbid BRSDs [238]. Benzodiazepine receptor agonists (BzRAs) such as zolpidem and eszopiclone, are FDA approved for insomnia with better side effect profile than benzodiazepines for treatment of insomnia. However, BzRAs have been associated with complex sleep-related behaviors such as sleepwalking and sleep eating. Severe zolpidem dependence has been associated with withdrawal seizures in multiple case reports, so regular use of zolpidem in epilepsy patients is probably best avoided as in the general population, although specific safety and efficacy trials for zolpidem and related hypnotics in this patient population remain lacking [278–281].

Melatonergic agents including ramelteon have been approved for treatment of insomnia. In a study including pediatric epilepsy patients with insomnia ($n = 10$), melatonin sustained release (9 mg) resulted in significant improvements in SOL and WASO as compared to placebo [282]. However, the results of this study may not be generalizable due to small sample size. Sedating antidepressants are used for insomnia treatment, especially in the presence of comorbid depression and anxiety disorders [238]. However, low risk (0.1%) of seizure exacerbation has been associated with antidepressants such as clomipramine (highest risk), followed by amitriptyline, venlafaxine, citalopram, sertraline, trazodone, mirtazapine, paroxetine, bupropion, and escitalopram. On the other hand, fluoxetine and duloxetine were associated with negligible exacerbation of seizure risk [283].

CBT-I is recognized as the standard and preferred initial modality for treatment of chronic insomnia. CBT-I incorporates techniques including stimulus control, sleep restriction, cognitive restructuring and relaxation. However, evidence is lacking for usefulness of CBT-I in epilepsy patients. CBT-I can be considered in treatment of insomnia in epilepsy patients with caution that sleep restriction can exacerbate seizures. Well-controlled studies are warranted to establish the safety and efficacy of CBT-I in management of insomnia in epilepsy patients [238].

Restless Legs Syndrome (RLS)

RLS is described as an uncomfortable and irresistible urge to move the legs, relieved by getting up to walk or any movement, with symptoms predominant in the evenings or during rest [284].

According to a Turkish epilepsy clinic sample, 13 (5.8%) of 225 patients were diagnosed with RLS by a clinical interview, with a mean International Restless Legs Syndrome Rating Scale score of 9.3 in terms of RLS symptom severity (range 6–18, consistent with mild to moderate symptoms), The authors found that RLS was not associated with any epilepsy-specific factors [285]. A higher frequency of RLS was found in 55 of 158 (35%) patients included in a Michigan epilepsy cohort study. The authors noted RLS to be a significant predictor of daytime sleepiness in epilepsy patients, using the ESS [252]. In an Iranian study, 32.3% of epilepsy patients had RLS compared to only 11.8% of controls [286].

Trotti and colleagues [284] suggested that sleep-related epilepsies can be confused with other sleep-related movement disorders like sleep-related leg cramps, sleep-related bruxism, propriospinal myoclonus at sleep onset (involving myoclonic flexion of the truncal muscles, with variable propagation to the upper body or limbs), and especially sleep-related rhythmic movement disorder, which is characterized by repetitive rhythmic movements at sleep–wake transition that may mimic clonic seizures [284]. Video PSG with EEG (VPSG-EEG) can be used reliably to distinguish sleep-related epilepsies from sleep-related movement disorders [238].

Aura symptoms without altered awareness, seen with focal seizures, can mimic RLS symptoms occasionally. Nocturnal unilateral left leg paresthesias and cramps, that preceded generalized tonic–clonic seizures, were treated very effectively with levetiracetam and carbamazepine in a patient with right posterior frontal focal cortical dysplasia [287]. On the other hand, zonisamide, an antiepileptic medication, has been implicated in causing RLS symptoms based on a few case reports [288, 289].

Management

Some of the nonpharmacological measures effective in treating minor or infrequent RLS symptoms include avoidance of RLS precipitants such as caffeine, nicotine, and alcohol. Use of counter-stimuli like using lavender oil for massage or taking temperate, hot, or cold baths and behavioral strategies including cognitive alerting, distraction and lifestyle modifications can be helpful [238]. Other practical approaches include eliminating or reducing the dose of antidepressants, which aggravate RLS. Iron-replacement therapy has shown to improve RLS symptoms after few weeks or months of treatment and should be considered in RLS patients, even with low-normal iron status (i.e., ferritin <75 mcg/L, transferrin percentage saturation <20%) [290]. First-line therapies for RLS include alpha-2-delta ligand agonists (gabapentin, pregabalin), dopamine agonists (pramipexole, ropinirole), and transdermal rotigotine patch [226, 290, 291].

Parasomnias

Parasomnias are described as abnormal and undesirable movement behaviors, dreams or perceptions either while going to sleep, during their sleep or waking up from sleep, which may be associated with daytime naps. Parasomnias are further divided in to two types- NREM and REM parasomnias. Somnambulism (sleepwalking), sleep terrors and confusion arousal are some of the main phenotypes of NREM parasomnias [292], that are characterized by abnormal arousal from the NREM sleep causing amnesia, confusion, and abnormal autonomic or motor behaviors. REM parasomnias include isolated sleep paralysis, nightmare disorder, and RBD [293]. Patients with isolated sleep paralysis experience brief muscle paralysis on either falling asleep or waking up from sleep associated with hypnagogic hallucinations in the absence of other features of narcolepsy like cataplexy and daytime sleepiness. Nightmare disorder is associated with frequent and frightful dreams causing uncomplicated arousal with lack of other symptoms except motor starts or brief vocalizations. RBD is diagnosed when patients have a complex motor or vocal behavior along with dream mentation (dream-enactment behaviors) associated with RSWA [294].

Nocturnal frontal lobe epilepsy (NFLE) is characterized by seizures with complex, often bizarre, and violent behaviors that arise only or mainly during sleep. It is difficult to distinguish NFLE seizures from other nonepileptic events, namely, parasomnias, as these unusual seizures and their occurrence during sleep are often accompanied by normal EEG tracings [295]. Additionally, as compared to controls, increased frequency of arousal parasomnias has been reported in relatives of patients with NFLE. The authors suggested an intrinsic link between parasomnias and NFLE and an abnormal arousal system as a possible common pathophysiological mechanism [296]. Among REM parasomnias, RBD has been associated with epilepsy in several studies. In a questionnaire-based study to assess subjective sleep disturbances, as compared to 6% of the controls, 12 % of the epilepsy patients endorsed symptoms suggestive of probable RBD ($p < 0.05$) [297]. In another study, video PSG confirmed idiopathic RBD coexisted in 12.5 % of the elderly epilepsy patients ($n = 80$). The authors noted that RBD was more prevalent in men and in those with cryptogenic epilepsy [298].

Frontal Lobe Epilepsy and Parasomnias (FLEP) scale has been proposed as a practical bedside tool to assist with distinction between parasomnias and sleep-related epilepsies. The FLEP scale includes several cardinal clinical features of the sleep-related hypermotor epilepsies and parasomnias and showed correct diagnosis of NFLE in all 31 patients with NFLE from another 31 with NREM parasomnias in one validation cohort, with an excellent sensitivity and specificity [298]. However, it performed less well in distinguishing REM parasomnias from NFLE in an Italian cohort, which also included RBD cases, suggesting that additional refinement of the FLEP is needed for its clinical use to differentiate between REM parasomnias and NFLE [300]. VPSG-EEG is indicated in patients with complex nocturnal behaviors when the routine EEG is nondiagnostic [301].

Management
Once the diagnosis is established, maintaining good sleep hygiene and prevention of sleep deprivation can be helpful initial steps in the management of NREM parasomnia behaviors. Use of benzodiazepines may be indicated in management of NREM parasomnias that are not responsive to conservative measures [302]. In addition

to bedroom safety, clonazepam (1–2 mg) or melatonin (3-12 mg) at bedtime is indicated for treatment of RBD.

SLEEP AND PSYCHOGENIC NONEPILEPTIC SPELLS (PNES)
PNES are defined as paroxysmal and apparently involuntary events characterized by changes in the patient's perceived level of consciousness, behavior, motor activity, or autonomic function without an ictal EEG signature of epileptic seizures occurring during the spell [303]. Psychological stress, exceeding an individual's coping capacity, often precedes PNES [304]. A majority of PNES cases (70%) develop between the second and fourth decades of life. In children, the risk of PNES is associated with older age, concurrent diagnosis of depression, family history of epilepsy and psychiatric illness, and an inadequate family environment [305]. At least 10% of PNES patients have concurrent epileptic seizures or have had epileptic seizures before the diagnosis of PNES [304]. Certain patient and seizure characteristics can help differentiate between PNES and epilepsy. These include long seizure duration (especially longer than 3–5 minutes), eye closure, asynchronous movements, intra-ictal awareness, lack of post ictal state, and frequent recurrence in the same context. Other features that raise suspicion for PNES include psychiatric comorbidities, history of abuse, cognitive impairment, and multiple nonspecific somatic complaints [303]. Less than 40% of PNES patients are expected to become seizure-free within 5 years after diagnosis [306].

PNES resemble epileptic seizures and are often misdiagnosed and mistreated as the latter while appropriate treatment is delayed. Reuber and colleagues [307] reported that PNES patients were diagnosed 7.2 years, on average, after initial manifestation. The authors noted that younger age, inter-ictal epileptiform potentials in the EEG, and anticonvulsant treatment were associated with longer delays in PNES diagnosis [307]. It can be challenging for clinicians to differentiate between PNES and epileptic seizures. Video EEG is the diagnostic gold standard for PNES, and a diagnosis is suspected when video EEG reveals no epileptiform activity before, during, or after the ictus [304]. However, video EEG is costly and not always easily accessible [308]. PNES occurs in approximately 25% to 40% of patients admitted to inpatient epilepsy monitoring units [309].

Sleep changes have been examined in PNES patients in comparison to those with epilepsy.

Bazil and colleagues [309] reported that, as compared to epilepsy patients (n = 10), PNES patients (n = 8) had significantly greater REM% and reduced REM latency (nonsignificant) [309]. Sleep architectural changes in PNES patients were similar to those found in patients with major depression. Benbadis et al. [310] noted that pre-ictal "pseudo-sleep" was associated with "ictal" events in 10 out 18 PNES patients, as compared to none of the epilepsy patients. The authors defined pre-ictal pseudo-sleep as a state that resembled normal sleep by behavioral criteria alone (patient with eyes closed and being motionless), while EEG showed evidence of wakefulness (alpha rhythm, active electromyography, and REMs) [310]. In another study, Seneviratne and colleagues [311] found a significant association between sleep and arousal such that the odds of PNES were four times higher when patients were awake (OR 4.27, 95% CI 2.44–7.48, p < 0.0001) as compared to while asleep. The authors retrospectively examined the seizure type (PNES vs. epileptic seizure), onset time of seizures, and the state of arousal (awake vs. sleep), and noted that the odds of having a PNES event were significantly higher if the seizure occurred with patients being awake at night. Based on these results, the authors suggested a complex interaction between the sleep–wake cycle and the 24-hour time cycle leading to PNES [311].

SLEEP DISORDERS AND TRAUMATIC BRAIN INJURY (TBI)

TBI is defined as injury occurring to the brain or skull, directly or indirectly affecting its function with some loss of consciousness. It is classified based on the type of injury as either focal or velocity injury. Focal injury describes the part of the brain injured and is further divided as open or closed type, whereas velocity injury is either acceleration or deceleration injury causing generalized damage. Approximately, 1.7 million individuals sustain a TBI of varying severity every year in the United States (500–600 per 100,000), and 16·3% of these injuries lead to hospital admissions.

According to World health organization, TBI secondary to road traffic accidents is going to be the third leading cause of disability after heart disease and depression in the world by 2020 [312]. The American Academy of Neurology categorized TBI based on time involving loss of consciousness, the presence of skull fracture, and Glasgow Coma Scale (GCS) [313, 314]. TBI is classified as mild, moderate, and severe as depicted in Table 26.1. TBI presentation can be so severe that it can lead to serious disabilities and even death. TBI-related symptoms are specific to the type and site of injury to the brain and commonly manifest as cognitive dysfunction, neurobehavioral disorders, somatosensory perceptive difficulties, somatic symptoms, and comorbid substance dependence.

Sleep is often disrupted following TBI, and disturbed sleep associated with TBI has the potential to severely undermine patient rehabilitation, recovery, and overall outcomes [315]. The underlying neurophysiological and neuropathological changes contributing to sleep disturbances associated with TBI are not well understood [316]. Evidence suggests that TBI severity does not predict the degree of sleep disturbances [317]; therefore, most patients with a TBI may be at risk to develop disturbed sleep [316]. According to a meta-analysis, approximately 50% of TBI patients suffer from sleep disturbance, and 25% to 29% of these patients are diagnosed with a sleep disorder [315]. In a study examining risk factors for sleep disturbances in mild-severe TBI patients (n = 98), the authors noted that symptoms including headaches, dizziness, anxiety, and depression were associated with insomnia, whereas GCS score was independently associated with hypersomnolence [318].

The results of a longitudinal observational study suggest that sleep disturbance in the acute TBI period has been associated with increased symptoms of depression, anxiety and apathy at 12 months post-injury follow-up [319]. Presence of sleep disorders can exacerbate other TBI symptoms such as fatigue, pain, and cognitive impairment [320]. Sleep disruption in TBI patients is

TABLE 26.1. CLASSIFICATION OF TRAUMATIC BRAIN INJURY (TBI)

Severity	Time of loss of consciousness (LOC)	Skull fracture	Glasgow coma scale (GCS)
Mild	< 30min	No skull fracture	13–15
Moderate	30min–24 hours	With or without skull fracture	9–12
Severe	>24 hours	Contusion, hematoma, fracture	< 8

associated with several cognitive deficits, including attention, memory, and executive function impairments, which can negatively affect activities of daily living [321], thus compromising long-term rehabilitation outcomes [322]. In this section, we focus on common TBI-related sleep disorders with an emphasis on frequency, risk factors, clinical implications, and their management.

Insomnia

Based on review of multiple studies of insomnia in TBI patients, approximately 40% (n = 2,816) reported symptoms of insomnia. Studies included in this review had varying methodologies, thus leading to varying frequencies for insomnia (15%–84%) in TBI patients [323]. Insomnia in TBI patients is likely multifactorial and can be caused by factors including TBI itself (direct injury to the brain), physical symptoms of TBI such as pain and headaches, and finally the neuropsychiatric consequences of TBI such as depression, anxiety, and PTSD [323]. Abnormalities of neurotransmitters involved in generation and maintenance of sleep and wakefulness including hypocretin, dopamine, and serotonin have been implicated in moderate or severe TBI [317, 324, 325]. Zhou and colleagues [326] reported an association between insomnia and hypothalamic–pituitary–adrenal (HPA) axis system in mild TBI patients. Compared to healthy controls, mild TBI patients experienced more serious subjective insomnia symptoms than assessed by objective measurement. The insomnia symptoms were associated with HPA dysfunction, which was measured with low-dose short synacthen test. In this test, tetracosactide, a chemical analogue of ACTH, is used to assess for possible adrenal insufficiency [326].

The risk factors associated with insomnia in TBI patients are less well understood [327]. In a prospective study from India, 40% of the TBI patients (n = 208) reported insomnia, and almost half of the TBI patients with insomnia had multiple cerebral contusions [327]. Patients with moderate TBI had significantly higher occurrence of insomnia as compared to those with mild TBI [327]. However, some studies have shown that those with mild TBI may have higher rates of insomnia as compared to those with more severe TBI [328, 329]. Severe TBI patients may also have memory and cognitive dysfunction, which may compromise the awareness and reporting of their sleep problems [323].

Khoury and colleagues [330] explored the relationship between pain and sleep in mild TBI patients using PSQI sleep architecture, and quantitative EEG (qEEG) brain activity after TBI. The average time between brain injury and study assessments was 45 days. Patients with mild TBI reported three times poorer subjective sleep quality than healthy controls. Patients with mild TBI had lower delta (deep sleep) and higher beta and gamma power (arousal) at certain EEG derivations than controls (p < 0.04). As compared to mild TBI patients without pain and healthy controls, mild TBI patients with pain showed greater increase in rapid EEG frequency bands, mostly during REM sleep, and beta bands in non-REM sleep (p < 0.001). Pain was associated with more rapid qEEG activity, mostly during REM sleep, suggesting that pain is associated with poor sleep in mild TBI patients [330].

Objective sleep changes in TBI have been corroborated with self-reported sleep quality, fatigue, and daytime sleepiness. Lu and colleagues [331] reported that poor sleep quality was associated with poor sleep efficiency, short duration of N2 sleep, and long duration of REM sleep, based on nocturnal PSG study [331]. In another study comparing mild-severe TBI and comorbid insomnia (n = 14) with healthy controls (n = 14), the authors noted that TBI patients had higher proportion of N1 sleep and unmedicated TBI patients had more awakenings and shorter REM latency [332]. Additionally, TBI patients had tendency to overestimate their sleep disturbance as compared to objective measures using PSG. Assessment of insomnia should be done using structured interviews and questionnaires including the PSQI and the ISI. However, given the previous findings, the interpretation of subjective insomnia in TBI deserves caution [333].

Management

Treatment of insomnia in TBI patients can be challenging due to lack of evidence-based guidelines. In a study with a randomized double-blind crossover design, mild-severe TBI patients (n = 33) reporting sleep disturbances were noted to have improved sleep quality and improved sleep efficiency with use of melatonin prolonged-release formulation (2 mg) 2 hours before bedtime, as compared to placebo. Melatonin use was associated with decreased anxiety and fatigue but had no significant effect on hypersomnolence in TBI patients [334]. In a randomized controlled, double-blind crossover trial, the authors found that amitriptyline (25 mg) and melatonin (5 mg) were equally effective and well tolerated in a small group of TBI patients with chronic sleep disturbances. As compared to baseline, TBI patients taking melatonin reported improved daytime alertness, whereas those taking amitriptyline reported increased sleep duration [335]. In another randomized controlled, double-blind crossover trial, lorazepam (0.5–1 mg) and zopiclone (3.75–7.5 mg) were equally effective in improving subjective sleep quality in patients with TBI and stroke [29]. However, benzodiazepines should be avoided when possible in patients with TBI, as cognitive side effects may be compounded in this population [336].

CBT-I, including stimulus control, sleep restriction, cognitive restructuring, sleep hygiene education, and fatigue management, for a period of 8 weeks has been shown to be effective in TBI patients ($n = 11$) in terms of improvements in sleep efficiency, reduction in total wake time, and reduction in general fatigue [337]. Addressing and treating psychiatric comorbidities such as mood disorders, anxiety, and PTSD in TBI patients can potentially improve insomnia outcomes.

Hypersomnolence

Several studies indicate a higher prevalence of hypersomnolence symptoms, including EDS and increased need for sleep per 24 hours, in TBI patients [317, 338, 339]. Findings from a meta-analysis suggest that hypersomnolence symptoms were among the most common and disturbing sleep problems in TBI patients [315]. The pathophysiology of hypersomnolence associated with TBI is not well established. However, injury to the wake-promoting systems, including ascending reticular activating system and hypocretin neurons, has been implicated [340, 341]. Watson and colleagues [342] compared 514 consecutive subjects with TBI, 132 noncranial trauma controls, and 102 trauma-free controls at 1 month and 1 year to assess natural history of sleepiness after TBI using subjective measures. The authors noted that more severe TBI was associated with increased sleepiness and two-thirds of TBI patients improved in terms of sleepiness over 1-year follow-up [342].

In a prospective study examining sleep–wake disturbances in TBI patients over 6 months, using objective sleep measurements, the authors noted that 57% of the TBI patients had EDS as compared to healthy controls. TBI patients had significantly reduced mean sleep onset latencies (8.7 ± 4.6 minutes) as compared to healthy controls (12.1 ± 4.7 min), based on MSLT [343]. Additionally, TBI patients underestimated the hypersomnolence symptoms, when using subjective assessment tools alone. The authors found that presence of intracranial hemorrhage had the most significant correlation for development of increased sleep need after TBI [343]. Masel and colleagues [338] examined the prevalence of hypersomnolence in TBI patients in a residential rehabilitation program using self-report and objective measures (PSG and MSLT). Mean sleep latency was ≤10 minutes in 47% and ≤5 minutes in 18.3% of the cohort. The authors reported that hypersomnolence is common in adults with TBI, with a relatively high prevalence of sleep apnea–hypopnea syndrome and PLMD. TBI patients had inability to perceive their hypersomnolence using self-report questionnaires.

Presence of hypersomnolence can affect cognitive recovery in TBI patients. The results of a prospective study, examining the effects of disturbed sleep on cognitive function after acute TBI, suggested that patients with moderate and severe TBI had longer daytime TST, as compared to those with mild TBI [344]. Additionally, the relationship between the TBI severity and the recovery of cognitive function was mediated by daytime TST in this study, although this effect may have likely been a proxy measure for severity of TBI.

Management
No specific guidelines exist for management of hypersomnolence associated with TBI.

Hypersomnia in patients with TBI probably has multiple contributors. Any underlying conditions that may contribute to hypersomnia should be treated, for example, treatment of depression, initiation of PAP therapy for OSA, treatment of any underlying circadian rhythm disturbances, treatment of RLS, reduction in dose or elimination of sedating medications if safe and feasible, and extension of sleep duration if there is insufficient sleep syndrome. For patients with persistent symptoms or no other identifiable causes, pharmacologic treatment options include wakefulness-promoting agents (modafinil, armodafinil), and stimulants such as methylphenidate. In a randomized, placebo-controlled, multicenter trial of 117 adults with a history of TBI, baseline ESS score ≥10, and sleep latency less than 8 minutes on a MSLT, patients treated with armodafinil 250 mg daily for 12 weeks showed significant improvement in sleep latency compared to placebo (+7.2 vs. +2.4 minutes) [345]. Subjective sleepiness was improved on some measures but not others at various doses of armodafinil (50, 150, or 250 mg/day). Similar results were reported in a smaller randomized trial of modafinil [346]. Except for headache, the most common side effect reported, both modafinil and armodafinil were well tolerated. Modafinil can be started at a dose of 100 mg twice daily (first dose upon awakening, second dose at mid-day) and can be titrated up to 200 mg twice daily as needed to achieve symptomatic benefit. Armodafinil has a longer half-life and is typically dosed at 50, 150, or 250 mg once daily in the morning. Methylphenidate is less well studied option for treatment of hypersomnia in TBI.

Morning bright light therapy has been studied as a nonpharmacologic treatment option in posttraumatic fatigue and may also provide some degree of wake promotion. In a small randomized trial of 30 patients with TBI and persistent fatigue, patients treated with high intensity blue light therapy showed reduced fatigue and daytime sleepiness after 4 weeks compared with lower intensity yellow light therapy and no treatment.

Modafinil treatment has also been associated with therapeutic improvement in fatigue in TBI patients [347]. In patients with mild-moderate TBI, as compared to placebo, armodafnil (250 mg/day) significantly improved mean SOL in patients with EDS on MSLT testing. However, subjective measurements of EDS did not differ between the two groups [345]. According to a randomized placebo-controlled study, high intensity blue light therapy (45-minute daily morning sessions over 4 weeks) appeared to be effective in alleviating fatigue and daytime sleepiness following TBI, as compared to yellow light therapy and no treatment group. Thus, light therapy may offer a safe nonpharmacological alternative for management of hypersomnolence in TBI patients [348]. Additionally, treatment of comorbid primary sleep disorders, such as OSA and PLMD, and mood disorders is recommended to improve hypersomnolence in TBI patients.

Breathing-Related Sleep Disorders (BRSDs)

Despite clinical symptoms of OSA such as cognitive dysfunction, fatigue and EDS, that are similar to TBI, limited research has been done examining the association between BRSDs and TBI [349]. Increased frequency of sleep disorders including OSA has been reported in patients with TBI. OSA has been associated with a wide range of cognitive deficits including vigilance, attention, arousal, memory, and executive functions. TBI-related cognitive deficits, which are significantly correlated with TBI severity [350], can be potentially exacerbated by presence of comorbid OSA. A study comparing TBI patients with and without OSA demonstrated that those with comorbid OSA ($n = 19$) performed significantly worse on verbal and visual delayed-recall measures, and comorbid OSA was associated with impairment of sustained attention and memory in TBI patients [351].

Webster and colleagues [349] reported that central apnea events were more frequently observed in TBI patients ($n = 28$) within 3 months post injury. No studies exist to determine the efficacy of PAP treatment, the first-line treatment for OSA, on sleep and cognitive outcomes in TBI patients with comorbid OSA. However, BRSDs should be adequately screened and optimally treated in TBI patients.

Other Sleep Disorders and TBI

Other sleep disorders including CRSDs, narcolepsy, sleep-related movement disorders and parasomnias have been less well studied in TBI patients. Ayalon and colleagues [352] examined prevalence of CRSDs in mild TBI patients with insomnia. All patients filled a self-reported Morningness-Eveningness Questionnaire to determine their circadian preference. Patients suspected of having CRSD underwent actigraphy, salivary melatonin, and oral temperature measurements, and PSG study. The authors noted that 15 of 42 (36%) mild TBI patients were diagnosed with CRSD. Eight patients displayed a delayed sleep phase syndrome, whereas seven displayed an irregular sleep–wake pattern [352]. Additionally, patients with severe TBI in an intensive care unit setting exhibited a disrupted pattern of melatonin secretion and reduced melatonin levels. These findings were associated with severity of TBI, as those with less severe TBI had a relatively intact diurnal rhythm of melatonin secretion [353].

Posttraumatic narcolepsy has been associated with injury of the ventral lower ascending reticular activating system between the pontine reticular formation and the hypothalamus in a young male TBI patient [354]. TBI has been rarely associated with parasomnias including sleepwalking, sleep terrors, and RBD [313]. Parasomnia overlap disorder comprising of both NREM and REM parasomnias has been reported with brain injury [355]. PLMD has been associated with TBI and may respond to treatments including dopamine agonists (pramipexole/ropinirole), gabapentin, pregabalin, and gabapentin encarbil [313].

CONCLUSIONS

Sleep disorders are considered to be both risk factors and consequences of various neurological disorders. The common sleep disorders in patients with neurologic disorders include BRSD, insomnia, hypersomnolence, CRSDs, sleep-related movement disorders, and parasomnia disorders. Presence of untreated comorbid sleep disorders can worsen neurological, cognitive, psychiatric, quality-of-life, and rehabilitation outcomes in neurological patients. Yet, sleep disorders are underrecognized and undertreated in clinical settings, and there is an imminent need for development of specific guidelines for management of sleep disorders to optimize overall clinical and quality-of-life outcomes in patients suffering from neurological disorders.

FUTURE DIRECTIONS

Specific evidence-based treatment guidelines need to be developed for management of primary sleep disorders comorbid with neurological disorders including stroke, PD, epilepsy, MS, and TBI. More research is warranted to establish the efficacy of CBT-I in treatment of insomnia in patients with neurological disorders given its safety and efficacy profile in treatment of primary insomnia. Hypersomnolence is often a treatment-refractory symptom in neurological disorders and there is an imminent need to develop safe and effective treatments to improve daytime alertness and overall functioning in patients with neurological disorders.

KEY CLINICAL PEARLS

- OSA is an independent and a modifiable risk factor for stroke, especially ischemic stroke.
- Patients with persistent insomnia have a higher 3-year cumulative incidence rate of stroke.
- RBD can be associated with brainstem infarctions in stroke patients.
- At least 10% of advanced PD patients consider sleep problems as their most bothersome symptom.
- Changes in sleep architecture in PD patients include decreased TST and decreased SWS (N3) relative to lighter sleep (increase in N1 and N2 sleep).
- PD patients taking dopamine agonists have a higher frequency of hypersomnolence as compared to those taking levodopa.

- Patients with advanced PD are more likely to experience daytime sleepiness as compared to early onset PD patients.
- Presence of OSA is predictive of shorter sleep onset latencies during daytime MSLT in PD patients. CPAP treatment of OSA is associated with reduced subjective and objective daytime sleepiness in PD patients.
- Risk factors for insomnia in PD include increased age, disease duration, comorbid depression, and female sex.
- DBS, an FDA approved treatment for medication refractory PD, has been associated with significant improvements in subjective and objective sleep quality in PD patients.
- PD-specific symptoms such as akathisia, motor restlessness, nocturnal leg restlessness, and sensory complaints can mimic RLS.
- RBD can precede or follow the onset of PD and it is considered as one of the strongest risk factors of future development of PD. Within a decade, approximately 50% to 70% of patients with idiopathic RBD will convert to a Parkinsonian disorder.
- MS patients, particularly those with brainstem involvement, have higher predilection for obstructive and central apnea events.
- MS patients presenting with severe RLS may present with disrupted sleep, daytime fatigue, and hypersomnolence.
- New-onset RBD in a known MS patient should be evaluated for signs of radiographic brainstem MS attack recurrence or progression.
- Majority of the sleep-related seizures occur during NREM, especially N2 sleep.
- Primary sleep disorders (e.g., sleep apnea and RLS) and not the epilepsy related factors (such as nocturnal seizures, AEDs, type of epilepsy) are significantly associated with hypersomnolence in epilepsy patients.
- Epilepsy patients who received CPAP treatment for OSA have a significantly higher likelihood to become seizure-free than the untreated patients.
- VNS is FDA-approved treatment of medication-refractory epilepsy, causes an increase in respiratory rate and a decrease in respiratory amplitude, tidal volume, and oxygen saturation during periods of VNS activation.

- Insomnia in TBI patients is likely multifactorial and can be caused by factors including TBI itself (direct injury to the brain), physical symptoms of TBI such as pain and headaches, and finally the neuropsychiatric consequences of TBI such as depression, anxiety, and PTSD.
- Severe TBI is associated with increased hypersomnolence and TBI patients underestimate hypersomnolence symptoms, when using subjective assessment tools alone.

SELF-ASSESSMENT QUESTIONS

1. A 58-year-old white man presents with recurrent dream enactment behaviors with accompanying self-injurious behaviors. Sleep history is negative for sleep apnea and restless legs syndrome. Psychiatric history is negative and patient currently does not take psychotropic medications. Neurological exam is within normal limits. This patient is at the highest risk of developing which of the following neurological disorders in the next 10 years?
   a. Multiple sclerosis
   b. Parkinson's disease
   c. Stroke
   d. Epilepsy

Answer: b

2. Most interictal epileptiform discharges (spikes) seen during sleep EEG occur during which of the following sleep stages?
   a. REM
   b. Stage N1
   c. Stage N2
   d. Stage N3

Answer: d

3. Which of the following factors is most associated with hypersomnolence in epilepsy patients?
   a. Primary sleep disorders
   b. Antiepileptic medications
   c. Type of epilepsy
   d. Nocturnal seizures

Answer: a

4. Which of the following statements is true about subjective sleep disturbance in patients with traumatic brain injury?
   a. Underestimate insomnia and overestimate hypersomnia
   b. Overestimate insomnia and underestimate hypersomnia
   c. Overestimate both insomnia and hypersomnia
   d. Underestimate both insomnia and hypersomnia

Answer: b

5. A 46-year-old white woman with a history of multiple sclerosis presents with new-onset excessive daytime sleepiness without any other new neurological symptoms or signs. She denies a history suggestive of snoring and restless legs syndrome. No history suggestive of depression is reported. Her sleepiness symptoms do not correlate with the use of current medications. What of the following diagnostic tests is most appropriate to consider?
   a. Multiple sleep latency test
   b. Serum ferritin
   c. CSF hypocretin
   d. MRI brain with and without contrast

Answer: d

REFERENCES

1. Lyons OD, Ryan CM. Sleep apnea and stroke. Can J Cardiol. 2015;31(7):918–927.
2. Knutson KL. Sleep duration and cardiometabolic risk: a review of the epidemiologic evidence. Best Pract Res Clin Endocrinol Metabol. 2010;24(5):731–743.
3. Cappuccio FP, Cooper D, D'Elia L, Strazzullo P, Miller MA. Sleep duration predicts cardiovascular outcomes: a systematic review and meta-analysis of prospective studies. Eur Heart J. 2011;32(12):1484–92.
4. Ge B, Guo X. Short and long sleep durations are both associated with increased risk of stroke: a meta-analysis of observational studies. Int J Stroke. 2015;10(2):177–184.
5. Yaggi HK, Concato J, Kernan WN, Lichtman JH, Brass LM, Mohsenin V. Obstructive sleep apnea as a risk factor for stroke and death. New Eng J Med. 2005;353(19):2034–2041.
6. Culebras A. Sleep apnea and stroke. Curr Neurol Neurosci Rep. 2015;15(1):503.
7. Koo DL, Nam H, Thomas RJ, Yun CH. Sleep disturbances as a risk factor for stroke. J Stroke. 2018;20(1):12–32.
8. Terzoudi A, Vorvolakos T, Heliopoulos I, Livaditis M, Vadikolias K, Piperidou H. Sleep architecture in stroke and relation to outcome. Eur Neurol. 2009;61(1):16–22.
9. Mims KN, Kirsch D. Sleep and stroke. Sleep Med Clin. 2016;11(1):39–51.
10. Johnson KG, Johnson DC. Frequency of sleep apnea in stroke and TIA patients: a meta-analysis. J Clin Sleep Med. 2010;6(2):131–137.

11. Bassetti CL, Milanova M, Gugger M. Sleep-disordered breathing and acute ischemic stroke: diagnosis, risk factors, treatment, evolution, and long-term clinical outcome. Stroke. 2006;37(4):967–972.

12. Peppard PE, Young T, Palta M, Skatrud J. Prospective study of the association between sleep-disordered breathing and hypertension. N Engl J Med. 2000;342(19):1378–1384.

13. Portela PC, Fumado JC, Garcia HQ, Borrego FR. Sleep-disordered breathing and acute stroke. Cerebrovasc Dis. 2009;27 Suppl 1:104–110.

14. Kaynak D, Goksan B, Kaynak H, Degirmenci N, Daglioglu S. Is there a link between the severity of sleep-disordered breathing and atherosclerotic disease of the carotid arteries? Eur J Neurol. 2003;10(5):487–493.

15. Baguet JP, Hammer L, Levy P, Pierre H, Launois S, Mallion JM, et al. The severity of oxygen desaturation is predictive of carotid wall thickening and plaque occurrence. Chest. 2005;128(5):3407–3412.

16. Scherbakov N, Sandek A, Ebner N, Valentova M, Nave AH, Jankowska EA, et al. Sleep-disordered breathing in acute ischemic stroke: a mechanistic link to peripheral endothelial dysfunction. J Am Heart Assoc. 2017;6(9).

17. Urbano F, Roux F, Schindler J, Mohsenin V. Impaired cerebral autoregulation in obstructive sleep apnea. J Appl Physiol (1985). 2008;105(6):1852–1857.

18. Wallace DM, Ramos AR, Rundek T. Sleep disorders and stroke. Int J Stroke. 2012;7(3):231–242.

19. Bassetti C, Aldrich MS. Sleep apnea in acute cerebrovascular diseases: final report on 128 patients. Sleep. 1999;22(2):217–223.

20. Bazzano LA, Khan Z, Reynolds K, He J. Effect of nocturnal nasal continuous positive airway pressure on blood pressure in obstructive sleep apnea. Hypertension. 2007;50(2):417–23.

21. Giles TL, Lasserson TJ, Smith BJ, White J, Wright J, Cates CJ. Continuous positive airways pressure for obstructive sleep apnoea in adults. Cochrane Database Syst Rev. 2006;(1):CD001106.

22. Leppavuori A, Pohjasvaara T, Vataja R, Kaste M, Erkinjuntti T. Insomnia in ischemic stroke patients. Cerebrovasc Dis (Basel, Switzerland). 2002;14(2):90–97.

23. Wu MP, Lin HJ, Weng SF, Ho CH, Wang JJ, Hsu YW. Insomnia subtypes and the subsequent risks of stroke: report from a nationally representative cohort. Stroke. 2014;45(5):1349–1354.

24. Chen YK, Lu JY, Mok VC, Ungvari GS, Chu WC, Wong KS, et al. Clinical and radiologic correlates of insomnia symptoms in ischemic stroke patients. Int J Ger Psychiatry. 2011;26(5):451–457.

25. Tang WK, Lu JY, Liang H, Chan TT, Mok V, Ungvari GS, et al. Is insomnia associated with suicidality in stroke? Arch Phys Med Rehab. 2011;92(12):2025–2027.

26. Tang WK, Lu JY, Mok V, Ungvari GS, Wong KS. Is fatigue associated with suicidality in stroke? Arch Phys Med Rehab. 2011;92(8):1336–1338.

27. Tang WK, Liang H, Mok V, Ungvari GS, Wong KS. Is pain associated with suicidality in stroke? Arch Phys Med Rehab. 2013;94(5):863–866.

28. Tang WK, Chen YK, Liang HJ, Chu WC, Mok VC, Ungvari GS, et al. Cerebral microbleeds and suicidality in stroke. Psychosomatics. 2012;53(5):439–445.

29. Li Pi Shan RS, Ashworth NL. Comparison of lorazepam and zopiclone for insomnia in patients with stroke and brain injury: a randomized, crossover, double-blinded trial. Am Phys Med Rehab. 2004;83(6):421–427.

30. Mayer G, Jennum P, Riemann D, Dauvilliers Y. Insomnia in central neurologic diseases: occurrence and management. Sleep Med Rev. 2011;15(6):369–378.

31. Herron K, Farquharson L, Wroe A, Sterr A. Development and Evaluation of a Cognitive Behavioural Intervention for Chronic Post-Stroke Insomnia. Behav Cogn Psychother. 2018;46(6):641–660.

32. Monk T. Shift work: basic principles. In: Kryger MR, T.; Dement, WC., eds. Principles and Practice of Sleep Medicine 4th ed. Philadelphia, PA: Elsevier; 2005. p. 673–680.

33. Brown DL, Feskanich D, Sanchez BN, Rexrode KM, Schernhammer ES, Lisabeth LD. Rotating night shift work and the risk of ischemic stroke. Am J Epidemiol. 2009;169(11):1370–1377.

34. Hermansson J, Gillander Gadin K, Karlsson B, Lindahl B, Stegmayr B, Knutsson A. Ischemic stroke and shift work. Scand J Work Environ Health. 2007;33(6):435–439.

35. Hermida RC, Ayala DE, Smolensky MH, Portaluppi F. Chronotherapy in hypertensive patients: administration-time dependent effects of treatment on blood pressure regulation. Expert Rev Cardiovasc Ther. 2007;5(3):463–475.

36. Routledge FS, McFetridge-Durdle JA, Dean CR, Canadian Hypertension S. Night-time blood pressure patterns and target organ damage: a review. Can J Cardiol. 2007;23(2):132–8.

37. Hermida RC, Ayala DE, Mojon A, Fernandez JR. Influence of circadian time of hypertension treatment on cardiovascular risk: results of the MAPEC study. Chronobiol Int. 2010;27(8):1629–1651.

38. Izzedine H, Launay-Vacher V, Deray G. Abnormal blood pressure circadian rhythm: a target organ damage? Int J Cardiol. 2006;107(3):343–349.

39. Ohkubo T, Hozawa A, Yamaguchi J, Kikuya M, Ohmori K, Michimata M, et al. Prognostic significance of the nocturnal decline in blood pressure in individuals with and without high 24-h blood pressure: the Ohasama study. J Hypertens. 2002;20(11):2183–2189.

40. Kario K, Shimada K, Pickering TG. Abnormal nocturnal blood pressure falls in elderly hypertension: clinical significance and determinants. J Cardiovasc Pharmacol. 2003;41 Suppl 1:S61–S66.

41. Kario K, Shimada K, Schwartz JE, Matsuo T, Hoshide S, Pickering TG. Silent and clinically overt stroke in older Japanese subjects with white-coat and sustained hypertension. J Am Coll Cardiol. 2001;38(1):238–245.

42. Kario K, Pickering TG, Umeda Y, Hoshide S, Hoshide Y, Morinari M, et al. Morning surge in blood pressure as a predictor of silent and clinical cerebrovascular disease in elderly hypertensives: a prospective study. Circulation. 2003;107(10):1401–1406.

43. Allen RP, Picchietti D, Hening WA, Trenkwalder C, Walters AS, Montplaisi J, et al. Restless legs syndrome: diagnostic criteria, special considerations, and epidemiology. a report from the restless legs syndrome diagnosis and epidemiology workshop at the National Institutes of Health. Sleep Med. 2003;4(2):101–119.

44. Ulfberg J, Nystrom B, Carter N, Edling C. Prevalence of restless legs syndrome among men aged 18 to 64 years: an association with somatic disease and neuropsychiatric symptoms. Mov Disord. 2001;16(6):1159–1163.

45. Winkelman JW, Finn L, Young T. Prevalence and correlates of restless legs syndrome symptoms in the Wisconsin Sleep Cohort. Sleep Med. 2006;7(7):545–552.

46. Allen RP, Walters AS, Montplaisir J, Hening W, Myers A, Bell TJ, et al. Restless legs syndrome prevalence and impact: REST general population study. Arch Intern Med. 2005;165(11):1286–1292.

47. Hogl B, Kiechl S, Willeit J, Saletu M, Frauscher B, Seppi K, et al. Restless legs syndrome: a community-based study of prevalence, severity, and risk factors. Neurology. 2005;64(11):1920–1924.

48. Trenkwalder C, Paulus W. Restless legs syndrome: pathophysiology, clinical presentation and management. Nat Rev Neurol. 2010;6(6):337–346.

49. Kang SY, Sohn YH, Lee IK, Kim JS. Unilateral periodic limb movement in sleep after supratentorial cerebral infarction. Parkinsonism Relat Disord. 2004;10(7):429–431.

50. Lee JS, Lee PH, Huh K. Periodic limb movements in sleep after a small deep subcortical infarct. Mov Disord. 2005;20(2):260–261.

51. Anderson KN, Bhatia KP, Losseff NA. A case of restless legs syndrome in association with stroke. Sleep. 2005;28(1):147–148.

52. Phillips B, Hening W, Britz P, Mannino D. Prevalence and correlates of restless legs syndrome: results from the 2005 National Sleep Foundation Poll. Chest. 2006;129(1):76–80.

53. Winkelman JW, Shahar E, Sharief I, Gottlieb DJ. Association of restless legs syndrome and cardiovascular disease in the Sleep Heart Health Study. Neurology. 2008;70(1):35–42.

54. Walters AS, Rye DB. Review of the relationship of restless legs syndrome and periodic limb movements in sleep to hypertension, heart disease, and stroke. Sleep. 2009;32(5):589–597.

55. Gupta A, Shukla G, Mohammed A, Goyal V, Behari M. Restless legs syndrome, a predictor of subcortical stroke: a prospective study in 346 stroke patients. Sleep medicine. 2017;29:61–67.

56. Woo HG, Lee D, Hwang KJ, Ahn TB. Post-stroke restless leg syndrome and periodic limb movements in sleep. Acta neurologica Scandinavica. 2017;135(2):204–210.

57. Boulos MI, Wan A, Black SE, Lim AS, Swartz RH, Murray BJ. Restless legs syndrome after high-risk TIA and minor stroke: association with reduced quality of life. Sleep medicine. 2017;37:135–140.

58. Hermann DM, Bassetti CL. Sleep-related breathing and sleep-wake disturbances in ischemic stroke. Neurology. 2009;73(16):1313–1322.

59. Garcia-Borreguero D, Silber MH, Winkelman JW, Hogl B, Bainbridge J, Buchfuhrer M, et al. Guidelines for the first-line treatment of restless legs syndrome/Willis-Ekbom disease, prevention and treatment of dopaminergic augmentation: a combined task force of the IRLSSG, EURLSSG, and the RLS-foundation. Sleep Med. 2016;21:1–11.

60. Silber MH, Becker PM, Buchfuhrer MJ, Earley CJ, Ondo WG, Walters AS, et al. The Appropriate Use of Opioids in the Treatment of Refractory Restless Legs Syndrome. Mayo Clin Proc. 2018;93(1):59–67.

61. Trotti LM. REM sleep behaviour disorder in older individuals: epidemiology, pathophysiology and management. Drugs Aging. 2010;27(6):457–70.

62. Boeve BF, Silber MH, Saper CB, Ferman TJ, Dickson DW, Parisi JE, et al. Pathophysiology of REM sleep behaviour disorder and relevance to neurodegenerative disease. Brain. 2007;130(Pt 11):2770–2788.

63. Tang WK, Hermann DM, Chen YK, Liang HJ, Liu XX, Chu WC, et al. Brainstem infarcts predict REM sleep behavior disorder in acute ischemic stroke. BMC Neurol. 2014;14:88.

64. Reynolds TQ, Roy A. Isolated cataplexy and REM sleep behavior disorder after pontine stroke. J Clin Sleep Med. 2011;7(2):211–213.

65. Culebras A, Moore JT. Magnetic resonance findings in REM sleep behavior disorder. Neurology. 1989;39(11):1519–1523.

66. Kimura K, Tachibana N, Kohyama J, Otsuka Y, Fukazawa S, Waki R. A discrete pontine ischemic lesion could cause REM sleep behavior disorder. Neurology. 2000;55(6):894–895.

67. Peter A, Hansen ML, Merkl A, Voigtlander S, Bajbouj M, Danker-Hopfe H. REM sleep behavior disorder and excessive startle reaction to visual stimuli in a patient with pontine lesions. Sleep Med. 2008;9(6):697–700.

68. Xi Z, Luning W. REM sleep behavior disorder in a patient with pontine stroke. Sleep Med. 2009;10(1):143–146.

69. Lees AJ, Blackburn NA, Campbell VL. The nighttime problems of Parkinson's disease. Clin Neuropharmacol. 1988;11(6):512–519.

70. Poryazova RG, Zachariev ZI. REM sleep behavior disorder in patients with Parkinson's disease. Folia Med (Plovdiv). 2005;47(1):5–10.

71. Junho BT, Kummer A, Cardoso FE, Teixeira AL, Rocha NP. Sleep quality is associated with the severity of clinical symptoms in Parkinson's disease. Acta neurologica Belgica. 2018;118(1):85–91.

72. Hsiao YH, Chen YT, Tseng CM, Wu LA, Perng DW, Chen YM, et al. Sleep disorders and an increased risk of Parkinson's disease in individuals with non-apnea sleep disorders: a population-based cohort study. J Sleep Res. 2017;26(5):623–628.

73. Chen JC, Tsai TY, Li CY, Hwang JH. Obstructive sleep apnea and risk of Parkinson's disease: a population-based cohort study. J Sleep Res. 2015;24(4):432–437.

74. Bergonzi P, Chiurulla C, Gambi D, Mennuni G, Pinto F. L-dopa plus dopa-decarboxylase inhibitor. Sleep organization in Parkinson's syndrome before and after treatment. Acta neurologica Belgica. 1975;75(1):5–10.

75. Mouret J. Differences in sleep in patients with Parkinson's disease. Electroencephal Clin Neurophysiol. 1975;38(6):653–657.

76. Latreille V, Carrier J, Lafortune M, Postuma RB, Bertrand JA, Panisset M, et al. Sleep spindles in Parkinson's disease may predict the development of dementia. Neurobiol Aging. 2015;36(2):1083–1090.

77. Maria B, Sophia S, Michalis M, Charalampos L, Andreas P, John ME, et al. Sleep breathing disorders in patients with idiopathic Parkinson's disease. Respir Med. 2003;97(10):1151–1157.

78. Diederich NJ, Vaillant M, Leischen M, Mancuso G, Golinval S, Nati R, et al. Sleep apnea syndrome in Parkinson's disease. A case-control study in 49 patients. Mov Disord. 2005;20(11):1413–1418.

79. Yong MH, Fook-Chong S, Pavanni R, Lim LL, Tan EK. Case control polysomnographic studies of sleep disorders in Parkinson's disease. PloS One. 2011;6(7):e22511.

80. Ferini-Strambi L, Franceschi M, Pinto P, Zucconi M, Smirne S. Respiration and heart rate variability during sleep in untreated Parkinson patients. Gerontology. 1992;38(1-2):92–98.

81. Trotti LM, Bliwise DL. No increased risk of obstructive sleep apnea in Parkinson's disease. Mov Disord. 2010;25(13):2246–2249.

82. Valko PO, Hauser S, Sommerauer M, Werth E, Baumann CR. Observations on sleep-disordered breathing in idiopathic Parkinson's disease. PloS One. 2014;9(6):e100828.

83. Gros P, Mery VP, Lafontaine AL, Robinson A, Benedetti A, Kimoff RJ, et al. Obstructive sleep apnea in Parkinson's disease patients: effect of Sinemet CR taken at bedtime. Sleep Breath/Schlaf Atmung. 2016;20(1):205–212.

84. Neikrug AB, Liu L, Avanzino JA, Maglione JE, Natarajan L, Bradley L, et al. Continuous positive airway pressure improves sleep and daytime sleepiness in patients with Parkinson disease and sleep apnea. Sleep. 2014;37(1):177–185.

85. Bittencourt LR, Lucchesi LM, Rueda AD, Garbuio SA, Palombini LO, Guilleminault C, et al. Placebo and modafinil effect on sleepiness in obstructive sleep apnea. Prog Neuropsychopharmacol Biol Psychiatry. 2008;32(2):552–559.

86. Kylstra WA, Aaronson JA, Hofman WF, Schmand BA. Neuropsychological functioning after CPAP treatment in obstructive sleep apnea: a meta-analysis. Sleep Med Rev. 2013;17(5):341–347.

87. Kushida CA, Nichols DA, Holmes TH, Quan SF, Walsh JK, Gottlieb DJ, et al. Effects of continuous positive airway pressure on neurocognitive function in obstructive sleep apnea patients: The Apnea Positive Pressure Long-term Efficacy Study (APPLES). Sleep. 2012;35(12):1593–1602.

88. Harmell AL, Neikrug AB, Palmer BW, Avanzino JA, Liu L, Maglione JE, et al. Obstructive sleep apnea and cognition in Parkinson's disease. Sleep Med. 2016;21:28–34.

89. Kaminska M, Mery VP, Lafontaine AL, Robinson A, Benedetti A, Gros P, et al. Change in Cognition and Other Non-Motor Symptoms With Obstructive Sleep Apnea Treatment in Parkinson Disease. Journal of clinical sleep medicine : JCSM : official publication of the American Academy of Sleep Medicine. 2018;14(5):819–828.

90. Chahine LM, Amara AW, Videnovic A. A systematic review of the literature on disorders of sleep and wakefulness in Parkinson's disease from 2005 to 2015. Sleep Med Rev. 2017;35:33–50.

91. Gjerstad MD, Alves G, Wentzel-Larsen T, Aarsland D, Larsen JP. Excessive daytime sleepiness in Parkinson disease: is it the drugs or the disease? Neurology. 2006;67(5):853–858.

92. Verbaan D, van Rooden SM, Visser M, Marinus J, van Hilten JJ. Nighttime sleep problems and daytime sleepiness in Parkinson's disease. Mov Disord. 2008;23(1):35–41.

93. Cochen De Cock V, Bayard S, Jaussent I, Charif M, Grini M, Langenier MC, et al. Daytime sleepiness in Parkinson's disease: a reappraisal. PloS One. 2014;9(9):e107278.

94. Wienecke M, Werth E, Poryazova R, Baumann-Vogel H, Bassetti CL, Weller M, et al. Progressive dopamine and hypocretin deficiencies in Parkinson's disease: is there an impact on sleep and wakefulness? J Sleep Res. 2012;21(6):710–717.

95. Chung S, Bohnen NI, Albin RL, Frey KA, Muller ML, Chervin RD. Insomnia and sleepiness in Parkinson disease: associations with symptoms and comorbidities. J Clin Sleep Med. 2013;9(11):1131–1137.

96. Hobson DE, Lang AE, Martin WR, Razmy A, Rivest J, Fleming J. Excessive daytime sleepiness and sudden-onset sleep in Parkinson disease: a survey by the Canadian Movement Disorders Group. JAMA. 2002;287(4):455–463.

97. Ondo WG, Dat Vuong K, Khan H, Atassi F, Kwak C, Jankovic J. Daytime sleepiness and other sleep disorders in Parkinson's disease. Neurology. 2001;57(8):1392–1396.

98. Sanjiv CC, Schulzer M, Mak E, Fleming J, Martin WR, Brown T, et al. Daytime somnolence in patients with Parkinson's disease. Parkinsonism Relat Disord. 2001;7(4):283–286.

99. Pal PK, Calne S, Samii A, Fleming JA. A review of normal sleep and its disturbances in Parkinson's disease. Parkinsonism Relat Disord. 1999;5(1-2):1–17.

100. Jahan I, Hauser RA, Sullivan KL, Miller A, Zesiewicz TA. Sleep disorders in Parkinson's disease. Neuropsychiatr Dis Treat. 2009;5:535–540.

101. Suzuki K, Okuma Y, Hattori N, Kamei S, Yoshii F, Utsumi H, et al. Characteristics of sleep disturbances in Japanese patients with Parkinson's disease. A study using Parkinson's disease sleep scale. Mov Disord. 2007;22(9):1245–1251.

102. Moller JC, Stiasny K, Hargutt V, Cassel W, Tietze H, Peter JH, et al. Evaluation of sleep and driving performance in six patients with Parkinson's disease reporting sudden onset of sleep under dopaminergic medication: a pilot study. Mov Disord. 2002;17(3):474–481.

103. Ondo WG, Fayle R, Atassi F, Jankovic J. Modafinil for daytime somnolence in Parkinson's disease: double blind, placebo controlled parallel trial. J Neurol Neurosurg Psychiatry. 2005;76(12):1636–1639.

104. Adler CH, Caviness JN, Hentz JG, Lind M, Tiede J. Randomized trial of modafinil for treating subjective daytime sleepiness in patients with Parkinson's disease. Mov Disord. 2003;18(3):287–293.

105. Hogl B, Saletu M, Brandauer E, Glatzl S, Frauscher B, Seppi K, et al. Modafinil for the treatment of daytime sleepiness in Parkinson's disease: a double-blind, randomized, crossover, placebo-controlled polygraphic trial. Sleep. 2002;25(8):905–909.

106. Ondo WG, Perkins T, Swick T, Hull KL, Jr., Jimenez JE, Garris TS, et al. Sodium oxybate for excessive daytime sleepiness in Parkinson disease: an open-label polysomnographic study. Arch Neurol. 2008;65(10):1337–40.

107. van Maanen A, Meijer AM, van der Heijden KB, Oort FJ. The effects of light therapy on sleep problems: a systematic review and meta-analysis. Sleep Med Rev. 2016;29:52–62.

108. Videnovic A, Klerman EB, Wang W, Marconi A, Kuhta T, Zee PC. Timed light therapy for sleep and daytime sleepiness associated with Parkinson disease: a randomized clinical trial. JAMA Neurol. 2017;74(4):411–418.

109. Gjerstad MD, Wentzel-Larsen T, Aarsland D, Larsen JP. Insomnia in Parkinson's disease: frequency and progression over time. J Neurol Neurosurg Psychiatry. 2007;78(5):476–479.

110. Factor SA, McAlarney T, Sanchez-Ramos JR, Weiner WJ. Sleep disorders and sleep effect in Parkinson's disease. Mov Disord. 1990;5(4):280–285.

111. Oerlemans WG, de Weerd AW. The prevalence of sleep disorders in patients with Parkinson's disease: a self-reported, community-based survey. Sleep Med. 2002;3(2):147–149.

112. Tse W, Liu Y, Barthlen GM, Halbig TD, Tolgyesi SV, Gracies JM, et al. Clinical usefulness of the Parkinson's disease sleep scale. Parkinsonism Rel Disord. 2005;11(5):317–321.

113. Porter B, Macfarlane R, Walker R. The frequency and nature of sleep disorders in a community-based population of patients with Parkinson's disease. Eur J Neurol. 2008;15(1):50–54.

114. Dhawan V, Dhoat S, Williams AJ, Dimarco A, Pal S, Forbes A, et al. The range and nature of sleep dysfunction in untreated Parkinson's disease (PD): a comparative controlled clinical

study using the Parkinson's disease sleep scale and selective polysomnography. J Neurol Sci. 2006;248(1-2):158–162.

115. Louter M, van Sloun RJ, Pevernagie DA, Arends JB, Cluitmans PJ, Bloem BR, et al. Subjectively impaired bed mobility in Parkinson disease affects sleep efficiency. Sleep Med. 2013;14(7):668–674.

116. Gomez-Esteban JC, Zarranz JJ, Lezcano E, Velasco F, Ciordia R, Rouco I, et al. Sleep complaints and their relation with drug treatment in patients suffering from Parkinson's disease. Mov Disord. 2006;21(7):983–988.

117. Suzuki K, Miyamoto M, Miyamoto T, Okuma Y, Hattori N, Kamei S, et al. Correlation between depressive symptoms and nocturnal disturbances in Japanese patients with Parkinson's disease. Parkinsonism Rel Disord. 2009;15(1):15–19.

118. Kulisevsky J, Roldan E. Hallucinations and sleep disturbances in Parkinson's disease. Neurology. 2004;63(8 Suppl 3):S28–S30.

119. Nomura T, Inoue Y, Mitani H, Kawahara R, Miyake M, Nakashima K. Visual hallucinations as REM sleep behavior disorders in patients with Parkinson's disease. Mov Disord. 2003;18(7):812–817.

120. Barone P, Antonini A, Colosimo C, Marconi R, Morgante L, Avarello TP, et al. The PRIAMO study: a multicenter assessment of nonmotor symptoms and their impact on quality of life in Parkinson's disease. Mov Disord. 2009;24(11):1641–1649.

121. Shearer J, Green C, Counsell CE, Zajicek JP. The impact of motor and non motor symptoms on health state values in newly diagnosed idiopathic Parkinson's disease. Journal of neurology. 2012;259(3):462–468.

122. Forsaa EB, Larsen JP, Wentzel-Larsen T, Herlofson K, Alves G. Predictors and course of health-related quality of life in Parkinson's disease. Mov Disord. 2008;23(10):1420–1427.

123. Duncan GW, Khoo TK, Yarnall AJ, O'Brien JT, Coleman SY, Brooks DJ, et al. Health-related quality of life in early Parkinson's disease: the impact of nonmotor symptoms. Mov Disord. 2014;29(2):195–202.

124. Politis M, Wu K, Molloy S, P GB, Chaudhuri KR, Piccini P. Parkinson's disease symptoms: the patient's perspective. Mov Disord. 2010;25(11):1646–1651.

125. Caap-Ahlgren M, Dehlin O. Insomnia and depressive symptoms in patients with Parkinson's disease: relationship to health-related quality of life. An interview study of patients living at home. Arch Gerontol Geriatr. 2001;32(1):23–33.

126. Seppi K, Weintraub D, Coelho M, Perez-Lloret S, Fox SH, Katzenschlager R, et al. The Movement Disorder Society evidence-based medicine review update: treatments for the non-motor symptoms of Parkinson's disease. Mov Disord. 2011;26 Suppl 3:S42–S80.

127. Menza M, Dobkin RD, Marin H, Gara M, Bienfait K, Dicke A, et al. Treatment of insomnia in Parkinson's disease: a controlled trial of eszopiclone and placebo. Mov Disord. 2010;25(11):1708–1714.

128. Medeiros CA, Carvalhedo de Bruin PF, Lopes LA, Magalhaes MC, de Lourdes Seabra M, de Bruin VM. Effect of exogenous melatonin on sleep and motor dysfunction in Parkinson's disease: a randomized, double blind, placebo-controlled study. J Neurol. 2007;254(4):459–464.

129. Trenkwalder C, Kies B, Rudzinska M, Fine J, Nikl J, Honczarenko K, et al. Rotigotine effects on early morning motor function and sleep in Parkinson's disease: a double-blind, randomized, placebo-controlled study (RECOVER). Mov Disord. 2011;26(1):90–99.

130. Monaca C, Ozsancak C, Jacquesson JM, Poirot I, Blond S, Destee A, et al. Effects of bilateral subthalamic stimulation on sleep in Parkinson's disease. Journal of neurology. 2004;251(2):214–218.

131. Iranzo A, Valldeoriola F, Santamaria J, Tolosa E, Rumia J. Sleep symptoms and polysomnographic architecture in advanced Parkinson's disease after chronic bilateral subthalamic stimulation. J Neurol Neurosurg Psychiatry. 2002;72(5):661–664.

132. Arnulf I, Bejjani BP, Garma L, Bonnet AM, Houeto JL, Damier P, et al. Improvement of sleep architecture in PD with subthalamic nucleus stimulation. Neurology. 2000;55(11):1732–1734.

133. Dobkin RD, Menza M, Bienfait KL, Gara M, Marin H, Mark MH, et al. Depression in Parkinson's disease: symptom improvement and residual symptoms after acute pharmacologic management. Am J Geriatr Psychiatry. 2011;19(3):222–229.

134. Menza M, Dobkin RD, Marin H, Mark MH, Gara M, Buyske S, et al. A controlled trial of antidepressants in patients with Parkinson disease and depression. Neurology. 2009;72(10):886–892.

135. Richard IH, McDermott MP, Kurlan R, Lyness JM, Como PG, Pearson N, et al. A randomized, double-blind, placebo-controlled trial of antidepressants in Parkinson disease. Neurology. 2012;78(16):1229–1236.

136. Szatmari S, Jr., Bereczki D, Fornadi K, Kalantar-Zadeh K, Kovesdy CP, Molnar MZ. Association of restless legs syndrome with incident Parkinson's disease. Sleep. 2017;40(2).

137. Ondo WG, Vuong KD, Jankovic J. Exploring the relationship between Parkinson disease and restless legs syndrome. Arch Neurol. 2002;59(3):421–424.

138. Lee JE, Shin HW, Kim KS, Sohn YH. Factors contributing to the development of restless legs syndrome in patients with Parkinson disease. Mov Disord. 2009;24(4):579–582.

139. Wetter TC, Collado-Seidel V, Pollmacher T, Yassouridis A, Trenkwalder C. Sleep and periodic leg movement patterns in drug-free patients with Parkinson's disease and multiple system atrophy. Sleep. 2000;23(3):361–367.

140. Turjanski N, Lees AJ, Brooks DJ. Striatal dopaminergic function in restless legs syndrome: 18F-dopa and 11C-raclopride PET studies. Neurology. 1999;52(5):932–937.

141. Linke R, Eisensehr I, Wetter TC, Gildehaus FJ, Popperl G, Trenkwalder C, et al. Presynaptic dopaminergic function in patients with restless legs syndrome: are there common features with early Parkinson's disease? Mov Disord. 2004;19(10):1158–1162.

142. Lahut S, Vadasz D, Depboylu C, Ries V, Krenzer M, Stiasny-Kolster K, et al. The PD-associated alpha-synuclein promoter Rep1 allele 2 shows diminished frequency in restless legs syndrome. Neurogenetics. 2014;15(3):189–192.

143. Shimohata T, Nishizawa M. Sleep disturbance in patients with Parkinson's disease presenting with leg motor restlessness. Parkinsonism Rel Disord. 2013;19(5):571–572.

144. Gjerstad MD, Tysnes OB, Larsen JP. Increased risk of leg motor restlessness but not RLS in early Parkinson disease. Neurology. 2011;77(22):1941–1946.

145. Boroojerdi B, Wolff HM, Braun M, Scheller DK. Rotigotine transdermal patch for the treatment of Parkinson's disease and restless legs syndrome. Drugs Today (Barcelona, Spain: 1998). 2010;46(7):483–505.

146. Neikrug AB, Maglione JE, Liu L, Natarajan L, Avanzino JA, Corey-Bloom J, et al. Effects of sleep disorders on the non-motor symptoms of Parkinson disease. J Clin Sleep Med. 2013;9(11):1119–1129.

147. Sixel-Doring F, Trautmann E, Mollenhauer B, Trenkwalder C. Associated factors for REM sleep behavior disorder in Parkinson disease. Neurology. 2011;77(11):1048–1054.

148. Postuma RB, Gagnon JF, Tuineaig M, Bertrand JA, Latreille V, Desjardins C, et al. Antidepressants and REM sleep behavior disorder: isolated side effect or neurodegenerative signal? Sleep. 2013;36(11):1579–1585.

149. Howell MJ, Schenck CH. Rapid Eye movement sleep behavior disorder and neurodegenerative disease. JAMA Neurol. 2015;72(6):707–712.

150. Schenck CH, Boeve BF, Mahowald MW. Delayed emergence of a parkinsonian disorder or dementia in 81% of older men initially diagnosed with idiopathic rapid eye movement sleep behavior disorder: a 16-year update on a previously reported series. Sleep Med. 2013;14(8):744–748.

151. Kim YE, Jeon BS. Clinical implication of REM sleep behavior disorder in Parkinson's disease. J Parkinsons Dis. 2014;4(2):237–244.

152. Gong Y, Xiong KP, Mao CJ, Shen Y, Hu WD, Huang JY, et al. Clinical manifestations of Parkinson disease and the onset of rapid eye movement sleep behavior disorder. Sleep Med. 2014;15(6):647–653.

153. Aurora RN, Zak RS, Maganti RK, Auerbach SH, Casey KR, Chowdhuri S, et al. Best practice guide for the treatment of REM sleep behavior disorder (RBD). J Clin Sleep Med. 2010;6(1):85–95.

154. Larsson V, Aarsland D, Ballard C, Minthon L, Londos E. The effect of memantine on sleep behaviour in dementia with Lewy bodies and Parkinson's disease dementia. Int J Geriat Psychiatry. 2010;25(10):1030–1038.

155. Braley TJ, Chervin RD. A practical approach to the diagnosis and management of sleep disorders in patients with multiple sclerosis. Therap Adv Neurol Disord. 2015;8(6):294–310.

156. Veauthier C, Radbruch H, Gaede G, Pfueller CF, Dorr J, Bellmann-Strobl J, et al. Fatigue in multiple sclerosis is closely related to sleep disorders: a polysomnographic cross-sectional study. Multiple Sclerosis (Houndmills, Basingstoke, England). 2011;17(5):613–22.

157. Edwards KA, Molton IR, Smith AE, Ehde DM, Bombardier CH, Battalio SL, et al. Relative importance of baseline pain, fatigue, sleep, and physical activity: predicting change in depression in adults with multiple sclerosis. Arch Phys Med Rehab. 2016;97(8):1309–1315.

158. Ghaem H, Borhani Haghighi A. The impact of disability, fatigue and sleep quality on the quality of life in multiple sclerosis. Ann Indian Acad Neurol. 2008;11(4):236–241.

159. Lobentanz IS, Asenbaum S, Vass K, Sauter C, Klosch G, Kollegger H, et al. Factors influencing quality of life in multiple sclerosis patients: disability, depressive mood, fatigue and sleep quality. Acta neurologica Scandinavica. 2004;110(1):6–13.

160. Brass SD, Li CS, Auerbach S. The underdiagnosis of sleep disorders in patients with multiple sclerosis. J Clin Sleep Med. 2014;10(9):1025–1031.

161. Steffen A, Hagenah J, Wollenberg B, Bruggemann N. [Central sleep apnea in multiple sclerosis]. HNO. 2010;58(4):405–408.

162. Hensen HA, Krishnan AV, Eckert DJ. Sleep-disordered breathing in people with multiple sclerosis: prevalence, pathophysiological mechanisms, and disease consequences. Front Neurol. 2017;8:740.

163. Kallaur AP, Oliveira SR, Colado Simao AN, Delicato de Almeida ER, Kaminami Morimoto H, Lopes J, et al. Cytokine profile in relapsingremitting multiple sclerosis patients and the association between progression and activity of the disease. Mol Med Rep. 2013;7(3):1010–1020.

164. Bergeron C, Kimoff J, Hamid Q. Obstructive sleep apnea syndrome and inflammation. J Allerg Clin Immunol. 2005;116(6):1393–1396.

165. Hatipoglu U, Rubinstein I. Inflammation and obstructive sleep apnea syndrome pathogenesis: a working hypothesis. Respiration. 2003;70(6):665–671.

166. Braley TJ, Segal BM, Chervin RD. Sleep-disordered breathing in multiple sclerosis. Neurology. 2012;79(9):929–936.

167. Auer RN, Rowlands CG, Perry SF, Remmers JE. Multiple sclerosis with medullary plaques and fatal sleep apnea (Ondine's curse). Clin Neuropathol. 1996;15(2):101–105.

168. Howard RS, Wiles CM, Hirsch NP, Loh L, Spencer GT, Newsom-Davis J. Respiratory involvement in multiple sclerosis. Brain. 1992;115(Pt 2):479–94.

169. Kaminska M, Kimoff RJ, Benedetti A, Robinson A, Bar-Or A, Lapierre Y, et al. Obstructive sleep apnea is associated with fatigue in multiple sclerosis. Mult Scler (Houndmills, Basingstoke, England). 2012;18(8):1159–1169.

170. Braley TJ, Segal BM, Chervin RD. Obstructive sleep apnea and fatigue in patients with multiple sclerosis. J Clin Sleep Med. 2014;10(2):155–162.

171. Trojan DA, Kaminska M, Bar-Or A, Benedetti A, Lapierre Y, Da Costa D, et al. Polysomnographic measures of disturbed sleep are associated with reduced quality of life in multiple sclerosis. J Neurol Sci. 2012;316(1-2):158–163.

172. Braley TJ, Kratz AL, Kaplish N, Chervin RD. Sleep and cognitive function in multiple sclerosis. Sleep. 2016;39(8):1525–1533.

173. Dias RA, Hardin KA, Rose H, Agius MA, Apperson ML, Brass SD. Sleepiness, fatigue, and risk of obstructive sleep apnea using the STOP-BANG questionnaire in multiple sclerosis: a pilot study. Sleep Breath/Schlaf Atmung. 2012;16(4):1255–1265.

174. Cote I, Trojan DA, Kaminska M, Cardoso M, Benedetti A, Weiss D, et al. Impact of sleep disorder treatment on fatigue in multiple sclerosis. Mult Scler (Houndmills, Basingstoke, England). 2013;19(4):480–489.

175. Vgontzas AN, Zoumakis E, Lin HM, Bixler EO, Trakada G, Chrousos GP. Marked decrease in sleepiness in patients with sleep apnea by etanercept, a tumor necrosis factor-alpha antagonist. J Clin Endocrinol Metab. 2004;89(9):4409–4413.

176. Dyken ME, Yamada T. Narcolepsy and disorders of excessive somnolence. Prim Care. 2005;32(2):389–413.

177. Morrison I, Riha RL. Excessive daytime sleepiness and narcolepsy: an approach to investigation and management. Eur J Intern Med. 2012;23(2):110–117.

178. Ripley B, Overeem S, Fujiki N, Nevsimalova S, Uchino M, Yesavage J, et al. CSF hypocretin/orexin levels in narcolepsy and other neurological conditions. Neurology. 2001;57(12):2253–2258.

179. Hor H, Kutalik Z, Dauvilliers Y, Valsesia A, Lammers GJ, Donjacour CEHM, et al. Genome-wide association study identifies new HLA class II haplotypes strongly protective against narcolepsy. Nature Gen. 2010;42:786.

180. Cvetkovic-Lopes V, Bayer L, Dorsaz S, Maret S, Pradervand S, Dauvilliers Y, et al. Elevated Tribbles homolog 2-specific antibody levels in narcolepsy patients. J Clin Investig. 2010;120(3):713–719.

181. Hallmayer J, Faraco J, Lin L, Hesselson S, Winkelmann J, Kawashima M, et al. Narcolepsy is strongly associated with the T-cell receptor alpha locus. Nature Gen. 2009;41:708.

182. Nishino S, Kanbayashi T. Symptomatic narcolepsy, cataplexy and hypersomnia, and their implications in the hypothalamic hypocretin/orexin system. Sleep Med Rev. 2005;9(4):269–310.

183. Oka Y, Kanbayashi T, Mezaki T, Iseki K, Matsubayashi J, Murakami G, et al. Low CSF hypocretin-1/orexin-A associated with hypersomnia secondary to hypothalamic lesion in a case of multiple sclerosis. J Neurol. 2004;251(7):885–886.

184. Berg O, Hanley J. Narcolepsy in two cases of multiple sclerosis. Acta Neurol Scand. 1963;39(3):252–256.

185. Vetrugno R, Stecchi S, Plazzi G, Lodi R, D'Angelo R, Alessandria M, et al. Narcolepsy-like syndrome in multiple sclerosis. Sleep Med. 2009;10(3):389–391.

186. Schrader H, Gotlibsen OB, Skomedal GN. Multiple sclerosis and narcolepsy/

cataplexy in a monozygotic twin. Neurology. 1980;30(1):105–108.

187. Nishino S, Okuro M. Emerging treatments for narcolepsy and its related disorders. Expert Opin Emerg Drugs. 2010;15(1):139–158.

188. Morrison I, Buskova J, Nevsimalova S, Douglas NJ, Riha RL. Diagnosing narcolepsy with cataplexy on history alone: challenging the International Classification of Sleep Disorders (ICSD-2) criteria. Eur J Neurol. 2011;18(7):1017–1020.

189. Billiard M, Bassetti C, Dauvilliers Y, Dolenc-Groselj L, Lammers GJ, Mayer G, et al. EFNS guidelines on management of narcolepsy. Eur J Neurol. 2006;13(10):1035–1048.

190. Alshaikh MK, Tricco AC, Tashkandi M, Mamdani M, Straus SE, BaHammam AS. Sodium oxybate for narcolepsy with cataplexy: systematic review and meta-analysis. J Clin Sleep Med. 2012;8(4):451–458.

191. Brass SD, Duquette P, Proulx-Therrien J, Auerbach S. Sleep disorders in patients with multiple sclerosis. Sleep Med Rev. 2010;14(2):121–129.

192. Bjorvatn B, Pallesen S. A practical approach to circadian rhythm sleep disorders. Sleep Med Rev. 2009;13(1):47–60.

193. Martinez D, Lenz Mdo C. Circadian rhythm sleep disorders. Indian J Med Res. 2010;131:141–149.

194. Taphoorn MJ, van Someren E, Snoek FJ, Strijers RL, Swaab DF, Visscher F, et al. Fatigue, sleep disturbances and circadian rhythm in multiple sclerosis. J Neurol. 1993;240(7):446–448.

195. Qiu W, Raven S, Wu JS, Bundell C, Hollingsworth P, Carroll WM, et al. Hypothalamic lesions in multiple sclerosis. J Neurol Neurosurg Psychiatry. 2011;82(7):819–822.

196. Huitinga I, Erkut ZA, van Beurden D, Swaab DF. Impaired hypothalamus-pituitary-adrenal axis activity and more severe multiple sclerosis with hypothalamic lesions. Ann Neurol. 2004;55(1):37–45.

197. Dyken ME, Afifi AK, Lin-Dyken DC. Sleep-related problems in neurologic diseases. Chest. 2012;141(2):528–544.

198. Viana P, Rodrigues E, Fernandes C, Matas A, Barreto R, Mendonca M, et al. InMS: Chronic insomnia disorder in multiple sclerosis: a Portuguese multicentre study on prevalence, subtypes, associated factors and impact on quality of life. Mult Scler Relat Disord. 2015;4(5):477–483.

199. Veauthier C, Gaede G, Radbruch H, Wernecke KD, Paul F. Sleep disorders reduce health-related quality of life in multiple sclerosis (Nottingham Health Profile Data in Patients with Multiple Sclerosis). Int J Mol Sci. 2015;16(7):16514–16528.

200. Kaynak H, Altintas A, Kaynak D, Uyanik O, Saip S, Agaoglu J, et al. Fatigue and sleep disturbance in multiple sclerosis. Eur J Neurol. 2006;13(12):1333–1339.

201. Boe Lunde HM, Aae TF, Indrevag W, Aarseth J, Bjorvatn B, Myhr KM, et al. Poor sleep in patients with multiple sclerosis. PloS One. 2012;7(11):e49996.

202. Mendozzi L, Tronci F, Garegnani M, Pugnetti L. Sleep disturbance and fatigue in mild relapsing remitting multiple sclerosis patients on chronic immunomodulant therapy: an actigraphic study. Mult Scler. 2010;16(2):238–247.

203. Nadjar Y, Coutelas E, Prouteau P, Panzer F, Paquet D, Saint-Val C, et al. Injection of interferon-beta in the morning decreases flu-like syndrome in many patients with multiple sclerosis. Clin Neurol Neurosurg. 2011;113(4):316–322.

204. Baron KG, Corden M, Jin L, Mohr DC. Impact of psychotherapy on insomnia symptoms in patients with depression and multiple sclerosis. J Behav Med. 2011;34(2):92–101.

205. Edinger JD, Wohlgemuth WK, Radtke RA, Marsh GR, Quillian RE. Cognitive behavioral therapy for treatment of chronic primary insomnia: a randomized controlled trial. JAMA. 2001;285(14):1856–1864.

206. Morin CM, Vallieres A, Guay B, Ivers H, Savard J, Merette C, et al. Cognitive behavioral therapy, singly and combined with medication, for persistent insomnia: a randomized controlled trial. JAMA. 2009;301(19):2005–2015.

207. Clancy M, Drerup M, Sullivan AB. Outcomes of cognitive-behavioral treatment for insomnia on insomnia, depression, and fatigue for individuals with multiple sclerosis: a case series. Int J MS Care. 2015;17(6):261–267.

208. Deriu M, Cossu G, Molari A, Murgia D, Mereu A, Ferrigno P, et al. Restless legs syndrome in multiple sclerosis: a case-control study. Mov Disord. 2009;24(5):697–701.

209. Ferini-Strambi L, Filippi M, Martinelli V, Oldani A, Rovaris M, Zucconi M, et al. Nocturnal sleep study in multiple sclerosis: correlations with clinical and brain magnetic resonance imaging findings. J Neurol Sci. 1994;125(2):194–7.

210. Buysse DJ, Reynolds CF, 3rd, Monk TH, Berman SR, Kupfer DJ. The Pittsburgh Sleep Quality Index: a new instrument for psychiatric practice and research. Psychiatry Res. 1989;28(2):193–213.

211. Dauvilliers Y, Winkelmann J. Restless legs syndrome: update on pathogenesis. Curr Opin Pulm Med. 2013;19(6):594–600.

212. Winkelman JW. Periodic limb movements in sleep: endophenotype for restless legs syndrome? N Engl J Med. 2007;357(7):703–705.

213. Winkelmann J, Schormair B, Lichtner P, Ripke S, Xiong L, Jalilzadeh S, et al. Genome-wide association study of restless legs syndrome identifies common variants in three genomic regions. Nat Genet. 2007;39(8):1000–1006.

214. Rosenberg RS, Van Hout S. The American Academy of Sleep Medicine inter-scorer reliability program: sleep stage scoring. J Clin Sleep Med. 2013;9(1):81–87.

215. Vavrova J, Kemlink D, Sonka K, Havrdova E, Horakova D, Pardini B, et al. Restless legs syndrome in Czech patients with multiple sclerosis: an epidemiological and genetic study. Sleep Med. 2012;13(7):848–851.

216. Auger C, Montplaisir J, Duquette P. Increased frequency of restless legs syndrome in a French-Canadian population with multiple sclerosis. Neurology. 2005;65(10):1652–1653.

217. Italian RSG, Manconi M, Ferini-Strambi L, Filippi M, Bonanni E, Iudice A, et al. Multicenter case-control study on restless legs syndrome in multiple sclerosis: the REMS study. Sleep. 2008;31(7):944–952.

218. Manconi M, Fabbrini M, Bonanni E, Filippi M, Rocca M, Murri L, et al. High prevalence of restless legs syndrome in multiple sclerosis. Eur J Neurol. 2007;14(5):534–539.

219. Manconi M, Rocca MA, Ferini-Strambi L, Tortorella P, Agosta F, Comi G, et al. Restless legs syndrome is a common finding in multiple sclerosis and correlates with cervical cord damage. Mult Scler. 2008;14(1):86–93.

220. Li Y, Munger KL, Batool-Anwar S, De Vito K, Ascherio A, Gao X. Association of multiple sclerosis with restless legs syndrome and other sleep disorders in women. Neurology. 2012;78(19):1500–1506.

221. Hartmann M, Pfister R, Pfadenhauer K. Restless legs syndrome associated with spinal cord lesions. J Neurol Neurosurg Psychiatry. 1999;66(5):688–9.

222. Manconi M, Ferini-Strambi L, Filippi M, Bonanni E, Iudice A, Murri L, et al. Multicenter case-control study on restless legs syndrome in multiple sclerosis: the REMS study. Sleep. 2008;31(7):944–52.

223. Lutz EG. Restless legs, anxiety and caffeinism. J Clin Psychiatry. 1978;39(9):693–8.

224. Aldrich MS, Shipley JE. Alcohol use and periodic limb movements of sleep. Alcohol Clin Exp Res. 1993;17(1):192–6.

225. Hoque R, Chesson AL, Jr. Pharmacologically induced/exacerbated restless legs syndrome, periodic limb movements of sleep, and REM behavior disorder/REM sleep without atonia: literature review, qualitative scoring, and comparative analysis. J Clin Sleep Med. 2010;6(1):79–83.

226. Allen RP, Chen C, Garcia-Borreguero D, Polo O, DuBrava S, Miceli J, et al. Comparison of pregabalin with pramipexole for restless legs syndrome. N Eng J Med. 2014;370(7):621–631.

227. McCarter SJ, Tippmann-Peikert M, Sandness DJ, Flanagan EP, Kantarci K, Boeve BF, et al. Neuroimaging-evident lesional pathology associated with REM sleep behavior disorder. Sleep Med. 2015;16(12):1502–1510.

228. Chen JH, Huang Y, Liu XQ, Sun HY. [Prevalence of REM sleep behavior disorder in patients with brainstem lesions]. Zhonghua yi xue za zhi. 2013;93(37):2942–2945.

229. Tippmann-Peikert M, Boeve BF, Keegan BM. REM sleep behavior disorder initiated by acute brainstem multiple sclerosis. Neurology. 2006;66(8):1277–1279.

230. Plazzi G, Montagna P. Remitting REM sleep behavior disorder as the initial sign of multiple sclerosis. Sleep Med. 2002;3(5):437–439.

231. Wang YQ, Zhang MQ, Li R, Qu WM, Huang ZL. The mutual interaction between sleep and epilepsy on the neurobiological basis and therapy. Curr Neuropharmacol. 2018;16(1):5–16.

232. Mirzoev A, Bercovici E, Stewart LS, Cortez MA, Snead OC, 3rd, Desrocher M. Circadian profiles of focal epileptic seizures: a need for reappraisal. Seizure. 2012;21(6):412–416.

233. Al-Biltagi MA. Childhood epilepsy and sleep. World J Clin Ped. 2014;3(3):45–53.

234. de Weerd A, de Haas S, Otte A, Trenite DK, van Erp G, Cohen A, et al. Subjective sleep disturbance in patients with partial epilepsy: a questionnaire-based study on prevalence and impact on quality of life. Epilepsia. 2004;45(11):1397–1404.

235. Khatami R, Zutter D, Siegel A, Mathis J, Donati F, Bassetti CL. Sleep–wake habits and disorders in a series of 100 adult epilepsy patients: a prospective study. Seizure. 2006;15(5):299–306.

236. Im HJ, Park SH, Baek SH, Chu MK, Yang KI, Kim WJ, et al. Associations of impaired sleep quality, insomnia, and sleepiness with epilepsy: A questionnaire-based case-control study. Epilep Behav. 2016;57(Pt A):55–59.

237. St Louis EK, Foldvary-Schaefer N. Sleep-Related Epilepsy Syndromes UpToDate; 2018. https://www.uptodate.com/contents/sleep-related-epilepsy-syndromes.

238. Latreille V, St Louis EK, Pavlova M. Co-morbid sleep disorders and epilepsy: A narrative review and case examples. Epilep Res. 2018;145:185–197.

239. St Louis EK. Sleep and Epilepsy: Strange Bedfellows No More. Minerva Pneumol. 2011;50(3):159–176.

240. Herman ST, Walczak TS, Bazil CW. Distribution of partial seizures during the sleep–wake cycle: differences by seizure onset site. Neurology. 2001;56(11):1453–1459.

241. Steriade M, McCormick DA, Sejnowski TJ. Thalamocortical oscillations in the sleeping and aroused brain. Science. 1993;262(5134):679–685.

242. Lin Z, Si Q, Xiaoyi Z. Obstructive sleep apnoea in patients with epilepsy: a meta-analysis. Sleep Breath. 2017;21(2):263–270.

243. Vendrame M, Jackson S, Syed S, Kothare SV, Auerbach SH. Central sleep apnea and complex sleep apnea in patients with epilepsy. Sleep Breath. 2014;18(1):119–124.

244. Khachatryan SG, Prosperetti C, Rossinelli A, Pedrazzi P, Agazzi P, Ratti PL, et al. Sleep-onset central apneas as triggers of severe nocturnal seizures. Sleep Med. 2015;16(8):1017–1019.

245. Latreille V, Abdennadher M, Dworetzky BA, Ramel J, White D, Katz E, et al. Nocturnal seizures are associated with more severe hypoxemia and increased risk of postictal generalized EEG suppression. Epilepsia. 2017;58(9):e127–e31.

246. Nadkarni MA, Friedman D, Devinsky O. Central apnea at complex partial seizure onset. Seizure. 2012;21(7):555–558.

247. Pavlova M, Singh K, Abdennadher M, Katz ES, Dworetzky BA, White DP, et al. Comparison of cardiorespiratory and EEG abnormalities with seizures in adults and children. Epilepsy Behav. 2013;29(3):537–541.

248. Schuele SU, Afshari M, Afshari ZS, Macken MP, Asconape J, Wolfe L, et al. Ictal central apnea as a predictor for sudden unexpected death in epilepsy. Epilepsy Behav. 2011;22(2):401–403.

249. Devinsky O, Hesdorffer DC, Thurman DJ, Lhatoo S, Richerson G. Sudden unexpected death in epilepsy: epidemiology, mechanisms, and prevention. Lancet Neurol. 2016;15(10):1075–1088.

250. Manni R, Terzaghi M, Arbasino C, Sartori I, Galimberti CA, Tartara A. Obstructive sleep apnea in a clinical series of adult epilepsy patients: frequency and features of the comorbidity. Epilepsia. 2003;44(6):836–840.

251. Gammino M, Zummo L, Bue AL, Urso L, Terruso V, Marrone O, et al. Excessive daytime sleepiness and sleep disorders in a population of patients with epilepsy: a case-control study. J Epilepsy Res. 2016;6(2):79–86.

252. Malow BA, Bowes RJ, Lin X. Predictors of sleepiness in epilepsy patients. Sleep. 1997;20(12):1105–1110.

253. Piperidou C, Karlovasitou A, Triantafyllou N, Terzoudi A, Constantinidis T, Vadikolias K, et al. Influence of sleep disturbance on quality of life of patients with epilepsy. Seizure. 2008;17(7):588–594.

254. Economou NT, Dikeos D, Andrews N, Foldvary-Schaefer N. Use of the Sleep Apnea Scale of the Sleep Disorders Questionnaire (SA-SDQ) in adults with epilepsy. Epilepsy Behav. 2014;31:123–126.

255. Weatherwax KJ, Lin X, Marzec ML, Malow BA. Obstructive sleep apnea in epilepsy patients: the Sleep Apnea Scale of the Sleep Disorders Questionnaire (SA-SDQ) is a useful screening instrument for obstructive sleep apnea in a disease-specific population. Sleep Med. 2003;4(6):517–521.

256. Sharma A, Molano J, Moseley BD. The STOP-BANG questionnaire improves the detection of epilepsy patients at risk for obstructive sleep apnea. Epilepsy Res. 2017;129:37–40.

257. Bazil CW. Sleep and epilepsy. Curr Opin Neurol. 2000;13(2):171–175.

258. Campos-Rodriguez F, Queipo-Corona C, Carmona-Bernal C, Jurado-Gamez B, Cordero-Guevara J, Reyes-Nunez N, et al. Continuous positive airway pressure improves quality of life in women with obstructive sleep apnea. a randomized controlled trial. Am J Respir Crit Care Med. 2016;194(10):1286–1294.

259. Dalmases M, Sole-Padulles C, Torres M, Embid C, Nunez MD, Martinez-Garcia MA, et al. Effect of CPAP on cognition, brain function, and structure among elderly patients with OSA: a randomized pilot study. Chest. 2015;148(5):1214–1223.

260. Rosenzweig I, Glasser M, Crum WR, Kempton MJ, Milosevic M, McMillan A, et al. Changes in neurocognitive architecture in patients with obstructive sleep apnea treated with continuous positive airway pressure. EBioMedicine. 2016;7:221–229.

261. Zhao YY, Redline S. Impact of continuous positive airway pressure on cardiovascular risk factors in high-risk patients. Curr Atheroscler Rep. 2015;17(11):62.

262. Li P, Ghadersohi S, Jafari B, Teter B, Sazgar M. Characteristics of refractory vs. medically controlled epilepsy patients with obstructive sleep apnea and their response to CPAP treatment. Seizure. 2012;21(9):717–721.

263. Oliveira AJ, Zamagni M, Dolso P, Bassetti MA, Gigli GL. Respiratory disorders during sleep in patients with epilepsy: effect of ventilatory therapy on EEG interictal epileptiform discharges. Clin Neurophysiol. 2000;111 Suppl 2:S141–S145.

264. Pornsriniyom D, Shinlapawittayatorn K, Fong J, Andrews ND, Foldvary-Schaefer N. Continuous positive airway pressure therapy for obstructive sleep apnea reduces interictal epileptiform discharges in adults with epilepsy. Epilepsy Behav. 2014;37:171–174.

265. Parhizgar F, Nugent K, Raj R. Obstructive sleep apnea and respiratory complications associated with vagus nerve stimulators. J Clin Sleep Med. 2011;7(4):401–407.

266. Ohayon MM. Epidemiology of insomnia: what we know and what we still need to learn. Sleep Med Rev. 2002;6(2):97–111.

267. Macedo P, Oliveira PS, Foldvary-Schaefer N, Gomes MDM. Insomnia in people with epilepsy: A review of insomnia prevalence, risk factors and associations with epilepsy-related factors. Epilepsy Res. 2017;135:158–167.

268. American Academy of Sleep Medicine. International Classification of Sleep Disorders. 3rd ed. Darien, IL: American Academy of Sleep Medicine; 2014.

269. Yang KI, Grigg-Damberger M, Andrews N, O'Rourke C, Bena J, Foldvary-Schaefer N. Severity of self-reported insomnia in adults with epilepsy is related to comorbid medical disorders and depressive symptoms. Epilep Behav. 2016;60:27–32.

270. Vendrame M, Yang B, Jackson S, Auerbach SH. Insomnia and epilepsy: a questionnaire-based study. J Clin Sleep Med. 2013;9(2):141–146.

271. Jain SV, Glauser TA. Effects of epilepsy treatments on sleep architecture and daytime sleepiness: an evidence-based review of objective sleep metrics. Epilepsia. 2014;55(1):26–37.

272. Voges BR, Schmitt FC, Hamel W, House PM, Kluge C, Moll CK, et al. Deep brain stimulation of anterior nucleus thalami disrupts sleep in epilepsy patients. Epilepsia. 2015;56(8):e99–e103.

273. Sanchez Fernandez I, Ramgopal S, Powell C, Gregas M, Zarowski M, Shah A, et al. Clinical evolution of seizures: distribution across time of day and sleep/wakefulness cycle. J Neurol. 2013;260(2):549–557.

274. Manni R, De Icco R, Cremascoli R, Ferrera G, Furia F, Zambrelli E, et al. Circadian phase typing in idiopathic generalized epilepsy: dim light melatonin onset and patterns of melatonin secretion-semicurve findings in adult patients. Epilep Behav. 2016;61:132–137.

275. Bazil CW, Dave J, Cole J, Stalvey J, Drake E. Pregabalin increases slow-wave sleep and may improve attention in patients with partial epilepsy and insomnia. Epilep Behav. 2012;23(4):422–425.

276. Hallbook T, Lundgren J, Kohler S, Blennow G, Stromblad LG, Rosen I. Beneficial effects on sleep of vagus nerve stimulation in children with therapy resistant epilepsy. Eur J Paed Neurol. 2005;9(6):399–407.

277. Malow BA, Edwards J, Marzec M, Sagher O, Ross D, Fromes G. Vagus nerve stimulation reduces daytime sleepiness in epilepsy patients. Neurology. 2001;57(5):879–884.

278. Wang LJ, Ree SC, Chu CL, Juang YY. Zolpidem dependence and withdrawal seizure: report of two cases. Psychiatria Danubina. 2011;23(1):76–78.

279. Sethi PK, Khandelwal DC. Zolpidem at supratherapeutic doses can cause drug abuse, dependence and withdrawal seizure. J Assoc Physicians India. 2005;53:139–140.

280. Pitchot W, Ansseau M. [Zolpidem dependence and withdrawal seizure]. Revue medicale de Liege. 2009;64(7-8):407–408.

281. Aragona M. Abuse, dependence, and epileptic seizures after zolpidem withdrawal: review and case report. Clin Neuropharmacol. 2000;23(5):281–283.

282. Jain SV, Horn PS, Simakajornboon N, Beebe DW, Holland K, Byars AW, et al. Melatonin improves sleep in children with epilepsy: a randomized, double-blind, crossover study. Sleep Med. 2015;16(5):637–644.

283. Steinert T, Froscher W. Epileptic Seizures Under Antidepressive Drug Treatment: Systematic Review. Pharmacopsychiatry. 2018;51(4):121–135.

284. Trotti LM. Restless legs syndrome and sleep-related movement disorders. Continuum. 2017;23(4):1005–1016.

285. Ozturk I, Aslan K, Bozdemir H, Foldvary-Schaefer N. frequency of restless legs syndrome in adults with epilepsy in Turkey. Epilepsy Behav. 2016;57(Pt A):192–195.

286. Yazdi Z, Sadeghniiat-Haghighi K, Naimian S, Zohal MA, Ghaniri M. Prevalence of sleep disorders and their effects on sleep quality in epileptic patients. Basic Clin Neurosci. 2013;4(1):36–41.

287. Arico I, Condurso R, Granata F, Nobili L, Bruni O, Silvestri R. Nocturnal frontal lobe epilepsy presenting with restless leg syndrome-like symptoms. Neurol Sci. 2011;32(2):313–5.

288. Velasco PE, Goiburu JA, Pinel RS. Restless legs syndrome induced by zonisamide. Mov Disord. 2007;22(10):1517–1518.

289. Chen JT, Garcia PA, Alldredge BK. Zonisamide-induced restless legs syndrome. Neurology. 2003;60(1):147.

290. Allen RP, Picchietti DL, Auerbach M, Cho YW, Connor JR, Earley CJ, et al. Evidence-based and consensus clinical practice guidelines for the iron treatment of restless legs syndrome/

Willis-Ekbom disease in adults and children: an IRLSSG task force report. Sleep Med. 2018;41:27–44.

291. Hening WA, Allen RP, Ondo WG, Walters AS, Winkelman JW, Becker P, et al. Rotigotine improves restless legs syndrome: a 6-month randomized, double-blind, placebo-controlled trial in the United States. Mov Disord. 2010;25(11):1675–1683.

292. Irfan M, Schenck CH, Howell MJ. Non-Rapid Eye Movement Sleep and Overlap Parasomnias. Continuum. 2017;23(4):1035–1050.

293. Hogl B, Iranzo A. Rapid eye movement sleep behavior disorder and other rapid eye movement sleep parasomnias. Continuum. 2017;23(4):1017–1034.

294. St Louis EK, Boeve BF. REM sleep behavior disorder: diagnosis, clinical implications, and future directions. Mayo Clin Proc. 2017;92(11):1723–1736.

295. Bisulli F, Vignatelli L, Provini F, Leta C, Lugaresi E, Tinuper P. Parasomnias and nocturnal frontal lobe epilepsy (NFLE): lights and shadows—controversial points in the differential diagnosis. Sleep Med. 2011;12 Suppl 2:S27–S32.

296. Bisulli F, Vignatelli L, Naldi I, Licchetta L, Provini F, Plazzi G, et al. Increased frequency of arousal parasomnias in families with nocturnal frontal lobe epilepsy: a common mechanism? Epilepsia. 2010;51(9):1852–1860.

297. Ismayilova V, Demir AU, Tezer FI. Subjective sleep disturbance in epilepsy patients at an outpatient clinic: a questionnaire-based study on prevalence. Epilepsy Res. 2015;115:119–125.

298. Manni R, Terzaghi M, Zambrelli E. REM sleep behaviour disorder in elderly subjects with epilepsy: frequency and clinical aspects of the comorbidity. Epilepsy Res. 2007;77(2-3):128–33.

299. Derry CP, Davey M, Johns M, Kron K, Glencross D, Marini C, et al. Distinguishing sleep disorders from seizures: diagnosing bumps in the night. Arch Neurol. 2006;63(5):705–709.

300. Manni R, Terzaghi M, Repetto A. The FLEP scale in diagnosing nocturnal frontal lobe epilepsy, NREM and REM parasomnias: data from a tertiary sleep and epilepsy unit. Epilepsia. 2008;49(9):1581–1585.

301. Foldvary-Schaefer N, Alsheikhtaha Z. Complex nocturnal behaviors: nocturnal seizures and parasomnias. Continuum. 2013;19(1 Sleep Disorders):104–31.

302. Drakatos P, Marples L, Muza R, Higgins S, Gildeh N, Macavei R, et al. NREM parasomnias: a treatment approach based upon a retrospective case series of 512 patients. Sleep Med. 2018.

303. Takasaki K, Diaz Stransky A, Miller G. Psychogenic Nonepileptic Seizures: Diagnosis, Management, and Bioethics. Ped Neurol. 2016;62:3–8.

304. Devinsky O, Gazzola D, LaFrance WC, Jr. Differentiating between nonepileptic and epileptic seizures. Nat Rev Neurol. 2011;7(4):210–220.

305. Vincentiis S, Valente KD, Thome-Souza S, Kuczinsky E, Fiore LA, Negrao N. Risk factors for psychogenic nonepileptic seizures in children and adolescents with epilepsy. Epilepsy Behav. 2006;8(1):294–8.

306. Asadi-Pooya AA. Psychogenic nonepileptic seizures: a concise review. Neurol Sci. 2017;38(6):935–940.

307. Reuber M, Fernandez G, Bauer J, Helmstaedter C, Elger CE. Diagnostic delay in psychogenic nonepileptic seizures. Neurology. 2002;58(3):493–495.

308. Mostacci B, Bisulli F, Alvisi L, Licchetta L, Baruzzi A, Tinuper P. Ictal characteristics of psychogenic nonepileptic seizures: what we have learned from video/EEG recordings: a literature review. Epilepsy Behav. 2011;22(2):144–153.

309. Bazil CW, Legros B, Kenny E. Sleep structure in patients with psychogenic nonepileptic seizures. Epilepsy Behav. 2003;4(4):395–398.

310. Benbadis SR, Lancman ME, King LM, Swanson SJ. Preictal pseudosleep: a new finding in psychogenic seizures. Neurology. 1996;47(1):63–67.

311. Seneviratne U, Minato E, Paul E. Seizures by the clock: temporal patterns of psychogenic nonepileptic seizures. Epilepsy Behav. 2017;76:71–75.

312. Maas AI. Traumatic brain injury: simple data collection will improve the outcome. Wien Klin Wochenschr. 2007;119(1-2):20–22.

313. Viola-Saltzman M, Musleh C. Traumatic brain injury-induced sleep disorders. Neuropsychiatr Dis Treat. 2016;12:339–348.

314. Teasdale G, Jennett B. Assessment of coma and impaired consciousness: a practical scale. Lancet. 1974;2(7872):81–84.

315. Mathias JL, Alvaro PK. Prevalence of sleep disturbances, disorders, and problems following traumatic brain injury: a meta-analysis. Sleep Med. 2012;13(7):898–905.

316. Sandsmark DK, Elliott JE, Lim MM. Sleep–wake disturbances after traumatic brain injury: synthesis of human and animal studies. Sleep. 2017;40(5).

317. Baumann CR, Werth E, Stocker R, Ludwig S, Bassetti CL. Sleep–wake disturbances 6 months after traumatic brain injury: a prospective study. Brain. 2007;130(Pt 7):1873–1883.

318. Hou L, Han X, Sheng P, Tong W, Li Z, Xu D, et al. Risk factors associated with sleep disturbance

following traumatic brain injury: clinical findings and questionnaire based study. PloS One. 2013;8(10):e76087.

319. Rao V, McCann U, Han D, Bergey A, Smith MT. Does acute TBI-related sleep disturbance predict subsequent neuropsychiatric disturbances? Brain Inj. 2014;28(1):20–26.

320. Ouellet MC, Beaulieu-Bonneau S, Morin CM. Sleep-wake disturbances after traumatic brain injury. Lancet Neurol. 2015;14(7):746–57.

321. Duclos C, Beauregard MP, Bottari C, Ouellet MC, Gosselin N. The impact of poor sleep on cognition and activities of daily living after traumatic brain injury: a review. Australian Occup Ther J. 2015;62(1):2–12.

322. Worthington AD, Melia Y. Rehabilitation is compromised by arousal and sleep disorders: results of a survey of rehabilitation centres. Brain Inj. 2006;20(3):327–332.

323. Zeitzer JM, Friedman L, O'Hara R. Insomnia in the context of traumatic brain injury. J Rehab Res Dev. 2009;46(6):827–836.

324. Donnemiller E, Brenneis C, Wissel J, Scherfler C, Poewe W, Riccabona G, et al. Impaired dopaminergic neurotransmission in patients with traumatic brain injury: a SPECT study using 123I-beta-CIT and 123I-IBZM. Eur Nuclear Med. 2000;27(9):1410–1414.

325. Porta M, Bareggi SR, Collice M, Assael BM, Selenati A, Calderini G, et al. Homovanillic acid and 5-hydroxyindole-acetic acid in the csf of patients after a severe head injury. II. Ventricular CSF concentrations in acute brain post-traumatic syndromes. Eur Neurol. 1975;13(6):545–554.

326. Zhou D, Zhao Y, Wan Y, Wang Y, Xie D, Lu Q, et al. Neuroendocrine dysfunction and insomniain in mild traumatic brain injury patients. Neurosci Lett. 2016;610:154–159.

327. Jain A, Mittal RS, Sharma A, Sharma A, Gupta ID. Study of insomnia and associated factors in traumatic brain injury. Asian J Psychiatry. 2014;8:99–103.

328. Beetar JT, Guilmette TJ, Sparadeo FR. Sleep and pain complaints in symptomatic traumatic brain injury and neurologic populations. Arch Phys Med Rehab. 1996;77(12):1298–1302.

329. Clinchot DM, Bogner J, Mysiw WJ, Fugate L, Corrigan J. Defining sleep disturbance after brain injury. Am Phys Med Rehab. 1998;77(4):291–295.

330. Khoury S, Chouchou F, Amzica F, Giguere JF, Denis R, Rouleau GA, et al. Rapid EEG activity during sleep dominates in mild traumatic brain injury patients with acute pain. J Neurotrauma. 2013;30(8):633–641.

331. Lu W, Cantor JB, Aurora RN, Gordon WA, Krellman JW, Nguyen M, et al. The relationship between self-reported sleep disturbance and polysomnography in individuals with traumatic brain injury. Brain Inj. 2015;29(11):1342–1350.

332. Ouellet MC, Morin CM. Subjective and objective measures of insomnia in the context of traumatic brain injury: a preliminary study. Sleep Med. 2006;7(6):486–497.

333. Baumann CR. Sleep and traumatic brain injury. Sleep Med Clin. 2016;11(1):19–23.

334. Grima NA, Rajaratnam SMW, Mansfield D, Sletten TL, Spitz G, Ponsford JL. Efficacy of melatonin for sleep disturbance following traumatic brain injury: a randomised controlled trial. BMC Med. 2018;16(1):8.

335. Kemp S, Biswas R, Neumann V, Coughlan A. The value of melatonin for sleep disorders occurring post-head injury: a pilot RCT. Brain Inj. 2004;18(9):911–919.

336. Buffett-Jerrott SE, Stewart SH. Cognitive and sedative effects of benzodiazepine use. Curr Pharma Design. 2002;8(1):45–58.

337. Ouellet MC, Morin CM. Efficacy of cognitive-behavioral therapy for insomnia associated with traumatic brain injury: a single-case experimental design. Arch Phys Med Rehab. 2007;88(12):1581–1592.

338. Masel BE, Scheibel RS, Kimbark T, Kuna ST. Excessive daytime sleepiness in adults with brain injuries. Arch Phys Med Rehab. 2001;82(11):1526–1532.

339. Castriotta RJ, Wilde MC, Lai JM, Atanasov S, Masel BE, Kuna ST. Prevalence and consequences of sleep disorders in traumatic brain injury. J Clin Sleep Med. 2007;3(4):349–356.

340. Jang SH, Kwon HG. Injury of the ascending reticular activating system in patients with fatigue and hypersomnia following mild traumatic brain injury: two case reports. Medicine. 2016;95(6):e2628.

341. Baumann CR, Stocker R, Imhof HG, Trentz O, Hersberger M, Mignot E, et al. Hypocretin-1 (orexin A) deficiency in acute traumatic brain injury. Neurology. 2005;65(1):147–149.

342. Watson NF, Dikmen S, Machamer J, Doherty M, Temkin N. Hypersomnia following traumatic brain injury. J Clin Sleep Med. 2007;3(4):363–368.

343. Imbach LL, Valko PO, Li T, Maric A, Symeonidou ER, Stover JF, et al. Increased sleep need and daytime sleepiness 6 months after traumatic brain injury: a prospective controlled clinical trial. Brain. 2015;138(Pt 3):726–735.

344. Chiu HY, Lo WC, Chiang YH, Tsai PS. The effects of sleep on the relationship between

brain injury severity and recovery of cognitive function: a prospective study. Int J Nurse Stud. 2014;51(6):892–899.

345. Menn SJ, Yang R, Lankford A. Armodafinil for the treatment of excessive sleepiness associated with mild or moderate closed traumatic brain injury: a 12-week, randomized, double-blind study followed by a 12-month open-label extension. J Clin Sleep Med. 2014;10(11):1181–1191.

346. Kaiser PR, Valko PO, Werth E, Thomann J, Meier J, Stocker R, et al. Modafinil ameliorates excessive daytime sleepiness after traumatic brain injury. Neurology. 2010;75(20):1780–1785.

347. Sheng P, Hou L, Wang X, Wang X, Huang C, Yu M, et al. Efficacy of modafinil on fatigue and excessive daytime sleepiness associated with neurological disorders: a systematic review and meta-analysis. PloS One. 2013;8(12):e81802.

348. Sinclair KL, Ponsford JL, Taffe J, Lockley SW, Rajaratnam SM. Randomized controlled trial of light therapy for fatigue following traumatic brain injury. Neurorehab Neural Repair. 2014;28(4):303–313.

349. Webster JB, Bell KR, Hussey JD, Natale TK, Lakshminarayan S. Sleep apnea in adults with traumatic brain injury: a preliminary investigation. Arch Phys Med Rehab. 2001;82(3):316–321.

350. Draper K, Ponsford J. Cognitive functioning ten years following traumatic brain injury and rehabilitation. Neuropsychology. 2008;22(5):618–625.

351. Wilde MC, Castriotta RJ, Lai JM, Atanasov S, Masel BE, Kuna ST. Cognitive impairment in patients with traumatic brain injury and obstructive sleep apnea. Arch Phys Med Rehab. 2007;88(10):1284–1288.

352. Ayalon L, Borodkin K, Dishon L, Kanety H, Dagan Y. Circadian rhythm sleep disorders following mild traumatic brain injury. Neurology. 2007;68(14):1136–1140.

353. Paparrigopoulos T, Melissaki A, Tsekou H, Efthymiou A, Kribeni G, Baziotis N, et al. Melatonin secretion after head injury: a pilot study. Brain Inj. 2006;20(8):873–878.

354. Jang SH, Seo WS, Kwon HG. Post-traumatic narcolepsy and injury of the ascending reticular activating system. Sleep Med. 2016;17:124–125.

355. Schenck CH, Boyd JL, Mahowald MW. A parasomnia overlap disorder involving sleepwalking, sleep terrors, and REM sleep behavior disorder in 33 polysomnographically confirmed cases. Sleep. 1997;20(11):972–981.

27

Pain Disorders

TIMOTHY ROEHRS AND THOMAS ROTH

INTRODUCTION

The Institute of Medicine has estimated that in the United States approximately 100 million adults experience chronic pain, and a World Health Organization survey found that 37% of adults in the 10 developed countries included in the study have chronic pain.[1] Furthermore, acute pain following injury or surgery is estimated to progress to chronic pain in 20% to 50% of patients.[2] While the mechanisms of this evolution are not well understood, suboptimal acute pain management is thought to be associated with the risk of developing chronic pain through sensitization of the nociceptive system.[2,3] However, important factors omitted in this hypothesis are the role of sleep, mood, and cognition on pain.

Information and appreciation regarding the role of insufficient sleep in pain, whether due to sleep disturbance or inadequate sleep opportunity, is now emerging. This emerging information clearly indicates the sleep–pain relation is bidirectional; that is, sleep inadequacy enhances pain and enhanced pain disrupts sleep. This latter proposition seems obvious. But, the issue is more complex. The experimental studies of pain sensitivity in humans without clinical pain, assessed using electroencephalography (EEG) arousal or electrocardiography acceleration responses during sleep to noxious versus nonnoxious stimuli suggest that sleep is protective with the nature and magnitude of response alteration varying as a function of sleep stage.[4] The question then arises as to whether or not and how the normal inhibitory effect of sleep on nociception is altered in chronic pain.

The other important factor is the role of mood/ anxiety and cognitive ruminations in chronic pain disorders. The overlap of mood or anxiety disturbance and chronic pain is well documented.[5,6] One cognitive factor that has been shown to mediate pain is referred to as "pain catastrophizing," which is characterized as ruminating on pain sensations.[7] In addition, mood and anxiety disorders and cognitive ruminations are known to be associated with sleep disturbance. Attempts to parse and understand the interactive effects of these factors in the sleep–pain nexus continue. An important clinical question is where the treatment efforts should be focused on sleep or pain and how effective they have been in improving clinical outcomes.

In this chapter, we will review the sleep, daytime sleepiness, and fatigue complaints reported by patients with chronic pain disorders and the nature of the specific sleep disturbances that have been documented in laboratory studies. To appreciate the bidirectional inactive effects of sleep and pain, we will describe experimental studies that have manipulated sleep and/or its continuity, while assessing pain thresholds and pain sensitivity. The moderating effects of mood/anxiety and cognitive rumination in the sleep–pain nexus are explored as well. Pharmacological and behavioral treatments for chronic pain disorders are reviewed. Finally, we will describe the hypothesized neurobiological mechanisms mediating the sleep-pain nexus.

METHODOLOGICAL ISSUES

The majority of the sleep–pain literature relies on self-report of both sleep and pain, which heightens the risk of response bias. In other words, reporting one symptom increases the likelihood of reporting the other and in society the general expectation is that pain disturbs sleep. The result is that reporting both sleep disturbance and pain disturbance is enhanced. Thus, the reader in evaluating the sleep–pain literature should place more weight on studies using an objective measure for at least one of the two or more self-report measures being collected in a given study and preferably both subjective and objective measures of both sleep and pain should be assessed in a given study.

Pain assessment is complex as pain is a *perception* of unpleasant or noxious sensation detected by nociceptive receptors, which can be modulated by sleepiness, attention, and emotion. Clinical studies, most typically, use self-report scales with demonstrated reliability such as the McGill Pain Inventory, the Brief Pain Inventory, or a variety of disease-specific pain inventories.[8] A common symptom in many chronic pain conditions is fatigue, which is assessed by the Fatigue Severity Scale (FSS).[9] The National Institutes of Health fostered the development of patient reported outcome scales for a variety of domains including pain, fatigue, and depression.[10] Experimental studies done in chronic pain patients and healthy volunteers without pain have assessed thresholds or sensitivity across multiple suprathreshold presentations of noxious hot, cold, and mechanical stimuli. Thresholds or sensitivity is established based on reports of pain or withdrawal responses. As well, investigators have done brain imaging and electrophysiological studies to assess evoked neural responses to painful stimuli.

In the sleep field, reliable and validated self-report scales include the Pittsburgh Sleep Quality Index[11] and the Insomnia Severity Index[12] for nocturnal sleep and the Epworth Sleepiness Scale (ESS)[13] for daytime sleepiness. It is now broadly recognized that sleepiness and fatigue are distinct physiological states, although patients will conflate the two symptoms. A recent study comparing objective and subjective measures among patients with fibromyalgia (FM), rheumatoid arthritis (RA), and age-matched healthy volunteers illustrates the overlap of sleepiness and fatigue in the patients.[14] The ESS (sleepiness) and FSS (fatigue) scores were correlated in both patient groups, but not the volunteers. The ESS scores were correlated with an objective measure of daytime sleepiness (multiple sleep latency test [MSLT]) in the volunteers, but not in the patient groups. The point being, volunteers without pain were able to make the distinction between fatigue and sleepiness, but patients were not.

The standard objective measurement of sleep is polysomnography (PSG), which involves the continuous monitoring of multiple physiological parameters including EEG, electromyography (EMG), and electrooculography (EOG). This methodology has been used since the 1950s and documents sleep versus wakefulness and the various sleep stages.[15] We previously noted that response to all stimuli including painful stimuli varies as a function of sleep stage and the loss of specific sleep stages *may be* critical to pain sensitivity. Depending on the pain condition or the nature of the sleep disturbance self-report can either overestimate or underestimate the duration of sleep and awakenings relative to PSG. Using PSG methods daytime sleepiness can be assessed objectively with the MSLT in which speed of sleep onset is measured in repeated tests across the day.[16] As previously noted, depending on the study population self-report of sleepiness can vary from the MSLT result.

A less expensive, burdensome, and labor-intensive methodology employed to measure sleep is actigraphy, which measures physical movement with a wrist-worn device and coupled with validated analytic software can document time to sleep onset and the duration of sleep versus wake over the recorded period. However, actigraphy has limitations as it can overestimate sleep time in some populations such elderly or patients with insomnia, while underestimating sleep time in various sleep disorders such as sleep apnea or periodic leg movements.[17] Actigraphy does not yield information regarding sleep stages, which, as noted, may be important in understanding sleep disturbance of various pain conditions.

PAIN DISORDERS

Primary Headache

The headache literature includes a variety of disorders with various symptom expressions and etiologies, and most headache disorders have an association with sleep disturbance. The *International Classification of Headache Disorders* (third edition, beta version; ICHD-3) identifies four major types of primary headache including migraine, tension-type headache, cluster headache, and hypnic headache.[18] Daily headache or awakening headache is reported in 4% to 6% of the general population and in patients that snore or have obstructive sleep apnea (OSA) the rates are 18% to 60% and 18% in patients with insomnia.[19]

Sleep duration and continuity are critical factors as specific sleep disorders fragment sleep (i.e., OSA, restless legs/periodic leg movements [RLS/PLMS]) and sleep loss due to insufficient opportunity or timing of sleep (i.e., circadian rhythm disorders) are known common triggers of headache.[20] A most common symptom of OSA is morning headache and the etiology of the headache in OSA is disputed. Every apnea event is terminated with brief EEG speeding which is evidence of fragmented and disrupted sleep continuity producing excessive daytime sleepiness, but each event is also associated with hypoxia and hypercapnia. Both factors, enhanced sleepiness and hypoxia/hypercapnia, are known to enhance pain (see the discussion later in this chapter).

The literature on migraine, cluster headache, and tension-type headache points to the importance of sleep duration and sleep–wake schedule. One migraine headache subtype is referred to as weekend migraine, a condition in which nighttime sleep is extended on weekends and is associated with migraine.[21] Notably, extended sleep on weekends is often a response to chronic insufficient sleep due to reduced time in bed (TIB) on week nights. Weekend oversleeping is one of the diagnostic features of insufficient sleep syndrome, a sleep disorder listed in the ICSD-3.[22] Consequently, accumulated sleep loss during weekdays may trigger the attack during the weekend extended sleep period. Increased slow-wave sleep is also reported in weekend migraine, and enhanced slow-wave sleep is consistent with insufficient sleep.

The role of specific sleep stages is equivocal. A specific diagnostic entity of the ICHD-3 is hypnic headache, which is a headache that occurs in the latter portion of the night. Hypnic headache was associated with arousal from slow-wave sleep in one study,[23] whereas it was associated with oxygen desaturation during rapid eye movement (REM) sleep in another study.[24] In migraine patients, the PSG is normal outside of the attack and during attacks studies report reduced sleep efficiency and slow-wave sleep. In contrast, some studies have reported an increase in slow-wave sleep just prior to an attack.[21] Increased slow-wave sleep is a known response to sleep loss and sleep loss is a known trigger for headache. Associations to REM sleep or transitions from non-REM (NREM) to REM sleep are reported in cluster headaches and tension-type headaches, although other studies suggest there is no sleep-stage specificity.[25,26]

The primary headache literature fails in documenting sleep duration and sleep schedule prior to the laboratory PSG studies, and the headache literature totally neglects consideration of daytime napping and various other compensatory behaviors (i.e., use of caffeine or other over-the-counter stimulants) that patients adopt to cope with their increased daytime sleepiness associated with their reduced or fragmented sleep. Later in the chapter, we discuss the impact of sleepiness on pain thresholds and sensitivity.

Musculoskeletal Pain
Rheumatoid Arthritis

RA is an autoimmune inflammatory disorder that primarily affects the joints and patients with RA experience sleep disturbance and pain. The sleep disturbance of RA has been characterized in PSG studies as sleep that is fragmented with increased wake caused by discrete, short arousals.[27,28] RA patients were also found to have multiple sleep-stage shifts and a higher occurrence, as compared to healthy volunteers, of periodic leg movements, which also fragment sleep.[27,29] A PSG study in RA patients with comorbid insomnia, but without other sleep or psychiatric disorders, reported reduced sleep efficiency and increased wakefulness during the sleep period, without the frequent brief arousals that do not progress to frank wakefulness and are associated with sleep disorders.[14] The persisting pain in RA patients is noteworthy in that sleep efficiency did not improve on a recovery night following a night of reduced bedtime (4 hours) as it did in patients with FM.[30] The difference may relate to the peripheral versus central origin of the pain in the two disorders.

Fatigue is a major daytime symptom of RA. As noted earlier, daytime sleepiness and fatigue are often conflated in patients with chronic pain. The fatigue may relate to the primary disease process, inflammatory cytokine activation. In fact, fatigue and pain are correlated in RA patients.[14] We discuss the possible mechanisms for the sleep-pain nexus later in this chapter. Cytokine activation present in various sleep, pain, and mood disorders is often accompanied by fatigue.

Fibromyalgia

Unlike the pain of RA, the pain of FM is widespread and not localized. Its etiology is not fully understood, but it is hypothesized that FM is a member of a class of chronic pain disorders, termed central sensitivity syndromes, which are characterized by intense enhancement of pain by central nervous system mechanisms.[31] FM is the most extensively PSG studied among the chronic pain disorders.

The first PSG study of FM dates to 1975, and that study found the amounts of slow-wave sleep, REM sleep, and total sleep duration were all reduced relative to healthy volunteers, and these findings have been replicated in numerous studies.[32,33] One additional anomaly reported in the 1975 study was the observation of intrusions of EEG alpha activity (8–12 Hz) in NREM sleep and the admixture of alpha activity with delta activity

(0.5–2.5 Hz). The anomaly was first reported in patients with depression and was termed *alpha-delta sleep*.[34] However, the clinical significance of alpha-intrusions is disputed as healthy volunteers also show alpha-intrusions, and some have suggested the intrusions are actually protective of sleep in that they are a sign of sleep maintaining processes.[35] To better characterize sleep–wake processes in FM a recent study tallied 30-second bouts of sleep and wake during the 8-hour sleep period in patients with FM, primary insomnia (PI), and healthy volunteers.[36] The study found both FM and PI subjects had shorter mean duration of sleep bouts compared with volunteers, but subjects with FM had significantly shorter and more frequent wake bouts than those with PI. Does the intrusion of frequent short wake bouts into sleep suggest disturbance of the sleep maintaining systems or an overactivation of waking systems?

A prominent daytime symptom in FM along with pain is daytime sleepiness and fatigue. As noted earlier sleepiness is measured objectively using the MSLT. Despite comparably disturbed nocturnal sleep to RA patients, FM patients had unusually high MSLT scores (i.e., greater alertness), even compared to healthy volunteers.[14] Of note, elevated MSLT scores coupled with low nocturnal sleep efficiencies have been reported in patients with PI and are considered a sign of hyperarousal.[37] The hyperarousal of FM is consistent with the hypothesized hypersensitization of sensory processing in FM.[31]

Temporomandibular Joint Disorder

Temporomandibular joint disorder (TMD) is characterized by episodic, masticatory muscle, and joint pain. As with other of the central sensitivity syndrome members its etiology is not completely known, but it shares the hypothesized central nervous system sensitization of nociceptive processing.[31] We are aware of one PSG study done in patients meeting diagnostic criteria for TMD; the study included concurrent objective daytime assessments of pressure and heat pain thresholds.[38] Multiple primary sleep disorders including insomnia, sleep apnea, and active sleep bruxism were found in this sample of TMD patients with 43% of the patients showing two or more sleep disorders. While insomnia disorder with mildly reduced PSG sleep efficiency (88%) was associated with reduced thermal and mechanical pain thresholds relative to controls, mild sleep disordered breathing (Respiratory Disturbance Index [RDI] 13.7) was associated with increased mechanical (i.e., less pain), but not thermal thresholds. The reason for this discrepancy is unclear.

Neuropathic Pain

The various neuropathic pain conditions are thought to involve a maladaptive response of the somatosensory nervous system to damage triggered by metabolic disorders (diabetes, vitamin B deficiency), infections (herpes zoster HIV), neurotoxins (alcohol, chemotherapy), and traumatic injury.[39] The symptomatic nature of the pain (sharp, dull, persisting, episodic) can vary and can depend on the specific nerves involved.

Orofacial Neuropathic Pain

Trigeminal neuralgia is associated with reported sleep disturbance in 60% of patients, where innocuous stimuli induce awakening.[20] No PSG studies have been done to document the extent of the sleep disturbance. Postherpetic trigeminal neuropathy is also associated with disturbed sleep and objective PSG studies have documented the disturbance. Sleep was fragmented with an overall reduction in sleep efficiency, reduced stages 3 and 4 and REM sleep and increased stage 1, light sleep, compared to controls.[40]

Peripheral Neuropathic Pain

There are a number of PSG studies in patients with diabetic or postherpetic peripheral neuropathies. The PSG studies are placebo-controlled pharmacological treatment trials. Some information on the extent of sleep disturbance in these patient is seen in the placebo data of the trials. But these studies have not compared peripheral neuropathic pain to other chronic pain conditions or age-matched healthy controls to determine the extent of sleep disturbance. One PSG study in patients with diabetic and postherpetic neuropathies found sleep efficiencies of 68% with sleep latencies of 34 minutes and wakefulness after sleep onset of 108 minutes.[41] This degree of sleep disturbance is quite similar to that seen in FM and RA patients.[30] In addition, 10 of the 35 patients had clinically significant sleep apnea (i.e., RDI ≥10). A PSG treatment study of patients with diabetic neuropathy showed in the placebo treatment condition average sleep efficiencies of 77% and 79%, and among these patients, the apnea–hypopnea index ranged from 3 to 6 and the periodic limb movements during sleep index from 16 to 20.[42] Thus, the reported fragmented sleep may be due to the sleep disorders and not the pain.

PAIN SENSITIVITY AND SLEEP

Total Sleep Deprivation

Initially, the point was made that the sleep–pain relation is bidirectional; that is, sleep inadequacy enhances pain and pain disturbs sleep. That relation is directly seen in studies that have manipulated sleep in either patients with chronic pain or volunteers without pain and then measured subsequent pain sensitivity and thresholds to noxious stimuli. Most studies in healthy volunteers show one night of total sleep deprivation enhances pain sensitivity and reduces pain thresholds.[43-45] One night of total sleep deprivation increased pain sensitivity (assessed by latency to finger withdrawal responses) by 27% over a range of radiant heat intensities.[43] Total sleep deprivation for 40 hours reduced the pain threshold to a mechanical pressure stimulus by 8%.[44] Thermal pain thresholds were reduced with total sleep deprivation, but the sleep deprivation had no effect on somatosensory thresholds to touch.[45] This is an important observation as it shows that the activation of nociception is specific and not a by-product of a general activation of all somatosensation.

Reduced Sleep Time

In daily life, total sleep deprivation is rare. The most frequent pattern in the general population is a reduction of TIB that consequently reduces the nightly amount of sleep. Studies in volunteers have reduced TIB to 4 or 5 hours, and the consequent sleep reduction relative to an 8-hour TIB enhances pain. In the previously discussed study using radiant heat assessment and total sleep deprivation, a 4-hour bedtime was associated with a 13.5% enhancement of pain sensitivity, 50% of that in the total deprivation.[43] In volunteers, 4 hours of sleep relative to habitual sleep increased pain ratings to a laser-generated heat stimulus by 30%.[46] Evoked potentials to the laser stimulation were also assessed and the N1 amplitude was *reduced* by approximately 30%. This result suggested to the authors that the observed sleep restriction-induced hyperalgesia is perceptual amplification rather than sensory amplification, in that the sensory-evoked potentials were reduced, not increased.

Few studies have experimentally reduced sleep time in chronic pain patients. One such study compared 8 to 4 hours TIB in RA patients and healthy volunteers.[47] Sleep restriction increased McGill pain ratings relative to the volunteers and to the RA patients own 8 hours TIB. The sleep restriction also increased Profile of Mood States ratings on the fatigue, depression, and anxiety scales. Later, we discuss the moderating effects of mood and anxiety in the pain–sleep nexus.

Sleep Fragmentation

The primary sleep disorders sleep apnea disorder and periodic leg movement disorder are not generally associated with reduced sleep time or prolonged awakenings. Rather, the continuity of sleep is disrupted with brief EEG (3–15 seconds) arousals following each event. Disruption of sleep continuity without frank awakening is referred to as sleep fragmentation. It was previously noted that these primary sleep disorders were observed in the various previously discussed chronic pain disorders. One study in healthy volunteers, while not specifically fragmenting sleep, did assess the role of multiple awakenings on pain.[48] Multiple awakenings during sleep compared to uninterrupted sleep reduced pain inhibition, a normal adaptive response to pain. Apnea patients with fragmented sleep pain sensitivity to a radiant heat stimulus were assessed before and after treatment with continuous positive airway pressure (CPAP).[49] CPAP reduced the RDI from 50 to 2 (i.e., improved sleep continuity) and reduced pain sensitivity by 29%.

Sleep Stage Deprivation
Slow-Wave Sleep Deprivation

In response to the early description of alpha delta sleep in patients with FM, a number of studies have focused on the selective deprivation of slow-wave sleep. The results of these studies are equivocal.[50] Discrepancy among the study results may relate to several factors. The deprivation procedure itself, which requires multiple awakenings to deprive slow-wave sleep, also reduces total sleep time. We previously pointed out that reducing sleep time or producing multiple awakenings has a hyperalgesic effect. Also as a person ages, the amount of slow-wave sleep declines and to the extent that studies differ in sample age greater or lesser hyperalgesic effects may be observed.

REM Sleep Deprivation

The unique sleep stage that may be important to nociceptive signaling is REM sleep. Later we discuss the overlap in the neurobiology of pain and sleep and specifically REM sleep. There is animal and human research that suggests specific deprivation of REM sleep has a hyperalgesic effect.[50] A correlational study in healthy women found percentage of REM sleep was correlated with ratings of thermal pain and frequency of unsolicited pain reports.[51] In a REM deprivation study in healthy volunteers, pain sensitivity to a radiant heat stimulus was increased compared to a yoked control NREM awakening condition in which the frequency and distribution of awakenings was similar to the REM condition, and pain sensitivity was similar to a 2-hour TIB.[43] Pain tolerance, not pain threshold or sensitivity, was unaffected by REM deprivation and minimally affected by total sleep deprivation.[44] Laser-evoked potential thresholds and pain perception were not affected by REM deprivation compared to 2 nights of total sleep deprivation.[52] But, these two negative studies failed to show adequate sensitivity to total sleep deprivation and neither controlled for the multiple awakenings required to produce the REM-specific deprivation.

MODULATORS/MEDIATORS OF THE SLEEP–PAIN NEXUS

Mood Factors

Cognitive and mood factors are likely to play a modulatory role in the sleep–pain nexus and may even serve as mediators of the relation. A number of studies have shown that total or partial sleep deprivation in healthy volunteers enhances mood measures of depression and anxiety. For example, 56 hours of sleep deprivation produced subclinical elevations of depression, anxiety, and somatic pain scales of the Personality Assessment Inventory,[53] and 30 hours of sleep deprivation elevated the fatigue and depression scales of the Profile of Mood States (POMS).[54] Reducing sleep time by one-third for 7 nights increased scores on all the POMS scales (e.g., anger, fatigue, depression, anxiety, vigor, confusion).[55] In assessing positive mood factors, a 50% reduction of sleep time reduced optimism and sociability on visual analog scales.[56]

Most of these healthy volunteer studies did not assess pain and the question remains whether or not the hyperalgesic effect of sleep loss is mediated by its effects on mood. In chronic pain patients, there is evidence that partial sleep deprivation (4 hours TIB) exacerbates fatigue, depression, anxiety, and pain compared to volunteers without pain.[57] In a large study of patients with various chronic pain conditions structural equation modeling analyses found a direct relation

between sleep disturbance and pain and negative mood mediated that relation.[58] On the other hand, in patients with FM sleep quality served as the mediator of the relation of depressive symptoms and pain.[59] Only large prospective studies in samples including multiple chronic pain conditions will help disentangle the relations of sleep, pain, and mood. Clinically, the important question is where to direct treatment efforts.

Cognitive Factors

Important cognitive factors that modulate pain have been identified. One important factor is referred to as "pain catastrophizing," which is characterized as rumination on pain sensations, exaggeration of the threat associated with pain, and feeling an inability to control pain.[7] For example, patients with osteoarthritis of the knee were followed for 24 months after arthroplasty. Their pain catastrophizing scores were predictive of the presence of pain on the McGill Pain Questionnaire over the 24 months.[7] A similar construct is applied in the insomnia literature regarding the presence of rumination around the inability to sleep.[60]

Another important cognitive factor modulating pain involves the attention–distraction dimension. Perception of pain is altered by the attentional focus of a person such that focus-on as opposed to distraction-from intensifies the pain. A study used pain-evoked EEG responses and reported pain thresholds to assess nociception (i.e., pain-evoked EEG) versus pain perception under two differing attention conditions, stimulus intensity discrimination (e.g., pain focus) and mental arithmetic (e.g., pain distraction).[46] Pain responses were assessed after habitual versus bedtime restriction to 4 hours. The sleep restriction reduced the amplitude of the evoked responses, but pain was enhanced by 30% in the focused condition. In other words, in this study, the sleep restriction reduced the nociceptive response (i.e., EEG-evoked response), but the perception of pain was enhanced by focus on the pain stimulus. Unlike previous sleep restriction and deprivation studies, this is the first study attempting to parse the nociceptive from the perceptive components of pain by manipulation of the perceptive component.

MECHANISMS

In this section we discuss the various central nervous system and peripheral nervous system mechanisms through which sleep and pain may have their bidirectional interactive effects. In discussing the neurobiology of the sleep–pain nexus, it should be noted that the source and etiology of the pain (i.e., peripheral vs. central, inflammatory vs. structural) may be important considerations.

Central Nervous System Opioid Systems

It is well established that pain is modulated by the opioid system. One inhibitory opioid system originates in the midbrain periaqueductal gray, projects to the nucleus raphe magnus in the pons, and then along the dorsolateral funiculus to the dorsal horn in the spinal cord, where nociceptive information is modulated.[50] Opioid receptors are intermingled among nuclei in these areas with nuclei that control sleep–wake. Preclinical studies have shown that sleep deprivation disrupts endogenous opioid function such that opioid receptor function is downregulated, and endogenous opioid levels are diminished.[61] Our study in healthy volunteers without pain supports this preclinical work.[62] Relative to placebo the analgesic effects of codeine, as measured by finger withdrawal latency to a radiant heat stimulus, was reduced in sleepy versus nonsleepy participants. The sleepiness/nonsleepiness of the participants was established by the MSLT and determined to be due to chronic insufficient sleep. When a 10-hour bedtime is enforced in such sleepy volunteers their MSLT is normalized and pain sensitivity is reduced,[63] and when a 10-hour bedtime is encouraged for the 7 nights just prior to elective hip and knee replacement surgeries their postsurgery morphine use is reduced by 30% relative to those patients remaining on their habitual sleep schedule, while pain ratings were improved.[64]

Acetylcholine

Both animal and human studies show acetylcholine is important in the sleep and nociception nexus. In animal studies, cholinomimetics (i.e., carbachol) have been shown to have an analgesic effect and cholinergic agonists (i.e., neostigmine) are used for pain control in the clinic.[50]

Acetylcholine is known to have a significant role in the generation of REM sleep and thus may promote both REM sleep and analgesia. Previously, we noted that selective REM sleep deprivation has a hyperalgesic effect.[43] On the other hand, opiates have been shown acutely to be REM-suppressing agents, and whether or not REM suppression lessens their analgesic activity is not known.

Other Transmitter Systems

Adenosine is considered to be the major neurochemical involved in sleep homeostasis.[65] Its brain levels accumulate during periods of sustained wakefulness, and during sleep, particularly slow-wave sleep, brain levels decrease. The activation of adenosine has been shown to produce analgesia in animal studies.[66] However, these findings are inconsistent with human sleep restriction studies in which pain thresholds are reduced and pain sensitivity is enhanced, and presumably the sleep restriction has enhanced adenosine levels.

Central dopamine and serotonin have also been implicated in chronic pain. It is hypothesized that serotonergic and dopaminergic cells in the raphe magnus, which reciprocally control alertness and modulate pain become dysregulated in chronic pain conditions.[67] Evidence supportive of this hypothesis is the observation that patients with chronic facial pain and FM have reduced cerebrospinal fluid levels of dopamine metabolites.[61] Also consistent with this hypothesis is our own data showing hyperarousal on the MSLT in patients with FM relative to age-matched pain-free volunteers and patients with RA.[14] The FM patient MSLT scores are similar to those patients with insomnia disorder that show hyperarousal on the MSLT; that is, their average daytime sleep latencies are unusually high particularly given sleeping 6 hours or less the previous night.

Peripheral Mechanisms

Accumulating evidence suggests that the sleep–pain nexus is mediated by activation of the proinflammatory cytokines (PIC). The early literature is equivocal regarding sleep loss and PIC activation,[68] but recent studies have shown total sleep deprivation and sleep restriction to 4 to 6 hours nightly produces elevated levels of interleukin 6 (IL-6) and less consistently tumor necrosis factor alpha (TNF-α).[69-73]

The association of sleepiness and PIC elevations can be concurrently reversed by either sleepiness improvement or PIC blockage. Increased IL-6 levels and sleepiness due to sleep restriction are both reversed by a midday nap, and sleepiness and elevated TNF-α levels in sleepy patients are both reversed by the TNF-α antagonist, etanercept.[74] TNF-α levels are elevated in sleepy children with OSA due to enlarged tonsils. Tonsillectomy reverses the OSA and sleepiness of the children and, importantly, also reduces TNF-α levels.[75]

An important linkage is that of PIC activation and pain. PICs in both the peripheral and central nervous system are known to play a key role in both acute and chronic pain conditions.[76] In the periphery the cytokines are released by macrophages in response to tissue injury. The local hyperalgesic effects of cytokine release were demonstrated in animal studies showing that local application of TNF-α or IL-1 increased pain sensitivity.[77] Also, administration of cytokine antagonists reversed the hyperalgesia.[77] In human chronic pain conditions, both IL-6 and TNF-α levels are elevated peripherally and their levels are correlated with the experienced pain and hyperalgesia.[78]

TREATMENT OF SLEEP AND PAIN

Behavioral Therapy

Behavioral Treatment for Insomnia

There is a rather large literature on various cognitive behavioral therapy for chronic pain (CBT-P) of various etiologies. These treatments are directed to the pain, and in some cases, sleep is assessed as a secondary outcome. We will not attempt to review these studies for this chapter. In contrast, cognitive behavioral treatment for insomnia (CBT-I) has been used as treatment in small number of studies conducted in patients with insomnia and comorbid chronic pain. These studies have produced equivocal results. Typically, as shown in studies of patients with insomnia disorder (formally termed PI), in patients with chronic pain and insomnia CBT-I reduces sleep latency, improves sleep efficiency (sleep time per TIB), and in some cases increases total sleep time. As described in the following text, the CBT-I did not consistently improve pain.

CBT-I improved sleep in patients with musculoskeletal pain but did not significantly improve pain.[80] In FM patients, CBT-I and a parallel sleep hygiene control both improved sleep, but pain reduction was only seen in the sleep hygiene control group.[81] CBT-I in patients with chronic neck and back pain improved sleep and "sleep interference by pain" ratings, but not pain severity.[82] An interesting large study (*n* = 150) compared CBT-I and CBT-P in patients with osteoarthritic pain.[83] CBT-I improved sleep relative to the CBT-P and control groups. But neither active treatment had an impact on pain severity ratings.

Of note, CBT-I usually has three components: cognitive therapy and sleep hygiene instructions, stimulus control, and sleep restriction. Both stimulus control and sleep restriction functionally reduce a patient's TIB. The consequent enhancement of sleep drive due to the restricted TIB thereby reduces sleep latency and improves sleep efficiency (i.e., its therapeutic effect), but it does not increase sleep time. Earlier we described studies showing that sleep restriction has a hyperalgesic effect, which may explain the equivocal effects of CBT-I on pain. Studies that enhance sleep time, as well as consolidating sleep, may be more successful in treating the various pain conditions.

Behavioral Treatment in Other Sleep Disorders

Persistently reduced TIB produces chronic excessive daytime sleepiness as documented by the MSLT, a condition identified in the *International Classification of Sleep Disorders* as chronic insufficient sleep syndrome.[22] Enforcing a 10-hour TIB for 1 to 2 weeks in sleepy people normalizes their daytime sleepiness/alertness.[16] Earlier we noted that a study in pain-free excessively sleepy people showed four consecutive nights of a 10-hour TIB reduced pain sensitivity to a radiant heat stimulus[63] and a 1-week extension of TIB prior to elective joint replacement reduced postsurgery pain and morphine use.[64] These studies point to the importance of identifying and correcting insufficient and irregular sleep behavior in chronic pain patients.

Pharmacological Therapy

Drugs from a variety of classes including analgesics, antidepressants, antiepileptics, and hypnotics have been used as therapies in the various chronic pain disorders. Pain is the primary focus in these studies and any sleep outcomes, when included as a secondary outcome, are typically assessed by self-reports. We previously discussed the danger of measurement bias in self-reporting both sleep and pain. In addition the impact of treatment on daytime function, specifically daytime sleepiness/fatigue, is often overlooked in studies or considered a side effect of the medication. Another issue is that the patient samples enrolled in these studies are not specifically selected for the presence of insomnia comorbid with the pain disorder. This potentially introduces greater heterogeneity around sleep in the study sample and diminishes the study's power to detect positive sleep effects.

Fibromyalgia

With the previously mentioned cautions, in a meta-analysis of randomized trials of the treatment of FM, the authors concluded there was "limited robust clinical data for some therapeutic classes including tricyclic antidepressants, analgesics, sedative hypnotics, and monoamine oxidase inhibitors"[84] (p. 472). This review also noted that trials of pregabalin and the two serotonin norepinephrine reuptake inhibitors, milnacipran and duloxetine, exhibited improved pain scores, but only pregabalin improved sleep ratings.

In a large ($N = 119$) clinical PSG trial of FM patients with complaints of comorbid sleep maintenance insomnia, pregabalin reduced the amount of wakefulness during sleep and modestly increased the percent of slow wave sleep.[85] Additionally daily pain and fatigue scores were reduced. In healthy volunteers, a PSG study found that pregabalin relative to placebo increased slow-wave sleep, but not sleep efficiency or sleep time, although one would not expect improved sleep efficiency in these volunteers without sleep disturbance.[86]

To determine whether the sleep–pain effects of pregabalin were primarily due to its effects on sleep or its effects on pain, a study conducted mediation analyses.[86] Data of two large FM studies in which significant pain effects and sleep effects were observed were combined for the analyses. The results showed 43% to 80% of the sleep effects were the result of the direct effects of pregabalin on sleep and not through pain relief.[87]

Neuropathic Pain

The International Association for the Study of Pain published a set of guidelines for the treatment of neuropathic pain.[88] Based on randomized clinical trials the first-line treatments included tricyclic antidepressants, dual serotonin and norepinephrine reuptake inhibitors, and the calcium channel alpha 2-delta ligands, gabapentin and pregabalin. These guidelines never mentioned sleep, and daytime sleepiness was only cited as a side effect. These guidelines did note the paucity of comparative studies. In that light, an interesting comparative study randomized patients with diabetic neuropathic pain to amitriptyline, duloxetine, and pregabalin.[42] Relative to placebo all treatments improved pain with no drug showing superiority, but the medications had differential effects on sleep measured by PSG. Pregabalin improved sleep continuity at both doses (300 and 600 mg daily), as did amitriptyline at the higher dose (75 mg daily), but duloxetine (60 and 120 mg daily) increased wake and reduced sleep time. The results of this study underscore the consideration of sleep in making clinical decisions for treatment of neuropathic pain.

Acute Post-Surgery Pain

In the introduction section (p. 474), it was noted that acute postsurgery pain can advance to chronic pain in 20% to 50% of individuals.[2] The presurgery study referred to earlier identified chronic insufficient sleep among hip and knee replacement patients and extended TIB the week before surgery.[64] Relative to patients remaining on their habitual sleep schedule, the sleep extension was associated with reduced in-patient daily pain ratings and morphine usage the 3 days after surgery.

Similar to our behavioral prophylactic presurgery sleep treatment study,[64] several studies have treated postsurgery sleep and reduced acute postsurgery pain and analgesia use. In patients undergoing knee arthroscopy, the hypnotic zolpidem (10 mg), relative to placebo, reduced postoperative pain scores and postoperative hydrocodone/acetaminophen consumption.[89] The anticonvulsant, gabapentin (1,200 mg), which acts at the alpha-2-delta subunit of N-type voltage-gated calcium channels, was shown to reduce postoperative pain and morphine consumption relative to placebo in women after hysterectomy.[90] Neither of these studies nor our behavioral study followed patients beyond the acute postsurgery period, but one might hypothesize that the risk of transitioning to chronic pain would be reduced by improving sleep around the surgery period.

Sedative Drugs and Chronic Pain

Standard hypnotics have been assessed in a number of chronic pain conditions with a pattern of mixed results. In FM patients zolpidem,[91] but not zopiclone,[92] improved some of the sleep measures, but neither drug improved pain. Triazolam improved pain and sleep in patients with RA,[93] whereas zopiclone only improved pain.[94] The S isomer of zopiclone, eszopiclone, was studied in a large study of patients with insomnia and comorbid RA.[95] Relative to placebo eszopiclone improved self-reported sleep and pain.

Cannabis and cannabinoids, while still illegal under US federal law, are available now in 29 states and the District of Columbia under various states laws and policies. Most of the state laws and policies allow for the use of cannabis and cannabinoids for a variety of medical conditions with chronic pain among them. The most current (2017) review of the scientific evidence regarding the analgesic effects of cannabis and cannabinoids concluded that inhaled cannabis is effective in reducing noncancer pain.[96] Oral cannabinoids in some chronic pain conditions seem to also improve sleep and quality of life. Due to the differing pathophysiologies and types of the various pain conditions cannabis and cannabinoids have not been shown to be effective in acute postoperative pain, abdominal chronic pain, or rheumatoid pain. Among the side effects are sedation and disturbances of attention and performance, both likely due to the sedation.

CONCLUSIONS

Sleep disturbance is a prominent symptom in people with chronic pain of various etiologies, and it has been objectively documented by PSG studies. The sleep–pain nexus has been modeled in healthy pain-free volunteers showing that sleep deprivation, restriction, and fragmentation can cause hyperalgesic effects. These studies have shown that the sleep–pain relation is likely bidirectional. Additionally, mood and cognitive factors modulate the sleep–pain relation. Both central and peripheral mechanisms have been identified that underlie the sleep–pain nexus. Some behavioral and pharmacological therapies specifically directed toward sleep have shown sleep improvement, which is associated with pain improvement.

FUTURE DIRECTIONS

Further research is necessary to better understand the normal physiology and pathophysiology of chronic pain, which will further enhance the clinician's ability to manage sleep and pain. Some of the questions that remain around the sleep–pain nexus include whether an increase in sleep time, irrespective of sleep stages, is sufficient to improve pain. How important is slow-wave sleep, given sleep is protective against painful stimulation and during slow-wave sleep arousal threshold is the highest (i.e., most protective against arousal from pain)? In contrast, arousal threshold is lowest during REM sleep, and antidepressants, used clinically with some success in chronic pain, are suppressive of REM sleep. Yet, some of the experimental pain literature suggests REM deprivation is hyperalgesic, although the chronicity of the REM deprivation may be critical. The experimental studies are acute, while antidepressant associated REM suppression is chronic.

From the pain side of the sleep–pain nexus, what is the significance of the etiology and the time course of the pain condition: peripheral versus central, inflammatory versus structural, and acute versus chronic? What central and peripheral adaptations occur as pain progresses from acute to chronic?

From a treatment perspective, is there differential treatment efficacy for specific drug classes in specific pain populations? Given most pain conditions are chronic, it is important to study treatment effects over chronic treatment periods; those studies currently are not available. The major problem with the behavioral treatment studies is that although sleep continuity was improved, sleep time was not increased. A major component of CBT-I is sleep restriction, and in healthy normals and pain patients, reducing sleep time enhances pain sensitivity. This would suggest consolidating sleep alone is not sufficient to improve pain. Increasing sleep time after having consolidated sleep is probably also necessary.

KEY CLINICAL PEARLS

- In managing acute and chronic pain the clinician should inquire about their patients' sleep as to its adequacy in duration, regularity, and continuity.
- Assessment for primary sleep disorders that may be disrupting sleep continuity and treating the identified sleep disorder should facilitate management of chronic pain.
- Identifying and treating sleep disorders prior to elective surgery may lessen the postsurgery pain and reduce the need for opiates.

ACKNOWLEDGMENTS
Roehrs is funded by NIDA grant # R01-DA013877 and Merck grant #53198 and has served as a consultant to Purdue Pharmaceuticals. Roth has served as a consultant to Merck, Flamel, Eisai, Purdue, Idorsia, GSK, Pfizer, Jazz, SEQ.

SELF-ASSESSMENT QUESTIONS

1. **In experimental pain models, restriction of which specific sleep stage appears to enhance pain?**
   a. Slow wave sleep
   b. REM
   c. Stage 2 NREM
   d. None of the above

   Answer: b

2. **The chronic pain condition fibromyalgia**
   a. is a wide spread and non-localized pain disorder.

b. is hypothesized to be a member of a class of disorders termed central sensitivity syndromes.

c. is characterized by alpha intrusions into REM sleep.

d. Both a and b

Answer: d

3. Among headache disorders,

a. reduced sleep duration may be the cause of the migraine headache subtype termed week-end migraine.

b. studies clearly indicate that headache subtypes are associated with specific sleep stages.

c. the rates of headache in insomnia are approximately 60%.

d. Both a and c

Answer: a

4. Mechanisms that may explain the bidirectional relation of sleep and pain are

a. histaminergic neurons of the tubercular mammillary nucleus.

b. GABA neurons of the ventral lateral preoptic area.

c. activation of pro-inflammatory cytokines.

d. Both a and b

Answer: c

5. Sleep fragmentation refers to

a. enhanced wakefulness during the sleep period.

b. the consequence of REM behavior disorder.

c. frequent brief EEG arousals during sleep.

d. alpha-delta sleep.

Answer: c

REFERENCES

1. Dzau, VJ, Pizzo, PA. Relieving pain in America: insights from an Institute of Medicine committee. *JAMA* 2014;312: 1507–1508.

2. Kehlet H, Jensen TS, Woolf CJ. Persistent postsurgical pain: risk factors and prevention. *Lancet* 2006;367:1618–1625.

3. Vanderah TW. Pathophysiology of pain. *Med Clin N Am* 2007;91:1–12.

4. Bentley AJ. Pain perception during sleep and circadian influences: the experimental evidence. In: Lavigne G, Sessle J, Choiniere M, Soja PJ, eds. *Sleep and pain*. Seattle WA: IASP Press; 2007:123–136.

5. McWilliams LA, Cox BJ, Ennis MW. Mood and anxiety disorder associated with chronic pain: an examination in a nationally representative sample. *Pain* 2003;106:127–133.

6. Gerrits M, Vogelzangs N, van Oppen P, van Marwijk H, van der Horst H, Penninx B. Impact of pain on the course of depressive and anxiety disorders. *Pain* 2012;153:429–436.

7. Forsythe ME, Dunbar MJ, Hennigar AW, Sullivan MJ, Gross M. Prospective relation between catastrophizing and residual pain following knee arthroplasty: two-year follow-up. *Pain Res Management* 2008;13:335–341.

8. Williams DA, Arnold LM. Measures of fibromyalgia. *Arth Care Res* 2011;63:S86–S97.

9. Schwartz JE, Jandorf L, Krupp LB. The measurement of fatigue: a new instrument. *J Psychosom Res* 1993;93:753–62.

10. Cella D, Yount S, Rothrock N, Gershon R, Cook K, Reeve B, Ader D, Fries JF, Bruce B, Rose M. The Patient-Reported Outcomes Measurement Information System (PROMIS): progress of an NIH Roadmap cooperative group during its first two years. *Med Care.* 2007;66:S3–S11.

11. Buysse DJ, Reynolds CF, Monk TH, et al. Pittsburgh Sleep Quality Index: a new instrument for psychiatric practice and research. *Psychiatry Res* 1989;28:193–213.

12. Bastien CH, Vallières A, Morin C M. Validation of the Insomnia Severity Index as an outcome measure for insomnia research. *Sleep Med* 2001;2:297–307.

13. Johns MW. Reliability and factor analysis of the Epworth Sleepiness Scale. *Sleep* 1992;15:376–381.

14. Roehrs T, Diederichs C, Gillis M, Burger AJ, Stout RA, Lumley MA, Roth T. Nocturnal sleep, daytime sleepiness and fatigue in fibromyalgia patients compared to rheumatoid arthritis patients and healthy controls: a preliminary study. *Sleep Med* 2013;14:109–115.

15. Keenan S, Hirshkowitz M. Monitoring and staging human sleep. In Kryger MH, Roth T, Dement WC, eds. *Principles and practice of sleep medicine.* 6th ed. Philadelphia PA: Elsevier, 2017:1567–1575.

16. Roehrs T, Carskadon MC, Dement WC, Roth T. Daytime sleepiness and alertness. In Kryger MH, Roth T, Dement WC, eds. *Principles and practice of sleep medicine.* 6th ed. Philadelphia PA: Elsevier, 2017:39–48.

17. Weiss AR, Johnson NL, Berger NA, Redline S. Validity of activity-based devices to estimate sleep. *J Clin Sleep Med* 2010;6:336–342.

18. Headache Classification Committee of the International Headache Society. The international classification of headache disorders, 3rd edition (beta version). *Cephalagia* 2013;33: 629–808.

19. Rains JC, Poceta JS, Penzien DB. Sleep and headaches. *Curr Neurol Neuosci Rep* 2008;8:167–175.

20. Almoznino G, Benoliel R, Sharav Y, Havis Y. Sleep disorders and chronic craniofacial pain: characteristics and management possibilities. *Sleep Med Rev* 2017;33:39–50.

21. Ong JC, Park M. Chronic headaches and insomnia: Working toward a bio-behavioral model. *Cephalagia* 2012;32:1059–1070.

22. American Academy of Sleep Medicine. *International classification of sleep disorders.* 3rd ed. Darien, IL: American Academy of Sleep Medicine; 2014.

23. Arjona JA, Jimenez-Jimenez FJ, Vela-Bueno A, Talon Barranco A. Hypnic headache associated with stage 3 slow wave sleep. *Headache* 2000;40:753–754.

24. Dodick DW. Polysomnography in hypnic headache syndrome. *Headache* 2000;40:748–752.

25. Jennum P, Jensen R. Sleep and headache. *Sleep Med* 2002;6:471–479.

26. Zaremba S, Holle D, Wessendorf TE, Diener HC, Katsarava Z, Oberman M. Cluster headache shows no association with rapid eye movement sleep. *Cephalalgia* 2012;32:289–296

27. Hirsch M, Carlander B, Verge M, Tafti M, Anaya J. Billiard M, Sany J. Objective and subjective sleep disturbances in patients with rheumatoid arthritis. *Arthritis Rheum* 1994;37:41–49.

28. Lavie P, Nahir M, Lorber M, Scharf Y. Nonsteroidal anti-inflammatory drug therapy in rheumatoid arthritis patients: lack of association between clinical improvement and effects on sleep. *Arthritis Rheum* 1991;34:655–659.

29. Drewes AM, Svedsen L, Taagholt J, Bjerregárd K, Neilsen KD, Hansen B. Sleep in rheumatoid arthritis: a comparison with healthy subjects and studies of sleep/wake interactions. *Brit J Rheumatology,* 1998;37:71–81.

30. Roehrs T, Diederichs C, Gillis M, Burger AJ, Stout RA, Lumley MA, Roth T. Effects of reduced time in bed on daytime sleepiness and recovery sleep in fibromyalgia and rheumatoid arthritis. *J Psychosom Res* 2015;79:27–31.

31. Yunus MB. Fibromyalgia and overlapping disorders: the unifying concept of central sensitivity syndromes. *Semin Arthritis Rheum* 2007;36:339–356.

32. Moldofsky H, Scarisbrick P, England R, Smythe H. Musculoskeletaly symptoms and non-REM sleep disturbances in patient with fibrositis syndrome and healthy subjects. *Psychosom Med* 1975;37:341–351.

33. Mahowald ML, Mahowald MW. Nighttime sleep and daytime functioning (sleepiness and fatigue) in less well defined chronic rheumatic diseases with particular reference to the alpha-delta NREM sleep anomaly. *Sleep Med* 2000;1:77–83.

34. Hauri P, Hawkins DR. Alpha-delta sleep. *Electroenceph Clin Neurophys* 1973;34:233–237.

35. Pivik kRT, Harman K. A reconcep0tualization of EEG alpha activity as an index of arousal during sleep: all alpha activity is not equal. *J Sleep Res* 1995;4:131–137.

36. Roth T, Bhadra-Brrown P, Pitman VW, Roehrs TA, Resnick EM. Characteristics of disturbed sleep in patients with fibromyalgia compared with insomnia or with pain-free volunteers. *Clin J Pain* 2016;32:302–307.

37. Roehrs TA, Randall S, Harris E, Maan R, Roth T. MSLT in primary insomnia: Stability and relation to nocturnal sleep. *Sleep* 2011;34: 1647–1652.

38. Smith MT, Wickwire EM, Grace EG, Edwards RR, Buenaver LF, Peterson S, Kick B, Hathornthwaite JA. Sleep disorders and their association with laboratory pain sensitivity in temporomandibular joint disorder. *Sleep* 2009;32:779–790.

39. Von Hehn CA, Baron R, Woolf CJ. Deconstructing the neuropathis pain phenotype to reveal neural mechanisms. *Neuron* 2012;73:638–652.

40. Roth T, van Seventer R, Murphy TK. The effect of pregabalin on pain-related sleep interference in diabetic neuropathy or postherpetic neuralgia: A review of nine clinical trials. *Curr Med Res Opin* 2010;26:2411–2419.

41. Hsu T, Roth T, Lamoreaux L, Martin S, HotaryL. Polysomnographic profile of patients with neuropathic pain and self-reported sleep disturbance. *Sleep* 2004;27:A33.

42. Boyle J, Erriksson MV, Gouni R, Johnsen S, Coppini DV, Kerr D. Randomized, placebo-controlled comparison of amitriptyline, duloxetine, and pregabalin in patients with chronic diabetic peripheral neuropathic pain. *Diabetes Care* 2012;35:2451–2458.

43. Roehrs TA, Hyde M, Blaisdell B, Greenwald M, Roth T. Sleep loss and REM sleep loss are hyperalgesic. *Sleep* 2006;29:145–151.

44. Onen SH, Alloui A, Gross A, Eschallier A, Dubray C. The effects of total sleep deprivation, selective sleep interruption and sleep recovery on pain tolerance thresholds in healthy subjects. *J Sleep Res* 2001;10:35–42.

45. Kundermann B, Spernal J, Huber MT, Krieg JC, Lautenbacher S. Sleep deprivation affects thermal pain thresholds but not somatosensory threshold in healthy volunteers. *Psychosom Med* 2004;66:932–937.

46. Tiede W, Mageri W, Baumgartner U, Durrer B, Ehlert U, Treede R. Sleep restriction attenuates amplitudes and attentional modulation of pain-evoked potentials, but augments pain ratings in healthy volunteers. *Pain* 2010;148:36–42.

47. Irwin MR, Olmstead R, Carrillo C, Sadeghi N, Fitzgerald JD, Ranganath VK. Sleep loss exacerbates fatigue, depression, and pain in rheumatoid arthritis. *Sleep* 2012;35:537–543.

48. Smith MT, Edwards RR, Stonerock GL, McCann UD, Haythornthwaite JA. The effects of sleep deprivation on pain inhibition and spontaneous pain in women. *Sleep* 2007;30:494–505.

49. Khalid I, Roehrs TA, Hudgel DW, Roth T. Continuous positive airway pressure in severe obstructive sleep apnea reduces pain sensitivity. *Sleep* 2011;34:1687–1691.

50. Roehrs T, Roth T. Sleep and pain, interaction of two vital functions. *Sem Neurology* 2005;25:106–116.

51. Smith MT, Edwards RR, Stonerock GL, McCann UD. Individual variation in rapid eye movement sleep is associated with pain perception in healthy 2women: Preliminary data. *Sleep* 2005;28:809–812.

52. Azevedo E, Manzano GM, Silva A, Martins R, Anersen ML, Tufik S. The effects of total and REM sleep deprivation on laser-evoked potential threshold and pain perception. *Pain* 2011;152:2052–2058.

53. Kahn-Green ET, Killgore DB, Maminori GH, Balkin TJ, Killgore WDS. The effects of sleep deprivation on symptoms of psychopathology in healthy adults. *Sleep Med* 2007;8:215–221.

54. Scott JPR, McNaughton LR, Polman RCJ. Effects of sleep deprivation and exercise on cognitive, motor performance, and mood. *Physio Behav* 2006;87:396–408.

55. Dinges DE, Pack F, Williams K, Gillen KA, Powell JW, Ott GE. Cumulative sleepiness, mood disturbance, and psychomotor vigilance performance decrements during a week of sleep restricted to 4–5 hours per night. *Sleep* 1997;20:267–277.

56. Haack M, Mullington JM. Sustained sleep restriction reduces emotional and physical well-being. *Pain* 2005;119:56–64.

57. Irwin MR, Olmstead R, Carrillo C, Sadeghi N, FitzGerald JD, Ranganath VK, Nicassio PM. *Sleep* 2012;35:537–543.

58. O'Brien EM, Waxenberg LB, Atchison JW, Gremillion HA, Staud RM, McCrae CS, Robinson ME. Negative mood mediates the effect of poor sleep on pain among chronic pain patients. *Clin J Pain* 2010;26:310–319.

59. Miro E, Martinez MP, Sanchez AI, Prados G, Medina A. When is pain related to emotional distress and daily functioning in fibromyalgia syndrome? The mediating roles of self-efficacy and sleep quality. *Br J Health Psychol* 2011;16:799–814.

60. Carney CE, Harris AL, Falco A, Edinger JD. The relation between insomnia symptoms, mood, and rumination about insomnia symptoms. *J Clin Sleep Med* 2013;9:567–575.

61. Finan PH, Goodin BR, Smith MT. The association of sleep and pain: an update and a path forward. *J Pain* 2013;12:1539–1552.

62. Steinmiller CL, Roehrs TA, Harris E, Hyde M, Greenwald MK, Roth T. Differential effect of codeine on thermal nociceptive sensitivity in sleepy versus nonsleepy healthy subjects. *Exp Clin Psychopharmacol* 2010;18:277–283.

63. Roehrs TA, Harris E, Randall S, Roth T. Pain sensitivity and recovery from mild chronic sleep loss. *Sleep* 2012;35:1667–1672.

64. Roehrs TA, Roth T. Increasing presurgery sleep reduces postsurgery pain and analgesic use following joint replacement: a feasibility study. *Sleep Med* 2017;33:109–113.

65. McGinty D, Szymusiak R. Neural control of sleep in mammals. In Kryger MH, Roth T, Dement WC, eds. *Principles and practice of sleep medicine.* 6th ed. Philadelphia PA: Elsevier, 2017:62–77.

66. Ribeiro JA, Sebastiao AM, deMendonca A. Adensoine receptors in the nervous system: pathophysiological implications. *Prog Neurobiol* 2002;68:377–392.

67. Foo H, Mason P. Brainstem modulation of pain during sleep and waking. *Sleep Med Rev* 2003;7:145–154.

68. Dinges DF, Douglas SD, Hamarman S, Zaugg L, Kapoor S. Sleep deprivation and human immune function. *Advan Neuroimmunol* 1995;5:97–110.

69. Shearer WT, Reuben JM, Mullington JM, Price NJ, Lee BN, Smith EO, Szuba MP, Van Dongen HPA, Dinges DF. Soluble TNFα receptor 1 and IL-6 plasma levels in humans subjected to the sleep deprivation model of spaceflight. *J Allergy Clin Immunol* 2001;107:165–170.

70. Vgontzas AN, Zoumakis E, Bixler EO, Lin HM, Follett H, Kales A, Chrousos GP. Adverse effects of modest sleep restriction on sleepiness, performance and inflammatory cytokines. *J Clin Endocrinol Metab.* 2004;89:2119–2126.

71. Haack M, Sanchez E, Mullington JM. Elevated inflammatory markers in response to prolonged sleep restriction are associated with increased pain experience in healthy volunteers. *Sleep.* 2007;30:1145–1152.

72. Irwin MR, Wang M, Campomayor CO, Collado-Hidalgo A, Cole S. Sleep deprivation and activation of morning levels of cellular and genomic markers of inflammation. *Arch Intern Med* 2006;166:1756–1762.

73. Vgontzas AN, Pejovic S, Zoumakis E, Lin HM, Bixler EO, Basta M, Fang J, Sarrigiannidis A, Chrousos GP. Daytime napping after a night of sleep loss decreases sleepiness, improves

performance, and causes beneficial changes in cortisol and interleukin-6 secretion. *Am J Physiol Endocrinol Metab.* 2007;292:E253–E261.

74. Vgontzas AN, Zoumakis E, Lin HM, Bixler EO, Trakada G, Chroussos GP. Marked decrease in sleepiness in patients with sleep apnea by Etanercept, a tumor necrosis factor-α antagonist. *J Clin Endocrinol Metab* 2004; 89:4409–4413.

75. Gozal D, Serperio LD, Kheirandish-Gozal L, Capdevila OC, Khalyfa A, Tauman R. Sleep measures and morning plasma TNF-α levels in children with sleep-disordered breathing. *Sleep* 2010;33:319–326.

76. Watkins LR, Milligan ED, Maier SF. Glial proinflammatory cyctokines mediate exaggerated pain states: Implications for clinical pain. *Adv Exp Med Biol.* 2003;521:1–21.

77. Cunha F, Poole S, Lorenzetti B, Ferreira S. The pivotal role of tumor necrosis factor alpa in the development of inflammatory hyperalgesia. *Br J Pharmacol.* 1992;107:660–664.

78. Cunha JM, Cunha S, Poole S, Ferreira SH. Cytokine-mediated inflammatory hyperalgesia limited by interleukin-1 receptor antagonist. *Br J Pharmacol.* 2000;130:1418–1424.

79. Sommer C, Kress M. Recent findings on how proinflammatory cytokines cause pain: peripheral mechanisms in inflammatory and neuropathic hyperalgesia. *Neurosci Lett.* 2004;361:184–187.

80. Currie SR, Wilson KG, Pontefract AJ, deLaplate L. Cognitive behavioral treatment of insomnia secondary to chronic pain. *J Consult Clin Psychology* 2000;68:407–416.

81. Edinger JD, Wohlgemuth WK, Krystal AD, Rice JR. Behaviorial insomnia therapy for fibromyalgia patients: a randomized clinical trial. *Arch Inter Med* 2005;165:2527–2535.

82. Jungquist CR, O'Brian C, Matteson-Rusby S, Smith MT, Pigeon WR. Xia Y. The efficacy of cognitive-behavioral therapy for insomnia in patients with chronic pain. *Sleep Med* 2010;11:302–309.

83. Vitiello MV, McCurry SM, Shortreed SM, Balderson BH, Baker LD, Keefe FJ. Cognitive-behavioral treatment for comorbid insomnia and osteoarthritis pain in primary care: The lifestyles randomized controlled trial. *J Am Ger Soc* 2013;61:947–956.

84. Choy E, Marshall D, Gabriel ZL, Mitchell SA, Gylee E, Dakin AA. A systematic review and mixed treatment comparison of the efficacy of pharmacological treatments for fibromyalgia. *Sem Arthritis Reumat* 2011;41:335–345.

85. Roth T, Lankford A, Bhadra P, Whalen E, Resnick EM. Effect of pregabalin on sleep in patients with

fibromyalgia and sleep maintenance disturbance: A randomized, placebo-controlled, 2-way crossover polysomnography study. *Arthrit Care Res* 2012;62:597–606.

86. Hindmarch I, Dawson J, Stanley N. A double-blind study in healthy volunteers to assess the effects on sleep of pregabalin compared with alprazolam and placebo. Sleep 2005;28:187–193.

87. Russel IJ, Crofford LJ, Leon T, Cappelleri JC, Bushmakin AG, Whalen E. The effects of pregabalin on sleep disturbance symptoms among individuals with fibromyalgia syndrome. *Sleep Med* 2009;10:604–610.

88. O'Connor AB, Dworkin RH. Treatment of neuropathic pain: An overview of recent guidelines. *Am J Med* 2009;122:S22–S32.

89. Tashjian RZ, Banerjee R, Bradley MP. Zolpidem reduces postoperative pain, fatigue, and narcotic consumption following knee arthroscopy: A prospective randomized placebo-controlled double-blinded study. *J Knee Surg* 2006;19:105–111.

90. Dierking G, Duedahl TH, Rasmussen ML. Effects of gabapentin on postoperative morphine consumption and pain after abdominal hysterectomy: a randomized, double-blind trial. *Acta Anaesthesiol Scand* 2004;98:1370–1373.

91. Moldofsky H, Luc FA, Mously C, Roth-Schechter B, Reynolds WJ. The effect of zolpidem in patients with fibromyalgia: a dose ranging, double-blind, placebo controlled, modified crossover study. *J Rheumatol* 1996;23:529–533.

92. Gronbald M, Nykanen J, Konttinen Y. Effect of zopiclone on sleep quality, morning stiffness, widespread tenderness and pain and general discomfort in primary fibromyalgia patients: a double-blind randomized trial. *Clin Rheumatol* 1993;12:186–191.

93. Walsh JK, Muehlbach MJ, Lauter SA, Hilliker A, Schweitzer PK. Effects of triazolam on sleep, daytime sleepiness, and morning stiffness in patients with rheumatoid arthritis. *J Rheumatol* 1996;23:245–252.

94. Drewes AM, Bjerregard K, Taaghold SJ. Zopiclone as night medication in rheumatoid arthritis. *Scand J Rheumatol* 1998;27:180–187.

95. Roth T, Price JM, Amato DA, Rubens RP, Roach JM, Schnitzer TJ. The effect of eszopiclone in patients with insomnia and coexisting rheumatoid arthritis: a pilot study. *Prim Care Comp J Clin Psychiat* 2009;11:291–301.

96. Romero-Sandoval EA, Kolano AL, Alvarado-Vazquez. Cannabis and cannabinoids for chronic pain. *Curr Rheumatol Rep* 2017;16:67–77.

28

Psychotropic Medications and Sleep

WILLIAM C. JANGRO AND DANIEL A. NEFF

INTRODUCTION

Data from the National Survey on Drug Use and Health from 2017 indicate that over 29 million respondents, correlating to 10% of the population, are exposed to medications for psychiatric purposes within a single year.[1] Coupled with people taking primarily psychiatric medications for other nonpsychiatric indications (such as selective serotonin reuptake inhibitors [SSRIs] in premature ejaculation), the total exposure to these medications is substantial. Common adverse effects of these medications include those affecting sleep: insomnia, sedation, limb movement disorders, and parasomnias. Patients make implicit cost–benefit analyses of medications, with greater concerns about medications correlating with decreased adherence.[2] As a result, providers need to possess a clear understanding of the occurrence, frequency, and management of sleep-related adverse effects of psychiatric medications.

This chapter focuses on describing the sleep-related side effects of psychotropic medications. We report on major psychiatric drug classes and, where available, specific medications within each class. When possible, we have incorporated studies focusing on the sleep effects of psychotropic medications in patients with psychiatric illnesses, and we have tried to limit the use of case reports. However, we have considered case reports when higher quality data are unavailable. Commonly used abbreviations are listed in Table 28.1.

ANTIDEPRESSANTS

People suffering from depressive disorders typically complain of difficulty falling asleep, frequent awakenings, early morning awakening, and nonrestorative sleep. Polysomnographic (PSG) studies of depressed persons have confirmed these findings and show reduced rapid eye movement (REM) latency, increased total time in REM sleep, reduced slow-wave sleep (SWS), and frequent awakenings throughout the night.[3] Not only do the majority of patients with depression suffer from sleep dysregulation, but sleep disturbance is also closely linked to mood dysregulation. Abnormalities in acetylcholine, neuropeptide, and monoamine neurotransmission are implicated in the pathophysiology of both mood and sleep dysregulation.

Antidepressants exert their effects on the sleep architecture of depressed people not only by alleviating the depression, but also through modulation of various monoamines and interactions with receptors such as histamine and muscarinic cholinergic receptors, all of which are involved in sleep–wake processes. Through these interactions, antidepressants can have a significant impact on sleep physiology. The effects of various antidepressants on sleep architecture are summarized in Table 28.2.

Selective Serotonin Reuptake Inhibitors (SSRIs)

Antidepressants are widely prescribed for mood and anxiety disorders. According to the National Health and Nutrition Examination Survey, 11% of Americans over the age of 12 are taking an antidepressant medication.[4] SSRIs, the most commonly prescribed antidepressants, are thought to exert their clinical effects by inhibiting the reuptake of serotonin. These medications have minimal effects on the reuptake of dopamine and norepinephrine.

Subjective complaints of both insomnia and daytime somnolence are common in people with depression being treated with SSRIs. Up to a quarter of subjects in clinical trials involving SSRIs complain of insomnia.[5] In a fixed-dose study comparing placebo and fluoxetine in the treatment of major depressive disorder (MDD), rates of activation or sedation were found to depend on the dose.[6] Rates of activation were stable between doses of 5 and 40 mg/day but increased at 60 mg/day. On the other hand, rates of sedation increased linearly up to doses of 40 mg/

TABLE 28.1. ABBREVIATIONS

Abbreviation	Definition
ADHD	Attention deficit-hyperactivity disorder
GABA	Gamma-aminobutyric acid
MAOI	Monoamine oxidase inhibitor
MDD	Major depressive disorder
NREM	Nonrapid eye movement
PLM	Periodic limb movements
PLMD	Periodic limb movement disorder
PSG	Polysomnography
REM	Rapid eye movement
RLS	Restless leg syndrome
SARI	Serotonin-2 receptor antagonist/serotonin reuptake inhibitor
SE	Sleep efficiency
SNRI	Serotonin-norepinephrine reuptake inhibitor
SOL	Sleep onset latency
SSRI	Selective serotonin reuptake inhibitor
SRED	Sleep-related eating disorder
SWS	Slow-wave sleep
TCA	Tricyclic antidepressant
TST	Total sleep time
VLPO	Ventrolateral preoptic nucleus
WASO	Wakefulness after sleep onset

day and then were comparable at 40 and 60 mg/day. In this study, it was also noted that activation tended to peak early and decline over time with all doses while occurrences of sedation also tended to peak early but may have declined less

TABLE 28.2. EFFECTS OF ANTIDEPRESSANTS ON SLEEP ARCHITECTURE

SSRI	REM suppression, ↑ REM latency
SNRI	REM suppression, ↑ REM latency
Trazodone	↓ SOL, ↑ SWS
Mirtazapine	↓ SOL, ↑ SWS
Bupropion	↓ REM latency, ↑ total REM time
TCA	REM suppression, ↑ REM latency, ↓ SOL
MAO-I	REM suppression, ↑ SOL, ↑ WASO

Abbreviations: MAOI, monoamine oxidase inhibitor; REM, rapid eye movement; SNRI, serotonin-norepinephrine reuptake inhibitor; SOL, sleep onset latency; SSRI, selective serotonin reuptake inhibitor; SWS, slow wave sleep; TCA, tricyclic antidepressant; WASO, wakefulness after sleep onset.

over time compared to occurrences of activation. A trial comparing fluoxetine and trazodone in outpatients with MDD found that more activation (agitation, anxiety, insomnia) occurred with those receiving fluoxetine and more sedation (somnolence, asthenia) occurred with those receiving trazodone. However, sedation was seen more frequently than activation when considering fluoxetine alone (21.5% sedation vs. 15.4% activation).[7]

Of the SSRIs currently indicated for the treatment of depression, fluoxetine's effects on sleep have been the most thoroughly studied. These effects may represent a class effect. Other SSRIs have shown similar subjective effects on sleep. A trial comparing fluvoxamine and paroxetine in outpatients with MDD reported 30% of those in the paroxetine group complaining of somnolence.[8] In those receiving fluvoxamine, 40% complained of somnolence while 30% complained of insomnia. In a double-blind comparison of citalopram and placebo in moderately to severely depressed outpatients who met the *Diagnostic and Statistical Manual of Mental Disorders* (third edition; DSM-III) criteria for either major depression or bipolar depression and also met criteria for melancholia, citalopram was given in a flexible dose of 20 to 80 mg/day.[9] Patients in the citalopram group exhibited significantly greater improvement on the Hamilton Rating Scale for Depression subscale of sleep disturbance compared to those receiving placebo. Citalopram was also associated with increased daytime somnolence compared to placebo. Rates of reported insomnia did not differ between the citalopram and placebo groups.

SSRIs have been shown to have numerous effects on sleep latency and measures of sleep continuity. Fluoxetine's effects on sleep in depressed patients include REM suppression,[10,11] decreased sleep efficiency (SE),[12] and increased number of awakenings after sleep onset (WASO).[13] Disruption in sleep continuity has been found to correlate with plasma levels of fluoxetine and its biologically active metabolite, norfluoxetine.[14] Thus, changes in sleep continuity may develop over time as plasma levels increase because of accumulation of the drug. Fluoxetine has also been shown to increase the number of oculomotor movements during non-REM (NREM) sleep, classically known as "Prozac eyes."[15,16] This finding may suggest a generalized increase in central arousal.

In healthy volunteers, paroxetine has been shown to decrease REM sleep and increase REM latency compared to placebo.[17] In the same study, it also increased the number of awakenings and reduced actual sleep time and efficiency. A double-blind trial compared paroxetine with amitriptyline after a 10-day placebo washout period and 4-week active treatment period.[18] Paroxetine increased number of awakenings and reduced SE but did not affect sleep onset latency (SOL) or total sleep time (TST). Both drugs decreased REM sleep with effects lasting at 1 week after withdrawal of the drug.

In a randomized double-blind trial, the effects of sertraline were compared to placebo with sleep studies that were completed before and 12 weeks after treatment.[19] Sertraline-treated patients experienced an increase in delta wave sleep in the first sleep cycle and prolonged REM latency compared to those given placebo. While sertraline decreased the number of REM periods from 3.86 to 2.40, the activity of REM periods 1 and 2 was significantly increased. Sertraline was associated with increased SOL but not associated with worsening of measures of sleep continuity. There were no significant sertraline–placebo differences in subjective sleepiness.

Serotonin–Norepinephrine Reuptake Inhibitors (SNRIs)

Serotonin–norepinephrine reuptake inhibitors (SNRIs) combine the serotonin reuptake inhibition of SSRIs with various levels of inhibition of the norepinephrine transporter. For example, venlafaxine, which functions primarily as an SSRI at lower doses, exhibits increasing levels of norepinephrine reuptake inhibition at higher doses. SNRIs are associated with frequent subjective complaints of insomnia and daytime somnolence as well as vivid dreams. Studies using PSG techniques have been limited. Most studies involve the use of the older SNRIs, venlafaxine and duloxetine.

A double-blind, placebo-controlled study evaluated the effects of venlafaxine on PSG variables in inpatients with MDD.[20] Patients were given a 1- to 2-week placebo washout period before starting active treatment versus placebo. Sleep evaluations took place at baseline, 1 week after treatment, and 1 month after treatment. Treatment with venlafaxine showed a decrease in sleep continuity, an increase in REM latency, and a decrease in total REM sleep duration. These effects were evident after 1 week of treatment and persisted after 1 month of treatment.

Treatment with venlafaxine has been associated with periodic limb movements (PLMs), which are repetitive involuntary movements of the extremities, typically the legs, occurring during sleep or just before falling asleep. This effect was seen in a study of eight normal volunteers who received 75 mg doses for 2 nights and then 150 mg for 2 nights.[21] The repetitive involuntary movements were recorded as periodic bursts of electromyographic (EMG) activity in the anterior tibialis electrodes of the lower extremities during PSG. Effects were continuous and tended to worsen over time, with rates of greater than 25 PLMs per hour. In some of the volunteers, these movements persisted for up to a week after discontinuation of treatment. The pathophysiologic basis of these movements, and venlafaxine's contribution to them, is unknown.

PSG studies done in 10 patients with MDD before and 7- to 14-days after treatment with duloxetine[22] revealed increased stage 3 sleep, increased REM latency, and decreased REM sleep. In healthy volunteers, two dosing regimens of duloxetine (60 mg twice per day or 80 mg once per day) were evaluated with sleep electroencephalography.[23] Both doses produced an increase in REM latency and decrease in total REM sleep duration. Compared to placebo, duloxetine 60 mg twice per day showed a reduction in sleep continuity whereas 80 mg once per day showed an improvement in the "getting to sleep" subscale on the Leeds Sleep Evaluation Questionnaire.

Serotonin-2 Receptor Antagonist/ Serotonin Reuptake Inhibitors (SARIs)

Selective serotonin receptor antagonist/serotonin reuptake inhibitors (SARIs) are weak inhibitors of serotonin reuptake compared to SSRIs but are potent inhibitors of $5\text{-}HT_2$ serotonin receptors, which have been implicated in the regulation of sleep. Trazodone's use as an antidepressant is often limited by its tendency to produce daytime somnolence. In that respect, it is often used, at low doses, as a sleep aid or co-administered with an SSRI to decrease the SSRIs' deleterious and disruptive effects on sleep. When administered as monotherapy to depressed patients, trazodone has been shown to increase TST, decrease SOL, reduce WASO, increase SWS, and increase REM latency.[24]

Serotonin-2/Serotonin-3/Alpha-2 Adrenergic Receptor Antagonists

Mirtazapine has multiple mechanisms of action including antagonism of central presynaptic α_2-adrenergic receptors and blockade of postsynaptic serotonin $5\text{-}HT_2$ and $5\text{-}HT_3$ receptors. The former leads to increased activity at norepinephrine and serotonin receptors, while the later can improve anxiety, insomnia, and appetite. It is also a potent antihistamine and a moderately potent antagonist of α_1-adrenergic and muscarinic-cholinergic receptors.

Daytime somnolence is a common adverse effect of mirtazapine. In clinical trials, up to 54% of patients treated with mirtazapine reported it as an adverse event.[25] Although insufficiently characterized in the literature, this effect can have utility in improving sleep disturbance in select populations. Mirtazapine produces predominantly sedating antihistaminergic effects at lower doses, compared with increasingly activating noradrenergic and serotonergic effects at higher doses.[26,27]

In depressed patients, mirtazapine has been shown to significantly increase TST and SE and to significantly reduce SOL, without significantly altering REM sleep parameters.[28] Although mirtazapine has typically been associated with beneficial effects on sleep, disturbing dreams and confusional states have been reported in clinical trials.[29] Compared to other antidepressants, mirtazapine may be more likely to induce or exacerbate restless leg syndrome (RLS) and PLMs. In a systematic review by Kolla et al.,[30] the authors found two open-label studies that indicated mirtazapine might be associated with an increased risk of RLS compared to other antidepressants (up to 28%). However, two other open-label studies that did not specifically ask patients about RLS showed that only 0.5% to 0.6% of patients spontaneously reported symptoms. The authors concluded that while RLS symptoms may be common in patients taking mirtazapine, they may seldom be clinically significant.

Norepinephrine/Dopamine Reuptake Inhibitors (NDRIs)

Bupropion works as norepinephrine and dopamine reuptake inhibitor (NDRI) while having no demonstrable effects on serotonin receptors. Its modulation and enhancement of dopamine may be beneficial in the treatment of RLS.[31] Bupropion is associated with reports of insomnia in patients treated for both depression and seasonal affective disorder with rates ranging from 11% to 20% depending on the dose, formulation, and condition being treated. However, electroencephalographic studies have shown bupropion to be one of the few antidepressants that actually shortens REM latency and increases total REM sleep time.[32] This finding is in contrast to most other antidepressants, which are prominent suppressants of REM sleep.

Tricyclic Antidepressants (TCAs)

TCAs block norepinephrine and serotonin transporters and also have a range of other secondary activities on muscarinic acetylcholine, histamine H_1, and α_1- and α_2-adrenergic receptors. Varying affinities for these receptors are what largely accounts for their side effect profile. Tertiary amine TCAs (amitriptyline, doxepin, clomipramine, imipramine, trimipramine), being relatively more potent antihistaminergic and anticholinergic agents, tend to be more sedating whereas secondary amine TCAs tend to be less sedating (nortriptyline, amoxapine) or even activating (desipramine, protriptyline).

Therefore, it may be easier to choose an agent in this class that will have the desired effect on sleep compared with other classes of antidepressants. Sedating, tertiary amine TCAs have been demonstrated to shorten SOL, improve sleep continuity and efficiency, and reduce WASO.[33-35] Activating, secondary amine TCAs, on the other hand, have been demonstrated to prolong SOL, reduce SE, and increase WASO.[36]

Doxepin, a tertiary amine TCA, first approved in 1969 for the management of major depression and anxiety and as a topical preparation (5% cream) for pruritus, was recently reformulated in lower oral doses (3 mg and 6 mg) with demonstrated efficacy for insomnia characterized by difficulties with sleep maintenance following sleep onset and early morning awakening.[37] In addition to subjective improvements in insomnia measures, PSG measures of WASO, TST, and SE have been shown to improve following its administration at bedtime. Plasma histamine levels are known to rise in the early morning hours.[38] Although the mechanism of action of doxepin is not known, it is presumed to promote sleep by antagonizing the histamine-based arousal pathways.[39,40]

All TCAs, with the exception of trimipramine, typically suppress REM sleep; this often manifests as an increase in REM latency and a decreased percentage of time spent in REM sleep.[41-43] At standard antidepressant doses, clomipramine appears to have the most potent REM suppressant effects, although comparative data are limited. Placebo and plasma concentration-controlled studies of maintenance nortriptyline therapy in depressed elderly patients have shown that REM suppression and increased REM latency persist, even in those with no recurrence of depression 1 year later.[44,45] In addition, patients on TCA therapy have reported intense, vivid dreams, and even nightmares. Recall of dreams may be due to the REM-disrupting effect of TCAs.

Monoamine Oxidase Inhibitors (MAOIs)

Treatment with monoamine oxidase inhibitors (MAOIs) is associated with frequent complaints of insomnia, especially with tranylcypromine, which is structurally similar to amphetamine and is more stimulating than other MAOIs. MAOIs tend to cause prolonged SOL, impaired sleep continuity, and increased WASO.[46,47] REM suppression is also common, possibly more so with irreversible MAOIs like tranylcypromine and phenelzine than with reversible MAOIs like moclobemide.[48] REM suppression typically occurs quickly after initiation and has been shown to persist for months into ongoing treatment. REM rebound occurs with discontinuation of therapy and can lead to intense and vivid dreams.

Newer Antidepressants

Several medications have recently been approved for the treatment of MDD. These medications include levomilnacipran (2013), vilazodone (2011), and vortioxetine (2013). Sleep disturbance was not listed as a common adverse effect in clinical studies for levomilnacipran.[49] Somnolence, insomnia, and abnormal dreams were listed as common adverse effects in clinical trials with vilazodone.[50] Abnormal dreams, but not insomnia or somnolence, were listed as a common adverse effect in clinical trials with vortioxetine.[51] Further studies, including PSG testing in patients taking these medications, are needed to better understand the effects of these newer agents on sleep.

Antidepressants and REM Sleep Behavior Disorder

REM sleep behavior disorder (RBD) is a parasomnia characterized by dream-enactment behaviors and loss of normal skeletal muscle atonia during REM sleep. Psychiatric disorders as well as antidepressants have been associated with RBD. In a cross-sectional study of 1,235 psychiatric outpatients, the estimated lifetime prevalence of RBD-like disorder was 5.8%. Among those patients taking SSRIs, the prevalence of RBD-like disorder was 5%.[52] In a study assessing REM sleep without atonia (RSWA) in patients receiving antidepressants, with and without RBD, antidepressants were associated with RSWA even in those without RBD. The authors concluded that it was antidepressants, not depression, that promoted RSWA.[53] While most cases of RBD or RSWA associated with antidepressants have been reported with TCAs and SSRIs, a case was reported in which RBD symptoms arose after the initiation of treatment with the SNRI, duloxetine. In the case, the patient experienced enactment behaviors with violent dreams that were associated with tonic or phasic chin EMG activity during REM sleep. The symptoms decreased and then completely resolved after discontinuation of the medication for 37 days.[54] Further prospective studies are needed to clarify the relationship between antidepressants, psychiatric disorder, and RBD.

ANTIPSYCHOTICS

Antipsychotics are indicated for the treatment of schizophrenia and other psychotic disorders. Many of the atypical antipsychotics also have indications for the treatment of bipolar disorder and adjunctive treatment of MDD. Insomnia is common in patients with schizophrenia and bipolar disorder and can be a prelude to a psychotic or manic episode.[55] PSG studies in individuals with schizophrenia not taking antipsychotics show increased SOL and decreased TST, SE, NREM sleep spindles. SWS, and REM latency. However, in many of these studies, patients have been without antipsychotics for only short periods of time. Therefore, some of these PSG findings may be from residual effects of the medication.[56] Antipsychotics are thought to exert much of their indicated effects through antagonism of dopamine receptors. Many typical and atypical antipsychotics also exert effects on various monoamines as well as histamine and muscarinic cholinergic receptors. These effects may increase the likelihood of both somnolence and insomnia and can also alter certain PSG sleep parameters. See Table 28.3 for a summary of the effects of antipsychotics on sleep architecture.

Atypical antipsychotics can produce subjective effects of both activation and sedation. A study by Citrome characterized the relative activation and sedation caused by these agents.[57] Predominantly activating agents included lurasidone and cariprazine, similarly activating and sedating agents (equal prevalence of akathisia vs. sedation) included risperidone and aripiprazole, and predominantly sedating agents included olanzapine, quetiapine (immediate and extended

TABLE 28.3. EFFECTS OF
ANTIPSYCHOTICS ON SLEEP
ARCHITECTURE

Typical	↑ TST, ↑sleep efficiency, ↓ SOL, ↓ WASO, ↑ REM latency, ↔ SWS
Atypical	↑ TST, ↑sleep efficiency, ↓ SOL, ↓ WASO, ↑ SWS

Abbreviations: REM, rapid eye movement; SOL, sleep onset latency; SWS, slow wave sleep; TST, total sleep time; WASO, wakefulness after sleep onset.

release formulations), ziprasidone, asenapine, and iloperidone. Paliperidone and brexpiprazole were neither activating nor sedating. A similar study by Fang et. al classified clozapine as having a high risk of causing somnolence; olanzapine, perphenazine, quetiapine, risperidone, and ziprasidone as having a moderate risk; and aripiprazole, asenapine, haloperidol, lurasidone, paliperidone, and cariprazine as having a low risk.[58] Rates of somnolence had a positive correlation to dose and duration for some, but not all antipsychotics. Since most of the cases of somnolence were reported as being mild to moderate, the authors suggested allowing tolerance to develop for at least 4 weeks before discontinuing the agent due to this adverse effect.

Typical antipsychotics can also produce subjective effects of both activation and sedation. High-potency antipsychotics are generally less sedating than lower potency agents. Activation in the form of akathisia is perhaps more common in older, typical antipsychotics compared with newer, atypical antipsychotics.[59] Studies evaluating the PSG effects of typical antipsychotic drugs in patients with schizophrenia are limited. Winokur and Kamath reviewed seven studies examining the effects of haloperidol, thiothixene, flupenthixol, and other typical antipsychotics by PSG.[60] The authors concluded that, in general, these agents increase TST and SE, shorten SOL, decrease WASO, and increase REM latency. without significantly altering SWS.

PSG studies involving atypical antipsychotics in patients with schizophrenia have shown clozapine, olanzapine, and paliperidone to have beneficial effects on sleep architecture. Clozapine has consistently been shown to improve TST by improving sleep continuity.[61–64] Several studies have shown consistent results in olanzapine's ability to reduce SOL and to increase TST, SE, and SWS.[65–67] Paliperidone has been shown to decrease SOL, improve TST and SE, and increase

SWS and REM sleep.[68] Interestingly, despite its well-known sedating effects, quetiapine has been shown to increase SOL, WASO, and REM latency and to reduce SWS and REM sleep in patients with schizophrenia.[69] Studies with risperidone have failed to show consistent effects on sleep variables in patients with schizophrenia.[70,71]

Antipsychotics and Restless Leg Syndrome/Periodic Limb Movement Disorder

A diagnosis of RLS is made clinically and is characterized by an urge to move, usually accompanied by unpleasant sensations in the legs, which emerges during periods of inactivity and is most prominent in the evening. It is temporarily relieved with voluntary movement. PLM disorder (PLMD), on the other hand, is diagnosed by PSG and requires more than 15 limb movements per hour of sleep. RLS and PLMD show improvement with the administration of dopamine agonists, and so dopamine deficiency is thought to play a part in their pathophysiology.[72]

Antipsychotics may exacerbate or induce RLS and/or PLMD due to their dopamine antagonism. Indeed, prevalence rates of RLS in patients with schizophrenia treated with antipsychotics have been reported to be twice that of healthy controls.[73] A case series of seven patients given low-dose quetiapine reported a dose-dependent provocation of RLS.[74] The investigators noted that most of these patients suffered from affective disorders and were on concomitant antidepressants. The prescribing information for quetiapine notes the occurrence of RLS in 2% of persons on quetiapine versus none on placebo.[75] RLS and PLMD have been documented in patients taking other atypical antipsychotics as well and can be difficult to differentiate from akathisia, another possible adverse effect of these medications. However, akathisia is less likely to be associated with unpleasant sensations localized solely to the legs and can be relieved by voluntary movement. Furthermore, unlike RLS, there is no circadian rhythmicity in akathisia.

Antipsychotics and NREM Parasomnias

Antipsychotics have been associated with NREM parasomnias. Typical antipsychotic-associated[76] (chlorprothixene, perphenazine, and thioridazine) as well as atypical antipsychotic-associated[77–81] (olanzapine and quetiapine) somnambulism have been mentioned in a number of case reports. Case reports have also associated quetiapine, olanzapine, and ziprasidone with sleep-related eating disorder (SRED).[82–84] Since multiple classes of medications,[85] and not just antipsychotics, have been associated with NREM parasomnias, prospective studies are needed to fully elucidate the impact that antipsychotics assert on these syndromes.

MOOD STABILIZERS

A common feature of mania and hypomania, as seen in bipolar and related disorders, is a period of increased energy and activity associated with a decreased need for sleep. Many of the medications indicated for the treatment of bipolar disorder are also indicated for the treatment of seizure disorders. These medications modulate neuronal excitability via effects on GABA and glutamate neurotransmitter systems. The most studied medications in this class in terms of effects on sleep physiology are gabapentin, pregabalin, and tiagabine. However, these three medications are not indicated for the treatment of psychiatric disorders such as bipolar disorder, and studies that have been performed have not necessarily been in the psychiatric patient population.

The effects of gabapentin on sleep and sleep physiology have been studied in healthy volunteers and certain patient populations including those with alcohol use disorders and RLS. In a placebo-controlled study of subjects with alcohol-related sleep disruption, gabapentin doses of 300 and 600 mg were shown to decrease WASO and increase SE compared to placebo.[86] The gabapentin 600 mg dose was associated with increased SWS, decreased arousals, and decreased REM sleep. In a double-blind crossover study, patients with RLS treated with gabapentin showed a significantly reduced PLM during sleep index; increased TST, SE, and SWS; and decreased stage 1 sleep compared to those receiving placebo.[87] The mean effective dose at the end of the 6-week treatment period was 1,855 mg, given twice daily in divided dose (one-third dose at 12:00 PM and two-thirds dose at 8:00 PM). The effects of pregabalin on sleep have been studied in healthy volunteers and certain patient populations. In a randomized crossover trial, the effects of pregabalin on sleep were compared to alprazolam and placebo in healthy volunteers.[88] As compared to placebo, treatment with pregabalin was associated with increased SWS, reduction in SOL, reduced REM latency, and decreased WASO.

Tiagabine has been shown to increase SWS and to decrease WASO. In a double-blind,

placebo-controlled study, the effects of single dose of tiagabine was assessed in 10 healthy elderly volunteers.[89] The tiagabine-treated group experienced significantly increased SE, decreased wakefulness, and increased SWS compared to the placebo group. In another study, patients meeting *Diagnostic and Statistical Manual for Mental Disorders* (fourth edition; DSM-IV) criteria for primary insomnia were randomized to tiagabine 4, 8, 12, or 16 mg versus placebo.[90] There was a significant dose-dependent increase in SWS and decrease in WASO at all doses. Doses up to 8 mg did not impair next-day alertness or psychomotor performance.

Lithium is one of the mainstays of bipolar disorder treatment both in the acute and maintenance phases. Lithium has been shown to have potent chronobiologic effects in animals, restoring circadian function and memory impairment after sleep deprivation (a model used to explore mania).[91] In humans, lithium is shown to decrease REM sleep and REM sleep latency, as well as delay circadian rhythm in both patients with bipolar or unipolar depression and controls.[92]

HYPNOTICS

Hypnotics include broad classes of compounds that promote sleep via distinct mechanisms. Among these are the traditional GABA-ergic benzodiazepines and barbiturates, as well as newer classes of medications with preferential binding to specific GABA receptor subunits. A newer agent, suvorexant, which is an orexin receptor antagonist, also has a primary indication for insomnia but avoids interaction at the GABA receptor site.

The newer agents, exhibiting tropism for ω1-type GABA receptors, are zolpidem, zopiclone, its enantiomer eszopiclone, and zaleplon, the so-called "z-drugs," or non-benzodiazepine hypnotics. The z-drugs, while offering comparable or similar hypnotic efficacy to benzodiazepines, offer several advantages: less disruptive effects on sleep architecture (Table 28.4), relatively limited daytime impairment, rare rebound insomnia, limited withdrawal symptoms, and minimal or no effects on respiratory parameters in chronic obstructive pulmonary disease and sleep apnea.[93]

While a rare adverse event, the popular association of z-drugs with parasomnias prompted the US Food and Drug Administration (FDA) to mandate adding a safety warning of this adverse effect to product labeling.[94] Commonly observed parasomnias include sexsomnia, SRED, somnambulism, and sleep driving. Most case reports

TABLE 28.4. EFFECTS OF BENZODIAZEPINE RECEPTOR AGONISTS ON SLEEP AS COMPARED TO BENZODIAZEPINES

Medication	Sleep Latency	Total Sleep Time	Nocturnal Awakenings	Sleep Quality
Zolpidem	Equivalent	Equivalent	Equivalent	Equivalent
Zopiclone	Superior or equivalent	Superior or equivalent	Superior or equivalent	Superior or equivalent
Zaleplon	Limited data	Limited data	Limited data	Limited data

involve polypharmacy with other sedative/hypnotics or supratherapeutic doses (greater than 10 mg dose of zolpidem per night). SCRED was most commonly experienced at drug initiation or titration and remitted on discontinuation.[95] The literature presents little evidence to support similar prevalence of parasomnias with eszopiclone use in general or psychiatric populations.[96] A similar dearth of reports exists with respect to zaleplon. While zolpidem appears to be the z-drug most commonly associated with parasomnias in the published literature, the absence of similar evidence for the other z-drugs cannot necessarily be taken as evidence of greater safety. Given the increased risks associated with polypharmacy in psychiatric patients using z-drugs for insomnia, there may be good cause for extra caution in using z-drugs in psychiatric population.

Suvorexant, acting with a novel mechanism, may have a different adverse effect profile than the z-drugs. In one large randomized double-blind placebo-controlled trial, suvorexant was associated with a single event of parasomnia compared to zero events for the control group.[97] Currently, there are no data specifically evaluating the safety or effects of suvorexant in psychiatric patients, which remains an area for further study.

Benzodiazepines function through allosteric modulation of the $GABA_A$ receptor, promoting chloride influx and hyperpolarization of neurons. While only some carry an FDA indication for primary insomnia (quazepam, estazolam, flurazepam, triazolam, temazepam), many others are often prescribed off-label for sleep-related disorders. Benzodiazepines as a class show similar effects on sleep including decreased SOL, increased TST, and acute REM suppression. In general, stage 1 sleep is reduced, while stage 2 sleep time and sleep spindles are increased with benzodiazepines.[98] Depending on the nature of the underlying sleep disorder, shorter- or longer-acting benzodiazepines may be preferable for specific insomnias. Benzodiazepines have been

popular in treating RLS but a recent Cochrane review found insufficient evidence to support their first-line use in this condition.[99]

The generalized respiratory depression seen with benzodiazepines has raised concerns that they may be contraindicated in patients with respiratory impairments. A Cochrane review found no significant increase in apnea–hypopnea index or oxygen desaturation index with brotizolam, flurazepam, nitrazepam, temazepam, or triazolam in obstructive sleep apnea, but central sleep apneas remain an area of concern.[100]

STIMULANTS

In psychiatric practice, stimulants are prescribed for a broad range of indications including attention deficit-hyperactivity disorder (ADHD) and to augment other agents used for mood disorders. While current practice has become more accepting of psychopharmacologic treatment of ADHD in the adult population, stimulants remain best studied in the child and adolescent population. Stimulants used for psychiatric indications include methylphenidate and amphetamine salts.

Studies of stimulants are complicated by the high baseline rates of sleep disturbance in ADHD. Unmedicated children with ADHD experience increased SOL, decreased TST and SE, and increased daytime sleepiness than non-ADHD controls with insomnia.[101] While less well studied, adults with ADHD also experience increases in time to sleep onset and excessive daytime sleepiness compared with non-ADHD controls. In children, methylphenidate has been associated with inconsistent effects that appear to vary widely with dosing, age, weight, length of medication use, and rate of titration.[102] The most consistent finding across studies was a delay in time to sleep onset. PSG findings in children with ADHD have been inconsistent, with studies of immediate-release formulations (methylphenidate) showing no changes in sleep architecture, while extended-release formulations (methylphenidate ER) were associated with increased percentage of stage 2 sleep and fewer awakenings.[103] Amphetamines also showed similar idiosyncratic effects with variations of dose, timing, and release formulation.[104,105] Small studies of stimulants in adults with ADHD show trends toward improvement in sleep quality, but remain underpowered and too methodologically diverse for generalized interpretation.[106] Patients with ADHD are thought to have arousal dysfunction.[107] Treatment with stimulants may improve sleep in people with ADHD by improving this arousal dysfunction, leading to wakefulness consolidation and subsequent improvements with sleep consolidation.[108]

MANAGEMENT OF PSYCHOTROPIC-INDUCED SLEEP DISTURBANCES

When there is clinical suspicion of psychotropic-induced sleep disturbances, a multimodal approach is appropriate. It may not always be clear, given complex regimens and illness phenotypes, whether a given sleep disturbance is secondary to medication or another process. As such, a strategy that seeks to weigh the risks and benefits of any response is paramount. Before making any medication changes, the provider should attempt, with the patient, to determine the clinical significance of any sleep disturbance and whether attempts to address it are warranted relative to the efficacy of the current regimen for primary target symptoms.

Often, off-target effects on sleep, such as subjective complaints of vivid dream recall, are insufficiently bothersome to patients to warrant therapeutic intervention. In many cases, conservative measures including psycho-education around medication administration and timing, sleep hygiene, and other behavioral management strategies are sufficient to manage mild off target effects. When necessary, psychopharmacologic changes including dose adjustment and a switch of agents within class or between classes (i.e., change from benzodiazepine to z-drug) can be effective strategies to continue treatment while minimizing sleep disturbances. When conservative measures fail, or when there are clear clinical indications, such as persistent insomnia, emergent sleep disordered breathing, and parasomnias to name a few, PSG remains the gold standard for diagnosis and treatment.

CONCLUSIONS

Psychotropic medications frequently result in sleep-related adverse effects, primarily insomnia and daytime somnolence. However, these effects have not been comprehensively evaluated. Data from placebo-controlled trials are available primarily in the form of spontaneous reports rather than systematic assessments. Where sleep-related effects have been specifically studied as end points, the data are limited by small sample sizes and methodological inconsistencies. In addition, comparative data between various agents are lacking. Nevertheless, the data available do provide some guidance regarding possible adverse effects on sleep and wakefulness, such that a therapeutic plan can be crafted for each patient's individual clinical situation.

FUTURE DIRECTIONS

Further research is needed to fully elucidate and disentangle the associations between psychotropic medications and sleep disorders in psychiatric patients. More research is needed to examine the sleep-related side effects of psychotropic medications in both psychiatric and non-psychiatric populations. While compelling, the quality of current literature on this subject is inadequate in proportion to the importance and number of people taking psychotropic medications.

CASE ILLUSTRATION

A 65-year-old woman with a history of MDD presented to her primary care physician complaining of low mood, difficulty enjoying her usual activities, poor sleep and appetite, and low energy. Symptoms had become progressively worse over the last month. Basic lab tests including a comprehensive metabolic panel, complete blood count, thyroid-stimulating hormone, and serum B12 and folate levels were all normal. She had been prescribed an antidepressant many years ago but could not remember its name. She recalled that it had helped her depressive symptoms, but that she had eventually stopped it when she felt better.

Her primary care physician decided to prescribe mirtazapine to help target the symptoms of insomnia and anorexia. Her mood slowly improved, and her appetite became quite robust. However, her sleep became worse. Whenever she tried to relax or wind down in bed at night, she would get an intense urge to move her legs. Walking up and down her hallway a few times relieved the urge for a short time, but the symptom would return as soon as she tried to go to sleep again.

She was referred to a sleep medicine clinic. Serum iron and ferritin levels were checked and came back within normal ranges. PSG showed 25 PLMs per hour. Potential causes of PLMs were ruled out including other sleep disorders, medical disorders, and substance use including caffeine and tobacco. A diagnosis of PLMD was made. Mirtazapine was suspected of being a major culprit in causing her PLMD.

Several medication treatment options were discussed, including dopamine agonists, alpha-2-delta calcium channel ligands, and benzodiazepines. Since her weight was continuing to increase on mirtazapine, it was decided that she would discontinue it and start bupropion. She was happy that to hear that bupropion was associated with weight loss and, due to its modulation and enhancement of dopamine, might help to eliminate her RLS and PLMs.

KEY CLINICAL PEARLS

- While both sedation and activation are associated with the use of antidepressants, sedation is much more common.
- Fluoxetine may produce changes in sleep continuity over time due to its long half-life and active metabolite, norfluoxetine.
- Trazodone can be helpful as a sleep aid and may help counteract deleterious effects on sleep produced by other antidepressants.
- Mirtazapine produces predominantly sedating antihistaminergic effects at lower doses and increasingly activating noradrenergic and serotonergic effects at higher doses. Although the dose inflection point is unclear, theoretically, lower doses of mirtazapine should be more beneficial for treating insomnia.
- While typically used in depressed patients with insomnia, mirtazapine may be more likely than other antidepressants to cause or exacerbate PLMs and RLS.
- Due to its dopamine reuptake inhibition, bupropion may be helpful in treating RLS.
- Tertiary amine TCAs tend to be more sedating than secondary amine TCAs. Some secondary amine TCAs are actually activating (desipramine, protriptyline).
- Although many antipsychotics are known to have sedating effects, PSG studies have shown that clozapine, olanzapine, and paliperidone have objectively beneficial effects on sleep.

- "Z-drugs" are commonly associated with parasomnias, especially in psychiatric populations involving polypharmacy and/or supratherapeutic doses. Extra caution is warranted in these cases.
- Stimulants may improve sleep in people with ADHD by improving a dysfunction in arousal systems, leading to wakefulness consolidation and subsequent improvements with sleep consolidation.

SELF-ASSESSMENT QUESTIONS

1. According to available literature, which antidepressant is most likely to produce or exacerbate restless leg syndrome?
   a. Bupropion
   b. Mirtazapine
   c. Vortioxetine
   d. Fluoxetine

Answer: b

2. Many antidepressants have been shown to increase REM latency when given to patients suffering from depressive disorders. Which antidepressant has been shown to actually shorten REM latency?
   a. Sertraline
   b. Venlafaxine
   c. Bupropion
   d. Trazodone

Answer: c

3. Antipsychotic medications have been associated with both restless leg syndrome and the onset of akathisia. Which of the following would put akathisia higher on the differential diagnosis?
   a. Symptoms more prominent in the evening
   b. Symptoms more prominent with inactivity
   c. Symptoms not relieved by voluntary movement
   d. Symptom onset immediately after starting an antipsychotic medication

Answer: c

4. Which medication used to treat insomnia is thought to produce its effect by acting as an orexin-receptor antagonist?
   a. Suvorexant
   b. Zolpidem
   c. Trazodone
   d. Gabapentin

Answer: a

5. Which tricyclic antidepressant would be least likely to produce sedating effects?

   a. Amitriptyline
   b. Doxepin
   c. Trimipramine
   d. Nortriptyline

Answer: d

REFERENCES

1. SAMHSA. *Substance Abuse and Mental Health Services Administration.* Retrieved from https://www.datafiles.samhsa.gov/study/national-survey-drug-use-and-health-nsduh-2017-nid17938

2. Horne, R., & Weinman, J. (1999). Patients' beliefs about prescribed medicines and their role in adherence to treatment in chronic physical illness. *Journal of Psychosomatic Research, 47*(6), 555–567. doi:S0022399999000574

3. Benca R. M., Obermeyer, W. H., Thisted, R. A., & Gillin, J. C. (1992). Sleep and psychiatric disorders: A meta-analysis. *Archives of General Psychiatry, 49*(8), 651–668; discussion 669–670.

4. Pratt, L. A., Brody, D. J., & Gu, Q. (2011). *Antidepressant Use in Persons Aged 12 and Over: United States, 2005–2008.* Hyattsville (MD): U.S. Department of Health and Human Services; Centers for Disease Control and Prevention; 2011. Retrieved from http://www.cdc.gov/nchs/data/databriefs/db76.pdf

5. Winokur, A., Gary, K. A., Rodner, S., Rae-Red, C., Fernando, A. T., & Szuba, M. P. (2001). Depression, sleep physiology, and antidepressant drugs. *Depression and Anxiety, 14*(1), 19–28. doi:10.1002/da.1043

6. Beasley, C. M., Jr, Sayler, M. E., Weiss, A. M., & Potvin, J. H. (1992). Fluoxetine: Activating and sedating effects at multiple fixed doses. *Journal of Clinical Psychopharmacology, 12*(5), 328–333

7. Beasley, C. M., Jr, Dornseif, B. E., Pultz, J. A., Bosomworth, J. C., & Sayler, M. E. (1991). Fluoxetine versus trazodone: Efficacy and activating-sedating effects. *Journal of Clinical Psychiatry, 52*(7), 294–299.

8. Kiev, A., & Feiger, A. (1997). A double-blind comparison of fluvoxamine and paroxetine in the treatment of depressed outpatients. *Journal of Clinical Psychiatry, 58*(4), 146–152.

9. Mendels, J., Kiev, A., & Fabre, L. F. (1999). Double-blind comparison of citalopram and placebo in depressed outpatients with melancholia. *Depression and Anxiety, 9*(2), 54–60. doi:10.1002/(SICI)1520-6394(1999)9:2<54::AID-DA2>3.0.CO;2-T

10. Kerkhofs, M., Rielaert, C., de Maertelaer, V., Linkowski, P., Czarka, M., & Mendlewicz, J. (1990). Fluoxetine in major depression: Efficacy, safety and effects on sleep polygraphic variables. *International Clinical Psychopharmacology, 5*(4), 253–260.

11. Hendrickse, W. A., Roffwarg, H. P., Grannemann, B. D., Orsulak, P. J., Armitage, R., Cain, J. W., et al. (1994). The effects of fluoxetine on the polysomnogram of depressed outpatients: A pilot study. *Neuropsychopharmacology, 10*(2), 85–91. doi:10.1038/npp.1994.10

12. Gillin, J. C., Rapaport, M., Erman, M. K., Winokur, A., & Albala, B. J. (1997). A comparison of nefazodone and fluoxetine on mood and on objective, subjective, and clinician-rated measures of sleep in depressed patients: A double-blind, 8-week clinical trial. *Journal of Clinical Psychiatry, 58*(5), 185–192.

13. Trivedi, M. H., Rush, A. J., Armitage, R., Gullion, C. M., Grannemann, B. D., Orsulak, P. J., et al. (1999). Effects of fluoxetine on the polysomnogram in outpatients with major depression. *Neuropsychopharmacology, 20*(5), 447–459. doi:S0893133X98001316

14. Keck, P. E., Jr, & McElroy, S. L. (1992). Ratio of plasma fluoxetine to norfluoxetine concentrations and associated sedation. *Journal of Clinical Psychiatry, 53*(4), 127–129.

15. Armitage, R., Trivedi, M., & Rush, A. J. (1995). Fluoxetine and oculomotor activity during sleep in depressed patients. *Neuropsychopharmacology, 12*(2), 159–165. doi:0893133X9400075B

16. Dorsey, C. M., Lukas, S. E., & Cunningham, S. L. (1996). Fluoxetine-induced sleep disturbance in depressed patients. *Neuropsychopharmacology, 14*(6), 437–442. doi:0893-133X(95)00148-47

17. Sharpley, A. L., Williamson, D. J., Attenburrow, M. E., Pearson, G., Sargent, P., & Cowen, P. J. (1996). The effects of paroxetine and nefazodone on sleep: A placebo controlled trial. *Psychopharmacology, 126*(1), 50–54.

18. Staner, L., Kerkhofs, M., Detroux, D., Leyman, S., Linkowski, P., & Mendlewicz, J. (1995). Acute, subchronic and withdrawal sleep EEG changes during treatment with paroxetine and amitriptyline: A double-blind randomized trial in major depression. *Sleep, 18*(6), 470–477.

19. Jindal, R. D., Friedman, E. S., Berman, S. R., Fasiczka, A. L., Howland, R. H., & Thase, M. E. (2003). Effects of sertraline on sleep architecture in patients with depression. *Journal of Clinical Psychopharmacology, 23*(6), 540–548. doi:10.1097/01.jcp.0000095345.32154.9a

20. Luthringer, R., Toussaint, M., Schaltenbrand, N., Bailey, P., Danjou, P. H., Hackett, D., et al. (1996). A double-blind, placebo-controlled evaluation of the effects of orally administered venlafaxine

on sleep in inpatients with major depression. *Psychopharmacology Bulletin, 32*(4), 637–646.

21. Salin-Pascual, R. J., Galicia-Polo, L., & Drucker-Colin, R. (1997). Sleep changes after 4 consecutive days of venlafaxine administration in normal volunteers. *Journal of Clinical Psychiatry, 58*(8), 348–350.

22. Kluge, M., Schussler, P., & Steiger, A. (2007). Duloxetine increases stage 3 sleep and suppresses rapid eye movement (REM) sleep in patients with major depression. *European Neuropsychopharmacology, 17*(8), 527–531. doi:S0924-977X(07)00019-3

23. Chalon, S., Pereira, A., Lainey, E., Vandenhende, F., Watkin, J. G., Staner, L., et al. (2005). Comparative effects of duloxetine and desipramine on sleep EEG in healthy subjects. *Psychopharmacology, 177*(4), 357–365. doi:10.1007/s00213-004-1961-0

24. Mouret, J., Lemoine, P., Minuit, M. P., Benkelfat, C., & Renardet, M. (1988). Effects of trazodone on the sleep of depressed subjects: A polygraphic study. *Psychopharmacology, 95 Suppl*, S37–S43.

25. Organon, Inc. (1996). Remeron—a novel pharmacological treatment for depression. West Orange, NJ: Organon, Inc.

26. Kent, J. M. (2000). SNaRIs, NaSSAs, and NaRIs: New agents for the treatment of depression. *Lancet, 355*(9207), 911–918. doi:S0140-6736(99)11381–11383

27. Grasmader, K., Verwohlt, P. L., Kuhn, K. U., Frahnert, C., Hiemke, C., Dragicevic, A., et al. (2005). Relationship between mirtazapine dose, plasma concentration, response, and side effects in clinical practice. *Pharmacopsychiatry, 38*(3), 113–117. doi:10.1055/s-2005-864120

28. Winokur, A., Sateia, M. J., Hayes, J. B., Bayles-Dazet, W., MacDonald, M. M., & Gary, K. A. (2000). Acute effects of mirtazapine on sleep continuity and sleep architecture in depressed patients: A pilot study. *Biological Psychiatry, 48*(1), 75–78. doi:S0006-3223(00)00882-9

29. Organon USA. (2007). Product information REMERON oral tablets, mirtazapine tablets. Roseland, NJ: Organon USA, Inc; 2007.

30. Kolla, B. P., Mansukhani, M. P., & Bostwick, J. M. (2017). The influence of antidepressants on restless legs syndrome and periodic limb movements: A systematic review. *Sleep Medicine Reviews*, doi:S1087-0792(17)30124-7

31. Kim, S. W., Shin, I. S., Kim, J. M., Yang S. J., Shin H. Y., & Yoon, J. S. (2005). Bupropion may improve restless legs syndrome: A report of three cases. *Clinical Neuropharmacology, 28*(6), 298–301.

32. Nofzinger, E. A., Reynolds, C. F., III, Thase M. E., Frank, E, Jennings, J. R., Fasiczka, A. L., et al.

(1995). REM sleep enhancement by bupropion in depressed men. *American Journal Psychiatry, 152*(2), 274–276.

33. Kupfer, D. J., Spiker, D. G., Rossi, A., Coble, P. A., Shaw, D., & Ulrich, R. (1982). Nortriptyline and EEG sleep in depressed patients. *Biological Psychiatry, 17*(5), 535–546.

34. Shipley, J. E., Kupfer, D. J., Dealy, R. S., Griffin, S. J., Coble, P. A., McEachran, A. B., & Grochocinski, V. J. (1984). Differential effects of amitriptyline and of zimelidine on the sleep electroencephalogram of depressed patients. *Clinical Pharmacology & Therapeutics, 36*(2), 251–259.

35. Ware, J. C., Brown, F. W., Moorad, P. J., Jr, Pittard, J. T., & Cobert, B. (1989). Effects on sleep: A double-blind study comparing trimipramine to imipramine in depressed insomniac patients. *Sleep, 12*(6), 537–549.

36. Kupfer, D. J., Perel, J. M., Pollock, B. G., Nathan, R. S., Grochocinski, V. J., Wilson, M. J., & McEachran, A. B. (1991). Fluvoxamine versus desipramine: Comparative polysomnographic effects. *Biological Psychiatry, 29*(1), 23–40.

37. Markov, D., & Doghramji, K. (2010). Doxepin for insomnia. *Current Psychiatry, 9*(10), 67–77.

38. Rehn, D., Reimann, H. J., von der Ohe, M., Schmidt, U., Schmel, A., & Hennings, G. (1987). Biorhythmic changes of plasma histamine levels in healthy volunteers. *Agents and Actions, 22*(1–2), 24–29.

39. Roth, T., Rogowski, R., Hull, S., Schwartz, H., Koshorek, G., Corser, B., et al. (2007). Efficacy and safety of doxepin 1 mg, 3 mg, and 6 mg in adults with primary insomnia. *Sleep, 30*(11), 1555–1561.

40. Scharf, M., Rogowski, R., Hull, S., Cohn, M., Mayleben, D., Feldman, N., et al. (2008). Efficacy and safety of doxepin 1 mg, 3 mg, and 6 mg in elderly patients with primary insomnia: A randomized, double-blind, placebo controlled crossover study. *Journal of Clinical Psychiatry, 69*, 1557–1564.

41. Vogel, G. W., Buffenstein, A., Minter, K., & Hennessey, A. (1990). Drug effects on REM sleep and on endogenous depression. *Neuroscience & Biobehavioral Reviews, 14*(1), 49–63.

42. Nofzinger, E. A., Schwartz, R. M., Reynolds, C. F., III, Thase, M. E., Jennings, J. R., Frank, E., et al. (1994). Affect intensity and phasic REM sleep in depressed men before and after treatment with cognitive-behavioral therapy. *Journal of Consulting and Clinical Psychology, 62*(1), 83–91.

43. Sharpley, A. L., & Cowen, P. J. (1995). Effect of pharmacologic treatments on the sleep of depressed patients. *Biological Psychiatry, 37*(2), 85–98.

44. Reynolds, C. F., III, Buysse, D. J., Brunner, D. P., Begley, A. E., Dew, M. A., Hoch, C. C., et al. (1997). Maintenance nortriptyline effects on electroencephalographic sleep in elderly patients with recurrent major depression: Double-blind, placebo- and plasma-level-controlled evaluation. *Biological Psychiatry, 42*(7), 560–567.

45. Taylor, M. P., Reynolds, C. F., III, Frank, E., Dew, M. A., Mazumdar, S., Houck, P. R., & Kupfer, D. J. (1999). EEG sleep measures in later-life bereavement depression: A randomized, double-blind, placebo-controlled evaluation of nortriptyline. *American Journal of Geriatric Psychiatry, 7*(1), 41–47.

46. Wyatt, R. J., Fram, D. H., Kupfer, D. J., & Snyder, F. (1971). Total prolonged drug-induced REM sleep suppression in anxious-depressed patients. *Archives of General Psychiatry, 24*(2), 145–155.

47. Kupfer, D. J., & Bowers, M. B., Jr. (1972). REM sleep and central monoamine oxidase inhibition. *Psychopharmacologia, 27*(3), 183–190.

48. Monti, J. M. (1989). Effect of a reversible monoamine oxidase-A inhibitor (moclobemide) on sleep of depressed patients. *British Journal of Psychiatry Supplement,* 6:61–65.

49. Forest Pharmaceuticals USA, Inc. (2013). Product information for FETZIMA (levomilnacipran) extended-release capsules. St Louis, MO: Forest Pharmaceuticals USA.

50. Forest Pharmaceuticals USA, Inc. (2015). Product information for VIIBRYD (vilazodone hydrochloride) tablets. Cincinnati, OH: Forest Pharmaceuticals USA.

51. Takeda Pharmaceuticals America, Inc. (2013). Product information for BRINTELLIX (vortioxetine) tablets. Deerfield, IL: Takeda Pharmaceuticals America.

52. Lam, S. P., Fong, S. Y., Ho, C. K., Yu, M. W., & Wing, Y. K. (2008). Parasomnia among psychiatric outpatients: A clinical, epidemiologic, cross-sectional study. *Journal of Clinical Psychiatry, 69*(9), 1374–1382. doi:ej08m03938.

53. McCarter, S. J., St Louis, E. K., Sandness, D. J., Arndt, K., Erickson, M., Tabatabai, G., et al. (2015). Antidepressants increase REM sleep muscle tone in patients with and without REM sleep behavior disorder. *Sleep, 38*(6), 907–917. doi:10.5665/sleep.4738.

54. Tan, L., Zhou, J., Yang, L., Ren, R., Zhang, Y., Li, T., & Tang, X. (2017). Duloxetine-induced rapid eye movement sleep behavior disorder: A case report. *BMC Psychiatry, 17*(1), 372. doi:10.1186/s12888-017-1535-4

55. Reeve, S., Sheaves, B., & Freeman, D. (2019). Sleep disorders in early psychosis: Incidence, severity, and association with clinical symptoms. *Schizophrenia Bulletin, 45*(2), 287–295. doi:10.1093/schbul/sby129

56. Lauer, C. J., Schreiber, W., Pollmacher, T., Holsboer, F., & Krieg, J. C. (1997). Sleep in schizophrenia: A polysomnographic study on drug-naive patients. *Neuropsychopharmacology, 16*(1), 51–60. doi:S0893-133X(96)00159-5

57. Citrome, L. (2017). Activating and sedating adverse effects of second-generation antipsychotics in the treatment of schizophrenia and major depressive disorder: Absolute risk increase and number needed to harm. *Journal of Clinical Psychopharmacology, 37*(2), 138–147. doi:10.1097/JCP.0000000000000665

58. Fang, F., Sun, H., Wang, Z., Ren, M., Calabrese, J. R., & Gao, K. (2016). Antipsychotic drug-induced somnolence: Incidence, mechanisms, and management. *CNS Drugs, 30*(9), 845–867. doi:10.1007/s40263-016-0352-5

59. Kumar, R., & Sachdev, P. S. (2009). Akathisia and second-generation antipsychotic drugs. *Current Opinions in Psychiatry, 22*(3), 293–299.

60. Winokur, A., & Kamath, J. (2008). The effect of typical and atypical antipsychotic drugs on sleep of schizophrenic patients. In J. Monti, S. R. Pandi-Peruma, B. L. Jacobs, & D. Nutt (Eds.), *Serotonin and sleep: olecular, functional and clinical aspects.* Basel, Switzerland: Birkhauser-Verlag; 2008.

61. Wetter, T. C., Lauer, C. J., Gillich, G., & Pollmacher, T. (1996). The electroencephalographic sleep pattern in schizophrenic patients treated with clozapine or classical antipsychotic drugs. *Journal of Psychiatric Research, 30*(6), 411–419. doi:S0022-3956(96)00022-2

62. Wetter, T. C., Lauer, C. J., Gillich, G., & Pollmacher, T. (1996). The electroencephalographic sleep pattern in schizophrenic patients treated with clozapine or classical antipsychotic drugs. *Journal of Psychiatric Research, 30*(6), 411–419. doi:S0022-3956(96)00022-2

63. Lee, J. H., Woo, J. I., & Meltzer, H. Y. (2001). Effects of clozapine on sleep measures and sleep-associated changes in growth hormone and cortisol in patients with schizophrenia. *Psychiatry Research, 103*(2–3), 157–166. doi:S0165-1781(01)00284-0

64. Lee, J. H., Woo, J. I., & Meltzer, H. Y. (2001). Effects of clozapine on sleep measures and sleep-associated changes in growth hormone and cortisol in patients with schizophrenia. *Psychiatry Research, 103*(2-3), 157–166. doi:S0165-1781(01)00284-0

65. Salin-Pascual, R. J., Herrera-Estrella, M., Galicia-Polo, L., & Laurrabaquio, M. R. (1999). Olanzapine acute administration in schizophrenic patients increases delta sleep and sleep

efficiency. *Biological Psychiatry*, *46*(1), 141–143. doi:S0006-3223(98)00372-2

66. Salin-Pascual, R. J., Herrera-Estrella, M., Galicia-Polo, L., Rosas, M., & Brunner, E. (2004). Low delta sleep predicted a good clinical response to olanzapine administration in schizophrenic patients. *Revista De Investigacion Clinica; Organo Del Hospital De Enfermedades De La Nutricion*, *56*(3), 345–350.

67. Muller, M. J., Rossbach, W., Mann, K., Roschke, J., Muller-Siecheneder, F., Blumler, M., et al. (2004). Subchronic effects of olanzapine on sleep EEG in schizophrenic patients with predominantly negative symptoms. *Pharmacopsychiatry*, *37*(4), 157–162. doi:10.1055/s-2004-827170

68. Luthringer, R., Staner, L., Noel, N., Muzet, M., Gassmann-Mayer, C., Talluri, K., et al. (2007). A double-blind, placebo-controlled, randomized study evaluating the effect of paliperidone extended-release tablets on sleep architecture in patients with schizophrenia. *International Clinical Psychopharmacology*, *22*(5), 299–308. doi:10.1097/YIC.0b013e3281c55f4f

69. Keshavan, M. S., Prasad, K. M., Montrose, D. M., Miewald, J. M., & Kupfer, D. J. (2007). Sleep quality and architecture in quetiapine, risperidone, or never-treated schizophrenia patients. *Journal of Clinical Psychopharmacology*, *27*(6), 703–705. doi:10.1097/jcp.0b013e31815a884d

70. Haffmans, P. M., Oolders, H. J., Hoencamp, E., & Schreiner, A. (2004). Sleep quality in schizophrenia and the effects of atypical antipsychotic medication. *Acta Neuropsychiatrica*, *16*(6), 281–289. doi:10.1111/j.0924-2708.2004.00103.x

71. Yamashita, H., Morinobu, S., Yamawaki, S., Horiguchi, J., & Nagao, M. (2002). Effect of risperidone on sleep in schizophrenia: A comparison with haloperidol. *Psychiatry Research*, *109*(2), 137–142. doi:S0165178102000094

72. Allen, R. P., & Earley, C. J. (2001). Restless legs syndrome: A review of clinical and pathophysiologic features. *Journal of Clinical Neurophysiology*, *18*(2), 128–147.

73. Kang, S. G., Lee, H. J., Jung, S. W., Cho, S. N., Han, C., Kim, Y. K., et al. (2007). Characteristics and clinical correlates of restless legs syndrome in schizophrenia. *Progress in Neuro-Psychopharmacology & Biological Psychiatry*, *31*(5), 1078–1083. doi:S0278-5846(07)00106-6

74. Rittmannsberger, H., & Werl, R. (2013). Restless legs syndrome induced by quetiapine: Report of seven cases and review of the literature. *International Journal of Neuropsychopharmacology*, *16*, 1427–31.

75. AstraZeneca Pharmaceuticals LP. (2009). Product information for SEROQUEL (quetiapine fumarate) tablets. Wilmington, DE: AstraZeneca Pharmaceuticals LP.

76. Huapaya, L. V. (1979). Seven cases of somnambulism induced by drugs. *American Journal of Psychiatry*, *136*(7):985–986. doi:10.1176/ajp.136.7.985

77. Kolivakis, T. T., Margolese, H. C., Beauclair, L., & Chouinard, G. (2001). Olanzapine-induced somnambulism. *American Journal of Psychiatry*, *158*(7), 1158. doi:10.1176/appi.ajp.158.7.1158

78. Chiu, Y. H., Chen, C. H., & Shen, W. (2008). Somnambulism secondary to olanzapine treatment in one patient with bipolar disorder. *Progress in Neuro-Psychopharmacology & Biological Psychiatry*, *32*(2), 581–582. doi:S0278-5846(07)00359-4

79. Faridhosseini, F., & Zamani, A. (2012). A case report of somnambulism associated with olanzapine. *Iranian Journal of Psychiatry and Behavioral Sciences*, *6*(1):72–74.

80. Hafeez, Z. H., & Kalinowski, C. M. (2007). Somnambulism induced by quetiapine: Two case reports and a review of the literature. *CNS Spectrum*, *12*(12), 910–912.

81. Raja, M., & Raja, S. (2013). Sleepwalking in four patients treated with quetiapine. *Psychiatria Danubina*, *25*(1), 80–83.

82. Tamanna, S., Ullah, M. I., Pope, C. R., Holloman, G., & Koch, C. A. (2012). Quetiapine-induced sleep-related eating disorder-like behavior: A case series. *Journal of Medical Case Reports*, *6*, 380. doi:10.1186/1752-1947-6-380

83. Paquet, V., Strul, J., Servais, L., Pelc, I., & Fossion, P. (2002). Sleep-related eating disorder induced by olanzapine. *Journal of Clinical Psychiatry*, *63*(7), 597.

84. Das P. (2016). A case of sleepwalking with sleep-related eating associated with ziprasidone therapy in a patient with schizoaffective disorder. *Journal of Clinical Psychopharmacology*, *36*(4), 393–394. doi:10.1097/JCP.0000000000000525

85. Stallman, H. M., Kohler, M., & White, J. (2018). Medication induced sleepwalking: A systematic review. *Sleep Medicine Reviews*, *37*, 105–113. doi:S1087-0792(17)30020-5

86. Bazil, C. W., Battista, J., & Basner, R. C. (2005). Gabapentin improves sleep in the presence of alcohol. *Journal of Clinical Sleep Medicine*, *1*(3), 284–287.

87. Garcia-Borreguero, D., Larrosa, O., de la Llave, Y., Verger, K., Masramon, X., & Hernandez, G. (2002). Treatment of restless legs syndrome with gabapentin: A double-blind, cross-over study. *Neurology*, *59*(10), 1573–1579.

88. Hindmarch, I., Dawson, J., & Stanley, N. (2005). A double-blind study in healthy volunteers to assess

the effects on sleep of pregabalin compared with alprazolam and placebo. *Sleep, 28*(2), 187–193.

89. Mathias, S., Wetter, T. C., Steiger, A., & Lancel, M. (2001). The GABA uptake inhibitor tiagabine promotes slow wave sleep in normal elderly subjects. *Neurobiology of Aging, 22*(2), 247–253. doi:S0197458000002323

90. Walsh, J. K., Zammit, G., Schweitzer, P. K., Ondrasik, J., & Roth, T. (2006). Tiagabine enhances slow wave sleep and sleep maintenance in primary insomnia. *Sleep Medicine, 7*(2), 155–161. doi:S1389-9457(05)00112-7

91. Ota, S. M., Moreira, K. D., Suchecki, D., Oliveira, M. G., Tiba, P. A. (2013). Lithium prevents REM sleep deprivation-induced impairments on memory consolidation. *Sleep, 36*(11), 1677–1684. doi:10.5665/sleep.3126

92. Billiard, M. (1987). Lithium carbonate: Effects on sleep patterns of normal and depressed subjects and its use in sleep-wake pathology. *Pharmacopsychiatry, 20*(5), 195–196. doi:10.1055/s-2007-1017102

93. Wagner, J., & Wagner, M. L. (2000). Non-benzodiazepines for the treatment of insomnia. *Sleep Medicine Review, 4*(6), 551–581. doi:S1087-0792(00)90126-6

94. Dolder, C. R., & Nelson, M. H. (2008). Hypnosedative-induced complex behaviours: Incidence, mechanisms and management. *CNS Drugs, 22*(12), 1021–1036. doi:10.2165/0023210-200822120-00005

95. Howell, M. J. (2012). Parasomnias: An updated review. *Neurotherapeutics, 9*(4), 753–775. doi:10.1007/s13311-012-0143-8

96. Pennington, J. G., & Guina, J. (2016). Eszopiclone-induced parasomnia with suicide attempt: A case report. *Innovations in Clinical Neuroscience, 13*(9–10), 44–48.

97. Kishi, T., Matsunaga, S., & Iwata, N. (2015). Suvorexant for primary insomnia: A systematic review and meta-analysis of randomized placebo-controlled trials. *PloS One, 10*(8), e0136910. doi:10.1371/journal.pone.0136910

98. Obermeyer, W. H., & Benca, R. M. (1996). Effects of drugs on sleep. *Neurologic Clinics, 14*(4), 827–840.

99. Carlos, K., Prado, G. F., Teixeira, C. D., Conti, C., de Oliveira, M. M., Prado, L. B., et al. (2017). Benzodiazepines for restless legs syndrome. *Cochrane Database of Systematic Reviews, 3*, CD006939. doi:10.1002/14651858.CD006939.pub2

100. Mason, M., Cates, C. J., & Smith, I. (2015). Effects of opioid, hypnotic and sedating medications on sleep-disordered breathing in adults with obstructive sleep apnoea. *Cochrane Database of Systematic Reviews, 7*, CD011090. doi:10.1002/14651858.CD011090.pub2

101. Cortese, S., Faraone, S. V., Konofal, E., & Lecendreux, M. (2009). Sleep in children with attention-deficit/hyperactivity disorder: Meta-analysis of subjective and objective studies. *Journal of the American Academy of Child and Adolescent Psychiatry, 48*(9), 894–908. doi:10.1097/CHI.0b013e3181ac09c9

102. Stein, M. A., Weiss, M., & Hlavaty, L. (2012). ADHD treatments, sleep, and sleep problems: Complex associations. *Neurotherapeutics, 9*(3), 509–517. doi:10.1007/s13311-012-0130-0

103. Kim, H. W., Yoon, I. Y., Cho, S. C., Kim, B. N., Chung, S., Lee, H., et al. (2010). The effect of OROS methylphenidate on the sleep of children with attention-deficit/hyperactivity disorder. *International Clinical Psychopharmacology, 25*(2), 107–115. doi:10.1097/YIC.0b013e3283364411

104. Stein, M. A., Waldman, I. D., Charney, E., Aryal, S., Sable, C., Gruber, R., et al. (2011). Dose effects and comparative effectiveness of extended release dexmethylphenidate and mixed amphetamine salts. *Journal of Child and Adolescent Psychopharmacology, 21*(6), 581–588. doi:10.1089/cap.2011.0018

105. Biederman, J., Krishnan, S., Zhang, Y., McGough, J. J., & Findling, R. L. (2007). Efficacy and tolerability of lisdexamfetamine dimesylate (NRP-104) in children with attention-deficit/hyperactivity disorder: A phase III, multicenter, randomized, double-blind, forced-dose, parallel-group study. *Clinical Therapeutics, 29*(3), 450–463. doi:S0149-2918(07)80083-X

106. Surman, C. B., & Roth, T. (2011). Impact of stimulant pharmacotherapy on sleep quality: Post hoc analyses of 2 large, double-blind, randomized, placebo-controlled trials. *Journal of Clinical Psychiatry, 72*(7), 903–908. doi:10.4088/JCP.11m06838

107. Kooij, J. J., Middelkoop, H. A., van Gils, K., & Buitelaar, J. K. (2001). The effect of stimulants on nocturnal motor activity and sleep quality in adults with ADHD: An open-label case-control study. *Journal of Clinical Psychiatry, 62*(12), 952–956.

108. Sobanski, E., Schredl, M., Kettler, N., & Alm, B. (2008). Sleep in adults with attention deficit hyperactivity disorder (ADHD) before and during treatment with methylphenidate: A controlled polysomnographic study. *Sleep, 31*(3), 375–381.

29

Forensic Sleep Medicine

KENNETH J. WEISS, CLARENCE WATSON, AND MARK R. PRESSMAN

INTRODUCTION

Clinical psychiatrists are aware that, for a variety of reasons and dynamics, patients have contact with the criminal justice system. Most such instances involve persons with serious mental illness, often lacking insight or resources, who run afoul of social norms or whose behavioral adaptations cause their diversion into jails and prisons. There are others whose symptomatology (e.g., delusional ideas) brings them into focus for determination of criminal responsibility. In the United States, all but four jurisdictions permit evidence of legal "insanity,"[1] usually in the form of a cognitive standard: whether at the time of the incident the person knew the wrongfulness of the conduct charged. The insanity defense represents an excuse for otherwise unlawful conduct and, when successful, may become the basis for civil commitment instead of imprisonment. Still, these individuals may be culpable, since the insanity defense is not often successful.

There is another principal in the criminal law: that a person cannot be held accountable for what would otherwise be criminal conduct if, at the time in question, that person lacks consciousness. Examples include persons who are medically unconscious due to gross brain impairment, those having an epileptic seizure or post-ictal (lacking conscious awareness), and persons who were asleep. It is the last group of individuals who will be the focus of this chapter.

If the inquiry into criminal responsibility is whether a mental illness deprived the defendant of the ability to judge wrongfulness, there is still the assumption that the actions were conducted by a conscious person albeit with discrete impairments. In the case of sleep disorders, by contrast, the question is whether full consciousness existed. If not, according to general principles of culpability, there was no culpable act (*actus reus*). And without *actus reus*, which the prosecution must establish, there is no basis for culpability. This is a time-honored principle embedded in the Latin phrase *In somno voluntas non erat libera* (a sleeping person has no free will). Accordingly, the role of the scientist is to shed light on whether the criminal defendant was asleep or conscious during the act in question—not a simple matter, given the often-ambiguous presentation of individuals with parasomnias or complex conditions affecting consciousness.

The inquiry into the nature, existence, genesis, and measurement of consciousness is an immense undertaking, spanning philosophy, neuroscience, clinical medicine, and legal determinations. Sample questions include the following: When is consciousness lost to sleep states? Are there partial losses of consciousness among parasomnias? How is it possible to know a person's state of awareness during an alleged parasomnia episode? What kinds of technology and expertise must be brought to bear on retrospective assessment? Can claims of sleep-related behaviors be taken at face value, or is there an inquiry into feigned conditions? Since it is clearly beyond the scope of this chapter to address the deeper questions of consciousness, and given the law's focus on assigning culpability where applicable, the following sections are practical considerations in the interface between sleep disorders and criminal responsibility.

APPROACH TO THE LEGAL CONSULTATION

Assessment of claims by criminal defendants that alleged violent behavior occurred during an episode of, or due to, a sleep disorder falls between the domains of mental health professionals and sleep specialists. However, many forensic psychiatrists and psychologists lack the clinical experience or expertise (both acceptable credentials) to evaluate the defendant with a parasomnia, and many sleep experts are reluctant to enter the legal arena. By contemporary standards, there is a core workup necessary to assess the validity of the claim.

While it is ideal to undertake a polysomno-graphic (PSG) assessment (see Chapter 7), there are practical problems assessing criminal defendants, especially when incarcerated. First is the practical issue of getting the data, even assuming a portable device can be employed. Second is the question of the frequency of the parasomnia in relation to case finding. Is it a nightly occurrence, or one that is rare and unpredictable? Third, if the parasomnia is detected, what can be inferred from its presence to illuminate the behavior at the time in question? And fourth, to what degree of certainty can an expert determine that the claim is authentic? The presence of PSG or similar objective findings that predate the incident is ideal, but the expert is still required to place the defendant within an episode (or not); such attributions are difficult and, for jurors, often counterintuitive.[2] Shedding light on the roots of behavior is the job of the expert witness, who must first be grounded in the ways of legal proceedings.

Courts, Rules, and Expert Testimony

For clinicians unacquainted with criminal justice, it is worthwhile to clarify some fundamentals that govern the presentation of expert opinions. Criminal justice is a system of assigning responsibility to wrongdoers, but only when the facts against them are proven beyond reasonable doubt. Thus, in the case of a person harming another during a parasomnic episode, the demonstration that the defendant was or was not in a state of pathological sleep can be argued. It is only the prosecutor and defense attorney who make arguments to the jury or judge—not witnesses. But attorneys are not permitted to give scientific evidence, because they are not qualified to do so; sleep medicine, for example, is not in their training or area of expertise. Instead, they can argue for guilt or innocence of the defendant by first presenting expert testimony. By contrast, expert witnesses never argue for guilt or innocence. Rather, they shed light, without biasing the judge or jury, on scientific matters beyond the understanding of ordinary citizens.

Who Is an Expert?

Expert witnesses are different from fact witnesses, who are not permitted to express opinions about the condition of the defendant (e.g., treating clinicians, police officers, and eyewitnesses). Expert witnesses must be "qualified" by the judge before their findings are permitted to be heard by the jury or court. This is often done in conjunction with rule of evidence, for example, Federal Rule of Evidence 702 or a state shadow rule. The rule states:

> A witness who is qualified as an expert by knowledge, skill, experience, training, or education may testify in the form of an opinion or otherwise if: (a) the expert's scientific, technical, or other specialized knowledge will help the trier of fact to understand the evidence or to determine a fact in issue; (b) the testimony is based on sufficient facts or data; (c) the testimony is the product of reliable principles and methods; and (d) the expert has reliably applied the principles and methods to the facts of the case.[3]

It is not a high threshold, since a professional who has studied the subject matter before the court is nearly always permitted to offer an opinion. Nevertheless, admissibility of scientific testimony is the domain of the judge, acting as "gatekeeper," as elaborated in the 1993 *Daubert* decision[4] and subsequent cases. This is not the only standard employed in American jurisdictions. Professionals serving as expert witnesses must check with their retaining attorneys to determine the legal standards in the case's jurisdiction.

The Expert's Role

There is generally no controversy around the necessity of expert testimony. However, when the expert is called to educate the "trier of fact" (jury or judge) about a matter that contains a novel theory, approach, or manner of inference, the court, as gatekeeper, may use discretion and bar the evidence because it lacks literature support or general acceptance within the professional community. Thus, for example, a court might bar testimony claiming that excessive mobile telephone use induced a state of pathological sleep and caused the defendant to commit a violent act—even though the testifying expert may be qualified based on ordinary Rule 702 criteria. It should be emphasized that expert's opinions must not be so persuasive as to "prejudice" the jury; rather, they must educate the factfinder sufficiently for them to weigh the evidence and arrive at a reasonable decision. Potential experts should also understand that, while they may believe their opinions represent the truth of the matter, the judge will instruct the jurors that they can accept or reject all or part of any expert opinion. It would be unethical for professionals of any type to attempt to opine on a matter beyond his or her training or expertise.

No expert opinion, by itself, answers the question before the court: guilt or innocence of the defendant. That is the exclusive province of the factfinder, a basic tenet of the justice system. Indeed, in criminal cases within jurisdictions using a form of Rule 704(b),[5] the expert may not be allowed to express an opinion on the ultimate issue before the court: "In a criminal case, an expert witness must not state an opinion about whether the defendant did or did not have a mental state or condition that constitutes an element of the crime charged or of a defense. Those matters are for the trier of fact alone." Here, "element" refers to intent (*mens rea*). However, since sleep states involve consciousness, the witness would be able to state that the defendant was not in a state of awareness to be culpable generally (*actus reus*).

Relating to the Legal System

The expert witness, on either side, will have been contacted to assess an aspect of the defendant. Examples include a defendant's current mental capacity to participate in the proceedings (trial competency), a defendant's state of mind at the time of the offense (criminal responsibility), or the presence or absence of a medical or psychological disorder that bears on the question of criminal culpability. With this question in mind, it is important that the expert transparently explain how the assessment sheds light on the question before the factfinder. For example, how the diagnosis of a parasomnia might explain observed behavior during the commission of the offense or how aspects of the behavior tend to indicate conscious awareness. And if awareness was present, there is a question of malingering—the intentional production of medical symptoms for external gain (avoidance of prosecution)—a matter that must be considered in every case.

It is also necessary that the potential expert witness be aware of local laws and legal decisions that provide guidance to the court. It would be a foolish undertaking, for example, to give an opinion on legal insanity without knowing how the legislature has defined *insanity* (a purely legal term), since the judge will read the definition to the jury. In this way, the expert's written report will have identified the question posed, acknowledged the legal process underlying the factfinder's task, and collated the clinical findings in forming an opinion. Expert opinions must be expressed within "reasonable certainty" or probability (more likely than not)—no more and no less.

TABLE 29.1. DIFFERENTIAL DIAGNOSIS FOR SLEEP-RELATED BEHAVIORS

Disorders of arousal	Nightmares
Confusional arousal	Nocturnal seizures
Sexual behavior in sleep	Hypnogogic/hypnopompic hallucinations
Sleepwalking	Somniloquy/sleep talking
Sleep driving	Dissociative states
Sleep terrors	PTSD
Sleep eating	Malingering

Reprinted by permission of Oxford University Press, USA, *Psychiatric Expert Testimony: Emerging Applications* (2015) ed. by Weiss & Watson. "Sleep Disorders and Criminal Responsibility" by Watson, Pressman & Weiss. p. 104.
Abbreviation: PTSD, posttraumatic stress disorder.

SLEEP, PARASOMNIAS, AND VIOLENCE

The most common scenario in the interface between sleep and criminal law is a claim made by a defendant that the act occurred during sleep generally or a parasomnic episode specifically. Potential candidates for disorders of sleep used in legal settings must derive from the classifications found in the *Diagnostic and Statistical Manual of Mental Disorders* (fifth edition; DSM-5)[5] or the *International Classification of Sleep Disorders* (third edition; ICSD-3).[6] Failure to do so will create confusion. Table 29.1 lists the parasomnias, described in detail elsewhere in this volume, along with other differential diagnoses, for which claims have been made for nonresponsibility. In addition, common conditions, such as excessive daytime sleepiness, narcolepsy, posttraumatic stress disorder (PTSD)-related nightmares, intoxications, delirium, head trauma, and medication-related conditions have been the subject of similar claims.

Historical Cases and Concepts

Historically, most attempts to use a clinical diagnosis of a sleep disorder as a defense against *actus reus* have involved somnambulism. Simply stated, a sleeping person cannot be held responsible. Cases of putative somnambulism-associated violence have been reported for hundreds of years.[7] Since the recognition of normative and pathological sleep architecture in the 20th century, there has been a substantial literature on the application of this knowledge to criminal matters.[8] Nevertheless, separating true from false claims remains a consistent issue. It is easy to imagine that persons with legitimate somnambulism can consciously break the law and may use the diagnosis to evade responsibility. This where clinicians and sleep experts must employ advanced differential diagnostic—detective, if you will—skills.

In the celebrated 1846 case of Albert Tirrell, the defense employed clinical evidence of sleepwalking (Box 29.1). This case was one of the first

---

BOX 29.1. THE CASE OF ALBERT TIRRELL, 1846

Albert Tirrell, 21, was charged with the murder of Mary Ann Bickford, 21. Both were married, had left their spouses and co-habited. Ms. Bickford had previously been known to be a prostitute. There was apparently considerable negative public opinion against their arrangement. At the time of the crime, Ms. Bickford was living in a Boston rooming house.

The prosecution's case was based on testimony that he had been seen at her rooming house that evening. Around 4 AM, a noise and a fall were heard. Thirty minutes later, someone left the rooming house. The owner's wife yelled "Fire"—which was located in Ms. Bickford's room. Ms. Bickford was found with her throat cut, a bloody razor nearby, and her straw mattress evidently set on fire.

Meanwhile, Mr. Tirrell fled the scene, eventually arriving in New Orleans where he was arrested several months later. There was testimony that as he was trying to leave the Boston area, he had stated someone tried to murder him. His appearance was described as disheveled and his manner as "peculiar and wild."

The prosecutor put on a mostly circumstantial case. However, one prosecution witness who testified he saw and talked with Tirrell after the incident stated, "He seemed to be in a strange state, as asleep or crazy." However, he did state his intent to go to Weymouth to get some clothing.

The defense made a number of arguments familiar in the present day: The evidence was circumstantial; Mr. Tirrell had already been convicted in the media; the death might have been the result of self-inflicted wounds; and Mr. Tirrell was not culpable due to his state of mind. Then there was the sleepwalking defense. Based on the medical science of the day, counsel argued sleepwalking was a common disorder and that violence could be an element of a sleepwalking episode. The defense relied primarily on published scientific articles, and medical witnesses provided general information about the nature of sleepwalking. However, a defense expert stated under oath that a sleepwalker could get dressed, murder someone, set a fire, and flee the scene. Once having established that sleepwalking violence was common and generally accepted by science, counsel proceeded to establish that Mr. Tirrell had the characteristics of a sleepwalker. He relied on the defendant's childhood history of sleepwalking. Witnesses confirmed this history as well as difficulty arousing him from sleep. Other witness testified that the defendant continued to sleepwalk as an adult and even showed sleep-related violence as a married adult, including that he attempted to smother his wife and beat her violently. The defense argued that Mr. Tirrell had a predisposition for sleepwalking, but that he was well aware of these tendencies and took steps to prevent them, including keeping a light on in his room. The defense, nevertheless, pressed the arguments that there was a lack of proof that Mr. Tirrell had committed the crime, that it could have been suicide, but if the jury concluded he had physically committed the act, he did not do so with willful intent.

The prosecutor argued that the suicide theory based on the evidence was not credible. He further argued that there was not real evidence that Mr. Tirrell had been sleepwalking, and even if such defense were permitted, it had not been proven.

The judge's charge to the jury in the homicide case allowed only for a finding of suicide or murder. The jury deliberated for 65 minutes before finding Mr. Tirrell not guilty. The jury foreman stated that the acquittal had not been on the basis of sleepwalking. The defendant was acquitted of arson in the same incident, using a similar defense, the next year.

highly publicized cases of alleged sleepwalking violence.[7] As the "O.J. Simpson" trial of its time, local newspapers sent reporters and stenographers to the trial.[9] As a result, a complete transcript of the trial exists,[10] compared to the brief newspaper stories of other alleged sleepwalking related episodes.

Despite the poor state of scientific knowledge about sleep and sleepwalking in 1846, this trial followed a similar pattern, to a degree, to modern sleepwalking defenses; in particular, the defendant's history of past sleepwalking episodes with testimony by numerous family members. However, there was no testimony on generally accepted features of sleepwalking, such as the priming role of sleep deprivation and stress or the presence of a trigger. In fact, Mr. Tirrell's defense never established if he had been asleep prior to the incident. Sleepwalking cannot occur directly from wakefulness. Additionally, the behaviors immediately following the death of Ms. Bickford would not likely be accepted as a continuation of sleepwalking. Setting fire to the victim's room would no doubt be regarded as an attempt to conceal evidence. Fleeing the scene of the crime would also indicate awareness and memory of the act—not possible with typical amnesia that follows sleepwalking. Finally, sleepwalking in adults is known to occur intermittently. In the absence of an eyewitness, it is only circumstantial evidence.

The *Tirrell* case illustrates the problems encountered by clinicians, expert witnesses, judges, and juries in coming to terms with claims made by an individual who may have a parasomnia history but presents with complex behavior. The case was full of intrigue and gruesome details[9] (Figure 29.1), drawing attention from an early forensic psychiatrist, Dr. Isaac Ray, who had written about somnambulism and feigned symptoms in 1838.[11] In Ray's opinion, Mr. Tirrell had been feigning symptoms. Tirrell's acquittal on murder and conviction on arson charges have puzzled commentators. It is interesting to note that the jurors claimed not to have given weight to the somnambulism claim. It is frequent today, in trials involving opposing expert opinions, for the opinions to nullify each other, leaving the jury to rely on other evidence, arguments, and ordinary common sense.

It is apparent that prescientific formulations of the authenticity of sleepwalking claims considered clinical factors that continue to form the basis for expert testimony. These include reliable history of childhood-onset somnambulism; the presence of amnesia for the episode; shock and remorse over the behavior by the defendant; objective observations of altered consciousness given by reliable sources; and absence of ordinary motives and dynamics that might otherwise explain the violent behavior if it had been done in clear consciousness. One would think that, with the advent of scientific studies of human sleep, technology would play a larger role in validating or disproving claims of sleep-related violence. However, the clinical approach relies more on clinical history, collateral or eyewitness accounts, and an understanding of typical parasomnic behaviors than it does on diagnostic studies of brain function.

Subsequent to the *Tirrell* case, American courts have used varied approaches to the sleepwalking defense.[12] In *Fain v. Commonwealth* (1879),[13] the Court of Appeals of Kentucky found that a defendant was unconscious when he shot and killed his victim during sleep and, accordingly, was unable to understand the consequences of his behavior. The sleepwalking defense was also regarded as an "unconsciousness defense" in a 1974 California case.[14] US courts have also permitted the "automatism defense" in sleepwalking cases. In *McClain v. Indiana* (1997),[15] the Supreme Court of Indiana held that a criminal defendant was entitled to present evidence of sleepwalking, highlighting the absence of a necessary component of the *actus reus*—the culpable act. Many American courts use the terms automatism defense and unconsciousness defense synonymously. Despite the use of these defenses and in various American jurisdictions, they are rarely employed.

CLINICAL APPROACH TO PARASOMNIAS AND CRIMINAL CHARGES

Since courts are skeptical of criminal defendants' claims that acts of violence were committed during sleep, all clinicians must be mindful of the typical presentation of a genuine condition. The clinical history should suggest a bona fide sleep disorder, compared with others seen or described in literature. Similar episodes, with benign or morbid outcome, will have occurred previously and can be documented by collateral accounts. Episodes are usually brief, although longer episodes may occur. However, the action in question, for example, violence, is usually abrupt, immediate, impulsive, and senseless—without apparent motivation. The behavior itself, although ostensibly purposeful, is completely inappropriate for the context as well as out of character for the individual.

THE BOSTON TRAGEDY.

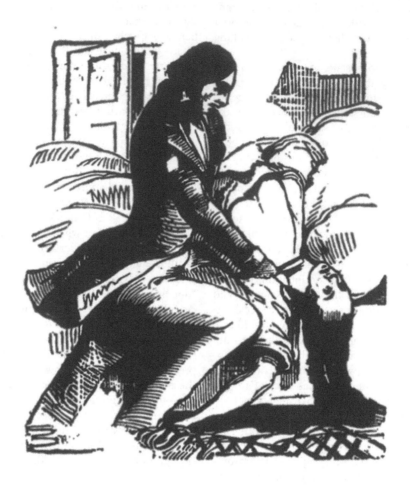

TIRRELL MURDERING MARIA A. BICKFORD,

WHILE IN A STATE OF SOMNAMBULISM.

FIGURE 29.1. Newspaper depiction of a somnambulistic homicide.[9]

Evidence of premeditation may not be needed in a given jurisdiction, but for forensic purposes, the question may be whether the behavior was *knowing* and *purposeful* (standard elements of culpability). In most instances, the victim is someone who happened to be in close proximity and who encountered, touched or blocked the sleeper's behavior. The victim's own behavior may have provoked the sleepwalker's response. Sleepwalkers do not seek out victims. As such, if that appears to be the case, a parasomnia must be regarded as less likely, if not impossible. In terms of mental state at the time in question, there should be no evidence of conscious awareness. Similarly, there should be no evidence of higher cognitive functioning—memory from before the episode, formation of memory during the episode, planning, intent, or social interaction. Episodes are generally followed by complete amnesia. Occasionally, sleepwalkers may have a memory of a brief, static dreamlike image that occurred during the episode, but no memory of their actual behaviors. After regaining consciousness, there is often bewilderment over what occurred and the sleeper's role in it; there is no attempt to conceal the behavior.[16]

Sleep-related violence does not occur directly from wakefulness. It most often occurs during deep (slow-wave, N3) sleep, 1 to 3 hours after sleep onset. Sleep deprivation and situational stress may be risk factors. The behavior can be associated with a trigger that causes arousal from sleep, such as sleep-disordered breathing, leg movements, sounds, or touch. However, as a rule, it is not associated with alcohol or alcohol intoxication. PSG (sleep studies) performed months or years after the index episode cannot determine if the individual was in a sleepwalking episode or related state at the time of the incident.

The work-up for disorders of arousal includes a sleep history (including family and personal history of sleep disorders and collateral history from the bed partner) and complete physical and neurologic examinations. Although a full-night PSG with audiovisual monitoring is warranted, it may not capture these episodes. For the purposes of a forensic evaluation of a disorder of arousal, Guilleminault and colleagues[17] recommend that the history include:

> 1) detailed description of the event and characterization of the degree of amnesia; 2) current, past, and family sleep disorders; 3) social habits, such as sleep deprivation, drug use, and alcohol intake; 4) current and past medical records and family medical history; 5) employment records (to check for difficulties related to sleep disorders); 6) determination of the frequency of abnormal behavior and its stereotypic nature. Furthermore, the history must include interviews with the spouse or bed partner and family members, questioning the following items: description of the event and prior ones; timing of the behavior; age of onset and associated life events or trauma; degree of amnesia noted; attitude after previous sleep-related disturbances (p. 335).

CLINICAL CONDITIONS

Behaviors of varying complexity have been attributed to individuals experiencing sleep abnormalities, as described elsewhere in this volume. There are rapid eye movement (REM) and non-REM (NREM) parasomnias (see Table 29.1), as well as other conditions, that can give the outward appearance of altered or absent consciousness. In the following section, these conditions will be described with attention to forensic applications.

REM Sleep Behavior Disorder

Since REM sleep, under normal conditions, is associated with tonic paralysis of skeletal muscles, it is highly unlikely that movement, let alone complex behavior, would give rise to violence. Yet, REM behavior disorder (RBD) is the exception. As described in Chapter 12, this rare condition has some traction in the courtroom, especially under the folk psychological formulation that the sleeper acted out a dream. RBD is a chronic condition, the signs of which will appear in the PSG on a nightly basis. However, the behaviors are likely to be much simpler than those attributed to the defendant. Therefore, the clinical approach involves verification of previous episodes, ideally reported to health professionals by reliable informants. The clinical features of RBD relevant to criminal justice are as follows: sudden and violent movements of the arms, legs and body striking anyone in close proximity only and pushing and pulling of anyone in close proximity occasionally results in their falling out of bed. This could lead to domestic violence complaints or criminal charges.

It is possible for person with RBD to remember a dream associated with an actual episode of violence. The rise of psychoanalytic theory, over 100 years ago, provided a theoretical framework for a connection between dreams and unconscious wishes.[7] However, under current scientific standards, this theory would not tend to persuade a jury. Indeed, such a claim made by defendant, who is expected to be amnestic for the incident, would likely be regarded as a sign of malingered illness. A jury would have the unenviable task of sorting it out.

In the event that an episode of RBD is detected on PSG, or otherwise validated by reliable observation, there is precedent for successful defense. In a Welsh case in which one of the authors (MRP) participated,[2] Brian Thomas had strangled his wife. He was acquitted by a jury after providing strong evidence of preincident sleep disturbance and other factors: long-standing sleepwalking, causing the couple to sleep apart; disturbing thoughts during the day; sleeping together in a camper van; nightmare in which he needed to fight to protect them; calling for help immediately on awakening; and character references. The defense expert included RBD in the differential, but ultimately the experts agreed it was a violent night terror at the time in question.

NREM Parasomnias

Several conditions have been associated with complex behaviors after the initiation of sleep (see Table 29.1). These include partial awakenings, somnambulism, sexsomnia, automatisms, and other conditions. The clinician's task is to verify and validate the presence of a qualifying sleep disorder that could be used to document lack of consciousness or to provide evidence to the contrary. In the absence of a PSG determination of the parasomnia, which is frequent, both sleep clinicians and forensic professionals may opine on the question of whether a criminal defendant was asleep or awake during the incident.

Partial Awakenings

In partial awakenings, which are sometimes captured during PSG studies with video, behaviors of varying complexity can occur. Unlike RBD, these episodes are associated with NREM sleep and, unlike somnambulism, rarely associated with sleepers' getting out of bed. Characteristics of NREM awakenings include those listed in Table 29.2.[18] These clinical indicators, abstracted from historical cases by Bonkalo,[18] aid investigators of claimed parasomnia-associated instances of violence.

Somnambulism

Easily the most famous of the parasomnias associated with complex behavior, sleepwalking has vexed the legal system, as it lies on the boundary of sleep and wakefulness.[8,19]

Among the most demanding tasks of the expert witness is to evaluate a claim of complex behavior associated with a parasomnia. As noted in the Tirrell case (see Box 29.1), it has long been known that claims of somnambulism have been used as ploys to evade criminal responsibility. Given the low yield of PSG studies to confirm infrequent behaviors, clinical methods, coupled with preincident history and reliable eyewitness observations, are essential in separating genuine from malingered episodes.

TABLE 29.2. CHARACTERISTICS OF TYPICAL PARTIAL AWAKENINGS WITH VIOLENCE

Impulsive act occurred on awakening

The arousal was forced, not spontaneous

Arousal is early in sleep, from deep sleep

Possibly a predisposition to act violently due to fear

Behavior appeared automatic; unmotivated and seemingly purposeful but out of context

Dazed appearance; eyes open; mechanical movements

Confusional states lasts seconds to minutes

The victim was random, usual the person causing the awakening

Full insight after awakening; no attempt to deny

Partial or total amnesia for the act

AUTOMATISM: ARE SLEEPWALKERS INSANE?

The sleepwalking defense has also been considered a variant of the insanity defense in the United States.[a] The insanity defense undermines the *mens rea* requirement by establishing that at the time of the crime, a mental disease or defect was present that impaired the defendant's ability to know or appreciate the nature of their act or to confirm their behavior to the requirements of the law. In *Tibbs v. Commonwealth* (1910), the Court of Appeals of Kentucky held that the only defense available for acts occurring during sleepwalking was the insanity defense.[20] In *Bradley v. State* (1925), the Court of Criminal Appeals of Texas overturned a murder conviction, holding that the trial court erred in not applying the insanity defense where the defendant claimed to be sleepwalking at the time of the crime.[21]

Later decisions clearly opposed the use of the insanity defense in sleepwalking cases. In *State v. Caddell*,[22] the Supreme Court of North Carolina, while acknowledging sleepwalking as a form of unconsciousness, stated that the defenses of insanity and unconsciousness are distinct because "unconsciousness at the time of the alleged

[a] This section is reprinted by permission of Oxford University Press, USA from *Psychiatric Expert Testimony: Emerging Applications* (2015) ed. by Weiss & Watson. "Sleep Disorders and Criminal Responsibility" by Watson, Pressman & Weiss. 112–114.

criminal act need not be the result of a disease or defect of the mind" (p. 360). The Supreme Court of Wyoming also made this distinction in *Fulcher v. State* (1981).[23] The Wyoming court reasoned that without such distinction a person who was unconscious but not mentally ill at the time of the crime would face commitment at a mental institution upon acquittal. The court stated that commitment of such an individual to a mental institution for rehabilitation would be of no value. The Supreme Court of Indiana, in *McClain v. Indiana*,[24] citing *Fulcher*, agreed with this distinction and held that the automatism defense was more appropriate than the insanity defense in sleepwalking cases.

Automatism and Sexual Behavior During Sleep

Sexual behaviors involving a sleeping person and an unwilling victim can be associated with NREM sleep. Such behaviors have been classified as variants of somnambulism or confusional arousals.[25] The behaviors vary in complexity from simple exposure to penetration and can include adult and child victims.[2,26] A well-known example of a sexsomnia-based defense to rape is the 2003 Canadian case of Jan Luedecke. Although the defense's facts were tainted by the defendant's being drunk prior to falling asleep beside the victim, Luedecke's clinical profile was compatible with sexsomnia. He was later acquitted, affirmed on appeal in 2008.[27,28]

Criminal cases implicating sexual behavior during sleep are a medicolegal conundrum: Was the actor awake or asleep? In Canadian jurisprudence, this behavior falls under automatism, described as "the state of a person who, though capable of action, is not conscious of what he is doing . . . in other words, an unconscious involuntary action."[29] The controversial nature of these cases is illustrated by the 2008 acquittal of Jan Luedecke in Ontario. Luedecke, a landscaper with a history of somnambulism as a child and adult, attended a party at which he drank alcohol to intoxication and fell asleep next to a woman who later accused him of rape. During the trial, he presented a "noninsane automatism" defense based on his claim that he suffered from sexsomnia. The court accepted Luedecke's defense based on a multitude of factors, including his history of somnambulism, precipitating factors (alcohol consumption and sleep deprivation), his PSG test results, the fact that this was his first criminal offense, and his cooperation with officials at

the time of the event. To the court's discredit, the extent to which drugs and alcohol played a role in his behavior was one of the factors that led to his acquittal. The defense's argument that the excessive consumption of alcohol can induce somnambulism is a controversial claim.[30] Also, the court was aware that Luedecke was wearing a condom during the incident, which could have served as an indicator of conscious awareness of his actions and the potential consequences of unprotected sex. Worse, there was no rebuttal expert testimony from the Crown; the court rejected the Crown's proposed expert on the basis of qualifications. In a subsequent Canadian case,[31] the sexsomnia defense was rejected after a defense expert provided unscientific opinions regarding the relationship between alcohol and sleepwalking, and credible rebuttal expert testimony was presented by the Crown.[32] Following the expert testimony in that case, the defendant abandoned his sexsomnia claim and then argued that the sex was consensual.

In the United States, several cases have involved the sexsomnia defense, although the judgments rarely favor the defense. In 2001, Adam Kieczykowski was charged with entering dormitory rooms at the University of Massachusetts without permission and inappropriately touching a woman.[33] He had a significant personal and family history of sleepwalking and had no recollection of the events. In addition to his defense claims, several of the victims were unable to identify Kieczykowski as the attacker, resulting in his acquittal.[34] In 2005, Richard Anderson of Chelmsford, Massachusetts, was accused of sexually molesting two adolescent girls on two different occasions.[35] At the grand jury hearing, one of the girls testified that he had to be sleeping during the event because he was snoring. Anderson pled guilty to lesser charges of assault and battery and served 3 years' probation, which included court-ordered sex-offender counseling. Here, *unconsciousness* negated the more severe charges and permitted plea negotiation.

Hypersomnolence and Driving

Disorders of excessive sleepiness (hypersomnolence) can be associated with unlawful behavior. In the latter case, an individual, often a driver, is involved in an accident in which someone is injured or killed.[36] Because a drowsy driver makes a conscious decision, while awake, to operate a motor vehicle, culpability would attach to the driver if, upon falling asleep at the wheel, harm comes to another person or property. This would tend to be true even in narcolepsy, where there may not be warning of a sleep attack, but the driver should have known not to drive and disregarded a risk of harm (recklessness).[36] Sleep physicians should always recommend that patients with narcolepsy not drive, except when it is documented that the condition has entirely abated. The Narcolepsy Network provides a state-by-state list of driving laws that may govern self- and physician-reported conditions.[37]

Sleep-driving is a phenomenon most likely related to the use of short-acting hypnotic medications, such as zolpidem.[38] In a New Jersey case involving use of alcohol and zolpidem in 2006, the driver was not legally intoxicated from alcohol. The court found that, since the driver had no knowledge of the possibility of sleep-driving, she was under involuntary intoxication (patient did not expect this type of interaction between zolpidem and alcohol) and therefore innocent.[39] Since 2007, however, when the US Food and Drug Administration issued a package-insert warning about odd behaviors associated with these medications, it has been difficult for affected drivers to claim ignorance of their effects (pathological/involuntary intoxication or unknown behavioral toxicity).[8pp203–211, 38,40] These cases are important for practitioners treating insomnia in instances where a patient wishes to attribute a driving problem to drug effects. It is difficult for patients to evade all responsibility for driving under the influence of a substance.

In addition to civil actions (personal injury lawsuits for negligence), a driver may be subject to criminal penalties for failure to use adequate precautions when the driver knew or should have known not to drive. Such situations can be associated with conditions ranging from simple sleep deprivation (insomnia, shift work, jetlag) to the effects of obstructive sleep apnea to narcolepsy. It would be negligent per se for a person to drive under the influence of sedating medications. Expert testimony would not be required except in the rare case of an unknown or unforeseeable reaction to a prescribed medication. Similarly, in already diagnosed conditions, such as obstructive sleep apnea and narcolepsy, the burden would tend to fall on the driver, especially if he or she has been counseled not to do so.

There is an intriguing question as to whether sleep clinicians have a reporting requirement to have driving privileges revoked when there is a public hazard, as is seen in epilepsy. The short answer is yes, clearly when there is a reporting requirement,[37] but also if local state law supports physician liability for acts committed by impaired patients.[2] Aside from the obvious standard of practice to counsel patients, reporting requirements tend to vary among jurisdictions. Accordingly, clinicians are advised to consult with authorities on this matter. In jurisdictions requiring physicians to report continued driving, against medical advice, the state motor vehicle bureau may have to be contacted. Box 29.2 suggests a risk-management approach to counseling patients.

BOX 29.2.   COUNSELING PATIENTS WITH EXCESSIVE SLEEPINESS ABOUT DRIVING

For patients with conditions such as sleep deprivation, obstructive sleep apnea, and narcolepsy, there is a risk of harm to self, others, and property from driving.

For risk-management purposes, keep the following in mind:

- State laws may bar persons with impairing conditions from driving; not all conditions are named.[37]
- All sleep disorder patients must be questioned about driving ability and counseled, regardless of whether the duty to report falls on the clinician or patient.
- All efforts to obtain accurate information must be documented in the clinical record.
- In states requiring self-reporting, the patient should be encouraged to do so.
- In states requiring clinician reporting, failure to report will increase liability, under the legal theory of duty to prevent harm to third parties.

THE EXPERT REPORT AND TESTIMONY

Expert witnesses, that is, professionals permitted to give opinions under the rules of evidence, are usually required to present their findings in written form. Open to scrutiny by all parties, such reports may be the most important element of the expert's role. A great deal has been written about expert reports as they apply to an array of medicolegal applications.[41] However, there are several generic elements of reports, summarized here.

The essential structure of the expert report contains (a) a statement of the question posed to the expert; for example, What was the defendant's state of mind at the time of the incident?; (b) listing of all activities and materials used in conducting the assessment; (c) detailed clinical and laboratory findings that are relevant to the question; and (d) the expert's opinion, based on the findings, that speaks to the question before the court Expert opinions are expressed within reasonable scientific certainty (or a local phrasing of the standard). Scientific studies, such as PSG, EEG, or home-based telemetry, must be made available to all parties. It is also essential that the expert provide a personal assessment of the data and then explain how it relates to the matter before the court. Opinions must not only be stated, but backed up with the bases for them. An expert will not be admitted with a "net opinion" such as, "I examined the defendant and conclude that she was asleep at the time of the crime."

Whereas in an adversarial system such as America's, expert witnesses provide testimony for the defense or the prosecution, the following should be borne in mind. First, there is no obligation, when assessing a criminal defendant, to arrive at opinions that are in keeping with the retaining attorney's point of view. If the opinion sought by defense counsel does not suit the defense position, no report is required. If there is a defense report and the prosecution asks for an independent opinion, the prosecution expert may agree wholly, in part, or not at all with the other side. In nations using expert advice in a nonadversarial schema, the only obligation is to be objective and transparent. Second, it is important to remember that experts must not be overly attached to their opinions, an attitude requiring flexibility, for example, in the face of facts not considered. And third, as previously noted, expert witnesses may be influential and necessary, but they do not decide the ultimate issue before the court: guilt or innocence.

Most criminal cases do not go to trial. Instead, they are settled by plea negotiation, whereby the defendant accepts criminal responsibility, usually in exchange for a reduced penalty. However, a guilty plea may result in a criminal record and associated stigma. In cases involving sleep-related events, such as violent or sexual acts, if experts can establish that the defendant was not fully conscious at the time in question, the charges may be resolved due to the preclusion of *actus reus*. However, prosecutors may be reluctant to drop the charges, especially when there is a victim of sexual assault, and judges may prefer to have the question of culpability addressed by a jury, which will have heard all the evidence. Then the case can be tried, and expert testimony, which can be polarized, becomes salient. The application of expert testimony to matters involving parasomnias and other phenomena is too large a topic for this chapter but can be found elsewhere.[12] For present purposes, the following illustrations of trials involving parasomnia defenses and expert testimony are intended to convey a sense of how experts operate in court. In an Arizona case, Scott Falater was charged with the murder of his wife of 20 years, Yarmilla. This case is remarkable for the presence of an eyewitness to most of the episode and the testimony of five sleep experts (Box 29.3).

Mr. Falater's case was one in which evidence of behavior—too complex to be credibly explained as somnambulistic—overwhelmed the defense. Although there were many pieces of evidence that strongly argued against sleepwalking, two in particular were most important. First, there has never been a documented episode of two attacks by the same sleepwalking individual separated by 20 minutes or so. Second, it is generally accepted that sleepwalkers do not seek out their victims; rather, the victim's encounter with the sleepwalker accidentally provokes defensive aggression. This might apply to the first episode of violence with the knife, although 44 stabs would seem to indicate rage, not found in sleepwalking. However, the second episode of drowning is not consistent; the victim had stopped moving and could not have provoked the second attack. Additionally, evidence concealment—hiding evidence in car trunk—strongly suggests conscious awareness of what had happened and a guilty mind.

CONCLUSIONS

As we learn more about the pathophysiology and clinical presentations of the parasomnias, both

---

BOX 29.3.   COMPLEX BEHAVIOR ATTRIBUTED TO SOMNAMBULISM

On January 16, 1997, the defendant and victim were at home. Around 9 PM, Mr. Falater went outside to check on the faulty pool pump. He attempted to repair it but did not finish due to the late hour. Around 10 PM, Mr. Falater went upstairs to bed, leaving his wife downstairs; the children had already gone to sleep. Mr. Falater later reported he had changed into his pajamas. Minutes later, the Falaters' next-door neighbor heard screaming and moaning. He walked to the back of his yard and looked over the cinderblock wall into the Falaters' property, where he saw a body near the pool. The body was still moving, rolled over, arms and legs moved and then was motionless.

The prosecution's evidence indicated the following: Mr. Falater got out bed, but it was not known if he had slept. He got dressed, left the bedroom, descended the stairs, located and retrieved a knife, a mouthpiece, and a flashlight. Exiting via the patio or garage door, he moved toward the pool pump and used the flash light—it was later found turned on. It was assumed that Yarmilla awakened, discovered her husband was not in the house and went outside looking for him. She approached the same pool area where her body was seen by the next-door neighbor. This portion of the incident was not observed. However, the coroner reported she was stabbed 44 times, including 12 defensive wounds to her hands. Many details of Mr. Falater's behavior were incriminating: Once outside again, he walked directly to his wife's body. Then, in an organized manner, he moved the body toward the swimming pool. First, he grabbed her feet and moved them toward the pool and then grabbed her arms and moved then toward the pool. He repeated this until the body was on the edge of the pool, and then pushed her in. He then came over to the edge of the pool and pushed her head under the water. He left the pool area and walked back to the garage and entered. He opened the trunk of his car, opened the black leaf back and placed the wet black work gloves inside—as these were later found by the police. Until this happened, the next-door neighbor was not sure what was happening. But now he re-entered his house and called 911. The police arrived and arrested Mr. Falater as he came down the stairs. The police determined that victim's wedding ring was missing and has never been found.

The defense presented a sleepwalking violence case, retaining two well-known sleep specialists. The prosecution also retained two well-known sleep specialists. The overall strategies of the defense and prosecution were quite different. The defense focused on circumstantial evidence: prior sleep deprivation, situational stress, amnesia, no apparent motivation, and apparently good relations prior to the episode. The prosecution focused on the events of that episode. It is quite rare have an eyewitness to an alleged sleepwalker's behaviors. These can be compared to what is known about the sleepwalker's cognitive abilities. In this case, the jury found these behaviors to be too complicated and after 6 hours of deliberation found him guilty. He was sentenced to natural life in prison. All subsequent appeals have failed.

---

clinicians and expert witnesses will likely benefit from understanding the boundaries of consciousness and sleep states. At present, science has much to offer to criminal justice, as long as we are modest in our claims and evaluate all cases thoroughly and objectively. Knowing about the range of REM and NREM disorders and their presentations will enable forensic professionals to distinguish legitimate from malingered cases. However, criminal matters require accurate, reliable, relevant, honest, and helpful expert testimony. Care must be taken not to prejudice jurors with scientific findings of dubious quality. Since all postarrest PSG studies reflect only present tendencies, at best, expert witnesses must be circumspect in drawing inferences about a state of consciousness during the commission of a crime. When inferences can be drawn, evidence should not be overstated but, rather, stated within reasonable scientific certainty. It is attorneys' role to argue the evidence one way or the other and the judge or jury's to draw ultimate conclusions regarding culpability from the evidence and arguments.

KEY CLINICAL PEARLS

- A sleeping person is generally not liable for harm to others.
- Somnambulism can be raised as a defense but tends to fail when the behavior is complex.
- Malingering should be in the differential diagnosis of persons raising a somnambulism defense.
- Descriptions of behavior and observations by others tend to be more meaningful than PSG results.
- There may be professional liability for failing to prevent a sleep-impaired patient from driving.

SELF-ASSESSMENT QUESTIONS

1. The best reason judges act as "gatekeepers" in deciding whether an expert should testify is
a. they know who gives the best testimony.
b. to determine the facts of the case.
c. to eliminate certain schools of thought in the case.
d. to ensure that the testimony is helpful to the jury, not prejudicial.
e. they want to engineer the outcome.

Answer: d

2. The standard by which expert witnesses state opinions in court is
a. reasonable scientific certainty.
b. beyond a reasonable doubt.
c. clear and convincing evidence.
d. None of the above
e. a, b, and c (they are all the same)

Answer: a

3. Which is true about harm caused by a sleepwalker?
a. The sleepwalker had a grudge against the victim.
b. Sleepwalkers do not seek out their victims.
c. It is usually accompanied by verbal threats.
d. The sleepwalker has a different version of events afterwards.
e. The sleepwalker makes an effort to conceal the harmful behavior.

Answer: b

4. The work-up for disorders of arousal should include
a. interviewing the bed partner.
b. personal and family history of sleep disorders.
c. physical, neurological, and PSG assessments.
d. substance use history.
e. All of the above

Answer: e

5. Sleep-related violence is most often associated with
a. hypnogogic hallucinations.
b. hypnopompic hallucinations.
c. slow-wave NREM sleep.
d. REM sleep.
e. intoxication.

Answer: c

REFERENCES

1. AAPL Task Force to revise the Guideline on Forensic Psychiatric Evaluation of Defendants Raising the Insanity Defense: AAPL practice guideline for forensic psychiatric evaluation of defendants raising the insanity defense. J Am Acad Psychiatry Law. 2014;42(4 Suppl):S1–S76.
2. Doghramji K, Bertoglia SM, Watson C. Forensic aspects of the parasomnias. In Kothare SV, Ivanenko A, eds. Parasomnias. New York: Springer; 2012:463–477. doi:10.1007/978-1-4614-7627-6_31.
3. Malone DM, Zwier P. Expert Rules. 3rd ed. Boulder, CO: National Institute for Trial Advocacy; 2012. Appendix A: Selected federal rules of evidence.
4. Daubert v. Merrell Dow Pharmaceuticals, Inc. 509 U.S. 579 (1993)
5. American Psychiatric Association. Diagnostic and Statistical Manual of Mental Disorders. 5th ed. Washington, DC: American Psychiatric Association; 2013.
6. American Academy of Sleep Medicine. International Classification of Sleep Disorders. 3rd ed. Darien, IL: American Academy of Sleep Medicine; 2014.
7. Weiss KJ, del Busto E. Early American jurisprudence of sleep violence. Sleep Clin. 2011;6(4):469–482. doi:10.1016/j.jsmc.2011.08.005.
8. Pressman MR. Sleepwalking, Criminal Behavior, and Reliable Scientific Evidence. Washington, DC: American Psychological Association; 2018.
9. Anonymous. Trial of Albert John Tirrell, for the murder of Mary Ann Bickford. Nat Pol Gaz. 1846 Apr 4;1(30):852.
10. Weeks JEP. Trial of Albert John Tirrell for the murder of Mary Ann Bickford. Boston: Boston Daily Times, 1846.

11. Ray I. A Treatise on the Medical Jurisprudence of Insanity. Boston, MA: Little & Brown; 1838: 398–400.
12. Weiss KJ, Watson C, eds. Psychiatric Expert Testimony: Emerging Applications. New York: Oxford University Press; 2015.
13. Fain v. Commonwealth, 78 Ky. 183 (1879).
14. People v. Sedeno, 518 P.2d 913 (Cal. 1974).
15. McClain v. Indiana, 678 N.E.2d 104 (Ind. 1997).
16. Cramer-Bornemann MA, Mahowald MW. Sleep forensics. In: Kryger MH, Roth T, Dement WC, eds. Principles and Practice of Sleep Medicine. 5th ed. St. Louis, MO: Elsevier Saunders; 2011: 725–737
17. Guilleminault C, Moscovitch A, Yuen K, Poyares D. Atypical sexual behavior during sleep. Psychosomatic Med. 2002; 64:328–336
18. Bonkalo A. Impulsive acts and confusional states during incomplete arousal from sleep: criminological and forensic implications. Psychiatric Q. 1974;48:400–409. doi:10.1007/BF01562162.
19. Cartwright R. Sleepwalking violence: a sleep disorder, a legal dilemma, and a psychological challenge. Am J Psychiatry. 161(7):1149–1158;2004.
20. Tibbs v. Commonwealth, 128 S.W. 871 (Ky. 1910).
21. Bradley v. State, 277 S.W. 147 (Tex. Crim. App. 1925).
22. State v. Caddell, 215 S.E.2d 348 (NC 1975).
23. Fulcher v. State, 633 P.2d 142 (Wy. 1981).
24. McClain v. Indiana, 678 N.E.2d 104 (Ind. 1997).
25. Schenck CH, Arnulf I, Mahowald MW. Sleep and sex: what can go wrong? A review of the literature on sleep related disorders and abnormal sexual behaviors and experiences. Sleep. 30(6):683–702;2007. doi:10.1093/sleep/30.6.683.
26. Shapiro CM, Trajanovic NN, Federoff JP. Sexsomnia—a new parasomnia? Can J Psychiatry. 48(5):311–317;2003. doi:10.1177/070674370304800506.
27. Kari S. Ontario court upholds "sexsomnia" acquittal. Canada.com. http://www.canada.com/health/Ontario+court+upholds+sexsomnia+acquittal/292924/story.html. February 7, 2008. Accessed on November 5, 2018.
28. R. v. Luedecke, 2005 ONCJ 294.
29. Buchanan A. Sleepwalking and indecent exposure. Medicine, Science and the Law. 1991;31:38–40.
30. Pressman MR, Mahowald MW, Schenck CH, Cramer-Bornemann MA. Alcohol-induced sleepwalking or confusional arousal as a defense to criminal behavior: a review of scientific evidence, methods and forensic considerations. J Sleep Res. 2007;16:198–212.
31. R. v. Teepell (2009). Walkerton 05-543.
32. Makin K. Judge rejects "sexsomnia" defence." The Globe and Mail (Toronto). May 2, 2009.
33. Morgan R. Are you raping your wife in your sleep? Details. http://www.details.com/sex-relationships/marriage-and-kids/200604/are-you-raping-your-wife-in-your-sleep. April 2006. Accessed November 14, 2013.
34. Lindsay J. Man charged with child molestations. The Milford (Massachusetts) Daily News. http://www.milforddailynews.com/archive/x1612084296. March 26, 2005. Accessed July 1, 2011.
35. Schenck CH. Sleep: The Mysteries, the Problems, and the Solutions. New York: Avery; 2007.
36. Venkateshiah SB, Hoque R, DelRosso LM, Collop NA. Legal and regulatory aspects of sleep disorders. Sleep Med Clin. 2017;12:149–160. doi:10.1016/j.jsmc.2016.10.002.
37. Narcolepsy Network. Narcolepsy and Driving Laws. https://narcolepsynetwork.org/narcolepsy-drivinglaws/. Accessed February 6, 2019.
38. Pressman MR. Sleep driving: sleepwalking variant or misuse of z-drugs? Sleep Med Rev. 15(5):285–292;2011. doi:10.1016/j.smrv.2010.12.004.
39. Weiss KJ, del Busto E. Sleep-driving and pathological intoxication: saved by the FDA? Am J Foren Psychiatry. 31(1):5–15;2010.
40. Daley C, McNiel DE, Binder RL. "I did what?" zolpidem and the courts. J Am Acad Psychiatry Law 39(4):535–542;2011.
41. Buchanan A, M. Norko M., eds. The Psychiatric Report. Cambridge, UK: Cambridge University Press; 2011.

30

Eating Disorders

ANOOP NARAHARI, RAMAN BAWEJA, PIYUSH DAS, AND AMIT CHOPRA

INTRODUCTION

Eating behavior is regulated by a complex inter-play of factors including peripheral endocrine stimuli, central neurotransmitter systems, circadian rhythms and environmental cues [1]. Sleep and eating behavior are complimentary homeo-static functions as evident by shared involvement of hypothalamic neuropeptides (orexin/hypocretin) in the regulation of sleep, appetite and endocrine function [2]. Research evidence suggests significant association between sleep loss and alterations in nutritional and metabolism and, therefore, adequate sleep is fundamental for the nutritional balance of the body [3]. Short sleep duration, poor sleep quality, and later bedtimes are all associated with increased food intake, poor diet quality, and excess body weight [4]. Lack of adequate sleep has been shown to increase snacking, the number of meals consumed per day, and the preference for energy-rich foods. The proposed mechanisms that explain increased caloric consumption in persons with inadequate sleep include more time and opportunities for eating, psychological distress, greater sensitivity to food reward, disinhibited eating, more energy needed to sustain extended wakefulness, and changes in appetite hormones. Excess energy intake associated with inadequate sleep seems to be preferentially driven by hedonic rather than homeostatic factors [4].

Sleep duration has been linked to development of obesity and abnormal eating patterns in children and adults. Hicks and Rozette [5] compared eating patterns in short and longer-sleeping college students and noted that short sleepers were five times more likely to exhibit abnormal eating patterns than the longer-sleeping group. Wrzosek and colleagues [6] reported that insomnia was most strongly correlated with daily consumption of snack foods in a sample of obese persons requiring bariatric surgery ($n = 361$), whereas, depressive symptoms were strongly associated with both

eating in response to ≥3 specific emotions as well as with daily consumption of snack foods. The study participants had to choose from emotions including being happy, lonely, depressed, bored, sad, angry, stressed, frightened, love, surprised, upset, and anxious. In a Dutch study ($n = 574$), as compared to those without eating disorder, the individuals screened positive for eating disorders ($n = 67$) reported significantly higher symptoms suggestive of sleep apnea, insomnia, circadian rhythm disorders, and impairment of daytime functioning [7]. Lombardo and colleagues [8] reported that the persistence of poor sleep quality at follow-up directly predicts the severity of the eating disorder symptoms both directly and through the mediation of depression. The authors suggest that the treatment of eating disorders may benefit from addressing poor sleep quality since the presence and persistence of poor sleep quality increase the comorbidity and attrition to the standard treatment.

On the other hand, aberrant eating behaviors can lead to sleep disturbances. Bos and colleagues [9] conducted a prospective study to investigate if disordered eating behaviors predicted the development of sleep disturbances. The authors reported that the global disordered eating behaviors at baseline predicted sleep disturbances including difficulty with sleep initiation and sleep maintenance at 1 and 3 year follow-up. It has been shown that obese women with binge eating (BE) report worse insomnia as compared to obese women without BE. Yeh and Brown [10] surveyed 330 participants about their height and weight, recent sleep quality, and recent experiences of BE and nighttime eating. Using multiple regression analyses, the authors reported that high body mass index (BMI) was related to shorter sleep duration, increased sleep latency, use of sleeping medications, and worse BE, whereas poor sleep quality was related to worse night-eating, even after controlling for depression and demographic factors. Using mediational analyses, BE was shown to partly mediate the relationship between worse sleep quality to higher body mass index (BMI), whereas night eating mediated the reverse association between high BMI to sleep quality.

Finally, sleep disturbances have been implicated in suicidal behaviors in patients with eating disorders. In a study determining the correlates of suicidal behavior in children with eating disorders ($n = 90$), including bulimia and anorexia nervosa (AN), the authors reported that suicidal ideation was more prevalent in children with bulimia nervosa (BN; 43%) as compared to children with AN (20%). Among children expressing suicidal ideation, all children with BN attempted suicide as compared to only 3% of children with AN who attempted suicide. The authors found externalizing behavior problems and sleep disturbances as correlates of "suicidal ideation." BN, self-induced vomiting, nightmares, and physical or sexual abuse were noted as correlates of "suicide attempts" [11].

It is beyond doubt that untreated sleep disturbances in patients with eating disorders are associated with significant morbidity and severe prognostic implications, including higher risk of suicide, and there is an imminent need to synthesize the current literature to further our understanding on this topic. AN and BN are two major groups of eating disorders. Besides these two groups, two additional entities are described in this chapter: Night eating syndrome (NES) and BE disorder (BED). This chapter focuses on pathophysiology, clinical approach, assessment, and management of sleep disturbances in patients with eating disorders. Sleep-related eating disorder (SRED), which is classified as a parasomnia disorder with a significant overlap of eating disorder, has also been discussed in detail in this chapter.

PATHOPHYSIOLOGY
In this section, we highlight the effects of diet on sleep and also outline the shared pathophysiological mechanisms that explain comorbidity of sleep and circadian rhythm dysfunction in eating disorders.

Nutrients
There is adequate research evidence showing sleep can influence dietary choices; however, research evidence assessing the impact of diet and nutrients on sleep is scarce. Sleep can be influenced by macronutrients and micronutrients in diet

via modulating neurotransmitters like serotonin, melatonin, GABA, adenosine, and nitric oxide. Carbohydrates, proteins, and fats can influence the quality of sleep by modulating the ratio of rapid eye movement (REM) and non-REM sleep. Research shows that that a high-carbohydrate and low-fat meal reduces deep slow-wave sleep (SWS; non-REM sleep) and increases the proportion of REM sleep, as compared to low-carbohydrate and high fat diet [12]. In a study ($n = 12$), Afaghi et al. [13] noticed shortened sleep onset latency by approximately 10 minutes after a carbohydrate-rich evening meal with a high glycemic index compared with a low-index meal, suggesting a difference between the variety of carbohydrates. Cholecystokinin (CCK) is secreted in response to dietary fats and is abundantly distributed in the brain [14]. Wells et al. [15] noticed that postprandial release of CCK induces sleepiness in healthy adult volunteers 2 to 3 hours after a high-fat, low-carbohydrate meal. In a study ($n = 14$), authors observed that diet very low in carbohydrates and rich in fat increased the proportion of deep SWS and reduced the percentage of REM sleep recorded by polysomnography (PSG) when compared to control diet high in carbohydrates and low in fat [16].

Similarly, micronutrients like magnesium, B vitamins, and tryptophan precursors influence the quality of sleep and sleep–wake rhythm by promoting the synthesis of melatonin and serotonin. The tranquilizing effect of cow's milk is due to α-Lactalbumin, a milk protein, which is a good source of tryptophan [17]. Magnesium acts as γ-aminobutyric acid (GABA) agonist and stimulates serotonin N-acetyltransferase activity, the key enzyme in melatonin synthesis. Vitamin B_6/pyridoxine is required for the synthesis of serotonin from tryptophan. In summary, foods impacting the availability of tryptophan, as well as the synthesis of serotonin and melatonin, may help promote sleep; however, the clinical relevance of this association needs further exploration [17].

Hormones
Evidence suggests a possibility that central nervous system (CNS) neuropeptide alterations may contribute to dysregulated secretion of the gonadal hormones, cortisol, thyroid hormones, and growth hormone (GH) in the eating disorders. However, most of the neuroendocrine and neuropeptide alterations, which are apparent during symptomatic episodes of AN and BN tend to normalize after recovery [18]. This suggests that

most of the CNS neuropeptide disturbances are consequences rather than causes of malnutrition, weight loss and/or altered meal patterns [18]. Orexins, leptin, and ghrelin have an important role in sleep–neuroendocrine interplay in terms of appetite regulation and their alterations in eating disorders will be discussed here.

Orexin (Hypocretin) System

Orexin-A and orexin-B (hypocretin-1 and hypocretin-2) are neuropeptides produced by a small group of neurons in the lateral hypothalamic and perifornical areas, the brain regions implicated in the control of mammalian feeding behavior [2]. Orexin neurons project throughout the CNS and play an important role in the control of feeding, maintenance of wakefulness, neuroendocrine homeostasis, and autonomic regulation [2]. Orexin neuropeptides play a critical role in the maintenance of wakefulness by activating two distinct receptors, the orexin-1 (OX1R) and the orexin-2 (OX2R) receptor that are widely distributed throughout the brain [19]. Orexin neurons are sensitive to both glucose and leptin (appetite suppressing hormone); elevated circulating glucose levels lead to reduced firing of orexin neurons, suggesting that orexins are part of a negative feedback loop [20], and leptin inhibits food intake by suppressing orexin neuronal activity [21].

Orexin stimulates both food intake and willingness to work for palatable food. Additionally, orexin neurons are activated during the anticipation of food reward and tend to promote a number of phenomena involved in successful foraging including food-anticipatory locomotor behavior, olfactory sensitivity, visual attention, spatial memory, and mastication [22]. Conversely, targeted disruption of the orexin gene produces excessive daytime sleepiness (EDS), cataplexy, and other pathological manifestations of the intrusion of REM sleep-related features into wakefulness; finally, orexin knockout mice are hypophagic suggesting a role of orexins in modulating energy metabolism [2]. Piccoli and [23] colleagues examined the efficacy of orexin receptor antagonists (OX1R, OX2R, and OX1/OX2R) in suppressing BE in rat model and found OX1R antagonists selectively reduced BE for highly palatable food without affecting standard food pellet intake and without inducing sleep. The authors suggested a major role of OX1R mechanisms in BE with the possibility that selective antagonism at OX1R could represent a novel pharmacological

treatment for BE and other eating disorders with a compulsive component [23].

In a Spanish study [24], comparing orexin levels in patients with AN (*n* = 48) and healthy controls (*n* = 98), the plasma concentration of orexin-A levels did not significantly differ between the AN and control groups. However, among women with AN, higher orexin-A concentrations correlated with poorer sleep quality, sleep efficiency, and total sleep quality. A possible hypothesis is that AN patients may have greater sleep impairment due to the dysregulation of orexin receptors secondary to chronic malnutrition. In patients with AN, orexin-A concentrations have been associated with greater sleep disturbances, poor sleep efficiency, and poorer overall sleep quality. Additionally, both elevated orexin-A concentrations and inadequate sleep predicted poorer treatment outcomes in AN [24].

Leptin

Leptin is secreted by adipocytes in proportion to the fat mass and acts on the hypothalamic regions of the brain, which control eating behavior, thus playing a significant role in maintaining body's metabolism. Leptin decreases food intake and increases energy expenditure by affecting the balance between orexigenic and anorexigenic hypothalamic pathways. During sleep, leptin increases to suppress the appetite, whereas sleep restriction results in decreased levels of leptin thus leading to increased hunger and appetite [25]. Decreased leptin is a key endocrine abnormality in AN due to loss of fat mass, and several symptoms in acute AN are related to the low circulating leptin levels including amenorrhea and semi-starvation-induced hyperactivity [26]. Hypoleptinemia is associated with downregulation of hypothalamic–pituitary–gonadal and thyroid axes and upregulation of the hypothalamic–pituitary–adrenal (HPA) axis [26]. During therapeutically induced weight gain, leptin levels can intermittently increase above normal concentrations in patients with AN [26]. Monteleone and colleagues [27] reported that BN patients with a significantly longer duration of the illness and a significantly higher number of daily BE/purging episodes had hypoleptinemia despite no significant modifications in their body weight.

Ghrelin

Ghrelin, a gastric-derived natural ligand of the GH secretagogue (GHS) receptor, is predominantly secreted by stomach and stimulates appetite thus triggering a positive energy balance [28]. In a study of 10 healthy male volunteers, authors measured plasma levels of ghrelin, cortisol, and human GH (hGH) during two experimental sessions of 24 hours each: once when the subjects were allowed to sleep between 11:00 PM and 7:00 AM and once when they were kept awake throughout the night. The authors found that nocturnal increase in ghrelin levels was more likely to be caused by sleep-associated processes rather than by circadian influences [29]. It is believed that ghrelin stimulates the activity of the HPA axis, thus affecting concentrations of GH and cortisol, both of which are involved in sleep regulation [30]. The endocrine effects of ghrelin may be age- and sex-dependent. Ghrelin increases slow-sleep wave and stage 2 sleep and decreases stage 1 sleep and REM sleep in elderly men but does not affect sleep in elderly women [31].

Ghrelin secretion is negatively modulated by food intake as fasting ghrelin levels are reduced in obesity, whereas ghrelin levels are elevated in AN, and ghrelin levels are restored by weight recovery in patients with AN. Chronic elevation of circulating ghrelin levels in AN has been associated with desensitization of the GHS receptor and reduction in the GH response to ghrelin [32]. Evidence from multiple studies reflects that individuals with AN have higher levels of fasting plasma ghrelin as compared to normal weight (NW) healthy controls [33–35]. Tolle and colleagues [36] reported that, as compared to NW and constitutionally thin women, individuals with AN have increased morning fasting plasma ghrelin concentrations in AN, which remained higher during rest of the day (measured every 4 hours in a 24-hour period), and these levels normalized after renutrition. The authors suggested that ghrelin levels in AN, in addition to being body weight-dependent, are also affected by acute nutritional status, and altered levels of ghrelin may be a consequence of disordered eating rather than a cause for AN [36].

The results of ghrelin levels in individuals with BN are mixed; however, Troisi and colleagues [37] found that women with AN had significantly higher fasting plasma ghrelin level than BN, BED, and control women. The authors reported that ghrelin concentrations of women with BE and purging behavior were significantly lower than those of women with AN, restricting type, and there was a negative relation between the frequency and severity of BE and purging behavior and ghrelin concentrations. The results of this study did not confirm the prior hypothesis that

ghrelin concentrations are higher in patients with binge-eating/purging forms of eating disorders. The authors suggested that, in women with eating disorders, ghrelin concentrations best reflect nutritional status rather than specific patterns of disordered eating behavior [37].

Endocannabinoid System

Endocannabinoids (ECS) are signaling molecules derived from long-chain fatty acids that display significant affinity to the cannabinoid (CB) receptors including CB1 and CB2 receptors [38, 39]. ECS is constituted by ECS together with their receptors and enzymes involved in synthesis and breakdown. ECS play an important role in a wide variety of biological processes, and there appears to be mounting evidence to suggest that ECS plays a central role in the modulation of both homeostatic and hedonic elements of appetite and food intake [38]. It has been reported that plasma and tissue concentrations of ECS and related lipid-derived signaling molecules are influenced by factors such as food intake, dietary pattern, and body weight [40, 41]. In humans, plasma levels show a circadian rhythm [42] and several lines of evidence suggest that obese persons have higher plasma levels of ECS as compared with lean individuals [41–44]. The 2-arachidonoylglycerol (2-AG) is an endogenous agonist of the CB1 receptor, which is widely expressed in the brain, including in reward centers, and in metabolic organs. Activation of CB1 receptor stimulates food intake and lipogenesis [45]. Sleep restriction has been associated with an increase in the peak and amplitude of the 24-hour daily rhythm in circulating concentrations of a key ECS 2-AG and its structural analogue, 2-oleoylglycerol (2-OG), without changes in the 24-hour mean levels [46]. Enhanced activity in the brain areas associated with reward in response to food stimuli, especially unhealthy foods, has been reported after sleep deprivation [47, 48].

Sleep Duration

In a prospective cohort study ($n = 14,800$), the authors reported a dose–response association between cumulative exposure to short sleep throughout adolescence and early adulthood and obesity outcomes. As compared to study participants with no instances of short sleep, those who reported short sleep duration at different points of 15-year study follow-up were approximately 1.5 times more likely to be obese and have an elevated waist circumference [49]. Sleep has an inhibitory effect on ghrelin release, which is consistent with the association of sleep and fasting [50]. On the other hand, sleep deprivation has been associated with a decrease in leptin, an appetite-suppressing hormone, and an accompanying increase in ghrelin, an appetite-stimulating hormone, which promotes continued consumption of food [50, 51]. These changes in leptin and ghrelin associated with short sleep duration likely contribute to the increased appetite and possibly the increased BMI [51].

Circadian Rhythm Abnormalities

Circadian system orchestrates metabolism in daily 24-hour cycle by anticipating recurring feeding–fasting cycles to increase metabolic efficiency [52]. In humans, circadian rhythms regulate glucose, insulin, glucose tolerance, lipid levels, energy expenditure, and appetite. Earlier in the daytime is optimal for food intake as several of these rhythms peak in the biological morning or around noon [52]. Circadian misalignment negatively impacts energy balance and increases the risk of weight gain in persons doing shift work [49]. Additionally, disturbances of the circadian variation in composition of the gut microbiome may be involved in the increased risk of obesity associated with insufficient sleep and circadian misalignment [49]. Finally, disturbances of sleep and circadian rhythms in children and young adults are considered to be risk factors for the development of lifelong obesity [49].

CLINICAL APPROACH

Sleep disturbance has been reported to be amongst the three most common reasons for initial psychiatric consultation in patients with eating disorders, in additional to eating/weight problems and emotional problems [53]. In this section, we outline the clinical assessment of nocturnal eating behaviors in terms of clinical features, psychiatric and sleep-related comorbidities, and finally the subjective and objective assessment methods for evaluation of nocturnal eating behaviors. In addition, we also focus on the assessment of key sleep disturbances associated with daytime eating disorders.

The nocturnal disordered eating behaviors are mainly categorized as NES and SRED. NES can be distinguished from SRED by complete awareness of nocturnal eating episodes in NES. SRED is characterized by recurrent episodes of eating after a partial arousal from sleep with partial or complete amnesia of eating [54]. According to the *Diagnostic and Statistical Manual of Mental Disorders* (fifth edition; DSM-5 classification), sleep-related eating is considered a variant of somnambulism, a parasomnia disorder; however, according to the *International Classification of Sleep Disorders* (third edition; ICSD-3) classification, it is considered as a separate parasomnia disorder, which is distinct from somnambulism. Some authors argue that NES and SRED represent the two ends of the spectrum of nocturnal eating behaviors and not two separate diagnostic categories. Moreover, both these conditions may respond successfully to pharmacological treatments such as topiramate [55].

Presence of nocturnal eating behaviors can lead to serious outcomes including weight gain, obesity, metabolic syndrome, and potential sleep-related injury in patients with SRED. These patients can accidentally harm themselves in the pursuit of food and by ingesting inedible and potentially dangerous foods. Despite the high prevalence and potentially serious consequences, the nocturnal eating behaviors are underreported by patients partly because of episodic nature of symptoms and due to lack of awareness of potentially serious consequences. Hence, clinicians should have high suspicion for nocturnal disordered eating behaviors. Both NES and SRED can coexist with eating disorders such as AN, BN, and BED. Therefore, evaluation of daytime eating disorders is recommended for a thorough assessment of patients with nocturnal eating behaviors, and vice-versa.

Screen for Comorbid Psychiatric Disorders

Eating disorders often coexist with other psychiatric disorders, most commonly affective illnesses and, particularly, major depressive disorder. Depressive disorder often develops simultaneously or following the onset of AN, with 75% to 85% of patients presenting for AN treatment having a lifetime prevalence of a major depressive episode [56]. Prevalence of affective disorders is increased in first- and second-degree relatives of eating disorder patients [57]. Antidepressant drugs have been shown to be effective in the treatment of eating disorders, particularly in BN. These findings, taken together, suggest a significant biological link between eating disorders and affective disorders.

Sleep disturbances in patients with eating disorders can be mediated by comorbid affective disorders such as major depression. Studies have shown that sleep disturbances (early morning awakening) and changes in sleep architecture are associated with severity of depressive symptoms [58]. Similarly, reduction in SWS among patients with AN has been associated with depressive symptoms [59]. Delvenne and colleagues [60] compared sleep electroencephalography (EEG) variables in adolescents with AN ($n = 11$), adolescents with depression ($n = 11$), and healthy controls ($n = 11$). The authors reported that in comparison with controls, those with AN showed less sleep efficiency, a higher length of awakenings, and less REM sleep. In addition, adolescents with AN differed from those with depression in terms of greater number and a higher length of awakenings [60]. These findings suggest that not all of the sleep problems among patients with eating disorder are mediated by comorbid depression.

Screen for Primary Sleep Disorders

Patients with eating disorders report a higher frequency of primary sleep disorders including sleep apnea, insomnia, and circadian rhythm disorders [7]. In a recent study among patients with AN ($n = 9$) and BN ($n = 14$), the authors reported that, as compared to controls, patients with eating disorders had significantly higher sleep disturbances including all types of insomnia (initial, middle, and terminal/late), daytime hypersomnolence, and parasomnias. The most commonly reported complaints were initial insomnia (56.5%), interrupted sleep (47.8%), daytime hypersomnolence (21.7%), and parasomnias (39%) [61]. Similar results were reported in another study with eating disorder patients ($n = 400$), where authors found that approximately 50% the patients, especially those with BE/purging subtypes reported sleep problems [62].

Olbrich and colleagues [63] examined the association between night eating, other forms of disordered eating, and obstructive sleep apnea (OSA). In a sample of 81 participants with OSA (20 women and 61 men; mean age 53.7 years), the authors found that 8.6% of the participants screened positive for NES. Additionally, 7.5% met criteria for daytime eating disorder. NES was significantly associated with diagnoses of depression, anxiety, and eating disorders along with impairment of mental quality of life (QOL) [63]. Restless legs syndrome (RLS), which causes fragmented sleep and the inability to stay in bed when awakened, may predispose individuals to nocturnal eating. Provini and colleagues [64] compared patients with RLS to healthy controls

in terms of eating disorder, obsessive-compulsive, depressive, poor subjective sleep quality, and EDS symptoms. The authors noted that, as compared with controls, RLS patients reported higher obsessive-compulsive symptoms and had greater nocturnal sleep disturbance and EDS. SRED was significantly more prevalent in RLS patients than controls (33% vs. 1%, $p < 0.001$). Medication use and higher obsessive-compulsive scores were more prevalent in RLS patients with SRED as compared to RLS patients without SRED [64]. Therefore, the clinicians are advised to conduct a comprehensive sleep assessment in individuals with nocturnal eating behaviors as the identification and management of primary sleep disorders, such as OSA and RLS, can lead to significant clinical improvements by reducing the number of arousals from sleep that may trigger nocturnal eating episodes.

Screen for Substance Use Disorders

Higher rates of substance use disorders were found among patients diagnosed with NES in psychiatric outpatients, as compared to those without NES [65]. In a similar study, the authors found a higher prevalence of nicotine dependence, in addition to depression and impulse control disorder, in psychiatric outpatients diagnosed with NES, as compared to those without NES [66]. Additionally, the combination of short sleep duration with disinhibited eating behavior has been associated with greater alcohol intake in adults [67]. Moreover, higher frequencies of BE and purging have been associated with higher frequencies of substance use in eating disorder patients [68]. Therefore, it is recommended to screen for coexisting substance use disorders in patients presenting with nocturnal eating behaviors.

Screen for Iatrogenic Causes

Psychotropic medications have been associated with complex sleep-related behaviors including SRED. Among psychotropic medications, sedative antidepressants (mirtazapine), sedative hypnotics (zolpidem), and atypical antipsychotics (quetiapine) have been associated with sleep related eating [69–73]. Komada and colleagues [74] reported that as compared to primary SRED, the clinical features of drug-induced SRED include a higher mean age of onset (40 years old in drug-induced SRED vs. 26 years old in primary SRED), significantly higher rate of patients who had total amnesia during most of their SRED episodes (75.0% vs

31.8%), significantly lower rate of comorbidity of NES (0% vs. 63.3%), and significantly lower rate of childhood history of sleepwalking (10.0% vs. 46.7%) [74].

Assessment

The Night Eating Questionnaire (NEQ) is a valid and an efficient measure to assess behavioral and psychological symptoms of NES [75]. Except for SRED, a combination of parasomnia and eating disorder, PSG study is not clinically warranted for further evaluation of sleep disturbances associated with other eating disorders. PSG can be very helpful to establish the diagnosis of idiopathic SRED and also identify comorbid sleep disorders such as OSA and periodic limb movement disorder (PLMD) that could lead to SRED episodes.

ANOREXIA NERVOSA

William Gull introduced the term "anorexia nervosa" in 1874. The female-to-male ratio is 18:1 in AN and 4:1 in BN. Among patients with AN, BE/purging type have more sleep disturbances and worse global sleep quality than AN patients with restricting type. A large retrospective study (N = 1,374) among patients with eating disorder in outpatient setting found that patients with BE/purging type AN experience more sleep disturbances than patients with restricting type [76]. Similarly, Kim and colleagues [62] also reported higher prevalence of sleep disturbances in AN—more in BE/purging type (70.8%) as compared to restricting type (15.8%). It has been shown that low-weight AN patients usually sleep less and are more restless especially during the last 4 hours of the night [77]. However, after weight gain, there was a significant increase in length of sleep and REM sleep in these patients. The authors suggested an association between various anabolic profiles and differing need for REM sleep [77].

Subjective Findings

In a study comparing AN patients with controls, the authors noted that the subjective sleep quality in severely underweight AN patients, as measured by the Pittsburgh Sleep Quality Index (PSQI), was generally poor. After weight restoration, patients reported significant improvement on all subscales of the subjective questionnaire [78]. In another study, Tanahashi and colleagues [76] compared patients with subtypes of AN (BE/purging type vs. restricting type) in terms of subjective sleep quality. The authors reported that AN patients with BE/purging type had worse global sleep quality and circadian rhythm disruption as compared to those with restricting type. Poor global sleep quality in patients with AN was associated with BE/purging type, vomiting, and duration of illness [76].

Objective Findings

Walsh and colleagues [79] found that patients with AN, mostly restrictive type, differed from NW patients with BN and healthy controls in terms of reduction of total sleep time and stage 1 of sleep [79]. Objective sleep studies using PSG have reported marked effects on sleep architecture among patients with an eating disorder (AN or BN) including significant lengthening of sleep latency and arousal index and reduction in sleep efficiency [61]. Another study showed increased sleep latency and reduced sleep efficiency in patients with AN, but no significant differences were noted in patients with BN as compared to controls [80].

In study of patients with AN (n = 6) and BN (n = 9) with no concomitant diagnosis of endogenous depression, the researchers did not find significant REM differences, such as shortened REM latency and increased REM density, between eating disorder patients and healthy control subjects. suggesting that REM sleep changes in patients with eating disorder are mediated by comorbid depression. Multiple studies have established that eating disorders are distinct from affective disorders in terms of sleep architectural changes. However, low-weight patients with AN did appear to have less SWS as compared to controls [80]. Reduced SWS has been noted to predict a longer time to recover from AN [78]. The authors proposed that this might be related to the changes in GH release in AN. Nobili and colleagues [82] found a positive correlation between BMI and slow-wave activity (SWA) in patients with AN and postulated that amount of SWA appears to be consistent with the neurobiological consequences of the malnutrition state [82].

Management

Weight restoration is the one of the most important steps in recovery among patients with AN. Previous studies have shown improvement in self-reported or subjective scores of sleep quality after weight restoration among patients with AN restricting type. El Ghoch and colleagues [83] assessed sleep patterns in female patients with AN, before and after weight restoration, by using an actigraph for objective sleep monitoring in female patients with AN ($n = 50$) and in healthy controls ($n = 25$). At baseline, patients with AN exhibited lower total sleep time and sleep onset latency than controls. The lower total sleep time was apparently associated with baseline BMI, duration of illness, and age. However, after weight restoration, total sleep time and sleep onset latency were similar to controls, despite the persistence of longer periods of wake after sleep onset. The authors reported that sleep disturbances including decreased total sleep time and sleep onset latency seem to be influenced by the duration and severity of malnutrition and appears to normalize with weight restoration [83]. However, in a different study using sleep questionnaires and PSG, only the subjective measures of sleep improved after weight restoration in patients with AN [78].

BULIMIA NERVOSA

For a long time, bulimic behavior was thought to be closely associated with AN and hence the terms "restricting anorexics" and "bulimic anorexics." Gerald Russell introduced the term "bulimia nervosa" and formulated specific diagnostic criteria, but also suggested this disorder to be a variant of AN [84]. A definite distinction between AN and BN was then proposed by the American Psychiatric Association in its third edition of *the Diagnostic and Statistical Manual of Mental Disorders*. BN is characterized by consuming an objectively large amount of food in a 2-hour period due to loss of control and coupled with inappropriate compensatory behaviors such as vomiting, laxative abuse, or excessive exercise to avoid weight gain. BE episodes and their subsequent compensatory behaviors must occur at least once per week for a period of 3 months for a diagnosis of BN. The nutritional status of patients with BN is heterogeneous from slightly underweight to obese.

Subjective Findings

Latzer and colleagues [85] compared sleep-wake patterns between patients with BN ($n = 29$) and healthy controls ($n = 18$) using self-report questionnaires and actigraphy for 1 week. The authors found that patients with BN, as compared to controls, reported significantly more sleep disturbances on subjective sleep questionnaires. Actigraphy results showed that patients with BN had a sleep onset and offset of 1 hour later, which may be related to BE–purging patterns during the day [85].

Objective Findings

Hudson and colleagues [86] examined sleep EEG characteristics of patients with BN ($n = 11$) and compared the findings with young females with major depression ($n = 44$) and young female healthy controls ($n = 20$). The authors noted that sleep EEGs of patients with BN were largely indistinguishable from those of the normal controls, except for a trend toward increased REM density in the first REM period among those with BN [86]. In contrast, those with major depression displayed marked sleep continuity disturbances with significantly increased REM intensity and REM density, as compared to healthy controls. Finally, no differences in any sleep EEG measures were observed between BN patients with and without major depression.

Management

There is a significant lack of evidence supporting the efficacy of conventional treatments, including psychotherapy and medications, on the sleep outcomes in patients with suffering from BN, and this clearly deserves further research. Comorbid primary sleep disorders such as OSA and parasomnias (nightmares) should be adequately recognized and treated for optimal sleep outcomes in patients with BN. Additionally, optimal treatment of comorbid psychiatric disorders including mood, anxiety, and substance use disorders in patients with BN is recommended to enhance sleep outcomes.

BINGE EATING DISORDER (BED)

BED is characterized by consuming an objectively large amount of food in a short period of time (≤ 2 hours) due to loss of control over eating but in the absence of compensatory behaviors. Individuals with BED often eat in the absence of hunger and typically experience significant psychological distress (i.e., guilt, shame) after BE episodes. BED is the most common eating disorders with a lifetime prevalence of 3.5% in women and 2.0% in men [87]. BED typically emerges in early adulthood [88] but may arise in adolescence [89] and persists beyond midlife [90]. Due to the absence of inappropriate compensatory behaviors, BED patients are overweight or obese, but persons of NW can also have BED. Individuals with severe obesity and those who are seeking obesity treatment are at a higher risk of BED [91, 92].

BED or BE behaviors have been associated with sleep disorders such as insomnia, hypersomnolence disorders, and OSA. In a study comparing adults with BED (*n* = 68) and no eating disorder (*n* = 78), the authors found that individuals with BED reported significantly higher insomnia symptoms, and this correlation was partially mediated by anxiety, whereas depression fully mediated the positive correlation between insomnia symptom severity and binge frequency in the BED group [93]. On the other hand, approximately one-fourth of the patients with narcolepsy/cataplexy (*n* = 60) were found to have clinical eating disorder suggestive of an incomplete form of BED, as compared to none of the controls (*n* = 120) [94]. In a Canadian retrospective study including bariatric surgery candidates (*n* = 1,099), the authors compared differences in psychopathology and QOL between four groups: OSA and BED, BED alone, OSA alone, and neither BED or OSA. The authors found that BE and depressive symptoms were significantly higher in patients with comorbid BED and OSA, as compared to patients with OSA alone or patients with no diagnosis of BED or OSA. Additionally, patients with comorbid BED and OSA had significantly lower physical and mental QOL as compared to patients with no diagnosis of BED or OSA [95]. These findings suggest that primary sleep disorders should be adequately assessed in patients with BED or BE behaviors.

In a study examining the psychiatric comorbidity of obese patients seeking bariatric surgery (*n* = 92), the authors used logistic regression to analyze associations between the presence of BED and the psychiatric comorbidity profiles [96]. The results showed that BED was significantly associated with two psychiatric comorbidity profiles: (a) bipolar and obsessive-compulsive disorder (odds ratio [OR] 7.7) and bipolar and panic disorder (OR 20.7). In a Swedish study, the authors analyzed longitudinal data to explore clinical characteristics at diagnosis, diagnostic flux, psychiatric comorbidity, and suicide attempts in individuals diagnosed BED (*n* = 850) [97]. The results showed that BED had considerable diagnostic flux with other eating disorders over time, and it carries significantly high psychiatric comorbidity burden with other eating disorders (OR 85.8, 95% confidence interval [CI] 61.6–119.4), major depressive disorder (OR 7.6, 95% CI: 6.2–9.3), bipolar disorder (OR 7.5, 95% CI 4.8–11.9), anxiety disorders (OR 5.2, 95% CI 4.2–6.4), and posttraumatic stress disorder (OR 4.3, 95% CI 3.2–5.7) [97]. Therefore, it is important to assess for psychiatric comorbidities, including other eating disorders, during sleep evaluation in BED patients.

Subjective Findings

Self-report questionnaires in children with primary obesity (*n* = 36), who were divided in to those with BE and those without BE groups, suggest significantly more sleep disturbances in both of these subgroups as compared to the control group consisting of 25 NW children [98]. Children with obesity and BE episodes demonstrated a marked decrease in sleep efficiency (using both objective and subjective measures of sleep) and reported more difficulty falling asleep, more mid-sleep awakenings, and more EDS than the obese subjects without BED, and NW controls [98].

Objective Findings

Tzischinsky and colleagues [99] evaluated sleep characteristics in obese BED patients in comparison to non-BED obese and nonbinging NW women using actigraphy. The ambulatory sleep data revealed that BED and obese subjects had significantly lower sleep efficiency and increased wake during sleep than the NW group.

Management

BED is the most common eating disorder but the best treatment options are still unclear [100]. A recent meta-analysis examined the efficacy of currently available treatments on four major outcomes in BED including BE and abstinence, eating-related psychopathology, weight, and general psychological and other outcomes. The authors noted that second-generation antidepressants, topiramate, and lisdexamfetamine were superior to placebo in achieving abstinence and reducing binge episodes and/or binge days and eating-related obsessions and compulsions [101]. The authors noted that second-generation antidepressants decreased depression, whereas topiramate and lisdexamfetamine produced weight reduction in study participants who were essentially overweight or obese. The authors reported that treatments including topiramate, fluvoxamine, and lisdexamfetamine were associated with sleep disturbance, including insomnia.

In the absence of evidence-based therapeutic interventions to enhance sleep in BED patients and most pharmacological interventions for BED causing sleep disturbances, there is an imminent need for further research to ascertain effective pharmacological and psychological treatments for management of sleep disturbances associated with BED. Additionally, optimal recognition and treatment of comorbid sleep and psychiatric disorders is likely to enhance sleep outcomes in patients with BED.

NIGHT EATING SYNDROME (NES)

NES is characterized by the clinical features of morning anorexia, evening hyperphagia, and insomnia with awakenings followed by nocturnal food ingestion [102]. NES is characterized by caloric intake ≥25% of total daily after dinner and/ or by two or more weekly nocturnal awakenings accompanied by food ingestion. The proposed criteria first appeared in the DSM-5 and listed in the category of eating disorders not otherwise specified [103]. NES can be distinguished from BN and BED by the timing of food intake, lack of associated compensatory behaviors, and smaller food ingestion rather than true BE episodes [102]. The prevalence of NES in the general population is estimated to be around 1.5%; however, it has been noted to be 27% in bariatric surgery patients [104]. The NEQ is an efficient and valid subjective questionnaire to assess behavioral and psychological symptoms of NES [105].

Delay in circadian timing of food intake appears to be the core clinical feature in NES [102]. Birketvedt et al. [106] studied neuroendocrine parameters in NES patients and reported that both nocturnal melatonin levels and the nocturnal rise in leptin were lower in NES subjects compared to controls. The authors suggested that dysregulation of these hormones may result in an inadequate suppression of appetite, impaired sleep consolidation, and could ultimately reflect underlying dysfunction of the HPA axis [106]. However, Allison et al. [102] failed to replicate these findings and found no significant differences in nocturnal melatonin or leptin levels when comparing NES patients to controls.

Kandeger and colleagues [107] examined the relationship between night eating symptoms and disordered eating attitudes by evaluating insomnia and chronotype differences in university students (n = 383) by using questionnaires including Morningness-Eveningness Questionnaire, Insomnia Severity Index, NEQ, and Eating Attitude Test. The authors found that both insomnia and night eating scores were associated with the evening chronotype, and these findings suggest that night eating symptoms exert a direct effect on the chronotype differences and insomnia and an indirect effect on disordered eating attitudes, by increasing insomnia scores. The authors concluded that NES may represent the misalignment

of food intake and may shift the circadian rhythm to delayed sleep phase [107]. Lundgren and colleagues [108] compared nonobese persons with NES (n = 19) to nonobese controls (n = 22) using 7-day, 24-hour prospective food and sleep diaries, the Eating Disorder Examination and the Structured Clinical Interview for DSM-IV fiagnoses interviews, and measures of disordered eating attitudes and behavior, mood, sleep, stress, and QOL. The authors noted that compared to controls, persons with NES reported significantly different circadian distribution of food intake, greater depressed mood, sleep disturbance, disordered eating and body image concerns, and perceived stress, along with more frequent psychiatric comorbidity, specifically anxiety, mood, and substance use disorders and decreased QOL [108].

Higher levels of serotonin transporter (SERT) binding in the temporal lobe of the midbrain have been reported in night eaters as compared to healthy controls [105]. Elevations in SERT binding can lead to dysfunctions in postsynaptic serotonin transmission, which may impair satiety and dysregulate circadian rhythms thereby leading to NES [109]. The selective serotonin reuptake inhibitors (SSRIs) like sertraline relieve NES by blocking SERT activity [100]. Lundgren and colleagues assessed the prevalence of NES in psychiatric outpatients (n = 399) using the NEQ. The authors found that 49 participants (12.3%) eventually had NES based on semistructured telephone interview and reported higher rates of substance use and obesity in patients with NES [65].

In another study, the authors found that 21.3% of the outpatients with depression (n = 155) reported NES. The authors noted that, as compared to non-NES patients, those with NES had significant differences in BMI, smoking, and poor sleep quality [110]. Palmese and colleagues [111] examined the frequency and clinical correlates of NES-related behaviors in a sample of obese patients with schizophrenia or schizoaffective disorder using NEQ and clinical interview. The authors found that 12% of these patients met criteria for NES on diagnostic interview and night eating behaviors were associated with increased insomnia and depression [111]. In a Turkish study, the authors determined the prevalence of NES in overweight or obese patients with schizophrenia, schizoaffective disorder, and bipolar disorder (n = 158). The authors found that 7.6% had NES based on clinical interview, and those with NES had worse insomnia scores and poor QOL as compared to the non-NES group [112].

Patients with NES may exhibit a comorbidity of PLM and RLS [113]. In a cross-sectional study, the authors reported that 17% of the RLS patients met criteria for NES, and RLS patients with night eating were older (67.2 ± 11.6 vs. 62.4 ± 11; p = 0.038) with higher BMI range (27.7 ± 3.8 vs. 26.1 ± 4.1 kg/m^2; p = 0.023), as compared to RLS patients without NES. The patients with RLS and NES were taking more drugs for concomitant diseases (89% vs. 72%; p = 0.031), were more likely to report insomnia (40% vs. 23%; p = 0.041), and were using more hypnotic agents (37.8% vs. 19.3%; p = 0.050) and dopaminergic drugs (65% vs. 46%; p = 0.041) [113]. Olbrich and colleagues [63] found that only 8.6% of patients with sleep apnea also exhibited night eating behavior and that NES was not related with the severity of sleep apnea. Thus, even though individuals with apnea experience frequent nocturnal awakenings, the desire to eat after these awakenings is not a typical reaction, and NES appears to be a distinct disorder [63].

Subjective Findings
Shorter sleep time and poor sleep quality, as determined by PSQI, have been associated with diagnosis of NES in a cross-sectional sample of undergraduate students. However, the authors suggested that further research is needed to clarify whether postevening hyperphagia in NES is a response to a lack of sleep, or vice versa [114]. Similarly, other authors have reported poorer sleep quality in patients with NES as compared to controls [105, 115].

Objective Findings
Nocturnal eaters were shown to have mild reduction in sleep efficiency and duration; however, percentage of each sleep stage was not significantly affected, as compared to gender-matched controls [116].

Management
The prevalence of obesity increases with NES as about half of the NES patients tend to report a NW status before the onset of the syndrome. Therefore, adequate treatment of NES is of importance clinically due to its association with obesity [102]. O'Reardon and colleagues examined the efficacy of sertraline (50–200 mg) in a double-blind, randomized controlled trial for treatment of NES over 8 weeks. The authors reported that, as compared to placebo, sertraline was associated with significant improvements in NES symptoms, QOL ratings, frequency of nocturnal awakenings

and ingestions, and caloric intake after the evening meal. Additionally, overweight and obese subjects in the sertraline group (n = 14) lost a significant amount of weight by week 8 (mean = –2.9 kg, SD = 3.8) compared to the overweight and obese subjects receiving placebo (n = 14) (mean = –0.3 kg, SD = 2.7) [65]. In a 12-week double-blind randomized controlled study of escitalopram (10–20 mg/day) in patients with NES (n = 40), the authors concluded that escitalopram was not superior to placebo in improving NES symptoms as measured by the NEQ [117]. It has been shown previously that patients with NES experience attenuation in the nocturnal rise of melatonin [106]; however, this finding was not replicated in the later research [118]. Two case studies have reported beneficial effect of agomelatine, a selective melatonin agonist and 5-HT2C antagonist, in treatment of NES with associated sleep disturbance and depressive symptoms without significant adverse effects [119, 120].

Topiramate, a GABA agonist and glutamatergic antagonist, has been shown to be effective in treatment of NES based on case reports [55, 121, 122]. The mechanism of action of topiramate in NES is unclear, but the anorexigenic effect of this medication may potentially improve NES symptoms and lead to reduction in weight. The NES symptoms can return after dose reduction or discontinuation of topiramate in these patients. Given the limited but promising evidence supporting the use of medications in patients with NES, there is a clear need for future randomized controlled trials to establish evidence-based pharmacological treatment modalities for NES [123]. Currently, there exist no guidelines for duration of pharmacological treatment of NES. It is recommended to continue the medication for at least 8 weeks prior to the medication trial being deemed as unsuccessful for NES treatment [123]. If the medication is effective for NES, then it should be continued for a period of at least 1 year prior to it being tapered off over a period of 2 to 3 months [123].

Evidence suggests that NES is associated with cognitive distortions such as one must eat to get to sleep [124], and patients with NES report specific food cravings and feeling anxious or agitated at night time [125]. Cognitive-behavioral therapy (CBT) protocols for BED and behavioral weight loss have been adapted by Allison and colleagues [103] for management of NES. In an open-label pilot study (n = 25), the participants received 10 CBT sessions for management of NES. The CBT intervention led to significant decreases in caloric intake after dinner (35.0% to 24.9%), number of nocturnal ingestions (8.7 to 2.6 per week), weight (82.5 to 79.4 kg), and Night Eating Symptom Scale score (28.7 to 16.3; all p values <0.0001). The authors reported that the number of awakenings per week, depressed mood, and QOL also improved significantly after CBT (p values <0.02) [103]. Core components of CBT include psychoeducation about NES and healthy eating, eating modification, relaxation strategies, establishing sleep hygiene, cognitive restructuring, improving physical activity, and establishing social support [126]. The primary aim of CBT is to correct the delay in circadian eating rhythms while targeting cognitive distortions associated with night eating and sleep in patients with NES [127]. Overall, CBT for NES appears to be a promising treatment; however, future randomized controlled trials with larger sample size are needed to establish the efficacy of this intervention in NES [127].

Progressive muscle relaxation (PMR) has been used for treatment of NES with success. In a 1-week trial of abbreviated PMR training, the authors reported decreased self-reported levels of state anxiety, perceived stress, evening appetite, and morning anorexia in patients with NES. Vander Wal and colleagues [128] recently examined the efficacy of PMR, education, and exercise for the treatment of NES in a randomized study. The authors noted that all the three interventions reduced the symptoms of NES [128].

Given that NES is considered a disorder of circadian misalignment, chronobiological treatments may be used for treatment of NES. In a pilot study, McCune and Lundgren [129] evaluated the efficacy of bright light therapy administered daily (1,000 lux for 2 weeks) in patients with NES (n = 15) and found that it caused significant pre-to-post treatment improvement in night eating symptomatology, mood disturbance, and sleep disturbance [129].

SLEEP-RELATED EATING DISORDER (SRED)

SERD is another important condition among nighttime eating spectrum disorders characterized by recurrent episodes of involuntary eating associated with varyingly diminished levels of consciousness during partial arousal from sleep. Level of consciousness during SRED episodes ranges from partial consciousness to dense unawareness typical of somnambulistic episodes. SRED episodes typically arise in the first half of the night, from NREM sleep stage (mostly N3), and for this reason, SRED is classified as a separate NREM parasomnia sleep disorder in the ICSD-3. Patients with SRED have several features in common with sleepwalkers such as high frequency of past or current sleepwalking, similar timing in the first half of the night, and frequent arousals from N3. Therefore, not surprisingly, SRED is considered a variant of sleepwalking per the DSM-5 classification criteria, and even ICSD-3 acknowledges that this is likely the case.

There are no current prevalence data on SRED in the general population and the reported prevalence results are inconsistent (0.5%–4.7%). However, the prevalence of SRED could be as high as 16.7% in patients who have daytime eating disorders (ICSD-3). SRED can be idiopathic or secondary where it can be associated with primary sleep disorder or use of psychotropic medications. Secondary SRED is usually more common, and therefore it is important to thoroughly assess secondary factors in patients presenting with SRED. Primary sleep disorders that are closely associated with SRED include sleepwalking, RLS, PLMD, OSA, and circadian rhythm sleep–wake disorders, particularly irregular sleep–wake pattern.

Schenck et al. [130] first described SRED in 1994. SRED can affect both sexes and all ages, generally starting in young adults, with a female predominance [131]. Idiopathic SRED can have insidious or precipitous onset, and its course is usually unremitting. Patients with SRED generally partially arise from sleep and eat within the first 1 to 3 hours after sleep onset. The eating episodes are generally characterized by rapid ingestion of food with preference for high caloric foods, but sometimes ingestion of nonedible or toxic items, such as cigarette butts and preservatives, has been reported. Injuries from careless food preparation and ingestion are dangerous implications of SRED.

Some authors consider NES and SRED to be situated at opposite poles of a disordered eating spectrum and the level of awareness during nocturnal food intake is the main distinguishing feature [132]. Compared to daytime eating disorders, patients with SRED lack inappropriate compensatory behaviors including self-induced vomiting, misuse of laxatives or other medications like diuretics, or purging behaviors. However, a person with daytime eating disorders can have coexisting SRED with eating episodes in context of confusional arousals but not associated with compensatory behaviors. Other differential diagnoses for SRED include medical and neurological disorders including hypoglycemic states, peptic ulcer disease, reflux esophagitis, and Kluver–Bucy syndrome.

In psychiatric literature, SRED has been mainly attributed to iatrogenic causes such as use of hypnotic medications, mainly zolpidem, based on case reports [71, 72, 133]. Takaesu et al. [134] examined the prevalence of SRED in psychiatric outpatients taking hypnotics ($n = 1048$). The authors found that 8.4% of the patients reported SRED based on screening questionnaire and clinical interviews. The major risk factors associated with SRED in this sample were younger age, higher dosage of hypnotics, and use of two or more types of antipsychotics [134]. There is emerging evidence that atypical antipsychotics are implicated in causation of SRED based on several case reports and case series [73, 135–137]. Our group is currently writing a literature review of atypical antipsychotic-induced SRED ($n = 15$), including four cases of SRED from our practice. We found that 11 out of 15 patients are males with a mean age of onset of SRED at 43.8 ± 12.6 years. Approximately 50% of these patients were diagnosed to have bipolar disorder, and only 2 out of 15 patients had a prior history of sleepwalking.

Subjective Findings

In a Chilean study examining the characteristics of patients with SRED ($n = 34$), insomnia (58.8%) and RLS (47%) were the most common subjective sleep complaints [138].

Objective Findings

The most common PSG finding is multiple confusional arousals, arising mainly from SWS, with or without eating episodes. The level of consciousness after the arousal from NREM sleep can range from virtual unconsciousness to varying levels of partial consciousness, despite the EEG pattern being predominantly awake, which is suggestive of dissociation between the level of consciousness and EEG pattern. Findings suggestive of OSA and recurrent PLM have been reported in patients with secondary SRED. Poor sleep quality and higher median night activity has been reported in patients with SRED using actigraphy monitoring [139].

Management

SRED can be idiopathic or more commonly associated with primary sleep disorders including sleepwalking, RLS, OSA, and use of psychotropic medications [140]. The first step in the management is to identify the underlying cause of SRED behaviors. Video PSG is generally indicated if comorbid primary sleep disorders that can lead to sleep fragmentation, such as RLS, PLMD, or OSA, are suspected. Optimal treatment of comorbid primary sleep disorders may improve SRED symptoms by reducing the number of arousals from sleep. Scheck and colleagues [131] reported successful outcomes in patients with SRED with use of dopaminergic agents in those with comorbid RLS/PLMD, and the use of nasal continuous positive airway pressure in those with comorbid OSA [131]. However, in double-blind, placebo-controlled crossover study ($n = 11$) of pramipexole (up to 0.36 mg per day), the SRED subjects demonstrated improvements in nocturnal activity monitored with actigraphy and subjective sleep quality but no improvements in eating outcomes related to SRED and no weight loss were observed [139].

In an open-label retrospective case series ($n = 25$), Winkelman reported that 68% of 25 patients with SRED responded to topiramate use (mean daily dose of 135 mg/day) and weight loss greater than 10% was observed in over one-quarter of responders. However, nearly half of the responders discontinued the medication after a mean of 12 months due to side effects such as dullness, paresthesias, and daytime sleepiness [141]. In a Chilean study, out of 20 patients with SRED treated with topiramate, 17 patients had adequate symptomatic responses with treatment [138]. The mechanism of action of topiramate in treatment of SRED is unclear; however, it has been hypothesized that this drug acts as an anorexigenic agent, either through glutamatergic antagonism or serotonergic agonism [55]. Additionally, topiramate may contribute to appetite regulation and weight loss by stimulating insulin release and increasing insulin sensitivity [142], [143].

Given commonalities between SRED and NES, and efficacy of SSRIs in the treatment of NES, it is plausible that SSRIs may have a beneficial role in treatment of SRED; however, no controlled trials exist to support the efficacy of SSRIs in the treatment of SRED. Varghese and colleagues [144] recently reported successful outcomes in treatment of idiopathic SRED in two male patients with use of low-dose sertraline (25 mg daily). Zapp and colleagues [145] reported successful outcome in treatment of severe SRED in a female patient with comorbid depression, panic disorder and sleep apnea with use of melatonergic agents including agomelatine and extended release melatonin.

In terms of iatrogenic causes, the major categories of psychotropic medications associated with SRED include selective benzodiazepine receptor agonists [71, 72, 146, 147], antidepressant (mirtazapine) [69, 70], and atypical antipsychotic use [135, 136, 148, 149]. Drug-induced SRED usually resolves with discontinuation of the offending medication. In some cases, reduction of dosage of the offending agent can be effective. In our case series and the literature review (pending submission for publication) examining the association of atypical antipsychotics with SRED ($n = 15$), the majority of the patients were taking quetiapine, and reduction of the atypical antipsychotic dosage or discontinuation of the offending agent led to complete cessation of SRED [150].

In case an antipsychotic needs to be continued due to superior efficacy in treatment of primary psychiatric disorder, then topiramate (50–200 mg/d) can be used to treat drug-induced SRED while continuing the antipsychotic. However, if topiramate is not well tolerated, then low-dose benzodiazepine (alprazolam 1–1.5 mg at nightly) may prove to be efficacious [14]. There is a clear need for future systematic research to find evidence-based treatments for optimal treatment of SRED and to understand the underlying pathophysiological mechanisms and risk factors associated with iatrogenic SRED. Patients should be counseled regarding possibility of emergence of SRED with use of certain psychotropic medications to enhance patient safety and prevent adverse metabolic outcomes that could result from SRED.

CONCLUSIONS

Sleep and eating behavior are complimentary homeostatic functions, and adequate sleep is fundamental for the nutritional balance of the body. Short sleep duration has been linked to development of obesity and abnormal eating patterns in children and adults. Individuals with eating disorders report significantly higher sleep disturbances including sleep apnea, insomnia, circadian rhythm disorders, and impairment of daytime functioning, as compared to controls. Sleep disturbances associated with AN are likely due to malnutrition and tend to improve after weight restoration. Nocturnal eating behaviors are mainly categorized as NES and SRED. NES can be distinguished from SRED by complete awareness of nocturnal eating episodes in NES. SRED manifests as a combination of eating disorder and NREM parasomnia disorder. Compared to daytime eating disorders, patients with NES and SRED lack inappropriate compensatory behaviors including self-induced vomiting, misuse of laxatives or diuretics, or purging behaviors. Potential treatment modalities for NES include SSRIs, topiramate, CBT, and bright light therapy. Idiopathic SRED may respond to topiramate, benzodiazepine, or SSRI treatment; however, for management of secondary SRED, identification and treatment of comorbid sleep disorders and addressing other iatrogenic causes like removal of offending hypnotic drug is recommended.

FUTURE DIRECTIONS

Greater focus on assessment of sleep disturbances in daytime eating disorders is warranted to assess the comorbidity and the impact of sleep disturbance in eating disorder outcomes. Effect of psychological and pharmacological treatment modalities for eating disorders on sleep disturbances needs to be thoroughly investigated to develop evidence based strategies that focus on improving sleep outcomes in this population. Clinical and research focus on nocturnal eating disorders is imminently needed in terms of assessment and evidence-based treatments of NES and SRED given their negative health and safety outcomes. Psychiatric clinician's familiarity with diagnostic assessment of primary sleep disorders such as OSA and RLS is likely to enhance recognition of secondary causes of SRED. Finally, knowledge of iatrogenic causes of SRED and understanding of potential pathophysiological mechanisms underlying iatrogenic SRED, with a particular focus on psychotropic medications, can significantly enhance patient safety and prevent adverse effects that can potentially result from sleep-related eating.

KEY CLINICAL PEARLS

- Sleep disturbances associated with AN are likely due to malnutrition and tend to improve after weight restoration.
- BE/purging subtype of AN has been associated with poor subjective sleep quality.
- Level of awareness during nocturnal food intake is the main distinguishing feature between NES and SRED.
- Night Eating Questionnaire is a valid and effective screening tool for assessment of NES.

- Sertraline has been found to be most effective for treatment of NES.
- SRED episodes arise mainly from N3 or SWS.
- For successful management of secondary SRED, treat comorbid sleep disorders including sleepwalking, OSA, RLS/PLMD, and address iatrogenic causes like use of hypnotic medications.

SELF-ASSESSMENT QUESTIONS

1. Sleep-related eating disorder is usually associated with arousal from which of the following sleep stages?
   a. N1
   b. N2
   c. N3
   d. REM

Answer: c

2. Night eating syndrome can be distinguished from sleep-related eating disorder by which of the following?
   a. Complete awareness of event
   b. Morning anorexia
   c. Poor sleep quality
   d. Weight gain

Answer: a

3. Which of the medications have been shown to be most effective in treatment of night eating syndrome?
   a. Fluoxetine
   b. Sertraline
   c. Escitalopram
   d. None of the above

Answer: b

4. Which of the following medications have been associated with sleep-related eating disorder?
   a. Zolpidem
   b. Quetiapine
   c. Mirtazapine
   d. All of the above

Answer: d

5. Secondary sleep-related eating disorder can be associated with which of the following sleep disorders?
   a. Obstructive sleep apnea
   b. Restless legs syndrome
   c. Sleepwalking
   d. All of the above

Answer: d

REFERENCES

1. Seftel, J., *Profile: Irene Pepperberg & Alex*, in *NOVA Science Video Podcast*, ed. N.d.G. Tyson. 2011, WGBH: Boston.
2. Willie, J.T., et al., *To eat or to sleep? Orexin in the regulation of feeding and wakefulness.* Annu Rev Neurosci, 2001. **24**: p. 429–458.
3. Crispim, C.A., et al., *The influence of sleep and sleep loss upon food intake and metabolism.* Nutr Res Rev, 2007. **20**(2): p. 195–212.
4. Chaput, J.P., *Sleep patterns, diet quality and energy balance.* Physiol Behav, 2014. **134**: p. 86–91.
5. Hicks, R.A. and E. Rozette, *Habitual sleep duration and eating disorders in college students.* Percept Mot Skills, 1986. **62**(1): p. 209–210.
6. Wrzosek, M., et al., *Insomnia and depressive symptoms in relation to unhealthy eating behaviors in bariatric surgery candidates.* BMC Psychiatry, 2018. **18**(1): p. 153.
7. Tromp, M.D., et al., *Sleep, eating disorder symptoms, and daytime functioning.* Nat Sci Sleep, 2016. **8**: p. 35–40.
8. Lombardo, C., et al., *Persistence of poor sleep predicts the severity of the clinical condition after 6months of standard treatment in patients with eating disorders.* Eat Behav, 2015. **18**: p. 16–19.
9. Bos, S.C., et al., *Disordered eating behaviors and sleep disturbances.* Eat Behav, 2013. **14**(2): p. 192–198.
10. Yeh, S.S. and R.F. Brown, *Disordered eating partly mediates the relationship between poor sleep quality and high body mass index.* Eat Behav, 2014. **15**(2): p. 291–297.
11. Mayes, S.D., et al., *Correlates of suicide ideation and attempts in children and adolescents with eating disorders.* Eat Disord, 2014. **22**(4): p. 352–366.
12. Phillips, F., et al., *Isocaloric diet changes and electroencephalographic sleep.* Lancet, 1975. **2**(7938): p. 723–725.
13. Afaghi, A., H. O'Connor, and C.M. Chow, *High-glycemic-index carbohydrate meals shorten sleep onset.* Am J Clin Nutr, 2007. **85**(2): p. 426–430.
14. Dockray, G.J., *Cholecystokinin and gut-brain signalling.* Regul Pept, 2009. **155**(1-3): p. 6–10.
15. Wells, A.S., et al., *Influences of fat and carbohydrate on postprandial sleepiness, mood, and hormones.* Physiol Behav, 1997. **61**(5): p. 679–686.
16. Afaghi, A., H. O'Connor, and C.M. Chow, *Acute effects of the very low carbohydrate diet on sleep indices.* Nutr Neurosci, 2008. **11**(4): p. 146–154.
17. Peuhkuri, K., N. Sihvola, and R. Korpela, *Diet promotes sleep duration and quality.* Nutr Res, 2012. **32**(5): p. 309–319.
18. Bailer, U.F. and W.H. Kaye, *A review of neuropeptide and neuroendocrine dysregulation in anorexia*

and bulimia nervosa. Curr Drug Targets CNS Neurol Disord, 2003. 2(1): p. 53–59.

19. de Lecea, L., et al., The hypocretins: hypothalamus-specific peptides with neuroexcitatory activity. Proc Natl Acad Sci U S A, 1998. 95(1): p. 322–327.

20. Burdakov, D. and J.A. Gonzalez, Physiological functions of glucose-inhibited neurones. Acta Physiol (Oxf), 2009. 195(1): p. 71–78.

21. Jequier, E., Leptin signaling, adiposity, and energy balance. Ann N Y Acad Sci, 2002. 967: p. 379–388.

22. Barson, J.R., Orexin/hypocretin and dysregulated eating: Promotion of foraging behavior. Brain Res, 2018.

23. Piccoli, L., et al., Role of orexin-1 receptor mechanisms on compulsive food consumption in a model of binge eating in female rats. Neuropsychopharmacology, 2012. 37(9): p. 1999–2011.

24. Sauchelli, S., et al., Orexin and sleep quality in anorexia nervosa: Clinical relevance and influence on treatment outcome. Psychoneuroendocrinology, 2016. 65: p. 102–8.

25. Leproult, R. and E. Van Cauter, Role of sleep and sleep loss in hormonal release and metabolism. Endocr Dev, 2010. 17: p. 11–21.

26. Muller, T.D., et al., Leptin-mediated neuroendocrine alterations in anorexia nervosa: somatic and behavioral implications. Child Adolesc Psychiatr Clin N Am, 2009. 18(1): p. 117–129.

27. Monteleone, P., et al., Leptin secretion is related to chronicity and severity of the illness in bulimia nervosa. Psychosom Med, 2002. 64(6): p. 874–879.

28. Atalayer, D., et al., Ghrelin and eating disorders. Prog Neuropsychopharmacol Biol Psychiatry, 2013. 40: p. 70–82.

29. Dzaja, A., et al., Sleep enhances nocturnal plasma ghrelin levels in healthy subjects. Am J Physiol Endocrinol Metab, 2004. 286(6): p. E963–E967.

30. Weikel, J.C., et al., Ghrelin promotes slow-wave sleep in humans. Am J Physiol Endocrinol Metab, 2003. 284(2): p. E407–E415.

31. Kluge, M., et al., Ghrelin increases slow wave sleep and stage 2 sleep and decreases stage 1 sleep and REM sleep in elderly men but does not affect sleep in elderly women. Psychoneuroendocrinology, 2010. 35(2): p. 297–304.

32. Broglio, F., et al., The endocrine response to acute ghrelin administration is blunted in patients with anorexia nervosa, a ghrelin hypersecretory state. Clin Endocrinol (Oxf), 2004. 60(5): p. 592–599.

33. Monteleone, P., et al., Plasma obestatin, ghrelin, and ghrelin/obestatin ratio are increased in underweight patients with anorexia nervosa but not in symptomatic patients with bulimia nervosa. J Clin Endocrinol Metab, 2008. 93(11): p. 4418–4421.

34. Nedvidkova, J., et al., Loss of meal-induced decrease in plasma ghrelin levels in patients with anorexia nervosa. J Clin Endocrinol Metab, 2003. 88(4): p. 1678–1682.

35. Otto, B., et al., Weight gain decreases elevated plasma ghrelin concentrations of patients with anorexia nervosa. Eur J Endocrinol, 2001. 145(5): p. 669–673.

36. Tolle, V., et al., Balance in ghrelin and leptin plasma levels in anorexia nervosa patients and constitutionally thin women. J Clin Endocrinol Metab, 2003. 88(1): p. 109–116.

37. Troisi, A., et al., Plasma ghrelin in anorexia, bulimia, and binge-eating disorder: relations with eating patterns and circulating concentrations of cortisol and thyroid hormones. Neuroendocrinology, 2005. 81(4): p. 259–266.

38. Jager, G. and R.F. Witkamp, The endocannabinoid system and appetite: relevance for food reward. Nutr Res Rev, 2014. 27(1): p. 172–185.

39. Pertwee, R.G., Receptors and channels targeted by synthetic cannabinoid receptor agonists and antagonists. Curr Med Chem, 2010. 17(14): p. 1360–1381.

40. Maccarrone, M., et al., The endocannabinoid system and its relevance for nutrition. Annu Rev Nutr, 2010. 30: p. 423–440.

41. Matias, I., B. Gatta-Cherifi, and D. Cota, Obesity and the endocannabinoid system: circulating endocannabinoids and obesity. Current Obesity Reports, 2012. 1(4): p. 229–235.

42. Vaughn, L.K., et al., Endocannabinoid signalling: has it got rhythm? Br J Pharmacol, 2010. 160(3): p. 530–543.

43. Matias, I., et al., Endocannabinoids measurement in human saliva as potential biomarker of obesity. PLoS One, 2012. 7(7): p. e42399.

44. Matias, I., et al., Regulation, function, and dysregulation of endocannabinoids in models of adipose and beta-pancreatic cells and in obesity and hyperglycemia. J Clin Endocrinol Metab, 2006. 91(8): p. 3171–3180.

45. Cota, D., et al., The endogenous cannabinoid system affects energy balance via central orexigenic drive and peripheral lipogenesis. J Clin Invest, 2003. 112(3): p. 423–431.

46. Hanlon, E.C., et al., Sleep restriction enhances the daily rhythm of circulating levels of endocannabinoid 2-arachidonoylglycerol. Sleep, 2016. 39(3): p. 653–664.

47. St-Onge, M.P., et al., Sleep restriction leads to increased activation of brain regions sensitive to food stimuli. Am J Clin Nutr, 2012. 95(4): p. 818–824.

48. St-Onge, M.P., et al., Sleep restriction increases the neuronal response to unhealthy food in normal-weight individuals. Int J Obes (Lond), 2014. 38(3): p. 411–416.

49. Broussard, J.L. and E. Van Cauter, Disturbances of sleep and circadian rhythms: novel risk factors

for obesity. Curr Opin Endocrinol Diabetes Obes, 2016. **23**(5): p. 353–359.

50. Spiegel, K., et al., *Twenty-four-hour profiles of acylated and total ghrelin: relationship with glucose levels and impact of time of day and sleep.* J Clin Endocrinol Metab, 2011. **96**(2): p. 486–493.

51. Taheri, S., et al., *Short sleep duration is associated with reduced leptin, elevated ghrelin, and increased body mass index.* PLoS Med, 2004. **1**(3): p. e62.

52. Poggiogalle, E., H. Jamshed, and C.M. Peterson, *Circadian regulation of glucose, lipid, and energy metabolism in humans.* Metabolism, 2018. **84**: p. 11–27.

53. Tseng, M.M., et al., *Variables influencing presenting symptoms of patients with eating disorders at psychiatric outpatient clinics.* Psychiatry Res, 2016. **238**: p. 338–344.

54. Howell, M.J., C.H. Schenck, and S.J. Crow, *A review of nighttime eating disorders.* Sleep Med Rev, 2009. **13**(1): p. 23–34.

55. Winkelman, J.W., *Treatment of nocturnal eating syndrome and sleep-related eating disorder with topiramate.* Sleep Med, 2003. **4**(3): p. 243–246.

56. Godart, N., et al., *Mood disorders in eating disorder patients: Prevalence and chronology of ONSET.* J Affect Disord, 2015. **185**: p. 115–122.

57. Swift, W.J., D. Andrews, and N.E. Barklage, *The relationship between affective disorder and eating disorders: a review of the literature.* Am J Psychiatry, 1986. **143**(3): p. 290–299.

58. Manber, R. and A.S. Chambers, *Insomnia and depression: a multifaceted interplay.* Curr Psychiatry Rep, 2009. **11**(6): p. 437–442.

59. Vieira, M.F. and P. Afonso, *Sleep disturbances in anorexia nervosa.* Eur Psychiatry, 2017. **41**: p. S561.

60. Delvenne, V., et al., *Sleep polygraphic variables in anorexia nervosa and depression: a comparative study in adolescents.* J Affect Disord, 1992. **25**(3): p. 167–72.

61. Asaad Abdou, T., et al., *Sleep profile in anorexia and bulimia nervosa female patients.* Sleep Med, 2018. **48**: p. 113–116.

62. Kim, K.R., et al., *Sleep disturbance in women with eating disorder: prevalence and clinical characteristics.* Psychiatry Res, 2010. **176**(1): p. 88–90.

63. Olbrich, K., et al., *Night eating, binge eating and related features in patients with obstructive sleep apnea syndrome.* Eur Eat Disord Rev, 2009. **17**(2): p. 120–127.

64. Provini, F., et al., *Association of restless legs syndrome with nocturnal eating: a case-control study.* Mov Disord, 2009. **24**(6): p. 871–877.

65. O'Reardon, J.P., et al., *A randomized, placebo-controlled trial of sertraline in the treatment of night eating syndrome.* Am J Psychiatry, 2006. **163**(5): p. 893–898.

66. Saracli, O., et al., *The prevalence and clinical features of the night eating syndrome in psychiatric out-patient population.* Compr Psychiatry, 2015. **57**: p. 79–84.

67. Chaput, J.P., et al., *Short sleep duration is associated with greater alcohol consumption in adults.* Appetite, 2012. **59**(3): p. 650–655.

68. Fouladi, F., et al., *Prevalence of alcohol and other substance use in patients with eating disorders.* Eur Eat Disord Rev, 2015. **23**(6): p. 531–536.

69. Shinith, D., et al., *Sleep-related eating disorder with mirtazapine.* BMJ Case Rep, 2018. **2018**.

70. Jeong, J.H. and W.M. Bahk, *Sleep-related eating disorder associated with mirtazapine.* J Clin Psychopharmacol, 2014. **34**(6): p. 752–753.

71. Nzwalo, H., et al., *Sleep-related eating disorder secondary to zolpidem.* BMJ Case Rep, 2013. **2013**.

72. Valiensi, S.M., et al., *[Sleep related eating disorders as a side effect of zolpidem].* Medicina (B Aires), 2010. **70**(3): p. 223–226.

73. Tamanna, S., et al., *Quetiapine-induced sleep-related eating disorder-like behavior: a case series.* J Med Case Rep, 2012. **6**: p. 380.

74. Komada, Y., et al., *Comparison of clinical features between primary and drug-induced sleep-related eating disorder.* Neuropsychiatr Dis Treat, 2016. **12**: p. 1275–1280.

75. Allison, K.C., et al., *The Night Eating Questionnaire (NEQ): psychometric properties of a measure of severity of the night eating syndrome.* Eat Behav, 2008. **9**(1): p. 62–72.

76. Tanahashi, T., et al., *Purging behaviors relate to impaired subjective sleep quality in female patients with anorexia nervosa: a prospective observational study.* Biopsychosoc Med, 2017. **11**: p. 22.

77. Lacey, J.H., et al., *Study of EEG sleep characteristics in patients with anorexia nervosa before and after restoration of matched population mean weight consequent on ingestion of a "normal" diet.* Postgrad Med J, 1976. **52**(603): p. 45–49.

78. Pieters, G., et al., *Sleep variables in anorexia nervosa: evolution with weight restoration.* Int J Eat Disord, 2004. **35**(3): p. 342–347.

79. Walsh, B.T., et al., *EEG-monitored sleep in anorexia nervosa and bulimia.* Biol Psychiatry, 1985. **20**(9): p. 947–956.

80. Levy, A.B., K.N. Dixon, and H. Schmidt, *Sleep architecture in anorexia nervosa and bulimia.* Biol Psychiatry, 1988. **23**(1): p. 99–101.

81. Levy, A.B., K.N. Dixon, and H. Schmidt, *REM and delta sleep in anorexia nervosa and bulimia.* Psychiatry Res, 1987. **20**(3): p. 189–197.

82. Nobili, L., et al., *A quantified analysis of sleep electroencephalography in anorectic adolescents.* Biol Psychiatry, 1999. **45**(6): p. 771–775.

83. El Ghoch, M., et al., *Sleep patterns before and after weight restoration in females with anorexia nervosa: a longitudinal controlled study.* Eur Eat Disord Rev, 2016. **24**(5): p. 425–429.

84. Russell, G., *Bulimia nervosa: an ominous variant of anorexia nervosa.* Psychol Med, 1979. **9**(3): p. 429–448.

85. Latzer, Y., et al., *Naturalistic sleep monitoring in women suffering from bulimia nervosa.* Int J Eat Disord, 1999. **26**(3): p. 315–321.

86. Hudson, J.I., et al., *Sleep EEG in bulimia.* Biol Psychiatry, 1987. **22**(7): p. 820–828.

87. Kessler, R.C., et al., *The prevalence and correlates of binge eating disorder in the World Health Organization World Mental Health Surveys.* Biol Psychiatry, 2013. **73**(9): p. 904–914.

88. Hudson, J.I., et al., *The prevalence and correlates of eating disorders in the National Comorbidity Survey Replication.* Biol Psychiatry, 2007. **61**(3): p. 348–358.

89. Swanson, S.A., et al., *Prevalence and correlates of eating disorders in adolescents. Results from the national comorbidity survey replication adolescent supplement.* Arch Gen Psychiatry, 2011. **68**(7): p. 714–723.

90. Guerdjikova, A.I., et al., *Binge eating disorder in elderly individuals.* Int J Eat Disord, 2012. **45**(7): p. 905–908.

91. Grucza, R.A., T.R. Przybeck, and C.R. Cloninger, *Prevalence and correlates of binge eating disorder in a community sample.* Compr Psychiatry, 2007. **48**(2): p. 124–131.

92. Nicdao, E.G., S. Hong, and D.T. Takeuchi, *Prevalence and correlates of eating disorders among Asian Americans: results from the National Latino and Asian American Study.* Int J Eat Disord, 2007. **40**(Suppl): p. S22–S226.

93. Kenny, T.E., et al., *An examination of the relationship between binge eating disorder and insomnia symptoms.* Eur Eat Disord Rev, 2018. **26**(3): p. 186–196.

94. Fortuyn, H.A., et al., *High prevalence of eating disorders in narcolepsy with cataplexy: a case-control study.* Sleep, 2008. **31**(3): p. 335–341.

95. Sockalingam, S., et al., *The relationship between eating psychopathology and obstructive sleep apnea in bariatric surgery candidates: a retrospective study.* Int J Eat Disord, 2017. **50**(7): p. 801–807.

96. Borges Da Silva, V., et al., *Association between binge eating disorder and psychiatric comorbidity profiles in patients with obesity seeking bariatric surgery.* Compr Psychiatry, 2018. **87**: p. 79–83.

97. Welch, E., et al., *Treatment-seeking patients with binge-eating disorder in the Swedish national registers: clinical course and psychiatric comorbidity.* BMC Psychiatry, 2016. **16**: p. 163.

98. Tzischinsky, O. and Y. Latzer, *Sleep-wake cycles in obese children with and without binge-eating*

episodes. J Paediatr Child Health, 2006. **42**(11): p. 688–693.

99. Tzischinsky, O., et al., *Sleep-wake cycles in women with binge eating disorder.* Int J Eat Disord, 2000. **27**(1): p. 43–48.

100. Brownley, K.A., et al., *Binge-eating disorder in adults: a systematic review and meta-analysis.* Ann Intern Med, 2016. **165**(6): p. 409–420.

101. Berkman, N.D., et al., *AHRQ Comparative effectiveness reviews*, in *Management and Outcomes of Binge-Eating Disorder.* 2015, Agency for Healthcare Research and Quality: Rockville, MD.

102. O'Reardon, J.P., A. Peshek, and K.C. Allison, *Night eating syndrome: diagnosis, epidemiology and management.* CNS Drugs, 2005. **19**(12): p. 997–1008.

103. Allison, K.C., et al., *Cognitive behavior therapy for night eating syndrome: a pilot study.* Am J Psychother, 2010. **64**(1): p. 91–106.

104. Vonk, J. and T.K. Shackelford, eds. *The Oxford handbook of comparative evolutionary psychology.* Oxford Library of Psychology, ed. P.E. Nathan. 2012, Oxford University Press: New York. 574.

105. Lundgren, J.D., et al., *123I-ADAM SPECT imaging of serotonin transporter binding in patients with night eating syndrome: a preliminary report.* Psychiatry Res, 2008. **162**(3): p. 214–20.

106. Birketvedt, G.S., et al., *Behavioral and neuroendocrine characteristics of the night-eating syndrome.* Jama, 1999. **282**(7): p. 657–663.

107. Kandeger, A., et al., *The relationship between night eating symptoms and disordered eating attitudes via insomnia and chronotype differences.* Psychiatry Res, 2018. **268**: p. 354–357.

108. Lundgren, J.D., et al., *A descriptive study of non-obese persons with night eating syndrome and a weight-matched comparison group.* Eat Behav, 2008. **9**(3): p. 343–351.

109. Stunkard, A.J., et al., *A biobehavioural model of the night eating syndrome.* Obes Rev, 2009. **10**(Suppl 2): p. 69–77.

110. Kucukgoncu, S., et al., *Clinical features of night eating syndrome among depressed patients.* Eur Eat Disord Rev, 2014. **22**(2): p. 102–108.

111. Palmese, L.B., et al., *Prevalence of night eating in obese individuals with schizophrenia and schizoaffective disorder.* Compr Psychiatry, 2013. **54**(3): p. 276–281.

112. Civil Arslan, F., et al., *[The prevalence of night eating syndrome among outpatient overweight or obese individuals with serious mental illness].* Turk Psikiyatri Derg, 2015. **26**(4): p. 242–248.

113. Antelmi, E., et al., *Nocturnal eating is part of the clinical spectrum of restless legs syndrome and*

an underestimated risk factor for increased body mass index. Sleep Med, 2014. **15**(2): p. 168–172.

114. Yahia, N., et al., *Night eating syndrome and its association with weight status, physical activity, eating habits, smoking status, and sleep patterns among college students.* Eat Weight Disord, 2017. **22**(3): p. 421–433.

115. Rogers, N.L., et al., *Assessment of sleep in women with night eating syndrome.* Sleep, 2006. **29**(6): p. 814–819.

116. Vinai, P., et al., *New data on psychological traits and sleep profiles of patients affected by nocturnal eating.* Sleep Med, 2015. **16**(6): p. 746–753.

117. Vander Wal, J.S., et al., *Escitalopram for treatment of night eating syndrome: a 12-week, randomized, placebo-controlled trial.* J Clin Psychopharmacol, 2012. **32**(3): p. 341–345.

118. Allison, K.C., et al., *Neuroendocrine profiles associated with energy intake, sleep, and stress in the night eating syndrome.* J Clin Endocrinol Metab, 2005. **90**(11): p. 6214–6217.

119. Milano, W., et al., *Agomelatine efficacy in the night eating syndrome.* Case Rep Med, 2013. **2013**: p. 867650.

120. Milano, W., et al., *Successful treatment with agomelatine in NES: a series of five cases.* Open Neurol J, 2013. **7**: p. 32–37.

121. Cooper-Kazaz, R., *Treatment of night eating syndrome with topiramate: dawn of a new day.* J Clin Psychopharmacol, 2012. **32**(1): p. 143–145.

122. Tucker, P., B. Masters, and O. Nawar, *Topiramate in the treatment of comorbid night eating syndrome and PTSD: a case study.* Eat Disord, 2004. **12**(1): p. 75–78.

123. Kucukgoncu, S., M. Midura, and C. Tek, *Optimal management of night eating syndrome: challenges and solutions.* Neuropsychiatr Dis Treat, 2015. **11**: p. 751–760.

124. Vinai, P., et al., *Clinical validity of the descriptor. "presence of a belief that one must eat in order to get to sleep" in diagnosing the night eating syndrome.* Appetite, 2014. **75**: p. 46–48.

125. Vinai, P., et al., *Psychopathology and treatment of night eating syndrome: a review.* Eat Weight Disord, 2008. **13**(2): p. 54–63.

126. Vander Wal, J.S., *Night eating syndrome: a critical review of the literature.* Clin Psychol Rev, 2012. **32**(1): p. 49–59.

127. Allison, K.C. and E.P. Tarves, *Treatment of night eating syndrome.* Psychiatr Clin North Am, 2011. **34**(4): p. 785–96.

128. Vander Wal, J.S., et al., *Education, progressive muscle relaxation therapy, and exercise for the treatment of night eating syndrome: a pilot study.* Appetite, 2015. **89**: p. 136–144.

129. McCune, A.M. and J.D. Lundgren, *Bright light therapy for the treatment of night eating syndrome: a pilot study.* Psychiatry Res, 2015. **229**(1-2): p. 577–579.

130. Schenck, C.H. and M.W. Mahowald, *Review of nocturnal sleep-related eating disorders.* Int J Eat Disord, 1994. **15**(4): p. 343–356.

131. Schenck, C.H., et al., *Additional categories of sleep-related eating disorders and the current status of treatment.* Sleep, 1993. **16**(5): p. 457–466.

132. Vinai, P., et al., *Defining the borders between sleep-related eating disorder and night eating syndrome.* Sleep Med, 2012. **13**(6): p. 686–690.

133. Najjar, M., *Zolpidem and amnestic sleep related eating disorder.* J Clin Sleep Med, 2007. **3**(6): p. 637–638.

134. Takaesu, Y., et al., *Prevalence of and factors associated with sleep-related eating disorder in psychiatric outpatients taking hypnotics.* J Clin Psychiatry, 2016. **77**(7): p. e892–e898.

135. Heathman, J.C., D.W. Neal, and C.R. Thomas, *Sleep-related eating disorder associated with quetiapine.* J Clin Psychopharmacol, 2014. **34**(5): p. 658–660.

136. Paquet, V., et al., *Sleep-related eating disorder induced by olanzapine.* J Clin Psychiatry, 2002. **63**(7): p. 597.

137. Lu, M.L. and W.W. Shen, *Sleep-related eating disorder induced by risperidone.* J Clin Psychiatry, 2004. **65**(2): p. 273–274.

138. Santin, J., et al., *Sleep-related eating disorder: a descriptive study in Chilean patients.* Sleep Med, 2014. **15**(2): p. 163–167.

139. Provini, F., et al., *A pilot double-blind placebo-controlled trial of low-dose pramipexole in sleep-related eating disorder.* Eur J Neurol, 2005. **12**(6): p. 432–436.

140. Chiaro, G., M.T. Caletti, and F. Provini, *Treatment of sleep-related eating disorder.* Curr Treat Options Neurol, 2015. **17**(8): p. 361.

141. Winkelman, J.W., *Efficacy and tolerability of open-label topiramate in the treatment of sleep-related eating disorder: a retrospective case series.* J Clin Psychiatry, 2006. **67**(11): p. 1729–1734.

142. Liang, Y., et al., *Topiramate ameliorates hyperglycaemia and improves glucose-stimulated insulin release in ZDF rats and db/db mice.* Diabetes Obes Metab, 2005. **7**(4): p. 360–369.

143. Wilkes, J.J., et al., *Topiramate is an insulin-sensitizing compound in vivo with direct effects on adipocytes in female ZDF rats.* Am J Physiol Endocrinol Metab, 2005. **288**(3): p. E617–E624.

144. Varghese, R., et al., *Two cases of sleep-related eating disorder responding promptly to low-dose sertraline therapy.* J Clin Sleep Med, 2018. **14**(10): p. 1805–1808.

145. Zapp, A.A., E.C. Fischer, and M. Deuschle, *The effect of agomelatine and melatonin on sleep-related eating: a case report.* J Med Case Rep, 2017. **11**(1): p. 275.

146. Hoque, R. and A.L. Chesson, Jr., *Zolpidem-induced sleepwalking, sleep related eating disorder, and sleep-driving: fluorine-18-flourodeoxyglucose positron emission tomography analysis, and a literature review of other unexpected clinical effects of zolpidem.* J Clin Sleep Med, 2009. **5**(5): p. 471–476.

147. Molina, S.M. and K.G. Joshi, *A case of zaleplon-induced amnestic sleep-related eating disorder.* J Clin Psychiatry, 2010. **71**(2): p. 210–211.

148. Chiu, Y.H., C.H. Chen, and W.W. Shen, *Somnambulism secondary to olanzapine treatment in one patient with bipolar disorder.* Prog Neuropsychopharmacol Biol Psychiatry, 2008. **32**(2): p. 581–582.

149. Kobayashi, N. and M. Takano, *Aripiprazole-induced sleep-related eating disorder: a case report.* J Med Case Rep, 2018. **12**(1): p. 91.

150. Chopra et al., [Poster presentation]. 2019. Society of Biological Psychiatry Meeting, Chicago.

31

Future of Sleep Medicine and Psychiatry

DAVID P. SHAHA, VINCENT F. CAPALDI II, SCOTT G. WILLIAMS,
BEVERLY FANG, AND EMERSON M. WICKWIRE

INTRODUCTION

As evidenced throughout this volume, sleep is intimately linked to healthy brain function as well as psychiatric disease. Indeed, insufficient and disturbed sleep can precede, exacerbate, and prolong virtually every psychiatric disorder. Furthermore, many of the most common psychiatric disorders (e.g., anxiety disorders, mood disorders, substance abuse disorders) include sleep disturbances among specific diagnostic criteria. Perhaps, most importantly, the sleep disorders incur worse outcomes in psychiatric patients, and evidence suggests that incorporating sleep treatments into psychiatric care can improve outcomes and patient quality of life.

Despite the frequent co-occurrence of sleep disturbances and psychiatric disorders, their additive negative effects, and availability of effective interventions, a very few psychiatrists receive formal training in sleep disorders medicine. As a result, most psychiatrists are unprepared to recognize, evaluate, or treat the broad range of sleep complaints common to their patients, and as a result, sleep disorders remain undiagnosed and untreated in psychiatric clinical practice. Thus, we believe that evaluation and management of sleep disorders represents an imminent clinical need and opportunity for growth within the field of psychiatry. The purpose of this chapter is to highlight several related trends and present a vision for the future of sleep and psychiatry.

EXPANDING SLEEP MEDICINE EDUCATION IN PSYCHIATRY TRAINING PROGRAMS

Due to the bidirectional relationship between sleep and psychiatric disorders, treatment for comorbid sleep and psychiatric disorders is most effective when both conditions are addressed simultaneously (1). However, despite this close association and potential therapeutic benefit, psychiatrists are often underprepared to recognize and treat sleep-related complaints (2). This is at least partially due to a lack of standardized requirements for sleep training in psychiatry residency programs in the United States with a subsequent lack in sleep education (2).

A recent survey of 39 chief residents of psychiatry residency programs in the Northeast United States showed that only 34% of programs surveyed even offered elective clinical sleep medicine rotations and that just 38% of these programs had board-certified sleep physicians on their faculty, as compared to 69% of neurology programs (2). While the data from this survey are limited by a relatively small sample size, it is consistent with a larger survey conducted in 2002 of 119 programs, which showed that while 82% of psychiatry programs had didactic lectures in sleep medicine, 55% had no actual sleep medicine specialist faculty to provide this instruction, and only 44% offered a sleep medicine elective (3). This shortage of sleep-trained psychiatrists extends beyond the walls of medical schools; in 2017, psychiatrists made up just 4.4% of all sleep medicine-boarded physicians (2).

Potential corrective measures for this trend away from sleep training in psychiatry include updating current curricula with modern treatment standards such as cognitive-behavioral treatment for insomnia and increasing the availability of sleep electives taught by board-certified sleep specialists (4). For programs without immediate access to psychiatry faculty trained in sleep medicine, telemedicine technology, webinars, and collaboration with sleep specialists from other fields may be pursued (2). Table 31.1 presents a broad range of recommendations to enhance sleep medicine education, with an emphasis on psychiatry.

TABLE 31.1. STRATEGIES TO INCREASE SLEEP TRAINING IN PSYCHIATRY

Level of Education	Pedagogical Strategies
Secondary	Incorporate sleep education into specific courses: • AP psychology (states of consciousness, stages and characteristics of the sleep cycle, theories of sleep and dreaming, symptoms and treatments of sleep disorders) • Health promotion class (normal sleep needs for appropriate states of growth and development) Increase advocacy for adolescent sleep health: • Start School Later (promotes later school start times)
Undergraduate	Model popular classes at leading institutions: • Harvard ("Time for Sleep") • Loyola ("Sleep, Health, and Behavior") • New York University ("While You Were Sleeping") • Stanford ("Sleep and Dreams") Increase education and intervention programs for students
Medical school	Incorporate sleep specific topics within appropriate rotations: • Neurology (Restless leg syndrome and period limb movement disorders) • Pediatrics (Normal sleep development) • Psychiatry (Insomnia disorders) • Pulmonary (Sleep apnea and hypoventilation)
Clinical internship	Expand sleep-specific training: • Fatigue management course • Duty hour restrictions
Psychiatry residency	Incorporate sleep specific topics into residency didactic and clinical training: • Sleep disturbances in major psychiatric disorders • Sleep disturbance as part of prodromal and risk of relapse in major psychiatric disorders • Effects of psychotropic medications on sleep • Medication management of insomnia • Management of side effects like insomnia and sedation related to psychiatric medications Sleep elective—done before PGY4 early enough to be able to apply for sleep fellowship
Sleep medicine fellowship	Integrate telemedicine and telepsychiatry into sleep fellowship training
Other psychiatry fellowships	Include sleep specific topics within other psychiatry fellowships: • Child and adolescent: normal sleep development, ADHD associated with sleep disordered breathing disorder, sleep management in autism spectrum disorder • Geriatric: normal sleep development, dementia and circadian rhythm disorders • Consultation and liaison: delirium vs. dementia • Addictions: sleep effects of drugs, along with intoxication, withdrawal • Forensic: parasomnias and legal implications
Continuing medical education	• Adopt self-assessment and performance improvement strategies, especially regarding insomnia evaluation and treatment • Include sleep-specific CME training for active military/VA psychiatrists: sleep in PTSD, TBI, and nightmares • Identify networking and sleep specialty opportunities (e.g., local societies, national conferences)

Abbreviations: ADHD, attention deficit-hyperactivity disorder; AP, advanced placement; CME, continuing medical education; PGY4, program year 4; PTSD, posttraumatic stress disorder; TBI, traumatic brain injury; VA, US Department of Veterans Affairs.

TARGETING SLEEP DISORDERS IN HIGH-RISK PSYCHIATRIC PATIENTS

Almost all psychiatric clinicians will interact with patients suffering from comorbid sleep and psychiatric disorders. Inpatient hospitalist teams are usually at the front line when it comes to balancing the management of acute exacerbations of physical illness accompanied with disrupted sleep–wake physiology. Inpatient behavioral health providers and consultation-liaison psychiatrists often encounter sleep disorders on a consistent basis, yet many are not trained to recognize and treat these conditions. Among inpatients in general hospital settings, sleep fragmentation is very common and can contribute to impaired wound healing and delirium (5). Despite the fact that insomnia is a risk factor for psychiatric disorders (6), patients are often reluctant to discuss their sleep problems during the limited time spent with their treatment team (7). Furthermore, many sleep disorders often masquerade as psychiatric conditions. For example, a large longitudinal study found that children with untreated sleep-disordered breathing were almost twice as likely to develop behavioral problems such as hyperactivity and inattention (8). Finally, sleep and psychiatric disorders are especially common among older adults (9) and among women (10), the two populations at particularly high risk for psychiatric disorders. In each of these populations, psychiatrists should assess overall sleep health, including sleep quality/satisfaction with sleep, sleep duration, and sleep parameters including sleep onset latency, wake after sleep onset, and night-to-night variability. In terms of screening for clinical sleep disorders, at minimum, patients should be asked if they snore or experience excessive daytime sleepiness. Detailed guidance regarding clinical assessment is provided elsewhere in this volume.

ADOPTING A BEHAVIORAL SLEEP MEDICINE APPROACH

For many sleep disorders, cognitive-behavioral interventions are considered first-line treatment approaches, with short-term effectiveness equal to pharmacotherapies, long-term effectiveness superior to pharmacotherapies, and dramatically reduced risks of side effects relative to pharmacotherapies. For example, the long-term effectiveness of cognitive-behavioral therapy for insomnia (CBT-I) is well-established, and CBT-I is recommended first-line treatment by the US National Institutes of Health (11), the American College of Physicians (12), the American Academy of Sleep Medicine (13), and the British Pharmacological Society (14). Similarly, only imagery rehearsal therapy has been recommended for trauma- and nontrauma-related nightmares (15). Evidence suggests that cognitive-behavioral approaches are also the most efficacious interventions to enhance adherence to positive airway pressure (PAP) therapy for obstructive sleep apnea (OSA) (16), and sleep scheduling—behavioral approach—is the cornerstone of care for shift work sleep disorder (17). Unfortunately, there is paucity of behavioral sleep medicine specialists nationwide and across the globe (18). As a result, online versions have been adopted to help increase access to certain behavioral sleep approaches, such as CBT-I (e.g., [19]). Such automated tools can be administered within the context of psychiatry care. Given the dominant emphasis on medication management in psychiatric practice, advancing collaboration between psychiatric practitioners and behavioral sleep specialists has great potential to improve sleep-related outcomes among psychiatric patients.

INCORPORATING NON-HARMACOLOGICAL INTERVENTIONS INTO SLEEP PSYCHIATRY

Given that the sleep researchers are still trying to understand the full impact of sleep on normal physiology, several groups are experimenting with devices to reduce the need for human sleep, thereby purportedly increasing the potential for waking productivity. Although still in the developmental stage, this technology aims at improving the restorative properties of slow-wave sleep. Formal full-scale trials are ongoing with initial promising results (20). In addition to enhancing slow-wave sleep, another key area of interest is non-pharmacologic treatment for insomnia. Recently, noninvasive photic and auditory technologies have shown promising results in treating chronic insomnia. One such approach, high-resolution, relational, resonance-based electro-encephalic mirroring (HIRREM) seeks to balance and calibrate neural oscillations (21). This technology seeks to balance problematic lateralization of autonomic function in the brain, in which right-sided activation is believed to produce downstream sympathetic effects, and left-sided activation is believed to produce downstream parasympathetic effects (21). Finally, near-infrared light has also been studied as a potential adjunct to promote intracellular healing in patients with chronic traumatic brain injury and insomnia. In a small trial, this approach resulted in significant improvement in depression rating scores and subjective reports of improved sleep quality (22).

Cranial electrotherapy stimulation (CES) has been studied in a variety of conditions ranging from anxiety, depression, chronic pain, and primary and comorbid insomnia in association with other sleep, medical, and psychiatric disorders (23, 24). It is important to note that the side effects of CES remain incompletely understood and can infrequently include physical side effects (e.g., skin burn) as well as impaired cognition. Neurofeedback, which seeks to train patients in recognizing and controlling autonomic activation, has also been studied for insomnia, and it is increasingly being marketed directly to consumers. A commercially available neurofeedback device in a healthy adult population showed modest benefits for attention and subjective well-being when compared to an active control group (25). For clinicians, it will be increasingly important to combine well-established pharmacotherapeutic approaches with the novel nonpharmacologic treatments for management of refractory insomnia. Future studies must address these combination treatments to optimize sleep outcomes in psychiatric patients.

ADVANCING DRUG DISCOVERY FOR SLEEP DISTURBANCES IN PSYCHIATRIC DISORDERS

As noted throughout this volume, sleep disruptions and insomnia are highly prevalent in almost every psychiatric condition. In the past, psychotropic medications treating insomnia symptoms were dominated by various compounds targeting the gamma-aminobutyric acid A ($GABA_A$)–benzodiazepine receptor complex. Other agents include melatonin receptor agonists such as ramelteon and histamine receptor antagonists such as doxepin. Given the considerable market share of these products, with more than 12 million people using sleep aids regularly (26) and the predicted US market value of $80.8 billion by 2020 (27), it is expected that novel pharmaceutical agents will continue to be developed to capitalize on this opportunity for growth.

Since the 1990s, the hypocretin-orexin system has been implicated in the pathophysiology of narcolepsy (28). At the beginning of the 21st century, several pharmaceutical manufacturers began to test compounds targeting orexin receptor-1 (OX1R) and orexin receptor-2 (OX2R) for both sleep and psychiatric indications. This receptor complex has opportunities for development in both the sleep and psychiatric realms as activation of OX1R is implicated in the development of anxiety and panic symptoms. In 2014, the US Food and Drug Administration (FDA) approved the first dual orexin receptor antagonist, suvorexant, for the treatment of insomnia [29].

Unlike other hypnotic-sedatives, (e.g., benzodiazepines and newer "z-drugs" such as zaleplon, eszopiclone, and zolpidem), dual orexin receptor antagonist class has been theorized to have less sleep inertia associated with chronic use and may be useful in treating patients with concurrent anxiety symptoms. Future medications related to this system may have greater OX1R affinity or may be produced in alternative formulations with multiple classes of medications (i.e. short-acting $GABA_A$ target with a longer-acting orexin receptor antagonist). Additionally, OX2R agonists may be useful as wake-promoting agents, especially for those with narcolepsy.

Other areas of development include medications targeted to treat nightmares associated with posttraumatic stress disorder (PTSD). In 2010, the $alpha_1$-noradrenergic antagonist, prazosin, was recommended in the American Academy of Sleep Medicine clinical practice guidelines following placebo-controlled trials showing efficacy in treating nightmares in several populations (30). Titration of this medication to therapeutic doses may be associated with undesirable side effects including orthostatic hypotension. Future work may focus on novel formulations such as sublingual or inhaled formulations that will target symptoms without a significant side effect profile. Novel compounds that target cannabinoid receptors may also prove to be helpful in decreasing PTSD-associated nightmares (31).

USE OF WEARABLES AND COMPLEMENTARY APPROACHES

Given that most humans spend approximately one-third of their lives asleep, it is no wonder why there has been a fascination with the phenomenon of sleep since the dawn of human civilization. During the 20th century, modern sleep medicine arguably found its roots with the publication of *The Interpretation of Dreams* by Sigmund Freud (32). Soon thereafter, the fascinations with sleep and scientific discovery lead to the development of the modern sleep laboratory and the growth of sleep medicine as a bone fide medical specialty. As is the trend with most areas of medicine, technological developments have allowed patients to take a more active role in measuring and optimizing their sleep, frequently with an emphasis on improved daytime performance.

The modern actigraph was developed by the US Army at Walter Reed Army Institute of Research in a series of experiments in the 1980s (33). Since that time the devices have become smaller, more rugged, and more easily interpretable by the average consumer. The vast majority of wearable devices make an attempt to use nighttime movement to characterize sleep parameters such as sleep onset latency, wake after sleep onset, and total sleep time and provide feedback to the wearer. The sampling rate of actigraph (i.e., the rate at which the device records the movements) currently separates laboratory specialized devices and those used within the consumer market. Relative to more expensive, research-grade devices, commercial devices tend to have lower sampling rates As compared to expensive clinical devices, consumer-based devices tend to underestimate sleep onset latency and the amount of time spent awake after sleep onset. In the field of psychiatry, more accurate characterization of sleep may be especially useful as sleep disturbance has been associated with the onset and exacerbation of psychiatric illness (34). Serial assessment of sleep can also provide valuable insight into the potential impact of psychotropic medications on subsequent psychiatric symptoms, including changes in mood (35).

Like other areas of medicine, complementary and alternative medicine (CAM) continues to be prevalent in the field of sleep and psychiatry. The FDA does not regulate herbal medications as it does other prescribed compounds; as such, the varying levels of active compound and other additive substances in formulations tends to vary by manufacturer and even production batch. For example, valerian continues to be one of the most widely used herbal supplements to treat insomnia symptoms. However, several studies have failed to demonstrate an improvement in symptoms greater than placebo (36, 37). Other forms of CAM utilized by consumers to treat fatigue and insomnia symptoms include tai chi, acupuncture, and yoga with limited clinical evidence regarding efficacy (38). Nonetheless, psychiatric practitioners should be aware that many patients enjoy or prefer exercise-based approaches, and such mind–body interventions might provide nonspecific clinical benefit from enhanced positive affect.

PROVIDING SLEEP PSYCHIATRIC CARE REMOTELY

Perhaps no two medical subspecialties are more amenable to telehealth care than sleep and psychiatry. The confluence of secure video consultation, ambulatory diagnostics, store and forward technologies such as asynchronous home sleep apnea tests (HSATs), and the advent of robust patient portals ensure that the vast majority of sleep and psychiatric patients can be managed remotely, thereby increasing access to specialty care across the United States and worldwide.

Consumer awareness of the consequences of OSA and decreased insurance reimbursement for providers have contributed to the ubiquitous deployment of home sleep apnea testing at most sleep centers (39). Because of dramatically reduced costs and reasonable diagnostic accuracy, sleep technologies like dry electrode technology and automated sleep scoring will likely dominate the field of sleep medicine in the future. Broadly, we consider HSAT and its related store-and-forward technologies, which enable asynchronous testing and remote sharing of records, as the key telehealth advancements in the sleep field during the modern era. These technologies are particularly amenable to "hub and spoke" approaches, whereby nonsleep clinicians can administer HSAT and refer to sleep specialty care for further evaluation and management as needed. For such approaches to succeed, it is essential that the front-line providers be thoroughly trained in screening, assessment, and initial management of patients with sleep disorders.

No less significant than diagnostic technologies, however, are the rapidly advancing remote monitoring technologies now commonplace among PAP devices. When combined with secure telemedicine and videoconferencing, most straightforward sleep apnea care can now be delivered remotely, including video-assisted physical exam. The American Academy of Sleep Medicine has published a formal position paper (40), as well as a sleep telemedicine implementation guide (41), to assist healthcare providers in incorporating both center-to-center and center-to-home sleep telemedicine into their practices. For in-depth considerations of these issues, readers are also referred to an overview of technology in sleep medicine (42), as well as a series of articles on benefits and risks of sleep telemedicine (43),

TABLE 31.2. ECONOMIC PERSPECTIVE IN SLEEP PSYCHIATRY

Perspective	Value-Based Outcome
Patient	Quality of life, ease of experience
Payer	Cost savings
Employer	Workplace productivity, accident risk mitigation
Health system	Revenue
Society	Aggregated costs and outcomes

TABLE 31.3. ACTIONABLE RECOMMENDATIONS FOR SLEEP PSYCHIATRY PROVIDERS

Domain	Recommendation
Clarify your objectives	What are your personal and organizational objectives? Where are you, career-wise? Where do you want to be in 2, 3, and 5 years?
Know your customer wants	Ask, who does sleep serve? Listen to uncover the outcomes that matter to your constituents. Make these your endpoints.
Develop customer-centric language	Develop value-based scripts. Rehearse them.
Understand trends in payments and technology	Is your region adopting bundled payments or paying more for improved outcomes? How might telemedicine or pre-authorization for sleep procedures and treatment impact your practice?
Know your numbers	Know your cost per patient, cost per test, cost per outcome, and lifetime value for patient.

starting a sleep telemedicine program (44), and advancing organizational objectives with sleep telemedicine (45).

ADOPTING A VALUE-BASED APPROACH TO SLEEP AND PSYCHIATRY

In the modern healthcare climate, with increasing costs on the one hand and limited resources on the other, the healthcare providers will experience an increased emphasis on economic aspects of care. Fortunately, evidence suggests economic benefit from treating sleep disorders, including reductions in healthcare utilization and cost-effectiveness of treatments for insomnia and other sleep disorders (1). However, important scientific questions remain regarding the health economics of sleep disorders and their treatments, such as, Which patients should be treated first? Which treatments are most cost-effective? Which providers should deliver sleep treatments? What is the optimal time horizon to assess cost-effectiveness and return on investment for sleep medicine care?

Further, many key economic stakeholders remain unconvinced of the economic value to sleep and psychiatric treatments. It is thus incumbent on sleep psychiatric providers to define, demonstrate, and maximize the value of the services provided. This will require an unwavering focus on the value received from sleep psychiatric care, which may be affected by multiple variables including the type of practice, payers, employers, health systems, and patients. As highlighted in Table 31.2, each of these constituent groups values different health and economic outcomes. Sleep psychiatry providers can follow specific action steps to improve patient outcomes and maximize value of services rendered (Table 31.3).

CONCLUSIONS

The need for management of sleep disorders in psychiatry has never been greater. Despite shared mechanistic underpinnings and high comorbidity, sleep disorders in psychiatric patients are frequently underdiagnosed and untreated. The major reason is that sleep medicine has not been insufficiently incorporated into all levels of psychiatric training and practice. Pillars of enhanced sleep and psychiatric care in the future include improved sleep training for psychiatric clinicians, increased provision of behavioral sleep medicine services in sleep and psychiatric clinics, discovery of new device-based interventions as well as novel pharmacologic compounds, an increased focus on telehealth, and an emphasis on value-based sleep psychiatric care. The future of sleep in psychiatry is bright.

REFERENCES

1. Krystal AD. Psychiatric Disorders and Sleep. Neurologic Clinics. 2012;30(4):1389–1413.
2. Khawaja IS, Dickmann PJ, Hurwitz TD, Thuras PD, Feinstein RE, Douglass AB, et al. The state of sleep medicine education in North American psychiatry residency training programs in 2013: chief resident's perspective. Primary Care Companion for CNS Disorders. 2017;19(04).
3. Krahn LE. Psychiatric residents' exposure to the field of sleep medicine: a survey of program directors. Academic Psychiatry. 2002;26(4):253–256.
4. Masters PA. Insomnia. Annals of Internal Medicine. 2014;161(7):ITC1.
5. Freedman NS, Gazendam J, Levan L, Pack AI, Schwab RJ. Abnormal sleep/wake cycles and the effect of environmental noise on sleep disruption in the intensive care unit. American Journal of Respiratory and Critical Care Medicine. 2001;163(2):451–457.
6. Breslau N, Roth T, Rosenthal L, Andreski P. Sleep disturbance and psychiatric disorders: a longitudinal epidemiological study of young Adults. Biological Psychiatry. 1996;39(6):411–418.
7. Ancoli-Israel S, Roth T. Characteristics of insomnia in the United States: results of the 1991 National Sleep Foundation Survey. I. Sleep. 1999;22 Suppl 2:S347–S53.
8. Bonuck K, Freeman K, Chervin RD, Xu L. Sleep-disordered breathing in a population-based cohort: behavioral outcomes at 4 and 7 years. Pediatrics. 2012;129(4):e857–e65.
9. Ancoli-Israel S. Sleep and its disorders in aging populations. Sleep Medicine. 2009;10:S7–S11.
10. Phillips BA, Collop NA, Drake C, Consens F, Vgontzas AN, Weaver TE. Sleep disorders and medical conditions in women: proceedings of the Women & Sleep Workshop, National Sleep Foundation, Washington, DC, March 5–6, 2007. J Womens Health (Larchmt). 2008;17(7):1191–1199.
11. NIH State-of-the-Science Conference Statement on manifestations and management of chronic insomnia in adults. NIH Consensus and State-of-the-Science Statements. 2005;22(2):1–30.
12. Qaseem A, Kansagara D, Forciea MA, Cooke M, Denberg TD. Management of chronic insomnia disorder in adults: a clinical practice guideline from the American College of Physicians. Annals of Internal Medicine. 2016;165(2):125–133.
13. Schutte-Rodin S, Broch L, Buysse D, Dorsey C, Sateia M. Clinical guideline for the evaluation and management of chronic insomnia in adults. Journal of Clinical Sleep Medicine. 2008;4(5):487–504.
14. Wilson SJ, Nutt DJ, Alford C, Argyropoulos SV, Baldwin DS, Bateson AN, et al. British Association for Psychopharmacology consensus statement on evidence-based treatment of insomnia, parasomnias and circadian rhythm disorders. Journal of Psychopharmacology (Oxford, England). 2010;24(11):1577–1601.
15. Morgenthaler TI, Auerbach S, Casey KR, Kristo D, Maganti R, Ramar K, et al. position paper for the treatment of nightmare disorder in adults: an American Academy of Sleep Medicine position paper. Journal of Clinical Sleep Medicine. 2018;14(6):1041–1055.
16. Wickwire EM, Lettieri CJ, Cairns AA, Collop NA. Maximizing positive airway pressure adherence in adults: a common-sense approach. Chest. 2013;144(2):680–693.
17. Wickwire EM, Geiger-Brown J, Scharf SM, Drake CL. Shift work and shift work sleep disorder: clinical and organizational perspectives. Chest. 2017;151(5):1156–1172.
18. Thomas A, Grandner M, Nowakowski S, Nesom G, Corbitt C, Perlis ML. Where are the behavioral sleep medicine providers and where are they needed? A geographic assessment. Behavioral Sleep Medicine. 2016;14(6):687–698.
19. Zachariae R, Lyby MS, Ritterband LM, O'Toole MS. Efficacy of internet-delivered cognitive-behavioral therapy for insomnia: a systematic review and meta-analysis of randomized controlled trials. Sleep Medicine Reviews. 2016;30:1–10.
20. Papalambros NA, Santostasi G, Malkani RG, Braun R, Weintraub S, Paller KA, et al. Acoustic enhancement of sleep slow oscillations and concomitant memory improvement in older adults. Frontiers in Human Neuroscience. 2017;11:109.
21. Lee SW, Gerdes L, Tegeler CL, Shaltout HA, Tegeler CH. A bihemispheric autonomic model for traumatic stress effects on health and behavior. Frontiers in Psychology. 2014;5:843.
22. Morries LD, Cassano P, Henderson TA. Treatments for traumatic brain injury with emphasis on transcranial near-infrared laser phototherapy. Neuropsychiatric Disease and Treatment. 2015;11:2159–2175.
23. Marksberry J, Kirsch D, Nichols F, Price LR, Platoni KT. Efficacy of cranial electrotherapy stimulation for anxiety, PTSD, insomnia and depression: military service members and veterans self reports. Brain Stimulation. 2015;8(2):311.
24. Lande RG, Gragnani C. Efficacy of cranial electric stimulation for the treatment of insomnia:

A randomized pilot study. Complementary Therapies in Medicine. 2013;21(1):8–13.

25. Bhayee S, Tomaszewski P, Lee DH, Moffat G, Pino L, Moreno S, et al. Attentional and affective consequences of technology supported mindfulness training: a randomised, active control, efficacy trial. BMC Psychology. 2016;4(1):60.

26. Chong Y, Fryar C, Gu Q. Prescription Sleep aid use among adults: United States, 2005–2010. US Department of Health and Human Services: Centers for Disease Control; August 2013.

27. Hare G. Global sleep aids market will reach US$80.8 bn by 2020: persistence market research. Persistence Market Research. https://globen-ewswire.com/news-release/2015/07/31/756724/10144080/en/Global-Sleep-Aids-Market-Will-Reach-US-80-8-Bn-by-2020-Persistence-Market-Research.html. 2015.

28. Nishino S, Ripley B, Overeem S, Lammers GJ, Mignot E. Hypocretin (orexin) deficiency in human narcolepsy. Lancet. 2000;355(9197):39–40.

29. Michelson D, Snyder E, Paradis E, Chengan-Liu M, Snavely DB, Hutzelmann J, et al. Safety and efficacy of suvorexant during 1-year treatment of insomnia with subsequent abrupt treatment discontinuation: a phase 3 randomised, double-blind, placebo-controlled trial. Lancet Neurology. 2014;13(5):461–471.

30. Sateia MJ, Buysse DJ, Krystal AD, Neubauer DN, Heald JL. Clinical practice guideline for the pharmacologic treatment of chronic insomnia in adults: an American Academy of Sleep Medicine clinical practice guideline. Journal of Clinical Sleep Medicine. 2017;13(2):307–349.

31. Jetly R, Heber A, Fraser G, Boisvert D. The efficacy of nabilone, a synthetic cannabinoid, in the treatment of PTSD-associated nightmares: a preliminary randomized, double-blind, placebo-controlled cross-over design study. Psychoneuroendocrinology. 2015;51:585–588.

32. Grubrich-Simitis I. Metamorphoses of the interpretation of dreams: Freud's conflicted relations with his book of the century. International Journal of Psycho-Analysis. 2000;81(Pt 6):1155–1183.

33. Kripke DF, Mullaney DJ, Messin S, Wyborney VG. Wrist actigraphic measures of sleep and rhythms. Electroencephalography and Clinical Neurophysiology. 1978;44(5):674–676.

34. Michaels MS, Balthrop T, Nadorff MR, Joiner TE. Total sleep time as a predictor of suicidal behaviour. Journal of Sleep Research. 2017;26(6):732–738.

35. Thase ME, Buysse DJ, Frank E, Cherry CR, Cornes CL, Mallinger AG, et al. Which depressed patients will respond to interpersonal psychotherapy? The role of abnormal EEG sleep profiles. American Journal of Psychiatry. 1997;154(4):502–509.

36. Lindahl O, Lindwall L. Double blind study of a valerian preparation. Pharmacology, Biochemistry, and Behavior. 1989;32(4):1065–1066.

37. Taibi DM, Vitiello MV, Barsness S, Elmer GW, Anderson GD, Landis CA. A randomized clinical trial of valerian fails to improve self-reported, polysomnographic, and actigraphic sleep in older women with insomnia. Sleep Medicine. 2009;10(3):319–328.

38. Xiang Y, Lu L, Chen X, Wen Z. Does Tai Chi relieve fatigue? A systematic review and meta-analysis of randomized controlled trials. PloS One. 2017;12(4):e0174872.

39. Wu P, Chen GT, Cui Y, Li JW, Kuo TBJ, Chang P. Development of home-based sleep monitoring system for obstructive sleep apnea. Studies in Health Technology and Informatics. 2017;245:268–272.

40. Singh J, Badr MS, Diebert W, Epstein L, Hwang D, Karres V, et al. American Academy of Sleep Medicine (AASM) position paper for the use of telemedicine for the diagnosis and treatment of sleep disorders. Journal of Clinical Sleep Medicine. 2015;11(10):1187–1198.

41. American Academy of Sleep Medicine. Sleep Telemedicine Implementation Guide. https://aasm.org/download-the-sleep-telemedicine-implementation-guide-a-free-resource-from-aasm/. 2017.

42. Wickwire EM. Sleep medicine for the 21st century: leveraging the internet to improve patient care. Sleep Review. 2012;13(7):14–19.

43. Wickwire E. Promises and pitfalls of telehealth. Sleep Review. 2014;15(4):44–48.

44. Wickwire EM. How to implement a telemedicine program in seven easy steps. Sleep Review. 2014;15(6):24–25.

45. Wickwire EM. Advancing organizational objectives with telehealth. Sleep Review. 2014;15(5):28–29.

INDEX

Tables, figures and boxes are indicated by *t*, *f* and *b* following the page number

For the benefit of digital users, indexed terms that span two pages (e.g., 52–53) may, on occasion, appear on only one of those pages.